volume 1 **Principles and Concepts**

Oxford Textbook of Primary Medical Care

Edited by
Roger Jones
Nicky Britten
Larry Culpepper
David A. Gass
Richard Grol
David Mant
and Chris Silagy

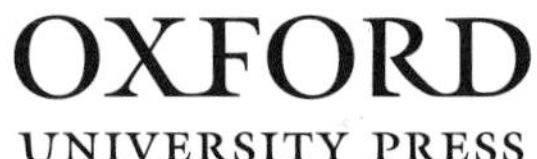
OXFORD
UNIVERSITY PRESS

OXFORD
UNIVERSITY PRESS

Great Clarendon Street, Oxford OX2 6DP

Oxford University Press is a department of the University of Oxford.
It furthers the University's objective of excellence in research, scholarship,
and education by publishing worldwide in

Oxford New York

Auckland Bangkok Buenos Aires Cape Town Chennai
Dar es Salaam Delhi Hong Kong Istanbul Karachi Kolkata
Kuala Lumpur Madrid Melbourne Mexico City Mumbai Nairobi
São Paulo Shanghai Taipei Tokyo Toronto

Oxford is a registered trade mark of Oxford University Press
in the UK and in certain other countries

Published in the United States
by Oxford University Press Inc., New York

First published 2004

British Library Cataloguing in Publication Data

Data available

ISBN 0 19 852963 5 (vol 1)
0 19 852964 3 (vol 2)
0 19 263219 1 (set)
(Available as a set only)

10 9 8 7 6 5 4 3 2 1

Typeset by Newgen Imaging Systems (P) Ltd, Chennai, India
Printed in Italy
on acid-free paper by Legoprint.

Section editors

Volume 1: Sections 1–16

Richard Baker
Professor, Clinical Governance Research and Development Unit, University of Leicester, Leicester General Hospital, Leicester, UK
Section 13: Quality improvement

Jozien Bensing
Director and Professor, NIVEL (Netherlands Institute for Health Services Research), Utrecht, The Netherlands
Section 5: The consultation

Nicky Britten
Professor of Applied Health Care Research, Institute of Clinical Education, Peninsula Medical School, Universities of Exeter and Plymouth, St Luke's Campus, Exeter, UK
Section 3: Reasons for consultation
Section 5: The consultation
Section 14: Research

Thomas L. Campbell
Professor, Family Medicine and Dentistry, University of Rochester School of Medicine and Dentistry, Rochester, New York, USA
Section 9: Family medicine

Larry Culpepper
Professor and Chairman of Family Medicine, Boston University, Boston, USA
Section 1: Primary medical care
Section 8: Integrated management
Section 9: Family medicine

Geert-Jan Dinant
Professor, University of Maastricht, Maastricht, The Netherlands
Section 6: Diagnosis and decision-making

Len Doyal
Professor of Medical Ethics, St Bartholomew's and The Royal London School of Medicine and Dentistry, Queen Mary College, University of London, UK
Section 16: Ethics and law

David A. Gass
Professor, Department of Family Medicine, Dalhousie University, Halifax, Canada
Section 15: Education and professional development
Section 16: Ethics and law

Richard Grol
Professor and Director, Centre for Quality of Care Research (WOK), Nijmegen University Medical Centre, Maastricht University, The Netherlands
Section 2: Primary care around the world
Section 8: Integrated management
Section 12: Practice management
Section 13: Quality improvement

Roger Jones
Wolfson Professor of General Practice and Primary Care, Guy's, King's and St Thomas' School of Medicine, London, UK
Section 1: Primary medical care
Section 2: Primary care around the world
Section 6: Diagnosis and decision-making

J.A. Knottnerus
Professor of General Practice, Netherlands School of Primary Care Research, Maastricht and President of the Health Council of the Netherlands, The Hague, The Netherlands
Section 4: Descriptive epidemiology

Michael M. Kochen
Professor of General Practice, University of Göttingen, Germany
Section 7: Management of individuals

David Mant
Professor of General Practice, University of Oxford, UK
Section 4: Descriptive epidemiology
Section 10: Managing the practice population
Section 11: Prevention and health promotion

Chris Silagy*
Professor and Director, Institute of Public Health and Health Services Research, Monash University, Monash Medical Centre, Clayton, Australia
Section 7: Management of individuals
Section 10: Managing the practice population
Section 11: Prevention and health promotion
Section 14: Research

Eloy H. van de Lisdonk
General Practitioner and Senior Lecturer, University of Nijmegen, Nijmegen, The Netherlands
Section 3: Reasons for consultation

Valerie Wass
Professor of Community Based Education, University of Manchester, School of Primary Care, Rusholme Health Centre, Manchester, UK
Section 15: Education and professional development

* It is with regret that we must report the death of Chris Silagy during the preparation of this Textbook.

Volume 2: Sections 1–17

Willem J.J. Assendelft
Head, Department of Guideline Development and Research Policy, Dutch College of General Practitioners, Utrecht, The Netherlands
Section 13: Musculoskeletal problems

Larry Culpepper
Professor and Chairman of Family Medicine, Boston University, Boston, USA
Section 3: Ear, nose, and throat problems
Section 5: Metabolic problems
Section 10: Child health

Niek J. de Wit
Senior Lecturer, General Practitioner, Julius Center for Health Sciences and Primary Care, University Medical Center, Utrecht, The Netherlands
Section 4: Digestive problems

Isser Dubinsky
Director of Emergency Services, The Toronto Hospital, Ontario, Canada
Section 14: Common emergencies and trauma

Peggy Frith
Consultant Medical Ophthalmologist, Oxford Eye Hospital, Radcliffe Infirmary, Oxford, UK
Section 12: Eye problems

David A. Gass
Professor, Department of Family Medicine, Dalhousie University, Halifax, Canada
Section 9: Mental health problems
Section 16: Old age
Section 17: Palliative care

Irene J. Higginson
Professor and Head, Department of Palliative Care and Policy, King's College London, Weston Education Centre, London, UK
Section 17: Palliative care

Richard Hobbs
Professor and Head of Primary Care and General Practice, Primary Care Clinical Sciences Building, University of Birmingham, Edgbaston, Birmingham, UK
Section 1: Cardiovascular problems

Roger Jones
Wolfson Professor of General Practice and Primary Care, Guy's, King's and St Thomas' School of Medicine, London, UK
Section 1: Cardiovascular problems
Section 4: Digestive problems
Section 7: Women's health
Section 8: Conception, pregnancy, and childbirth
Section 14: Common emergencies and trauma

Tony Kendrick
Professor of Primary Medical Care, Director of Community Clinical Sciences Division, University of Southampton Medical School, Aldermoor Health Centre, Southampton, UK
Section 9: Mental health problems

Michael C. Klein
Professor of Family Practice and Paediatrics and Head, Division of Maternity and Newborn Care, University of British Columbia, Vancouver, Canada
Section 8: Conception, pregnancy, and childbirth

David Mant
Professor of General Practice, University of Oxford, Oxford, UK
Section 12: Eye problems
Section 13: Musculoskeletal problems
Section 15: Skin and soft tissue problems

Kenneth Marshall
Professor of Family Medicine (retired), University of Western Ontario, Ontario, Canada
Section 3: Ear, nose, and throat problems
Section 6: Genito-urinary problems

Thomas Nicholas
Department of Family Medicine, University of Missouri Kansas City, Missouri, USA
Section 15: Skin and soft tissue problems

Mary Pierce
Senior Lecturer in General Practice, University of Warwick, UK
Section 5: Metabolic problems

Leone Ridsdale
Senior Lecturer in Neurology and Reader in General Practice, Guy's, King's, and St Thomas' School of Medicine, King's College School of Medicine, London, UK
Section 11: Neurological problems

Walter W. Rosser
Chair, Department of Family Medicine, Queens University, Kingston, Ontario, Canada
Section 10: Child health

Chris Silagy*
Professor and Director, Institute of Public Health and Health Services Research, Monash University, Monash Medical Centre, Clayton, Australia
Section 2: Respiratory problems
Section 6: Genito-urinary problems
Section 11: Neurological problems

Paul Wallace
Professor of Primary Health Care, University College London, London, UK
Section 16: Old age

Chris van Weel
Professor and Chairman, University Medical Center, Nijmegen, The Netherlands
Section 2: Respiratory problems

Ruth Wilson
Professor, Department of Family Medicine, Queen's University, Kingston, Ontario, Canada
Section 7: Women's health

*It is with regret that we must report the death of Chris Silagy during the preparation of this Textbook.

Summary of contents

Volume 1: Principles and Concepts

Volume 2: Clinical Management

Contents

Volume 1: Principles and Concepts

Volume 2: Clinical Management

Section 4 Digestive problems

Section 5 Metabolic problems

Section 6 Genito-urinary problems

Section 7 Women's health

Section 15 Skin and soft tissue problems

Section 16 Old age

Section 17 Palliative care

Preface

The concept of a definitive textbook for primary care physicians, general practitioners, and family physicians, published by Oxford University Press, has been under discussion for many years. The present work is the result of these detailed deliberations and the hard work of an almost unprecedented number of editors and authors, representing primary care medical expertise from around the globe. The final decision to produce the Textbook was based on a broad consensus that a fixed reference point in the maelstrom of information about primary medical care and primary care services was essential. Whilst many have argued that the volume and constantly changing content of information may render traditional paper-based textbooks redundant, in many ways it is the very extent of this information, and the difficulties of finding a way through it, that persuaded us to embark on this ambitious project.

Over the three or four years that it has taken to produce the Textbook, the need for it has become even more apparent. Paradoxically, in health care systems with well-developed primary care sectors, there has been a recent tendency to 'de-construct' primary care and general practice through the provision of multiple points of entry into the primary and secondary care systems, changing roles for primary care professionals, fragmentation of both personal and organizational continuity of care, and a policy focus on activity and volume rather than on quality and patient-centred outcomes. At the same time, the value of a strong primary care sector is increasingly appreciated in developing health care systems, where the generalist function in medicine is recognized as crucial to the delivery of effective and efficient care for populations.

Design issues

Even before drawing up the terms of reference that would inform the content of the Textbook, the editors spent many hours agonizing about the title, which would predicate these. 'General practice' is well-understood to be pretty well synonymous with primary medical care in northern European countries, and in parts of Australasia and the Pacific rim, but has a different connotation in North America. 'Family medicine' has a specific North American connotation, which is not widely shared and which, in other settings, has a specific, restrictive meaning. 'Primary care' was judged to be over-inclusive, with implications for public health, community development, and political structures and initiatives. We believe that 'primary medical care' sits reasonably comfortably at the interstices between these terms, and provides a conceptual framework that is both broad enough to ensure that primary care physicians and their teams practising medicine in a range of health care and geographical settings will find the book valuable, whilst being sufficiently focused to ensure adequate coverage of key topics within manageable constraints of space and cost.

We were particularly concerned to assemble a core Editorial Board, which, through selection of appropriate topics and authors, would ensure full coverage of the field from multiple disciplinary and cultural perspectives. This has resulted in the engagement of 400 authors from some 20 different countries.

The decision to produce this Textbook in two distinct volumes, of approximately equal length, stems from the need to adequately describe both the principles underlying the establishment and delivery of high-quality primary care and the clinical information and skills required for patient management in that setting. The first volume describes the fundamentals of primary care and the second focuses on clinical management in primary care, taking an approach based on the management of presenting symptoms, embedded in a systems-based framework.

Principles and concepts

The first volume, 'Principles and Concepts', provides a systematic overview of the nature, structure and functions of primary medical care, with a strong focus on the consultation and the doctor–patient interactions that are at the core of primary care medicine. We have described both individual and population approaches to the delivery of primary medical care and emphasized the wide range of disciplines involved. As well as clinical sciences, the basic sciences of primary medical care include medical sociology, health psychology, epidemiology, and the principles of organizational management. We have highlighted the importance of ensuring and enhancing the quality of care and provide concise, detailed sections on research, education, and ethics and law.

In many ways, the essays that make up the first volume of the Textbook represent the 'eternal verities' of primary medical care. Although health care systems and political priorities will shift and change, new diseases will emerge, patients will become increasingly well-informed and empowered, and the traditional role of primary health care professionals will be transformed, many of the fundamental principles of doctor–patient interaction within the consultation, and the means of studying and teaching them, will doubtless endure.

Clinical management

In the second volume of the Textbook, we have taken an approach based on presenting problems within a comprehensive systems framework. In our guidance to authors we emphasized the importance of taking a broad perspective on each topic, attempting to assure its relevance for physicians and health care systems at different levels of development, emphasizing core clinical principles of diagnosis and management and considering the broader public health and health economic implications of each problem. We identified, through section co-editors, individuals in a number of countries who were able to provide an expert primary care perspective on each problem, often by writing in conjunction with specialist colleagues. We recognize that this contemporary account of good practice in primary care medicine will, inevitably, change as new diagnostic technologies and therapeutic interventions are developed, and the introductory essay on genomic medicine reflects the pace of change in medical science and looks ahead at the extraordinary potential that it possesses for improving health and health care in the future.

Using the Textbook

The *Oxford Textbook of Primary Medical Care* has been written as a definitive account of primary care medical practice, and to act as a reference point for all those involved in teaching, learning, researching, and delivering primary medical care. We hope that practising physicians around the world will find the clinical sections a valuable source of contemporary advice and guidance, and that undergraduate medical students—tomorrow's doctors—will find not only the clinical problems directly relevant to their studies, but will also benefit from reading many of the sections in the 'Principles and Concepts' volume, providing them with a broadly based understanding of primary care medicine.

We would like to think that the Textbook will find its way into all those practices where undergraduate and postgraduate teaching and training are carried out. Vocational trainees, in particular, should find the level of detail in both volumes appropriate for their studies, and undergraduate teachers and postgraduate trainers will, we hope, find much here to inform and inspire the development and delivery of their curricula. There is much here too, we believe, for university departments of general practice and family practice; many of the essays in 'Principles and Concepts' are state-of-the-art, in-depth and fully referenced sources on key topics. The sections on research and education provide a substantial basis for engaging with the academic facets of primary care medical practice. Planners and policy makers will find valuable guidance in the Textbook about the essential components of high-quality primary care and its role within health services.

Acknowledgements

Any new literary venture, T.S. Eliot pointed out, is no more or less than an attempt to re-discover 'what has been lost and found and lost again and again' by those 'whom one cannot hope to emulate'. Whilst the authorship of this Textbook includes many of the most influential figures in primary medical care—and we are particularly proud that Professor Ian McWhinney has written its Foreword—we pay tribute to other giants of primary medical care who have not been able to contribute. We were privileged to have numbered Professor Chris Silagy amongst our core editorial team, and his death during the preparation of the Textbook represented a massive blow to primary care across the world.

I would like to take this opportunity to acknowledge the tremendous support and commitment that I have received from my co-editors, Professors Nicky Britten, Larry Culpepper, David Gass, Richard Grol, David Mant, and Chris Silagy and from all the section editors who joined us in putting together the second volume of the Textbook. I would also like to express profound thanks to all the authors involved in producing this Textbook, and to acknowledge their contributions of wisdom, expertise, experience, and passion.

It has been a pleasure working with Oxford University Press. Special thanks are due to Janet Whitehouse, the project administrator for the Textbook, who has displayed remarkable patience and tenacity coupled with highly developed author management skills, and Alison Langton, Editorial Director for Medicine at Oxford University Press, who was a constant source of wisdom, encouragement, and firm guidance. None of us could have contemplated undertaking this work without administrative and secretarial support from our own institutions but I would like to say a very special thank you, on behalf of all of us, to Pat Taylor, my personal assistant at King's College, London, without whom this enterprise would have been impossible.

Roger Jones
London, 2003

Foreword

Ian R. McWhinney

Emeritus Professor of Family Medicine, the University of Western Ontario

Recognition of a scientific discipline or body of knowledge by the academic community requires that it should not be entirely derived from other disciplines, that it should have its own scholarly and scientific literature, and that research should be generated within the discipline. The publication of scientific textbooks marks the articulation of a newly defined body of knowledge. The same could be said of the creation of new academic units and of listings in indices compiled by academic libraries. Kuhn[1] described the publication of textbooks as marking the emergence of a dominant paradigm, his term for the tacit assumptions and theoretical principles that form the basis of research and the organization of knowledge. According to Kuhn, textbooks usually treat the new paradigm as given, systematically disguising the scientific revolution which gave rise to it. Textbooks thus begin by 'truncating the scientist's sense of [the] discipline's history and then proceed to supply a substitute for what they have eliminated'. Osler's *Textbook of Medicine*, published in 1892, marked the culmination of almost a century of descriptive research, clinical and pathological, based on the revolution in medical thought that took place around the turn of the nineteenth century. Today, we might call it 'the medical model'. Osler saw no need to inform his readers about the origins of this paradigm, or to explain its concepts and vocabulary. Chapter 1 of Osler's textbook launches immediately into a description of infectious diseases and all the other chapters have diseases as their subject matter. For all his interest in the history of medicine, Osler in his textbook presented a medicine that was both unhistorical and a theoretical. This book promises to be different.

In his seminal lectures on diagnosis in 1926, Crookshank[2] remarked that every discipline sooner or later must define its fundamental concepts, and that for medicine the need was imperative. The medicine of Crookshank's time, and after, might well have been considered derivative from the laboratory sciences and therefore not a truly independent discipline. However, experience showed that no knowledge of basic science could predict all the phenomena of human illness: the application of this knowledge depended on a great body of taxonomic clinical knowledge accumulated over the years. Medicine derives from the laboratory sciences, but is also a descriptive science in its own right.

For many years, general practice was considered entirely derivative. It was assumed that the methods learned in one context—the teaching hospital—could be applied unmodified in the very different context of general practice. Even in these days, there were some who challenged these assumptions. In *The Future of Medicine*, Mackenzie[3] described the experience of the general practitioner as unique and maintained that general practice should be represented in the medical school. Mackenzie's research on the natural history of heart disease depended on such features of general practice as experience of the earliest stages of illness, observation over long periods, and personal knowledge of patients. His books became foundation texts for the emerging discipline of cardiology and his *Symptoms and their Interpretation*[4] could be regarded as a precursor text of general practice, even though it dealt only with one particular aspect.

From general practice to primary medical care

The first British textbooks of general practice appeared in the 1950s, a time when increasing specialization, and the need to teach the new trainee assistants, was forcing general practitioners to define their body of knowledge. When I entered general practice in 1954, two textbooks had recently become available. Both of these broke new ground and were remarkable achievements.[5,6] They were written by general practitioners using their own experience, backed up by data collected in their own practices. Both were insistent on the unique perspective of general practice, but there was little conceptual analysis, or indication that general practice might have distinctive methods and modes of thought. Both texts were organized according to conventional disease categories and nomenclature.

In the years since publication of these early texts, many more books have appeared, some of them research-based monographs on specific aspects of general practice, others covering the field as a whole. It is now customary to refer to the field as primary medical care, rather than general or family practice. The Institute of Medicine in the United States has described the four cornerstones of primary care as accessibility, comprehensiveness, continuity, and coordination. In some jurisdictions, general paediatrics and internal medicine share these features with general practice. Emergency medicine shares accessibility but not continuity. Bringing them together under one roof has administrative and pedagogic utility, but it would be a mistake to allow these disciplines to be submerged and disappear into a loose confederation. As well as sharing a great deal, each has a distinct culture, which is worth preserving. General practice, for example, has a long tradition and a unique outlook on medicine. It is not simply an amalgam of all the specialties, nor is it simply clinical medicine, plus epidemiology plus sociology. Its essence is an unconditional commitment to patients whatever may befall them. The commitment is to a person, not to a person with a certain disease. Since they cannot foresee all their patients' future needs, family doctors have to be generalists. Being generalists does not preclude a special interest in a single aspect of practice. Indeed, we need generalists who can speak with authority at consensus conferences, and who can write clinical chapters in textbooks. But generalists who make their patients their body of knowledge should be valued no less.

Primary care paediatricians and internists restrict their practices by age, but continue to be generalists capable of providing comprehensive care. If, however, primary care were to split into disease-specific specialties and become a mirror image of hospital medicine, two of the cornerstones (comprehensiveness and coordination) would collapse and the logic of a primary care sector would no longer apply.

Undifferentiated illness

Any textbook of general practice or primary care medicine faces a difficult problem. Family doctors are usually the first physicians to assess their patients' illnesses. These present as undifferentiated symptoms and, as Mackenzie understood, their assessment is a different process from the diagnosis of disease in its typical and fully developed form. In many patients the symptoms are self-limiting illnesses or short-lived responses to life's traumas, in some they are the earliest harbingers of a chronic illness, in others they are danger signals of an acute and life-threatening disease. The primary care physician must be adept at differentiating these conditions. A diagnosis of a spurious disease at this stage may set the stage for life-long invalidism. Misdiagnosis of an acute curable condition may result in disability or death. The importance of the primary assessment of symptoms, in the context of their meaning for the patient, cannot be overemphasized. Primary care physicians have to work at all levels of abstraction and all levels of certainty, though paucity of data in the early stages of illness often obliges them to make clinical judgements in conditions of high uncertainty. High uncertainty requires fail-safe strategies, such as robust rule-out tests and watchful waiting.

Necessary as they are in a textbook, the conventional divisions into the abstractions of disease and system categories do not fully represent the experience of the family doctor. Moreover, it is not sufficient for the textbook to include only the commoner diseases. If a patient with pheochromocytoma or cranial arteritis is misdiagnosed, it is no excuse to say that the disease is rare.

If a textbook of primary care has to be so inclusive, how can it avoid looking like a watered down textbook of internal medicine? Only by taking the perspective of the primary care clinician. Much progress has been made in our understanding of such aspects as clinical method, critical appraisal, preventive practice, doctor–patient relationships, working relationships with other professions, home care, and practice management.

Clinical epidemiology has given us tools for evaluating the relevance of evidence. We cannot assume that assessment or management protocols developed in other fields are appropriate in primary care. The predictive value of symptoms and tests varies with the prevalence of the target disorder. The harm done to disease-free patients who test positive may outweigh, in the primary care population, the benefits to patients with the target disorder. The sensitivity of a test varies with the stage of the illness. A test that is a good 'rule-out' test in a fully developed illness may not be sensitive enough in the early stages seen by the family doctor. Textbooks of internal medicine tend to deal with the later stages of illness.

Primary care clinicians have to be critical in their application of guidelines derived from randomized controlled trials. Clinical trials are done in highly selected populations. The elderly, the uneducated, the non-compliant, and patients with co-morbidity or borderline conditions are under-represented: yet these are common in primary care. Clinical trials are rarely long enough or large enough to reveal the long-term effects of drugs. To be useful in primary care, evidence-based guidelines should pass the scrutiny of well-informed primary care clinicians. We should expect this in a textbook such as this one. Even when evidence is universally accepted, it is often interpreted differently in different countries. An international text has the difficult task of dealing with such issues as the critical levels for prescription of cholesterol-lowering and antihypertension drugs, the management of otitis media, and the indications for a PSA test. A set of guidelines that makes sense in terms of one specialty may look very different when added to those of all the other specialties and viewed from the perspective of the primary care physician who has to apply them.

The importance of relationships

In most fields of primary medical practice, relationships are of prime importance. These may be relationships with patients, with families, with colleagues in other professions, and with communities. These values are embodied in the concept of continuity of care, by a physician or small practice team who know the patient. They are based on the well-founded belief that a personal relationship, when combined with professional competence, provides the best context for long-term care. Every new illness or episode is then interpreted in the context of knowledge of the patient. Continuity of care is now under siege from many quarters: from fragmentation of care, from consumer and commercial values, from the difficulty of reconciling accessibility with continuity.

To be healers for their patients, family doctors have to be involved, person to person. But there are right ways and wrong ways of being involved. The wrong way is to be involved at the level of the doctor's unexamined negative emotions: fear, helplessness, self-interest, likes and dislikes, self-centred attachments. The right way is to reconcile the seeming opposites of involvement and detachment.

Primary care physicians usually work closely with members of other professions, often in small close-knit teams, at other times by referral and collaboration. The nurse–physician relationship is important in the medical centre, the home, and the community, as are relationships with social workers, counsellors, psychologists, and others, especially for practices in areas of deprivation. Although primary care medicine includes only physicians, a textbook must address these roles and relationships, and convey the skills and attitudes required of team members.

Of all fields of medicine, general practice has traditionally been closest to where people live, and therefore vividly aware of the impact of poverty on health and on access to medical care. Although physicians cannot directly determine social policy, they can address difficulties of access, support their patients in obtaining their entitlements, and help them to adopt preventative practices.

A different world view

A primary care text should provide an alternative to the paradigm that still dominates biology and medicine. General practice, for example, has never fitted well into the low context, mechanistic, and reductionist approach to medicine. The person is not a machine, even though the body has some machine-like features. We can for practical purposes reduce a patient's problem to a simple linear causal chain, as when we prescribe an antibiotic or diagnose appendicitis. Medicine has achieved great success by treating the body as a machine, but everything we do for patients depends on their qualities as organisms. Mechanistic and organismic thinking are complementary not mutually exclusive—two perspectives on the same reality. Organisms have qualities possessed by no machine: growth, regeneration, learning, healing, intentionality, and self-transcendence. At its most successful, medicine works by supporting these natural processes. Our therapy often consists of removing the obstacles to healing whether they are psychological or physical. The traditional regimens of balanced nutrition, rest, sound sleep, exercise, relief of pain, personal support, and peace of mind are all measures that support the organism's natural healing powers. Immunization, the most effective of all scientific advances, strengthens the body's own powers of resistance. There is now convincing evidence that personal support works in the same way, justifying our belief in the power of the doctor–patient relationship.

An organism reacts to the traumas of life as a whole. 'The manner in which an organism copes with a defect is always characteristic of its individual nature.'[7] All significant illness affects the organism at every level, from the molecular to the cognitive and affective. The essence of the clinical method in general practice is that the body, the emotions, and the patient's experience of illness are attended to in every case, the degree of attention obviously depending on the individual circumstances. General practice is at the same time a clinical and existential medicine. The patient-centred clinical method requires us to make a clinical diagnosis and to attend to the patient's experience. A large part of general practice is helping patients to cope with and adapt to chronic illness and disability. No two patients are the same in their response. If we are to be healers, we have to understand the meaning of the illness in the life of each patient, and often in the life of the family. General practice has led the way in including the human experience of illness as a necessary part of medical knowledge. There is now a rich literature on the experience of illness and a textbook of primary care should find a place for it. It can teach us what it is like to become blind, to have multiple sclerosis, or to care for a spouse with

Alzheimer's disease or a child with diabetes. A textbook can mine this literature for the meanings that are common to all or most patients with a specific disability or disease; it can describe the tools and devices available to the disabled; and, by including case reports, it can stimulate the imagination of readers and help them to empathize with their patients. It is more difficult for a textbook addressed to a global readership to deal adequately with the power of a patient's and family's culture of origin to shape the meaning illness has for them. At least it should sensitize readers to the importance of culture.

The transition from mechanistic to organismic thinking requires a radical change in our notion of disease causation. Medicine has been dominated by a doctrine of specific aetiology: a cause for each disease. We have learned to think of a causal agent as a force acting in linear fashion on a passive object. In self-organizing systems such as organisms, causation is non-linear. The multiple feedback loops between patient and environment, and between all levels of the patient as organism, require us to think in causal networks, not straight lines. Moreover, the patient as organism is not a passive object. The 'specific cause' of an illness may only be the trigger, which releases a process that is already a potential of the organism. The causes that maintain an illness and inhibit healing may be different from the causes that initiated it, and these may include the patient's own maladaptive behaviours, or even the doctor's actions.

Organismic thinking is thinking in terms of complementarity rather than duality: both/and rather than either/or. As organismic thinkers, either/or questions, such as 'is migraine organic or psychogenic?' become meaningless to us.(8) In this context, it is disappointing to see tiredness and fatigue, sleeping disorders and somatization—all of them complex and multifactorial illnesses—categorized as mental health problems. What message will this convey to our trainees? Primary care physicians have to know where they are on the scale of the complementarities between organismic and mechanistic, uncertainty and precision, involvement and detachment, concrete and abstract, and the particular and the general. The dominance of the mechanistic, reductionist world view has not been unchallenged. An undercurrent of organismic thought has continued and is now finding new acceptance in the sciences of complexity.(7,9,10) Publication of the *Oxford Textbook of Primary Medical Care* will, I hope, be a milestone in the development of primary care medicine.

Acknowledgements

I thank the Canadian Library of Family Medicine for bibliographic support and Joanna L. Asuncion for preparing the manuscript.

References

1. **Kuhn, T.S.** *The Structure of Scientific Revolutions.* Chicago: University of Chicago Press, 1967.
2. **Crookshank, F.G.** (1926). The theory of diagnosis. *Lancet* **2**, 939.
3. **Mackenzie, J.** *The Future of Medicine.* London: Henry Frowde, Hodder and Stoughton, 1919.
4. **Mackenzie, J.** *Symptoms and their Interpretation.* London: Shaw, 1920.
5. **Fry, J.**, ed. *Clinical Medicine in General Practice.* London: J&A Churchill, 1954.
6. **Craddock, D.** *A Short Textbook of General Practice.* London: HK Lewis, 1953.
7. **Goldstein, K.** *The Organism.* New York: Zone Books, 1995.
8. **McWhinney, I.R.** (1996). The importance of being different. *British Journal of General Practice* **46**, 433–6.
9. **Dubos, R.** *Man Adapting.* London: Yale University Press, 1965.
10. **Boyd, C.A.R. and Noble, D.**, ed. *The Logic of Life: The Challenge of Integrative Physiology.* Oxford: Oxford University Press, 1993.

Contributors

Samuel B. Adkins Residency Director, East Carolina University, Greenville, South Carolina, USA
Volume 2: 13.6 Hip problems

Bert Aertgeerts Associate Professor, University of Leuven, Leuven, Belgium
Volume 2: 6.2 Haematuria and proteinuria

Mohammed Ali Lecturer, Centre for International Health, Curtin University of Technology, Perth, Western Australia
Volume 1: 1.8 First contact care in developing health care systems

Keith P. Allison Specialist Registrar in Plastic Surgery and Burns, University Hospital Birmingham, NHS Trust, Birmingham, UK
Volume 2: 14.6 Burns

Jeremy Anderson Professor of Epidemiology and Biostatistics, School of Population Health, University of Melbourne, Melbourne, Australia
Volume 1: 10.5 Community interventions—mental health

Richard Anstett Professor of Dermatology, University of Wisconsin-Madison, Wisconsin, USA
Volume 2: 15.6 Chronic skin rashes

Willem J.J. Assendelft Head, Department of Guideline Development and Research Policy, Dutch College of General Practitioners, Utrecht, The Netherlands
Volume 2: 13.8 Tennis elbow

Jo Baggen University of Maastricht, Maastricht, The Netherlands
Volume 1: 8.4 Clinical specialization

Macaran A. Baird Department Head, Family Practice and Community Health, University of Minnesota, USA
Volume 1: 9.3 Family interviewing and assessment
Volume 1: 10.7 Allocating and managing resources

Richard Baker Professor, Clinical Governance Research and Development Unit, University of Leicester, Leicester General Hospital, Leicester, UK
Volume 1: 13.1 Principles and models for quality improvement

Sally Baldwin Research Professor, The University of York, Heslington, York, UK
Volume 1: 10.6 Social care and its place in primary care

Kevin Barraclough General Practitioner, Painswick, Gloucestershire, UK
Volume 2: 1.3 Palpitations and silent arrhythmias

Marie-Dominique Beaulieu Professeur titulaire Chaire Dr Sadok Besrour en Medecine Familiale, Département de Médecine Familiale et Centre de Recherche du CHUM, Université de Montréal, Montréal, Quebec, Canada
Volume 2: 7.12 Screening for cancer in women

Justin Beilby Professor of General Practice, University of Adelaide, Adelaide, Australia
Volume 2: 2.3 Acute non-infective respiratory disorders

Kathleen A. Bell-Irving Clinical Instructor, University of British Columbia, Vancouver, Canada
Volume 2: 16.7 Functional assessment of the elderly

Eugene Bereza Director, Medical Ethics Program, Faculty of Medicine, McGill University, Montréal, Canada
Volume 1: 16.3 Truth-telling in family medicine

Howard Bergman The Dr Joseph Kaufmann Professor of Geriatric Medicine, McGill University, Jewish General Hospital, Montréal, Canada
Volume 2: 16.4 Non-specific presentations of illness
Volume 2: 16.5 Dementia

Thomas M. Best Associate Professor of Orthopedics and Rehabilitation and Family Medicine, University of Wisconsin Medical School, Madison, Wisconsin, USA
Volume 2: 13.3 Acute joint pain

Jo Betterton Team Leader, Consultancy Liaison Service, Hurley Clinic, London, UK
Volume 2: 9.5 Alcohol misuse and primary care

Alison Blenkinsopp Professor of the Practice of Pharmacy, Keele University, Staffs, UK
Volume 1: 3.5 Self-care and self-medication

Wienke G.W. Boerma Senior Researcher, NIVEL (The Netherlands Institute for Health Services Research), Utrecht, The Netherlands
Volume 1: 2.1 Health care systems: understanding the stages of development
Volume 1: 12.7 General practitioners' use of time and time management

Christine Bond Professor of Primary Care, Head of Teaching, University of Aberdeen, Foresterhill Health Centre, Aberdeen, UK
Volume 1: 3.5 Self-care and self-medication

Jeffrey M. Borkan Sackler Faculty of Medicine, Tel Aviv University, Tel Aviv, Israel
Volume 1: 1.4 Community primary care
Volume 1: 9.5 Working with families with chronic medical disorders

Peter Bower Senior Research Fellow, National Primary Care Research and Development Centre, University of Manchester, UK
Volume 1: 1.3 The health care team

Colin Bradley Professor of General Practice, University College Cork, Cork, Ireland
Volume 1: 16.6 Ethics of resource allocation

Suzanne F. Bradley Associate Professor of Internal Medicine, University of Michigan and Veterans Affairs, Ann Arbor Healthcare System, Ann Arbor, Michigan, USA
Volume 2: 16.3 Infections

Nicky Britten Professor of Applied Health Care Research, Institute of Clinical Education, Peninsula Medical School, Universities of Exeter and Plymouth, St Luke's Campus, Exeter, UK
Volume 1: 7.5 Concordance and compliance

Howard Brody Professor, Family Practice and Center for Ethics and Humanities in the Life Sciences, Michigan State University, Michigan, USA
Volume 1: 16.7 End-of-life decisions

Carlos Brotons Unitat d'Epidemiologia, Hospital General Vall d'Hebron, Barcelona, Spain
Volume 1: 11.7 Anticipatory care of established illness: vascular disease

Judith Belle Brown Professor, Center for Studies in Family Medicine, UWO Research Park, Ontario, Canada
Volume 1: 5.6 Time and the consultation

Frank Buntinx Professor, Catholic University of Leuven, Belgium, University of Maastricht, The Netherlands
Volume 2: 6.2 Haematuria and proteinuria

Frederick I. Burge Faculty of Medicine, Dalhousie University, Halifax, Canada
Volume 2: 17.5 Hospice and home care

Sandra K. Burge Professor, University of Texas Health Science Center, San Antonio, Texas, USA
Volume 1: 9.6 Family violence

Peter Burke General Practitioner, St Bartholomew's Medical Centre, Oxford, UK
Volume 1: 11.3 Screening

John L. Campbell Professor of General Practice and Primary Care, Peninsula Medical School, Postgraduate Medical Centre, Exeter, UK
Volume 1: 2.6 Primary care and general practice in Europe: West and South
Volume 1: 12.5 Organization of services

Thomas L. Campbell Professor, Family Medicine and Dentistry, University of Rochester School of Medicine and Dentistry, Rochester, New York, USA
Volume 1: 9.1 Working with families in primary care

Yvonne H. Carter Professor of General Practice & Primary Care, Director, Institute of Community Health Sciences, Barts and the London, Queen Mary's School of Medicine and Dentistry, London, UK
Volume 1: 14.1 History and structure

Francoise P. Chagnon Director of Professional Services, McGill University Health Centre, Montréal, Canada
Volume 2: 3.1 Epistaxis
Volume 2: 3.5 Hoarseness and voice change

Carlos A. Charles Wound Healing Fellow, University of Miami School of Medicine, Florida, USA
Volume 2: 15.4 Pigmented skin lesions

Ian Charlton Associate Professor of Medicine, Newcastle University; Chairman, Asthma Watch, NSW Central Coast, New South Wales, Australia
Volume 2: 2.4 Asthma

Rodger Charlton Director of General Practice, Undergraduate Medical Education, Warwick Medical School, University of Warwick, Coventry, UK
Volume 2: 17.2 Pain concepts and pain control in palliative care

Howard Chertkow Director, Bloomfield Centre for Research in Aging, Lady Davis Institute for Medical Research, S.M.B.D. Jewish General Hospital, Montréal, Canada
Volume 2: 16.5 Dementia

G. Kheng Chew Subspecialty Fellow, Aberdeen Royal Infirmary, Aberdeen, UK
Volume 2: 7.10 Abnormal cervical smear

Joseph L. Chin Professor and Chair, Division of Urology, University of Western Ontario, London Health Sciences Centre, Ontario, Canada
Volume 2: 6.3 Acute urinary retention in adults
Volume 2: 6.4 Testicular and scrotal problems

Katia Cikurel Consultant Neurologist, King's College Hospital, London, UK
Volume 2: 11.7 Coma

A. Mark Clarfield Chief of Geriatrics, Soroka Hospital; Professor and Sidonie Hecht Chair of Gerontology, Faculty of Health Sciences, Ben Gurion University of the Negev, Beersheva, Israel
Volume 2: 16.4 Non-specific presentations of illness
Volume 2: 16.5 Dementia

Lyn Clearihan Senior Lecturer, Monash University, Melbourne, Australia
Volume 2: 15.5 Acute skin rashes
Volume 2: 15.7 Acne

Matthew K. Cline AnMed Family Practice Center, Anderson, South Carolina, USA
Volume 2: 8.8 Caring for women in labour

Kathleen Cole-Kelly Professor, Family Medicine, Case Western Reserve University School of Medicine, Cleveland, Ohio, USA
Volume 1: 9.5 Working with families with chronic medical disorders

Colin Coles Professor, Institute of Health and Community Studies, Bournemouth University, Hampshire, UK
Volume 1: 15.4 Personal growth and professional development

Matthew W. Cooke Reader in Emergency Care, Warwick Medical School, University of Warwick, Warwick, UK
Volume 2: 14.4 Head and neck injuries

Massimo Costantini Senior Epidemiologist, Hospice Medical Director, Servizio di Epidemiologia Clinica, Istituto Nazionale per la Ricerca sul Cancro, Genova, Italy
Volume 1: 7.8 Terminal and palliative care
Volume 2: 17.1 The dying patient and their family

Angela Coulter Chief Executive, Picker Institute Europe, Oxford, UK
Volume 1: 3.4 Medicine and the media

Sarah Cox Consultant in Palliative Medicine, Chelsea and Westminster Hospital, London, UK
Volume 1: 7.8 Terminal and palliative care
Volume 2: 17.6 Symptoms and palliation

Benjamin F. Crabtree Professor and Research Director, University of Medicine and Dentistry of New Jersey, Robert Wood Johnson Medical School, New Brunswick, USA
Volume 1: 14.2 Methods: qualitative

Marilyn A. Craven Associate Clinical Professor, McMaster University, Hamilton, Ontario, Canada
Volume 2: 9.2 Anxiety

Margaret E. Cruickshank Senior Lecturer in Gynaecology and Oncology, Aberdeen Maternity Hospital, Aberdeen, UK
Volume 2: 7.10 Abnormal cervical smear

Alicia Curtin Clinical Assistant Professor, Brown University School of Medicine, Memorial Hospital of Rhode Island, Pawtucket, Rhode Island, USA
Volume 2: 16.1 Falls in the elderly

Jeremy Dale Professor of Primary Care, Warwick Medical School (LWMS), University of Warwick, Coventry, UK
Volume 1: 1.5 Primary care in the emergency department

Maaike Dautzenberg Senior Researcher, Centre for Quality of Care Research (WOK), Universiteit Maastricht/Universitair Medisch Centrum, Nijmegen, The Netherlands
Volume 1: 8.7 Collaboration between professional and lay care

David Davis Associate Dean, University of Toronto, Ontario, Canada
Volume 1: 15.3 The professional development of the family physician: managing knowledge

Jan de Maeseneer Professor and Head of Department, Department of General Practice and Primary Health Care, Ghent University, Gent, Belgium
Volume 1: 4.5 Socio-economic differences in health

Ruut A. de Melker Former Head of the Department of Family Medicine, Emeritus Professor of General Practice, University of Utrecht, Utrecht, The Netherlands
Volume 1: 4.1 The iceberg of illness

Marc De Meyere Vakgroep Huisartsgeneeskunde, Gent, Belgium
Volume 2: 2.5 Chronic lower respiratory disorders

Peter A.G.M. de Smet Clinical Pharmacologist and Professor in Pharmaceutical Care, Scientific Institute Dutch Pharmacists, The Hague, The Netherlands
Volume 1: 1.6 Traditional healers as health care providers: Africa as an example

An de Sutter Department of General Practice and Primary Health Care, Ghent University, Ghent, Belgium
Volume 2: 2.5 Chronic lower respiratory disorders

Niek J. de Wit Senior Lecturer, General Practitioner, Julius Center for Health Sciences and Primary Care, University Medical Center, Utrecht, The Netherlands
Volume 2: 4.3 Acute abdominal pain
Volume 2: 4.11 Constipation

Chris Del Mar Professor and Director, Centre for General Practice, Medical School, University of Queensland, Queensland, Australia
Volume 2: 3.2 Ear pain in adults

F.W. Dijkers General Practitioner, Teacher in Practice Organization, Leiden University Medical Center, Leiden, The Netherlands
Volume 1: 12.3 Equipment and premises in general practice

Geert-Jan Dinant Professor, University of Maastricht, Maastricht, The Netherlands
Volume 1: 6.1 Undifferentiated illness and uncertainty in diagnosis and management
Volume 1: 6.2 Clinical diagnosis: hypothetico-deductive reasoning and other theoretical frameworks

Sean Dinneen Community Diabetologist, Addenbrooke's Hospital, Cambridge, UK
Volume 2: 5.2 Diabetes—Type 1 and Type 2

Anna Donald Chief Executive, Bazian Ltd, London, UK
Volume 1: 13.3 Evidence-based medicine as a tool in quality improvement

Len Doyal Professor of Medical Ethics, St Bartholomew's and The Royal London School of Medicine and Dentistry, Queen Mary College, University of London, UK
Volume 1: 16.1 Ethics in primary care

Gordon W. Duff Florey Professor of Molecular Medicine, Director, Division of Genomic Medicine, School of Medicine and Biomedical Science, University of Sheffield, UK
Volume 2: Introduction—genomic medicine

Tzvi Dwolatzky Director, Geriatric Department, Mental Health Hospital, Beersheva, Israel
Volume 2: 16.4 Non-specific presentations of illness

Kathi Earles Assistant Director of Pediatric Residency Program, Morehouse School of Medicine, SW Atlanta, Georgia, USA
Volume 2: 10.2 Childhood respiratory infections

Martin Eccles Professor of Clinical Effectiveness and The William Leech Professor of Primary Care Research, Centre for Health Services Research, University of Newcastle, Newcastle upon Tyne, UK
Volume 1: 13.4 Using and developing clinical guidelines

Polly Edmonds Consultant/Honorary Senior Lecturer, Palliative Care Team, King's College Hospital, London, UK
Volume 1: 7.8 Terminal and palliative care
Volume 2: 17.1 The dying patient and their family
Volume 2: 17.6 Symptoms and palliation

Adrian Edwards Reader, Primary Care Group, Swansea Clinical School, University of Wales Swansea, Swansea, UK
Volume 1: 5.5 Shared decision-making in clinical practice
Volume 1: 7.3 Communication about risks and benefits of treatment and care options

Helena Elkington Research Fellow and General Practitioner, Guy's, King's and St Thomas' School of Medicine, King's College, London, UK
Volume 2: 2.6 Chronic cough

Glyn Elwyn Senior Lecturer in General Practice, University of Wales College of Medicine, Llanedeyrn Health Centre, Cardiff, UK
Volume 1: 5.5 Shared decision-making in clinical practice
Volume 1: 7.3 Communication about risks and benefits of treatment and care options
Volume 1: 14.1 History and structure

Jon Emery Cancer Research UK, Clinician Scientist General Practice & Primary Care Research Unit, University of Cambridge, Institute of Public Health, Cambridge, UK
Volume 1: 6.6 Computerized decision support
Volume 1: 9.4 Assessment and management of genetic risk

Michael Francis Evans Principal Investigator, Knowledge Translation Program, Assistant Professor and Research Scholar, Family & Community Medicine, University of Toronto, Toronto, Canada
Volume 1: 15.3 The professional development of the family physician: managing knowledge

Wes E. Fabb Honorary Clinical Associate Professor, Department of General Practice, Monash University, Melbourne, Australia
Volume 1: 2.13 International organizations

Tom Fahey Professor of Primary Care Medicine, Tayside Centre for General Practice, University of Dundee, Dundee, UK
Volume 2: 1.10 High blood pressure
Volume 2: 2.7 Haemoptysis

Steven R. Feldman Professor of Dermatology, Pathology, and Public Health Sciences, Wake Forest University School of Medicine, Medical Center Boulevard, North Carolina, USA
Volume 2: 15.8 Psoriasis

Ian S. Fentiman Professor of Surgical Oncology, Guy's Hospital, London, UK
Volume 2: 7.11 Abnormal mammogram

Richard A. Figler Assistant Clinical Instructor, Assistant Clinical Professor, Co-coordinator of Procedural Skills, East Carolina University School of Medicine, Brody School of Medicine, East Carolina University, North Carolina, USA
Volume 2: 13.7 Foot problems

Gerda Fijten General Practitioner and Medical Teacher, Skillslab, University of Maastricht, Maastricht, The Netherlands
Volume 2: 4.8 Rectal bleeding

Denise Findlay Caulfield Community Care Centre, Victoria, Australia
Volume 2: 1.8 Varicose veins
Volume 2: 1.9 Leg ulcers

David A. Fitzmaurice Professor of General Practice, The University of Birmingham Medical School, Birmingham, UK
Volume 1: 6.5 Diagnostic tests and use of technology
Volume 2: 1.6 Thrombosis and thromboembolism

Douglas M. Fleming Director, Birmingham Research Unit, Royal College of General Practitioners, Birmingham, UK
Volume 1: 10.3 Health surveillance

Sander Flikweert Senior Scientific Staff Member of Dutch College of General Practitioners (Nederlands Huisartsen Genootschap (NHG)), Utrecht, The Netherlands
Volume 2: 8.6 Vaginal bleeding in early pregnancy

Signe Flottorp Researcher, Directorate for Health and Social Affairs, Oslo, Norway
Volume 1: 13.5 Tools for quality improvement and change in practice

Colleen Fogarty Assistant Professor and Director of Psychosocial Medicine, Department of Family Medicine, Boston University Medical Center, Boston, Massachusetts, USA
Volume 1: 9.6 Family violence

Walter A. Forred Director, Family Practice Residency Program, Kansas City, USA
Volume 2: 15.3 Pruritus

Robbie Foy Clinical Senior Lecturer in Primary Care, Centre for Health Services Research, University of Newcastle upon Tyne, Newcastle, UK
Volume 1: 14.3 Methods: quantitative

Gerri Frager Medical Director, Pediatric Palliative Care, IWK Health Centre, Halifax, Nova Scotia, Canada
Volume 2: 17.4 Death of a child

Deborah A. Frank Professor of Pediatrics, Boston University School of Medicine, Boston, Masssachusetts, USA
Volume 2: 10.5 Failure to thrive

Caroline Free Research Fellow, Guy's, King's, and St Thomas's School of Medicine, Department of General Practice and Primary Care, London, UK
Volume 2: 8.5 Teenage pregnancy

George K. Freeman Professor of General Practice, Centre for Primary Care and Social Medicine, Imperial College London, London, UK
Volume 1: 8.1 Coordination and continuity of care

Peggy Frith Consultant Medical Ophthalmologist, Oxford Eye Hospital, Radcliffe Infirmary, Oxford, UK
Volume 2: 12.4 Ptosis and unequal pupils

Yvonne Fry Chief, Maternal and Child Health Team, Instructor of Clinical Pediatrics, National Center for Primary Care, Morehouse School of Medicine, Atlanta, Georgia, USA
Volume 2: 10.2 Childhood respiratory infections

George E. Fryer Analyst, The Robert Graham Center for Policy Studies in Family Practice and Primary Care, Washington DC, USA
Volume 1: 1.1 The nature of primary medical care

John M. Galloway General Practitioner, St James' House Surgery, Norfolk, UK
Volume 2: 4.2 Dysphagia

Goh Lee Gan Associate Professor, Department of Community, Occupational, and Family Medicine, National University of Singapore, Singapore
Volume 1: 2.3 Primary care and general practice in East and Southeast Asia

B.C. Gee Specialist Registrar in Dermatology, Queen's Medical Centre, Nottingham, UK
Volume 2: 15.1 Hair-related problems

Clare Gerada Director, Royal College of General Practitioners Drugs Training Programme; General Practitioner, London, UK
Volume 2: 9.4 Drug misuse and dependence
Volume 2: 9.5 Alcohol misuse and primary care

Dwenda Kay Gjerdingen University of Minnesota, St Paul, Minneapolis, USA
Volume 2: 8.11 Postpartum care

Hein G. Gooszen Professor of Surgery, University Medical Centre, Utrecht, The Netherlands
Volume 2: 4.5 Abdominal mass

Amy A. Gorin Assistant Professor of Psychiatry and Human Behavior, Brown Medical School, Weight Control and Diabetes Research Center, The Miriam Hospital, Providence, Rhode Island, USA
Volume 2: 5.1 Obesity

Kees J. Gorter General Practitioner, Lecturer and Senior Researcher, Julius Center for Health Sciences and Primary Care, University Medical Center (UMC), Utrecht, The Netherlands
Volume 2: 13.7 Foot problems

Th.M.E. Govaert formerly General Practitioner; formerly member of the Research Department of General Practice, University of Maastricht, Stein, The Netherlands
Volume 2: 16.9 Influenza

Sandra Gower Practice Manager and Executive Partner, Hemel Hempstead, UK
Volume 1: 12.5 Organization of services

Jan Grace Subspecialty Trainee in Reproductive Medicine, Guy's and St Thomas' Hospitals Trust, Assisted Conception Unit, Guy's Hospital, London, UK
Volume 2: 8.2 Sub-fertility

Roger Gray Consultant Ophthalmologist, Taunton and Somerset NHS Trust, Taunton and Somerset Hospital, Somerset, UK
Volume 2: 12.7 Eye trauma

Edward C. Green Senior Research Scientist, Harvard University, Center for Population and Development Studies, Boston, USA
Volume 1: 1.6 Traditional healers as health care providers: Africa as an example

Larry A. Green Professor and Director, The Robert Graham Center for Policy Studies in Family Practice and Primary Care, Washington DC, USA
Volume 1: 1.1 The nature of primary medical care

Sally Green Associate Professor, Monash Institute of Health Services Research, Monash University, Melbourne, Australia
Volume 2: 13.8 Tennis elbow

Trisha Greenhalgh Professor of Primary Health Care, University College London, London, UK
Volume 1: 13.3 Evidence-based medicine as a tool in quality improvement

R. Stephen Griffith Associate Professor & Chairman, University of Missouri Kansas City, Kansas City, Missouri, USA
Volume 2: 15.11 Bruising and purpura

Jeremy Grimshaw Professor and Director, Clinical Epidemiology Programme, Ottawa Health Research Institute, University of Ottawa, Canada
Volume 1: 13.4 Using and developing clinical guidelines
Volume 1: 13.5 Tools for quality improvement and change in practice

Peter P. Groenewegen Head of Research Department, Professor of Social and Geographical Aspects of Health and Health care, Utrecht University, NIVEL (The Netherlands Institute for Health Services Research), Utrecht, The Netherlands
Volume 1: 12.7 General practitioners' use of time and time management

Richard Grol Professor and Director, Centre for Quality of Care Research (WOK), Nijmegen University Medical Centre, Maastricht University, The Netherlands
Volume 1: 13.1 Principles and models for quality improvement
Volume 1: 13.6 Total quality management and continuous quality improvement
Volume 1: 13.7 The patient's role in improving quality

Stefan Grzybowski Children's and Women's Health Center of British Columbia, Vancouver, Canada
Volume 2: 8.1 Pre-conception care

Jane Gunn Associate Professor, University of Melbourne, Victoria, Australia
Volume 1: 14.3 Methods: quantitative

Allan C. Halpern Chief, Dermatology Service, Memorial Sloan-Kettering Cancer Center, New York, USA
Volume 2: 15.4 Pigmented skin lesions

Hilary Haman Fellow of The Chartered Institute of Personnel & Development, Organisational Management, Personnel Adviser, Cardiff, UK
Volume 1: 12.2 Staff

Philip Hannaford Grampian Health Board Professor of Primary Care, University of Aberdeen, Aberdeen, UK
Volume 1: 10.1 The individual and the population

Mark Harris Professor of General Practice, School of Public Health and Community Medicine, University of New South Wales, Sydney, Australia
Volume 1: 14.6 Outcomes

Susan Harris Head, Department of Family Practice, Children's and Women's Health Centre of British Columbia, Vancouver, Canada
Volume 2: 8.3 Contraception

Yvonne Hart Consultant Neurologist, Radcliffe Infirmary, Oxford, UK
Volume 2: 11.2 Epilepsy

M. Jawad Hashim Program Director, Primary Care Pakistan, Islamabad, Pakistan
Volume 1: 2.10 Primary care and general practice in Pakistan

Richard Hays Chair of General Practice and Rural Medicine, James Cook University, Queensland, Australia
Volume 1: 15.2 Vocational and postgraduate training

Jane Haywood Clinical Nurse Specialist, CLAS Team, Hurley Clinic, London, UK
Volume 2: 9.4 Drug misuse and dependence

M.S. Darrell Henderson Health Policy Analyst, American Academy of Family Physicians, Leawood, Kansas, USA
Volume 1: 2.12 Primary care and general practice in North America

John Henry Professor of Accident and Emergency Medicine, Imperial College Faculty of Medicine, St Mary's Hospital, London, UK
Volume 2: 14.7 Poisoning

John M. Hickner Professor of Family Practice, Michigan State University, Michigan, USA
Volume 2: 3.6 Acute sinusitis

Irene J. Higginson Professor and Head, Department of Palliative Care and Policy, King's College London, Weston Education Centre, London, UK
Volume 1: 7.8 Terminal and palliative care
Volume 2: 17.1 The dying patient and their family

Roger Higgs Professor of General Practice, Guy's, King's and St Thomas' School of Medicine, London, UK
Volume 1: 16.4 Confidentiality

Wolfgang Himmel Medical Sociologist, University of Göttingen, Göttingen, Germany
Volume 1: 7.1 Principles of patient management

Per Hjortdahl Professor of General Practice, University of Oslo, Oslo, Norway
Volume 1: 7.6 Continuity of care
Volume 1: 12.4 The office laboratory

Richard Hobbs Professor and Head of Primary Care and General Practice, Primary Care Clinical Sciences Building, University of Birmingham, Edgbaston, Birmingham, UK
Volume 2: 1.2 Heart failure
Volume 2: 1.11 Dyslipidaemia and cardiovascular disease

David B. Hogan Professor and Brenda Strafford Foundation Chair in Geriatric Medicine, University of Calgary Health Sciences Centre, Alberta, Canada
Volume 2: 16.5 Dementia

Mary P. Hogan Home Care and Office-based Nurse, Case Western University School of Medicine, Ohio, USA
Volume 1: 9.5 Working with families with chronic medical disorders

Tony Hope Professor of Medical Ethics, ETHOX (The Oxford Centre for Ethics and Communication in Health Care Practice), University of Oxford, Oxford, UK
Volume 1: 16.5 Ethics of research

Jan Lucas Hoving Senior Research Fellow, Monash University, Melbourne, Australia
Volume 2: 13.2 Neck pain

William Howlett Consultant Neurologist and Honorary Senior Lecturer in Neurology, King's College Hospital, London, UK
Volume 2: 11.8 Meningitis and CNS infections

Suber S. Huang Director, Vitreoretinal Diseases and Surgery, University Hospitals of Cleveland; Associate Professor of Ophthalmology, Case Western Reserve University, Cleveland, Ohio, USA
Volume 2: 12.6 Blindness

Pali Hungin Professor of Primary Care and General Practice, University of Durham, Durham, UK
Volume 1: 6.4 The therapeutic illusion: self-limiting illness
Volume 2: 4.7 Haematemesis and melaena

Brian Hurwitz D'Oyly Carte Professor of Medicine and the Arts, King's College, London, UK
Volume 1: 13.4 Using and developing clinical guidelines
Volume 1: 16.8 Medico-legal issues
Volume 2: 11.3 Movement disorders

Sally Irvine Haman and Irvine Associates, Morpeth, Northumberland, UK
Volume 1: 12.1 Practice structures

Neill Iscoe Toronto-Sunnybrook Regional Cancer Centre, Ontario, Canada
Volume 2: 6.11 Prostate cancer

D. Anna Jarvis Professor of Paediatrics, University of Toronto, The Hospital for Sick Children, Toronto, Canada
Volume 2: 14.8 Drowning and inhalations
Volume 2: 14.9 Electrical injuries

David Jewell Editor, British Journal of General Practice; Honorary Senior Lecturer in Primary Care, University of Bristol, Bristol, UK
Volume 1: 14.7 Publishing primary care research

Sandra Marchese Johnson Clnical Trials Unit Director, Dermatology, University of Arkansas, Arkansas, USA
Volume 2: 15.13 Photosensitivity

Roger Jones Wolfson Professor of General Practice and Primary Care, Guy's, King's and St Thomas' School of Medicine, London, UK
Volume 1: 1.4 Community primary care
Volume 1: 8.4 Clinical specialization
Volume 1: 12.3 Equipment and premises in general practice
Volume 1: 14.7 Publishing primary care research
Volume 2: 4.1 Dyspepsia

Norman B. Kahn Jr Vice-President, Science and Education, American Academy of Family Physicians, Leawood, USA
Volume 1: 2.12 Primary care and general practice in North America

Joe Kai Professor of Primary Care, School of Community Health Sciences, University of Nottingham, Nottingham, UK
Volume 2: 10.1 Approach to the sick infant

Victoria S. Kaprielian Clinical Professor, Duke University Medical Center, Durham, North Carolina, USA
Volume 1: 1.9 Management and leadership

Michael P. Kelly Director of Research and Information, Health Development Agency, London, UK
Volume 1: 5.4 Doctors' perceptions of their patients

Tony Kendrick Professor of Primary Medical Care, Director of Community Clinical Sciences Division, University of Southampton Medical School, Aldermoor Health Centre, Southampton, UK
Volume 1: 11.8 Anticipatory care of mental health problems
Volume 2: 9.1 Depression

Ngaire Kerse Senior Lecturer, University of Auckland, Auckland, New Zealand
Volume 1: 2.4 Primary care and general practice in Australia and New Zealand

Michael Richard Kidd Professor of General Practice, University of Sydney and President, Royal Australian College of General Practitioners, Sydney, Australia
Volume 1: 5.7 Computers in the consultation
Volume 2: 6.7 HIV/AIDS

George E. Kikano Chairman, Department of Family Medicine, Case Western Reserve University, Ohio, USA
Volume 2: 12.6 Blindness

Ann Louise Kinmonth Professor and Head, General Practice and Primary Care Research Unit, Institute of Public Health, University of Cambridge, Cambridge, UK
Volume 1: 5.1 The patient–doctor relationship
Volume 2: 5.2 Diabetes—Type 1 and Type 2

Colleen Kirkham Clinical Associate Professor, University of British Columbia, Vancouver, Canada
Volume 2: 8.1 Pre-conception care

Maarten Klomp General Practitioner, Center for Primary Care Achtse Barrier, Eindhoven, The Netherlands
Volume 2: 6.10 Benign prostate disorders

Arie Knuistingh Neven General Practitioner/Epidemiologist, Leiden University Medical Centre, Leiden, The Netherlands; Centre for Sleep Wake Disorders, MCH Westeinde Hospital, The Hague, The Netherlands
Volume 2: 9.9 Sleep disorders

Michael M. Kochen Professor of General Practice and Head, University of Göttingen, Germany
Volume 1: 7.1 Principles of patient management

Lakshmi Kolagotla Boston University Medical Center, Boston, Massachussetts, USA
Volume 2: 10.5 Failure to thrive

Eliana C. Korin Senior Associate and Director of Behavioral Science, Department of Family and Social Medicine, Montefiore Medical Center and Albert Einstein College of Medicine, New York, USA
Volume 1: 9.2 Families, health, and cultural diversity

Madelon W. Kroneman Researcher, International Health Care Systems, NIVEL (The Netherlands Institute for Health Services Research), Utrecht, The Netherlands
Volume 1: 2.1 Health care systems: understanding the stages of development

Phillipa M. Kyle Consultant in Maternal and Fetal Medicine, St Michael's Hospital, Bristol, UK
Volume 2: 8.8 Caring for women in labour

Toine Lagro-Janssen General Practitioner and Professor, Women's Studies Medicine University Medical Center, Nijmegen, The Netherlands
Volume 2: 7.6 Urinary incontinence
Volume 2: 16.6 Urinary incontinence

Henk Lamberts Professor of General/Family Practice, Division of Clinical Methods & Public Health, Academic Medical Center, University of Amsterdam, Amsterdam, The Netherlands
Volume 1: 4.3 Classification and the domain of family practice

Tim Lancaster Clinical Reader in General Practice, Department of Primary Health Care, Oxford University, Oxford, UK
Volume 1: 11.4 Changing behaviour: smoking
Volume 1: 14.5 Secondary research

Pekka Larivaara Professor in Systemic Family Medicine, University of Oulu, Finland
Volume 1: 9.1 Working with families in primary care

Hilary Lavender General Practitioner, London, UK
Volume 2: 1.12 Anaemia

Patricia Lebensohn Associate Professor of Clinical, Family and Community Medicine, Family Practice Residency Program, University of Arizona, Tucson, Arizona, USA
Volume 1: 9.2 Families, health, and cultural diversity

Barbara Lent Associate Professor, University of Western Ontario, London, Ontario, Canada
Volume 2: 7.13 Violence as a women's health issue

Alexander K.C. Leung Clinical Associate Professor of Paediatrics, The University of Calgary, Calgary, Canada
Volume 2: 12.2 Sticky eye

Morten Lindbak Associate Professor, Department of General Practice, University of Oslo, Oslo, Norway
Volume 2: 3.6 Acute sinusitis

Christos Lionis Associate Professor, University of Crete, Faculty of Medicine, Crete, Greece
Volume 2: 4.9 Jaundice

Verity Livingstone Associate Professor, University of British Columbia, Canada
Volume 2: 8.9 Breastfeeding

Irvine Loudon Medical historian (previously General Practitioner), Green College and Wellcome Unit for the History of Medicine, University of Oxford, UK
Volume 1: 1.2 From general practice to primary care, 1700–1980

Julie Lumeng Instructor of Pediatrics, Boston University School of Medicine, Boston, USA
Volume 2: 10.9 Developmental delay

Denise Mabey Consultant Ophthalmologist, St Thomas' Hospital, London, UK
Volume 2: 12.3 Loss of vision

Vincent E. MacDonald Grief Counselor, Private Practice, Nova Scotia, Canada
Volume 2: 17.4 Death of a child

Jane Macnaughton Centre for Arts and Humanities in Medicine, University of Durham, Durham, UK
Volume 1: 6.3 Clinical judgement

Antonio Maiques Primary Health Centre, Valencia, Spain
Volume 1: 11.7 Anticipatory care of established illness: vascular disease

David Mant Professor of General Practice, University of Oxford, UK
Volume 1: 11.1 Principles of prevention

Alon P.A. Margalit Atzmon Post Misgav, Israel
Volume 1: 9.3 Family interviewing and assessment

Ashfaq A. Marghoob Assistant Attending Physician, Memorial Sloan-Kettering Cancer Center, New York, USA
Volume 2: 15.4 Pigmented skin lesions

Marjukka Mäkelä Head, Finnish Office for Health Care Technology Assessment, Helsinki, Finland
Volume 1: 13.5 Tools for quality improvement and change in practice

Andrew K. Marsden Consultant Medical Director, Scottish Ambulance Service, Edinburgh, UK
Volume 2: 14.1 Out-of-hospital cardiac arrest

Martin Marshall Professor, National Primary Care Research and Development Centre, University of Manchester, Manchester, UK
Volume 1: 13.2 Measuring the quality of primary medical care

James Mason Professor of Health Economics, Centre for Health Services Research, University of Newcastle Upon Tyne, Newcastle upon Tyne, UK
Volume 1: 13.4 Using and developing clinical guidelines

Danielle Mazza Formerly Associate Professor, International Medical University, Kuala Lumpur, Malaysia
Volume 2: 7.4 Amenorrhoea
Volume 2: 7.9 Dyspareunia

Ronald McCoy General Practitioner and HIV Educator, Melbourne, Australia
Volume 2: 6.7 HIV/AIDS

Gary W. McEwen Associate Clinical Professor, Lee's Summit, Missouri, USA
Volume 2: 15.10 Skin infections

Ian R. McWhinney Emeritus Professor of Family Medicine, The University of Western Ontario, Centre for Studies in Family Medicine, London, Ontario, Canada
Foreword

Jack H. Medalie Dorothy Jones Weatherhead Professor Emeritus of Family Medicine, School of Medicine, Case Western Reserve University, Ohio, USA
Volume 1: 9.5 Working with families with chronic medical disorders

Villy Meineche-Schmidt General Practitioner, Copenhagen, Denmark
Volume 2: 4.11 Constipation

Juan Mendive La Mina Health Centre, Barcelona, Spain
Volume 1: 2.6 Primary care and general practice in Europe: West and South
Volume 2: 4.6 Nausea, vomiting, and loss of appetite

Job F.M. Metsemakers University of Maastricht, Maastricht, The Netherlands
Volume 1: 12.6 The medical record

Thomas M. Mettee Family Practitioner, Clinical Associate Professor, Case Western University School of Medicine, Ohio, USA
Volume 1: 9.5 Working with families with chronic medical disorders

Betty Meyboom-de Jong Professor and Chair, Department of General Practice, Groningen University, Groningen, The Netherlands
Volume 1: 4.4 Age and gender

Peter E. Mezciems Senior Staff Physician, Homewood Health Center, Guelph, Ontario, Canada
Volume 1: 15.7 Addictions and mental illness in physicians

Michael J. Michell Consultant Radiologist/Clinical Director, South East London Breast Screening Programme, King's Healthcare NHS Trust, King's College Hospital, London, UK
Volume 2: 7.11 Abnormal mammogram

J. Lloyd Michener Clinical Professor and Chairman, Duke University Medical Center, North Carolina, USA
Volume 1: 1.9 Management and leadership

William L. Miller Chair, Department of Family Medicine, Lehigh Valley Hospital, Allentown, Pennsylvania, USA
Volume 1: 14.2 Methods: qualitative

Louise M. Millward Research and Development Specialist, Health Development Agency, London, UK
Volume 1: 5.4 Doctors' perceptions of their patients

Rosie Moon General Practice Professorial Unit, University of Sydney, Manly Hospital, Manly, Australia
Volume 1: 2.4 Primary care and general practice in Australia and New Zealand

Charles Mouton Associate Professor and Associate Chief, Division of Community Geriatrics, University of Texas Health Science Center, Texas, USA
Volume 1: 9.6 Family violence

Robert D. Murray Research Fellow in Endocrinology, Christie Hospital, Manchester, UK
Volume 2: 5.7 Endocrine problems (calcium, water, and adrenal)

T. Jock Murray Professor of Medical Humanities, Tupper Link, Halifax, Canada
Volume 2: 11.6 Progressive neurological illnesses: multiple sclerosis and amyotrophic lateral sclerosis

John Murtagh Adjunct Professor of General Practice, Monash University, Melbourne, Australia
Volume 2: 11.1 Headache and facial pain

Lawrence Mynors-Wallis Consultant Psychiatrist, Dorset Healthcare NHS Trust, Alderney Community Hospital, Dorset, UK
Volume 2: 9.10 Psychological treatments for mental health problems

Irwin Nazareth Professor of Primary Care and Population Sciences, Royal Free and University College Medical School, London, UK
Volume 2: 11.4 Dizziness

John Newton Unit of Health Care Epidemiology, Institute of Health Sciences, Oxford, UK
Volume 1: 10.2 Defining the population: registration and record linkage

Richard A. Nicholas Denver, Colorado, USA
Volume 2: 15.9 Eczema and dermatitis

Mattijs E. Numans General Practitioner and Senior Staff Member, Julius Center for Health Sciences and Primary Care, University Medical Utrecht, Utrecht, The Netherlands
Volume 2: 4.4 Chronic abdominal pain

Natalie O'Dea Director, EdAct Pty. Ltd, Willoughby, Australia
Volume 1: 3.3 Health beliefs

Norma O'Flynn Lecturer in General Practice, Imperial College London, UK
Volume 2: 7.7 Menstrual disorders: menorrhagia
Volume 2: 7.8 Menstrual disorders: dysmenorrhoea

Karen S. Ogle Professor, Family Practice, Michigan State University, Michigan, USA
Volume 1: 16.7 End-of-life decisions

Inge M. Okkes Senior Researcher, Division of Clinical Methods & Public Health, Academic Medical Center, University of Amsterdam, Amsterdam, The Netherlands
Volume 1: 4.3 Classification and the domain of family practice

Frede Olesen Research Unit for General Practice, University of Aarhus, Aarhus C, Denmark
Volume 1: 2.8 General practice in Europe: Scandinavia
Volume 1: 8.3 Generalists in hospitals

Daniel J. Ostergaard Vice President, International and Interprofessional Activities, American Academy of Family Physicians, Kansas, USA
Volume 1: 2.12 Primary care and general practice in North America

Tim Overton Consultant Obstetrician and Gynaecologist, Norfolk and Norwich University Hospital, NHS Trust, Norfolk, UK
Volume 2: 8.7 Complications of pregnancy

Alan Owen Senior Research Fellow, Centre for Health Service Development, Faculty of Commerce, University of Wollongong, Australia
Volume 1: 1.8 First contact care in developing health care systems

James F. Pagel Assistant Clinical Professor, University of Colorado Medical School; Director, Sleep Disorders Center of Southern Colorado & Rocky Mt. Sleep Pueblo/Colorado Springs, Colorado, USA
Volume 2: 10.10 Sleep disorders in children

Claire Parker General Practitioner, Jericho Health Centre, Oxford, UK
Volume 1: 11.2 Immunization and vaccination

Steven Parker Associate Professor, Boston University School of Medicine, Boston Medical Center, Boston University, Boston, USA
Volume 2: 10.9 Developmental delay

Christopher Patterson Professor, Division of Geriatric Medicine, McMaster University, Hamilton, Ontario, Canada
Volume 2: 16.5 Dementia

Debra M. Phillips Professor, Family and Community Medicine, Southern Illinois University School of Medicine, Quincy, Illinois, USA
Volume 2: 10.12 School issues

William R. Phillips Clinical Professor, University of Washington, Seattle, Washington, USA
Volume 2: 10.3 Otitis media

Robert L. Phillips Jr Assistant Director, The Robert Graham Center: Policy Studies in Family Practice and Primary Care, Washington DC, USA
Volume 1: 1.1 The nature of primary medical care

Munir Pirmohamed Professor of Clinical Pharmacology and Consultant Physician, The University of Liverpool and the Royal Liverpool University Hospitals, Liverpool, UK
Volume 2: 16.8 Drugs in the elderly

Leon Piterman Professor of General Practice, Head of School of Primary Health Care, Monash University, Melbourne, Victoria, Australia
Volume 1: 7.2 Patient education, advice, and counselling
Volume 2: 1.1 Chest pain and myocardial infarction

Paul E. Plsek Consultant in Quality Management, Paul E. Plsek & Associates, Inc., Atlanta, Georgia, USA
Volume 1: 13.6 Total quality management and continuous quality improvement

Victor J. Pop Professor of Primary Health Care, Tilburg University, Tilburg, The Netherlands
Volume 2: 5.5 Thyroid disorders

David Portnoy Assistant Professor, McGill University, Montréal General Hospital, Montréal, Quebec, Canada
Volume 2: 6.5 Genital ulcers and warts
Volume 2: 6.6 Gonorrhoea and chlamydial infections

Jennifer Powell Consultant Dermatologist, Churchill Hospital, Oxford, UK
Volume 2: 15.1 Hair-related problems
Volume 2: 15.14 Genital disorders

David Price Assistant Professor, McMaster University, Stonechurch Family Health Centre, Ontario, Canada
Volume 2: 8.4 Normal pregnancy

Mike Pringle Professor of General Practice and Head of School of Community Health Sciences, Division of Primary Care, University of Nottingham, Newark, UK
Volume 1: 12.1 Practice structures

Luis E. Quiroga Medical School, UMSS, Cochabamba, Bolivia
Volume 2: 2.2 Lower respiratory tract infections

Anan S. Raghunath General Practitioner and Honorary Research Fellow, St Andrews Group Practice, Maramaduke Health Centre, University of Hull, UK
Volume 1: 2.9 Primary care and general practice in India

Alexander H. Rajput Associate Professor of Neurology, University of Saskatchewan, Royal University Hospital, Saskatoon, Canada
Volume 2: 16.2 Gait and movement disorders

Ali H. Rajput Professor Emeritus (Neurology), University of Saskatchewan, Royal University Hospital, Saskatoon, Canada
Volume 2: 16.2 Gait and movement disorders

A.S. Ramanujam Chief Medical Officer, Lal Bahadur Shastri Hospital, New Delhi, India
Volume 1: 2.9 Primary care and general practice in India

Victoria H. Raveis Associate Professor of Clinical Sociomedical Sciences, Columbia University, Mailman School of Public Health, New York, USA
Volume 2: 17.3 Bereavement and grief

Gerald M. Reaven Falk CVRC, Stanford Medical Center, Stanford, California, USA
Volume 2: 5.3 Insulin resistance/syndrome X

Shelley Rechner Assistant Clinical Professor, Faculty of Health Sciences, McMaster University, Southwest Family Health Centre, Hamilton, Ontario, Canada
Volume 2: 9.11 Adult survivors of sexual abuse

Graham J. Reid Assistant Professor, Bill and Anne Brock Family Professor in Child Health, Psychology and Family Medicine, University of Western Ontario, Ontario, Canada
Volume 2: 10.11 Behaviour problems in children

Melody Rhydderch Organisational Psychologist and NHS Research Training Fellow, Primary Care Group, The Clinical School, University of Wales Swansea, Swansea, UK
Volume 1: 5.5 Shared decision-making in clinical practice

David G. Riddell Clinical Professor of Pediatrics, University of British Columbia, Vancouver, Canada
Volume 2: 8.10 Feeding problems in infants and young children

Leone Ridsdale Senior Lecturer in Neurology and Reader in General Practice, Guy's, King's, and St Thomas' School of Medicine, King's College School of Medicine, London, UK
Volume 2: 9.8 Fatigue
Volume 2: 11.2 Epilepsy

Zoltan Rihmer National Institute for Psychiatry and Neurology, Budapest, Hungary
Volume 2: 9.3 Suicide and attempted suicide

Alan Riley Professor of Sexual Medicine, Cwmann, Wales, UK
Volume 2: 6.9 Female sexual dysfunction

Isabel Rodrigues Professeur adjoint de Clinique, Université de Montréal, CLSC-CHSLD du Marigot, Québec, Canada
Volume 2: 7.12 Screening for cancer in women

Anja Rogausch Psychologist, University of Göttingen, Göttingen, Germany
Volume 1: 7.1 Principles of patient management

Martin Roland Professor and Director, National Primary Care Research and Development Centre, University of Manchester, Manchester, UK
Volume 1: 8.2 The primary–secondary care interface
Volume 1: 13.2 Measuring the quality of primary medical care

Lewis C. Rose Associate Professor of Family Medicine, University of Texas Health Science Center, Texas, USA
Volume 2: 10.7 Disorders of growth

Peter Rose University Lecturer, University of Oxford, Institute of Health Sciences, Oxford, UK
Volume 1: 9.4 Assessment and management of genetic risk

Andrew Ross General Practitioner, Northfield Health Centre, Birmingham, UK
Volume 1: 10.3 Health surveillance

Walter W. Rosser Professor and Chair, Department of Family Medicine, Queens University, Kingston, Ontario, Canada
Volume 2: 10.4 Fever and common childhood infections
Volume 2: 10.6 Anticipatory guidance and prevention

James T.B. Rourke Assistant Dean, Rural and Regional Medicine, The University of Western Ontario, Director, Southwestern Ontario Rural Regional Medicine Education Research and Development Network, Canada
Volume 1: 1.7 Rural primary care

Greg Rubin Professor of Primary Care, University of Sunderland School of Sciences, Sunderland, UK
Volume 2: 4.10 Diarrhoea

Anthony G. Rudd Consultant Stroke Physician, Guy's and St Thomas' Hospital, London, UK
Volume 2: 1.7 Stroke and transient ischaemia

George Rust Professor of Family Medicine and Deputy Director, National Center for Primary Care at Morehouse School of Medicine, Atlanta, Georgia, USA
Volume 2: 10.2 Childhood respiratory infections

Jerry G. Ryan Associate Professor, University of Wisconsin–Madison, Madison, Wisconsin, USA
Volume 2: 13.3 Acute joint pain

Janice Rymer Senior Lecturer/Consultant in Obstetrics and Gynaecology, Guy's, King's and St Thomas' School of Medicine, Guy's and St Thomas' Hospital Trust, London, UK
Volume 2: 7.5 The menopause

Rebecca B. Saenz Associate Professor of Family Medicine, University of Mississippi Medical Center, Mississippi, USA
Volume 2: 7.2 Nipple discharge

Alena Salim Dermatologist, Royal Berkshire Hospital, Reading, UK
Volume 2: 15.14 Genital disorders

Robert B. Salter Professor Emeritus of Orthopaedic Surgery and Senior Scientist Emeritus, The Research Institute, The Hospital for Sick Children, Ontario, Canada
Volume 2: 10.8 The child with a limp

Deborah C. Saltman Professor of General Practice, University of Sydney, Australia
Volume 1: 2.4 Primary care and general practice in Australia and New Zealand
Volume 1: 3.3 Health beliefs

Sverre Sandberg Professor, NOKLUS, Division for General Practice and Laboratory of Clinical Biochemistry, Haukeland University Hospital, University of Bergen, Bergen, Norway
Volume 1: 12.4 The office laboratory

Kanwaljit Sandhu Specialist Registrar in Nephrology, St George's Hospital, London, UK
Volume 2: 6.2 Haematuria and proteinuria

Brenda Sawyer Adviser to the Institute of Healthcare Management; GP Tutor in South West and Mid Hampshire; Independent Management Consultant, UK
Volume 1: 12.7 General practitioners' use of time and time management

Arun Sayal Emergency Physician and Lecturer, North York General Hospital, University of Toronto, Toronto, Canada
Volume 2: 14.2 Fractures and limb trauma

François G. Schellevis Research Coordinator, NIVEL (The Netherlands Institute for Health Services Research), Utrecht, The Netherlands
Volume 1: 4.2 Physical and mental illness

H.J. Schers General Practitioner, University Medical Centre, St Radboud, Nijmegen, The Netherlands
Volume 1: 12.3 Equipment and premises in general practice

Theo Schofield Director of Communication, ETHOX (The Oxford Centre for Ethics and Communication in Health Care Practice), University of Oxford, Oxford, UK
Volume 1: 5.3 Communication skills

Knut Schroeder Clinical Lecturer, University of Bristol, Bristol, UK
Volume 2: 1.10 High blood pressure
Volume 2: 2.7 Haemoptysis

Brian Schwartz Assistant Professor, University of Toronto, Toronto, Ontario, Canada
Volume 2: 14.5 Non-accidental injuries

E. Robert Schwartz Professor and Chair, University of Miami, Miami, Florida, USA
Volume 2: 12.5 Visual disturbances

Martin Schwartz Consultant Neurologist, Atkinson Morley Hospital, London, UK
Volume 2: 11.5 Peripheral neuropathies

Roberta Schwartz Lecturer, Faculty of Medicine, University of Toronto, Toronto, Canada
Volume 2: 14.5 Non-accidental injuries

Gunjan Sharma Medicine/Pediatrics Resident, University of Massachusetts Medical Centre, Worcester, USA
Volume 2: 15.12 Lumps in and under the skin

Deborah J. Sharp Professor of Primary Health Care, University of Bristol, Bristol, UK
Volume 2: 9.13 Post-natal depression

Elizabeth Shaw McMaster University Medical Center, Hamilton, Ontario, Canada
Volume 2: 8.4 Normal pregnancy

Paul Shekelle Senior Research Associate, Veterans Affairs Health Services Research and Development Service, Greater Los Angeles Health Care System, California, USA
Volume 1: 13.4 Using and developing clinical guidelines

Andrew Shennan Professor of Obstetrics, St Thomas' Hospital, London, UK
Volume 2: 8.7 Complications of pregnancy

Pesach Shvartzman Chairman, Division of Community Health, Ben-Gurion University of the Negev, Beersheva, Israel
Volume 1: 2.11 Primary care and general practice in the Middle East

Bonnie Sibbald Professor, National Primary Care Research and Development Centre, The University of Manchester, Manchester, UK
Volume 1: 1.3 The health care team

Douglas E. Sinclair Chair of Emergency Medicine, Dalhousie University, Nova Scotia, Canada
Volume 2: 9.7 Psychiatric emergencies

Anne Slowther Research Fellow, ETHOX (Oxford Centre for Ethics and Communication in Health Care Practice), University of Oxford, Institute of Health Sciences, Oxford, UK
Volume 1: 16.5 Ethics of research

Gary Smith Research Assistant, The Surgery, Solihull, UK
Volume 2: 17.2 Pain concepts and pain control in palliative care

Gillian Smith Registrar, Department of Plastic Surgery, City General Hospital, Staffordshire, UK
Volume 2: 14.6 Burns

A. Patricia Smith Honorary Lecturer, Aberdeen Maternity Hospital, Aberdeen, UK
Volume 2: 7.10 Abnormal cervical smear

Leif I. Solberg Associate Medical Director for Care Improvement Research, HealthPartners Research Foundation, Minneapolis, USA
Volume 1: 8.6 Getting beyond disease-specific management
Volume 1: 13.6 Total quality management and continuous quality improvement

Peter Sonksen Emeritus Professor of Medicine, St Thomas' Hospital, London, UK
Volume 2: 5.6 Endocrine problems (pituitary and sex hormones)

Stephen J. Spann Professor and Chairman, Baylor College of Medicine, Texas, USA
Volume 1: 2.5 Primary care and general practice in Latin America

Bruce L.W. Sparks Faculty of Health Sciences, University of Witwatersrand, Johannesburg, South Africa
Volume 1: 2.2 Primary care and general practice in Africa

M.P. Springer General Practitioner; Professor of General Practice, Leiden University Medical Centre, Leiden, The Netherlands
Volume 2: 9.9 Sleep disorders

Yvonne Steinert Clinical Psychologist and Professor of Family Medicine, McGill University, Montréal, Canada
Volume 1: 15.6 Multi-professional education

Moira Stewart Professor and Director, Centre for Studies in Family Medicine, The University of Western Ontario, Ontario, Canada
Volume 1: 5.1 The patient–doctor relationship

Jelle Stoffers Associate Professor of General Practice, University of Maastricht, Public Health Research Institute (CAPHRI), Maastricht, The Netherlands
Volume 2: 1.5 Peripheral arterial disease

Tim Stokes Senior Lecturer in General Practice, University of Leicester, Leicester General Hospital, Leicester, UK
Volume 2: 7.3 Vaginal discharge

Nigel C.H. Stott Professor of General Practice, University of Wales College of Medicine, Cardiff, UK
Volume 1: 5.2 Consultation tasks

Derek Summerfield Honorary Senior Lecturer, Institute of Psychiatry, King's College, London, UK
Volume 2: 9.12 Post-traumatic stress disorder

Patricia Sunaert Assistant, Department of General Practice and Primary Health Care, Ghent University, Ghent, Belgium
Volume 2: 15.2 Nail disorders

Robert Sweet Assistant Professor Department of Otolaryngology, McGill University Health Centre, Montréal, Canada
Volume 2: 3.4 Hearing loss

Richard P. Swinson Morgan Firestone Chair in Psychiatry, McMaster University, Ontario, Canada
Volume 2: 9.2 Anxiety

Howard Tandeter Ben-Gurion University, Israel
Volume 1: 2.11 Primary care and general practice in the Middle East

Danny Tayar Family Physician, The Mifne Centre, Israel
Volume 1: 12.6 The medical record

Alison Taylor Consultant in Gynaecology and Reproductive Medicine, Assisted Conception Unit, Guy's and St Thomas' Hospitals Trust, London, UK
Volume 2: 8.2 Sub-fertility

Ted L. Tewfik Professor of Otolaryngology, McGill University; Director of Otolaryngology, Montréal Children's Hospital, Montréal, Quebec, Canada
Volume 2: 3.3 The discharging ear
Volume 2: 3.4 Hearing loss

Kate Thomas Deputy Director, Medical Care Research Unit, School of Health and Related Research, University of Sheffield, Sheffield, UK
Volume 1: 3.6 Alternative sources of advice: traditional and complementary medicine

Sharon Thomson The University of British Columbia Family Practice Centre, British Columbia, Canada
Volume 2: 8.3 Contraception

Geir Thue General Practitioner, NOKLUS, University of Bergen, Bergen, Norway
Volume 1: 12.4 The office laboratory

Arno Timmermans Executive Director, Dutch College of General Practitioners, Utrecht, The Netherlands
Volume 1: 2.6 Primary care and general practice in Europe: West and South

John M. Tomlinson Director, Men's Health Clinic, Royal Hampshire County Hospital, Winchester, UK
Volume 2: 6.8 Sexual dysfunction in men

Les Toop Pegasus Professor of General Practice, Christchurch School of Medicine, Christchurch, New Zealand
Volume 1: 7.4 Principles of drug prescribing

Simon Travis Consultant Gastroenterologist, John Radcliffe Hospital, Oxford, UK
Volume 2: 4.12 Perianal disease

Julian Tudor Hart Retired General Practitioner, Glyncorrwg, Swansea, Wales, UK
Volume 1: 10.4 Community interventions—physical health

André Tylee Professor of Primary Care Mental Health, Institute of Psychiatry, London, UK
Volume 2: 9.3 Suicide and attempted suicide

Martin Underwood Professor of General Practice, Barts and The London, Queen Mary's School of Medicine and Dentistry, Queen Mary University of London, London, UK
Volume 2: 5.4 Hyperuricaemia

Peter Underwood Professor of Public and International Health, Murdoch University, Murdoch, West Australia
Volume 1: 1.8 First contact care in developing health care systems

Richard P. Usatine Professor and Vice-Chair for Education, University of Texas Health Science Center, Texas, USA
Volume 2: 15.12 Lumps in and under the skin

Jaap J. van Binsbergen General Practitioner; Professor of Nutrition and Family Medicine, University Medical Centre Nijmegen, Nijmegen, The Netherlands
Volume 1: 11.5 Changing behaviour: diet and exercise

Eloy H. van de Lisdonk General Practitioner and Senior Lecturer, University of Nijmegen, Nijmegen, The Netherlands
Volume 1: 3.2 Illness behaviour
Volume 1: 14.4 Primary care research networks

Wil J.H.M. van den Bosch General Practitioner and Professor of General Practice, University Medical Centre, Nijmegen, The Netherlands
Volume 1: 8.1 Coordination and continuity of care
Volume 2: 13.4 Chronic joint pain

Pieter van den Hombergh Senior Research Assistant Working Party on Quality of Care Research (WOK), University of Nijmegen; Staff member, Dutch College of General Practitioners (NHG), Utrecht, The Netherlands
Volume 1: 12.2 Staff
Volume 1: 12.3 Equipment and premises in general practice

Willem Jan van der Veen Registratie Netwerk Groningen, Faculteit Medische Wetenschappen, Groningen, The Netherlands
Volume 1: 4.4 Age and gender

Danielle A.W.M. van der Windt Associate Professor, Department of General Practice, Institute for Research in Extramural Medicine, VU University Medical Centre, Amsterdam, The Netherlands
Volume 2: 13.5 Shoulder pain

Jouke van der Zee NIVEL (The Netherlands Institute for Health Services Research), Utrecht, The Netherlands
Volume 1: 2.1 Health care systems: understanding the stages of development

G.A. van Essen General Practitioner, Accredited to the Julius Centre for Health Sciences and Primary Care, University Medical Centre, Utrecht, The Netherlands
Volume 2: 16.9 Influenza

Peter van Hasselt Family Physician and Senior Lecturer, Utrecht University, The Netherlands
Volume 1: 2.7 Primary care and general practice in Europe: Central and East
Volume 1: 15.5 Reaccreditation and recertification

Eric van Hecke Professor of Dermatology, University Hospital Ghent, Belgium
Volume 2: 15.2 Nail disorders

Yvonne D. van Leeuwen Director of Postgraduate Training for General Practice, University of Maastricht, Maastricht, The Netherlands
Volume 1: 6.2 Clinical diagnosis: hypothetico-deductive reasoning and other theoretical frameworks
Volume 1: 8.4 Clinical specialization

Jan W. van Ree General Practitioner/Professor in General Practice, Maastricht University, Maastricht, The Netherlands
Volume 1: 1.10 The role of primary care in public health

Maurits W. van Tulder Senior Investigator Health Technology Assessment, Institute for Research in Extramural Medicine, VU University Medical Center, Amsterdam, The Netherlands
Volume 2: 13.1 Low back pain and sciatica

Chris van Weel Professor and Chairman, University Medical Center, Nijmegen, The Netherlands
Volume 1: 2.13 International organizations
Volume 1: 11.5 Changing behaviour: diet and exercise

Gregg K. VandeKieft Clinical Faculty, Providence St Peter Hospital Family Practice Residency Program, Olympia, USA
Volume 1: 16.7 End-of-life decisions

Theo J.M. Verheij Professor of General Practice, Julius Centre for Health Sciences and Primary Care, University Medical Centre Utrecht, Utrecht, The Netherlands
Volume 2: 2.1 Upper respiratory tract infections
Volume 2: 2.2 Lower respiratory tract infections

Myrra Vernooij-Dassen Coordinator, Alzheimer Centre, Nijmegen University; Senior Researcher, Centre for Quality of Care Research, Nijmegen, The Netherlands
Volume 1: 8.7 Collaboration between professional and lay care

Andrew Vickers Assistant Attending Research Methodologist, Integrative Medicine Service, Memorial Sloan–Kettering Cancer Center, New York, USA
Volume 1: 7.7 Complementary therapies

Paola Viterbori Unit of Clinical Epidemiology and Trials, National Cancer Institute, Genova, Italy
Volume 1: 7.8 Terminal and palliative care
Volume 2: 17.1 The dying patient and their family

Theo Voorn Professor of General Practice, University Medical Centre, Utrecht, The Netherlands
Volume 2: 12.1 Acute red eye

Patrick C.A.J. Vroomen Neurologist, Maastricht University Hospital, Maastricht, The Netherlands; Austin & Repatriation Medical Centre, Melbourne, Australia
Volume 2: 13.1 Low back pain and sciatica

Paul Wallace Professor of Primary Health Care, University College London, London, UK
Volume 1: 8.5 Interprofessional communication

Christopher Ward Professor of Rehabilitation Medicine, Head of the Division of Rehabilitation and Ageing, University of Nottingham Rehabilitation Research Unit, Derby City General Hospital, Derby, UK
Volume 2: 11.3 Movement disorders

Gary Ward Coventry and Warwickshire Hospital, Coventry, UK
Volume 2: 14.3 Control of haemorrhage

Helen Ward Clinical Senior Lecturer in Epidemiology and Public Health; Honorary Consultant in Genitourinary Medicine, Imperial College, London, UK
Volume 1: 11.6 Changing behaviour: promoting sexual health

John H. Wasson Dartmouth Medical School, New Hampshire, USA
Volume 1: 8.6 Getting beyond disease-specific management

Mary-Lynn Watson Assistant Professor, Dalhousie University, Halifax, Nova Scotia, Canada
Volume 2: 9.7 Psychiatric emergencies

David P. Weller Professor and Head, Department of General Practice, University of Edinburgh, Edinburgh, Scotland, UK
Volume 1: 14.3 Methods: quantitative
Volume 1: 14.4 Primary care research networks

Dennis Y. Wen Associate Professor, University of Missouri, Columbia, USA
Volume 2: 13.9 Hand and forearm problems

Michel Wensing Senior Researcher, University Medical Centre St Radboud, Nijmegen, The Netherlands
Volume 1: 3.7 Patients' expectations of treatment
Volume 1: 13.7 The patient's role in improving quality

W. Wayne Weston Byron Family Medicine Center, Ontario, Canada
Volume 1: 16.2 The doctor–patient relationship—ethical perspectives

Patrick White Senior Lecturer in General Practice, Guy's, King's and St Thomas' School of Medicine, King's College, London, UK
Volume 2: 1.4 Ankle swelling and breathlessness
Volume 2: 2.4 Asthma
Volume 2: 2.6 Chronic cough

Paula Whitty Senior Lecturer in Epidemiology and Public Health, Centre for Health Services Research, University of Newcastle, UK
Volume 1: 13.4 Using and developing clinical guidelines

Kimberley A. Widger Clinical Nurse Specialist, Pediatric Palliative Care Service, IWK Health Centre, Nova Scotia, Canada
Volume 2: 17.4 Death of a child

Ellen Wiebe Clinical Professor, University of British Columbia, Vancouver, British Columbia, Canada
Volume 2: 8.12 Unwanted pregnancy and termination of pregnancy

Tjerk Wiersma Senior Scientific Staff Member, Dutch College of General Practitioners, Utrecht, The Netherlands
Volume 2: 6.1 Urinary tract infections
Volume 2: 8.6 Vaginal bleeding in early pregnancy

Sara Willems Researcher, Department of General Practice and Primary Health Care, Ghent University, Belgium
Volume 1: 4.5 Socio-economic differences in health

Nefyn H. Williams Senior Clinical Fellow, University of Wales College of Medicine, Wrexham, Wales, UK
Volume 2: 13.2 Neck pain

Robert L. Williams Professor, University of New Mexico, Albuquerque, New Mexico, USA
Volume 1: 1.4 Community primary care

Adam Windak Head of Department of Family Medicine, Jagiellonian University Medical College, Krakow, Poland
Volume 1: 2.7 Primary care and general practice in Europe: Central and East
Volume 1: 15.5 Reaccreditation and recertification

Rena R. Wing Weight Control and Diabetes Center, Providence, Rhode Island, USA
Volume 2: 5.1 Obesity

Ron Winkens Associate Professor for Integrated Care Research, University Hospital Maastricht & Maastricht University, Maastricht, The Netherlands
Volume 1: 8.5 Interprofessional communication

Jan C. Winters General Practitioner, Department of Family Practice, University of Groningen, Groningen, The Netherlands
Volume 2: 13.5 Shoulder pain

Charles Wolfe Professor of Public Health Medicine, Guy's, King's, and St Thomas' School of Medicine, London, UK
Volume 2: 1.7 Stroke and transient ischaemia

Steven H. Woolf Virginia Commonwealth University, Virginia, USA
Volume 1: 13.4 Using and developing clinical guidelines

Robert F. Woollard Professor of Family Practice, Royal Canadian Legion Chair and Head, Department of Family Practice, University of British Columbia, Vancouver, Canada
Volume 1: 15.1 Medical education: the contribution of primary care

Lawrence R. Wu Medical Director, Marshall Pickens Family Medicine Center, Duke University, Durham, North Carolina, USA
Volume 1: 1.9 Management and leadership

Sally Wyke Professor and Director, Scottish School of Health Sciences, University of Edinburgh, Edinburgh, UK
Volume 1: 3.1 Use of health services

Michael Yelland Senior Lecturer in General Practice, Centre for General Practice, University of Queensland; Inala Health Centre General Practice, Queensland, Australia
Volume 2: 3.2 Ear pain in adults

Doris Young Professor and Head, Department of General Practice, University of Melbourne, Parkville, Australia
Volume 2: 9.6 Eating disorders

Catherine E. Zollman General Practitioner, Montpelier Health Centre, Bristol, UK
Volume 1: 7.7 Complementary therapies

Helen Zorbas Clinical Director, National Breast Cancer Centre, Camperdown, Australia
Volume 2: 7.1 Breast pain and lumps

1

Primary medical care

1 Primary medical care

1.1 The nature of primary medical care

Larry A. Green, Robert L. Phillips, Jr., and George E. Fryer

The term 'primary care' is widely used, as if it is a precise, well-understood term. This is not the case. The term may not be found in ordinary or epidemiological dictionaries, and its origin is uncertain. There is a wide spectrum of opinion about what is and is not primary care.

The famous study of the ecology of medical care by White et al. in 1961 did not use the exact term, but it did crystallize the importance of what has become known as primary care by quantifying for a population the distribution of people across different levels of care and creating a visual image that provoked thinking about the spectrum and balance of services necessary in a health care system.(1) Within this framework of the health care experiences of 1000 adults in an average month, primary care could be understood to comprise the 250 adult patients who consulted a physician and the interfaces among various sites of health care. This relatively large number of individuals stood in contrast to nine persons admitted to hospitals, five referred to other physicians, and a single person who received care in an academic medical centre hospital. These relationships have been subsequently verified and expanded to include children and other health care settings and continue to provide a framework for understanding the position and the roles of primary care in a health care system (Fig. 1).(2)

The purpose of this chapter is to define and describe primary care from several perspectives, summarize why it is so valuable, and suggest in general terms, potential future directions likely to require the further development of primary care.

History and context

Among the historical milestones of primary care, the Dawson Report from the United Kingdom in 1920 is often cited because it distinguished three levels of health care services: primary health centres, secondary health centres, and teaching hospitals.(3) The Millis and Willard reports in the United States during the 1960s are sometimes cited as sources of the term primary care, but neither formulated an explicit notion called primary care. Millis referred to the need of every individual for a primary physician,(4) and Willard focused on family medicine as a corrective force to redress a decline in general practice and an over-emphasis on medical specialization.(5)

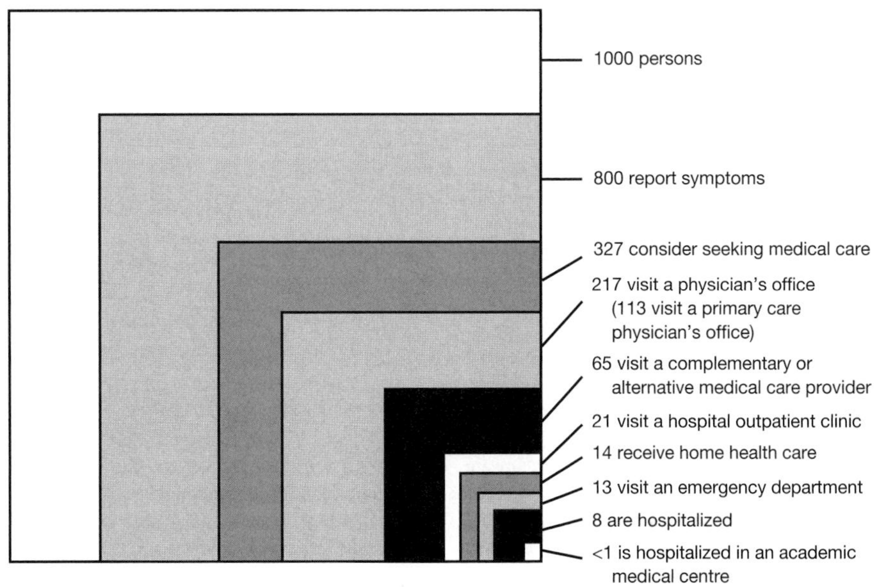
1000 persons
800 report symptoms
327 consider seeking medical care
217 visit a physician's office (113 visit a primary care physician's office)
65 visit a complementary or alternative medical care provider
21 visit a hospital outpatient clinic
14 receive home health care
13 visit an emergency department
8 are hospitalized
<1 is hospitalized in an academic medical centre

Fig. 1 The ecology of medical care revisited. (Used with permission from Green, L.A. et al. (2001). The ecology of medical care revisited. *New England Journal of Medicine* **344**, 2021–5. Copyright © 2001, Massachusetts Medical Society. All rights reserved.)

The Lalonde Report from Canada[6] was another landmark event influencing primary care. This report emphasized the importance of health promotion and disease prevention, including strategies focused on individuals within the health care system. The identification of opportunities to prevent important diseases and enhance health through strategies achievable in primary care served as another stimulus for strengthening primary care through the incorporation of defined preventive services.

The World Health Organization had a major impact on thinking about primary care in 1978 when it defined 'primary *health* care' at the International Conference on Primary Health Care held in the former Soviet Union. This definition in The Declaration of Alma-Ata was subsequently affirmed at the World Health Assembly's meeting in May of 1979:[7]

> Primary health care is essential health care based on practical, scientifically sound and socially acceptable methods and technology made universally accessible to individuals and families in the community through their full participation and at a cost that the community and the country can afford . . . It forms an integral part of both the country's health system, of which it is the central function and main focus, and the overall social economic development of the community. It is the first level of contact of individuals, the family and the community with the national health system, bringing health care as close as possible to where people live and work and constitutes the first element of a continuing health care process.

This definition was elaborated to indicate that primary health care is broad in scope and includes at least the following:

1. education concerning prevailing health problems and the methods of preventing or controlling them;
2. promotion of food supply and proper nutrition;
3. an adequate supply of safe water and basic sanitation;
4. maternal and child health care, including family planning;
5. immunization against major infectious diseases;
6. prevention and control of locally endemic diseases;
7. appropriate treatment of common diseases and injuries;
8. provision of essential drugs.

The World Health Organization's definition fuelled interest in primary care and had international impact.[8] However, it intermingled functions considered to be part of public health and personal health services and left some confusion about who was responsible for achieving this 'essential health care'. The definition was not unexpectedly interpreted differently by countries depending on their level of industrialization, philosophy of government, evolution of health care services and the amount and distribution of wealth. It inspired interest in primary care in some countries and permitted other countries to be dismissive of primary care, assuming that once essential services such as clean water were established, that primary health care could be considered to be achieved. Then, attention and resources could be devoted to other levels of personal health care services instead of primary care. In some instances, primary health care was equated with health care for poor people but not necessary for everyone, and in others primary care designated the effort to focus less on diseases and molecular mechanisms and more on health and people. Starfield later resolved some of this confusion by asserting that 'primary care connotes conventional primary medical care striving to achieve the goals of primary health care'.[9]

The concept of 'Community-Oriented Primary Care' (COPC) represents a major effort to meld primary medical and primary health care services. COPC was initially developed and promulgated by Sidney Kark and others in South Africa and later in Israel and the United States. It was characterized as a strategy whereby elements of primary care and community medicine are systematically united in coordinated practice.[10,11] COPC has been defined as the provision of primary care services to a defined community, coupled with systematic efforts to identify and address the major health problems of that community through effective modifications both of the primary care services and other appropriate community health programmes.[12] The practical skills necessary to implement the theory of COPC have been identified and assembled for everyday use.[13] This iterative process, focused on defining the community to be served, engaging that community, and defining strategies responsive to that particular community's needs, was an important landmark in the development of primary care.

Another key development in the evolution of thinking about primary care emerged through the identification of key attributes of primary care. The Institute of Medicine (IoM) in the United States proposed in 1978 that accessibility, comprehensiveness, coordination, continuity and accountability were essential attributes of primary care.[14] These were consistent with other analyses that also emphasized first contact and longitudinality as key features of primary care.[15,16] Sometimes 'affordability' was added to the list of critical attributes, calling attention to the balancing act expected of primary care between optimizing health and judiciously and equitably distributing always limited resources. There is widespread agreement that the assessment of primary care can legitimately focus on these attributes: the three 'As' (accessibility, accountability, affordability) and the three 'Cs' (comprehensiveness, continuity, coordination).

Despite these and many other reports and publications and dedicated efforts by many throughout the world, primary care did not totally thrive during the last half of the twentieth century. In some environments, it struggled to exist, hardly the central function and main focus of the health care system. The World Development Report published by the World Bank in 1993 called for targeted investments to enhance health. It recommended reduced government investment in tertiary facilities and sub-specialist training and more investment in public health and essential services needed by everyone.[17] This recommendation was consistent with the results of an historic collaboration between the World Health Organization and the World Organization of Family Doctors in 1994 that resulted in a seminal working paper that concluded:[18]

> To meet people's needs, fundamental changes must occur in the health care system, in the medical profession, and in medical schools and other educational institutions. The family doctor (general practitioner/family physician) should have a central role in the achievement of quality, cost effectiveness, and equity in health care systems. To fulfill this responsibility, the family doctor must be highly competent in patient care and must integrate individual and community health care.

While the history and specific manifestations of primary care vary from country to country, the need for primary care seems to be universal. Its role and place in modern health care systems is appropriately in persistent evolution, adapting to the needs of particular communities in every country.

A contemporary definition

In the United States, interest in re-organizing and 'managing' care resurrected interest in primary care and led to another comprehensive study of primary care by the IoM.[19] The IoM's primary care study committee found it necessary to revisit the definition of primary care to guide the study. It found reports and studies in the world literature in which primary care was considered to be whatever a certain group of health care providers did. In other studies, primary care was considered to be a set of activities, a level of care or setting, a set of attributes, or an organizational strategy. Finding none of these to incorporate the full dimensions intended by the term, the study committee formulated the following definition that has become an authoritative definition:

> Primary care is the provision of integrated, accessible health care services by clinicians who are accountable for addressing a large majority of personal health care needs, developing a sustained partnership with patients, and practicing in the context of family and community.

This definition establishes without equivocation that primary care is a *function*. It is not a discipline nor a specialty, although there are clearly special groups of providers who do primary care, for example, general practitioners and family physicians.[20,21] Health care professionals using knowledge and skills from various sources can contribute to achieving this function, and often the best primary care is delivered by teams comprised of individuals with a spectrum of expertise sufficient to respond to the needs and demands of their specific community. These teams may include nurses, physicians, administrators, receptionists, information assistants, social workers, physician assistants, mental health specialists, and other persons with expertise relevant to the challenges faced by the persons served by the primary care enterprise.

The IoM study group concluded that:[19]

1. Primary care is the logical foundation of an effective health care system because it can address the large majority of the health problems present in the population.
2. Primary care is essential to achieving the objectives that together constitute value in health care: high quality of care, including achievement of desired health outcomes; patient satisfaction; and efficient use of resources.
3. Personal interactions that include trust and partnership between patients and clinicians are central to primary care.
4. Primary care is an important instrument for achieving stronger emphasis on both ends of the spectrum of care: (a) health promotion and disease prevention; and (b) care of the chronically ill, especially among the elderly with multiple problems.
5. The trend toward integrated health care systems in a managed care environment will continue and will provide both opportunities and challenges for primary care.

Each term in the definition was carefully examined and explained.[19] The word 'integrated' was used to encompass comprehensive, coordinated, and continuous services in a seamless process, combining events and information from disparate settings and levels of care. 'Accessible' referred to the ease with which an individual could initiate an interaction for any health problem with a clinician. Access involves financial, geographic, cultural, language, and temporal considerations. 'Health care services' referred to all settings of care from home to hospital. 'Clinician' implied an expert using a recognized body of scientific knowledge and having authority to direct the delivery of personal health care services. 'Accountable' applied to both individual clinicians and the systems in which they work and included responsibility for the quality of care, patient satisfaction, efficient use of resources, and ethical behaviour. 'Majority of personal health care needs' clarified an essential characteristic of primary care clinicians: they receive whatever patients bring to them unrestricted by problem or organ system, including physical, emotional, mental, and social concerns. Effective primary care physicians refer relatively infrequently, for example, 6.3 per cent of visiting patients, based on United States 1999 National Ambulatory Medical Care Survey data. 'Sustained partnership' referred to the centrality of the relationship established between patients and their personal clinicians and the expectation that the relationship will continue over time, predicated on mutual trust, respect, and responsibility. 'Context of family and community' referred to the need to understand the patient's living conditions, family dynamics, and cultural background; and 'community' could be a geopolitical unit or refer to neighbours who share values, experiences, language, religion, and/or culture. The focus on community also implied responsibility to the entire population, whether they are patients or not.

Unlike health care limited to a particular organ system or disease, primary care cannot be defined by the problem(s) it addresses. By definition, all health problems exist in primary care, and often more than one problem exists simultaneously. Thus, the content and nature of primary care varies according to the needs and demands of specific individuals in their communities. The typical content of a primary care practice is knowable for a particular community, and different countries often have similar patterns. A profile of visits to the offices of US primary care physicians appears in Tables 1–3. Based on data from the National Ambulatory Medical Care Surveys (NAMCS) covering 1995–1999 in the United States, the 30 most frequent reasons patients visited a primary care physician in the office setting and the 30 most frequent primary diagnoses made during these visits are shown in Tables 1 and 2. The 30 entries in Table 1 accounted for the reason for visit in 55.7 per cent of visits, and the 30 entries in Table 2 accounted for the primary diagnosis made during 47.3 per cent of all office visits to primary care physicians in the United States. The top 10 reasons for visit and top 10 diagnoses for six age groups, for males and females, are shown in Table 3. Only 37 diagnoses and 35 reasons for visit were required for this entire profile. NAMCS is conducted annually by the United States National Center for Health Statistics (NCHS) of the Centers for Disease Control and Prevention (CDC). These data have been weighted to produce national estimates of ambulatory care services provided by the primary care physicians of the United States, that is, family physicians, general practitioners, general internists, and general paediatricians.

Similar lists are known for other countries[22–24] and represent from a 'problem perspective' a large portion of the primary care enterprise that can be mastered and dealt with expertly. A critical skill manifest through excellent primary care is recognizing the limits of what can be achieved in primary care and the rest of the health care system and to expedite care as *needed and useful* for a particular patient in other settings by sub-specialty clinicians and other community resources. Some problems require consultation, others referral, and all are welcomed into the 'sustained partnership'.

There are other characteristics of primary care that in the aggregate distinguish it.[19] Excellent primary care is grounded in both the biomedical and the social sciences and is supportable by relevant technologies. Clinical

Table 1 Most frequent reasons for visits to the offices of US primary care physicians (1995–1999)

Reason for visit	Per 1000 visits
General medical examination	83.84
Cough	56.16
Sore throat	34.80
Well baby examination	34.56
Follow-up visit nos	29.69
Fever	28.40
Earache	21.80
Hypertension	21.20
Head cold, upper respiratory infection	19.20
Skin rash	18.66
Nasal congestion	17.78
Back pain, ache, discomfort	17.63
Blood pressure check	16.63
Headache	16.10
New/renewed medication nos	13.75
Diabetes mellitus	13.04
Chest pain nos	12.11
Abdominal pain nos	10.44
Vaccinations/immunizations	9.56
Vertigo, dizziness	9.40
Knee pain, ache, discomfort	8.51
Low back pain, ache, discomfort	8.42
Tiredness, exhaustion	8.27
Test results	7.55
Shoulder pain, ache, discomfort	6.97
Diarrhoea	6.79
Shortness of breath	6.61
Depression	6.58
Neck pain, ache, discomfort	6.50
Ear symptoms nos	6.34

nos, not otherwise specified.

Table 2 Most frequent diagnoses for visits to the offices of US primary care physicians (1995–1999)

Diagnosis	Per 1000 visits
Routine child health exam	62.35
Hypertension nos	57.23
Acute uri nos	47.05
Otitis media nos	33.82
Type II diabetes	27.10
Chronic sinusitis nos	24.83
Chronic bronchitis nos	22.06
Acute pharyngitis	20.60
Routine medical exam	19.34
Asthma nos	15.37
Allergic rhinitis nos	11.00
Urinary tract infection nos	10.29
Viral infection nos	9.50
Dermatitis nos	9.23
Depression nos	8.72
Coronary artery disease	8.69
Gastroenteritis	7.69
Obesity nos	7.39
Chronic obstruct lung disease	6.94
Osteoarthritis nos	6.51
Acute tonsillitis	6.39
Hyperlipidaemia nos	6.19
Influenza nos	6.18
Pneumonia nos	5.93
Acute bronchitis	5.61
Elev blood press w/o hypertn	5.45
Abdominal pain unspcf site	5.44
Med exam admin purpose	5.44
Congestive heart failure	5.39
Strep throat	5.23

nos, not otherwise specified; uri, upper respiratory infection; elev, elevated; press, pressure; w/o, without; hypertn, hypertension; unspcf, unspecified; med, medical.

decision making in primary care frequently differs from that in referral specialties, having a strong emphasis on prognostication. Primary care clinicians work with probabilities and test performance characteristics based on 'unfiltered' population-based prevalences. This means that knowledge from other health care settings may not translate automatically into primary care in a manner that is responsive or even relevant, revealing why a research enterprise is essential for primary care. It also means that primary care clinicians must weigh the probability of iatrogenic injury from referrals, screening tests, and interventions against population-based prevalences to protect patients from harm—another reason research is essential for primary care. In primary care, mental health is extraordinarily important and cannot be separated from physical health. Opportunities to promote health and prevent disease are prevalent, and these opportunities may be missed without primary care.

Escalating health care costs challenged all health care systems in the 1990s. Many countries viewed the functions, capacity, and opportunities in primary care as key ingredients for an effective, affordable, and sustainable health care system. Unfortunately, proponents of 'managed care', a set of strategies deployed to organize health care more efficiently, focused heavily on the potential for primary care to contain costs (see Chapter 8.6). Primary care physicians were often given increased status and labelled 'gatekeepers' and valued because of their contributions to cost containment. This emphasis frequently created the reality or appearance of conflicts between the best interests of patients and the best interests of those working in the health care system. Being a gatekeeper did not necessarily promote and sustain trusting relationships nor support balancing personal and public needs inherent in sorting out and responding to the complex problems abundant in primary care. Consequently, the gatekeeper role, emphasized as such, had a tendency to erode the trusting relationship on which salutary effects of primary care were based.

The failings of 'managed care' in the 1990s are further evidence that some clinicians and policy-makers do not recognize the complexity and particular opportunities of primary care, for example, the breadth of problems encountered; the unfiltered presentations of disease; the interactions of biomedical, social, and psychological issues; and the insight that comes from understanding the context of various situations. Within this complexity are opportunities not accessible at other levels of health care to promote health, prevent disease and understand the origins of health and disease. Understood in this manner, it is possible to assess the value of primary care.

The value of primary care

Primary care *provides a place* to which people can bring a wide range of health problems and expect in most instances that their problems will be resolved without referral. It *guides people* through increasingly complex health care systems, including appropriate referrals for services from other health professionals and sectors. Primary care *facilitates an ongoing relationship* between patients and clinicians and *fosters participation* by people in decision making about their own care. Primary care *opens opportunities* for disease prevention and health promotion as well as early detection of problems. It is a *bridge* between personal health care and patients' families and communities.(19)

The United States provides a natural laboratory to assess primary care because it has had considerable variation in health care arrangements that have resulted in a dispersion of outcomes within a single country. Multiple investigators from various disciplines have assessed the effects of primary care, and this body of work supports the following conclusions:

1. When people have access to primary care, treatment occurs before evolution to more severe problems.(25–28)
2. Emergency department utilization and hospital admissions decrease when people have primary care.(29–36)
3. Primary care clinicians use fewer tests and spend less money.(37–42)
4. Particularly for the poor, access to primary care is associated with improved vision, more complete immunization, better blood pressure control, enhanced dental status, and reduced estimated mortality.(43–45)
5. Primary care and sub-specialty clinicians both fail to achieve preventive service guidelines, but people with a regular source of primary care receive more preventive services.(46–48)
6. Higher levels of primary care in a geographic area are associated with lower mortality rates, after controlling for important effects of urban–rural difference, poverty rates, education, and lifestyle factors.(49–53)

Starfield's landmark work showed that countries with health systems more oriented toward primary care generally achieve better health status (e.g. in terms of low birth weight, neonatal mortality, life-expectancy, years of potential life lost) with higher patient satisfaction, lower per capita expenditures, and lower medication use.(9,54) Contemporary interest in medical errors and patient safety(55) and recommendations to make care safer(56) indicate a critical role for primary care in protecting people from

Table 3 Most frequent reasons for visits by patient gender and age group to the offices of US primary care physicians (1995–1999)

Age group	Female		Male	
	Reason	**Per 1000 visits**	**Reason**	**Per 1000 visits**
Under 15	Well baby examination	127.54	Well baby examination	118.25
	Cough	94.49	Cough	100.69
	General medical examination	86.24	General medical examination	90.44
	Fever	82.87	Fever	86.54
	Sore throat	52.89	Earache	50.14
	Earache	50.24	Sore throat	46.33
	Nasal congestion	38.35	Nasal congestion	34.22
	Head cold, upper resp infection	31.88	Skin rash	29.34
	Skin rash	31.63	Head cold, upper resp infection	27.45
	Vaccination/immunization	17.65	Ear symptoms nos	20.98
15–24	Sore throat	81.08	Sore throat	103.11
	General medical examination	62.25	General medical examination	70.89
	Routine prenatal examination	61.56	Cough	64.35
	Cough	45.26	Sports/camp physical exam	35.15
	Headache	28.81	Skin rash	25.44
	Abdominal pain nos	24.09	Head cold, upper resp infection	20.92
	Skin rash	21.84	Back pain, ache, discomfort	20.12
	Head cold, upper resp infection	21.68	Headache	18.87
	Sports/camp physical exam	19.78	Required school physical exam	18.63
	Earache	18.53	Nasal congestion	18.48
25–44	General medical examination	53.20	General medical examination	64.27
	Cough	43.08	Cough	41.42
	Sore throat	42.61	Sore throat	40.78
	Headache	30.43	Back pain, ache, discomfort	34.64
	Routine prenatal examination	26.29	Follow-up visit nos	26.41
	Back pain, ache, discomfort	26.28	Low back pain, ache, discomfort	23.23
	Head cold, upper resp infection	20.67	Skin rash	20.34
	Earache	18.51	Headache	19.85
	Skin rash	17.88	Chest pain nos	18.55
	Follow-up visit nos	17.32	Blood pressure check	17.92
45–64	General medical examination	86.82	General medical examination	103.75
	Hypertension	39.67	Hypertension	43.33
	Cough	37.81	Follow-up visit nos	40.58
	Follow-up visit nos	35.27	Cough	36.55
	Blood pressure check	28.89	Blood pressure check	33.21
	Back pain, ache, discomfort	25.97	Diabetes mellitus	32.48
	New/renewed medication nos	24.51	Back pain, ache, discomfort	27.59
	Headache	21.63	New/renewed medication nos	23.98
	Sore throat	17.85	Chest pain nos	23.76
	Diabetes mellitus	17.33	Head cold, upper resp infection	17.11
65–74	General medical examination	94.99	General medical examination	106.42
	Follow-up visit nos	53.98	Follow-up visit nos	50.42
	Hypertension	46.51	Hypertension	47.46
	Cough	42.09	Cough	33.03
	Blood pressure check	37.31	Blood pressure check	30.49
	Diabetes mellitus	30.11	Diabetes mellitus	28.32
	New/renewed medication nos	23.88	Chest pain nos	20.08
	Back pain, ache, discomfort	19.53	Knee pain, ache, discomfort	17.86
	Vertigo, dizziness	18.48	Skin rash	16.18
	Knee pain, ache, discomfort	17.61	New/renewed medication nos	16.08
75+	General medical examination	95.55	General medical examination	102.65
	Follow-up visit nos	66.17	Follow-up visit nos	73.24
	Hypertension	42.72	Hypertension	29.30
	Cough	35.47	Cough	27.67
	Blood pressure check	34.41	Vertigo, dizziness	27.02
	Vertigo, dizziness	23.73	Diabetes mellitus	26.37
	Diabetes mellitus	19.73	Shortness of breath	21.95
	Back pain, ache, discomfort	19.26	Blood pressure check	19.82
	New/renewed medication nos	19.14	Back pain, ache, discomfort	18.18
	Leg pain, ache, discomfort	16.24	General weakness	17.03

nos, not otherwise specified; resp, respiratory.

harm in their health care systems, by improving primary care and often by not engaging in risky endeavours of little or no value, avoiding a toxic cascade effect.[57–60]

Another measure of how primary care is valued is seen by an assessment of what people did in the United States when they had the choice of visiting their primary care clinician or going directly to other types of specialists. Forrest et al. found that 93–96 per cent of individuals who chose to enroll in and pay extra for health plans with an option to obtain sub-specialty care via self-referral did *not* exercise it. When self-referral occurred, it was more likely for individuals with chronic and orthopaedic conditions and less continuity with their regular physician. Interestingly in this particular study, a slightly higher proportion of people self-referred to a generalist than a sub-specialist, possibly doing so to retain their relationships with their regular doctor in a system permitting or promoting fragmentation instead of integration.[61] This study indicates that even when individuals are in a position to go wherever they want, they choose to go first to their regular doctor. This desire to maintain a relationship has been documented elsewhere, such as the United Kingdom, and is associated with trust which patients' value highly.[62]

Of course, there are data about the limitations of primary care and legitimate criticism of studies done to evaluate it.[19,63,64] Nonetheless, decades of investigations in multiple settings, when taken together, provide a web of evidence that supports the value and role of primary care. In summary, primary care is valued because it provides people with access to appropriate services, at reduced costs, with satisfying results. It enhances the performance of health care systems. It is not the solution to every health-related problem, but few, if any, health-related problems can be adequately addressed without excellent primary care.

Further development of primary care

No country seems to be fully satisfied with its health care system, and experimentation abounds. Because of the centrality of primary care in health care systems, primary care is affected by policy changes directed not only at primary care but also the rest of the health care system. For example, the United Kingdom introduced primary care groups in 1999 bringing together doctors, nurses, and other health and social care professionals to plan and implement health care services, improve health of local communities, and establish mechanisms of accountability.[65] These developments are accompanied by concern that such re-organization of the National Health Service may weaken its primary care enterprise[66,67] possibly to the detriment of people. Since 1995, Australia, a country providing universal insurance coverage through a compulsory public programme delivered by a large private sector, has promoted private health insurance through changes in contracting, government subsidies for health insurance, and moving away from pure community rating.[68,69] After some 30 years of innovations in Canada, there are aspects of primary care that have changed little and significant progress in reform seems unlikely absent major investments by government in primary care infrastructures.[70]

While each country wrestles with its challenges in its own way, there are themes and directions that cut across national boundaries. Modern health care systems are expected to be safe, effective, patient-centred, timely, efficient, and equitable.[56] These aims are directly in the realm of primary care. It is difficult to imagine their achievement without a robust primary care enterprise, and thus it will be difficult if not impossible to achieve them without a vigorous commitment to further primary care research and development.[71,72]

An imminent shift from old ways of thinking and delivering health care toward a new world of health care occurring in the information age has been glimpsed and characterized:[56]

1. Care based on visits will yield to care based on continuous healing relationships.
2. Instead of professional autonomy driving variability, care will be customized according to the needs and values of patients.
3. Patients, more than professionals, will be the source of control of care.
4. Information will cease being a mere record, and knowledge will be shared and information will flow freely.
5. Decisions will be based less on training and experience and more on evidence.
6. Instead of 'do no harm' being an individual responsibility, it will be the responsibility and a property of the entire health care system.
7. Secrecy will give way to transparency as a necessity.
8. The health care system will not just react to demands and needs; it will anticipate needs.
9. Instead of seeking reductions in cost, waste will be continually decreased.
10. Rather than professional roles trumping system performance, cooperation among clinicians will be the priority.

Such a vision begs for more and better primary care. The future of primary care depends now on constructing its place in evolving health care systems in every country, and to an important extent, the success of each country's health care system depends upon the adequacy of its primary care system.

Conclusion

Former Colorado Governor Richard D. Lamm[73] has written:

> Modern medicine has outgrown its metaphors. It is no longer possible for a physician to do everything 'beneficial' for every patient, and clearly physicians cannot say that costs should 'never be a consideration.' Everything a . . . payer does for one patient prevents it from doing something else for another. The price of modern medicine is the painful necessity to set limits, make tradeoffs, set priorities. Someone must place health care needs in the larger context of other patient needs and other social needs.[73]

Placing health care into context and setting priorities is the realm of primary care. Primary care is essential to effective, sustainable health care systems. Its importance and salutary effects are supported by evidence. As the information age emerges, primary care is a frontier full of challenge, in the midst of further development and exploration. Its future is sure because primary care is necessary. Indeed, primary care is primary in the sense of being care that is first, foremost, and fundamental.

References

1. **White, K.L., Williams, T.F., and Greenberg, B.** (1961). The ecology of medical care. *New England Journal of Medicine* **265**, 885–92.
2. **Green, L.A., Fryer, G.E., Yawn, B.P., Lanier, D., and Dovey, S.M.** (2001). The ecology of medical care revisited. *New England Journal of Medicine* **344**, 2021–5.
3. **Lord Dawson of Penn. Interim Report on the Future Provisions of Medical and Allied Services.** United Kingdom Ministry of Health. Consultative Council on Medical Allied Services. London: Her Majesty's Stationery Offices, 1920.
4. **Citizens Commission on Graduate Medical Education,** Millis, J.S., Chairman. *The Graduate Education of Physicians.* Chicago IL: American Medical Association, 1966.
5. **Ad Hoc Committee on Education for Family Practice, Willard Committee.** *Meeting the Challenge of Family Practice.* Chicago IL: American Medical Association, 1966.
6. **Lalonde, M.** *A New Perspective on the Health of Canadians.* Ottawa: Ministry of National Health and Welfare, 1974.
7. **World Health Organization.** Alma-Ata 1978: Primary Health Care. *Report of the International Conference on Primary Health Care,* Alma-Ata, Union of Soviet Socialist Republics, 6–12 September 1978. Geneva: World Health Organization, 1978.

8. **World Health Organization.** *Global Strategy for Health for All by the Year 2000.* Geneva: World Health Organization, 1981.
9. **Starfield, B.** *Primary Care. Concept, Evaluation, and Policy.* New York: Oxford University Press, 1992, pp. 6, 213–35.
10. **Nutting, P.A.**, ed. *Community-Oriented Primary Care: From Principle to Practice.* US Department of Health and Human Services. Health Resources and Services Administration. Office of Primary Care Studies. Washington DC: US Government Printing Office, 1987.
11. **Abramson, J.H. and Kark, S.L.** (1983). Community oriented primary care; meaning and scope. In *Community Oriented Primary Care—New Directions for Health Services* (ed. E.D. Conner and F. Mullan), pp. 21–59. Washington DC: National Academy Press.
12. **Institute of Medicine.** *Community Oriented Primary Care: A Practical Assessment, Vol. 1: The Committee Report.* Washington DC: National Academy Press, 1984.
13. **Rhyne, R., Bogue, R., Kukulka, G., and Fulmer, H.** *Community-Oriented Primary Care: Health Care for the 21st Century.* Washington DC: American Public Health Association, 1998.
14. **Institute of Medicine.** *A Manpower Policy for Primary Health Care.* Report of a Study. Washington DC: National Academy Press, 1978.
15. **Alpert, J.J. and Charney, E.** *The Education of Physicians for Primary Care.* Publication No. (HRA)74-3113. Rockville MD: US Department of Health Education, and Welfare, 1973.
16. **Parker, A.** (1974). The dimensions of primary care: blueprints for change. In *Primary Care: Where Medicine Fails* (ed. S. Andreopoulos). New York: John Wiley and Sons.
17. **The International Bank for Reconstruction and Development/The World Bank.** World Development Report 1993. *Investing in Health. World Development Indictors.* New York: Oxford University Press, 1993, p. 6.
18. **World Health Organization and The World Organization of Family Doctors.** Making medical practice and education more relevant to people's needs: the contribution of the family doctor (ed. M.L. Rivo and J.E. Heck). The Joint WHO-WONCA Conference in Ontario, Canada, November 6–8, 1994. Geneva: World Health Organization, 1994.
19. **Institute of Medicine. Donaldson, J.S., Yordy, K.D., Lohr, K.N., and Vanselow, N.A.**, ed. *Primary Care: America's Health in a New Era.* Washington DC: National Academy Press, 1996, pp. 18, 27–34, 53, 71–2, 80–1.
20. **Olesen, F., Dickinson, J., Hjortdahl, P.** (2000). General practice—a time for a new definition. *British Medical Journal* **320**, 354–7.
21. **Heath, I., Evans, P., and van Weel, C.** (2000). The specialist of the discipline of general practice. *British Medical Journal* **320**, 326–7.
22. **Lamberts, H. and Hofman-Okkes, I.M.** (1996). Episode of care: a core concept in family practice. *Journal of Family Practice* **42**, 161–7.
23. **Lamberts, H., Wood, M., and Hofmans-Okkes, I.M.**, ed. *The International Classification of Primary Care in the European Community.* With a multi-language layer. Oxford: Oxford University Press, 1993.
24. **Okkes, I.M., Polderman, G.O., Fryer, G.E., Yamada, T., Bujak, M., Oskam, S.K., Green, L.A., and Lamberts, H.** (2002). The role of family practice in different health care systems. A comparison of reasons for encounter, diagnoses, and interventions in primary care populations in the Netherlands, Japan, Poland, and the United States. *Journal of Family Practice* **51**, 72–3. http://www.jfponline.com
25. **Gonnella, J.** et al. (1977). Use of outcome measures in ambulatory care evaluation. In *Ambulatory Medical Care—Quality Assurance* (ed. G. Gebink, N. White, and E. Short). La Jolla CA: La Jolla Health Science Publications.
26. **Shea, S.** et al. (1992). Predisposing factors for severe, uncontrolled hypertension in an inner-city minority population. *New England Journal of Medicine* **327**, 776–81.
27. **Ferrante, J.M., Gonzales, E.C., Pal, N., and Roetzheim, R.G.** (2000). Effects of physician supply on early detection of breast cancer. *Journal of the American Board of Family Practice* **13**, 408–14.
28. **Gadomski, A. and Jenkins, P.** (2001). Ruptured appendicitis among children as an indicator of access to care. *Health Services Research* **36**, 129–42.
29. **Hochheiser, L.I., Woodward, K., and Charney, E.** (1971). Effect of the neighborhood health center on the use of pediatric emergency departments in Rochester, New York. *New England Journal of Medicine* **285**, 148–52.
30. **Alpert, J.J.** et al. (1976). Delivery of health care for children: report of an experiment. *Pediatrics* **57**, 917–30.
31. **Wasson, J.H.** et al. (1984). Continuity of outpatient medical care in elderly men: a randomized trial. *Journal of the American Medical Association* **252**, 2413–17.
32. **Hurley, R.E., Freund, D.A., and Taylor, D.E.** (1988). Emergency room use and primary care case management: evidence from four medicaid demonstration programs. *American Journal of Public Health* **79**, 843–6.
33. **Fryer, G.E.** Evaluation of the primary care physician program. Unpublished report to the Colorado Department of Social Services. Denver CO: Colorado Department of Social Service, 1991.
34. **Parchman, M.L. and Culler, S.** (1994). Primary care physicians and avoidable hospitalization. *Journal of Family Practice* **39**, 123–8.
35. **Bindman, A.B.** et al. (1995). Preventable hospitalizations and access to health care. *Journal of the American Medical Association* **274**, 305–11.
36. **Starfield, B.** (1995). Access—perceived or real, and to what? *Journal of American Medical Association* **274**, 346–7.
37. **Manu, P. and Swartz, S.E.** (1983). Patterns of diagnostic testing in the academic setting: the influence of medical attendings' subspecialty training. *Social Science and Medicine* **17**, 1339–42.
38. **Cherkin, D.C.** et al. (1987). The use of medical resources by residency trained family physicians and general internists. *Medical Care* **25**, 455–68.
39. **Dor, A. and Holahan, J.** (1990). Urban–rural differences in medicaid physician expenditures. *Inquiry* **27**, 307–18.
40. **Greenfield, S.** et al. (1992). Variations in resource utilization among medical specialties and systems of care: results from the medical outcomes study. *Journal of the American Medical Association* **267**, 1624–30.
41. **Welch, W.P.** et al. (1993). Geographic variation in expenditures for physicians' services in the United States. *New England Journal of Medicine* **328**, 621–7.
42. **Mark, D.H.** et al. Medicare costs and the supply of primary care physicians. Unpublished document. Milwaukee WI: D.H. Mark, Medical College of Wisconsin, 1995.
43. **Lohr, K.N.** et al. (1986). Use of medical care in the Rand Health Insurance Experiment: diagnosis- and service-specific analyses in a randomized controlled trial. *Medical Care* **24**, S1–87.
44. **Goldberg, G.A. and Newhouse, J.P.** (1987). Effects of cost sharing on physiological health, health practices, and worry. *Health Services Research* **22**, 279–306.
45. **Newhouse, J.P. and the Health Insurance Group.** *Free for All? Lessons from the RAND Health Insurance Experiment.* Cambridge MA: Harvard University Press, 1993.
46. **Dietrich, A.J. and Goldberg, H.** (1984). Preventive content of adult primary care: do generalists and subspecialists differ? *American Journal of Public Health* **74**, 223–7.
47. **Bindman, A.B.** et al. (1996). Primary care and receipt of preventive services. *Journal of General Internal Medicine* **11**, 269–76.
48. **Dovey, S., Green, L.A., and Fryer, G.E.** (2000). Educating doctors to provide counseling and preventive care: turning 20th century professional values head over heels. *Education for Health* **13**, 307–16.
49. **Farmer, F.L., Stokes, C.S., Fiser, R.H., and Papini, D.P.** (1991). Poverty, primary care and age-specific mortality. *Journal of Rural Health* **7**, 153–69.
50. **Shi, L.** (1992). The relationship between primary care and life chances. *Journal of Health Care for the Poor and Underserved* **3**, 321–35.
51. **Vogel, R.L. and Ackermann, R.J.** (1998). Is primary care physician supply correlated with health outcomes? *International Journal of Health Services* **28**, 183–96.
52. **Shi, L., Starfield, B., Kennedy, B., and Ichiro, K.** (1999). Income inequality, primary care, and health indicators. *Journal of Family Practice* **48**, 275–84.
53. **Franks, P. and Fiscella, K.** (1998). Primary care physicians and specialists as personal physicians. Health care expenditures and mortality experience. *Journal of Family Practice* **47**, 105–9.
54. **Starfield, B.** (1991). Primary care and health. a cross-national comparison. *Journal of the American Medical Association* **266**, 2268–71.
55. **Institute of Medicine.** Kohn, L.T., Corrigan, J.M., and Donaldson, M.S., ed. *To Err is Human: Building a Safer Health System.* Washington DC: National Academy Press, 2000.

56. **Institute of Medicine.** Committee on Quality of Health Care in America. *Crossing the Quality Chasm: A New Health System for the 21st Century.* Washington DC: National Academy Press, 2001, pp. 41–94.
57. **Mold, J. and Stein, H.** (1986). The cascade effect in the clinical care of patients. *New England Journal of Medicine* **314**, 512–14.
58. **Starfield, B.** (2000). Is US health really the best in the world? *Journal of the American Medical Association* **284**, 483–5.
59. **The Robert Graham Center** (2001). Toxic cascades: a comprehensive way to think about medical errors. *American Family Physician* **63**, 847.
60. **The Robert Graham Center** (2001). The patient safety grid: toxic cascades in health care settings. *American Family Physician* **63**, 1047.
61. **Forrest, C.B., Weiner, J.P., Fowles, J., Vogeli, C., Frick, K.D., Lemke, K.W., and Starfield, B.** (2001). Self-referral in point-of-service health plans. *Journal of the American Medical Association* **285**, 2223–31.
62. **Mainous, A.G., Baker, R., Lvoe, M.M., Gray, D.P., and Gill, J.M.** (2001). Continuity of care and trust in one's physician: evidence from primary care in the United States and the United Kingdom. *Family Medicine* **33**, 22–7.
63. **Harrold, L.R., Field, T.S., and Gurwitz, J.H.** (1999). Knowledge, patterns of care, and outcomes of care for generalists and specialists. *Journal of General Internal Medicine* **14**, 499–511.
64. **Bickell, N.A. and Siu, A.L.** (2001). Why do delays in treatment occur? Lessons from ruptured appendicitis. *Health Services Research* **36**, 1–5.
65. **Bindman, A.B., Weiner, J.P., and Majeed, A.** (2001). Primary care groups in the United Kingdom: quality and accountability. *Health Affairs* **20**, 132–45.
66. **Kperski, M.** (2000). The state of primary care in the United States of America and lessons for primary care groups in the United Kingdom. *British Journal of General Practice* **50**, 319–22.
67. **Pollock, A.M.** (2001). Will primary care trusts lead to US-style health care? *British Medical Journal* **322**, 964–7.
68. **Iglehart, J.K.** (2001). An activist health minister in a conservative government. *Health Affairs* **20** (3), 146–51.
69. **Willcox, S.** (2001). Promoting private health insurance in Australia. *Health Affairs* **20** (3), 152–61.
70. **Hutchison, B., Abelson, J., and Lavis, J.** (2001). Primary care in Canada: so much innovation, so little change. *Health Affairs* **20** (3), 116–31.
71. **Green, L.A.** (1996). Science and the future of primary care. *Journal of Family Practice* **42**, 119–22.
72. **Norton, P.G., Stewart, M., Tudiver, F., Bass, M., and Dunn, E.**, ed. *Primary Care Research. Traditional and Innovative Approaches. Vol. 1.* London: Sage Publications, 1991.
73. **Lamm, R.D.** (2001). Medicine and the arts. *Academic Medicine* **76**, 256.

1.2 From general practice to primary care, 1700–1980

Irvine Loudon

In the winter of 1699/1700, John Seale, a butcher in Hungerford market (London), fell ill. He was treated by William Rose, a London apothecary. The butcher, who was 'never the better but much worse' for his treatment, was so angry when presented with an outrageous bill for £50, that he complained to the Royal College of Physicians, which, at that time, had a legal monopoly of the 'practice of physic' in London. This meant that apothecaries, who had evolved from the Company of Grocers, were supposed to stay in their shops and dispense prescriptions written by physicians. They were not allowed to 'practise physic': that is, to act as doctors and treat patients.

Rose was prosecuted and found guilty of 'practising physic'. But the verdict was quashed by the House of Lords partly because what Rose had done—treating a patient—was already being done by many apothecaries; partly because the poor, who could not afford a physician, would suffer; and partly because their Lordships were aware that many physicians 'would not attend when at dinner or abed' and they might be unable to obtain an apothecary for an 'out-of-hours' emergency. So the Lords ruled that apothecaries could indeed treat all illnesses, whether slight or grave; but they placated the physicians by adding that apothecaries could only charge for medicines, not for attendance or advice.[1]

The birth of the surgeon-apothecary

The Rose case is historically important because it revealed a change that was taking place anyway in the late seventeenth century: a change that, to my mind, marked the beginning of the general practitioner. By 1700, not only were many apothecaries selling medicines directly to patients 'over the counter', and visiting the sick in their homes. They were also treating surgical cases that came their way. This may sound odd until we recall that major ('capital') operations were then rare events. Surgery in the eighteenth century consisted to a very great extent of dealing with injuries, local infections like abscesses, leg ulcers, eye diseases (other than cataracts), skin diseases, toothache, and similar conditions that did not call for the special surgical skills. A few apothecaries stuck to their original tasks, but a rapidly growing majority became a new kind of practitioner, known as the 'surgeon-apothecary'.

From about 1740, these practitioners, added midwifery to their services and sometimes adopted the cumbrous title, 'surgeon-apothecary and man-midwife'. This was part of a radical change. At the beginning of the eighteenth century midwifery was not part of the medical curriculum. Only a tiny minority of births were attended by medical men of any description, and usually only for some severe complication such as obstructed labour. By the end of the century, however, about half of all deliveries in England, normal and abnormal, were attended by medical practitioners of whom a large majority were surgeon-apothecaries, and the other half were delivered by midwives. Surgeon-apothecaries took to midwifery like ducks to water for one very good reason: it was essential for building a practice. 'Deliver the babies and you will have the family as patients for life' was an article of faith in general practice until the mid-twentieth century.[2]

Historians often differ on when general practitioners as we know them today first appeared. Some point to the Apothecaries Act of 1815, others to the Medical Act of 1858. I believe the question should be resolved by reference to the mode and extent of medical practice rather than parliamentary Acts. In my view, the surgeon-apothecaries of the eighteenth century were general practitioners in all but name.[3] They became increasingly numerous not only in cities, but in market towns and villages all over the country, proudly boasting that when called out they could deal with any kind of case, whether medical, surgical, or obstetrical. They only needed assistance from physicians or 'pure' surgeons when faced with occasional complex cases, or major operations such as amputation or cutting for stone.

So far I have considered the birth of the general practitioner in the United Kingdom. What happened in other countries? Here one meets two major difficulties. First, the difficulty of identifying medical practitioners in other countries during, for instance, the eighteenth or nineteenth century, for whom the label 'general practitioner' is appropriate. Secondly, the paucity of historical research on international aspects of general practice. One can, however, make an informed guess that all of the countries we now call 'developed' possessed doctors who at least resembled general practitioners. They were typically the only doctors for rural and sparsely populated areas that could not support a specialist, and urban doctors for the poorer patients who could not afford a university-trained physician. We will return briefly to international comparisons of general practice/primary care in the second half of the twentieth century at the end of the chapter.

In England and Wales, the medical education of the eighteenth-century surgeon-apothecary was apprenticeship, supplemented in the second half of the century by attendance at medical lectures in hospitals and private medical schools. Some surgeon-apothecaries were rough, ignorant, and

Table 1 UK, 1951–1995. Total population, number of hospital medical staff (whole time equivalents) and number of general practitioners in the National Health Service, and the ratio of hospital staff and general practitioners to population

Year	Population UK (thousands)	Number of hospital medical staff	Ratio of hospital medical staff to population	Number of general medical practitioners	Ratio of general practitioners to population*
1951	50225	14393	1:3489	22478	1:2234
1961	52709	19816	1:2659	23603	1:2233
1971	55515	28102	1:1975	24998	1:2220
1981	58848	40386	1:1382	30182	1:1850
1991	56467	51060	1:1105	34449	1:1639

* This ratio is often referred to in general practice as the 'average list size'.

Notes: It can be seen that the number of medical staff per head of population has increased much more rapidly for hospital staff (column 4) than for general practitioners (column 6); and that the increase in numbers of general practitioners relative to the population only began to increase after 1971.

Source: Office of Health Economics, Compendium of Health Statistics, 9th edn., 1995, table 4.7.

scraped a living, but many—at a guess a majority—had a good school education, were quite widely read and thoughtful men who owned medical books, attended medical meetings, and dined out with attorneys, the upper ranks of the clergy, and the local squire. The surgeon-apothecaries thrived because they treated a wide range of social classes and pandered to the extraordinary propensity of the eighteenth-century public to swallow medicines in astonishing quantities, not only when ill but also to fend off disease or just make themselves feel better (ref. 3, Chapters 1–5). There are many examples of this, but one will do.

Bernard Baine, a Somerset surgeon-apothecary, was the regular medical attendant to a rich Somerset family. Although the family suffered no more than a few minor complaints, in just one year (1755) Baine provided this family and its servants with a total of 687 items of medicine, delivered almost every day. The family's medical bill for that year was £154.5.7½ d., roughly half an average country practitioner's annual income at the time. Baine never charged for attendance; only for medicines and the occasional venesection.[1] The potential profits of pharmacy were indeed formidable, and when it came to prescribing in bulk, the most profligate general practitioner in the NHS cannot hold a candle to his eighteenth-century predecessors (ref. 3, Chapter 3, footnote 4, pp. 54–72).

The trouble was, however, that the more the surgeon-apothecaries prospered the more they worried about the competition from 'the vile quacks with which this country is infected'.[(4)] These were not just itinerant healers, travelling from one market place to another, although a few of these existed. They were usually such people as butchers, grocers, blacksmiths, the wives of the clergy, and many others who dabbled in medicine and acquired local reputations as healers, and the numerous sellers of patent medicines. Worst of all, however, were the dispensing chemists (the predecessors of today's pharmacists) who, from about the 1780s, suddenly appeared all over the country, set up their shops, and sold medicines at a much lower price than the orthodox practitioners. The rage of the surgeon-apothecaries at the perceived increase in quackery in general (whether it was really increasing is a moot point) and dispensing chemists in particular, was the driving force behind what has become known as the 'period of medical reform' from about the 1780s to the Medical Act of 1858.[(5)]

The period of medical reform

The aims of reform were simple: to outlaw quackery and improve the standard of medicine by introducing a formal system of medical education, examination, and licensing. Only then would the public be able to tell the trained practitioners from the quacks, the orthodox from the unorthodox. But the progress of medical reform was anything but smooth. Numerous plans were put forward (some of them excellent) only to be rejected by the Royal Colleges of Physicians and Surgeons who saw every attempt to improve the quality of the rank and file practitioners as a threat to their status at the top of the medical tree (ref. 3, footnote 4, pp. 129–51). The first tangible result of medical reform was the highly unsatisfactory Apothecaries Act of 1815 after which all new entrants to general practice had to sit for the examination of the Licence of the Society of Apothecaries (the LSA) (ref. 3, pp. 152–70). The majority also acquired Membership of the Royal College of Surgeons so that the dual qualification, MRCS LSA, became the hallmark of general practitioners, the sign of professional men with letters after their name. As Dr Jobling said in Martin Chuzzlewit:

> We know a few secrets in our profession, sir. Of course we do. We study for that. We pass the Hall and the College for that: and we take our station in society *by* that.[(6)]

Some 300–400 students a year took the LSA in the 1830s and 1840s. General practice rapidly became so popular that there was no shortage of candidates. On the contrary, there were soon bitter complaints of an overcrowded profession. What was to be done about it?

Physicians and surgeons derived political power, high status, and leadership through their Royal Colleges. But the Society of Apothecaries was a failure as far as leadership and standards were concerned. The Provincial Medical and Surgical Association, which was founded in 1832 and became the British Medical Association in 1855, was an institution to which general practitioners could belong, but it was not enough. So a few enterprising people founded The National Association of General Practitioners in 1844, which rapidly recruited 4000 members with the single ambitious aim of founding a Royal College of General Practitioners. This association received strong support from Sir James Graham, the Home Secretary, and very nearly succeeded, only to fall at the final fence when the Royal College of Surgeons brutally crushed the proposal (ref. 3, footnote 4, pp. 282–96). It is interesting, but futile, to speculate how general practice might have developed had the plan succeeded.

The complaints about an overcrowded profession were not exaggerated. In the middle of the nineteenth century, there was approximately one general practitioner to every 1200 of the population in England and Wales, compared with around 1 to 2000 under the NHS (see Table 1). Imagine a provincial town of about 25 000 people in the middle of the nineteenth century that was roughly the population of Gloucester, Cardiff, Exeter, or Oxford in 1850. Such a town would probably have 25 medical practitioners of whom two would be physicians, three surgeons, and 20 general practitioners. Most towns of this size or over would have a general (voluntary) hospital, a dispensary, and a poor-law medical service.

The physicians would have lived partly by consulting practice, but were also the general practitioners for some of the richest people in town. The surgeons would have been general practitioners with a special interest in surgery and an appointment as honorary surgeon to the local infirmary (nepotism was often rife in such appointments). The general practitioners would have competed for private patients and also for lucrative posts such as factory doctor, poor-law medical officer, medical officers of sickness clubs,

[1] Somerset County Record Office, Taunton. Bill from Mr Baine, surgeon-apothecary to Thomas Carew, DD/TB box 14/20.

insurance doctor, and so on. In the second half of the nineteenth century, their standard income was about £600 a year; but the poorer general practitioners would have struggled on about £300 a year and a few with the best practices might have produced an income close to £1000 a year.(7)

The principle of referral

Between 1881 and 1911, when the population of England and Wales increased by 27 per cent, the number of clergy increased by 20 per cent and lawyers by 23 per cent; but doctors increased by 63 per cent (ref. 7, table 2.2, p. 30). Competition for patients was intense and incomes were falling when a new threat arose from a little known but extraordinary change in hospitals for which there is no easy explanation. Suddenly, in the middle of the nineteenth century, hospitals became so popular with the mass of the people that there was a massive increase in the number of self-referred out-patients or 'casualties'. These consisted of the poor (and some supposedly poor) who flooded into hospital casualty departments to obtain free medical relief, whether their complaints were medical or surgical, severe or minor, real or imagined. It is essential to appreciate that they were *not* referred by general practitioners.(8)

This happened at hospitals in London and the provinces. At the Liverpool Royal Infirmary, for instance, between 1750 and 1860 there were no more than 1000–2000 out-patient attendances a year. After 1860, there was a sudden rise with out-patient attendances climbing to 25 000 a year by the end of the century. But for sheer numbers the London Hospital, Whitechapel, won first prize. Here the annual number of new out-patient attendances rose from 5000 a year in the 1820s, to 52 000 in the 1870s, and finally to the astonishing peak of 221 781 in 1910. If you exclude Sundays and Christmas Day, this works out at about 700 patients a day who were seen by junior medical staff at the impossible rate of one or two patients a minute.[2] The hospitals permitted—even welcomed—this shameful parody of primary care to continue because it provided a huge reservoir for selecting 'good teaching cases', and because they could use it to advertise the extent of their service to the poor.

The effect on general practitioners in the vicinity of large hospitals was devastating. Many were bankrupted by the scandal of 'the out-patient problem' (this phrase was used at the time). General practitioners demanded something that I must emphasize was quite new: namely, that hospitals would only see out-patients who were sent by general practitioners with an accompanying letter. This was the origin of the peculiarly British system of referral: the gate-keeper role of the general practitioner. It slowly became accepted practice, but it always was and still is an ethical principle, not a law or regulation. The principle of referral, universally accepted in the United Kingdom, is often praised on clinical grounds; but it was introduced quite simply because general practitioners were going broke in large numbers.

National Health Insurance (NHI), 1911

The National Health Insurance Act of 1911, which came into operation in 1913, meant that employees earning less than £160 a year were entitled to free medical care from the general practitioners who had signed up to take part in the scheme.[3] Of the three possible ways of paying the doctors for NHI work—by salary, by 'item of service' whereby every visit, attendance at a surgery or bottle of medicine would attract a fee, or by the 'capitation' method—the capitation system was adopted. It is still in operation and explains why every eligible patient has to be registered with a particular general practitioner, and why general practitioners are still paid (at least in large part) by the number of patients on their list.[4] The average income of general practitioners in the early decades of the twentieth century began to rise because of NHI, and partly because this was the period when motor cars and telephones were introduced.(10) As their income rose, the total numbers attending hospital out-patients fell, with a growing proportion of out-patients being referred from general practice.

General practice under the National Health Service (NHS)

It is often said that the greatest achievement of the NHS was the introduction of high standards of hospital care to all parts of the country. General practice, however, was relatively unchanged, for three features of general practice were already so deeply entrenched that they were simply adopted by the NHS. These were the capitation system of payment, valued by general practitioners as a guarantee (or so it was thought) of clinical independence; the principle of referral, which meant, as one historian famously wrote, that 'the physician and surgeon retained the hospital but the general practitioner retained the patient';(11) and thirdly, a national system of administration of general practice through Local Medical Committees that was introduced in 1913.

Because of the perceived success of the 'panel' system (over 40 per cent of the population were 'panel patients' by 1938) there seemed no need for radical changes in general practice. It is only a slight over-simplification to say that as far as general practice was concerned the NHS did little more than extend the system of National Health Insurance, lock, stock, and barrel, to the whole instead of a part of the population. The continued use of the dreadfully inadequate medical record envelope as the official system of record-keeping in general practice symbolized the absence of change.

Few even bothered to look at the state of general practice until an explosive report was published in the *Lancet* in 1950. The report was written by Joseph Collings (1918–1971), an Australian doctor who toured around Britain visiting numerous practices. Many were in a deplorable state. 'Few skilled craftsmen' wrote Collings, 'be they plumbers, butchers or motor mechanics, would be prepared to work under such conditions or with equipment so bad . . .' And the standard of clinical care was often as dire as the practice equipment and premises.(12) It was true that there were excellent practices here and there. Collings found one in Scotland, where a general practitioner had built his own laboratory and provided a 'quality of service . . . far above anything his colleagues could offer'. But his colleagues 'regarded this doctor as crazy . . .' because he was in danger of being forced out of practice by the cost of providing a high quality of service. The worst aspect of the legacies of the past was that the whole system of general practice in the early years of the NHS could almost have been designed to discourage change, innovation, and progress.

Just at the time, therefore, when the hospital service was beginning to forge ahead in a state of high optimism as a result of the therapeutic revolution, general practice was stagnant. Post-graduate education was virtually non-existent. All too often, general practitioners, who were poorly paid, lacked self-respect and showed little or no ambition to improve either their standards of practice or knowledge.

Most of us who entered general practice in or before the 1950s (in my own case it was 1952) believe that the Collings Report was on the whole correct, and certainly salutary. But many of us have lived to see a rise in standards and morale amounting to a transformation of general practice between 1948 and 1980. Although this is seldom appreciated outside the world of general practice, the extent of the transformation is, in retrospect, little less than astonishing. It has been due to many factors that can only be discussed very briefly in this chapter.(13)

[2] Records of the Liverpool Royal Infirmary, Liverpool Record Office, and the archives of the Royal London Hospital. See also ref. 9.

[3] The income limit was raised in stages to £420 by 1942. National Health Insurance never, of course, covered dependents so that wives and children had to pay fees for medical attention from general practitioners.

[4] Although the National Health Insurance patients were known as 'panel patients' the origin of the term 'panel', which simply means a list, was first used to describe the list (or 'panel') of general practitioners who agreed to take patients under the National Health Insurance scheme. But the term soon became attached to the patients who were referred to as being 'on the panel'.

Although general practitioners are sometimes accused of an obsession with money, there would have been no transformation without improvements in pay and conditions of service. These occurred mainly through the Danckwerts Award of 1952 and the Family Doctor's Charter in 1966. Perhaps the most important factors in the transformation were the foundation of the College (later the Royal College) of General Practitioners in 1952, the establishment of university departments of general practice (the first was in Edinburgh in 1963), the introduction of vocational training, and the growing volume of research from general practice.

As morale improved, some of the brightest medical students put general practice as their first choice as a career and brought a new spirit of energy, enthusiasm, and criticism to the discipline. With no shortage of recruits, the ratio of general practitioners to population began to rise after 1971 (Table 1) and the recruits were entering a new world in three respects. First, the rapid growth of group practice, shown vividly in Fig. 1. Secondly, the increasing number of health centres provided by local health authorities and privately owned, purpose-built, general practice premises of high quality. The third and absolutely vital factor for change was dependent on the other two: this was the attachment of district (community) nurses, health visitors, midwives, and sometimes social workers to group practices. Teamwork, in other words. There is a downside to most changes, and some would argue that teamwork reduced continuity of care and the much-treasured concept of the personal doctor. When one remembers, however, that in the 1940s, a majority of general practitioners were single-handed, that they practised surgery in their homes or a converted shop and had minimal contacts with community nursing staff, the gains from teamwork far out-weigh the losses. Whatever the actual origin of the term 'Primary Care', the essence of it and the justification for using it, lies in the changes outlined above.

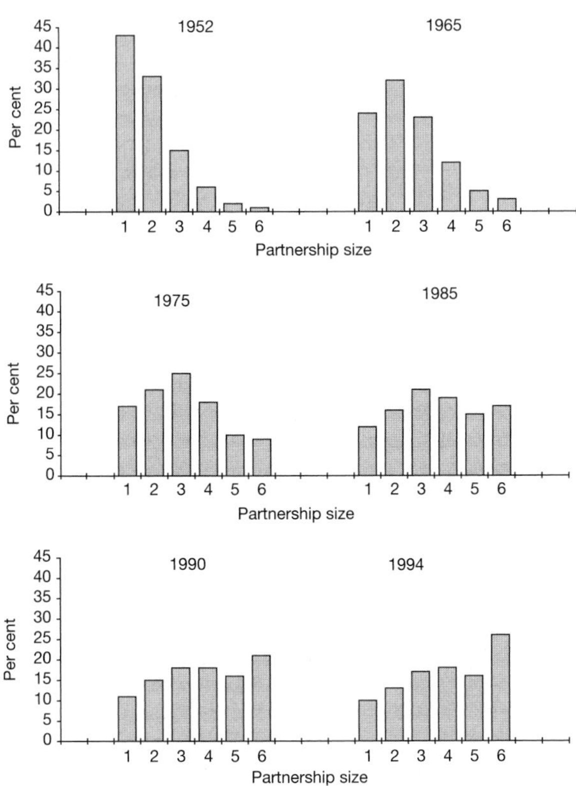

Fig. 1 Percentage distribution of unrestricted general practitioners by number of partners in a practice ranging from single-handed practice to groups of six or more partners. (*Source:* Department of Health, Health and Personal Social Services Statistics, and Office of Health Economics, *Compendium of Health Statistics*, 9th edn., 1995, table 4.16.)

International comparisons

Those of us who live and work in the United Kingdom are apt to assume that ours is the only country that has a substantial number of general practitioners, and the only one with the process of referral by which access to specialists is always (or nearly always) obtained through referral by their general practitioners. But the facts of the matter are more complex.(14)

If we look at the number of medically qualified personnel per 100 000 population in a selection of developed countries in 1990, we find that Germany came at the top with about 280 per 100 000; next came Sweden, Denmark, and France with about 260 followed by the Netherlands, Sweden, and the United States of America with around 200–230. Finally, way down at the bottom is the United Kingdom with around 170 per 100 000 (ref. 13, p. 262).

But what we want to know is the *proportion* of medically qualified personnel who are registered as general practitioners. Here the order is quite different. In 1980, for instance, Canada, France, and the United Kingdom had almost exactly the same proportion of general practitioners in their medical professions (about 42 per cent of the total). They were separated by quite a big gap from Sweden, Denmark, the Netherlands and Germany (about 22 per cent), with the United States of America at the bottom of the list with about 10 per cent of the medical profession working as general practitioners. The country with the largest number of general practitioners per 100 000 population is, by quite a long way, France (with just under 150), not Britain (which has just over 100 general practitioners per 100 000 population). At the other end of the spectrum, the United States of America has only about 10 general practitioners per 100 000 population (ref. 13, p. 265).

But what about direct access of patients to specialists, the so-called gate-keeping role of the general practitioner that we tend to think of as a unique feature of medicine in the United Kingdom? In the 1980s and 1990s, the tendency of patients to go directly to specialists (for instance, women going directly to gynaecologists or taking their children directly to paediatricians) is very high in Germany, high in France and Sweden, less so in Denmark and the Netherlands. It is nil in the NHS in the United Kingdom apart from a small number of special 'open access' hospital clinics and accident and emergency departments. The United States of America, of course, is the country where direct access to specialists is the rule (ref. 13, p. 266).

The more one examines the histories of different medical professions and systems of health care, the more one realizes that such systems have seldom evolved solely, or even mainly, by a series of rational, deliberate, step-by-step decisions. Accidental events and cultural factors, whose influence was not always obvious at the time, played a much larger part.

In the United Kingdom, the principle of referral to hospitals was introduced in the late nineteenth century, as explained above. This reinforced the existing system whereby general practitioners were excluded from the hospitals and the world of specialization.

When National Health Insurance was introduced by the Act of 1911, if general practitioners had chosen to be paid by salary or item of service things might have been very different. But they chose to be paid by capitation fee—so much per patient per year—which was only possible if every (panel) patient was *registered* with a general practitioner. Thus, every (panel) patient had his or her own general practitioner or 'family doctor', *because of the system of payment*, and this became a major factor in reinforcing the central role of general practitioners in the provision of medical care. This system was adopted with very little change with the introduction of the National Health Service in 1948, with the result that general practitioners alone are not salaried doctors but independent contractors.

In other countries, the development of current systems of health care will reflect histories of different medical, cultural, economic, and other factors. There would be a great deal to learn from detailed studies of the development of health care in general, and the role of the general practitioner in particular, in a wide variety of countries. That is a study which has yet to be undertaken.

In this chapter, many aspects of the history of general practice have not even been mentioned, let alone discussed. I have written about England and Wales, and failed to deal with the differences in Scotland or Ireland. I have said little about the importance of continuity of care and the concept of the personal ('family') doctor, or the role of the General Medical Services Committee (a sub-committee of the British Medical Assocation). General practice today owes a debt to certain key figures such as Sir George Godber (Chief Medical Officer to the Ministry of Health 1960–1973), Sir Kenneth Robinson (Minister of Health at the time of the Doctor's Charter in 1966), and many others. I have deliberately excluded such recent changes in primary care as fund-holding, out-of-hours services, and primary care groups and trusts. The reason for these and many other omissions is simply lack of space.

References

1. **Clark, G.** *A History of the Royal College of Physicians* Vol. 2. Oxford: Clarendon Press, 1966, pp. 476–9.
2. **Loudon, I.** *Death in Childbirth. An International Study of Maternal Care and Maternal Mortality, 1800–1950.* Oxford: Clarendon Press, 1992, pp. 166–71.
3. **Loudon, I.** *Medical Care and the General Practitioner, 1750–1850.* Oxford: Clarendon Press, 1986, pp. 152–88. (The term 'general practitioner' first appeared in 1813 and gradually displaced 'surgeon-apothecary' over the next two to three decades.)
4. This phrase appeared in print in 1846: **Forbes J.** (1846). On the patronage of quacks and impostors by the upper classes of society. *British and Foreign Medical Review* **21**, 533–40. But it expressed exactly the views of the late eighteenth century.
5. **Loudon, I.** (1987). The vile race of quacks. In *Medical Fringe and Medical Orthodoxy 1750–1850* (ed. W.F. Bynum and R. Porter). London: Croom Helm.
6. **Dickens, C.** *The Life and Adventures of Martin Chuzzlewit.* London: Chapman and Hall, 1843–40. (The College and Hall were of course the Royal College of Surgeons and the Apothecaries Hall.)
7. **Digby, A.** (1999). *The Evolution of British General Practice 1850–1948.* Oxford: Oxford University Press, 1999, Fig. 5.1, p. 111.
8. **Bridges, R.** (1878). An account of the casualty department. *St. Bartholomew's Hospital Reports* **14**, 167–82. (This account by the young Robert Bridges, who soon abandoned medicine and later became Poet Laureate, is one of the most vivid accounts of hospital care in the nineteenth century by any author.)
9. **Loudon, I.** (1978). Historical importance of out-patients. *British Medical Journal* **6118** (1), 974–7.
10. **Loudon, I.** (2001). Doctors and their transport, 1700–1914. *Medical History* **45** (2), 185–206.
11. **Stevens, R.** *Medical Practice in Modern England.* New Haven: Yale University Press, 1996, p. 33.
12. **Collings, J.S.** (1950). General practice in England today: a reconnaisance. *Lancet* **1**, 555–85.
13. Accounts of the extent and nature of this transformation can be found in: **Loudon, I., Horder, J., and Webster, C.** *General Practice under the National Health Service, 1948–1997.* Oxford: Clarendon Press, 1998.
14. The best recent account of this aspect of primary care is: **Horder, J.** (1998). Developments in other countries. In *General Practice under the National Health Service, 1948–1997* Chapter 11 (ed. I. Loudon, J. Horder, and C. Webster), pp. 247–77. Oxford: Clarendon Press.

1.3 The health care team

Peter Bower and Bonnie Sibbald

Teamwork is increasingly seen as crucial for the effective delivery of primary health care. Good teamworking is believed to enhance the quality of care, constrain costs, and make best use of limited human resources. But what is a primary care team and how does it achieve these benefits?

What is a team?

Definitions of a 'team' may be either functional or structural, though none clearly defines the boundaries of a team (Fig. 1).

Structure of teams

Primary care physicians work in partnerships of varying sizes and employ varying numbers of clinical and non-clinical support staff. In developed countries, these support staff potentially include nurses, midwives, therapists, and the professions allied to medicine, together with their administrative support staff. Primary care clinicians may additionally work in partnership with professionals from other sectors, such as social care and hospital care. Individuals may be members of more than one team, working with different people to fulfil different tasks. Depending on the task, this may or may not necessitate working across organizational boundaries. The fuzzy nature of team boundaries is typical of primary care teams everywhere.

Figure 2 shows there is a considerable range in the size and composition of general practice teams both within and between countries.

Why do doctors work in teams?

The growth of larger and multidisciplinary teams has been encouraged in many countries as a means of improving quality while constraining costs. Quality improvements are sought through enhanced coordination of care delivery and by the opportunity for specialization within larger teams. Cost savings can be attained through economies of scale and scope, and by shifting care from expensive to cheaper health care professionals. An added consideration is the need to make best use of scarce human resources by breaking down the disciplinary boundaries that prevent professionals being deployed where their skills can best be utilized. Variation between countries in team structure largely reflects variation in the financial inducements in place, which encourage or discourage the development of teams.

Functional definitions

A group of people who make different contributions towards the achievement of a common goal.[1]

An interdependent group of general medical practitioners and secretaries and/or receptionists, health visitors, district nurses, midwives (and other nursing staff, i.e. practice nurses) who share a common purpose and responsibility, each member clearly understanding his/her own function and those of the other members, so that they all pool skills and knowledge to provide an effective primary health care service.[2]

Structural definitions

Staff comprising an organizational unit with responsibility for primary care provision. This is usually a practice or health centre.

The team may be further differentiated into a 'core', comprising the doctor and his/her employed staff, and the 'extended' team, which includes health professionals, employed by other organizations, who work in close association with the practice.

Fig. 1 What is a team?

In Australia, larger group practices are cheaper to run per physician and more profitable than solo practices.[3] Larger practices are able to employ a wider range of staff; for example, 61 per cent of large practices have a practice manager, compared with 30 per cent of small practices and 23 per cent of solo physicians. However, the staff to physician ratios are higher in solo practices (1.5 staff per GP) as compared with group practices (1.1 per GP). In other words, larger practices are able to benefit from economies in scale in their operating costs. Advantages such as these have stimulated growth in partnership size.[9]

In the United Kingdom, successive reforms of the national general medical practitioner contract during the 1990s also favoured growth in partnership size. For example, the introduction of payments for delivering preventive health care to an agreed proportion of the population could more easily be achieved by larger practices, which could afford the resources (e.g. computerized registers, call–recall systems, and nurses) needed to deliver the requisite service. The effect on partnership size was pronounced. In 1989, about 45 per cent of practitioners were in partnerships of three or fewer, compared with about 36 per cent by 1999. In contrast, the number of practitioners in partnerships of six or more increased by 54 per cent from 5535 to 8510.[6]

Organizational reforms, backed by financial incentives, had a similar impact on the numbers of staff employed by primary care physicians in the United Kingdom. General practitioner contract reforms in the 1970s reimbursed GPs 70 per cent of the salary costs of employing practice nurses, fuelling rapid expansion in nursing numbers. In the 1990s, further reforms enabled 'fundholding' general practices to purchase the services of community nurses and other health professionals.[10] Primary care nurses were encouraged to undertake extended roles, largely in the areas of health promotion and chronic disease follow-up.[11,12] Hospital physicians and other specialists, notably mental health counsellors, were brought into general practice to provide new services.[13,14] The impact on the size and composition of general practice teams was enormous. In the decade to 1995, there was a fivefold increase in practice-employed nurses and administrative staff doubled in number.[15] The new contract for general practitioners in the United Kingdom, which makes the practice rather than the practitioner the recipient of payment, is likely to further strengthen team working.

Apart from financial inducements, professional regulatory systems also influence team composition. In the United States of America, regulations governing the prescribing freedoms and supervision arrangements for 'mid-level' providers (such as nurse practitioners and physician assistants) vary from state to state. Needless to say, those states with the least restrictive arrangements attract the highest proportion of providers. A second concern is whether payers can be billed for the services delivered by mid-level providers or whether the costs must instead be subsumed as a physician overhead. The ability to bill for services rendered by mid-level providers again encourages higher proportions of such providers.[16,17]

Country	GP partnership size	Other staff
Australia	Single handed—30%; 1–4 doctors—35–40%; 5+ doctors—30–35%, average 2.5 doctors[3]	Little involvement of nurses or allied health professions[3]
United States	1–2 doctors—38%; 3–9 doctors—17%; >10 doctors—11% Others include: 5% medical school based; 14% hospital based; and 9% other[4]	46% non-health professions; 15% other physicians; 14% nurses; 3% lab technicians; 22% other health professions[5]
United Kingdom	Single handed—10%; 2–5 doctors— 60%; 6+ doctors—30%,[6] average 3.2 doctors[7]	Average 11.8 employed staff (mainly receptionists, nurse, managers) plus 6.33 'attached' staff (mainly district nurses, health visitors, midwives)[7]
Netherlands	54% single handed, remainder typically in small partnerships[8]	Group practices typically employ district nurses and physiotherapists[8]
France	Most work alone, small number in health centers[8]	Usually no other clinical staff
Finland	Most employed in large health centres[8]	Large multidisciplinary teams incorporating dentistry, lab facilities, maternity services, etc.[8]

Fig. 2 Team size and composition.

Characteristics of good teamworking

The larger size and more diverse composition of primary health care teams create opportunities for teamworking. However, there is a potential gap between having an appropriate team structure and the development of genuine teamwork.[18] How does a group of health care professionals come to function as a team?

Teamworking has been defined in terms of the processes within a team that enable them to achieve their goals. These processes include:[19,20]

1. *Shared vision and objectives*, as might be found in a mission statement.
2. *Participative safety*, such that all staff feel supported and motivated to participate in decision-making.
3. *Commitment to excellence*, a shared concern with the quality of the team's task performance. Examples might involve evaluations of team performance and critical appraisals.
4. *Support for innovation*, such that new ways of working and improved practices are encouraged and supported.
5. *Reflexivity*, the degree to which the team reflects on objectives, processes, and strategies.
6. *Communication*, both in informal interactions, and more formal settings such as team meetings.

One key issue in teamworking is the degree to which perceptions of these processes are *shared* between members of the team.[20] These shared perceptions are known as 'climate', and represent team members' views of organizational policies, practices, and procedures.[19] Lack of such shared perceptions may be a significant problem. There may be differences among team members in their definition of teamwork, some seeing it in terms of hierarchy and leadership, some concerned with collaboration and equality, while others work autonomously and use the group only when perceived to be required.[21,22] One study found that doctors were less positive than nurses and pharmacists about the benefits of teamworking in terms of the quality and cost of patient care.[23]

Benefits of effective teamworking

Teamworking is generally based on the idea that the *combination* of appropriate structural conditions (e.g. mix of staff and skills) and effective teamwork will be required in order to improve outcomes (Fig. 3). Without effective teamwork, increasing the number and range of staff may mean that patients have access to a wider range of clinical skills, but the benefit may not be realized if the processes are not in place to encourage effective sharing of clinical tasks.

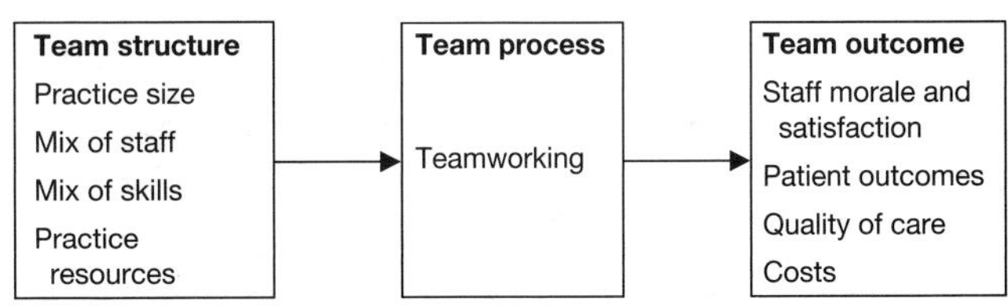

Fig. 3 Inter-relationship of structure, process, and outcome.

The outcomes of team structure and process may be of three broad types:

1. *Task effectiveness—the success of the team in achieving its task-related objectives.* The key task of the primary health care team is improving the health and well-being of the practice population, and a number of potential benefits to the patient have been identified. The gold-standard outcome is obviously improved patient health (or increased cost-effectiveness of care). For example, access to specialist medical and psychosocial skills in a team may improve the management of complex problems such as somatization.[24] However, the focus should not be restricted to health outcomes alone, given that proving a link between diffuse processes such as teamworking and eventual health status may be difficult.[25] Other important outcomes include patient satisfaction; increased access to appropriate skills; and improvements in the process of care, such as adherence of health professionals to clinical guidelines.
2. *Mental health—the morale, well-being, and professional satisfaction of team members.* Stress is known to be highly prevalent among health professionals, related to high workload and exposure to demanding situations during patient care.[26] Although stress and low morale may lead to increases in medical errors and other outcomes influencing patient health,[27] it is legitimate to view improvements in the morale of staff as an appropriate outcome in itself.
3. *Team viability—the degree to which the team will continue to function effectively over time.* Changes in the structure and organization of health care systems are occurring constantly, and primary health care teams are increasingly at the forefront of such changes. Effective teamworking may facilitate continued excellence and effective adaptation in response to such changes. This may be achieved through increased innovation within the health care team in response to emerging challenges. Aspects of team climate may predict innovation in primary care.[28]

Disadvantages of teams

The research base supporting the development of larger, multidisciplinary teams is meagre and occasionally unsupportive. As mentioned above, there is evidence to suggest that larger teams are able to achieve economies of scale in costs and promote specialization. However, there is little research into the benefits of adding specialists to primary care teams. In those areas where more rigorous evaluations have been carried out (i.e. mental health counsellors and hospital outreach clinics), the findings suggest that there may be limited or no gains in cost-effectiveness.[29–31] Effective change may require the introduction of a more complex system of care, where specialist support to the primary care team is highly integrated and augmented by additional interventions.[32] Evidence from controlled trials of doctor–nurse substitution suggests nurses can achieve as good health care outcomes as doctors and may have superior interpersonal skills.[33–37] However, their productivity is lower, making cost-savings highly dependent on salary differentials.[33,37]

Another issue that has been given little attention is the possible negative consequences of teamworking. Increases in the numbers of team members involved in patient care may threaten fundamental aspects of primary health care delivery, such as the individual doctor–patient relationship[38,39] and continuity of care.[24,40,41] 'Groupthink', the tendency of groups to make more extreme or radical decisions than their constituent members, may impair effective decision-making, while the development of teams may lead to anxieties concerning independence and autonomy.[42]

Factors that encourage or inhibit teamworking

What factors assist in making a disparate group of health professionals into an effective team? As suggested above, teamwork has the following prerequisites:[43]

1. the team must have a meaningful, clearly defined task;
2. there should be clear team objectives;
3. team members should have unique and meaningful tasks;
4. there should be regular feedback on the team's success in meeting objectives.

Other factors include the importance of leadership, and restrictions on the size of the team—performance of teams may decline with more than 8–10 members. However, even if such prerequisites are satisfied, there are other barriers of more specific importance to the primary care context, including:[44]

1. The large size of teams and the time constraints experienced by all health professionals may reduce the opportunities for effective communication and participation. Part-time working may further reduce communication and involvement.
2. Management by multiple agencies may cause conflict if there are differences in policies, aims, and objectives. There may be confusion over whether staff are accountable to their line managers or the team.
3. There may be a lack of agreement over task definition, which is not overcome by vague mission statements.
4. Staff may lack training and experience of working in multidisciplinary teams.
5. GPs and community staff may work with different patient populations.
6. There may be no clear definition as to who works as part of the team.

A number of surveys have examined the barriers as perceived by staff actually working in primary care. Surveys of nurses' experiences of teamwork through attachment to general practice found barriers to include lack of preparation for the attachments, poor communication (despite physical proximity), and conflicts over roles.[45,46]

A qualitative interview study with nurses working in primary care (midwives, health visitors, district nurses, and practice nurses) found six key issues relating to teamwork: team identity (i.e. feeling a member of a team); leadership (associated with power and status, rather than specifically providing direction to the team); access to general practitioners; philosophies of care (where health visitors and midwives were most likely to report differences); understanding of team members' roles and responsibilities; and disagreements regarding roles and responsibilities.[47] The experiences of the different nursing groups reflected recent changes in the organization of primary care that has threatened some nurses' roles (e.g. health visitors) and strengthened others (e.g. practice nurses).

At a more fundamental level, problems in developing effective teamwork may relate to class and gender differences between health professionals, the corresponding status associated with the different health professionals, and the ways in which these are evidenced in terms of assumptions about power and control, attitudes to cooperation,[22] and beliefs about how health and illness are best understood.[48]

Interventions to enhance teamworking

The previous section has indicated a number of important barriers to the development of effective teamwork in primary care. How are these barriers to be overcome?

Some barriers may require structural and regulatory changes. For example, current remuneration procedures in the United Kingdom might be counter-productive, as GPs are rewarded individually for outcomes related to the work of the whole team.[49] Specific organizational rewards for teams may be required in order to facilitate the development of genuine teamworking. Other regulatory changes also have the potential to improve teamwork—for example, changes in the provision of primary care in the United Kingdom have led to the possibility of multidisciplinary management of primary care organizations, rather than traditional unidisciplinary arrangements based on the GP partnership.[50]

Another issue is training for teamwork. Such training is rarely a feature of professional development: indeed, the socialization procedures that professionals undergo are possibly more likely to develop attitudes that inhibit teamworking.[49] Teamworking is a complex social process, and it cannot be assumed that it will simply develop in the absence of specific training and experience. The development of multidisciplinary teaching early in the curricula of staff may enhance later teamworking performance.[51]

For pre-existing teams, process assistance may be required, that is, specific help in overcoming barriers to teamwork and difficulties in communication. One method has involved the use of teamworking workshops, where team members are removed from their everyday work context and assisted in discussing and working through teamworking issues. One study carried out interviews with primary health care team members about their experiences of teamwork before and after such a workshop.[52] Before the workshop, the team identified a number of familiar barriers: the exact composition of the team; role perceptions; and concerns about communication, leadership, and hierarchy. Reported benefits of the workshop included improved communication and implementation of practical changes, although issues concerning leadership, hierarchy, and interpersonal processes proved more enduring.

Another study used a slightly different approach, the analysis of a 'significant event' concerning the care of a critically ill patient to examine issues around teamworking among members of the patient's primary care team.[53] Both these approaches were reported to be effective in dealing with some of these issues, although no 'hard' outcome measures were available.

The relationship between teamworking and outcomes

Testing the relationship between teamworking and outcomes is complicated, because teamworking is a difficult concept to measure, the appropriate outcome measures are not always clear,[54] and some aspects of research design (e.g. randomization) may be more difficult to implement at the level of the team. However, a number of studies have examined the relationships between teamworking and outcomes by using cross-sectional designs that look at the associations between measures of teamworking and team outcomes.

One study examined the relationship between team structure (e.g. size, fundholding status), team process (i.e. team climate), and team outcomes in a sample of 528 members of 68 primary care teams.[20] Outcome measures were teamworking, quality of professional practice, patient-centred care, and an overall measure of team effectiveness. Analyses indicated that 'shared objectives' was the best predictor of team effectiveness, and that team processes had more explanatory power than aspects of practice structure. However, a major limitation of this study was the similarity of measures of teamworking and team effectiveness. Both used self-report from the practice staff themselves, and thus the results of the study can only be considered preliminary evidence of the hypothesized relationships. Another potential problem was that the teams were involved in training workshops and thus had an active commitment to teamwork, so they may not be a very representative sample.

Two studies have examined the relationship between teamworking and effectiveness in primary health care teams in Spain.[55,56] Both found that aspects of teamworking were related to outcomes such as job satisfaction, efficacy, and quality as rated by users of the service. However, most outcome measures were also supplied by the team, which means these studies are vulnerable to the same criticism as the previous study.

These limitations were overcome, in part, by another study from the United Kingdom, which examined quality of care in 60 practices and used measures based on objective criteria (e.g. ratings of the quality of clinical care for chronic conditions) or patient evaluations of aspects of the practice (such as access to care and staff communication skills). Practices where staff rated team climate highly provided better quality clinical care for some conditions and received more favourable evaluations of their practice from patients.[57]

Another study examined the relationship between team structure and process and staff morale (e.g. job satisfaction, retention).[49] Team process and stress was measured in 71 teams. Poor reported team climate was associated with higher scores among the team on the General Health Questionnaire, a measure of physical and psychological symptoms. These authors then went on to conduct interventions in 10 primary health care teams, which provides a stronger basis for inferring cause and effect than the simple cross-sectional approach. This was a 6-month intervention, including six 1-day workshops, and involved defining objectives using health needs analysis, improving participation through devolving managerial responsibility to other members of the team, and improving team meetings. At the end of the intervention, there were significant changes in team processes and a significant drop in scores on the General Health Questionnaire. However, the lack of a control group means that other potential causes of these changes cannot be ruled out.

A study in Israel examined the effects of regular meetings between doctors and nurses engaged in the care of hypertension, facilitated by a doctor specifically trained in teaching team behaviour. This approach was associated with improvements in hypertension care compared with the care provided by teams in neighbouring areas who received no intervention.[58]

Research on the relationship between teamworking and outcomes is at a very preliminary stage. There is some evidence that better teamworking is associated with better outcomes for both staff and patients, and that changes in teamworking may lead to changes in staff morale. These initial findings should provide an impetus to further work in this area, with a focus on valid measurement of teamworking and objective outcome measurement. If teamworking is found to be a consistent predictor of outcomes, studies of interventions to improve teamworking will be an important part of the research agenda of the future.

Conclusions

The clear policy emphasis on the development of effective teams in health care means that the issues surrounding teamworking are likely to take on increasing importance in the future. However, at present, the available evidence concerning teamworking in primary health care is relatively limited. A significant research programme is required in order to determine the benefits and costs of teamworking, and the most effective ways of developing teams to maximize those benefits.

References

1. **Pritchard, P. and Pritchard, J.** (1994). Section 1: the nature and purpose of teamwork. In *Teamwork for Primary and Shared Care. A Practical Workbook*, pp. 13–31. Oxford: Oxford University Press.
2. **Standing Medical Advisory Committee and the Standing Nursing and Midwifery Advisory Committee.** *The Primary Health Care Team.* London: Department of Health and Social Security, 1981.
3. **Commonwealth Department of Health and Family Services** (1996). The organisation of general practice. In *General Practice in Australia: 1996*, pp. 107–34. Canberra: Commonwealth Department of Health and Family Services.
4. **Reschovsky, J.** et al. (2001). Physicians' assessments of their ability to provide high-quality care in a changing health care system. *Medical Care* **39**, 254–69.
5. **Bureau of Health Professions** (2000). *HRSA State Health Workforce Profile.* Rockville: National Centre for Health and Workforce Information & Analysis, Health Resources and Services Administration, US Department of Health and Human Services.
6. **Department of Health.** *Statistics for General Medical Practitioners.* Department of Health, 2000.
7. **Usherwood, T., Long, S., and Joesbury, H.** (1997). Who works in primary health care teams in England and Wales? *Journal of Interprofessional Care* **11**, 225–7.
8. **Boerma, W., de Jong, F., and Mulder, P.** *Health Care and General Practice Across Europe.* Utrecht: NIVEL, Netherlands Institute of Primary Health Care, 1993.

9. **Australian Medical Workforce Advisory Committee.** *The General Practice Workforce in Australia.* AMWAC 2000.2. Sydney: Australian Medical Workforce Advisory Committee, 2000.
10. **NHS Management Executive.** *New World, New Opportunities.* Report of a task group on nursing in primary care. London: NHS Management Executive, 1993.
11. **Atkin, K.** et al. (1994). The role and self-perceived training needs of nurses employed in general practice: observations from a national census of practice nurses in England and Wales. *Journal of Advanced Nursing* **20**, 46–52.
12. **Jewell, D. and Turton, P.** (1994). What's happening to practice nursing? *British Medical Journal* **308**, 735–6.
13. **Bailey, J., Black, M., and Wilkin, D.** (1994). The special branch. *Health Service Journal,* 28 July, 30–1.
14. **Sibbald, B.** et al. (1993). Counsellors in English and Welsh general practice: their nature and distribution. *British Medical Journal* **306**, 247–77.
15. **Health Policy and Economic Research Unit.** *Quarterly Bulletin* Vol. 11 (No. 3). London: British Medical Association, 1996.
16. **Sekcenski, E.** et al. (1994). State practice environments and the supply of physician assistants, nurse practitioners, and certified nurse-midwives. *New England Journal of Medicine* **331**, 1266–71.
17. **Weissert, C.** (1996). The political context of state regulation of the health professions. In *The US Health Workforce. Power, Politics, and Policy* (ed. M. Osterweis et al.) pp. 81–91. Washington: Association of Academic Health Centers.
18. **Jones, R.** (1992). Teamwork in primary care: how much do we know about it? *Journal of Interprofessional Care* **6**, 25–9.
19. **Anderson, N. and West, M.** *Team Climate Inventory—Manual and User's Guide.* Windsor: NFER-Nelson, 1994.
20. **Poulton, B. and West, M.** (1999). The determinants of effectiveness in primary health care teams. *Journal of Interprofessional Care* **13**, 7–18.
21. **Freeman, M., Miller, C., and Ross, N.** (2000). The impact of individual philosophies of teamwork on multiprofessional practice and the implications for education. *Journal of Interprofessional Care* **14**, 237–47.
22. **Dingwall, R.** (1980). Problems of teamwork in primary care. In *Teamwork in the Personal Social Services and Health Care* (ed. S. Lonsdale, A. Webb, and T. Briggs), pp. 111–37. London: Croom Helm.
23. **Brown, G. and Chamberlin, G.** (1996). Attitudes towards quality, costs and physician centrality in healthcare teams. *Journal of Interprofessional Care* **10**, 63–72.
24. **Van Weel, C.** (1994). Teamwork. *Lancet* **344**, 1276–9.
25. **Crombie, I. and Davies, H.** (1998). Beyond health outcomes: the advantage of measuring process. *Journal of Evaluation in Clinical Practice* **4**, 31–8.
26. **Howie, J. and Porter, M.** (1999). Stress and interventions for stress in general practitioners. In *Stress in Health Professionals: Psychological and Organisational Causes and Interventions* (ed. J. Firth-Cozens and R. Payne), pp. 163–76. Chichester: John Wiley and Sons.
27. **Vincent, C.** (1999). Fallibility, uncertainty, and the impact of mistakes and litigation. In *Stress in Health Professionals: Psychological and Organisational Causes and Interventions* (ed. J. Firth-Cozens, R. Payne), pp. 63–76. Chichester: John Wiley and Sons.
28. **West, M. and Wallace, M.** (1991). Innovation in health care teams. *European Journal of Social Psychology* **21**, 303–15.
29. **Black, M.** et al. *The Costs and Benefits of Specialist Outreach Clinics in General Practice in Two Specialties.* Manchester: National Primary Care Research and Development Centre, 1996.
30. **Bond, M.** et al. (2000). Evaluation of outreach clinics held by specialists in general practices in England. *Journal of Epidemiology and Community Health* **54**, 149–57.
31. **Bower, P. and Sibbald, B.** (2000). Systematic review of the effect of on-site mental health professionals on the clinical behaviour of general practitioners. *British Medical Journal* **320**, 614–17.
32. **Von Korff, M. and Goldberg, D.** (2001). Improving outcomes in depression. *British Medical Journal* **323**, 948–9.
33. **Venning, P.** et al. (2000). Randomised controlled trial comparing cost effectiveness of general practitioners and nurse practitioners in primary care. *British Medical Journal* **320**, 1048–53.
34. **Kinnersley, P.** et al. (2000). Randomised controlled trial of nurse practitioner versus general practitioner care for patients requesting 'same day' consultations in primary care. *British Medical Journal* **320**, 1043–8.
35. **Shum, C.** et al. (2000). Nurse management of patients with minor illness in general practice: multicentre, randomised controlled trial. *British Medical Journal* **320**, 1038–43.
36. **Mundinger, M.** et al. (2000). Primary care outcomes in patients treated by nurse practitioners or physicians. *Journal of the American Medical Association* **283**, 59–68.
37. **Sptizer, W.** et al. (1974). The Burlington randomized trial of the nurse practitioner. *New England Journal of Medicine* **290**, 251–6.
38. **Balint, M.** *The Doctor, His Patient and the Illness.* London: Pitman Medical, 1964.
39. **Barnard, D.** (1987). The viability of the concept of a primary health care team: a view from the medical humanities. *Social Science and Medicine* **25**, 741–6.
40. **Campbell, J.** (1996). The reported availability of general practitioners and the influence of practice list size. *British Journal of General Practice* **46**, 465–8.
41. **Freeman, G. and Richards, S.C.** (1990). How much personal care in four group practices? *British Medical Journal* **301**, 1028–30.
42. **Firth-Cozens, J.** (1998). Celebrating teamwork. *Quality in Health Care* **7** (Suppl.), S3–7.
43. **Guzzo, R. and Shea, G.** (1992). Group performance and intergroup relations in organizations. In *Handbook of Industrial and Organisational Psychology,* (ed. M. Dunnette and L. Hough). Palo Alto CA: Consulting Psychologists' Press.
44. **Jones Elwyn, G., Rapport, F., and Kinnersley, P.** (1998). Primary health care teams re-engineered. *Journal of Interprofessional Care* **12**, 189–98.
45. **McClure, L.** (1984). Teamwork, myth or reality: community nurses' experience with general practice attachment. *Journal of Epidemiology and Community Health* **38**, 68–74.
46. **Bond, J.** et al. (1987). Interprofessional collaboration in primary health care. *Journal of the Royal College of General Practitioners* **37**, 158–61.
47. **Wiles, R. and Robison, J.** (1994). Teamwork in primary care: the views and experiences of nurses, midwives and health visitors. *Journal of Advanced Nursing* **20**, 324–30.
48. **Beattie, A.** (1995). War and peace among the health tribes. In *Interprofessional Relations in Health Care* (ed. K. Soothill, L. Mackay, and C. Webb), pp. 11–26. London: Edward Arnold.
49. **Carter, A. and West, M.** (1999). Sharing the burden: teamwork in health care settings. In *Stress in Health Professionals: Psychological and Organisational Causes and Interventions* (ed. J. Firth-Cozens and R. Payne), pp. 191–202. Chichester: John Wiley and Sons.
50. **Sheaff, R., Holbourne, A., and Khong, C.** *Personal Medical Services Contracts: A Handbook.* Manchester: NPCRDC, 2001.
51. **Thomas, M.** (1995). Learning to be a better team-player: initiatives in continuing education in primary health care. In *Interprofessional Relations in Health Care* (ed. K. Soothill, L. Mackay, and C. Webb), pp. 194–215. London: Edward Arnold.
52. **Long, S.** (1996). Primary health care team workshops. *Journal of Advanced Nursing* **23**, 935–41.
53. **Benett, I. and Danczak, A.** (1999). Terminal care: improving teamwork in primary care using Significant Event Analysis. *European Journal of Cancer Care* **3**, 54–7.
54. **Poulton, B. and West, M.** (1993). Primary health care team effectiveness: developing a constituency approach. *Health and Social Care* **2**, 77–84.
55. **Goni, S.** (1999). An analysis of the effectiveness of Spanish primary health care teams. *Health Policy* **48**, 107–17.
56. **Peiro, J., Gonzalez-Roma, V., and Ramos, J.** (1992). The influence of work-team climate on role stress, tension, satisfaction and leadership perceptions. *European Review of Applied Psychology* **42**, 49–56.
57. **Campbell, S.** et al. (2001). Identifying predictors of high quality care in English general practice: observational study. *British Medical Journal* **323**, 1–6.
58. **Adorian, D.** et al. (1990). Group discussions with the health care team—a method of improving care of hypertension in general practice. *Journal of Human Hypertension* **4**, 265–8.

1.4 Community primary care

Robert L. Williams, Jeffrey M. Borkan, and Roger Jones

Dr B. and several nurse practitioners take care of the health needs of a group of small villages in a rural, arid region. About ten years ago the health team began to see sporadic cases of a disfiguring rash that appeared on exposed skin areas, composed of single or multiple oozing, erythematous ulcerations. These wounds showed up spontaneously and went through cycles of crusting and re-ulceration over the course of several months, until they finally healed, generally with significant scaring. Through biopsy they were diagnosed as cutaneous leishmaniasis, a protozoan infection spread by small, biting, sand flies of the genus *Phlebotomus*. As the years progressed, more and more cases occurred in all the villages, commonly on the faces of children, often leaving unsightful scars.

In response to community pressure, the public health office in the area began to spray houses with pesticide, attempting to kill the sand flies. Much to the consternation of residents, not only did more cases occur, but also the pesticide turned out to be DDT, a harmful and largely outlawed pesticide that lasts in the soil for decades. Several individuals formed an ad hoc committee, coordinated with the medical and nursing staff. After a joint public meeting, it was decided to take local action.

A national authority on the disease and its vectors was invited to an open seminar. He described the epidemiology, pattern of infection, and natural history of the disease. As it turned out, the reservoir for the sand fly carriers were rodents that lived in a specific type of reed-like bush that had recently increased in prevalence as irrigation had increased. More effective and less ecologically toxic solutions than spraying the houses with pesticides were suggested. These measures included changing community behaviours, such as sitting on the lawns near sunset when the sand flies' activity level was highest, using insect repellents, fixing screens, and removing the habitats of the rodents close to the communities.

Through further planning and collaboration between the medical staff and the community group, a system of tracking new cases was set up. In addition, a grant was written, and funds were received from the local council for removing rodent habitats. Individuals were trained for the job of identification and elimination. A public education campaign, spearheaded by the medical staff, informed the communities about what could be done. Pesticide use dropped by 80 per cent, and within a year the number of cases diminished by 40 per cent.

Primary care and the community

As this anecdote vividly points out, the aetiology, diagnosis, and management of health and disease are often not limited to the office or hospital setting. Medical science and its practitioners, however, tend to follow a linear, cause and effect model—pursuing single biological determinants generally within the body of the patient, and then isolating and attacking the offending agent. This approach tends to lead in turn to an exclusive focus on the individual within the office or hospital setting as the centre of attention. Thus, for example, strategies for preventing cardiovascular disease among primary care physicians emphasize reducing cholesterol levels with diet or medication, rather than changing the composition of locally consumed foodstuffs or organizing community walking groups. Low back pain is treated with analgesics and muscle relaxants rather than redesigning work environments.

When the issue is examined closely, it is apparent that most conditions are the result of complex interactions among a host of factors. Success with treating diseases requires that we begin to think of health and illness, and our roles in treating ill health, as extending from the practice into the community and society. Tuberculosis may be caused by a single pathogen, but poverty and crowding are just as important when considering its impact and spread. AIDS may be a result of infection with HIV, but socio-economic and behavioural considerations largely determine who becomes infected and how the disease progresses. Indeed, behavioural, community-based, and societal factors play key roles in much of human disease and have increasingly assumed dominant roles in determining health and illness around the world. Without an integrated approach at all levels of disease causation—the individual, family, community, and society—it is unlikely that significant progress in improving health can be made.

The primary care clinician is ideally situated to adopt and act on this broader perspective. Functioning at the interface between the individual and the health care system, the primary care provider is also best positioned to see the relationships between the person, the disease and the community. The first and perhaps most significant step in the process is to begin to 'think big'—to look beyond the patient sitting across from you. This demands a change in frame from the usual focus on the individual patient or family to the larger community and social ecosystem. Such a shift may seem more natural when one realizes that only a small proportion of persons in the community with symptoms actually reach the primary care practitioner,[1] and that many epidemiological risk factors (e.g. exposure to pollution, vectors of disease, exercise or eating habits, etc.) are shared among members of a community.

There are other reasons for the primary care practitioner to include the community in efforts to improve the health of individuals. Treating multiple persons with the same problem is inefficient and unsatisfying when critical causes outside of the office walls are not addressed. Extending preventive services from the practice to the community can reach people not otherwise receiving care. By extending the reach of preventive care, the overall costs of care for a community are ultimately reduced. Many would argue as well that apart from these pragmatic reasons, there is a moral argument for a community to be included in the planning and delivery of its health care.

What is 'community'?

While the word 'community' may seem as if it needs no explanation, when viewed from the primary care practice, community can have several meanings. Traditionally, it has meant the geographic area from which a practice's patients come. Many practices, though, serve a community that is better defined by its cultural or socio-economic characteristics (ethnic group, low-income, etc.), and that may or may not also have geographic definitions. Still other 'communities' may be defined by their common source of employment, or by shared values or religious beliefs. Future 'virtual' communities, some of which exist today, may be defined by their interconnection on the Internet or their use of similar transportation or communication. Occasionally, it may be difficult to describe the community with which a practice is affiliated, and an alternative is to define a practice's 'community' as its active and inactive patients together.[2]

Regardless of the way in which a practice defines its community, it is important to remain aware that a community is not a single, homogeneous entity. It is a dynamic composite of groupings that are constantly shifting. One segment of the community may be most concerned with the health effects of substance abuse, and later come to focus on domestic violence as a priority, while another portion may be more impacted by cardiovascular disease. Community leaders, both informal and formal, may differ in their views not only among themselves, but also with portions of the community most affected by particular health problems. For the primary care clinician, recognition of the fluid nature of communities is key to successfully working outside of the office setting.

Types of community involvement

Primary care practitioners can become involved in their communities in a number of ways. Pathman et al. have provided a convenient categorization of some of those ways.[3] They describe four types of involvement: (a) co-ordinating community health resources on behalf of patients; (b) providing culturally relevant health care; (c) assimilating into the community and its organizations; and (d) identifying and intervening in a community's health problems.[3] Each type of involvement along this spectrum is important, but it is the final category for which generalists, more than other clinicians, are particularly well suited. This final category might also be initiated by members of the community itself.

History of generalist involvement in community health

Generalist physicians have long played a key role in recognizing and acting on community patterns of disease. Pickles, a British generalist using observations from his country practice in the early 1900s, was able to elucidate key aspects of the epidemiology of hepatitis A through his experiences in his community.[4] Halley Stott, a generalist practicing in a Zulu area of South Africa, recognized the critical role of nutritional deficits among his patients, and began a community gardening programme and established a non-governmental organization dedicated to improving the nutritional status and health of local residents.[5] Also in South Africa in the 1940s, Sidney and Emily Kark and associates developed primary care practices that integrated community- and practice-based interventions on high-priority health problems using a model that later came to be known as community-oriented primary care (COPC).[6] Key members of this group later established similar models in Israel, and influenced the development of the community health centres initiative in the United States of America.[7] Elsewhere in the United States of America, primary care of Native Americans has often been based on similar linkages.[8]

Community-oriented primary care

With increasing realization that many of the causes of ill-health have roots in individuals' behaviour, community, and society, there has been a growth of interest in extending primary care to impact all levels of causation of ill-health. Community-oriented primary care, as an example of such an approach, has drawn particular interest.[9,10] Community-oriented primary care is best thought of as a process for integrating primary care practices with their communities. As depicted in Fig. 1, COPC begins with an assessment of community health needs and resources by a community and a primary care practice. Interventions both in the community and in the practice are developed for priority health needs, and the effects of the interventions are then evaluated.

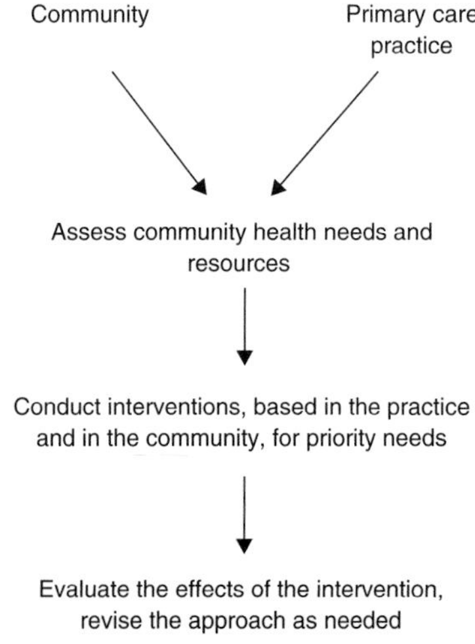

Fig. 1 Diagram of the community-oriented primary care process.

Many examples of steps of the COPC process have been published. One of the more complete examples of the entire COPC process was described by Bayer and Fiscella.[11] In an inner-city community and associated family practice in Rochester, New York, understanding about diabetes, tobacco addiction, and cervical and breast cancer screening were determined to be priority health needs by a patient advisory committee working with the practice staff. Combined practice and community-based actions targeting each of these areas of concern led to significant improvements in the markers for each condition.

Examples such as this and others published from around the world have spurred interest in expanding the application of the COPC model. By extending prevention and education from the practice into the community, COPC offers the opportunity to bridge the gap between public health and primary care, while increasing the role of community members in decisions about their health care. In moving beyond the office setting, COPC can reach persons not otherwise being seen in primary care. Finally, by targeting efforts at priority needs, COPC also offers the promise of efficient utilization of scarce resources.

Despite its very attractive potential, COPC has not yet been widely adopted. A key problem has been financing. Despite the potential for long-term cost savings, most health care systems have not provided adequate compensation for essential activities of the process, such as the community needs assessment. Furthermore, a number of examples of COPC in the literature have described a labour- and resource-intensive process that has seemed unachievable to many busy primary care practitioners. Coupled with the fact that many clinicians feel ill-prepared to carry out some of the activities of the process, and that most examples have been driven almost entirely by energetic clinicians, COPC has seemed unapproachable to many.

Recent developments may make COPC more practical, however. Trends in financing of health care are beginning to create incentives for improving the health of populations as well as that of individuals. Implementing COPC as a teamwork effort in which not only the primary care clinician but also other professionals and non-professionals throughout the community take part makes it less dependent on a single person to drive the process. Such strategies make it more realistic for primary care clinicians to engage and succeed in COPC.

'Tools' for COPC

Another key element for putting COPC within reach of more primary care clinicians is availability of feasible methods to carry out COPC in busy primary care practices. Conducting a community needs and resources assessment is at the heart of the COPC process, yet until recent years this process could be quite time consuming and expensive. Substantial progress has been made in recent years in this area.

To fully understand the needs and resources of a community requires both objective health data about the community as well as perspectives of community members; put another way, it requires both quantitative and qualitative data about the community. These methods should be seen as complementary, allowing a richer understanding of health needs and resources. On the quantitative side, it is important to know how well the health problems seen in the practice reflect those that are present in the broader community. Are there problems in the community that are not being seen in the practice, suggesting the need to modify the practice in some way? It is also important to understand the distribution of health problems through the community. Are there portions of the community at higher risk for certain health conditions or in greater need for particular services, suggesting the possibility of targeting outreach and intervention efforts to that segment of the community?

Rapid developments in health information technology are reducing both the time and cost of quantitative community assessment. A particularly dramatic advance has been the linking of health indicator data with geographic location. When this is available, geographic information system software can now produce maps that clearly depict the distribution of these indicators in a local area. With this capability, primary care practitioners can compare practice and community patterns of health and disease as part of the process of community assessment. As more of these community data become available to local users through the Internet, the feasibility of using it as part of a COPC community assessment improves.

On the qualitative side of the assessment, it is often important to understand community member perspectives on why particular patterns of disease or utilization exist, how much importance is attributed to specific problems, or on how to best resolve identified health problems. These qualitative data can often produce unexpected insights. Community members are often aware of or able to mobilize resources to assist with a problem in which the clinician may not be. Several methods of systematically, yet rapidly, gathering information from community members have been developed. These approaches include focus groups, mail and telephone surveys, participant observation, and key informants. Each of these approaches has particular strengths and weaknesses; they are most effective when matched to informational need and community type.[12] Various rapid appraisal/assessment techniques have also been developed that provide quick preliminary understandings of a situation.[13–15]

Getting started

The essential first step is to begin to think of the problems that are being seen in one's daily practice in their broader context. How is this patient's illness related to the community and how can action at the community level improve the situation? Look for patterns in the problems being seen, and for potential opportunities to link preventive care in the practice to action in the community. Examine the practice population, its demographic characteristics, and the common or unusual problems seen in the practice. Speak to patients about the community and its health concerns.

In looking beyond the practice, it is important to be realistic about one's goals at the community level, considering the time and resources available. Although the steps in conducting COPC may be similar in theory regardless of location, much of the process of linking the practice and the community is highly dependent on local circumstances. Identify partners to work with who bring interest, resources, or expertise to the effort. Examine what health-related data about the community are readily available and relevant. In many locations, census data may be the most readily available and can provide key information with which to profile the practice. In other areas, a broader range of health data may be available, such as specific disease rates, data on hospitalized patients, or on public health interventions. Target your search and use of community data to specific questions, and spend time developing mapping capabilities only if they will provide essential information.

The process of gathering views of community members should be guided by the type of information needed and the portion of the community for which the information is most relevant. To enhance the validity of the information obtained, more than one approach to gathering the data should be used where possible. However, it is important to balance efforts to obtain valid, unbiased qualitative data with the need for practicality in collecting that data.

In creating a picture of the community's health needs and resources through these processes, it is also important to recognize the limits of the data. Quantitative data about small geographic areas are subject to random variation, and patterns of distribution of health indicators may be more apparent than real. Qualitative data are prone to selection bias since not all community members will be represented. Nevertheless, keeping these limitations in mind, this information can still give the primary care clinician valuable direction.

Generally, a sense of priority will become apparent as a result of assessing the needs of a community, or the interests of the clinician will drive further work aimed at a specific need. However, it is important that members of the community be involved in prioritization, planning, and implementing of an intervention. A teamwork approach will not only enhance the feasibility of extending efforts of the practice into the community, but will also assure that the plans are well fitted to the community.

The steps of getting involved in the community's health can be summarized with the acronym CAP-IT:

- *C*ollect information.
- *A*ssess the problem, its aetiology, impact, and consequences.
- *P*rovide interventions in a systems manner.
- *I*nvolve the community in every step.
- *T*ight follow-up.

The process starts with collecting information—keeping your 'ear to the ground' for diseases, risk factors, or threats that concern you, your staff, and the community you treat. These hints may come in the form of sudden insights, as the shaping of a pattern from seemingly random occurrences. Assessing the problem involves taking a wide overview of the aetiology, impact, and consequences. Searching for interconnections is critical, both between individual, family, and community factors, and between types of risk factors. For example, reducing the community burden of asthma may involve examining the prevalence of smoking, adherence to medical regimens, access to services, and even sources of air pollution.

The practitioner must also think on a systems level in regard to interventions. The community should be involved in every aspect of the plan, from identifying problems, setting priorities, choosing interventions, executing plans, and carrying out follow-up. Follow-up is critical since outcomes are the ultimate measure of success and rarely can problems be solved with a single 'magic pill' or one-time intervention. Evaluating the process and impacts of interventions can lead to modifications in the approaches taken, to enhanced efficacy of the intervention, and to identification of opportunities for additional interventions.

Population-based care

The role of the community throughout the process described above is a key distinction between COPC and what has been termed population-based care. While the latter, in common with COPC, aims to link the care of the individual with the health of the larger community, or population, in population-based care, the community plays a more passive role. Prioritization, planning, and interventions are predominantly in the control of health care providers. As a concept that has risen with managed care, population-based care has its roots in efforts to use incentives to achieve desired health outcomes.

Related developments

Recent developments in the United Kingdom have served to strengthen the link between primary care and the community it serves. Traditionally, the work of general practitioners was focused on a small geographical catchment area, within which relationships with social, housing, and education services were often patchy and erratic. In an attempt to integrate these services with primary care, Primary Care Trusts are being set up in the United Kingdom, based on population units of around 100 000, in which the administrative geography of medical and social care are co-terminous, facilitating communication and interaction between agencies. Patient participation in service appraisal and planning will be important within Primary Care Trusts, which, for the first time, will have a commitment to providing integrated primary and secondary care services for a substantial, defined population.[16,17]

Beyond the United Kingdom, the World Health Organization in 1999 began its 'Toward Unity For Health' initiative. This worldwide programme is aimed at promoting models of health care that integrate primary care with community-based and relevant initiatives.

Summary

A new paradigm is slowly emerging in health care. Behavioural, community, and societal factors are becoming predominant influences in human health and disease at the same time as increasing scrutiny is being given to how health care resources are being used. Together, these trends are leading to a rethinking of the long-standing split between primary care and public health. Health and health care are increasingly recognized as a continuum running from the molecular to the societal levels. By adopting this new perspective and by applying simple tools for action at the community level, primary care practitioners can have a greater impact on the health of the people they serve.

References

1. **Green, L.A.** et al. (2001). The ecology of medical care revisited. *New England Journal of Medicine* **344**, 2021–5.
2. **Nutting, P.A., Nagle, J., and Dudley, T.** (1991). Epidemiology and practice management: an example of community-oriented primary care. *Family Medicine* **23**, 218–26.
3. **Pathman, D.E.** et al. (1998). The four community dimensions of primary care practice. *The Journal of Family Practice* **46**, 293–303.
4. **Pickles, W.N.** *Epidemiology in Country Practice.* Baltimore: Williams and Wilkins, 1939.
5. **Stott, H.H.** (1972). The Valley Trust experiment in raising the nutritional standards of a less-developed rural community. *South African Medical Journal* **46**, 1572–4.
6. **Tollman, S.M.** (1994). The Pholela Health Centre—the origins of community-oriented primary care (COPC). *South African Medical Journal* **84**, 653–8.
7. **Tollman, S.M.** (1991). Community oriented primary care: origins, evolution, applications. *Social Science & Medicine* **32**, 633–42.
8. **Williams, R.L.** (1985). Vehicular carbon monoxide screening: identification in a cross-cultural setting of a substantial public health risk factor. *American Journal of Public Health* **75**, 85–6.
9. **Rhyne, R.** et al., ed. *Community-Oriented Primary Care: Health Care for the 21st Century.* Washington DC: American Public Health Association, 1998.
10. **Nutting, P.A.**, ed. *Community-Oriented Primary Care: From Principle to Practice.* Albuquerque: University of New Mexico Press, 1987.
11. **Bayer, W.H. and Fiscella, K.** (1999). Patients and community together: a family medicine community-oriented primary care project in an urban private practice. *Archives of Family Medicine* **8**, 546–9.
12. **Williams, R.L.** et al. (1999). Practical tools for qualitative community-oriented primary care community assessment. *Family Medicine* **31**, 488–94.
13. **Beebe, J.** (1995). Basic concepts and techniques of rapid appraisal. *Human Organization* **54**, 42–51.
14. **Murray, S.A.** (1999). Experiences with 'rapid appraisal' in primary care: involving the public in assessing health needs, orientating staff, and educating medical students. *British Medical Journal* **318**, 440–4.
15. **Dale, J.** et al. (1996). Creating a shared vision of out of hours care: using rapid appraisal methods to create an interagency, community oriented, approach to service development. *British Medical Journal* **312**, 1206–10.
16. **Wilkin, D., Dowswell, T., and Leese, B.** (2001). Primary care groups: modernising primary and community health services. *British Medical Journal* **322**, 1522–4.
17. **Bojke, C., Gravelle, H., and Wilkin, D.** (2001). Is bigger better for primary care groups and trusts? *British Medical Journal* **322**, 599–602.

1.5 Primary care in the emergency department

Jeremy Dale

Demand at emergency departments continues to grow inexorably. This trend is international, and has persisted for decades. The growth in demand does not reflect changes in the prevalence of trauma and clinical emergencies. In the United Kingdom, for example, those with serious injuries or conditions that require immediate care or emergency admission comprise only a minority (approximately 15–20 per cent) of emergency department attenders.[1] Less than 0.1 per cent of patients present with severe multisystem injuries.[2] Instead, demand appears mostly to be fuelled by the large numbers of patients who attend emergency departments with minor injuries and conditions that are suited to the skills and facilities of primary medical care. In large part, this pattern of emergency department use reflects the ambiguous role that emergency departments have long had at the interface between hospital services and primary care.

Emergency departments have a vital gate-keeping role in all health care systems. Ideally, they should help patients in need of immediate treatment to receive timely and effective care, while protecting others with non-urgent and self-limiting problems from the potentially detrimental consequences of being over-investigated and over-treated. They should seek to encourage continuity of care, wherever possible, through setting limits on unnecessary intervention. However, there is increasing evidence that the traditional organization, structures, and resourcing of emergency departments make the provision of such care elusive. As discussed later in this chapter, the orientation of emergency medicine is directed towards the pursuit of diagnosis, but a consequence of the resultant intolerance of uncertainty is that needless investigations and treatments seem often to occur. This, it has been suggested is 'the antithesis of family practice'; incomplete, fragmented care at high cost.[3]

In this chapter, the interface between primary care and emergency department care will be considered, together with evidence from the United Kingdom, United States of America, Scandinavia, and Australia that supports alternative approaches to managing the demand for primary medical care at emergency departments.

Appropriate attenders

Estimates of the proportion of attenders who are appropriate to emergency departments vary widely: in the United Kingdom from 18[4] to 97 per cent;[5] in the United States of America, from 28[6] to 95 per cent,[7] while recent federal reports have estimated it to be between 45 and 60 per cent.[8,9] This variation reflects various factors relating to the organization of health care systems, the populations served, the characteristics of emergency departments, and, most importantly, the criteria used for classifying appropriateness.

There are numerous perspectives on what constitutes 'appropriate' attendance. The term is most often used to describe patients who present with injuries or ailments that on clinical assessment are judged not to require urgent hospital intervention.[10,11] There is, though, little agreement about how to judge appropriateness.[12–14] As stated by Foldes et al. 'professional consensus on what to call an emergency and where to treat it may be more a matter of physician training, specialty and beliefs than of scientific certainty'.[15]

One study in the United States compared seven different systems of classifying attendances and found that they resulted in between 10 (based on patients' own assessment of need) and 90 per cent (based on whether hospitalization occurred) as inappropriate, with the other five indicators ranging from 21 to 37 per cent.[16] A British study demonstrated that while 21 per cent of patients who considered their condition to be urgent were classified by emergency department staff as non-urgent, conversely 14 per cent of patients who considered their condition to be non-urgent were classified as needing emergency department care.[17] With the benefit of hindsight, the need for care often appears to be less urgent than when the patient first presents.

Why do patients attend emergency departments with non-urgent problems?

The decision to seek care often reflects a complex social process. Socio-demographic characteristics, individual health beliefs, experiences and expectations, and health service organizational barriers and arrangements may all influence the decision-making process. Furthermore, multiple interactions between these factors are likely. Almost all types of physical or emotional problem can in some circumstances result in a person feeling immediately in need of attention.

Based on an extensive review of the literature, Padgett and Brodsky proposed a three-stage model of the factors determining patients' emergency department use (Fig. 1).[18] The model differentiates between factors involved in problem recognition, the decision to seek help, and the decision to use the emergency department. Each of these may be influenced by a range of predisposing factors (such as age, sex, previous health care experience), enabling factors (such as accessibility and availability of care, access to private transport, costs), and factors associated with the patient's clinical condition.

The most important determinants appear to be the person's situation when the need arises; the perceived availability and accessibility of alternative providers of care; the patient or an adviser's view of urgency and the care that may be required; and perceptions of the costs and benefits involved in attending the emergency department or other services. In the United States of America, 'lack of primary care provider' or barriers to accessing alternative sources of health care are the most common reason given by patients for attending emergency departments with non-urgent problems.[11]

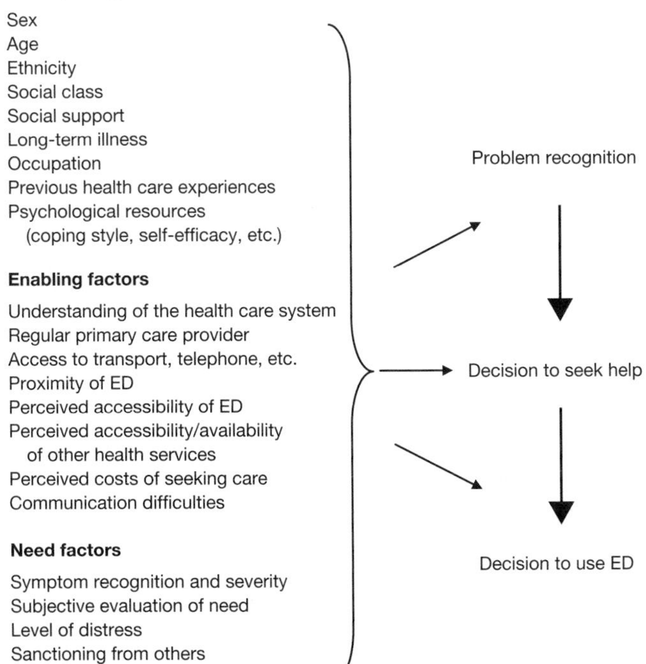

Fig. 1 Three-stage model of determinants of ED use: examples of factors that have been found to influence demand (modified from Padgett and Brodsky[18]).

Concerns about the appropriateness of care

The quality of care provided to patients who attend emergency departments with non-urgent needs has been questioned and criticized for being unduly interventionist. In the United Kingdom, there is evidence that emergency department medical staff have difficulty eliciting and responding to the psycho-social concerns of patients,[19,20] and important clinical matters and significant psycho-social problems may be overlooked. Even when psycho-social problems are recognized, therapeutic options and follow-up are seldom discussed with the patient.[21]

The failure to carefully determine why patients have presented to the emergency department, including the extent to which worry is a factor or a symptom, may result in unnecessary initiation or duplication of activities, procedures, and referrals to specialist teams and outpatient clinics. There is some evidence that continuity of care may be harmed and that follow-up of patients' needs is poor.[22]

Interventionist care is not only costly, but can also confirm in the patient's mind the validity of their fears, encourage fixation on their somatic symptoms, and so may increase, rather than relieve, anxiety and the perception of threat. The provision of such care may contribute to raising public expectations for high-technology medicine, and so encourage future dependency on emergency departments.

Responses to the demand for primary care in the emergency department

Given the range of variables that influence the decision to seek care from an emergency department, it is not surprising that advertising, sign-posting, and public information campaigns, although often advocated as means of helping the public understand the 'true' purpose of emergency departments, do not appear to have a significant impact on demand.

One means of reducing demand is to reduce the accessibility of a service. In the United States of America, financial disincentives have been shown to have this effect. Many emergency departments in the United States now have to seek pre-authorization from the patients' insurer before treatment can be provided. For example, it has been shown that emergency department use responds to cost-sharing between the patient and their health care insurer, but the effects of co-payments are greatest on those who are financially less well off.[23] In the United States many managed-care organizations have also implemented telephone triage systems that require patients to seek pre-authorization before the emergency department is used by the insured person.[24]

However, several reports indicate the hazards that may be involved in denying patients care.[10,25–27] Any intervention that risks deterring some patients with urgent clinical needs from seeking care is likely to encounter clinical, ethical, and possibly legal objections.

In the United Kingdom, increasing accessibility to telephone advice and triage has also been proposed as a means of increasing the accessibility of health care information and advice. NHS Direct has recently been introduced as a national nurse-led telephone advice service, although no evidence of an effect on emergency department demand was demonstrated over its first 24 months of operation.[28]

An alternative approach to reducing demand is through increasing the availability of other primary care services. Patients with access to a regular source of primary care appear to use emergency departments less frequently for non-urgent problems.[29] However, the evidence of the impact of improving access to primary care on emergency department demand is varied.

While some such initiatives have been shown to result in reduced demand at emergency departments,[13,21,30] others have failed to demonstrate significant decreases in attendance rates.[31] As already discussed in this chapter, the demand for emergency department care is not just a function of lack of alternative primary care provision; the relationship between the two is far more complex. The scope for influencing patient behaviour through primary care-based interventions may be limited in countries where primary care coverage is already well developed. Furthermore, there is likely to be a considerable time lag between changes in the availability and accessibility of primary care and changes in the knowledge and attitudes of patients.

Meeting demand more effectively

A range of approaches to meeting demand more effectively has been advocated. These range from interventions intended to re-direct patients attending with non-urgent needs away from the emergency department at the point of triage, to making the clinical service more responsive to primary care needs. Although few of these have been evaluated robustly, as discussed below primary care-trained health professionals can usefully play a role in meeting the needs of emergency department attenders, so enabling improvements in quality and continuity. Their experience and problem-solving skills may enable a large proportion of patients to be seen without resorting to investigations, referrals, and other costly interventions.

Re-directing patients at triage to alternative sources of primary care, such as general practitioners, has been widely proposed. Many departments in the United Kingdom have an informal policy of advising patients with non-urgent needs to seek alternative care, particularly when waiting times are long. Patient education opportunities can be maximized to encourage future first aid and use of over-the-counter medication, as well as advice about when to return to the department.(32)

In the United States a more stringent approach has been strongly advocated by Derlet and Nishio.(33) They recommend that triage nurses should have the authority to refuse care to patients. Although they have produced evidence to support the safety and effectiveness of this policy,(34) concerns have been raised about the lack of replicability of Derlet and Nishio's criteria for 'non-emergencies'(35,36) and the clinical, moral, ethical, economic, and legal problems associated with denying patients care.(37) Triage nurses' decision-making has been shown to lack consistency and reliability in many trials.(38,39)

Urgent medical problems may not be apparent without full assessment. The position statement of the Society of Academic Emergency Medicine identified that 'triage policies that refuse care to individuals meeting specific criteria put some of these patients at risk of further harm'.(37) Furthermore, it has been argued that once a brief history had been taken and vital signs checked by the triage nurse, completing the assessment and treatment does not take much more time for the types of patient who are refused care.

Alternative approaches

A number of interventions have been described that are based on increasing the availability of staff with primary care skills who can respond to the patient's immediate health care needs with the minimum of intervention, and re-direct the patient back to community-based primary care services for follow-up as required.

Hansagi et al. described a system in Stockholm where specially trained 'nurse-advisers' assess patients who had been triaged as non-urgent, offered them advice and, if necessary, assisted them in making an appointment for an alternative source of health care.(21) Of those seen by nurse-advisers, 55 per cent were referred to services outside the hospital or given self-care advice; the remainder were felt to require emergency department intervention. There were no reported adverse outcomes.

There is much evidence from the United States of America that nurse practitioners can manage many groups of emergency department patients effectively, and they are being employed in increasing numbers of departments to provide 'fast track' care to patients with non-urgent problems. Likewise, in the United Kingdom, nurse practitioners are increasingly being employed in emergency departments. However, emergency nurse practitioners tend to manage a narrower range of presenting problems than emergency department doctors, and their caseloads contain more trauma.(40) They also tend to be slower than doctors at assessing and treating patients.

For many years, suggestions have been made in the United Kingdom that general practitioners could be employed in emergency departments to treat patients presenting with primary care needs. The approaches used by GPs to problem-solve, elicit needs within a psycho-social context, cope with diagnostic uncertainty and risk-taking, and encourage continuity of care have all been identified as being highly relevant to managing primary care needs in an emergency department setting.

These views were reflected by the Royal Commission on the National Health Service (1978), which stated that 'where the tradition of using (emergency departments as a walk-in GP surgery) is strong, it may be preferable for the hospital to accept this role and make specific arrangements for fulfilling it, rather than to try and resist established local preferences'.(41)

In Australia, in the 1970s and 1980s, the feasibility of employing GPs in emergency departments was demonstrated.(42,43) The model was further developed at King's College Hospital, London, where around 40 per cent of emergency department attenders were categorized at triage as 'primary care', and hence suited to being managed by GPs.(44) The service was initially evaluated as part of a controlled prospective trial, and consistent differences were found between the care provided by GPs and the other emergency department doctors for patients who had been classified as 'primary care'.(45) For example, compared to the GPs, emergency department staff ordered radiographs more than twice as frequently, and ordered blood tests around six times as often. Referrals to hospital outpatient clinics or on-call teams occurred almost three times as frequently. This greater level of intervention was not associated with differences in outcome or patient satisfaction, and the yield of clinically important findings appeared to be similar for all groups.

The analysis of average costs indicated considerable potential savings.(46) Employing GPs in the emergency department appeared to lead to more effective use of available human and capital resources, contributing to immediate and potential longer-term benefits for patients and the health service. The experience and problem-solving strategies employed by GPs appeared to enable a greater proportion of patients to be seen without resorting to investigations, referrals, and other costly interventions. GPs reported that working in the emergency department led to overall increased job satisfaction, greater variation in their pattern of work, and new opportunities for professional development.

Several studies from the United States of America have demonstrated similar differences between specialists and family physicians. Compared to

Table 1 Key reasons for employing health care professionals skilled in primary medical care in emergency departments

Patients often present at EDs with vague, undifferentiated problems that are unrelated to particular systems or disease processes
While the episodic care provided in EDs may be detrimental for certain patients (such as those with on-going problems or psycho-social needs), for many acute self-limiting problems the convenience of being seen in EDs may outweigh this
Few medical or nursing staff in EDs have traditionally received training to develop effective primary care consultation skills to assess the relative importance of symptoms and signs at early stages of illness, to cope with diagnostic uncertainty and define the appropriate level of care that each patient requires
GPs have been shown to provide less interventionist, more cost-effective care in the ED for patients that present with primary care problems
Doctors skilled in primary medical care are more likely to be familiar with the health services available in their local community, including how to refer to them and make best use of them, and so should encourage greater continuity of care
This may contribute to improving relations between hospital- and community-based services, improved communication, and the provision of more seamless care

general internists, family physicians appear to order fewer diagnostic tests, make referrals less often, and admit patients less frequently.(47–50)

The case for employing GPs in emergency departments as primary care physicians is summarized in Table 1. Evidence supporting the applicability of the King's model of emergency department primary care to other settings has emerged from a number of studies in the United Kingdom and Ireland that demonstrated broadly similar differences between care provided by GPs and care provided by emergency department physicians.(51,52)

Several emergency departments in the United Kingdom now employ GPs as primary care physicians. The approach appears likely to have greatest relevance and applicability to large, inner city departments serving commuting, tourist, and/or socially deprived and homeless populations.(52,53)

Conclusion

In the last decade, there has been increasing interest in developing more primary care-oriented responses at emergency departments and for taking more of a whole systems view when considering the interface been emergency department and primary medical care. Service innovations that involve the employment of primary care-skilled nurses or doctors in emergency departments have been shown to be an effective use of human and capital resources, and might contribute to potential long-term benefits for patients and the wider health service. The approaches used by primary care-trained physicians to problem-solve, elicit patients' needs, cope with diagnostic uncertainty and risk-taking, and ensure continuity of care all appear to be highly relevant to managing primary care needs within an emergency department setting. There is also evidence that junior doctors working in emergency departments value receiving training to enhance the way they manage patients with non-urgent needs.(54,55) Together, this offers ways of responding to the need to manage the interface between primary medical care and emergency departments that should allow departments to meet patients' needs more efficiently and effectively than in the past.

References

1. **Audit Commission.** *By Accident or Design: Improving A&E Services in England and Wales.* London: HMSO, 1996.
2. **Burdett-Smith, P.** (1992). Estimating trauma centre workload. *Journal of the Royal College of Surgeons of Edinburgh* **37** (2), 128–30.
3. **Caplan, C.** (1975). Emergency room use by patients from a family practice. *Journal of Family Practice* **2**, 271–6.
4. **Crombie, D.L.** (1959). A casualty survey. *Journal of the College of General Practitioners* **2**, 346–56.
5. **Burke, D.P. and Rashid, N.** (1995). Primary care in accident and emergency departments: cost of employing general practitioners in department may outweigh savings. *British Medical Journal* **311**, 1438.
6. **Haddy, R.I., Schmaler, M.E., and Epting, R.J.** (1987). Non-emergency emergency room use in patients with and without primary care physicians. *Journal of Family Practice* **24**, 389–92.
7. **Stratmann, W.C. and Ullman, R.** (1975). A study of consumer attitudes about health care: the role of the emergency room. *Medical Care* **8**, 1033–43.
8. **McCaig, L.F.** *National Hospital Ambulatory Medical Care Survey: 1992 Emergency Department Summary: Advance Data from Vital and Health Statistics.* Hyattsville MD: National Center for Health Statistics, no. 245, DHSS publication no. (PHS) 94-1250, 1994.
9. **Nadel, M.** Report to the Chairman, Subcommittee on Health for Families and the Uninsured, Committee on Finance, US Senate. *Emergency Departments: Unevenly Affected by Growth and Change in Patient Use.* Washington DC: US General Accounting Office, publication no GAO/HRD-93-4, 1993.
10. **Lowe, R.A. and Young, G.P.** *Adverse Outcome of Managed Gatekeeping.* Washington DC: American College of Emergency Physicians Scientific Assembly, 1995.
11. **Grumbach, K., Keane, D., and Bindman, A.** (1993). Primary care and public emergency department overcrowding. *American Journal of Public Health* **83** (3), 372–8.
12. **Bindman, A.B.** (1995). Triage in accident and emergency departments (editorial). *British Medical Journal* **311**, 404.
13. **Gill, J.M. and Diamond, J.J.** (1996). Effect of primary care referral on emergency department use: evaluation of a statewide Medicaid program. *Family Medicine* **28**, 178–82.
14. **Green, J. and Dale, J.** (1992). Primary care in accident and emergency and general practice: a comparison. *Social Science and Medicine* **35**, 987–95.
15. **Foldes, S.S., Fischer, L.R., and Kaminsky, K.** (1994). What is an emergency? The judgements of two physicians. *Annals of Emergency Medicine* **23** (4), 833–40.
16. **Lowe, R.A., Bindman, A.B., Ulrich, S.K., Scaletta, T.A., Norman, G., and Grumbach, K.** (1993). What is an appropriate emergency department visit? An explanation for the failure to agree. *Annals of Emergency Medicine* **22**, 951.
17. **Driscoll, P.A., Vincent, C.A., and Wilkinson, M.** (1987). The use of the accident and emergency department. *Archives of Emergency Medicine* **4**, 77–82.
18. **Padgett, D.K. and Brodsky, B.** (1992). Psychosocial factors influencing non-urgent use of the emergency room: a review of the literature and recommendations for research and improved service delivery. *Social Science and Medicine* **35** (9), 1189–97.
19. **Bell, G., Reinstein, D.Z., Rajiyah, G., and Rosser, R.** (1991). Psychiatric screening of admissions to an accident and emergency ward. *British Journal of Psychiatry* **158**, 554–7.
20. **Williams, S., Dale, J., Glucksman, E., and Wellesley, A.** (1997). Senior house officers' work-related stressors, psychological distress and confidence in performing clinical tasks in accident and emergency. *British Medical Journal* **314**, 713–18.
21. **Hansagi, H., Edhag, O., and Alleback, P.** (1991). High consumers of health care in emergency units: how to improve their quality of care. *Quality Assurance in Health Care* **3** (1), 51–62.
22. **Magnussen, R.A., Hedges, J.R., Vanko, M., McCarten, K., and Moorhead, J.C.** (1993). Follow-up compliance after emergency department evaluation. *Annals of Emergency Medicine* **22**, 560–7.
23. **Selby, J.V., Fireman, B.H., and Swain, S.B.E.** (1996). Effect of a copayment on use of the emergency department in a health maintenance organization. *New England Journal of Medicine* **334**, 635–41.
24. **Franks, P., Clancy, C., and Nutting, P.** (1992). Gatekeeping revisited: protecting patients from overtreatment. *New England Journal of Medicine* **327**, 424–9.
25. **Osborn, H.H.** (1996). Health maintenance organizations: managed care or mismanaged care? *Annals of Emergency Medicine* **27**, 225–8.
26. **Wrenn, K. and Slovis, C.M.** (1996). TennCare in the emergency department: the first 18 months. *Annals of Emergency Medicine* **27**, 231–3.
27. **Knopp, R.K.** (1996). Health care reforms and the safety net. *Annals of Emergency Medicine* **27**, 234–6.
28. **Munro, J., Nicholl, J., O'Cathain, A., and Knowles, E.** (2000). Impact of NHS Direct on demand for immediate care: observational study. *British Medical Journal* **321**, 150–3.
29. **Shesser, R., Kirsch, T., Smith, J., and Hirsch, R.** (1991). An analysis of emergency department use by patients with minor illness. *Annals of Emergency Medicine* **20**, 743–8.
30. **Sjonell, G.** (1986). Effect of establishing a primary health care centre on the utilisation of primary health care and other outpatient care in a Swedish urban area. *Family Practice* **3**, 148–54.
31. **Douglass, R.L. and Torres, R.E.** (1994). Evaluation of a managed care programme for the non-Medicaid urban poor. *Journal of Health of the Poor and Underserved* **5**, 83–98.
32. **Kelly, K.A.** (1994). Referring patients from triage out of the emergency department to primary care settings: one successful emergency department experience. *Journal of Emergency Nursing* **20**, 458–63.
33. **Derlet, R.W. and Nishio, D.A.** (1990). Refusing care to patients who present to an emergency department. *Annals of Emergency Medicine* **1**, 262–7.
34. **Derlet, R.W., Kinser, D., Ray, L., Hamilton, B., and McKenzie, J.** (1995). Prospective identification and triage of non-emergency patients out of an

emergency department: a five year study. *Annals of Emergency Medicine* **25**, 215–23.

35. **Lowe, R.A., Bindman, A.B., Ulrich, S.K., Norman, G., Scaletta, T.A., Keane, D., Washington, D., and Grumbach, K.** (1994). Refusing care to emergency department of patients: evaluation of published triage guidelines. *Annals of Emergency Medicine* **23** (2), 286–93.
36. **Birnbaum, A., Gallagher, E.J., Utkewicz, M., Gennis, P., and Carter, W.** (1994). Failure to validate a predictive model for refusal of care to ED patients. *Academic Emergency Medicine* **1**, 213–17.
37. **Schmidt, T.A., Iserson, K.V., Freas, G.C., Adams, J.G., Burke, T.F., Derse, A.R., Goldfrank, L., Kalbfleisch, N.D., Keim, S.M., Krimm, J.R., and Larkin, G.L.** (1995). Ethics of emergency department triage: SAEM (Society for Academic Emergency Medicine) position statement. *Academic Emergency Medicine* **2**, 990–5.
38. **DiPasquale, J.T., Nichols, J.A., and Runge, J.W.** (1994). Can patients requiring a single physician evaluation be predicted at triage? *Academic Emergency Medicine* A2.
39. **Brillman, J.C., Doezema, D., Tandberg, D., Sklar, D.P., Davis, K.D., Simms, S., and Skipper, B.J.** (1996). Triage: limitations in predicting need for emergent care and hospital admission. *Annals of Emergency Medicine* **27**, 93–500.
40. **Read, S.M., Jones, N.M., and Williams, B.T.** (1992). Nurse practitioners in accident and emergency departments: what do they do? *British Medical Journal* **305**, 1466–70.
41. **Royal Commission's Report on the NHS.** *Chapter 10: Accident and Emergency Services.* London: HMSO, 1978.
42. **Catchlove, B.R.** (1974). Community requirements and the modern casualty department. *Medical Journal of Australia* **1**, 937–8.
43. **Andersen, N.A. and Gaudry, P.L.** (1984). Patients attending an accident and emergency department for primary medical care. *Family Practice* **1** (2), 79–85.
44. **Dale, J., Green, J., Reid, F., and Glucksman, E.** (1995). Primary care in the accident and emergency department: I. Prospective identification of patients. *British Medical Journal* **311**, 423–6.
45. **Dale, J., Green, J., Reid, F., Glucksman, E., and Higgs, R.** (1995). Primary care in the accident and emergency department: II. Comparison of general practitioners and hospital doctors. *British Medical Journal* **311**, 427–30.
46. **Dale, J., Lang, H., Roberts, J., Green, J., and Glucksman, E.** (1996). Cost effectiveness of treating primary care patients in accident and emergency: a comparison between general practitioners, senior house officers and registrars. *British Medical Journal* **312**, 1340–4.
47. **Cherkin, D.C., Rosenblatt, R.A., Hart, L.G., Schneeweiss, R., and LoGerfo, J.** (1987). The use of medical resources by residency trained family physicians and general internists: is there a difference? *Medical Care* **25**, 455–69.
48. **Greenfield, S., Nelson, E., Zubkoff, M., Manning, W., Rogers, W., Kravitz, R., Keller, A., Tarlov, A., and Ware, J.** (1992). Variations in resource use among medical specialties and systems of care: results from the medical outcomes study. *Journal of the American Medical Association* **267**, 1624–30.
49. **Bertaklis, K.D. and Robbins, J.A.** (1987). Gatekeeping in primary care: a comparison of internal medicine and family practice. *Journal of Family Practice* **24**, 305–9.
50. **Starfield, B., Powe, N.R., Weiner, J.R., Stuart, M., Steinwachs, D., Scholle, S.H., and Gerstenberger, A.** (1994). Costs versus quality in different types of primary care settings. *Journal of the American Medical Association* **272**, 1903–8.
51. **Murphy, A.W., Bury, G., Plunkett, P.K., Gibney, D., Smith, M., Mullan, E., and Johnson, Z.** (1996). Randomised controlled trial of general practitioner versus usual medical care in an urban accident and emergency department: process, outcome, and comparative cost. *British Medical Journal* **312**, 1135–42.
52. **Ward, P. and Huddy, H.** (1996). Primary care in London: an evaluation of general practitioners working in an inner city accident and emergency department. *Journal of Accident and Emergency Medicine* **13**, 11–15.
53. **Owens, C.W.I., Ben-Shlomo, Y., and Moore, F.P.** (1993). A&E in London: better primary care won't affect self referrals. *British Medical Journal* **306**, 1751.
54. **Dale, J., Davies, M., Vasant, K., and Glucksman, E.** (1997). Primary care consultation skills training in an accident and emergency department: implementing a new training programme. *Medical Education* **31**, 243–9.
55. **Dale, J., Williams, S., Wellesley, A., and Glucksman, E.** (1999). Training and supervision needs and experience: a longitudinal cross-sectional survey of A&E senior house officers. *Postgraduate Medical Journal* **75** (880), 86–9.

1.6 Traditional healers as health care providers: Africa as an example

Peter A.G.M. de Smet and Edward C. Green

Preface

There are many different traditional medical cultures around the world, which do not always have more in common with each other than with modern Western medicine.[1] In this chapter, we have not discussed traditional healers in general, but have restricted ourselves to a description of African traditional healers, as an example of the issues involved in the complex relationships between individual patients, families, and communities, and traditional and Western medicine healers.

Nature of African healing

In any place and at any time, conceptions of healing are based on beliefs about health and disease, which in their turn are rooted in fundamental ideas about life itself. This means that one has to study the African view of life to understand the nature of African healing. Traditional Africans tend to believe that everything is invested with a life force. This spirit or power is the essence of every living creature, deceased ancestor, inanimate object, and natural event, such as a thunderstorm. Preservation or restoration of health cannot be pursued without involving these life forces, all of which have their own personality and cosmic place. It is common to see an African healer talking to a tree so that he may control and use the life force within for the benefit of his patient. A healer's power is not determined by the number of medicinal tree barks he knows, but by his ability to apply his understanding of the intricate relations between all things for the good of the patient and the whole community.

A doctor trained in Western biomedicine concerns himself in the first place with the natural causes and bodily manifestations of disease, without intervening or sharing in the patient's social fabric. In contrast, traditional African healers interpret illness within the broader context of life forces at work. They look for the cause of the patient's misfortune in the relations between the patient and his social and physical environment. For instance, healers of the Congolese Yaka people attempt to master the origin of the disease and turn it against itself. At the same time, they seek to rehabilitate the patient within the group by expelling the conflict that has produced his symptoms. Their cult objects, herbal decoctions, food taboos, and cupping horns are merely tools in an intricate ritual drama, in which the healer's attention is directed towards the metaphysical equivalent of the biophysical problem. This way of African healing is an inextricable part of African religion, and turns the act of healing into a religious act. When African patients receive a herbal infusion, they expect to benefit from the life force of its ingredients and from the power of the ancestors or any other spirits invoked. This spiritual significance tends to be more important than the bioactive properties of the remedy.

Although this is often presented as the predominant model of illness and healing in traditional Africa, it is not the only model. Many Africans recognize common complaints (e.g. headache, cough, diarrhoea, skin ulcer, joint pain) as problems due to natural causes and treat these symptoms at the household level. Magical practices are only resorted to for other illnesses or if the common complaint persists. In many parts of Africa, even serious communicable diseases (malaria, tuberculosis, schistosomiasis, amoebic dysenstery, AIDS, etc.) are interpreted in a way that is more natural than supernatural. People do not fall ill because some avenging spirit or malevolent sorcerer has singled them out for misfortune, but because they have come into contact with something that anyone could come into contact with (e.g. a mystical contagion or pollution or an environmental danger, such an 'illness in the air' spread by the wind).[2]

African healers

It is difficult to characterize African healers without stereotyping, because there are many different kinds, and the cultural diversity and complexity of their practices are encyclopaedic, when considered in detail. Many healers have in common, however, the characteristic of describing and explaining most illnesses in terms of social interaction and act on the belief that religion permeates every aspect of human existence. Other prominent features of traditional African healers are a deep personal involvement in the healing process, the protection of therapeutic knowledge by keeping it secret, and being rewarded for their services. The social context of the therapeutic process requires reciprocity and some form of payment is believed to contribute to the effectiveness of the treatment. Over the years, the types and methods of payments for traditional healing have changed. Practitioners are increasingly demanding monetary payments, especially in urban settings.

Some healers have learnt their trade by undergoing treatment as a patient. Upon their recovery, they decided to become practitioners themselves. Another way of recruitment is through spiritual calling, in which case the healer's diagnoses and treatments are strictly determined by the supernatural. A third route is through informal learning from a close family member. A fourth possibility is through a long formal apprenticeship under an established practitioner, for which a fee is paid.

Urbanization

Urbanization has increasingly concentrated large numbers of Africans in an environment where there is stronger competition from Western medicine, which is more readily available in towns than in rural areas. Traditional healing is also flourishing in urban settings, however, because it adapts itself to these new surroundings. In other words, African traditional medicine is more than a static and inflexible institution that cannot survive the test of time.

In a case study in Kenya, the main growth of traditionally based medicine was found in urban areas and not in rural villages, and this expansion may continue to occur regardless of the availability of Western health services. In rural areas, the number of traditional practitioners was decreasing, not only because of a diminishing number of people becoming new practitioners, but also because of the migration of practitioners from the villages to the cities. The important incentive for this migration was that there were more patients and more money available in the city. Contrary to their rural counterparts, urban practitioners were more entrepeneurial and operated almost entirely on a fee-for-service basis. Their core practices and the expectations of their patients were still firmly rooted in tradition but had adapted dynamically to urban circumstances, for instance, by borrowing components from Western medicine (e.g. disease labelling, hygiene, or use of antibiotics). Such new elements had been gathered in a fragmented way but the practitioners expressed a desire to improve their biomedical knowledge and to cooperate with professionals trained in Western medicine.[3]

Different practitioners

In some African societies, one type of healer provides several or all therapeutic services, but others have separate practitioners for different functions. The different health care providers of the West African Hausa people may serve as an example of the latter (Table 1).

Diviners are generally listed as one of the most important or highest status types of traditional African healers. This is not surprising, since divination and healing are often practised by the same individual who has the powers to deal with the spiritual realm. Diviners are seers who are consulted to find out what has gone wrong, and they employ their skills to find lost objects or farm stock, to discover thieves, and to interpret the cause or meaning of diseases. Unlike Western fortune tellers, who are preoccupied

Table 1 Traditional health care providers among the Hausa people of Northern Nigeria[4]

Hausa name	Description
Boka	Herbal healer who acts as a consulting herbal practitioner. Patients come to the *boka* for consultation, advice, and treatment, sometimes from a considerable distance
Kantankar	Seller of herbal medicines who generally lives in the area in which he works and makes part of his living as a seller of herbal medicines for home cures in local marketplaces
Magori	Itinerant herbal salesman, who seldom spends much time in any one place; often sells love filtres, aphrodisiacs, and similar preparations
Ungozoma	Traditional birth attendant; usually an old woman who is a relative or friend of the family. Among her tasks is the cutting of the umbilical cord and subsequent disposal of the umbilical cord and afterbirth
Wanzami	Combines the function of barber and surgeon. He regularly shaves the heads of men and boys, but also performs a number of minor surgical procedures, such as cupping, circumcision, uvulectomy, and tattooing
Ma'dori	Bonesetter, who treats human as well as veterinary cases. He has a high reputation and is usually favoured over Western treatment
Mallam	His ability to read Arabic gives him access to esoteric Islamic mysteries that remain hidden for illiterate men and women. He is the custodian of spiritual power, which increases as his knowledge increases, and which can be tapped for healing purposes. He may act as a counsellor, diviner, astrologer, fortune teller, spiritual adviser, herbalist, and therapist. He operates by peering into his books—the repositories of his secrets
Bori	Adept of the *bori* possession cult who has access to special knowledge, which can be used to treat illness. The *bori* adept is most often a woman, who has undergone a rite of initiation to establish control over a spirit-induced illness. By regulating her relationship with the spirit, she becomes an interface between the human and spirit world, and she may use this new status to build up a practice as a healer. The performance of possession dances during *bori* ceremonies permits her to mimic a role of power and authority that might otherwise be unattainable in a society dominated by men

with the prediction of the future, they look for disturbing events in the past, which will cause or would continue to cause misfortune, if left untreated.

A predominant type of *faith healer* is the professed Christian faith healer, who has broken away from an overseas Western church or who belongs to an independent African church. The Christian type of faith healing has become particularly popular in South Africa, where it is practised in the African Initiated Churches. It is estimated that there are at least 6000 such churches today with a total membership of about 8.5 million people. The churches are autonomous and unaffiliated to any mission or mainline white church. The healing in these churches rests on a synthesis of early Christian healing practices and traditional indigenous practices, which both treat illness through purification and the elimination of evil spirits.[5]

Biomedical skills

The magio-religious inclination of African traditional medicine takes nothing away from the fact that many healers are experienced and skilled in biomedical components of their profession. They have an array of biomedical methods at their disposal, ranging from fasting and dieting to herbal therapies, and from bathing and massage to surgical procedures. The most important African healers with biomedical skills are herbalists, midwives, and surgeons.

Herbalists and patients have numerous different medicinal plants at their disposal. Readers interested in comprehensive information are referred to the general references at the end as well as a recent index of books about African herbs.[6] Some medicinal herbs are gathered and used without ceremony by everyone, whereas other herbs must be hand-picked in a special way or are known only to professional healers. This range is mirrored in the different types of herbalists that may be encountered in African societies. Some are itinerant or resident suppliers of herbs for the self-treatment of a well-known symptom (e.g. headache), whereas others are knowledgeable in the supernatural causes of illness and in the countermoves against these forces. The Nigerian Yoruba people make a distinction between divining herbalists (*babalawo*) and non-divining ones (*onisegun*). The latter are more inclined to carry out physical examinations, but such tests are usually limited to visual observation and smelling (urine being the most commonly examined item).[7]

Midwives or traditional birth attendants attend up to 80 per cent of all births in Africa. The majority are elderly women, whose skills and procedures are on the whole rational and not very different from midwifery practices elsewhere in the world. They only receive a small, usually nonmonetary, reward for their services and do not rely on this for subsistence. They see themselves as contributing to the good of their society, because a woman who is pregnant or in labour is the responsibility of the whole community. Many traditional birth attendants share a cultural heritage with the women and their families, and communication with the supernatural world may be an essential part of their expertise. They know which rituals, food taboos, and local herbs are needed before, during, and after delivery. Midwives may also act as consultants on diseases of women and small children and on traditional methods of contraception and fertility-promoting actions.

Surgeons in Africa tend to perform only minor surgery, such as bloodletting, incisions and excisions, tooth extraction, and the cutting of the umbilical cord. Major surgery as it is known in Western medicine does not stand out in African traditional medicine. Most often, bonesetting is the only traditional procedure, which can be classified as such, but some other forms have been found among certain Eastern African peoples, such as wound treatment and amputation among the Masai[8] and craniotomy among the Kisii.[9] These localized practices have not greatly influenced the status of traditional African surgery as a whole. The major reason why African surgery did not advance further seems to have been its supernatural orientation, which did little to abolish anatomical ignorance. An additional point may have been that in various areas bodily mutilation was dreaded because of its detrimental influence in the future life on one's ghost. In areas where mutilation was a customary form of punishment (e.g. in Ethiopia), people disliked operations with external sequelae because this would make them look like criminals.

Assets of traditional healers

Surveys of traditional African healers have consistently shown that they are willing to learn more about Western medicine and collaborate with Western-trained health care professionals, if only because this may increase their prestige and income.[10] There is also long-standing international support for their deployment in African biomedical health care. In 1978, WHO and UNICEF issued the so-called Alma Ata resolutions to support the use of indigenous health practitioners in government-sponsored health programmes. In 1994, a WHO declaration emphasized that due recognition should be given to the value of indigenous people's knowledge and expertise in traditional medicines and practices and that indigenous health care should be based on practical, socially, and culturally acceptable methods.[11]

Traditional African healers can offer several advantages over their Western-trained counterparts:

- They constitute the principal or only professional form of health care services for the large majority of Africans. Their services are particularly important in rural villages, where the nearest Western hospital may be too distant to be reached in time. Traditional healers are also an important option in the cities, however, because they show a culturally appropriate concern for their patients or because biomedical care is too expensive. Many urban Africans prefer traditional healers, and many consult a traditional healer before, during, or after biomedical treatment.
- They are often more accessible and more affordable than Western-type doctors. They enjoy credibility and respect in their local communities, and patients are willing to seek their advice and to pay privately for their services. Traditional healers do not make a biomedical distinction between body, mind, and spirit, and this holistic perspective makes them particularly apt to deal with psychological and sociocultural problems, in which the provision of care must be concordant with the patient's worldview. In the case of mental health, it is the spiritually based practitioner who can provide many Africans with a much needed specialist service.
- They outnumber biomedical doctors by hundreds to one. It is unlikely that African policy makers can realize all their country-wide health goals in the foreseeable future without involving traditional healers.
- Part of their traditional remedies may have therapeutic value based on real bioactive properties (see Table 2 for examples of African plants, for which there is some evidence up to the clinical level that they could be therapeutically useful).
- Co-operation with traditional healers suits the primary health care philosophy of self-reliance, which advocates that, where possible, dependence on external services should be replaced by reliance on local resources.

Some of the early collaborative programmes between biomedical and African indigenous health practitioners had a successful start. For instance, a programme in Swaziland focused on healers who gave herbal enemas to children with acute diarrhoea, thereby introducing a life-threatening risk of exacerbating their dehydration. Initially, there was evidence to suggest that healers were abandoning their traditional enemas and adopted oral rehydration therapy instead.[20] Ultimately, however, the project was no longer functioning, and other promising projects have met with the same fate. Various programmes faltered or were discontinued, and usually they have not been replicated on a national scale.[21] The following factors have been identified as powerful countervailing forces:

- The general arguments in favour of collaboration between Western-trained health care professionals and traditional African healers tend to reflect outsiders' views rather than the perspective of local communities.

Table 2 Examples of potentially effective herbs used in traditional African medicine[12,13]

Herb	Ethnobotanical data	Chemical and pharmacological data
Cryptolepis sanguinolenta	The root and root bark of this liana are employed in West and Central Africa for the treatment of infectious diseases. Traditional healers in Ghana use an aqueous root extract to treat symptoms that could occur in diabetes (e.g. fungal infections)	The root contains cryptolepine and related alkaloids. Cryptolepine has antibacterial, antimalarial, and antidiabetic activities in non-human test models. A blood glucose lowering effect of the aqueous root extract has been observed in human patients with type 2 (non-insulin dependent) diabetes[14]
Harpagophytum procumbens	Native Africans have used this plant for various health problems, ranging from indigestion, fever, and headaches to liver and kidney disorders and rheumatism	The secondary root, which is the medicinal plant part, contains iridoids (such as harpagoside). Studies in human patients suggest that it may provide some symptomatic benefit in the treatment of rheumatic disorders[15]
Neorautanenia mitis	Rwandese natives use the plant as a folk medicine for scabies in calves	Contains isoflavones (such as 12a-hydroxyrotenone) with antiscabies activity. Topical preparations from the powdered tuber have been tested in humans for the treatment of scabies[16]
Pygeum africanum	African natives use this plant for various medicinal purposes, including urinary complaints	In Western phytotherapy, bark extracts are widely used for benign prostatic hyperplasia. Clinical studies suggest modest improvements in urologic symptoms and flow measures[17]
Rauwolfia vomitoria	West African natives value the root for its depressant effects on the central nervous system. Traditional Nigerian healers use the root for the treatment of psychoses, while small doses of the root bark are given as a sedative to children in Ivory Coast	The root contains reserpine and other alkaloids, most of which are located in the root bark. Reserpine has well-established antipsychotic and sedative properties[18]
Ricinus communis	The West African Hausa people use the seeds of *R. communis* var. *minor* as an oral contraceptive	Contraceptive activity has been observed in animal and human experiments[19]

Table 3 Examples of possibly harmful practices in traditional African medicine[22]

The use of herbal enemas to prevent or treat childhood diarrhoea may sometimes exacerbate life-threatening dehydration
The induction of vomiting may be dangerous for patients who are already weakened
Some types of herbal medicines may be dangerous by themselves.[23,24] A notorious South African example is the tuberous rootstock of the *impila* plant (*Callilepis laureola*), a traditional Zulu remedy capable of causing serious hepatic and renal toxicity.[25] The risk that traditional remedies may be dangerous if taken at the same time as Western medicines should also be considered[26]
Herbal eye medicines may damage the eye not only by a direct action of toxic substances introduced into the conjunctival sac, but also by the introduction of microorganisms leading to infection or by physical trauma resulting from the application[27]
Certain traditional practices are performed with unclean instruments (e.g. vaccination, incision, scarification) and may therefore result in the transmission of infectious diseases, such as tetanus, hepatitis, and HIV[28,29]
Complications of fracture treatment by traditional healers, such as gangrene due to venous occlusion and immobilization; overwhelming sepsis leading to diaphyseal sequestration[30]
The provision of dangerous advice. A recent example is the encouragement to have sexual intercourse with a virgin as an alleged cure for HIV/AIDS infection.[31] While this popular belief has been reported, it may not reflect the usual view of traditional healers

- Indigenous practitioners and medically educated Africans and their expatriate advisors embrace different, rather contrasting, worldviews or paradigms of illness. Government officials and foreign doctors usually have little understanding of the worldview that African healers represent. They tend to think of traditional healing as an archaic system that should be overcome if there is to be progress. What such a view fails to recognize is that traditional systems are genuinely functioning and may be well-suited to the social and psychological needs of participants in these systems.
- Traditional African healers are egalitarian and deeply suspicious of any peer who claims to be superior and wishes to exercise authority. If a collaborative programme tries to incorporate traditional healers into the biomedical health care system as community health workers, the traditional healers have to accept the superiority of Western medicine and their role becomes a reduced, secondary one. The Western setting may alienate them from their traditional roots and their clients may feel that they no longer have control over the total healing process, which erodes their ancestral and social legitimation.
- Professional elitism on the side of Western-trained medical professionals, which may be rooted, at least partially, in a genuine concern that indigenous healing practices are potentially harmful. There is good evidence to suggest that certain traditional African practices may indeed do harm (see Table 3 for examples). Unfortunately, most rerefences about this subject merely offer case reports or case series, and reliable epidemiological data about the actual incidence of such iatrogenic sequelae are still hard to find. Besides direct health risks, there is also the indirect problem that there is little or no evidence of the biomedical effectiveness of many traditional African treatment methods. For instance, a recent study from Mali shows that the results of traditional couching are quite inferior to those of Western cataract surgery.[32] Another example is that all the evidence for the effectiveness of traditional African remedies in major communicable diseases (e.g. malaria, measles, tuberculosis) comes from inconclusive subclinical studies and small uncontrolled pilot trials. So far, no randomized controlled trials have shown irrefutably that traditional African remedies are as effective as Western antimicrobials in the prevention or treatment of such major diseases.
- Fear of economic and prestige competition for patients and social status. This may help to explain why many collaborative programmes throughout Africa have involved traditional birth attendants rather than traditional

Table 4 Maternal services in Dormaa District Hospital, Ghana[11]

Year	TBA coverage[a] (%)	Still births (%)	Maternal deaths (%)	Neonatal deaths (%)
1990	11	7.4	0.2	2.2
1991	25	5.7	0.6	0.5
1992	31	2.1	0.09	0.6

[a] Mothers delivered by trained TBAs (the training began in 1990).

Reproduced with permission from Hoff, W. (1997). Traditional health practitioners as primary health care workers. *Tropical Doctor* **27** (Suppl.1), 52–5.

healers in general. Traditional birth attendants often perform their services without cash compensation, their activities focus on childbirth and events immediately surrounding it, and their prestige does not typically rival that of doctors and nurses.

- Resentment of indigenous practitioners by African medical professionals may have been furthered by the formation of professional organizations of traditional healers which may wield political power. However, one of the more recent training programmes, which started with the recruitment of traditional healers through their formal organizations, found that such organizations did not cover all types of traditional healers and that they were unstable due to power struggles, politics, and problems of financial management.[10]

Besides these constraining factors, there is also the concern that little evaluation has been reported on how effective projects have been in terms of their actual impact on communities. Many projects have not been evaluated formally, and when evaluations have been reported, they are usually limited to the knowledge and attitude of traditional healers before and after training and/or self-reported changes in health care behaviour.[11,20] One of the few collaborating programmes, for which information about clinical outcome is available, is a Ghanese project of training traditional birth attendants. Statistical data suggested a reduction of stillbirths and maternal and neonatal deaths over a 3-year period in the areas where the trained traditional birth attendants had worked (see Table 4). One should be cautious in interpreting these results, because no good baseline data were available and no control group was included, so other factors could have contributed to the reported changes.[11]

Involvement in HIV/AIDS prevention

In recent years, concern about the spread of certain contagious diseases in Africa has rekindled interest in the involvement of traditional African healers in biomedical health care. Although some programmes are aimed at improving control of tuberculosis,[33] most focus on curbing the HIV/AIDS epidemic among Africans. Traditional healers are not only available and credible for this purpose, but also offer the advantage that in many rural communities they are the first to be consulted for sexually transmitted diseases, which necessitate greater sensitivity than a typical Western health facility may afford.[10] Several African countries have, therefore, started programmes to train traditional healers in the prevention of HIV infection. The training topics not only comprise culturally appropriate information about AIDS and condom promotion, but may also include how to prevent HIV transmission during traditional practices and how to prevent and treat sexually transmitted diseases in general (because of evidence that improved STD management is associated with a reduction in HIV incidence). Judging by some published evidence, such training programmes may improve the short-term knowledge, attitude, and self-reported behaviour of traditional healers.[10,21,29,34–36] However, there appears to be room for further improvement. In one of the studies, a one-shot training did not achieve the desired level of performance in trainees, which led to the conclusion that a repetitive model for training is probably preferable.[29] So far, none of the collaborative HIV/AIDS prevention programmes has been evaluated in terms of long-term changes or clinical outcome (i.e. a reduction in HIV/AIDS incidence).

Concluding remarks

Western biomedicine and African traditional medicine will probably remain apart as two parallel systems, because different paradigms of health and illness stand in the way of real amalgamation. This medical pluralism is also flourishing in our Western society, and it is probably not a bad situation. A comprehensive integration of biomedical and traditional services may not be of great interest to many African patients, because by and large they know where to go for a particular health problem. If they are suffering from a particular complaint, they are aware of the different health care options available to them, and they would normally make a well-considered choice between these, if they can afford that treatment option and reach it in time.

However, there is scope for cross-fertilization between the two different systems. On the one hand, traditional herbal medicines could be incorporated into biomedical health care, provided that there is robust evidence of efficacy and safety. Promoting and incorporating herbal medicines is easier than incorporating the traditional healers themselves (see the section on collaborative programmes). Herbal medicines are readily accepted and widely used, and offer the economic advantage that they are much less costly than Western synthetic pharmaceuticals. On the other hand, there is evidence to suggest that training traditional healers in certain aspects of Western health care may be useful as well. Promising developments in this domain are the training of traditional healers in the prevention and treatment of sexually transmitted diseases (such as AIDS) and the training of traditional birth attendants in Western-based hygiene and obstetric skills. Hopefully, future evaluations of such projects will not remain limited to intermediary cognitive and behavourial outcomes, but will also comprise a critical assessment of clinical endpoints.

References

1. **Young, A.** (1983). The relevance of traditional medical cultures to modern primary health care. *Social Science and Medicine* **17**, 205–11.
2. **Green, E.C.** (1997). Is there a basis for modern-traditional cooperation in African health promotion? *Journal of Alternative and Complementary Medicine* **3**, 311–14.
3. **Good, C.M.** *Ethnomedical Systems in Africa. Patterns of Traditional Medicine in Rural and Urban Kenya.* New York: The Guilford Press, 1987.
4. **Wall, L.L.** *Hausa Medicine. Illness and Well-being in a West-African Culture.* Durham: Duke University Press, 1988.
5. **Steyn, H.C.** (1996). Spiritual healing: a comparison between New Age groups and African Initiated Churches in South Africa. *Religion & Theology* **3**, 109–34.
6. **Neuwinger, H.D.** *African Traditional Medicine.* Stuttgart: Medpharm Scientific Publishers, 2000.
7. **Oyebola, D.D.** (1979). Methods of diagnosis and investigation of diseases by Yoruba traditional healers of Nigeria. *Journal of Tropical Medicine and Hygiene* **82**, 24–9.
8. **Merker, M.** *Die Masai. Ethnographische Monographie eines ostafrikanischen Semitenvolkes. 2. Auflage.* Berlin: Dietrich Reimer, 1910.
9. **Furnas, D.W., Sheikh, M.A., van den Hombergh, P., Froeling, F., and Nunda, I.M.** (1985). Traditional craniotomies of the Kisii tribe of Kenya. *Annals of Plastic Surgery* **15**, 538–56.
10. **Green, E.C.** *AIDS and STDs in Africa: Bridging the Gap Between Traditional Healers and Modern Medicine.* Boulder: Westview Press, 1994.
11. **Hoff, W.** (1997). Traditional health practitioners as primary health care workers. *Tropical Doctor* **27** (Suppl. 1), 52–5.
12. **De Smet, P.A.G.M.** (1998). Traditional pharmacology and medicine in Africa. Ethnopharmacological themes in sub-Saharan art objects and utensils. *Journal of Ethnopharmacology* **63**, 1–179.

13. **De Smet, P.A.G.M.** *Herbs, Health and Healers. Africa as Ethnopharmacological Treasury*. Berg en Dal: Afrika Museum, 1999.
14. **Luo, J.** et al. (1998). Cryptolepine, a potentially useful new antihyperglycemic agent isolated from *Cryptolepis sanguinolenta*: an example of the ethnobotanical approach to drug discovery. *Diabetic Medicine* **15**, 367–74.
15. **Long, L., Soeken, K., and Ernst, E.** (2001). Herbal medicines for the treatment of osteoarthritis: a systematic review. *Rheumatology (Oxford)* **40**, 779–93.
16. **Van Puyvelde, L.** (1995). Ontwikkeling van geneesmiddelen op basis van traditionele geneesmiddelen in Rwanda. *Foliola* **no. 2**, 37–62.
17. **Ishani, A., MacDonald, R., Nelson, D., Rutks, I., and Wilt, T.J.** (2000). *Pygeum africanum* for the treatment of patients with benign prostatic hyperplasia: a systematic review and quantitative meta-analysis. *American Journal of Medicine* **109**, 654–64.
18. **Obembe, A., Sokomba, E.N., Sijuwola, O.A., Olorunfemi, P.O., Alemika, T.O.E., Isichei, C.O., and Ogunkeye, O.O.** (1994). Antipsychotic effects and tolerance of crude *Rauvolfia vomitoria* in Nigerian psychiatric inpatients. *Phytotherapy Research* **8**, 218–23.
19. **Okwuasaba, F.K., Das, S.C., Isichei, C.O., Ekwenchi, M.M., Onoruvwe, O., Olayinka, A.O., Uguru, V.E., Dafur, S.J., Ekwere, E.O., and Parry, O.** (2001). Pharmacological studies on the antifertility effects of RICOM-1013-J from *Ricinus communis* var *minor* and preliminary clinical studies on women volunteers. *Phytotherapy Research* **11**, 547–51.
20. **Green, E.C.** (1988). Can collaborative programs between biomedical and African indigenous health practitioners succeed? *Social Science and Medicine* **27**, 1125–30.
21. **Green, E.C., Zokwe, B., and Dupree, J.D.** (1995). The experience of an AIDS prevention program focused on South African traditional healers. *Social Science and Medicine* **40**, 503–15.
22. **Green, E.C. and Makhubu, L.** (1984). Traditional healers in Swaziland: toward improved cooperation between the traditional and modern health sectors. *Social Science and Medicine* **18**, 1071–9.
23. **Buchanan, N. and Cane, R.D.** (1976). Poisoning associated with witchdoctor attendance. *South African Medical Journal* **50**, 1138–40.
24. **Nyazema, N.Z.** (1984). Poisoning due to traditional remedies. *Central African Journal of Medicine* **30**, 80–3.
25. **Popat, A.** et al. (2001). The toxicity of Callilepis laureola, a South African traditional herbal medicine. *Clinical Biochemistry* **34**, 229–36.
26. **Fugh-Berman, A.** (2000). Herb–drug interactions. *Lancet* **355**, 134–8.
27. **Yorston, D. and Foster, A.** (1994). Traditional eye medicines and corneal ulceration in Tanzania. *Journal of Tropical Health and Hygiene* **97**, 211–14.
28. **Kew, M.C., Reis, P., Macnab, G.M., Seftel, H.C., and Bersohn, I.** (1973). The witch-doctor and tribal scarification of the skin and the hepatitis B antigen. *South African Medical Journal* **47**, 2419–20.
29. **Somsé, P.** et al. (1998). Evaluation of an AIDS training program for traditional healers in the Central African Republic. *AIDS Education and Prevention* **10**, 558–64.
30. **Ofiaeli, R.O.** (1991). Complications of methods of fracture treatment used by traditional healers: a report of three cases necessitating amputation at Ihiala, Nigeria. *Tropical Doctor* **21**, 182–3.
31. **Ahmad, K.** (2001). Namibian government to prosecute healers. *Lancet* **357**, 371.
32. **Schemann, J.F., Bakayoko, S., and Coulibaly, S.** (2000). Traditional couching is not an effective alternative procedure for cataract surgery in Mali. *Ophthalmic Epidemiology* **7**, 271–83.
33. **Jones, J.S.** (1998). Bringing traditional healers into TB control. *South African Medical Journal* **88**, 929.
34. **Berger, R.A.** et al. (1994). Traditional healers in AIDS control. *AIDS* **8**, 1511–12.
35. **Green, E.C.** (1997). The participation of African traditional healers in AIDS/STD prevention programmes. *Tropical Doctor* **27** (Suppl. 1), 56–9.
36. **Green, E.C.** (2000). Traditional healers and AIDS in Uganda. *Journal of Alternative and Complementary Medicine* **6**, 1–2.

Further reading

The general descriptions of traditional healing in Africa have been largely derived from the exhibition catalogue 'Herbs, Health and Healers. Africa as Ethnopharmacological Treasury', which was written by the first author and published by the Afrika Museum in Berg en Dal (The Netherlands) in 1999. The most important general references underlying this publication were:

De Smet, P.A.G.M. (1998). Traditional pharmacology and medicine in Africa. Ethnopharmacological themes in sub-Saharan art objects and utensils. *Journal of Ethnopharmacology* **63**, 1–179.

Devisch, R. *Weaving the Threads of Life. The Khita Gyn-Eco-Logical Healing Cult among the Yaka*. Chicago: University of Chicago Press, 1993.

Green, E.C. (1998). Can collaborative programs between biomedical and African indigenous health practitioners succeed? *Social Science and Medicine* **27**, 1125–30.

Harley, G.W. *Native African Medicine. With Special Reference to its Practice in the Mano Tribe of Liberia*. London: Frank Cass & Co. Ltd., 1970.

Imperato, P.J. *African Folk Medicine. Practices and Beliefs of the Bambara and Other People*. Baltimore: York Press, Inc., 1977.

Iwu, M.M. *Handbook of African Medicinal Plants*. Boca Raton: CRC Press, 1993.

Kale, R. (1995). Traditional healers in South Africa: a parallel health care system. *British Medical Journal* **310**, 1182–5.

Sofowora, A. *Medicinal Plants and Traditional Medicine in Africa*. Chichester: John Wiley and Sons Ltd., 1982.

Tsey, K. (1997). Traditional medicine in comtemporary Ghana: a public health analysis. *Social Science and Medicine* **45**, 1065–74.

Van der Geest, S. (1997). Is there a role for traditional medicine in basic health services in Africa? A plea for a community perspective. *Tropical Medicine and International Health* **2**, 903–11.

1.7 Rural primary care

James T.B. Rourke

> You must give something to your fellow man. Even if it's a little thing, do something for those who have need of man's help, something for which you get no pay but the privilege of doing it.
>
> Albert Schweitzer * (1)

Introduction

What is rural primary medical care? A useful definition is the promotion of good health and the prevention, diagnosis, and treatment of illness, mainly provided by general practitioners (GPs) and family physicians (FPs) (or other primary care physicians) for people who live at a distance from urban centres and resources. Each setting for rural primary medical care is unique and is determined or affected by the geography of each country or region, rural peoples' health status and health care needs, overall health care system structure, and the number, mix, and distribution of the health care workforce and support structures. These factors vary tremendously from country to country and from region to region within countries. Most remarkable, however, is the similarity of the issues and challenges in providing medical care in rural areas around the world. These issues have stimulated discussions and the sharing of solutions at the World Rural Health Conferences held in

* A pioneer rural doctor, who was also a philosopher, theologian, musician, and Nobel Prize Winner, Dr Schweitzer distinguished himself by the medical work which he and his wife, a trained nurse, undertook in the early 20th century in Gabon, West Equatorial Africa.

China in 1996, South Africa in 1997, Malaysia in 1999, Canada in 2000, Australia in 2002 and Spain, 2003 organized by the World Organisation of Family Doctors (WONCA) Working Party on Rural Practice.[2–9]

The Durban Declaration (2nd World Rural Health Conference) calls for a 'Global initiative to achieve health for all rural people, by the year 2020'.[3,10] The World Health Organization's (WHO) 'Health for All in the 21st Century' targets include safe drinking water, adequate sanitation, food, and shelter, and access for all people throughout their lives to comprehensive essential quality health care supported by essential public health functions.[11] These targets will be most difficult to achieve in rural areas, particularly in the poorest countries. Primary care is essential to achieving health for all.[11]

This chapter discusses rural primary medical care in terms of rural context, rural health status and health care needs, and health care systems. It then goes on to describe rural medical practice, including education for rural medical practice, and finally addresses quality issues.

The rural context

A variety of geographic definitions are used around the world to define 'rural'.[12] Most include communities of up to 10 000 (upper limit ranges from 2500 to 20 000) people who are not close to larger cities. The worldwide context is illustrated by the following statements: '20 per cent of UK residents (11 million people) live in rural areas, but little attention has been paid to their health needs.'[13] 'One particularly challenging issue for rural America is its access to health services. The 1990 census counted 61 658 330 "rural" people (24.8 per cent of the total US population).'[14] 'We can never accept the notion of limited access to care for the one third of Canadians who live in rural Canada. Geography cannot become an excuse for inequity.'[15] 'Over half (52 per cent) of the population of South Africa live in rural areas. Rural areas in South Africa are populated by the very young and the elderly and most employable men and women are not present as they are finding work in the cities. This has serious consequences for the health of rural families.'[16] 'China has a population of 1.2 billion people, or almost 25 per cent of the total population of the world. About 80 per cent of China's population lives in rural communities. In China, the size of the country, the large number of people, and the nature of the agrarian economy present a special challenge for the practice of rural health care.'[17]

The rural geographic realities of a low population density separated by time and distance from concentrated urban populations and resources have an enormous direct impact on rural primary medical care. Even if primary medical care were equitably distributed, rural patients would still face geographic barriers of time and distance in accessing secondary and tertiary specialized medical care and resources.

Geographic barriers, weather, floods, and lack of transportation infrastructure compound the time and distance barriers for both rural people and their health care providers. This effect is most profound on the rural poor, who cannot afford private automobiles or expensive airplane fares, and must rely on public transportation that is often very inadequate and limited.

Rural health status and health care needs

Health determinants include economic resources, education, the environment, health care, and the involvement and support of family, friends, and society (Fig. 1). Rural people are particularly at risk. Many of the world's poorest people with the least access to economic resources are found in rural areas. In developing countries, rural people tend to be most affected by drought, famine, and lack of basic housing and sanitation. Educational opportunities to break the poverty cycle are often limited and of poor quality locally, and difficult to access at a distance. Those rural students who attend higher education usually do not return to rural areas because of urban employment and other opportunities. Employment in rural areas frequently involves farming, fishing, forestry, and mining; all industries with a high risk of serious occupational injuries that often occur at a remote distance from life- or limb-saving medical care.

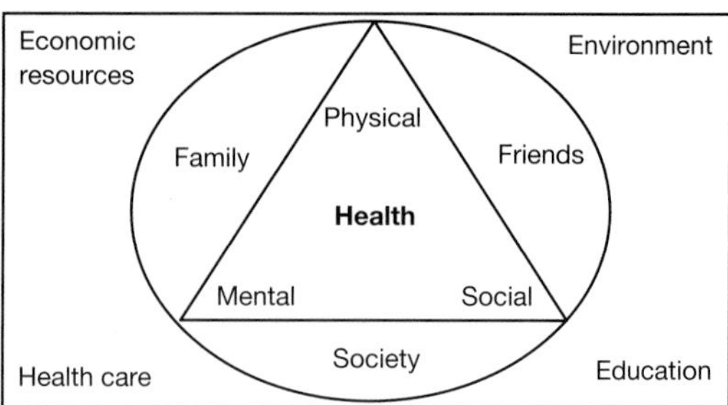

Fig. 1 The health matrix. (Rourke 2001)

Poor maternal and newborn outcomes in rural areas reflect the lack of availability of maternal and newborn care, especially for complications of pregnancy and birth in many rural parts of the world. Time and distance barriers are particularly difficult for rural people with physical and mental disabilities for whom there is often a paucity of local resources and social supports.

The disease and illness pattern in rural areas and hence health care needs, particularly among indigenous people, is often different than that of the general population. Indigenous people represent a special needs group. In most countries, their culture, and indeed their very survival, is at risk. Even in developed countries such as Canada, United States, Australia, and New Zealand, their health determinants, health status, health care access, and health outcomes, including life expectancy, are much worse than the general population.

The Kuching Statement (3rd World Rural Health Conference) affirms the right of indigenous people to health and equitable access to health care, and the need for the involvement of the indigenous population as well as health professionals to achieve these goals.[4,18]

The health care system

Barbara Starfeld has found that '... countries with a strong primary care base to their health care system achieve better outcomes, and at lower costs than countries in which the primary care base is weaker. The absence of a policy to distribute health personnel and facilities to areas of greatest need leads to a concentration of these resources in areas of least need because they are the areas that are most in a position to pay for their presence'.[19]

Health care infrastructure and support for rural primary care varies dramatically from country to country, depending on the country's health care system and resources. The health care system determines the number, mix, education, and distribution of a country's health care providers and thus has a profound effect on rural primary medical care. The role of the rural physician, whether as an independent private practitioner or as a member of a multidisciplinary, integrated team of nurses, nurse practitioners, midwives, physiotherapists, social workers, and other allied health professionals, is largely determined by the existent health care system. All of these personnel as well as traditional healers play important roles in primary health care, interacting closely with both patients and doctors. This chapter will focus, however, on primary medical care provided by rural doctors, rather than the broader primary health care team.

No health care system has been successful at reaching the ideal goal of providing rural people with equitable access to primary medical care. Strong publicly funded health care systems with active programmes to educate, recruit, and support rural physicians tend to be more successful in distributing primary care medical resources than those that rely solely on private enterprise health care market forces. In a patient-pay, private enterprise market force model, the relatively poor rural patient population, combined with the time and distance factors associated with low population density, tends to make rural practice economically unattractive in addition to all the other challenges and difficulties compared with urban practice. The trickle-down theory—increase the number of doctors in a country and some will spill over into the rural areas—has not been successful because of the insatiable health care demands of urban populations combined with the many attractive features of urban practice and living. The council on graduate medical education in the United States found that 'the number of physicians in many rural areas remains inadequate despite the rapid expansion of the nation's physician supply and that expansion of the total physician supply is a very inefficient way of addressing the problem of geographic distribution'.[(20)]

Rural medical practice

Rural medical practice can be defined as 'practice in a non-urban area where most medical care is provided by a few GPs or family doctors with limited or distant access to specialist resources and high technology health care facilities'.[(21)] The rural context of patient care needs, combined with geographic realities of time and distance, and limited or distant specialist and high tech resources, requires many rural physicians to apply a broad scope of practice in relative isolation. An Australian definition describes rural practice as 'medical practice outside urban areas, where the location of the practice obliges some general practitioners to have, or acquire, procedural and other skills not usually required in urban practice'.[(22)] A South African definition of rural medical practice is: 'Health care provided by generalist medical practitioners whose scope of practice includes care that would be provided by specialists in urban areas. It is appropriate technology health care, appropriate to the needs of particular communities that are served. It usually includes elements of family/general practice, public health, and extended procedural work, within the context of primary health care and the Primary Health Care team.'[(23)] 'The practice of medicine in rural America is different from medical practice in urban or suburban America. Rural physicians are called upon to care for a broad range of problems with a limited number of available technological, nursing, and consultant resources.'[(24)]

Rural family physicians have a different practice pattern than urban family physicians. In Canada, for example, in addition to office-based clinic family practice, rural physicians are more likely than urban physicians to do emergency department work, obstetric deliveries, and general anaesthetics, and are more likely to have more than 10 per cent of their practice devoted to aboriginal care.[(25–27)]

Often, the distinction between primary, secondary, and tertiary levels of medical care becomes blurred. For example, in caring for a rural family for many years, a rural family physician may provide office/clinic-based preventive and illness care including immunization and birth control planning, as well as hospital-based maternity care, for the births of the children, emergency care of fractures and lacerations, coronary care for the husband's myocardial infarction, and general anaesthesia for operations like appendectomy, tubal ligation, and cholecystectomy, and then provide house-calls for home-based palliative care of aging parents. In addition, some rural general practitioners perform major intra-abdominal surgery including Caesarean sections.

Many rural physicians provide care in smaller remote villages or areas without a hospital. This may involve long trips for either the patient or the physician or both, and/or distant supervision of care provided by village nurses or nurse practitioners. In many developing countries, the rural general practitioner is involved in public health medicine. Caring for patients with AIDS, both at home and in hospital, has become an increasingly common component of rural primary care in some parts of the world.

John Berger, in *A Fortunate Man*, described the life of John Sassall, a GP in a rural area in the west of England:

> Sassall is accepted by the villagers and foresters as a man who, in the full sense of the term, lives with them. Face to face with him, whatever the circumstances, there is no need for shame or complex explanations: he will understand . . . In general his patients think of Sassall as 'belonging' to their community . . . He is trusted . . . He does more than treat them when they are ill; he is the objective witness of their lives . . . He never separates an illness from the total personality of the patient—in this sense, he is the opposite of a specialist.[(28)]

Rural primary care most often involves living and working in rural communities where, over a period of many years, the rural family physician gets to know patients very well, providing the broad range of care from cradle to death in the office, on house calls, and in the hospital. This provides the opportunity for an extremely varied, intensely personal, and immensely rewarding practice. The author and his wife have had a rural practice in the same community for over 20 years; this has involved obstetric deliveries, emergency department shifts, and the care of a wide variety of in-hospital patients, in addition to their office family practice, house-calls, and nursing home visits. They recognize that the joys of rural practice are also often the greatest challenges, including developing and maintaining the knowledge and skills to provide and teach the broad scope of rural family practice. Often, rural physicians know many of their patients socially as friends or in other roles. This contributes to the richness of rural practice, but also adds a dimension of potential interpersonal challenge, particularly when dealing with critical or personal health care issues in friends as patients.[(29)]

Rural medical practice is full of joys and challenges, often both sides of the same coin. The joy of knowing your patients well, the challenge of knowing your neighbour as your patient; the joy of delivering babies, the challenge of managing serious emergencies with little local specialist backup; the joy of living in cottage country, the challenge of finding time to enjoy it; the joy of raising children in a safe, quiet small town, the challenge of finding educational opportunities to develop each child's potential; the joy of working close enough to home to have lunch with your children, the challenge of limiting on-call to avoid too much family disruption.[(30)]

By its very definition, rural practice is based outside urban areas, and in many cases in quite remote areas. While in some settings this means that rural physicians get to practise and live where others come for recreational holidays, it can also lead to a sense of isolation for rural physicians and their families, particularly in more remote rural locations. For single rural physicians, the prospective pool of potential mates can be depressingly limited, particularly in small and more remote locations. Limited professional job opportunities for spouses of rural physicians and educational opportunities for their children is a factor that deters many physicians from rural practice, and is a factor in the decision of some rural physicians to move to urban practice.

Primary medical care/family physician services should be evenly distributed, and available and accessible for the entire population. The challenge of providing primary rural medical care in both developed and developing countries is compounded by the urban/rural maldistribution of physicians with a worldwide shortage of rural physicians. In the United States, for example, rural counties have about half to two-thirds as many primary care physicians active in patient care, compared with large metropolitan counties.[(31)] In some developing countries, the shortage is extreme. This shortage is compounded by the factor that because many rural family physicians provide hospital-based medical services that are not provided by their urban counterparts, they thus have less time to provide traditional office-based primary medical care. In that regard, an even distribution of primary medical resources would require a higher number of family physicians per capita in rural areas than in urban areas.

A shortage of rural physicians results in a cascade of adverse effects that directly and indirectly affect rural primary care, including reduced patient access to primary care, and the shifting of the provision of rural primary medical care to nurses, nurse practitioners, allied health professionals, and other health care workers. Beyond direct service provision, a shortage results in an increased workload and increased on-call burden for existing rural family physicians. The high work load and burden of on-call can create significant personal and family stress. This can lead to burn-out and transfer to a more sustainable urban-based career, and is also seen as a deterrent for those considering rural practice as a career. Efforts to restrict the amount of on-call time are seen as very important by rural physicians, their families, and prospective rural physicians in training.[(8,32)] Rural communities provide a wonderful opportunity for enjoying small town living and community involvement, yet achieving a professional, personal, and family balance can be a major challenge, given the demands of rural practice.

The education, recruitment, and support of rural physicians are all tied together in developing and sustaining an effective primary care workforce. Given the worldwide shortage of rural physicians and the barriers to rural practice, the development of active programmes to recruit and support rural practice is needed to develop and maintain a sufficient and stable rural primary care workforce.[5] Key components include excellent clinic facilities and support staff team, the limitation of on-call duties, the provision of a reasonable but not overwhelming workload, and financial incentives that include attractive payment models, funded leave for continuing medical education (CME), and long service incentives. Return-of-service contracts may have a limited role, but not as a substitute for improved working conditions, remuneration, and training. Some countries have relied on geographic restrictive licenses for foreign-trained doctors. This is not a sustainable worldwide solution as it encourages doctors to leave developing countries where they are desperately needed, for better pay in developed nations.[33]

Education for rural medical practice

> . . . the country doctor has only himself to rely on: he cannot in every pinch hail specialist, expert and nurse. On his own skill, knowledge, resourcefulness, the welfare of his patient altogether depends. The rural district is therefore entitled to the best trained physician that can be induced to go there.[34]

It is an enormous challenge to educate a sufficient number of physicians with the skills, knowledge, and interest to choose rural practice where they will then apply a broad scope of practice with limited or distant specialist or high-tech resources. Studies of practising rural physicians have found that rural background, rural undergraduate learning experience, and postgraduate rural medical training experiences are associated with rural practice.[35] Medical schools that are located within a large rural region, have a rural focus, encourage admission of rural background students, and provide early and repeated undergraduate rural medical education learning experiences, are most successful at graduating physicians who will choose rural practice as a career. Twelve out of 121 medical schools in the United States produced over 25 per cent of the 15 335 graduates entering rural practice in the United States over a 10-year period.[36] The organization, location, and mission of medical schools is closely related to the propensity of their graduates to select rural practice.[36] International examples of rural-focused medical schools range from the Tromso Medical School in northern Norway, Jichi Medical School in Japan, and Memorial Medical School in Canada.[37–39] The James Cook Medical School in Townsville, Queensland, Australia, began its first enrolment with a rural and Aboriginal focus in January 2000.[40] A Northern Ontario Rural Medical School is being developed in Canada and will be the first new medical school in that country in 40 years.[41]

Rural medical education continues after graduation at the postgraduate training level. Traditionally, students who have graduated and wish to pursue a career in rural practice did a combination of rural family medicine training with some individually arranged electives or programmes to develop additional skills for rural practice. In Australia, Canada, and the United States, however, specific postgraduate rural family medicine training streams have been developed and are currently being expanded to meet the need to train more physicians for rural family practice.[25,27,39,42–44] The specifics of the training for rural family medicine will vary from country to country depending on the roles and skills that the rural family physician will need.

Some developing countries, most notably China, have developed alternative training programmes that begin much earlier (after 9 years of basic education) and are much shorter, to produce 'barefoot physicians' (12 months training) and 'diploma physicians' (3–4 years training). Their practice is then limited to villages, local clinics, and outpatient clinics in rural areas and they are ineligible to practice in cities.[17] This provides a practical reality of some primary medical care for the rural areas but falls short of the theoretical goal of equity of access to quality primary medical care for all.

Continuing medical education remains a challenge for rural family physicians, particularly given the need to develop and maintain the broad scope of skills required, and the time and travel required to attend traditional medical education. Distance learning, the Internet, and telemedicine have produced a wonderful increase in the accessibility of information for the rural family physician. The necessity and value of going away to specific update courses remain. In many countries, continuing medical education courses specifically designed for rural family physicians have been developed, often with the prompting of societies of rural physicians. Advanced Trauma Life Support was developed in northern Nebraska by a rural general surgeon to improve the level of trauma care and has become a worldwide model for practical hands-on skills courses that are useful to rural physicians.[45] Similar courses now exist for obstetric care, neonatal resuscitation, cardiac life support, and other rural emergencies in a variety of formats around the world.

Conclusion

WHO indicators of the quality of primary care include 'accessibility, effectiveness, utilization and the degree of integration into a broad referral system, and performance indicators for essential public health functions'.[11]

Measures of quality of rural primary care can include health status and outcome measures, health care services and workforce measures, and health care consumer access and satisfaction.[46] Effective rural primary medical care can prevent or improve the course of many illnesses, and impact on health status and morbidity and mortality outcome measures. Immunization, pregnancy care, and diabetes management are very different examples that produce measurable outcomes that can be compared to national and international norms. Health care services can be easily measured. Reduced utilization of primary medical services by rural people compared to national levels often indicates difficult access and an inequitable distribution of health care resources. Workforce measures of number and distribution of FP/GPs usually indicate a rural shortage, compared to urban areas, that contributes to reduced quality of primary care. All these measures indicate the worldwide need for major rural health care initiatives to reach the WHO target: 'By 2010 all people will have access throughout their lives to comprehensive, essential, quality health care supported by essential public health functions.'[11]

Strong rural primary medical care is needed to achieve the goal of health for all rural people. The broad scope of practice and responsibilities make rural medical practice one of the most exciting fields of medicine. Rural-oriented medical education is being developed around the world to meet the need to educate and train more physicians with the knowledge, skills, and interest to become rural physicians. Rural practice presents a unique combination of joys and challenges based on population needs, geographic realities, and a broad scope of practice combined with rural life.

Acknowledgements

The author would like to thank Dr Leslie Rourke, Diane Gauley, and Mary Ann Kennard for their assistance with the research and preparation of this chapter.

References

1. **Jones, E.B.** (1997). Historical rural practitioners: role models for the future (Albert Schweitzer). *South African Family Practice* **18** (5), 6.
2. **Reid, S.** (Guest editor) (1997). A positive approach to rural practice. *South African Family Practice* **18** (5), 1–25.
3. **Rourke, J.** et al. (1998). Report from the Second World Rural Health Congress—Durban, South Africa. *The Journal of Rural Health* **14**, 87–90.

4. **Topps, D. and Rourke, J.** (2000). From third world to fourth: third WONCA World Conference on Rural Health in Kuching, Malaysia; fourth in Calgary. *Canadian Family Physician* **46**, 2065.
5. **World Organisation of Family Doctors (WONCA) Working Party on Training for Rural Practice.** *Policy on Training for Rural Practice.* Endorsed by WONCA World Council Meeting on 9 June 1995, Australia (http://www.globalfamilydoctor.com/aboutWonca/working_groups/rural_training/documents.htm).
6. **World Organisation of Family Doctors (WONCA) Working Party on Training for Rural Practice** (1996). Policy on training for rural practice. *Canadian Family Physician* **42**, 1181–3.
7. **World Organisation of Family Doctors (WONCA) Rural Information Technology Exchange (WRITE)**, a subcommittee of the WONCA Working Party on Rural Practice. *Policy on Using Information Technology to Improve Rural Health Care.* Endorsed by the WONCA World Council Meeting on 12 June 1996, Australia 1998 (http://www.globalfamilydoctor.com/aboutWonca/working_groups/rural_training/documents.htm).
8. **World Organisation of Family Doctors (WONCA) Working Party on Rural Practice.** *Policy on Rural Practice and Rural Health.* World Organisation of Family Doctors, Australia 1999 (http://www.globalfamilydoctor.com/aboutWonca/working_groups/rural_training/documents.htm).
9. **World Organisation of Family Doctors (WONCA) Working Party on Rural Practice.** *Calgary Commitment to Women in Rural Family Medical Practice.* Adopted at the 4th World Rural Health Conference in Calgary, Canada, August 2000 (http://www.globalfamilydoctor.com/aboutWonca/working_groups/rural_training/documents.htm).
10. **World Organisation of Family Doctors (WONCA) Working Party on Rural Practice.** 2nd World Rural Health Conference. Health for all Rural People: The Durban Declaration—17 September 1997, Durban, South Africa. *South African Family Practice* **18** (5) inside front cover (http://www.globalfamilydoctor.com/aboutWonca/working_groups/rural_training/documents.htm).
11. **World Health Organization.** *Health for all in the Twenty-First Century.* Geneva: World Health Organization, 2000 (http://www.who.int/archives/hfa/policy.htm).
12. **Pong, R. and Pitblado, R.** (1999). Don't take 'geography' for granted! Some methodological issues in measuring geographic distribution of physicians. *Canadian Journal of Rural Medicine* **6**, 103–12.
13. **Cox, J. and Mungall, I.** (1999). Preface and introduction. In *Rural Healthcare* (ed. J. Cox and I. Mungall), pp. 1–5. Abingdon UK: Radcliffe Medical Press.
14. **Ricketts, T., Johnson-Webb, K., and Randolph, R.** (1999). Populations and places in rural America. In *Rural Health in the United States* (ed. T. Ricketts), pp. 7–24. New York: Oxford University Press.
15. **Rock, A.** Speech by Allan Rock, the Canadian Minister of Health, 132nd Annual General Meeting of the Canadian Medical Association, 23 August 1999, Ottawa, Canada.
16. **Reid, S., Couper, I., and Noble, V.** (2001). Rural medical practice in South Africa. In *Textbook of Rural Medicine* (ed. J. Geyman, T. Norris, and G. Hart), pp. 436–7. Toronto: McGraw-Hill.
17. **Schwarz, R.** et al. (2001). Rural Practice in China. In *Textbook of Rural Medicine*, pp. 449–71. Toronto: McGraw-Hill.
18. **WONCA Working Party on Rural Practice.** *The Health of Indigenous Peoples: The Kuching Statement.* Adopted at the 3rd World Rural Health Congress, Kuching, Malaysia, 1999 (http://www.wonca.org/working_groups/rural_training/kuching_statement.htm).
19. **Starfield, B.** *Primary Care: Balancing Health Needs, Services, and Technology.* Toronto: Oxford University Press, 1998, p. 401.
20. **United States. Department of Health and Human Services Council on Graduate Medical Education** (1998). Physician distribution health care challenges in rural and inner city areas. The Department, Washington, DC.
21. **Rourke, J.** (1997). In search of a definition of 'rural'. *Canadian Journal of Rural Medicine* **2**, 113–15.
22. **Strasser, R.** (1995). Rural general practice: is it a distinct discipline? *Australian Family Physician* **24**, 870–6.
23. **Couper, I.** *Definitions of Rural and Underserviced. Rural Health Task Force (RuDASA) Team—Discussion Document.* Rural Doctors' Association, South Africa: 2001.
24. **Yawn, B., Bushy, A., and Yawn, R.** (1994). Preface. In *Exploring Rural Medicine: Current Issues and Concepts* (ed. B. Yawn, A. Bushy, and R. Yawn), pp. xix–xx. Thousand Oaks USA: Sage Publications.
25. **Rourke, J.** (2000). Rural practice in Canada. In *Textbook of Rural Medicine* (ed. J. Geyman, T. Norris, and G. Hart), pp. 395–409. Toronto: McGraw-Hill.
26. **College of Family Physicians of Canada.** *CFPC JANUS Project: Family Physicians Meeting the Needs of Tomorrow's Society.* Mississauga, 1997.
27. **College of Family Physicians of Canada Working Group on Rural Family Medicine Education** (Rourke, J., Chair) (1999). *Postgraduate Education for Rural Family Practice: Vision and Recommendations for the New Millennium.* The College, Mississauga. *Canadian Family Physician* **45**, 2698–704. (http://www.cfpc.ca/education/rural/ruralpaperfull.asp)
28. **Berger, J. and Mohr, J.** *A Fortunate Man.* New York: Pantheon Books, 1967, pp. 100, 101, 109, 113.
29. **Rourke, L. and Rourke, J.** (1998). Close friends as patients in rural practice. *Canadian Family Physician* **44**, 1208–10.
30. **Rourke, J.** *The Future of Rural Family Medicine.* D.I. Rice Lecture, St. John's, Canada, 7 September, 2001.
31. **Larson, E. and Hart, G.** (2001). The rural physician. In *Textbook of Rural Medicine* (ed. J. Geyman, T. Norris, and G. Hart), pp. 27–40. Toronto: McGraw-Hill.
32. **Canadian Medical Association** (2000). Rural and remote practice issues. *Canadian Medical Association Journal* **163**, 1047–50.
33. **Bundred, P. and Levitt, C.** (2000). Medical migration: who are the real losers? *The Lancet* **356**, 245–6.
34. **Flexner, A.** *Medical Education in the United States and Canada: A Report to the Carnegie Foundation for the Advancement of Teaching.* New York: Carnegie Foundation for the Advancement of Teaching, Bulletin 4, 1910, pp. 47–8.
35. **Rourke, J.** *Education for Rural Medical Practice: Goals and Opportunities, an Annotated Bibliography.* Moe, Australia: Monash University, 1996.
36. **Rosenblatt, R.** et al. (1992). Which medical schools produce rural physicians? *Journal of the American Medical Association* **268**, 1559–65.
37. **Magnus, J. and Tollan, A.** (1993). Rural doctor recruitment: does medical education in rural districts recruit doctors to rural areas? *Medical Education* **27**, 250–3.
38. **Inoue, K., Hirayama, Y., and Igarashi, M.** (1997). A medical school for rural areas. *Medical Education* **31**, 430–4.
39. **Rourke, J. and Strasser, R.** (1996). Education for rural practice in Canada and Australia. *Academic Medicine* **71**, 464–9.
40. **Hays, R.** (2001). Australia's new medical school. *Medical Education* **35**, 500.
41. **Rourke, J.** (2002). Building the new Northern Ontario Rural Medical School. *Australian Journal of Rural Health* **10**, 112–16.
42. **Hays, R.** (2001). Rural Practice in Australia. In *Textbook of Rural Medicine* (ed. J. Geyman, T. Norris, and G. Hart), pp. 411–21. Toronto: McGraw-Hill.
43 **Rosenthal, T.**, ed. (2000). Special issue: Rural-based graduate medical education. *The Journal of Rural Health* **16**, 181–306.
44. **Rourke, J., Newbery, P., and Topps, D.** (2000). Training an adequate number of rural family physicians. *Canadian Family Physician* **46**, 1245–8.
45. **Collicott, P.** (1979). Advanced Trauma Life Support Course, an improvement in rural trauma care. *Nebraska Medical Journal* **64**, 279–80.
46. **World Organisation of Family Doctors (WONCA) Working Party on Rural Practice.** Document: policy on quality and effectiveness of rural health care. WONCA Council, 2002. (www.globalfamilydoctor.com/aboutWonca/working_groups/rural_training/quality/Quality_of_Rural_Healthcare.htm)

1.8 First contact care in developing health care systems

Peter Underwood, Mohammed Ali, and Alan Owen

In important ways, all health systems suffer from under-development, not just those in 'developing' countries. If equity of access is not guaranteed, the most affluent health spending will not result in improved health for all. Equitable opportunities for improved health have to be built in at the point where help is most needed. In this chapter we focus on the situation in the poorer, or developing, countries and examine the range of persons who are consulted at 'first contact' by a sick person, where the primary medical practitioner is only one of a range of likely contacts.

Since developing countries are far from homogeneous, and vary dramatically in their social structure, the health systems that grow out of them also vary. Further, these countries are in a state of unprecedented flux, and these fundamental changes influence disease, health and health seeking in a multitude of ways. Nevertheless, some broad patterns are common, and it is these we try to draw out in this chapter. This involves some preliminary generalizations, with specific examples drawn from several widely different developing countries. Our purpose is to add a sense of the diversity of these societies, and some human colour and pathos.

This chapter has four sections. The first outlines the social and economic features of Third World societies. In particular, it involves consideration of what is meant by 'developing societies', and how and why these are changing so rapidly. The second section looks more specifically at the health improvements that some, and not other, poor societies have experienced. Thirdly, we look more closely at a case study of what happens when the poor get sick. Finally, the chapter examines some of the barriers—local, national, and global—standing in the way of better health, and better primary health care services.

'Developing countries': what are they?

The term 'developing' is often used interchangeably with 'Third World', or 'South' or 'Non-Western'. We use the term 'developing' here to mean poor, with an emphasis on the problems of those most poor residing in the poorer countries. This qualification of the word 'developing' acknowledges the serious consequences of 'development' to the ecosystems on which our whole species depends.

To sketch the context, let us jump backwards to Africa, nearly half a century ago; it was then that David Morley, a young British paediatrician, took up a post in the hinterland of Nigeria. As well as clinical duties, he led a small research team that followed up all the babies born in a local village. The experience changed the way he understood disease and the services designed to combat it—within a poor and 'emerging' country.

Fifteen years later in 1973, he wrote *Paediatric Priorities in the Developing World*,[1] which set out the essential facts about the developing world, its health, and the role and limitations of doctors and health services. He concluded that medical services—primary, secondary, and tertiary—were largely inappropriate, and needed radical restructuring. Much of what Morley had to say then is relevant and challenging now, and a useful starting point for an examination of primary care in the developing world.

He began by describing the salient social, economic, and demographic characteristics of developing countries, noting that these factors—which govern not only the prevalent pattern of illness, but also their health services—had been strangely neglected by planners. 'Poor, rural, and young' were the features that stood out as distinguishing the peoples of 'developing' countries from those more affluent. Health services designed for populations that were wealthier, older, and mainly lived in industrial cities, as is the case in the West, were simply out of place.

Morley placed the health problems of developing countries clearly into a global context. With nearly 80 per cent of the world's (then) population of 4.5 billion living in the developing world, he noted mortality rates particularly among the young were further skewed, with deaths for under fives in developing countries accounting for over 95 per cent of global under fives' deaths.

Almost 30 years later, and after many changes, how poor, rural, young, and burdened by disease are the developing countries now?

Twenty years on, McMichael wrote *Planetary Overload*,[2] which marks a watershed. In 1993, with the world population rising to about 5.3 billion, about 820 million or 16 per cent could be called rich, with an average income of about US$20 000. The very poor, with an average per capita income as low as US$330, mainly reside in the huge regions of South Asia or Sub-Saharan Africa. Those classified as middle income, with average annual incomes ranging from US$1800 to 2400, are those mainly in the Middle Eastern, Eastern European, or South American regions.

Overall the world's population had risen, and so had its wealth, with some developing countries rising from poor to middle-income status. But many countries had not moved forward. McMichael notes that, while the number of persons living in 'absolute poverty', defined as an annual income of less than US$370, had shown a slight relative decline over the previous 20 years, actual numbers had risen. In the developing countries, which then made up 3.7 billion or 70 per cent of the world's total, about 30 per cent could be classified as living in absolute poverty. This means that about one in five of the world's inhabitants still lived in conditions so degraded by poverty to remain—in the words of former World Bank President McNamara as quoted by McMichael—'beneath any reasonable definition of human decency'.[2]

By 2002, the world population has risen further to 6.1 billion.[3] However, the number of the poorest amounts to 1.2 billion, and has changed little.[4] Not only does poverty remain the biggest problem, but the relative youth of developing countries has also not changed: for those very poor, almost half of those living in absolute poverty remain less than 15 years old.[5]

However, important changes have occurred. The poorest of the poor are not as 'rural' as they were when David Morley left Lagos for Nigeria's hinterland in 1956: they are in Lagos itself, and the dozens of vast cities sprouting in other developing countries. The last 30 years has been marked by massive migrations of communities from the countryside to the city. This process of urbanization now means that while the majority of the populations of developing countries can still be classified as rural, the proportion is falling, and many of the poorest—fleeing poverty, famine, and war—are now to be found in vast cities like Lagos and Dhaka. Lagos has grown by 6 per cent, and Dhaka by 7 per cent per year since 1975, so that the population of Lagos has increased fourfold, and Dhaka sixfold, so that by 2000 both had populations exceeding 10 million, so joining the class of mega-cities.[3]

While some migrants have 'made good' in the cities, whole generations of slum dwellers remain, inheriting many of the unhealthy conditions of their rural cousins—poor food and water, and little medical care. Adding problems more specific to the city, including those arising from overcrowding, and the stresses of drugs and violence, increases the disease burdens on the poor. The attenuation of older and more traditional social structures also means it may be harder to pass on limited but useful indi-genous healing and support practices. Work too is different: the new city dwellers—or the more fortunate of them—can now find work in factories making clothing, textiles, or machinery, as global capital moves in search of cheaper labour.[6]

Morley's other distinguishing characteristic of the people of the developing world—their overwhelming share of the burden of disease—remains. Table 1, showing some representative data on several selected low, middle, and high income countries, indicates not only the much lower life expectancy in the poorer countries, but also their peoples' even more greatly reduced chance of a life—as measured as a 'healthy life'—relatively free of disability and disease. Note also the higher proportion of the older population, and lower fertility rates of the richer countries.

Table 1 Demographic and health parameters of low, middle, and high income countries

Country	Gross national income/capita in US$	% Pop >60 years	Total fertility rate (%)	Life expectancy at birth (years)		Healthy life expectancy at birth (years)	
				M	F	M	F
Low income countries							
Laos	290	5.6	5.1	52.2	56.1	43.7	45.7
Central African Republic	290	6.1	5.1	41.6	42.6	34.7	33.6
Bolivia	1 000	6.2	4.1	60.9	63.6	51.4	51.4
Middle income countries							
Thailand	2 010	8.1	2.1	66.0	72.4	57.7	61.8
Malaysia	3 380	6.6	3.1	68.3	74.1	59.7	63.4
Mexico	5 080	6.9	2.6	71.0	76.2	63.1	65.3
High income countries							
Australia	20 530	16.3	1.8	76.6	82.1	69.6	73.3
UK	24 500	20.6	1.7	74.8	79.9	69.9	71.4
USA	34 260	16.1	2.0	73.9	79.5	67.2	68.8

Adapted from: (1) World Health Organization (2001). *World Health Report 2001*. Geneva: WHO. (2) World Bank (2001). *World Development Indicators 2001*. Washington DC: World Bank.

Looking beyond the figures, let us now consider what they mean in every day terms for the 1000 million living in 'absolute poverty' in 'developing countries'. It is these people that carry by far the greatest burden of the world's disease, and the greatest challenge to health planners and practitioners—just as Morley concluded in 1973. Further, while an increasing number fill the slums of the great conurbations of the Third World, more than half of these people still live in rural areas, in thousands of villages scattered across Asia, or Africa and South America, living a hand-to-mouth existence as subsistence farmers or landless labourers.

The multiple burdens consist of fitful and insufficient disposable income, poor and unhygienic living conditions, food deficient in quantity and quality, large family size, low education, and poor access to basic health services. These combine to produce a web of direct and indirect forces which together create the conditions where disease is fomented. Preventive and curative responses to disease are also hindered: thus such persons cannot, to quote the recent WHO jargon,[7] join the 'rising curve of health' that others more fortunate are joining, both in their own countries, and in the West.

Changing patterns of health and disease in developing countries

Despite the dismal picture for the majority of the poorer populations of the world, it is clear that for some, health has improved greatly. This section examines reasons for this.

In the broadest and simplest terms, health status can be measured by life expectancy, and by mortality rates; in particular the infant mortality rate (IMR) has often been used as a way to measure the relative level of prevailing health between countries, and within countries over time. As indicated in Table 1, in general life expectancy rises, and mortality rates tend to fall as income rises. Fertility rates follow the pattern of mortality rates.

The demography of most poor countries can be characterized as being high mortality, high fertility, low life expectancy; in richer countries the pattern is the opposite—low fertility, low mortality, high life expectancy. We now know that the change from one pattern to another, now called the demographic transition, has already occurred in western countries over the period from about the mid-nineteenth to the mid-twentieth century. In many of the poorer countries, the process is occurring much later.

It is only recently that the shape of this transition process, and the underlying reasons for it, are becoming understood. Such an analysis is not just of academic interest, it is vital for understanding the influence of health care, and of the key role of primary care within it.

Figure 1, taken from the 1999 WHO Annual Report[7] links time, income, and IMR: it complements the relatively simple picture arising from Table 1.

Figure 1 shows that in both the upper curve for 1952, and the lower curve for 1992, IMR falls as income rises. However, for any given level of income, in the 40-year period between the curves, IMR has almost halved, indicating that factors other than income are playing a major role in mortality reduction. The report goes on to draw on this and other evidence now available, indicating that however important income may be, these other factors—including access to health technology, and female education—are crucial.

In understanding this transition process, a further area has recently come into prominence. Marmot and Wilkinson[8] highlight the emergence—or more accurately the re-emergence—of key *social* determinants of health. This research is now beginning to establish that after the earliest stages of the health transition, human autonomy—individual and community—and equitable human relationships are fundamental to human mental and physical health: without them, we are almost as badly off as if we had nothing to eat.

In summary, the health transition, which follows the demographic transition, now appears to arise from several inter-related factors. Rising income is essential to lift the poorest from their dreadful base, so they can join 'the rising curve of health'. But it is capacity building—'social capital'—investments in education, in public health and housing, in equitable distributions and services—including basic health services—that then builds the fertile conditions that make sturdy those millions of little plants, our human lives. And in particular, researchers such as Starfield have defined how medical care, and especially primary medical care, influence patterns of health and disease.[9]

Against this backdrop, how do the primary care systems of the developing world fit into a process of health system development?

First contact: what happens when the poor get sick

We now move from the big picture to an individual human story—the story of a woman we call Kulsum, and as recorded by a researcher, Dr Amatul Uzma,[10] investigating the health care seeking behaviour of post-partum mothers living in a slum in Dhaka, the capital of Bangladesh.

The reader should first try to picture the slum: a swampy plot of about 2 ha containing over 5000 squatters, packed into over 700 flimsy structures

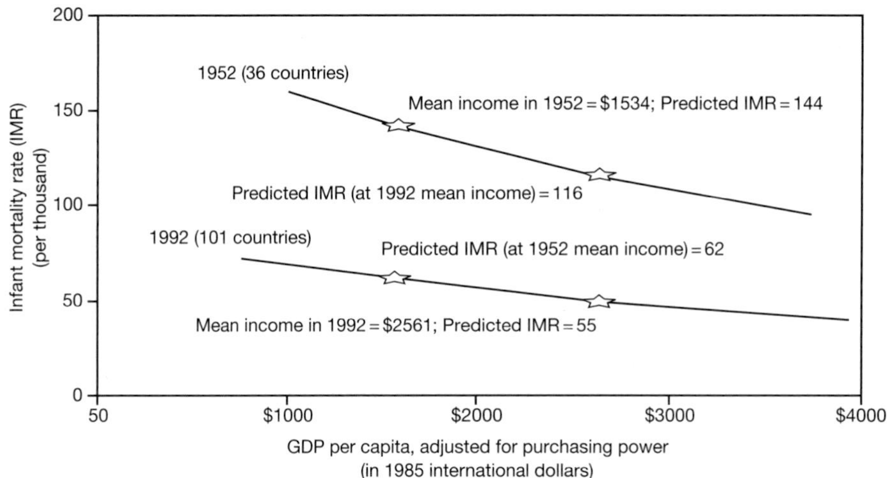

Fig. 1 The role of improvements in income in reducing infant mortality rates. (Reprinted from: World Health Organization (1999). Health and development in the 20th Century. In *World Health Report 1999*. Geneva: WHO, p. 5.)

with no running water or power, ranging from a few bits of tattered cloth, to a tiny shack of tin and boards. In the case below, our own comments are added in square brackets.

Kulsum had spent the first 13 years of her life in a poor rural village; her father was a landless farmer, and she was one of seven living children. Before puberty she was married off to Suruj Mia, and two years later, a thin 15 year old, she gave birth to her first son.

Eventually her husband reported, 'She was too thin to be a wife. I thought she would get big after having kids but it was the other way round. The more she had children, the more she became thin.' Suruj Mia stated that Kulsum was ill for all of her pregnancies, and could not adequately undertake her domestic tasks.

Her fragility became worse with each pregnancy. Said her husband: 'My mother told me that there is an *asor* (bad spirit) with Kulsum, and we did everything to get rid of it. You won't understand this. You are town people. There are lots of bad spirits. We treated her with *kabiraji* (herbal medicine), and used the *mowlanas* (spiritual healer). (But) . . . she had a strong *asor*.'

(During her first four pregnancies, all in the rural village, she never consulted either a doctor, or a 'western care provider,' relying on her family, and the local healers, here the herbalist and spiritual healer. Together they provided care at delivery and various herbs, potions and rituals.)

At aged 20, (escaping rural poverty and natural disaster), the (nuclear) family moved to Dhaka, and the slum. Three further pregnancies followed. There she visited the local TBA (Traditional Birth Attendant, who practises a mixture of traditional and some western care, and conducts most of the births in the slum for a small fee). Further, during the sixth of her 8 pregnancies, for the first time she had consulted a western doctor: escorted by a (government) health worker from a local clinic, she had attended a government hospital, and received tetanus toxoid. And, further, she had been told she had a serious disease, and needed urgent treatment.

'The doctors said that she had *jokkah* (local dialect for tuberculosis),' said her husband, 'and that she had to take medicines for 18 months, and should never get pregnant again. They asked her to deliver the baby in hospital, and they would do something to make her sterile. They wanted me to take her to another hospital (Dhaka Chest Hospital). I have never heard of a disease for which you are supposed to take medicine for 18 months and for which you should not get pregnant. Pregnancy . . . is controlled by God . . . I think she was responsible for what had happened . . . . She never listened to me or my mother . . . her movements during her pregnancies were wild . . . She attracted evil spirits . . .'

(As a result of these beliefs, and also because of cost, despite her own apparent willingness, Kulsum did not attend the chest hospital, and did not receive treatment for her tuberculosis). During her eighth, and final pregnancy, despite further herbal and traditional treatments, she became increasingly ill. Eventually she went into labour, but became distressed, and the TBA was called. Soon after her arrival, the patient collapsed into coma. She was transferred by 'baby taxi' (motorised three wheeler) to the local government hospital, but died in hospital immediately after the birth of a live baby.

Kulsum was then 26 years old. She left 7 living children, including the newborn, a husband Suruj Mia, a rickshaw puller, in their one room shack in the slum of Dhaka.

This single case history illustrates many of the characteristics of developing societies outlined above: Kulsum is poor, and young, a rural migrant to the great city, and cut off by poverty, lack of knowledge and personal autonomy from care that could have saved her life. Her poignant trajectory illustrates clearly the nature of 'first contact' care as experienced by many of the world's poorest.

Influenced by a host of inter-related factors, Kulsum seeks care from a wide variety of persons. These include: proximity and availability; cost; gender and appropriateness to her (and crucially her husband's) understanding of her illness; and the severity and stage of her symptoms. 'First contact care'—the first set of persons chosen by the patient and their family to attend them in their illness—is an intricate, dynamic and individualized process. While complex, it can be understood, and we now have a better picture of the way it works.

Helman's approachable text[(11)] reminds us that any society's health system is an integral part of the society itself: it grows from it. Landy[(12)] points out that a health system has two inter-related aspects, *cultural* and *social*. The *cultural* includes basic ideas, normative practices and shared modes of perception; the *social* includes the specified roles of carer and cared, and the rules governing these settings in different places, such as the home, health centre, and hospital.

In the West, our example might be reduced to 'the natural history of a case of TB'. Yet essentially Kulsum moves through a set of cultural and social encounters as she, and those around her, pursue a response that might help them, and one that matches their understanding of the problem, and the resources available.

Another way of building an understandable model of this experience is offered by Kleinman.[(13)] He suggests that in any system, three overlapping and interconnected sectors are operating: *the popular, folk*, and *professional*. Here, we see the first group to which Kulsum turns is the *popular* sector; this is the lay or non-professional domain. The dominant options here are self-treatment, or advice or care from relatives. While Kulsum herself did not engage in much self-treatment, or appear to make use of medicines from the thriving bunch of drug stores on the edge of the slum, Uzma's research[10] demonstrates their crucial role in the 'medical system' of the slum, a point of far-reaching importance explored later.

Kleinman's second domain, the *folk* sector, at one stage seemed to dominate only in developing societies, but now is re-emerging strongly as 'alternative medicine' in Western countries. Here individuals specialize in forms of healing that are either sacred (Kulsum's *mowlanas*) or secular (the *kabiraji*). These folk healers form a heterogeneous group, with extraordinary cultural variation in style, outlook, type of payment, and rules of entry and training.[11]

But essential in understanding the pluralism of newly emerging service providers is to note how many groups—particularly the folk healers—are beginning to fuse 'alternative' components to their more traditional treatments—including key allopathic medications rising from Western bio-medicine. This has been called the 'indigenization of Western medicine',[14] a process potentially fertile for outcomes both useful and harmful to health.

The following example, taken from the early work of one of the authors,[15] and as quoted by Helman, provides a case that illustrates a striking version of this process as seen in a country emerging from centuries of isolation. 'An example of a . . . secular (folk) healer, is the *sahi* as described by the Underwoods in Raymah, in the Yemen Arab Republic. These healers have only appeared . . . in recent years, and their practice consists (almost entirely) of giving injections of western drugs. They have little training . . . and limited diagnostic (or) counselling skills. To the inhabitant of Raymah, however, the *sahi* practises what is considered to be the quintessence of western medicine—'the treatment of illness by injections.'[11]

The original description went on to note that the recent arrival of the *sahi* is a mixed blessing for the poor *Raymis*. While some individuals benefit from the injections, particularly injections of antibiotics, the service is not only expensive but often actually dangerous. It also diverts understanding from the actual causes of ill-health.[15]

Helman notes the growing popularity of injections (and *injectionists*) in many other Third World countries. In Kenya, for instance, 'untrained bush doctors administer medicines and injections', and 'street and bus-depot doctor boys' hustle antibiotic capsules.[11] In a useful recent description from South Africa, Cocks and Dold[14] report the use of indigenous and indigenized Western medicine integrated into the local and 'traditional' *amayeza* system.

Kleinman's third sector—the *professional*—represents those persons organized and legally sanctioned as medical and paramedical members of the system. As Kulsum's story shows, even in a country as poor as Bangladesh, the government-sponsored health system does have outreach to the poorest. At one stage, the sick woman reached a local health centre worker, who referred her to a hospital and eventually to an allopathic 'Western' trained physician. There she received a crucial piece of information—a diagnosis of a serious but treatable disease. However, fatefully, this life-saving knowledge was not acted upon.

The *professional* sector has until recently been the focus for health planners, as they seek to combat the terrible health indices of the poor in developing countries. Yet a growing recognition of the pluralism of the health system—and particularly of the burgeoning growth of the 'private sector' in both the folk and professional sectors—has led many to revise this emphasis on the professional sector in general, and that part of it sponsored through government in particular.

An example of this approach comes from the work of Berman.[16] He argues that many people—not just the poor like Kulsum, but many more fortunate in wealth and education—'vote with their feet'. They attend a bewildering range of private healers who vary from private Western allopaths, to the drug stores of Dhaka's slums, the *amayeza* practitioners of South Africa, or the *sahi* of Yemen. This private sector provides something like half the health care of the sick of the developing world—and so can no longer be neglected by planners and researchers.

Despite appearances to the contrary, there is a consistent logic in this: like Morley 30 years before, Berman is saying—let us see what is there, and where the problems are, and direct our scarce resources accordingly. Such an emphasis should not be seen to allocate special privileges to the 'hidden hand' of the 'competitive market'—for it 'assigns priority to social development, not to the consumption-driven throughput of energy and materials.[6]

Summary: overcoming barriers to improved health services in developing counties

In this chapter, we began by outlining the distinguishing features of developing countries, and of the health problems they face. We cited evidence to indicate that the poorest still share an overwhelming burden of the world's disease, and that they require basic economic improvements to lift them onto the 'curve of rising health'. Nevertheless health services, as one of several key investments in 'social capital', can contribute significantly to move the poorest people along the curve, and so towards a longer, and a healthier life. It is now becoming clearer that it is primary care—providing the crucial interface with most of the sick—that offers the best returns from investment in health services. The miasma of poverty, a diseased environment, lack of education, and personal powerlessness, build insurmountable barriers between the sick person and what Schumacher[17] called so powerfully, 'the useful knowledge' that can preserve life.

What then can be done to lower some of these barriers to improved health for the poorest of the world's poor? Schumacher outlined the ingredients of a way forward at the same time Morley published his Nigerian prescription. He described the importance of questioning conventional economics and principles of growth, sought small-scale structures and solutions, promoted intermediate technologies, and taught reverence for the earth: these, we feel, are now even more relevant as the social basis of health is understood better.

Finally, we present three recommendations designed to focus the issues for readers of a textbook of primary medical care: they are not narrowly medical, drawing on the larger context that has been the emphasis of this chapter.

First, in every forum, as health workers we must speak up for the *big issues*, for it is they that make the biggest difference to health. A society whose wealth is evenly spread, that is fair, and peaceful, and in which all members play a respected role, and whose institutions are robust, participatory and accessible, will build healthier individuals and communities. Systems built on these core principles will be 'cheaper' to run, less invasive and more sustainable.

Second, within our clinics, health centres, hospitals, and teaching and research institutions, we should work at reforming the health sector so that it should be—as both Morley and Schumacher recommended so long ago—distributed better to where the people, and particularly the poorer people, are. That means systems that are more 'generalized' to address the basic and common and treatable health problems of the many. It also implies trade-offs within health systems to make them less specialized towards the rarer and less treatable conditions of the few, and more focused on prevention and care. This recognizes the central contribution that primary care—still so often the poor relation of health services—can make to improvements in health.

Third, while professional medicine has developed many effective therapies, it does not, nor should it, own them. First contact care has a rich range, of which 'professional' Western-based primary medical care is only a part. Improving the way the parts work together needs increased research and investment. We now know something of the therapies that work; many of these are already in the private and folk sectors which provide half the care to the world's sick. If primary health care is to become the core of the system, not just the entry point to a conduit into specialized and expensive interventions, it needs greater attention. Despite difficulties great and small, primary care for the poorest can be made more accessible, appropriate, participatory and sustaining of human community, itself the wellspring of physical and mental health.

After these recommendations comes the warning.

Here, we have emphasized the importance of recognizing the burden of ill-health that, in a global sense falls on the world's poor. But, since it threatens the whole species, the environmental crisis must also be recognized as the *biggest issue*. In reference to McMichael,[2] we used the term 'watershed'. The turning point it marks is the recognition that not only are the ecosystems of the earth—on which we all depend—'overloaded', but much of the cause is not the poor, but the minority of the rich who produce three quarters of the planet's pollution. His further analysis in 2001 recommends a 'more far-sighted approach ... (where) efficiency, fairness and sustainability should become the joint and interdependent goals of our social and economic policies.[6]

Thus, in an ironic twist, while in the shorter term it is the poor that are over-burdened with disease, in the longer term it is the rich that are burdening, indeed making sick, the very planet which provides us all with our sustenance. And it is 'development'—particularly that coarse version that is dependent on the exhaustion of the planet's reserves and the pollution of its systems—which is largely responsible. Globally, the pursuit of health should best start with those humans most in need. Yet while this is necessary, it is not sufficient—and so the focus must be widened beyond her children to include the well-being of Mother Earth herself.

We conclude that the examination of 'first contact care in developing countries', our vital starting point, should encourage us to work also at improving our contact with the Earth. Nurturing both this Earth and those humans who are poor and marginalized is not simply being kindly, it is practical good sense, and good public health. And is a true investment, paying off manifold for all of us.[18]

References

1. **Morley, D.** *Paediatric Priorities in the Developing World.* London: Butterworth, 1973.
2. **McMichael, A.J.** *Planetary Overload. Global Environmental Change and the Health of the Human Species.* Cambridge: Cambridge University Press, 1993.
3. **United Nations Department of Economic and Social Affairs Population Division.** *Population, Environment and Development. The Concise Report.* E/CN.9/2001/2. New York: United Nations, 2001.
4. **World Bank.** *World Development Report 2000/2001. Attacking Poverty.* New York: Oxford University Press, 2000.
5. **Fornos, W.** (1998). No vacancy: curbing the population explosion. *The Humanist* **58** (4), 15–18.
6. **McMichael, T.** *Human Frontiers, Environments and Disease. Past Patterns, Uncertain Futures.* Cambridge: Cambridge University Press, 2001, p. 337.
7. **World Health Organization.** Health and development in the 20th century. In *World Health Report 1999*, pp. 1–12. Geneva: WHO, 1999.
8. **Marmot, M. and Wilkinson, R.** *Social Determinants of Health.* New York: Oxford University Press, 1999.
9. **Starfield, B.** *Primary Care: Balancing Health Needs, Services and Technology.* New York: Oxford University Press, 1998.
10. **Uzma, A.** (1996). Mothers' health during the postpartum period in an urban slum of Dhaka, Bangladesh. Unpublished MMedSci thesis. University of Western Australia. Nedlands.
11. **Helman, C.** *Culture, Health and Illness* 4th edn. Oxford: Butterworth/Heinemann, 2000.
12. **Landy, D.** (1977). Medical systems in transcultural perspective. In *Culture, Disease and Healing: Studies in Medical Anthropology* (ed. D. Landy). London: Macmillan.
13. **Kleinman, A.** *Patients and Healers in the Context of Culture.* San Francisco CA: University of California Press, 1980.
14. **Cocks, M. and Dold, A.** (2000). The role of 'African chemists' in the health care system of the Eastern Cape province in South Africa. *Social Science and Medicine* **51**, 1505–15.
15. **Underwood, P. and Underwood, Z.** (1981). New spells for old: expectations and realities of Western Medicine in a remote tribal society in Yemen, Arabia. In *Changing Disease Patterns and Human Behaviour* (ed. N.F. Stanley and R.A. Joske). London: Academic Press.
16. **Berman, P.** (2000). Organization of ambulatory care provision: a critical determinant of health system performance in developing countries. *Bulletin of the World Health Organization* **78**, 791–802.
17. **Schumacher, E.F.** Small is Beautiful. A Study of Economics as if People Mattered. London: Sphere Books, 1973.
18. **McMichael, A. and Beaglehole, R.** (2000). The changing global context of public health. *Lancet* **356**, 495–9.

1.9 Management and leadership

J. Lloyd Michener, Lawrence R. Wu, and Victoria S. Kaprielian

Introduction

Family physicians are often called on to improve care for patients beyond those they see in day-to-day practice. Familiarity with multiple medical disciplines makes family physicians particularly well suited for leadership roles. Unfortunately, these are also roles that many find difficult and perplexing. This chapter will explore the ways in which leadership of health care systems differs from the normal role of clinicians, review the skills needed for management and leadership positions, outline some common errors, and offer suggestions for succeeding as a leader.

The role of the clinical leader has a number of similarities to the role of the clinician. Both have to listen carefully, develop hypotheses, gather information, obtain consent, implement plans, periodically confirm plans are working, and make changes as needed. However, the apparent similarity with clinical care is deceptive.

Clinical care generally occurs in the familiar environment of the office, with patients and staff whose roles are understood. Success is earned by managing individual patients well, one at a time. Leadership positions require stepping out of this comfortable environment into settings where the roles are unclear, problems are rooted in poorly functioning systems or work culture, and the expertise and authority of the physician is not assumed. Success in leadership positions is earned by managing systems of care (rather than individual patients), and leading teams of coworkers.

Leadership roles have two components. The *manager role* oversees and solves day-to-day problems, such as assuring that a clinic is adequately staffed, and hiring and giving feedback to colleagues. In contrast, the *leadership role* requires changing the structure and course of an organization. In practice, the two roles often overlap. A successful leader will often master the managerial role, then use that experience to lead wider change.

Breaking these roles into tasks and needed skills can simplify life for those who are new to the roles. The following examples are common management tasks that one is likely to encounter in practice.

Tasks of the clinical manager

Delivery of services

Each organization has operations to manage. While physicians are familiar with care of individual patients, the physician manager must become familiar with the steps by which patients make appointments, register, the length of time they wait, and how they are prepared for the physician visit. The physician manager must be able to coordinate services so they work well for patients as well as for the staff and physicians.

Decision-making

The success of a health care team depends on agreement among the team members. Questions ranging from the types of drugs to stock in a clinic to the frequency of on-call coverage require decision-making processes that the manager must initiate and supervise. Methods of decision-making include routine meetings of the health care team, executive decisions, task forces, and decision by a third party such as a board of directors. When the answer is obvious to everyone and/or has little consequence, process matters less and the manager can often decide unilaterally. When the issue is controversial or the consequences important, agreeing to a decision process is critical. A good manager will try to involve peers in these instances.

Assessing medical quality

Periodic accreditation of the clinic operations by an external group such as, in the United States, the Joint Commission on Accreditation of Healthcare Organizations, can be a benchmark of quality, highly regarded by purchasers and patients. To achieve such accreditation, the manager must develop and enforce policies and participate in quality improvement activities.

Personnel issues

The quality of the team depends on the selection and training of the people who make up the team. The physician leader needs to be able to recruit and retain high-quality colleagues through interviewing, selection, and salary negotiation. Once recruited, the physician leader must assure that the new physicians are oriented to the workplace.

The physician manager is the most credible agent in giving feedback to peers. Persistent trends such as being late for the first consultation, delinquent medical records, or patient complaints about attitudes or communication are instances when feedback to a clinician peer is warranted. Proper feedback focuses on behaviours that can be changed, is timely, and is communicated privately. Even more effective is praise when a peer or staff does something right.

Finances

Clinical managers must make decisions or provide input to the yearly budget. In private practice settings, physicians may seek to increase revenue collection. When resources are scarce, costs must be managed wisely. A knowledgeable clinician can assist administrative personnel in prioritizing spending needs, and help the practice live within its budget.

Administrative time

Managing operations and working with staff requires undivided attention, just as does individual patient care. Even though many physician managers continue to provide clinical care, some time dedicated to administration is vital. Making managerial decisions during patient care sessions is to be avoided.

Managing with the system

In larger health organizations, the physician leader answers to an executive leader, who is often another physician. Superiors and subordinates may differ in style of management, values and objectives. A clinical manager must be willing at times to subordinate his interests, timing, and priority to adapt to his superior and organization, while still gracefully advocating for the needs of the practice and its patients.

Self-management

Of all the tasks and challenges of the clinical manager, the hardest is managing oneself. Physicians receive years of training in managing patients, but rarely receive guidance in managing demanding colleagues, dysfunctional staff, or failing budgets. Worse, while patients are often appreciative of advice, this is rarely true of colleagues. Self-control in stressful situations is a necessity for clinical leaders.

Control over time and tasks are equally important. Patients may wait for an hour, but the clinical leader who is late for a meeting has wasted the time of the group and lost credibility.

Avoiding common mistakes

The new clinician

The office in which one works can be a relatively safe area to practice managerial and basic leadership skills. Early in their careers, aspiring leaders can recognize and learn to avoid many common mistakes.

Physicians joining a practice should spend the first several months 'joining the system' by learning the practice and its strengths and weaknesses. New physicians should show that they are willing to help the practice by assisting with and accepting small assignments.

If possible, clinicians new to a practice should wait 3–6 months before recommending any major changes, as their assessment of the problems will change and become clearer during that time. After problems crystallize, no more than two to three areas should be selected for potential interventions. Choose problems that have a reasonable probability of success over a few months. Review progress frequently and get support from a senior physician of your practice. As a project succeeds, celebrate! If there is no success within 12 months, it is time to reassess.

Practice leadership

Family physicians who survive and thrive in improving an aspect of a practice often find themselves thrust into a more formal leadership role. This role, often called a 'medical director' has a similar set of issues and pitfalls to those that arise when joining a practice. However, the larger role brings with it the risk of being overwhelmed by the number and complexity of issues.

New medical directors are challenged in more subtle ways as well. No longer members of the rank and file, they may be ostracized by their colleagues as a demonstration that they have joined 'management'. Sometimes, this separation is exacerbated by the behaviour of the new medical director, who seeks to remind his previous colleagues of his new role and the respect now due. A wiser strategy is to renew collaborative interests with colleagues by acknowledging the changing roles, but seeking the continued working relationship that both have enjoyed.

Being a medical director can be extremely fatiguing. The role seems so easy—the medical director just needs to tell people what to do, and it is only months later that the realization dawns that this is hard work, that little is achieved by issuing directives, and that clinical leaders earn their role by the respect granted to them by their colleagues. Many leadership qualities are 'soft' people skills; it is helpful to have a mentor who can give you non-judgmental feedback on newly developed skills and help you match your ambitions to the opportunities at hand.

The leader as an agent of change

Those who succeed in improving day-to-day operations of a practice can begin leading wider change in an organization, and may wish to consider service as the head of a department or operating unit. Change in organizations is often necessary to improve processes of clinical care, to adapt to growth/

contraction of a clinical practice, and to adopt new medical technology. As a result, the need for clinical leaders is great. However, the shift into these larger clinical leadership positions requires an additional set of skills.

Vision

Good clinical leaders have a clear perception of how some part of health care could be better. Being able to clearly and succinctly describe that vision is the first skill in these larger roles.

Assessment

An accurate accessment of the group's strengths and weaknesses, achievements, and threats is a necessity. Much as clinicians are unlikely to intervene in a patient with multi-organ failure without understanding the pathophysiology of the illness, clinical leaders need to understand the pathophysiology of their own organization before they attempt to fix the problem. Attention to patient and staff complaints can provide critical data, as can formal reports, patient surveys, and analyses by colleagues and constituents.

Similarly, an understanding of national long-term health care trends is needed, as these trends will shape the challenges and opportunities the group will face in the decades to come. A clinical leader will anticipate the effects of these forces and help the group prepare for possible changes.

Strategy

Groups can tolerate only a limited amount of change at a time, so a clinical leader must identify the two or three most important tasks or problems that the group faces. In choosing issues for targeted attention, leaders seek opportunities that will move the organization in a desired direction, are within the ability of the group to achieve, and are important enough to justify the risk and cost.

Funding and resources

Most projects require funding. If new funding is required, expectations for enhanced revenues or decreased expenses must be identified. If there is an expectation for a return on the investment, then the time to break even and the required rate must be determined. While many organizations will accept a rough financial analysis of costs and revenue, larger organizations may require formal financial analysis. Unless one has had training in finance, assistance by someone who has had such training and who knows the organizational rules and expectations is essential.

Action plan

Successful projects evolve through a series of methodical steps. Planning the initial step is particularly important, as failure at the beginning is often fatal to the project, and sometimes to the career of the aspiring leader. It is usually best to plan a small first step that has a high likelihood of success (a pilot or demonstration project). Subsequent steps should each have good probability of succeeding.

In most organizations it should be possible to identify the individuals or groups whose approval or consent is required. The more unusual the idea, the more likely it will be to cross organizational boundaries, and require a higher degree of acceptance and additional levels of approval. Often, multiple levels of approval by groups or people previously unknown will be required as the project proceeds.

Leaders consider how the proposal could help resolve larger problems. Identify influential allies whose support may be persuasive. Plot the process for achieving approval, including each person to be contacted, who is to do the contacting, and what points need to be made. Finally, make sure your staff and colleagues have the skills to provide the new services and are able to support the change. Align incentives to reinforce the new behaviour.

Negotiation

Successful negotiations require careful planning. Ideally, both sides leave the negotiation with a sense of having achieved what they most desired, of having given up nothing they could not afford, and conclude with a sense of renewed dedication to working through the remaining steps. Such an outcome requires knowing what one wishes to achieve, what is needed, what is unnecessary, and a willingness to find common ground. Successful negotiation also requires the ability to walk away when no agreement is possible, and when the process of negotiation has become destructive.

Managing conflict

In negotiating and implementing change, consensus is not always possible, and determined opposition is common. The ability to weigh strongly held conflicting advice from colleagues is a skill that family physicians often learn in clinical practice, and find equally useful in leadership roles. As in clinical practice, listen to the varying perspectives, and select the strategies best for the organization.

Delegation and supervision

Physician leaders are rarely able to carry out plans on their own. Being able to delegate and supervise effectively is an essential skill for clinical leaders. Delegation is the art of assigning a task to another individual so that both are in agreement on the goal to be achieved, the steps to be taken, deadlines to be met, resources available, and the points at which additional consultation are to be sought. It is rare for delegation to be detailed and specific; commonly, only the major elements are described, with considerable latitude provided for achievement of the task.

Supervision is the process of monitoring tasks that have been delegated. Senior leaders of experienced teams can rely on informal delegation and supervision, while new leaders, and new subordinates, require greater detail about expectations and more specific plans for follow-up. High risk and very important tasks will often require formal supervision, often including regular scheduled meetings, with review of steps taken, barriers encountered, and renegotiations of the next steps.

Evaluation

New programmes should be evaluated regularly to ensure they are on schedule. Identifying anticipated achievements at 1, 3, 6, and 12 months after implementation is common, with the items to be measured and the level of expected performance determined in advance. Setting goals with 'cut points' can help assure that a group stays focused on its task, and perseveres after the initial excitement of start-up.

There are few experiences more lonely than leading a failing project, nor one more crowded than leading one that succeeds. Projects that begin to fail are quickly held at arm's length, while success leads to a startling crowd of those who now proclaim their critical support. Sharing success is a useful way of building goodwill for the next, and perhaps harder, project.

Leadership as a full-time activity

Family physicians who discover they have a talent and ability to lead can choose to spend most or all of their professional efforts in leadership positions. While clinical care may still be part of their activities, it is generally a small part of the time, albeit symbolic and often emotionally important. The opportunities at this level are exciting: to shape future generations of health care trainees; to restructure health care so it is more humane and responsive; to return to society with thanks some of what it has invested in oneself. The issues are also more complex and entangled, and the techniques more subtle. Being able to choose and implement strategies through key lieutenants is critical, as often it is the traditions and structures, the 'institutional culture' that needs to be modified. Happily, the tenets of careful planning that one learned in patient care work here as well. Organizational leadership roles can be exciting and productive for those who mastered the earlier steps.

Family physicians can also have major roles in working with communities to improve health. Community action requires a different approach, as communities must balance a wider array of issues, and health care is not always the leading concern. Community change requires time for coalition building, respect for differing opinions, and willingness to set one's own agenda aside when the group wishes to focus on other concerns. Nevertheless, the give and take of community politics will often feel familiar to family physicians, especially those who have a similar interactive style with their patients.

Conclusion

Over the span of their careers, family physicians are called upon to serve in a variety of leadership roles. For many, taking on a leadership position is a natural outgrowth of the desire to help that initially led them into the profession. Leadership positions can be fulfilling, and the years of practice as a clinician can provide helpful experience in problem analysis and the need for personal action. Additional reading and reflection, a mentoring relationship with a successful colleague, and participation in local and professional training programmes in leadership can be extremely valuable. For those who found providing care to individuals and families to be satisfying, being able to help health care systems meet the needs of entire communities can be equally rewarding, and makes the challenges of leadership roles worthwhile.

References

1. **Sebenius, J.K.** (April, 2001). Six habits of merely effective negotiators. *Harvard Business Review* **79** (4), 87–95.
2. **Tangalos, E.G.** et al. (1998). Mayo leadership programs for physicians. *Mayo Clinic Proceedings* **73**, 279–84.
3. **Kotter, J.P.** (March, 1995). Leading change: why transformation efforts fail. *Harvard Business Review* **73** (2), 59–67.
4. **Reinertsen, J.L.** (1998). Physicians as leaders in the improvement of health care systems. *Annals of Internal Medicine* **128**, 833–8.
5. **Bodenheimer, T. and Casalino, L.** (1999). Executives with white coats—the work and world view of managed-care medical directors. *New England Journal of Medicine* **341**, 1945–8, 2029–31.
6. **McCall, M.W. and Clair, J.A.** (1990). Why physician managers fail—Part Two. *Physician Executive* **16**, 8–12.
7. **Ninomiya, J.S.** (April, 1988). Wagon masters and lesser managers. *Harvard Business Review* **66** (2), 84–90.
8. **Thomason, S.** (1999). Becoming a physician executive: where to look before making the leap. *Family Practice Management* **6**, 37–40.

1.10 The role of primary care in public health

Jan W. van Ree

Introduction

The development of medical science in the twentieth century has been characterized by increasing differentiation in the tasks of doctors. Although the different roles of hospital- and community-based physicians began to develop long before the twentieth century, the growing body of knowledge and technology has resulted in the development of a range of medical disciplines. At one end of the scale are doctors with a generalist task, often working outside the hospitals, fulfilling a primary role in the prevention of diseases in populations, and charged with caring for the health of populations. At the other end of that scale are specialists, more and more focused in narrow areas of health care, developing great expertise in specific disorders of certain parts of the human body. These disease-oriented specialists and sub-specialists have concentrated their practices in hospital settings. Interestingly, despite the wide gap between public health care and hospital-based care, in a number of Western countries academic departments of general practice and primary care have developed out of existing departments of public health sciences.

Primary health care, provided by the general practitioner (GP) as a specific medical professional, occupies an interesting position because, whilst in many countries, GPs operate entirely outside the hospital, in the United States they also retain a hospital base, providing a bridge between hospital and community. Indeed, remaining connected with the community is one of the key issues defining the roles of both primary care and public health physicians. GPs occupy a further unique position in which they can play a linking role between individual health care and care for the community that includes their practice population. Community-oriented primary health care is likely to play an increasing role in addressing some of the health problems we will face in the future. The society of the future will be an ageing society, with the concomitant burden of degenerative diseases, while high-risk behaviour will influence the health of populations and the levels of psychological stress. High rates of population growth and increasing poverty in large parts of the world will have a major impact on health status.

The 'Health for All' call, made by the WHO conference in Alma Ata in 1978,[(1)] with the aim of achieving this approach to health care, has failed to achieve many of its aims in the intervening 25 years. One important reason for this may be that we need to further improve and delineate the role of the general practitioner in public health care if we wish to achieve Health for All.[(2)]

The emphasis in health care should be shifted back to public health, since the individualist, high-cost hospital-based care system will not be able to deal with the problems we are going to face in the future. An effective approach to these new health problems requires a change in the structure of the hospital-based health care system in many countries, especially in developing and poorer countries, towards a public health oriented, community-based structure.

Developments in public health care

New insights into the causes and spread of diseases have in the past led to the discovery of the relation between nutritional deficiencies food and diseases such as the links between scurvy and vitamin C deficiency and between beri-beri and vitamin B deficiency. A similar discovery was that of the importance of hygienic measures to prevent diseases; a well-known example is the prevention of cholera in the inner city of London when John Snow closed the Broad Street public water pump in 1854. The growing body of knowledge about the emergence and spread of diseases as a result of unhealthy habits (poor quality food, widespread alcoholism, smoking) and poor working and living conditions has underlined the importance of disease prevention and the role of health education. Thus, public health care can be defined as 'the science of preventing diseases, prolonging life and promoting health through organised actions of society'. Measures to prevent diseases could be aimed at the entire community or parts of it, and success has been achieved by improved education aimed at the general population. Population-based health care has become a task for national or local authorities, resulting in the development of independent public health care organizations paid for from with public funds. This general public task of preventing diseases in populations has meanwhile been laid down in official legislation on population-oriented prevention.

These institutions were able to organize systematically and perform specific preventive tasks better than the hospital-based physicians, especially in cases where a systematic approach was essential to achieve adequate prevention. For example, preventing childhood diseases requires a minimum level of vaccination coverage in a population to block their spread. Thus, for those cases a systematic vaccination programme is needed, which aims to targets all children in a population.

Prevention of diseases in the population or in groups is the main task of public health physicians. In a community-based health care system, epidemiology becomes more specifically 'public health epidemiology'. It can contribute to primary health care by collecting scientific information about the health status of a community and the impact on individuals in that population. Public health epidemiology can also contribute to the future health system by studying methods to improve the outcome of care.[3]

The 'New Public Health', emerging in recent years has taken this thinking further. The New Public Health is not so much a concept as it is a philosophy which endeavors to broaden the older understanding of public health so that, for example, it includes the health of the individual in addition to the health populations, and seeks to address such contemporary health issues as are concerned with equitable access to health services, the environment, political governance, and social and economical development. It seeks to put health in the development framework to ensure that health is protected in public policy. Above all, the New Public Health is concerned with action. It is concerned with finding a blueprint to address many of the burning issues of our time, but also with identifying implementable strategies in the endeavour to solve these problems.[4]

Developments in general practice

The position and tasks of GPs have had a long development and a general practitioner is nowadays very different from a public health doctor. After World War II, many Western countries saw a revival of the tasks and position of the GP. Nowadays, GPs are specialists, with a very specific task and a central position in the health care system in many countries. They are the only general medical doctors in primary care and they provide continuing care for individuals and their families in all phases of life, within the social context and society, recognizing the environmental circumstances. This definition has great consequences for the position of GPs, the content of their daily work and for the scientific discipline and research.

The position of GPs in the health care system is not the same in all countries. Even within Europe, there are major differences in their position between the various countries. The position of GPs depends strongly on the structure and principles of a country's health care system, that is, on whether it has a hospital-based system or a public health based system. In a public health based system, GPs are the gatekeepers to the hospital system.[5] One of their main tasks is that of preventive medicine aimed at individuals and families, rather than at populations, and individual prevention is still an essential part of their work.

There are, however, a few examples of GPs taking on an explicit public health role. The work of Julian Tudor Hart in South Wales in the 1960s and 1970s, when he adopted a population approach to the prevention as well as treatment of cardiovascular and pulmonary disease, is a celebrated example of a single-handed GP adopting a public health role.[6]

Collective working but different approaches

Several publications have drawn attention to the considerable gaps between these two branches of medicine, but have also emphasized the need for collaboration, because they are increasingly working to the same agenda.[7] Bhopal has summarized the resources of public health and primary care and also the common agenda to which they work and has provided illustrations of the two differing, yet complementary, approaches (Tables 1 and 2).[7]

There are many arguments favouring such collaboration, including the close correlation between personal health and lifestyles in a population, the increasing interdependence between the quality of life of individuals and environmental factors, and the attention that must be given to prevention in communities, to health promotion aiming at groups, to medical risk reduction in high-risk groups and to the curative treatment of patients.

Table 1 The resources of public health and primary health care

Public health	Primary care
Perspective	
Care of populations	Care of individual patients on practice list
Environmental, social, organizational, and legislative interventions are of dominant importance	Medical interventions are of dominant importance
Professional attitudes	
Health requires the organized efforts of society	The consultation is the fundamental basis of health care
Prevention is better than cure	The care of the sick is the prime role, and prevention has a role
Knowledge	
Public health sciences (e.g. epidemiology/medical statistics)	Broad, clinical knowledge
Organizational and management issues	Local patterns of disease
Policy making	Communication with individuals
Administrative networks	Personal circumstances of families/individuals
Health status of large population/area	Local community and its services
Skills	
Epidemiological and health services investigation/research	Investigation and management of clinical problems
Report and policy writing	Consultation/communication
Administration	Small group leadership skills
Communication with professional	Practice management
Committee services work	Medical audit
Information and material	
Information on populations and their health in large areas	The practice register and disease register
Access to health authority resources	Information on individuals
Access to non-medical staff, such as finance, computing, etc.	Access to local networks and primary careteams

Modified from Bhopal, R.J. (1995). *Journal of Epidemiology and Community Health* **49**, 113–16, by permission.

It has become increasingly clear that programmes at the population level are much more successful if they are supported at the individual level. Cooperation between the public health authorities and the GPs is therefore a prerequisite.[8] Such collaboration can achieve quality, equity, relevance, and cost-effectiveness in health care.[9]

Many countries are struggling with the concept of community-oriented health care system and the position of the GP in such a system.[10,11] At the same time, primary care doctors/GPs in rural areas and in the poorer parts of these countries already have far more community-oriented tasks, because the organizational structure of such areas precludes the development of institutionalised public health organizations. The combination of certain population-oriented tasks (such as vaccination programmes) and individually oriented tasks (such as treating diseases) is the most appropriate approach in this situation. Application of the principles of community-oriented care can also be successful in the setting of a private general practice; a public setting is not an absolute precondition.[12]

Bridging the gap between the disciplines

The process of bridging the gap between GPs and public health doctors is facilitated by the fact that both strive to improve people's health, but at the

Table 2 The common agenda of public health and primary health care

Public health approach	Agenda	Primary care approach
Serve whole population Combination of methods including social and environmental policy change Mass approaches to education Education educators and policy makers Seek expansion of funding base for prevention Take responsibility for organizational aspects at a district/regional level	Improve health and prevent disease	Serve patients on register Focus on patients' illnesses and risk factors Prevent by medical intervention Lifestyle change by education Undertake specific, but increasing range of activities in prevention
Evaluation of the structure, process and outcome of services Based primarily on epidemiological and demographic data, and on economic concepts	Effectiveness and efficiency of services	Audit of clinical work and practice organization Based partly on subjective views of staff and patients
Emphasis on needs of those who make no demand	Assessment of health needs	Based mainly on demands of patients and contractual obligations
Focus on disease causes; means of disease prevention, and on processes and outcomes of health care	Research	Focus on management of common health problems, and on structures and processes of primary health care
Develop local health polich and adapt and implement national and regional health policy	Policy making and implementation	Develop practice policy, and adopt and implement health authority policy

Modified from Bhopal, R.J. (1995). *Journal of Epidemiology and Community Health* **49**, 113–16, by permission.

same time it is impeded by the fact that they tend to use different means and to work from different positions. Collaboration is made problematic by some of the fundamental differences between the two disciplines.[7] These differences are clearly reflected in the definitions of the core business of each of these disciplines, and we must consider these differences as serious practical and conceptual barriers to collaboration. GPs are focused on individual personal care, on consultation and on the questions raised by specific patients. In the process of improving health and preventing disease, GPs work with individuals visiting their practices, concentrating on illnesses and individual risk factors, and starting preventive therapies (e.g. by prescribing anti-hypertensives).

The foundations of the knowledge and research of public health are epidemiology, the health status of populations, statistical data on risks in populations, and the demand for medical care. The public health approach concentrates on educating the public, and on social and environmental causes. Public health doctors try to influence those factors which threaten the health status of a population, such as unhealthy habits or environmental pollution.

For public health doctors, stimulating and implementing preventive activities in the community is their core business, which they regard as more important than cure. For GPs, curing and caring for individual sick persons is fundamental. Although prevention is gaining importance in primary health care, it often takes the character of early disease diagnosis and secondary prevention. The core of the GP's work is clinical knowledge, knowledge of diseases and their natural course, and doctor–patient communication, taking into account personal factors like work and family circumstances. The skills of GPs also involve the management of clinical problems, communication regarding such problems and the organization of the care process. The skills of public health doctors include writing reports, keeping careful records for the purpose of evaluating health services, and doing epidemiological research.

It is understandable that there are serious barriers to collaboration between public health care and general practice. Such barriers are caused by the failure to achieve a mutual understanding of each other's roles and goals, by rivalries between professions because of overlapping tasks and by not understanding the differences between public health care and general practice in terms of need-based care versus demand-based care. These are other obstacles to the delivery of a common primary care: public health agenda have been summarized by Bhopal (Table 3).[7]

Table 3 Obstacles to the achievement of a common agenda

Inter-professional
Persistence of historical rivalries
Failure to achieve mutual understanding of roles and goals
Inequality of esteem—perceived or actual
Unrealistic expectations
Administrative
Mismatch between the geographical areas served by public health doctors and general practitioners
Tension created by the overlap in the role of public health doctors and general practitioners as purchasers
Philosophical and ethical
Conflict between need-based and demand-based approaches to care
Conflict between immediate needs of the patient and those of potential patients
Conflict between priority setting and rationing, and doing the best for the patient
Practical
Shortage of staff in public health medicine in relation to needs at primary care level
Rapidly increasing sphere of responsibility of general practitioners

Modified from Bhopal, R.J. (1995). *Journal of Epidemiology and Community Health* **49**, 113–16, by permission.

Why bridge the gap?

Because GPs work and usually also live in the area where their practice is located, they get direct or indirect information from their patients regarding aspects of the community. Practicing GPs tend to know very well what is happening in the area where their patients live. GPs know the negative consequences of poor housing circumstances, alcohol abuse, tensions between community groups, poverty and unemployment. This is precisely the kind of information about the community or parts of it that public health doctors need for their epidemiological research and health care planning. It is also logical that registration data from general practices could be used for public health activities and planning. It is unfortunate that, for instance, information about morbidity from general practices is rarely used for local community development purposes. The increase in the number of patients presenting to the GP with pulmonary problems, as a result of increased pollution or poor housing circumstances, could be used to develop early measures. Exchanging information on specific aspects of health and health-related circumstances could lead to an improved understanding of the health situation of people and their families in the context of their own community. This might result in a 'community diagnosis',[13] which could be a source of inspiration for GPs and primary health care teams to become involved in public health aspects of patient care and for public health doctors to support GPs in their everyday work.

Across-the-board cooperation between primary health care and public health care could produce better outcomes and much greater value for individuals as well as the community. Such cooperation requires fundamental agreement between the disciplines regarding their principles. Biological, clinical, and social sciences have the potential to prevent illness as well as cure it. Collaboration must focus on these goals, using the specific advantages of both health care disciplines. A recent example of the need for collaboration between primary care and public care is the terrible HIV disaster developing in large parts of the world. It is clear that the required health care for more than 35 million people, more than 23 million of them living in the southern part of Africa, cannot be provided by the often hospital-based medical system in these countries. Instead, people need community-based health care teams to provide care and cure, but especially preventive activities to halt this dreadful epidemic.

Can we bridge the gap?

We will not be able to bridge the gap by trying to transform GPs into public health physicians or vice versa. Primary care doctors and public health doctors have been conditioned by their education and training. They do their work as they have learned to do and they have been infused with the mode of thought that is characteristic of their discipline. We know that it is not easy to change such modes of thought or to learn entirely new skills.

Both general practice and public health care have proved to be equally important disciplines for the optimization of health care in the community. Both have proved to be very successful in their respective areas of care. But they are using different principles and different tools. Both play their own important roles, which cannot easily be taken over by the other discipline. In my view, only collaboration, including the sharing of knowledge and skills, can lead to optimized care, produce better outcomes and add more value both for individuals and for society as a whole.

Prerequisites for future developments

Closer collaboration between these two disciplines and informing doctors of each other's roles and strengths requires that university medical schools take their responsibility. They should offer their students curricula and training that are less disease- and hospital-centred and programmes that include community health related subjects.[14] There is only a relatively small number of medical schools that are basically community-oriented and express this in their curricula. Most of these universities are members of the Network Community Partnerships for Health through innovative education, service, and research. Many traditional medical curricula still do not emphasis the importance of community-related aspects of health. Subjects like medical sociology, health promotion skills, and epidemiology are often not included in the curricula, and insofar as they are included, they are often not the most popular parts of the curriculum for medical students and teaching staff. Training programmes should focus on collaboration and communications between the disciplines. However, it has been found that joint educational programmes teaching general practice residents and public health students to work together can produce good results.[15]

Another prerequisite for a greater involvement of primary care in public health is to clarify the position of GPs and their role in the health care system. To play this role, GPs must be the gatekeepers of the health care system and preferably have defined patient lists.[16] This allows them to get to know the people in the community and to take responsibility for a group of persons and their families over longer periods of time, taking into account the nature of the community in which their patients live. Only then can they take responsibility for general health aspects of the community and support the community-oriented primary care principle.

Examples of the current role of GPs in public health

It has been known for a long time that the involvement of GPs in attempts to improve people's participation in community prevention programmes is often crucial for the success of such programmes.[16] This is related to the specific function of GPs, that of caring for individual persons over longer periods of time, allowing them to detect if patients do not participate in preventive activities initiated by public health organizations. GPs can help to make cervical cancer prevention programmes a success by carrying out the smears at their own office. It is a well-known problem that certain groups do not respond to the invitation to have a cervical smear made for the early detection of cervical cancer. The much closer relation between GPs and their patients and the more familiar situation of the doctor's own office are important elements making it more acceptable to undergo this procedure. This approach has been found to be very successful. Many countries have been running extensive programmes over many years, in which the public health authorities systematically invite women of certain age groups to have cervical smears at their GP's office. GPs can also support systematic vaccination programmes for the prevention of childhood diseases by administering the vaccinations to children invited by a public health organization. They can play a supportive role in general public health campaigns, for example, to get pregnant women to give up smoking.

Israel has a long tradition in developing primary care and especially building primary health care teams. These teams have achieved the integration of community health care with the care for individuals and families. Prevention of cardiovascular diseases by this approach has been found to be very successful.[17] The above activities often feature GPs in supportive roles, and their contribution has turned out to be essential in improving the outcome of public health programmes. In Cuba, a large cadre of family doctors has been created, possessing an unusual combination of clinical and public health functions.

It is increasingly being recognized that the contribution of GPs in public health care programmes is crucial for the success of the programme. It would be better if primary health care, that is, general practitioners functioning as team members, become involved in the design and planning of public health programmes at an early stage.

One promising example of the integration of public health care and private medical care is currently being implemented in the Netherlands, namely the Hartslag Limburg (Limburg Heartbeat) programme in the Maastricht region. This project has been selected by WHO as a demonstration project to study the collaboration between public health care and general practice in the field of cardiovascular prevention.

In the Hartslag Limburg programme, we have designed a model in which the public health activities are combined with (private) primary health care activities, in collaboration with cardiologists at the local hospital. This structure allowed us to promote continuity of care from the community, via GPs, to the level of the cardiologists. We also stated the need for individual and population-based interventions to achieve optimized prevention at all levels of care. It is known that people from lower social levels have a higher risk of cardiovascular disease because of their risky lifestyles and eating habits, making the populations in some of the poorer areas of large cities high cardiovascular risk groups. Interventions using health education and health-promotion activities at the community level therefore tend to focus on these areas. In addition to the preventive activities in selected city areas, GPs working in these areas are treating high-risk patients individually, as well as referring them to, for example, antismoking clinics and local sports clubs.

An essential element of the programme is the attempt to achieve collaboration between all partners, medical or otherwise, in order to create win-win situations. The partners are also expected to work together at an operational level over a prolonged period of time. In order to induce the partners in care to collaborate, we accepted the differences between the various types of participants in the programme and we explicitly made no attempts to change the roles of the disciplines involved. All participants were thus allowed to retain their own identity. A prerequisite for this collaboration over longer periods of time is that the goals of the preventive programme are accepted by all partners, allowing community workers, public health doctors and general practitioners to recognize their own identity in the activities of the programme.

Conclusions

Although public health doctors and GPs stem from the same medical roots, specific scientific and technical developments over the last century have created a serious gap between primary care and public health care. Because both need each other's support and since they share the same area of interest, they need to work together. Future developments in the community will underline the need to cooperate and to provide a community-oriented health care system, as the hospital-based health care system that currently exists in many countries will not be able to solve the problems of health care in the future. Only by collaboration between public health care and individual, personal health care will it be possible to achieve health for all people. It is impossible to bridge the gap between doctors of these two disciplines by trying to change one into the other. Collaboration requires mutual trust, win-win situations and agreement on the principles of health promotion programmes. In the near future, institutes offering medical training programmes will have to take responsibility for this development and teach medical students about this need for cooperation.

References

1. **World Health Organization** (1978). Primary health care. Report of the International Conference on Primary Health Care, Alma-Ata, USSR, 6–12 September 1978. Geneva: World Health Organization.
2. **Making medical practice and education more relevant to people's need: the contribution of the family doctors.** WHO/WONCA Conference 1994, London, Ontario, Canada (document available on request from WHO, 1211 Geneva 27, Switzerland).
3. **Mackenbach, J.P.** (1995). Public health epidemiology. *Journal of Epidemiology and Community Health* **49**, 333–4.
4. **Ncayiyana, D., Goldstein, G., Goon, E., and Yack, D.** (1995). In New Public Health and the WHO's Ninth General Program of Work: A Discussion Paper. Geneva: World Health Organization.
5. **Fleming, D.** The European study of referrals from primary to secondary care. Thesis, Maastricht, The Netherlands, 1993.
6. **Hart, J.T.** *A New Kind of Doctor.* London: Merlin Press, 1989.
7. **Bhopal, R.J.** (1995). Public health medicine and primary health care: convergent, divergent, or parallel paths? *Journal of Epidemiology and Community Health* **49**, 113–16 (editorial).
8. **Perkins, J.E., Jolley, D., and Dunt, D.R.** (1998). Recruitment of women by GPs for pap tests: a meta analyses. *British Journal of General Practice* **48** (434), 1603–7.
9. **Boelen, C.** Towards unity for health (TUFH). *Challenges and Opportunities for Partnership in Health Development.* A working paper. Geneva: WHO, 2000.
10. **Starfield, B.** (1996). Public health and primary care: a framework for proposed linkages. *American Journal of Public Health* **86** (10), 1365–9.
11. **Wright, R.A.** (1993). Community oriented primary care. The cornerstone of health care reform. *Journal of the American Medical Association* **269** (19), 2544–7.
12. **Bayer, W.H. and Fischella, K.** (1999). Patients and communities together. A family medicine community oriented primary care projects in an urban private practice. *Archives of Family Medicine* **8** (6), 550–2.
13. **Maeseneer, J.D. and Derese, A.** (1998). Community oriented primary care. *European Journal of General Practice* **4**, 49–50 (editorial).
14. **Boelen, C. and Heck, J.E.** Defining and measuring the social accountability of medical schools. World Heath Organisation WHO/RHR/95, Geneva: WHO, 1995.
15. **Thomson, R., Haber, D., Fanuiel, L., Krohn, K., and Chambers, C.** (1996). Community oriented primary care in a family practice residency program. *Family Medicine* **28** (5), 326–30.
16. **Olesen, F. and Fleming, D.** (1998). Patient registration and controlled access to secondary care. Prerequisites for intergrated care. *European Journal of General Practice* **4**, 81–3.
17. **Abrahamson, J.H., Gofin, J., Hopp, C., Schein, M.H., and Naveh, P.** (1994). The CHAD program for the control of cardiovascular risk factors in a Jerusalem community: a 24 year retrospect. *Israel Journal of Medical Science* **30** (1), 108–19.

2

Primary care around the world

2 Primary care around the world

2.1 Health care systems: understanding the stages of development

Jouke van der Zee, Wienke G.W. Boerma, and Madelon W. Kroneman

Introduction

A health care system is the organized response to the health problems of a society. In mature economies, like the members of the Organization of Economic Cooperation and Development (OECD), the health sector absorbs around 10 per cent of their gross domestic product (GDP) and it can be considered as a major force in the economies of these countries.[1] Also in developing economies health (care) absorbs a substantial, albeit lower proportion of a country's wealth; approximately 5 per cent of the GDP.[2] Health system analysis is the scientific approach to understanding the relationship between the structure of health care and a country's economic level of development, taking into account the needs of the population. In this chapter, first a section will be devoted to the 'system' part of the concept 'health system'. The following two sections will focus on the crucial relationship between 'health' and 'wealth'. The next section will describe the growth of health care systems, as part of the development of the modern welfare state. This historical approach is relevant for those countries, and many are now in transition from mainly agricultural economies to industrial and service economies. At a certain stage in this transition process, these countries should decide what role the state should have, and what role should be played by social security and by private organizations in health care funding and provision. The last section ends with an analysis of a second important option: the choice between a primary care led or hospital-based health care system.

Health care system: a question of degree

Health care is usually referred to as a 'system' without paying much attention to the meaning of this term. In this chapter, however, 'system' is not just an equivalent of 'sector'; in studying health care one should realize that it is a concept with specific characteristics. Philipsen,[3] who studied the neighbouring but rather contrasting Dutch and Belgian health care systems, stated that these can successfully be compared as varying in the degree in which they have the characteristics of a system. Some systems are more 'systematic' than others. Based on Habermas, Philipsen characterized health care systems by:

- functional specificity: the existence of shared operational goals;
- structural differentiation: a division of labour;
- coordination, planning and evaluation: coherence among the elements;
- autonomy: identification and maintenance of—relatively open—borders with other systems.

These features provide a framework to understand health care developments and problems that have occurred in the past decades in Western countries. Progress in medical technology has strongly increased the division of labour and the organization of services has become more and more complex. Many new medical and paramedical disciplines, that entered health care in the past decades, required a multi-disciplinary approach and teamwork. Growing complexity is a threat to the extent that operational goals are shared. Coherence between primary, secondary, and tertiary care, between curative and preventive services or between somatic and mental health care are more difficult to maintain. Many countries have met with problems of system control; from the highly centralized British National Health Service to the Swiss health care system, which has been strongly decentralized in the 26 Cantons. Comparison of health care systems is hampered by the problem of unclear or different boundaries. Although within the health sector the borders of particular sub-systems may be clear and strong, for instance those of the medical professions, borders with sectors adjacent to health care, such as those with welfare, social security, and education, may not be well defined and different from country to country. So, determining the 'systemicness' of a certain system according to the four criteria mentioned above is useful in health care system analysis because it can reveal weaknesses, frictions, and inefficiencies and can offer possibilities for change.

Health care and societal transition: a basic framework

A shared central goal in any health care system is to reduce the population's health problems. So, the composition and the design of the health care system should, to a certain extent, reflect the general character of these health problems, which, for their part, are influenced by the country's specific demographic situation. Health systems aiming to cope with a high prevalence of infectious diseases that endanger the lives of infants, will set priorities with nutrition, public hygiene, and immunization. If, in contrast, chronic, degenerative health problems are the dominant conditions, other solutions will be required, relying more on medical specialization, hospitals and nursing homes and (expensive) medication. In reality, health care systems always lag behind changing patterns of need in the population. Many health reforms in the countries of western Europe are the result of changing needs and demands of their ageing populations.

It is evident, that more sophisticated and individualized health care systems, in terms of a more advanced division of labour, greater complexity, and more structures for coordination and planning, require an increasing volume of resources. The extent to which resources can be generated for health care depends on the stage of development of the economy. Only advanced economies will be able to reserve sufficient proportions of their income for health. So, it may be concluded that there are three—interacting—major determinants of a health care system: the socio-economic level of development, the demographic state, and the epidemiological situation. Each of these can be considered as the main dynamic factor and, consequently, each can be taken as the starting point for the analysis and a description of consequences for the design of health care.

Taking socio-economic indicators as the starting point, the following development can be identified. After societies have passed the hunting stage, they develop from agricultural economies, mainly focused on survival and self-sustenance of the smallholder and his (extended) family, towards economies creating surpluses (wealth) and added value to products that can be traded for other products that cannot be produced locally (see Scheme 1). Generated surpluses are used for creating and maintaining roles which are not directly productive, such as soldiers, healers, teachers, tax collectors, retailers, policemen, and researchers. History has learned that surpluses tend to grow in a long-lasting process, in which periods of prosperity alternate with periods of recession due to war, famine, pandemics. As society develops, more and more structures and institutions are created that diminish the traditional risks of life. The usual individual arrangements to cope with these risks are gradually supplemented and partly replaced by collective arrangements.[(4)] One of the effects of these changes is a reduction of the population's fertility. In modern society, for instance, it is no longer necessary to have many children as a provision against old age poverty if social security, includes a public pension scheme. In addition to these collective arrangements, the surpluses can be used to foster further economic growth by extending educational facilities, creating more teachers, health care providers, lawyers, and engineers.

These collective facilities and services are financed from revenues which can be collected with increasing amounts as countries develop, also proportionally.[(5)] Low income countries tend to collect up to 20 per cent of their GDP as taxes, while in the high income group of countries this percentage varies between 40 and 60 per cent.

With societies transforming from agricultural to industrial to service economies, there is not only a reduction in birth rates, but also the structure of families changes from rural, three generation units to urban nuclear families and an increasing proportion of single person households. Focusing on health, the societal transition implies changes from prevalent infectious diseases to developing chronic and non-communicable diseases in addition (see lower half of Scheme 1). The focus of care follows this development and evolves from attention to hygiene and other public health matters, such as safe water and vaccination, via the rise of curative care to a complex of highly specialized and long-term care services. There is a clear and stable link between health and wealth. Growing wealth results in more and more varied nutrition and a prolonged life expectancy, which leads to the epidemiological transition from mainly infectious diseases to an increasing prevalence of chronic diseases. As a consequence, more resources are needed to satisfy the changed health needs of the population. Treatment of chronic conditions requires the application of long-lasting curative care, the continuing use of drugs and repeated specialized medical interventions, often in a hospital. This can only be provided to broader sections of the population under favourable economic conditions. The state of the economy sets the limits for the availability of 'surplus resources' for health. That is why we consider economic growth, or wealth, as a major driv-ing power of societal development and, more particularly, of the development of health care systems. For an adequate analysis of health systems, it is not enough to have insight in the dominant health problems of a population. One should also have information on the stage of development of the economy.

An economic view on health system development

The influence of economic development on health and health care can best be illustrated by showing the well-known graph published in the World Bank Development Report 1993, where the average life expectancy (in years) was plotted against the average income per capita in a large number of countries with a generation's interval for the years 1900, 1930, 1960, and 1990.[(6)] The financial data were made comparable by expressing them as 1990 dollars and taking inflation into account (see Fig. 1).

What can this graph teach us? First, that there has been a general growth of the wealth of nations during the twentieth century. In 1900 there were no national per capita incomes over 5000 dollars (expressed as 1991 dollars), but in 1990 there were a considerable number. The second observation is that the greatest gain in life expectancy is found at the lower income range. Life expectancy differences are most marked when countries shift from poor to a little less poor. It is not a gradual increase in life expectancy that is taking place, but the profound impact of a relatively small increase in wealth. Measures aiming at a reduction in infant mortality, achieved at relatively low costs, are mainly responsible for this improvement. Thirdly, the top section of the graph clearly shows that, after a certain income level has been reached, further increase in wealth does not coincide with increasing life expectancy any more. Apparently, the effect of increasing wealth gradually peters out; diseases related to a more affluent lifestyle seem to form a ceiling for further growth of the life expectancy. So it is obviously much

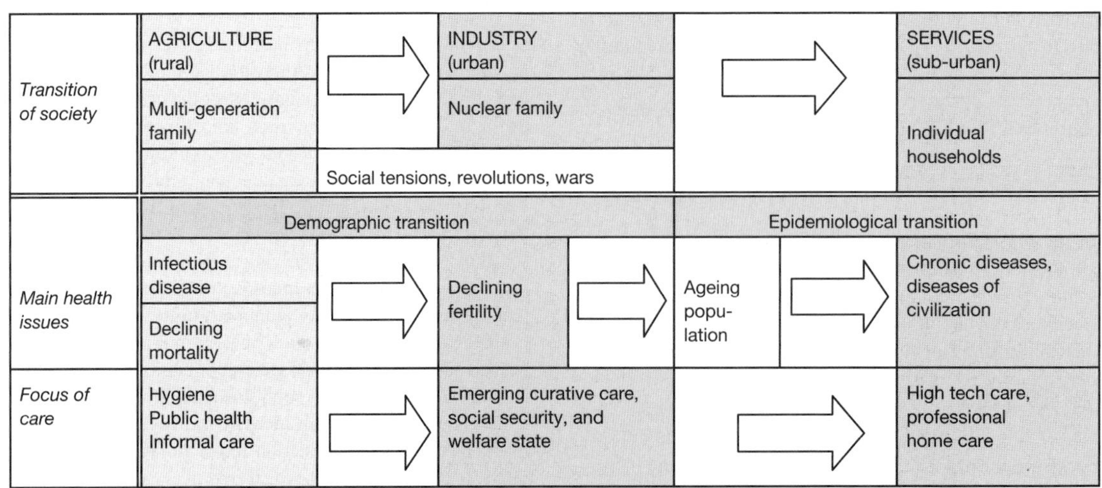

Scheme 1 Societal transitions and dominant health issues.

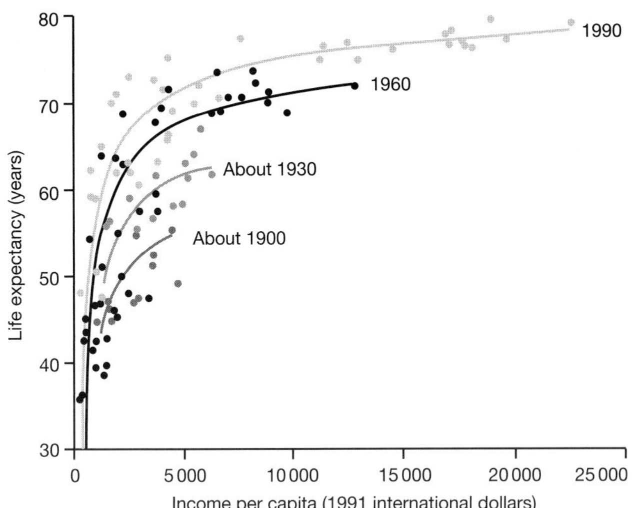

Fig. 1 Life expectancy and income per capita for selected countries and periods.[6]

more difficult to prolong life expectancy by increasing wealth in mature economies than it is in developing economies.

What are the implications of all this for health system analysis? First, countries should be distinguished according to the income level. In distinguishing three categories, the low income group would consist of countries with an average annual income of US$700 or less per inhabitant (in 1991). In these countries, hygiene, sanitation, improvement of nutrition, vaccination, and immunization are the core elements of health care. The government, aided by indigenous and foreign non-governmental bodies, plays the central role in the organization. Health is largely determined by factors outside the health system. Curative care is provided by local healers and there are some hospitals for those who can afford it. Rich people may seek medical treatment abroad. In the medium income group with an average annual income of up to about US$8000, the funding and organization of the expanding curative care is the main area of policy making. Health systems in the highest income countries are coping with the consequences of the epidemiological transition: rising costs resulting from an increased demand for chronic care with ageing populations. Health system analysis in the middle income countries is highly relevant because these countries are in a process of full transition and are obliged to take fundamental decisions about the structure of society and the design of collective arrangements, including health care.

Creating health care systems; policy options for middle income countries

Since the growth of wealth is usually not equally distributed over a country, health patterns of the population as well as the demand for health services may differ as well. The most dynamic growth will take place in the centre of a society (the capital, other big cities) where an increasing number of people accumulate wealth and thus can afford and require more expensive and more sophisticated health services. In this situation population groups with common interests may unite to compensate for loss of income due to bad health and disability and organize adequate health care for their members. Sooner or later, other categories in society may also find themselves as having common interests in proper health care; for instance, civil servants, the army, railway employees, or residents of wealthier neighbourhoods. In this way new—curative—health care arrangements will 'crystallize' around funding possibilities. The army will build hospitals for its officers; the ruling elite will create health facilities for its loyal servants, and affluent neighbourhoods can raise money for their own local health centre. Typical of this stage, which is found for instance in Egypt, is an uneven and unequal growth of categorical facilities with restricted access which together appear as isolated and scattered sub-systems, rather than a developing coherent structure. Contrasts are sharp between the urban centres and the periphery, where growth is weaker, but also within the urban centres, between well-to-do areas and slums. When a society becomes richer and more room is created for the extension of services to a broader population, the state may intervene, and will often do so in order to reduce the potential destabilizing effect of inequalities. However, the degree and character of the interference will vary strongly. The role of the state in health care regulation is a typifying characteristic of a country's health care system. Although state involvement is a continuum, the strand of actions can be characterized by three broad strategies, namely: (a) comprehensive state funding and provision; (b) harmonizing the arrangements that grew between groups of citizens; and (c) a policy of non-intervention: no comprehensive health care system and leaving room for substantial private insurance and care provision.

(a) The first strategy could be dubbed the State model or the Beveridge model, named after the British health minister who introduced the National Health Service in Great Britain in 1948. The state provides health services, offered free to the population and funded by taxation. As taxation, generally, has an equalizing effect (strongest shoulders carrying the heaviest burden), countries that value equity often opt for this model.[7] An earlier version of a state health care system, even more strongly dominated by state regulation, was introduced in the Soviet Union by Lenin's health minister Semashko in the 1920s.[8,9] Variations of the Beveridge model are currently found in southern Europe and Scandinavia.

(b) As part of a second strategy, state regulation aims to harmonize and expand existing mutual societies and other categorical arrangements among and between groups of citizens, mostly around their work or craft and aimed at the protection against loss of income due to severe illness or disability. The state has the function of mending the patchwork of numerous arrangements and extending the coverage to all groups of employees and to independently working citizens. This is the introduction of a social security based health care system, the so-called Bismarck model, named after the German Chancellor who established the first examples of this model in the late nineteenth century in Germany. Later it was introduced in Austria, the Netherlands, France, Belgium and Luxemburg (by force, during the German occupation in World War II, and never abolished afterwards). Services are funded by premiums that employees pay as part of their wages.[10] These proportional premiums indicate a sense of income redistribution comparable to proportional taxation. An important difference is that the premiums are earmarked for funding health services, while, in theory, in a taxation system health expenditures have to compete with education, infrastructure and defence. In the social security model health care provision is mostly left to private (usually not-for-profit) institutions and/or personal providers.

(c) Thirdly, a state can follow a policy of non-intervention and limit its interference in health care matters to the bare essentials, leaving the rest to private funding and provision. This can be considered as the 'American way'.[11] In the United States, federal schemes exist for the indigent (Medicaid) and the elderly (Medicare); for the rest federal and state intervention is minimal. Private funding and insurance (both for profit and not-for-profit) fill the gap, to some extent. The United States has 15 per cent of its population either uninsured or insufficiently covered against health care costs and loss of income due to illness and disability.

The three very general 'models', in reality to be found in many varieties, can be considered as descriptions of the final outcome of historical processes. That is not similar to the term 'options', used in the title of the section, which implies a more active process of choice. The point to make here is, that, at some moment in the development of countries towards a welfare state, decisions need to be taken aiming at a more coherent ordering at a national level of the organization and provision of health care. The choices made in the first half of the twentieth century in the highly developed economies of today, are still available as options for developing economies or for economies that trade one model of society for another. An example of the latter is the former Soviet Union, including its former satellite countries, that changed the Soviet model towards market capitalism. Any state intervention in health care of developing economies will increase its 'system character', but, depending on the strategy, to different degrees. System features are most clearly found in the centralized national health service approach. In the Bismarckian strategy, traces of the original patchwork cannot be wiped out completely which results in a less coherent structure. Obviously, the 'laissez-faire' strategy is the least systemic one, since it does not make the step to equal access and large population coverage. Which of the two first mentioned strategies, as outlined above, will be chosen, does not really matter in terms of health outcomes and not even in terms of costs. In the top 20 countries in the ranking list that appeared in the World Health Report 2000,[(12)] which is mainly based on health outcomes, there is a fair balance between the national health systems and countries with a social security-based health care system. With France (social security), Italy (NHS), San Marino (NHS), Andorra (social security), and Malta (NHS) in leading positions, the Mediterranean diet is perhaps a more important determinant of health outcomes than the type of health care system. Evans[(7)] shows that an option for Bismarck or Beveridge is not crucial for health care costs; France and Germany's health care is costly but so is Sweden's. No state intervention does not seem to be a good option, as the soaring health care costs in the United States show. Countries that experienced the results of the epidemiological transition are forced to find a way to stem the tide of rising costs.

Primary care led versus hospital-based services

As a result of the ageing of their populations, the Western market economies experienced, an apparent unbounded increase in the demand for long-term care, at home or in nursing homes, and more expensive health services, such as specialist monitoring, operations in hospital, and long-term use of drugs. In western Europe, this has happened in the 1960s and 1970s; in some countries this process continued through the 1980s and 1990s. Every self-respecting community built a well-equipped hospital and, for instance, hospital stays of at least 1 year were included in benefit packages for an ever extending group of beneficiaries. Since health care cost started absorbing a larger and larger proportion of the national economies, policy measures were needed to curb costs and regulate access. The way countries responded to this challenge and dealt with the issues of accessibility and efficiency is a second major sub-division in health care systems. An accepted distinction is between health care systems based on primary care and those which are more hospital based (also referred to as pluralistic systems). Some countries, such as the United Kingdom, The Netherlands, Spain, Denmark, and Norway, have prevented excess utilization of expensive secondary care services (specialist and hospital) by the introduction of a referral system, mostly with a general practitioner (GP) in a gate-keeping role. In these countries, patients only have access to hospital in- and out-patient services by means of referral. Other countries, most with social security systems such as France and Germany, maintained parallel access to GPs and medical specialists and used other means to ration the use of services, for instance through co-payments and other financial disincentives.

As with the distinction between national health systems and social security based systems, the central question is whether it makes a difference either to have or not to have a gate keeping or referral system. According to a study conducted by Starfield[(13)] primary care led health care systems are not only cheaper than systems with direct access to hospitals and medical specialists, but their health outcomes are better, too. Evidence on this matter, however, is not unequivocal. Replication studies, both in middle income countries and in 18 OECD countries, failed to reach similar conclusions.[(14,15)] The study of Delnoij,[(14)] in OECD countries, only found that gate-keeping health care systems were better able to control costs of ambulatory care. In the four studies, reviewed by the Cochrane Collaboration,[(15)] no clear evidence was found that more integrated primary health care services improved the delivery of services or the population's health status. Since these studies admitted to have had a limited scope, it is noted that more research is necessary to understand micro level mechanisms and to beter distinguish the primary care effects, such as gate keeping, from those of other structural features of a health care system.

Conclusions

Any health care system develops in response to the health problems of a population. We have argued that economic growth is a major force behind both the development and the accommodation of health problems. In low income countries, health care is not the major determinant of health; variations in health systems are limited. When countries transform from low to middle income economies, more variety in health care systems occurs. They have to cope with chronic instead of infectious diseases and there can be a greater variety in the organization of health care. Roughly speaking, societies that do not want to abstain from interference can opt either for extending and amending work-based arrangements in a social security approach, or develop a system with state funding and provision, a national health service. Rising costs, as a consequence of the epidemiological transition, can be curbed either by regulating access to specialized services (gate keeping or referral system), or by introducing more general disincentives for utilization of services. In terms of health outcomes, it does not appear to make a crucial difference; in terms of costs, gate-keeping systems seem somewhat less expensive. And what about the system character? Obviously the laissez-faire approach does not score high on this dimension. A centralized NHS-like system seems to offer good conditions for coordination, a proper division of labour, and the maintenance of shared operational goals; at least theoretically, because these conditions can be spoiled by bureaucracy and too much regulation. In a social security environment decision making and coordination are more difficult, but, with effective (dis)incentives, coherence and efficiency can be sufficiently maintained. Merely by its design the one system cannot be declared superior to the other.

References

1. **OECD** health data files, 2001.
2. **World Health Organization.** World Health Indicators, CD-ROM, 2001.
3. **Philipsen, H.** (1985). Gezondheid en gezondheidszorg in België en Nederland. Enige addertjes onder het zo groen gewaande gras van een systeemvergelijking. (Health and health care in The Netherlands and Belgium. Some little snakes in the believed green grass of a system comparison.) *Gezondheid & Samenleving* **4**, 223–32.
4. **De Swaan, A.** *In Care of the State. Health Care, Education and Welfare in Europe and the USA in the Modern Era.* Cambridge: Polity Press, 1988.
5. **World Bank.** *Health, Nutrition and Population.* Washington DC: World Bank, 1997.
6. **World Bank.** World Development Report. Investing in Health: World Development Indicators. Washington DC: World Bank, 1993.
7. **Evans, R.G.** (2002). Financing health care: taxation and the alternatives. In *Funding Health Care: Options for Europe* (ed. E. Mossialos), pp. 31–58. Buckingham/Philadelphia: Open University Press.
8. **Marrée, J. and Groenewegen, P.P.** *Back to Bismarck: Eastern European Health Care Systems in Transition.* Aldershot: Avebury, 1997.
9. **Mossialos, E.,** ed. *Funding Health Care: Options for Europe.* Buckingham/Philadelphia: Open University Press, 2002.
10. **Blanpain, J.E.** *National Health Insurance and Health Resources: The European Experience.* Cambridge MA: Harvard University Press, 1978.

11. **Navarro, V.** *Why the United States does not have a National Health Program.* Amityville NY: Baywood Publishing Company, 1992.
12. **World Health Organization.** The World Health Report 2000. Health systems: improving performance. Geneva: WHO, 2000.
13. **Starfield, B.** (1994). Is primary care essential? *Lancet* **344**, 1129–33.
14. **Delnoij, D., Van Merode, G., and Groenewegen, P.P.** (2000). Does general practitioner gatekeeping curb health care expenditure? *Journal of Health Services Research and Policy* **1**, 22–6.
15. **Briggs, C.J., Capdegelle, P., and Garner, P.** (2002). Strategies for integrating primary health services in middle and low-income countries: effects on performance, costs and patient outcomes (Cochrane Review). In *The Cochrane Library* Issue 1. Oxford: Update Software.

2.2 Primary care and general practice in Africa

Bruce L.W. Sparks

Africa is a vast continent consisting of over 55 countries and dependencies. Countries such as Algeria, Sudan, Angola, and the Democratic Republic of Congo are individually larger than the whole of Western Europe excluding Scandinavia. The United Kingdom could easily fit 16 times into the area of South Africa and her immediate neighbours. It is impossible, then, to do justice to the continent in this short summary. Accurate and assessable health-related data are often difficult to come by, and planners often rely on outside agencies for reliable statistical information.

Geography and demography

Africa is, in general, an undeveloped continent, where political unrest, chronic poverty, and poor medical services are common. It can be divided for geographical and cultural purposes into two distinct regions. That in the north includes the Islamic states that fringe the Mediterranean and north Atlantic coasts. These countries are united by their shared Islamic past and a common language. Most have fertile coastal regions and economies based on oil production.

The other region stretches some 7500 km from the Sahara Desert to the southern tip of the continent. It is more diverse geographically than the north, and is united by having a mainly Negroid population, who have gained independence from colonial rule. Some countries are subjected to periodic droughts, floods, and famines while others have been de-stabilized by wars and tribal conflict, which are often the legacies of inappropriate and unnatural borders drawn on maps in the nineteenth-century drawing rooms of Europe. Chronic poverty, low health status, lack of safe drinking water, and limited access to health services for the majority of the people contribute to a low life expectancy. The average life expectancy at birth in the sub-Saharan region is 48.4 years for both sexes compared to 67.2 years in the north and the infant mortality rate is 90.3 per 1000 live births in the south compared to 51.0 in the north.(1)

Major health issues

The greatest health challenge facing the continent is probably the HIV/AIDS pandemic, which is set to devastate the families and communities of the sub-Saharan region, producing societies with many AIDS orphans, fewer adults in the work-force, and health services often depleted of funds to care for patients with other conditions. Of the 33.6 million people living with HIV/AIDS in the world in 1999, 23.3 million (69 per cent) lived in sub-Saharan Africa, and 84 per cent of the 16.3 million global AIDS-related deaths occurred in the sub-Saharan region.(2) The HIV prevalence rate for 15–49-year-old adults in Botswana was 35.8 per cent. A recent report from the South African Medical Research Council indicates that 40 per cent of adult deaths in 15–49-year-olds in South Africa in 2000 were due to HIV/AIDS, with the syndrome accounting for 20 per cent of deaths overall.(3) The challenges to family practitioners and other primary health care workers in the region are considerable. With the limited access to anti-retroviral drugs and management services, and the unlikely impact of vaccines on presently infected individuals, the numbers of expected deaths in the continent are horrifying. In South Africa alone it is expected that the cumulative AIDS deaths by 2010 will be 5–7 million (nearly 18 per cent of the present population).(3)

Apart from the scourge of HIV/AIDS, an environment of malnutrition, poverty, sparse health facilities, and unhygienic living conditions often affects the health status of children. Children below the age of 5 years die mainly from preventable diseases or from diseases that could be cured if diagnosed and treated early.(4) Diarrhoea and respiratory infections are still leading killers, despite increased use of oral rehydration treatment and availability of antibiotics. Malaria too kills many children under the age of 5. Teenagers are at severe risk of contracting HIV/AIDS, while sexually transmitted infections, tuberculosis, motor vehicle accidents, violence, teenage pregnancy, and substance abuse are major contributors to morbidity and mortality.

Pregnancy and childbirth still constitutes a major threat to the lives of women aged between 15 and 45 years. Sixteen of the 19 countries globally with 'very high' reproductive risk indices are in sub-Saharan Africa. Eight have maternal death rates over 1200 deaths per 100 000 live births, well above those of Cuba (95), United Kingdom (9), and United States of America (12).(5)

African citizens are also victims of high incidences of other tropical and infectious diseases, such as tuberculosis, river blindness, hepatitis B and C, malaria, typhoid fever, sleeping sickness, leprosy, filariasis, bilharzias, typhus, trachoma, and human papilloma virus, to mention a few.(6) Tuberculosis, in particular, is more prevalent than ever, being one of the commonest presentations in HIV/AIDS.(7) Multiple drug resistance too is making the battle against TB an almost impossible one. The incidence of sexually transmitted infections is also very high, and is thought to enable infection by the HIV virus. The prevalences of hypertension, diabetes, and atherosclerosis are increasing with the introduction of 'western' diet and life styles. Malignancies often present too late for definitive management, particularly those of the breast, cervix, and liver.

Health care systems

The health care services of Africa vary enormously between and within countries—from highly sophisticated 'state-of-the-art' hospitals and plush well-equipped private general practices in some, to almost no medical care in some poorer countries. Almost half the 55 states have less than 10 doctors per 100 000 population, compared to countries such as Cuba (530), Italy (554), United Kingdom (164), and United States of America (279).(8) Many people have never had access to a medically trained health care worker, and the vast distances and relatively poor transport systems often make access to services more difficult.

General practitioners exist, especially in ex-British colonies such as Kenya, Nigeria, Zimbabwe, South Africa, Ghana and Uganda, and have both private- and public-sector family practitioners. Some Francophone and ex-Portuguese states only recently introduced family doctors. Generalist oriented doctors (medical officers) working in state clinics or hospitals usually do not consider themselves family practitioners. Most countries are reliant on nurses, medical assistants, and semi-trained community health workers for the delivery of primary health care services to their communities. It is not uncommon for medical personnel from Europe, North America, and elsewhere to work in underserved areas supported by international aid agencies, Church missions, and non-governmental organizations.

Professional organizations

Many countries have multidisciplinary, medico-political societies and associations that organize continuing medical education programmes, but formal postgraduate training in family medicine in the sub-Saharan region is limited to a few countries, such as Zimbabwe, South Africa, and the English speaking countries of West Africa (Nigeria, Ghana, Sierra Leone, the Gambia, Liberia). These countries have postgraduate colleges and professional accreditation. South Africa has also established masters degrees in family medicine at all universities, attended by candidates from African countries and some Indian Ocean Islands. Recently, distance education of masters degrees have been organized in the Democratic Republic of the Congo, from South Africa.

Teaching and training

In most states, undergraduate or basic medical training of medical students does not include family medicine training. In South Africa, the discipline has a well-established presence in the curricula of medical schools. Zimbabwe is attempting to achieve this in Harare as well. Most other medical schools in Africa have programmes in primary care/public health that incorporate some of what could be called family practice teaching.

Colleges of General Practice/Family Practitioners have been slow to develop in Africa. In South Africa, a chapter of the RCGP existed from the early 1950s. In 1958, The College of General Practitioners of South Africa was founded. Zimbabwe formed its College in 1973, and the West African College of Physicians was established in 1976, consisting of members from the five Anglophone countries mentioned above and spread across six faculties, including General Medical Practice. Much of the resistance to forming GP colleges and interest groups in Africa has come from the specialist groupings within the 'medical associations'—perhaps a legacy of the specialist dominance of medical education in global health systems.

Primary care

The primary care doctors or generalists in Africa, particularly those in rural and underdeveloped areas, require a wide range of competencies and skills to practise. Not only is he/she the clinician in the practice or health service, often required to attend to over 120 patients each day, operate, and give anaesthetics, but also in many instances required to be a health service manager, financial controller, teacher, district surgeon/coroner, public health planner and strategist, community leader, epidemiologist, confidante, and sometimes local priest. Many learn 'on the job', often using newer technologies for distance education. Some (the minority) are specifically trained individuals with suitable qualifications.

Traditional healers play a significant role in the health care of African communities. Clients consult these healers, not necessarily as an alternative to 'western' medicine, but as a complementary system of care. These practitioners often deal very effectively with the spiritual and contextual aspects of a patient's life—often better than a 'western' GP. However, many patients are seen at clinics and hospitals with toxic reactions to traditional remedies, plant extracts, and herbs. Attempts are being made in many states to incorporate the services of traditional healers into the management of psychiatric conditions, HIV/AIDS, and tuberculosis, where their holistic health belief models are being synergistically incorporated into the conventional care offered by the GP.

Challenges for primary care

Among the numerous challenges facing primary medical care and family practice in Africa, perhaps the greatest immediate problem is how the practitioner can influence the HIV/AIDS pandemic and give palliative care to the thousands of patients within the community (hospitals are too full). The age–sex pyramids of most sub-Saharan countries are changing dramatically with fewer economically active adults, and a relatively larger older population who must care for more orphans and also assist in the work force.[1] Most pyramids demonstrate fewer emerging young people to become the workers of the future. Health services and their budgets are strained to meet these increased needs. The work of the practitioner will of necessity change with greater community orientation and more ambulatory and domiciliary palliative and terminal care. Private practice too may be threatened as health economies adjust. Research to develop and refine new models is essential.

Despite the tremendous challenges in health care, and sometimes working against great odds, the primary care generalists of Africa are generally dedicated to their tasks and do the best they can with the facilities at their disposal for the communities that they serve. The stresses are often profound but the rewards emotionally rich. Said one GP, 'I will never forget the terror in the eyes of a 17 year-old girl with advanced AIDS and cryptococcal meningitis, and the immense trust she placed in her helpers. She survived this episode, and the joy in her face will stay with me forever'.

References

1. **US Bureau of the Census.** *International Data Base.* Washington DC: International Programs Centre, October 2000 (http://www.census.gov/ipc/www).
2. **UNAIDS.** *AIDS Epidemic Update.* Geneva: UNAIDS, December 1999.
3. **Dorrington, R.** et al. (2001). The impact of HIV/AIDS on adult mortality in South Africa. Technical report from the Burden of Disease Research Unit. Cape Town: Medical Research Council (http://www.mrc.ac.za/bod/index.htm).
4. **World Health Organization.** World Health Report 1998: Life in the 21st Century. A Vision For All. Geneva: WHO, 1998 (http://www.who.int/whr/2001/archives/1998/index.htm).
5. **Population Action International.** Report Card 2001: The Reproductive Risk Index. Washington: PIA, 2001.
6. **Brundtland, G.H.** *Address to Regional Committee for Africa.* Geneva: WHO, August 1998.
7. **UNAIDS.** *Press Release: HIV Threatens Progress against Worsening Global Tuberculosis Epidemic.* Geneva: UNAIDS, 1998.
8. **World Health Organization.** *WHO Estimates of Health Personnel.* Geneva: WHO, September 2001 (http://www-nt.who.int/whosis/statistics/health_personnel/health_personnel.cfm.).

2.3 Primary care and general practice in East and Southeast Asia

Goh Lee Gan

Introduction

Primary care and general practice in East and Southeast Asia is a polyglot. The rural areas are likely to be underserved. Primary care is provided as part of public health, some of it by the state and the rest by communities themselves. Non-government organizations (NGOs) may be a welcome source of care but this is often transient. Urban areas have many competing providers, including the state and a number of private and charitable organizations. General practices, similar to those seen in Western countries, are found in the urban areas. Besides these providers, there are the so-called complementary and alternative medicine (CAM) providers with such varied treatment techniques as herbal medicine, massage, moxibustion, and acupuncture.

The region

Asia can be divided into four sub-regions: Middle East (also called Asia Minor in the past), South Asia, East Asia, and Southeast Asia. This chapter focuses on the last two sub-regions and the countries in these sub-regions are:

- East Asia (China, Hong Kong, Japan, Macau, Mongolia, North Korea, South Korea, and Taiwan);
- Southeast Asia (Brunei Darussalam, East Timor, Indonesia, Laos, Malaysia, Myanmar (Burma), Philippines, Singapore, Thailand, and Vietnam).

Postgraduate training and professional development

Postgraduate training in general practice in Asia had steadily increased over the past 30 years. The system of postgraduate training is varied, depending in part on the political development, colonial past and the relationship with a particular Western country or countries, for example, the United Kingdom with Thailand, the United States with the Philippines, and Australia with Singapore. The Royal Australian College of General Practitioners has played a key role in sustaining the interest and in the dissemination of the principles and practice of Family Medicine in the Asia Pacific Region.[1]

In the last decade, WONCA (see Chapter 2.13) has also exerted some unifying influence in family medicine content and core values worldwide and also had an effect in the development of this discipline in Asia. The organization, working in concert with the general practice organizations in Canada, Hong Kong, Israel, Taiwan, and Singapore, was instrumental in bringing family medicine into China at the time when it was replacing its system of barefoot doctors with doctors trained in Western medicine. In 1998, the Central Government of China took an official decision to develop a community-based health care delivery system, a health insurance system, and general practice/family medicine oriented education and training programmes.[2]

A few generalizations may be made about the systems of family medicine training in this part of the world:

- In East Asia—Korea and Taiwan have the United States type of residency system of family medicine training of 3 years duration. Japan has a United States type of residency system in two medical schools, one in Kawasaki Medical School and the other at Jichi Medical School. The latter is aimed at training physicians for rural practice.[3]
- In Southeast Asia—Singapore, Malaysia, and Hong Kong have the British model of vocational training, with 3 years in Singapore and 4 years in Malaysia and Hong Kong; Philippines has a United States model of residency training of 3 years; Vietnam is beginning to have family medicine programme as a first level specialty in Hanoi and Ho Chi Min City.

Accreditation and professional organizations

In Southeast Asia—colleges of general practice/family physicians have been established in most countries. College Diploma examinations are conducted in countries like Hong Kong, Malaysia, and Singapore. Myanmar has initiated 1-year courses leading to a certificate in Family Medicine. A Master of Medicine degree is awarded in Singapore and Malaysia.

In East Asia—colleges of family medicine are also present. The courses in South Korea, Taiwan, and Japan lead to a Board Certification.

Quality improvement systems

Quality improvement systems are beginning to be developed. Efforts to introduce quality into practice are seen in several countries like Hong Kong, Malaysia, Taiwan, Korea, Philippines, and Singapore. Efforts to keep better medical records, reduce waiting times, prevent medical prescription errors and keep in view drug allergy history are common quality assurance topics. Clinical practice guidelines are beginning to appear. In order to make these freely available, some countries like Singapore have these available on the Internet.[4] With regards to the development of clinical guidelines, inviting family physicians to be part of the drafting committees, and exploration of the barriers to implementation are important steps. The likelihood of adoption of such clinical guidelines will be better.

Audit is the next level of development of quality improvement systems. There is as much need to audit individual performance as the need to audit systems. Failures in the provision of care often stem from systems that could be made safe. Checking on drug allergy is a case in point.

The Hong Kong College of General Practitioners has introduced a quality assurance programme for its members since 1999. It focuses on continuous professional development which covers activities such as supervising younger peers, examination and research, clinical self-audit activities on referrals, investigations, prevention activities continuing medical education with MCQ assessment.

Administrative arrangements

In all the countries, primary care is provided partly by the state and by the private sector and sometimes by NGOs. In countries like Indonesia, Thailand, and Myanmar, government doctors carry out private practice in primary care in the afternoons. This type of arrangement may lead to suboptimal care because time has to be divided between government or public practice in the mornings and private practice in the afternoons. It might be more efficient to work towards either major public service employment or major private service work.

Key policy developments

A key policy development with great impact on countries in Asia was the adoption in 1978 by all countries in Asia of the WHO's Declaration of Alma Ata's Health For All by 2000. The year 2000 has passed by but the spirit of working towards health for all continues. The work of the WHO continues to be focused on health promotion and disease prevention and disease control through primary care. One such preventive strategy is the reduction of morbidity and mortality of the under-fives through the Integrated Management of Childhood Infections (IMCI).

The WHO World Health Report for 2000[5] introduced three concepts for national health systems development that all countries, rich or poor, need to achieve, namely improving the health of the population they serve; responding to people's expectations; and providing financial protection against the costs of ill-health. Progress towards them depends crucially on how well systems carry out the four vital functions of *service provision, resource generation, financing,* and *stewardship.* It places special emphasis on stewardship, which has a profound influence on the other three. Hopefully, this will constitute the next wave of development.

Medical education and academic general practice

The United Kingdom's General Medical Council's document *Tomorrow's Doctors,* with the emphasis on more teaching of general practice, disease prevention and health promotion is being implemented in many countries in Asia. This document is likely to be impactful over time. Those countries whose medical education systems are recognized by the General Medical Council will be implementing its recommendations, if they have not already done so. For the countries outside the General Medical Council in the Asia Pacific, they too may consider such changes in the course of sharing of developments either as the result of a bilateral country exchanges or collaboration at the level of WONCA.

Academic general practice is beginning to take root and expand in medical schools throughout Asia. It is well established in Taiwan, Hong Kong, and Philippines. Textbooks of general practice have been written in Taiwan and Korea.

Specific primary care initiatives

The WHO's initiatives in its Southeast Asia Region and the Western Pacific Region provide governments with information and skills in dealing with its major health problems through primary care. The Western Pacific Regional Office, which deals with most of the countries of East and Southeast Asia, has four themes in its current work-plan: combating communicable diseases; building healthy communities and populations; health sector development; and reaching out to initiatives to the region. Lack of health services for large rural communities is a major problem in Asia. The Rural Health Initiative is therefore a key component of the Memorandum of Agreement between WONCA and WHO signed in October 1998. This commits WONCA and WHO to include the special needs of rural populations in all health plans.

Overview of current position of general practice

Public health provides much of the general practice services in most of the countries in East and Southeast Asia. Exceptions are found in the most developed countries in the region like Korea, Taiwan, Hong Kong, Malaysia, Singapore, and Philippines where Western style general practice has been established. In many of the urban centres in the region, specialists fill the vacuum of the lack of general practitioners. Also, in countries like Indonesia, doctors work in the morning in the government medical institutions as civil servants and become general practitioners in the afternoon and at night in their own practices. Reliable figures on the number of general practitioners are therefore not available. It is a fast changing scene and with the efforts of WONCA, general practice is being introduced into every country in the region. Some of the specialists in these countries have become champions of general practice.

China, in particular, has shown much progress in the last 10 years, following an invitation by the Chinese Government for WONCA to undertake a study and give recommendations on family medicine development. Bilateral relations also provided much of the technology transfer to introduce general practice knowledge, skills, and values into the recipient countries. Thus, Philippines has been in contact with Vietnam and Mongolia, and Indonesia with Singapore in the transfer of general practice technology. As in all countries, general practice has an image problem. There is still much work to be done to sway the minds of the people and hospital specialists on the role that general practice can play in the reduction of disease burden and the promotion of health. Curative medicine and high technology medicine remain overly seductive. Part of general practice development must include efforts towards the integration of hospital care and primary care in a seamless way. The general practice community may need to take the first step towards this.

Future plans for developing primary care in Asia

Future plans for developing primary care in Asia may be grouped into broad strategies and specific strategies. In the former, two can be identified. The first is the continuing effort of the Health for All movement by the governments of individual countries, working through the public health route initiated by WHO in the 1970s. The second is the family physician development route championed by WONCA. This organization has three decades of experience and represents a considerable source of influence around the world.

In the specific strategy category, several national and area specific plans can be identified. The first is the continuing attention to vulnerable population groups. The work of WHO, UNICEF, and other VWOs in the care of vulnerable population groups continues. The IMCI for children; family planning for reproductive women and, increasingly, multi-sectoral approaches to the care of elderly patients, are examples of future plans. The second is the primary care strategy to reduce the burden of endemic diseases like tuberculosis and malaria through specific disease control programmes.

Primary care represents the way forward in Asia. A strong primary health care sector staffed by sufficient numbers of well-trained doctors and other health workers and supported by equally well-trained specialists with their technical resources, is a model for the most effective, efficient and economic health care service in both developed and developing countries. Those responsible for education and training must ensure that they provide the community with the correct number of doctors trained to meet the needs of the community, and those responsible for the health care system must ensure that these doctors are enabled to provide the health care for which they were trained.[6]

References

1. **Goh, L.G. and Fabb, W.** (2001). Family medicine development in Asia Pacific Region. *Singapore Family Physician* **27** (3), 31–6.
2. **Fabb, W.** Family practice in the globe. Workshop on Follow-up on Making Medical Practice & Education more Relevant to People's Needs. A WONCA-WHO Statement, 1994, pp. 57–63.
3. **Smith, B., Demers, R., and Garcia-Shelton, L.** (1997). Family medicine in Japan. *Archives of Family Medicine* **6**, 59–62.
4. **Ministry of Health,** Singapore. Clinical Practice Guidelines—various topics. Available at http://www.moh.gov.sg—select 'publications' and 'Clinical Practice Guidelines'.
5. **World Health Organization.** World Annual Report 2000. Geneva: WHO, 2001, p. 6.
6. **Fabb, W. and Fry, J.** (1994). The past, the present and future. In *Principles and Practice of Primary Care and Family Medicine: Asia Pacific Perspectives* (ed. J. Fry and N. Yuen). Oxford: Radcliffe Medical Press.

2.4 Primary care and general practice in Australia and New Zealand

Rosie Moon, Ngaire Kerse, and Deborah C. Saltman

Introduction

In Australia and New Zealand, the last 20 years have seen substantial changes in all aspects of primary care service requirements, delivery, and funding arrangements. Reforms are now focusing on promoting a system of integrated care with collaborative methods across the health spectrum. A key component has been the emergence of general practice as a specialist discipline of medicine in its own right with specific postgraduate training programmes, ongoing quality assurance requirements, and academic infrastructure, both in Australia and New Zealand.(1)

In Australia, the 1990s saw two major Governmental General Practice reviews, the latter in 1998 putting forward 174 recommendations that are currently being addressed. In New Zealand, the New Zealand Primary Health Care Strategy was published in 2001 outlining substantial changes to the present system. Both countries are placing importance on a move towards integrated and coordinated care services.

Australia

Funding

Australia has a universal health insurance scheme, 'Medicare', funded by contributions from taxes and a levy (1.5 per cent of post-tax income) on individual taxpayers, providing access to free care as a public patient in a public hospital and free or subsidized treatment by GPs and medical consultants. Medical practitioners operate on a fee-for-service basis and charge fees that they consider are suitable for the services they provide. Reimbursements are then paid based on a percentage of the Medicare Schedule fee (usually 85 per cent) from the Treasury.

A private sector exists through private health insurance, operating on a community-rating scheme where all premium holders pay the same premium, regardless of age or pre-existing conditions. The community rating of health insurance has resulted in a substantial increase in insurance premiums and subsequent reduction in membership of private health insurance schemes. As an incentive to hold private insurance, the Government has introduced a tax rebate on 30 per cent of the premium, hoping to diminish the burden on the Medicare system.

Doctors' fees established under the fee-for-service system discriminate in favour of procedural consultants. In an effort to redress the imbalance between proceduralists and generalists, the Government initiated a review of GP services and fees. One of the main outcomes of the review was a differential fee scale for GPs who had undergone training and were prepared to undergo continuing quality assessment.

Organizations

Both the Royal Australian College of General Practitioners (RACGP) and the Royal New Zealand College of General Practitioners (RNZCGP) grew out of their English equivalent over a period of many years. The RACGP is the largest organization for GPs in Australia with over 10 500 members. RNZCGP's membership of over 3000 represents approximately 95 per cent of all New Zealand GPs.(2) Both are the national bodies concerned with standards of general practice and education for GPs. They also represent the views of their members through submissions, lobbying, and public statements.(3)

Education and training

For over 20 years, the major vocational training body for general practice in Australia has been the RACGP. However, a recent Ministerial review resulted in the formation of a Commonwealth controlled company, the Board of General Practice Education and Training Ltd, responsible for managing general practice vocational training. The major general practice stakeholders will be represented on this board.

There are 10 medical schools in Australia with a distinct general practice discipline. Recently, $117.6 million of Government funds have been committed over 4 years to establishing nine new rural clinical schools and two new university departments of Rural Health. This, combined with the Primary Care Research and Development initiative (which will contribute over $200 000 to each academic Department of General Practice to develop the infrastructure for research) is expected to result in considerable development of the academic base for rural and urban general practice in Australia. There is no corresponding investment in development of the academic arm of the discipline in New Zealand.

Vocational registration

Mandatory Vocational Training and Registration was introduced to register GPs separately, for Medicare purposes, from other non-specialist practitioners, and their services attract a higher rate of Medicare benefits than those of non-registered GPs. The requirements for vocational registration remove the capacity for doctors to become GPs without specific training(4) and include:

- completion of a formal general practice training programme;
- attainment of a Fellowship of the RACGP by examination;
- demonstration of ongoing involvement in continuing education and quality assurance activities;
- agreement to participate in peer review through an independent peer-review organization.

To maintain access to higher rebates, GPs must participate in ongoing quality assurance and continuing education. The RACGP Quality Assurance and Continuing Education Program is presently the only organization recognized to certify this process.

Standards and accreditation of general practices

Subsequent to initiating changes in the way individual practitioners were trained and reimbursed, entry standards for general practices were developed by the RACGP. Five categories are used to assess practices against validated, acceptable standards:

- practice services,
- the rights and needs of patients,
- quality assurance and education,
- practice administration,
- physical factors.

An independent body (Australian General Practice Accreditation Ltd —AGPAL), owned and managed by the profession, has been established to accredit general practices based on the standards. A practice must participate in a 3-year cycle, which includes a 12-month preparation period based on a self-assessment kit, followed by a peer-review survey with continuous quality improvement for the remainder of the period.(5) By December 1999, just over 60 per cent of general practices had registered for accreditation.(6)

Medical workforce

In 1999, there were 24 176 non-specialist medical practitioners billing Medicare.(7) In February 2001, there were 17 500 vocationally registered doctors in the Quality Assurance General Practice Program.(8) Australia-wide the estimated ratio of one GP to approximately 900 heads of population does not tell the full story. Maldistribution of GPs remains a major problem—an oversupply in urban centres and concomitant undersupply in rural and remote areas. Seventy-seven per cent of all practices are located in metropolitan areas, 20 per cent in rural regions, and 3 per cent in remote regions.[9]

Some attempts to address rural workforce issues have included:

- increasing numbers of temporary resident doctors to service remote communities defined as 'areas of need' by State Governments;
- access to registration and Medicare benefits to suitably qualified permanent resident overseas trained doctors willing to work in rural areas;
- rural retention incentive schemes.

In addition, the newly formed Australian College of Rural and Remote Medicine will assist in the development of a comprehensive package to help meet the needs of rural GPs in 2001, including a professional development programme for rural and remote GPs and training and support programmes for rural medical educators.

Aboriginal and Torres Strait Islander health

The health status of indigenous Australians remains very poor and the rate of improvement unacceptably slow, despite endeavours to improve the situation. There have been several major inquiries into the health of Aboriginal people over the last 20 years, the most recent in 1999. In the 1999–2000 Budget, the Government provided an additional $78 million over 4 years to improve the access of Aboriginal and Torres Strait Islander peoples to comprehensive health care services. The Department's approach to improving the health of indigenous Australians recognizes that a long-term partnership is required to achieve sustainable gains in health status.[10]

Aboriginal Community Controlled Health Services (ACCHSs) are culturally appropriate, autonomous primary health services initiated, planned, and governed by local Aboriginal communities.[11] ACCHSs vary in size and function and service delivery is constrained by under-resourcing. Larger ACCHSs typically employ several doctors and significant numbers of Aboriginal health workers. In smaller ACCHSs, Aboriginal health workers play a leading role in clinical and other work and on-site medical, dental, or nursing care is not available.

The RACGP, in partnership with the National Aboriginal Community Controlled Health Organisation (NACCHO), has developed the Training Program in Aboriginal Health curriculum in response to Governmental recommendations. All Registrars are provided with training in Aboriginal health, undertaken in partnership with Aboriginal educators. Registrars can undertake attachments to ACCHs or to a clinical setting with significant numbers of Aboriginal patients.[12]

Divisions of general practice

Designed to forge better links between GPs and other health agencies, Divisions were established in the 1990s and are defined by geographical areas and population size. Nationally, there are 123 Divisions with variation in size, activity, organizational structures (private companies to government agencies), and degree of collaboration with community and other health care providers. In 1999, 80 per cent of GPs were members of a Division.[6] However, the term 'membership' is not synonymous with active involvement and anecdotal evidence suggests that less than 10 per cent of GPs are active in the work of the Divisions.

To increase involvement and focus on health outcomes, funding for Divisions has moved from focusing on project development to supporting the achievement of community health outcomes. A number of levels of bureaucracy support Divisions, for example, State-based Organizations, have responsibility for providing support and coordinating cross-divisional activities and Rural Workforce Agencies support and coordinate initiatives in rural and remote general practice. Support and Evaluation Resource Units (SERUs), established in Universities, provide support and advice to Divisions on the development, implementation, and evaluation of their projects.

Coordinated care trials

General practitioners experience considerable obstacles in integrating patient care through the maze of services. Separate Commonwealth and State funding streams within the Australian health care system are a significant contributor to the fragmentation between the primary care services of GPs and the hospitals and their specialist services.[13] A number of Coordinated Care Trials have been set up with a budget composed of pooled Commonwealth and State funds to test whether it is possible to achieve a more effective allocation of resources and better quality of care for people with complex health care needs by creating a single fund holder. Evaluation of the trials continues.

New Zealand

General practitioners , in general, are self-employed and provide consultations in general practice on a fee-for-service basis. Visits to GPs in New Zealand are subsidized by the Government to variable degrees for children and those on a low income. The subsidy is paid for tax-generated Government funds, claimed by the doctor on behalf of the patient, and an additional fee is charged to the patient at the doctor's discretion. In a similar way, the Accident Compensation Corporation of New Zealand (a national accident and work-related injury insurance programme) subsidises general practice consultations for accident casualties. Between 30 and 50 per cent of the practice income, depending on the socio-demographic mix of patients, is derived from government funds, the remainder from the patients' out of pocket payments. The ratio of doctors to patients was previously modulated by supply and demand.

The 1990s and early 2000s saw the development of Independent Practitioner Associations (IPAs), organizations aimed at assisting GPs with contractual and educational needs. Other GP organizations developed alongside IPAs including Health Care Aotearoa, with a Community governance focus, and Maori Provider Organizations. Contracts for GP services were regulated on a regional basis, to encourage redistribution of GPs from 'overdoctored' areas to underserved and rural areas. The New Zealand Public Health and Disability Act 2000 created 21 District Health Boards (DHBs), holding population-based funds for primary and secondary care. For the first time in New Zealand, budgets for both primary and secondary care will be administered at a local level by the same Chief Executive Officer, a controversial move actively debated by GP organizations. Reservation about the move has been expressed as it is feared that the primary health care budget may come under pressure.

Prior to and throughout this period of professional development within general practice, the RNZCGP guided the discipline to become a specialty in its own right:

- the Medical Council of New Zealand holds the Vocational Register, designating general practice as a branch of medicine;
- an approved training and professional accreditation process leads to admission to the Vocational Register;
- the Maintenance of Professional Standards (MOPS) process, via the RNZCGP, is the main way to maintain Vocational Registration for General Practice.

The New Zealand Health Strategy 2000 and the Primary Health Care Strategy 2001 outline proposed reforms for this millennium. A further move to population-based funding will promote the organization of services based on the needs of a defined group of people. Primary Health Organizations (PHOs) deliver essential primary health care services and achieve health goals locally. Enrolment with the PHO will be encouraged through local providers. The strategy aims to increase Government funding for primary care and decrease out of pocket payments in order to improve access to primary health care.

Independent practitioners associations

In New Zealand, IPAs were created in 1992–1993 and by 1999 32 IPAs had more than 2000 members.[14,15] The majority are owned and controlled by the practitioners themselves although many organizations include Maori and consumer representation at board level. IPAs are largely responsible for contractual responsibilities with the funding authorities, educational needs, and quality assurance for their members.

Many IPAs hold the budget for pharmaceutical and laboratory expenditure, and the savings have been used at the discretion of the IPA, under strict

Health Funding Authority oversight, to enhance patients' services, provide education for GPs and practice teams, and fund population-based health promotion programmes.[16,17] Associations have established: comprehensive information systems; computerized practice registers; personalized feedback on prescribing and pathology ordering; and peer-group discussion of guidelines.

There is increasing interest in payment by capitation for general medical services.[16] In 1997, 45 per cent of GPs in one region of New Zealand were capitated and between 4.8 and 12 per cent of GPs were capitated in other parts of the country.[18] Capitation payments only cover the government subsidy contribution to medical services, between 30 and 50 per cent of practice revenues. Enrolment in a practice is a relatively novel concept for New Zealand citizens and does not meet with unanimous approval.

Associated initiatives

Maori and Pacific people's health lags behind that of others in the population. In recent years, Maori and Pacific Island peoples have begun to develop specific culturally competent health services for their own people.[19] It is hoped that improvements for these groups will be achieved through Maori and Pacific provider development as well as by improving the delivery of mainstream services.

Demonstration models of primary care delivery have been successfully tried in areas of high need and poor access. Salaried doctors deliver flexible services in collaboration with nursing, allied health, pharmacy, dentistry, and other health providers at reduced cost to particularly Maori, Pacific Islands people, migrants, and refugees with a high index of deprivation. Models of primary care practice achieved in these successful programmes may be disseminated more widely within the context of the current health reforms.

Medical workforce

In 2000, there were 3166 GPs in New Zealand serving a population of approximately 3.8 million persons. The average ratio of GPs per 100 000 population was 82.4 with regional variation in this ratio from 69.9 (Taranaki) to 90.8 (Canterbury-West Coast).[20]

The majority (66.6 per cent) of GPs operated in group practice, two or more GPs sharing cost , with one-third being in solo practice. The majority of GPs are male (63.2 per cent) but female GPs have steadily made up larger proportions of the GP workforce from less than 10 per cent in the 1980s. Overseas graduates make up about 34.5 per cent of New Zealand general practice. The majority of GPs are of European origin (79.6 per cent) with only 2 per cent being Maori and 0.9 per cent of Pacific Island ethnicity.

As in other nations, publicity has highlighted workforce issues and suggested low morale and increased work pressures for New Zealand GPs. While overall GPs are satisfied with their jobs, levels of psychological symptoms are of concern, particularly for rural and solo practitioners.[21]

Rural issues

Despite considerable progress since recommendations for rural health were made by the RNZCGP in 1999,[22,23] the plight of rural general practice in New Zealand is perceived to be dire.[24] The RNZCGP has a rural committee and representative on Council and the Rural GP Network. Other important initiatives include development of two Centres for Rural Health with multidisciplinary directors. Strategies to increase recruitment and retention in rural general practice have not improved the workforce shortages and the Ministry of Health has announced an intention to develop a coherent policy and package of assistance for rural communities.[19]

Training

Vocational training in general practice, the General Practice Education Program (GPEP), a 3-year programme commencing after 2 years of approved hospital-based experience is provided by the RNZCGP and prepares doctors for general practice and to attain Fellowship of the College (FRNZCGP), the recognized postgraduate qualification for general practice in New Zealand. This education has been accepted by the Australian Medical Council for vocational registration and the right to independent practice under the Medical Practitioners Act (1995).

Future trends

Evidence-based medicine

Australia and New Zealand are no exceptions in the worldwide trend towards the practice of evidence-based medicine based on identifying the best evidence in the literature and applying the information to clinical practice. The University Department of Evidence Based Care and General Practice in South Australia is a leader in the field to strategically plan for, develop, and conduct quantitative and qualitative research in general practice and to assist others in doing the same.

Use of evidence-based databases is low in New Zealand (14 per cent of GPs used the Cochrane database) and very low in Australia. Although 75 per cent of New Zealand GPs have access to the Internet regularly, only 40 per cent have access at the surgery and about half of New Zealand GPs have used the Internet for patient care.[25]

Collaborative practice

In New Zealand, there has been a long tradition of collaborative practice, with practice nurses supported by the practice nurse subsidy since 1970, working alongside GPs. Nurses have responsibility for immunization programmes, recall schedules, cervical screening if certified, and other areas depending on experience and expertise.[26] Because of Government subsidies, New Zealand has a higher ratio of practice nurses to population than many other countries.[19] Independent midwifery practice has been common in New Zealand since 1998.

In Australia, the advent of the use of nurse practitioners within the general practice setting will undoubtedly create changes, particularly in the rural areas where both Australia and New Zealand show serious shortages of GPs. There is a move towards nurses being trained in the prescribing of medications that will also impact on roles within primary medical care.[27]

References

1. **Fry, D. and Furler, J.** (2000). General practice, primary health care and population health interface. In *General Practice in Australia: 2000*, p. 389. Canberra: Commonwealth Department of Health and Aged Care.
2. **Royal New Zealand College of General Practitioners,** Wellington, New Zealand (online), available from http://www.rnzcgp.org.nz.
3. **Wright-St. Clair, R.E.** *A History of General Practice and of the Royal New Zealand College of General Practitioners.* Wellington, New Zealand, 1989.
4. **Mott, K., Kidd, M., and Weller, D.** (2000). Quality and outcomes in general practice. In *General Practice in Australia: 2000*, p. 284. Canberra: Commonwealth Department of Health and Aged Care.
5. **General Practice Strategy Review** (1998). General practice: changing the future through partnership. Report of the GP Strategy Review Group (1998). Canberra: Commonwealth of Australia.
6. **Rudd, C. and Steed, D.** (2000). The structural organisation of general practice. In *General Practice in Australia: 2000*, pp. 210, 220. Canberra: Commonwealth Department of Health and Aged Care.
7. **Harding, J.** *General Practice in Australia: 2000.* Canberra: Commonwealth Department of Health and Aged Care, 2000, pp. 45, 64.
8. **Royal Australian College of General Practitioners.** Personal communication. RACGP, Melbourne: RACGP, 2001.
9. **Campbell Research & Consulting** (1997). The general practices profile study: a national survey of Australian general practices. Prepared for the General Practice Branch, Department of Health and Family Services, Canberra, Australia.
10. **Australian Department of Health and Aged Care:** Budget Portfolio Statements, 2000 (www.health.gov.au:80/hfs/pubs/budget200/partc_7.htm).

11. **Bell, K.** et al. *General Practice in Australia: 2000.* Canberra: Commonwealth Department of Health and Aged Care, 2000, p. 75.
12. **Royal Australian College of General Practitioners.** Position Statement 'Aboriginal Health' endorsed by Council 42/15. Melbourne: RACGP, 2000.
13. **Blight, R.** (1998). Beyond coordinated care: the merging of general practices. *Healthcover* June–July.
14. **King, A.** *The Future Shape of Primary Health Care: A Discussion Document.* Wellington NZ: New Zealand Ministry of Health, 2000.
15. **Malcolm, L., Wright, L., and Barnett, P.** *The Development of Primary Care Organizations in NZ.* Wellington NZ: Ministry of Health, 1999.
16. **Malcolm, L. and Mays, N.** (1999). New Zealand's independent practitioner associations; a working model of clinical governance in primary care? *British Medical Journal* **317**, 1354–60.
17. **Kerr, D., Malcolm, L., Schousboe, J., and Pimm, F.** (1996). Successful implementation of laboratory budget holding by Pegasus Medical Group. *NZ Medical Journal* **109**, 334–7.
18. **Cumming, J.** *Funding Population Based Primary Health Care in New Zealand.* Report for the National Health Committee. Wellington NZ: Ministry of Health, 1999.
19. **King, A.** *The Primary Health Care Strategy.* Wellington NZ: Ministry of Health, 2001.
20. **NZHIS** (2001) *New Zealand Medical Practitioners 2000.* NZHIS, Wellington NZ (online), available from http://www.nzhis.govt.nz.
21. **Dowell, A.C., Hamilton, S., and McLeod, D.K.** (2000). Job satisfaction, psychological morbidity and job stress among New Zealand general practitioners. *New Zealand Medical Journal* **113**, 269–72.
22. **Burton, J.** *Rural Health Care in New Zealand; RNZCGP Recommendation.* Occasional Paper Number 4. Wellington NZ: RNZCGP, 1999.
23. **Royal New Zealand College of General Practitioners.** *General Practice into the Future; a Primary Health Care Strategy.* Report on the Presidential Task Force. Occasional Paper Number 5. Wellington NZ: RNZCGP, 1999.
24. **Janes, R.** *RNZCGP Rural Representative's Report: June.* Wellington NZ: RNZCGP, 2001.
25. **Kerse, N.M., Arroll, B., Lloyd, T., Young, J., and Ward, J.** (2001). Evidence databases and general practitioners: the NZ story. *New Zealand Medical Journal* **114**, 9–11.
26. **Docherty, B.** *Nursing in General Practice; a New Zealand Perspective.* Christchurch NZ: Barbara Docherty, 1996.
27. **Royal Australian College of General Practitioners.** Nurse Practitioners—Position Statement endorsed by Council 42/3. Melbourne: RACGP, 1999.

2.5 Primary care and general practice in Latin America

Stephen J. Spann

Introduction

The development of medical specialism in Latin America closely mirrored that which took place in the United States in the first half of the twentieth century. The development of Family Medicine as a special field of medical practice requiring a defined postgraduate residency training programme, and as an academic discipline, began in the early 1970s, starting with Mexico and slowly diffusing to the rest of the region. This development was stimulated in a major way during the 1980s by the International Center for Family Medicine (ICFM). Founded in 1981 under the leadership of Dr Julio Ceitlin, the ICFM's focus during its first decade was the promotion and development of Family Medicine throughout Latin America, Spain, and Portugal.

By the early 1990s, most of the countries in Latin America had developed postgraduate residency training programmes and national associations or colleges of Family Medicine. However, residency-trained family doctors continue to constitute a very small percentage of the physician workforce in the region, with the exception of Mexico and Cuba. Until very recently, the prevailing view of the medical schools and ministries of health in the region had been that graduation from medical school was sufficient training for general practitioners; Family Medicine residency training was felt to be unaffordable, and unnecessary.

Because of policies of open admissions to medical schools, most Latin American countries produce an excess number of physicians, many more than the available postgraduate residency training positions. This has resulted in physician underemployment, and a large number of general practitioners with no postgraduate training. As in many other parts of the world, specialists have traditionally been remunerated at significantly higher levels than primary care physicians. It is not surprising that general practice has been viewed historically as an undesirable, low prestige career choice for physicians in this region. Because of the excess production of physicians, in many Latin American countries physician specializing in Internal Medicine, Paediatrics, and Obstetrics–Gynaecology function mainly as primary care physicians; even medical and surgical sub-specialists do some primary care in their private practices in order to enhance practice income.

The region

Though geographically very diverse, the Latin American region, typically defined to include Mexico, the countries of Central and South America and Cuba, Puerto Rico, and the Dominican Republic in the Caribbean, share a common heritage, culture and, for the most part, language. All countries, with the exception of Cuba, currently enjoy a democratic form of government. Many of the countries in the region (Argentina, Chile, Cuba, Uruguay) have epidemiological characteristics similar to those of North America and Western Europe; the majority of the other countries in the region are in epidemiological transition from a predominance of acute, infectious disease morbidity/mortality towards one of chronic and degenerative diseases. The health care systems of these countries share certain similarities. In most countries of the region, the majority of health care is rendered in the public sector, either through public health care systems run by the ministries of health, or through national social security programmes which provide health care to workers and their families. Private health care is typically available to only a small portion of the population. Most physicians work in the public sector, and have a private practice as well.

Postgraduate training, accreditation, professional development, and national organizations

Postgraduate training programmes in Family Medicine are now available in all countries of the region except for Guatemala, Honduras, Guyana, and Suriname. Table 1 shows the year in which Family Medicine residencies were started, and the current number of such training programmes in each country. The duration of training is 3 years in all countries. Family Medicine is currently a recognized medical specialty in the great majority of these countries; many of these require the physician to pass a certifying examination. Most have one or more national associations of Family Medicine, as well (Table 2). National as well as regional, meetings involving neighbouring countries, constitute an important source of continuing medical education for family physicians.

Table 1 Family Medicine residency training in Latin America[(1)]

Country	Year FM started	Current number of FM residencies
Argentina	1970[a]	90
Bolivia	1976	3
Chile	1981	7
Colombia	1984	3[b]
Costa Rica	1987	1
Cuba	1985	1
Dominican Republic	1981	1
Ecuador	1987	4
El Salvador	1971	1
Guatemala[c]		
Guyana[c]		
Honduras[c]		
Mexico	1971	13
Nicaragua	1986	1
Panama	1976	1
Paraguay	1987	2
Peru	1991	3
Puerto Rico	1974	5
Suriname[c]		
Uruguay	1997	1
Venezuela	1980	11

[a] In 1970, Argentina established postgraduate residency training in General Medicine; Family Medicine residency programmes started in 1980.

[b] Two additional residency programmes in Family Medicine have been approved in Colombia, but are not currently in operation.

[c] Does not have any established Family Medicine residency programme.

Note: no data are available for Belize and Brazil.

Table 2 Specialty status, certification examinations, and national associations of Family Medicine in Latin America[(1)]

Country	Recognized specialty?	Certification examination?	National association?
Argentina	Yes	Yes	Yes
Bolivia	Yes	Yes	Yes
Chile	Yes	Yes	Yes
Colombia	Yes	Yes	Yes
Costa Rica	Yes	No	Yes
Cuba	Yes	Yes	Yes
Dominican Republic	Yes	Yes	Yes
Ecuador	Yes	No	Yes
El Salvador	No		No
Guatemala	No		No
Guyana	No		No
Honduras	No		No
Mexico	Yes	Yes	Yes
Nicaragua	Yes	Yes	Yes
Panama	Yes	No	Yes
Paraguay	Yes	No	Yes
Peru	Yes	No	Yes
Puerto Rico	Yes	Yes	Yes
Suriname	No		No
Uruguay	No		Yes
Venezuela	Yes	No	Yes

Note: no data are available for Belize and Brazil.

Quality improvement systems

There is a growing interest in quality improvement among family physicians of the region. This is typically implemented at a health care system, or institutional, level and typically focuses on prevention, maternal–child health, and chronic diseases. National academies/societies have generally not developed such systems.

Administrative arrangements

Family physicians employed by the public health care sector are typically paid on a salary basis. There are exceptions: the ministry of health of Uruguay compensates its family physicians based on a capitation method, according to the number of patients enrolled in their practices. In their private practices, family physicians are typically reimbursed on a fee-for-service basis. In some countries such as Argentina, Chile, and Colombia, there is a growing trend towards privatization of health care delivery. In these countries, family physicians are increasingly being recruited by private health care entities; compensation methods range from salary, to fee-for-service, to capitation. In the private health care sector, primary care physicians are generally compensated at a significantly lower level than procedurally-oriented specialists.

Key policy developments

A few health care systems in the region have made the policy decision to establish family physicians as the base of their delivery system. There are three outstanding examples: the Cuban health care system, the Mexican Institute of Social Security (IMSS), and the health care system operated by the Construction Workers' Union of Argentina (OSPECON). Beginning in 1984, the government of Cuba began to place family physicians in practice in communities where they have responsibility for a population of patients (120 families, 600–800 patients) living in a defined geographic area. A family physician/nurse team lives and practices in the community they serve. Mornings are typically spent providing acute care in the office; afternoons are spent making home visits in the community, with a focus on disease prevention/health promotion. Each team constructs an epidemiological map of the community served, stratifying the population according to health and risk status. Residency training is community based and follows an apprenticeship model.[(2)] There are currently over 30 000 family doctors in Cuba.[(3)] The country's health indices and epidemiological profile are similar to those of North America and Western Europe. The Mexican Institute of Social Security (IMSS), which provides care to most non-federal employees of that country, developed a programme using general practitioners for providing longitudinal health care to families in 1954.[(4)] Currently, 43 per cent of the physicians within IMSS are family physicians; these provide the primary medical care to the bulk of the IMSS patient population.[(3)]

In Argentina, where the social security system provides care to workers and their families through labour union-run health care systems, the Construction Workers' Union system (OSPECON) began transforming its delivery model in 1991 to one in which family doctors constitute the primary care base. This resulted in decreased health care costs and increased patient satisfaction, and OSPECON has served as a stimulus to other union-run systems to follow their lead.[5] Perhaps as a result of these successful health care models, the Pan American Health Organization (PAHO), the branch of the World Health Organization (WHO) serving the Americas and Caribbean region, has recently become much more interested in and supportive of the development of Family Medicine in the region. This shift in policy will undoubtedly have an effect on the health manpower policies of the ministries of health in the countries of the region.

Medical education and academic general practice

The introduction of Family Medicine into the medical school curriculum is proceeding slowly but surely within the Latin American region. A minority of the medical schools in most countries have departments of Family Medicine, except for Cuba, Puerto Rico, and Venezuela, where all medical schools have such departments. Some medical schools offer elective courses in Family Medicine, and a few schools have required courses in the discipline (Table 3). In most of the countries, research in Family Medicine is still at a very primitive stage. Most studies to date have been descriptive in nature.

Specific primary care initiatives

The public health care systems in many of the countries have primary care initiatives focused around certain health problems and/or age groups. Examples include maternal care including pregnancy and family planning, well child care/immunizations, care of specific chronic diseases (diabetes, hypertension) and care of certain infectious diseases (tuberculosis, STDs). This approach to care often flies in the face of the continuous, comprehensive, family-oriented care model typically offered by family doctors, and can discourage family physicians from practicing in these systems.

Current position and future development of family medicine in Latin America

Because the countries in the Latin American region are still developing from an economical standpoint, they cannot afford to waste precious health care resources. Family Medicine offers an ideal model of care, which has been shown to enhance the quality of care, while decreasing costs and enhancing the satisfaction of the population with their health care.[6] Family Medicine has a tenuous foothold in the health care systems of this region but medical specialism still holds a firm grip on both medical practice, and medical education in these countries. However, the same forces that are driving health care reform in the rest of the world are present in this region: inadequate access to care (despite an excess of physicians in many countries), escalating health care costs, sub-optimal quality of health care, and inequitable distribution of health care. A health care system with a strong primary care base comprised of well-trained family doctors can readily address these problems. Cuba has already implemented this solution. In other countries, such as Argentina, there is a growing demand for residency-trained family doctors. External funding agencies such as the

Table 3 Family Medicine presence in medical schools in Latin America[1]

Country	Number of medical schools	Medical schools with a department of Family Medicine	Medical schools with a required Family Medicine course	Medical schools with an elective Family Medicine course
Argentina	23	1	4	3
Bolivia	9	0	0	0
Chile	12	4	0	0
Colombia	42	3	9	3
Costa Rica	7	1	4	0
Cuba	21	21	21	0
Dominican Republic	9	2	2	0
Ecuador	9	1	2	1
El Salvador	6	2	0	0
Guatemala	3	2	2	0
Guyana	2	0	0	0
Honduras	1	0	0	0
Mexico	59	2	0	2
Nicaragua	3	0	0	0
Panama	3	1	3	0
Paraguay	5	0	0	0
Peru	21	0	0	0
Puerto Rico	4	4	3	1
Suriname	1	0	0	0
Uruguay	2	1	1	0
Venezuela	8	8	2	0

Note: no data are available for Belize and Brazil.

Inter-American Development Bank and the World Bank are stimulating the strengthening of primary medical care in these countries, including funding for increasing/improving training programmes in Family Medicine.

One important threat to the ongoing development of Family Medicine in the region is the possibility that health care system demand for well-trained family physicians will outstrip the supply. A number of programmes have sprung up in some countries to 're-train' physicians in other specialties, and non-residency trained general practitioners, to become family physicians. It will be important that these programmes provide rigorous, high quality training, in order to ensure high quality family physician graduates. Another important threat to Family Medicine development is the resistance of many medical schools to establish academic departments of Family Medicine. These are needed to expose medical students to family physician role models, and to assure the intellectual growth of the discipline through research.

References

1. **Parkerson, G.** et al. The status of family health care and family medicine in the region of the Americas. A joint project of the Pan American Health Organization and the Department of Family and Community Medicine of Baylor College of Medicine. Unpublished report submitted to the Pan American Health Organization, 2001.
2. **Ordoñez Carceller, C.** (1997). La insertión de la medicina familiar en Cuba. In *Medicina de familia: la clave de un nuevo modelo* (ed. J. Ceitlin and T. Gómez Gascón), pp. 293–301. Madrid: IM&C.
3. **Ceitlin, J.** (2001). Desarrollo de la medicina familiar en América Latina y España. In *Medicina familiar y práctica ambulatoria* (ed. A. Rubinstein, S. Terrasa, E. Durante, E. Rubinstein, and P. Carrete), pp. 18–22. Editorial Médica Panamericana, Buenos Aires: Editorial Médica Panamericana.
4. **del Olmo, J.** (1997). La inserción de la medicina familiar en México. In *Medicina de familia: la clave de un nuevo modelo* (ed. J. Ceitlin and T. Gómez Gascón), pp. 315–20. Madrid: IM&C.
5. **Cacace, J.** (1997). La seguridad social en Argentina: el caso OSPeCON. In *Medicina de familia: la clave de un nuevo modelo* (ed. J. Ceitlin and T. Gómez Gascón), pp. 309–14. Madrid: IM&C.
6. **Starfield, B.** (1991). Primary care and health. A cross-national comparison. *Journal of the American Medical Association* **268**, 2032–3.

2.6 Primary care and general practice in Europe: West and South

John L. Campbell, Juan Mendive, and Arno Timmermans

In this chapter we describe primary health care in the United Kingdom and the Netherlands in some detail, because of their strong primary care-led system of health care. Of necessity, we have been selective, and describe primary health care in other western European countries as an overview.

United Kingdom

Starfield's recent examination of the position of primary health care amongst Western industrialized nations showed that a primary care orientation of a country's health service system is associated with lower costs of care, higher satisfaction of the population with its health services, better health levels, and lower medication use.[1] In that analysis, the health care system of the United Kingdom was identified as being the most primary care oriented amongst 11 countries examined.

The United Kingdom National Health Service represents a comprehensive, centrally funded system of health care in which over 99 per cent of the population are registered with general practitioners who provide 24-h access to care and a range of other preventative, diagnostic, and curative services. Over 90 per cent of health care contacts take place within the context of this system. The total number of UK general practitioners providing care in 1999 was 38 009. Over 33 000 of these general practitioners were 'Principals', providing unrestricted primary care services, the remainder acting as assistants, general practitioner registrars in training, or a very small number providing a restricted range of services. Between 1983 and 1999, there was a doubling in the proportion of female general practitioners to 32 per cent. Under present arrangements, general practitioners are required to retire from NHS service at the age of 70—in 1999, 67 per cent of all general practitioners in England and Wales were aged between 30 and 49. Current data indicate that 84 per cent of general practitioner principals work full time, and of the remaining 16 per cent, 75 per cent are females. General practitioners have guarded their 'independent contractor' status—the general practitioner being self-employed but contracting with the NHS to provide general medical services for a named population of patients. Recent years have seen the introduction of 'personal medical services' contracts allowing for some general practitioners to be directly employed to deliver clinical services to patients.

Workload

Eighty-seven per cent of general practitioners have a full-time contract. An important feature of the NHS is the list system in which all individuals are registered with a named general practitioner who has responsibility for their care. The average number of patients cared for by unrestricted principals in the United Kingdom has fallen from 2011 (1985) to 1807 (1997). UK general practitioners carry out around 283 million consultations each year, a figure that has increased by 45 million since 1983. The average person consults a general practitioner five times a year, although this figure is higher for children under 4 years of age (7) and for patients over 65 (6.5).[2] Patients may be seen in the practice (71 per cent), at home (13 per cent), or spoken with on the telephone (12 per cent). Several alternative means of accessing primary care have been introduced in recent years, and are likely to change this pattern of service usage.

Medical education, postgraduate training, and professional development

'Tomorrow's Doctors'[3] was a milestone publication influencing undergraduate medical education in the United Kingdom. In most medical schools, students now have community based clinical exposure and attachment from the earliest years of the medical curriculum, with up to 20 per cent of the undergraduate curriculum being taught in the community in some institutions.

The 5 years spent in undergraduate medical education are followed by a year spent as a 'house officer' before full registration with the General Medical Council, and pursuit of specialist or generalist training. Doctors entering general practice must undertake a further 3 years of vocational training. At least 2 years of this are spent in hospital posts approved for the purpose. A further year is spent as a general practice registrar involving working and training in general practice with a recognized trainer. Successful completion of vocational training involves (since 1998) summative assessment of competencies. The competencies assessed are outlined in Box 1.

Summative assessment involves a multiple choice questionnaire, video assessment of consultation skills, written submission of practical work, and a report submitted by the registrar's training doctor. Until recently, the process of vocational training has been overseen by the Joint Committee for Postgraduate in General Practice, a body which will be replaced by the

Box 1 Competencies assessed at summative assessment

1. Factual medical knowledge.
2. The ability to apply factual medical knowledge to the management of problems presented by patients.
3. Effective communication.
4. Satisfactory consultation skills.
5. The ability to review and critically analyse the practitioner's own working practices.
6. Clinical skills.
7. The ability to synthesize these competencies and apply them in a general practice setting.

Postgraduate Medical Education Training Board. These bodies are presently considering extension of the general-practice-based component of training to a 24-month period.

Continuing professional development

The aim of continuing professional development is to sustain lifelong learning among general practitioners and help them to provide high-quality patient care throughout their careers. The postgraduate education allowance scheme encourages established general practitioners to keep up to date with developments in clinical practice. To claim the full allowance (£2695 in 2000/01), the general practitioner must (within the preceding year) have completed at least two courses covering 5 days of educational activity approved by the Director of Postgraduate General Practice Education for the region in which the course is held.

Revalidation

Revalidation has been described as the 'regular demonstration by doctors that they remain fit to practice'. There are presently no legal requirements to continue training once a doctor has qualified as a general practitioner. This is changing, however, and the General Medical Council has introduced proposals for the revalidation of doctors' registration on a regular basis—current proposals suggest that it is likely that this procedure will take place on a 5-yearly cyclical basis.

Professional organizations

To practice medicine, all doctors must be registered with the General Medical Council. The British Medical Association provides union and workforce representation on behalf of doctors in the United Kingdom, whilst the Royal College of General Practitioners (RCGP) is one of a number of UK medical royal colleges representing professional sub-groups. Membership and Fellowship of the college are open to general practitioners who sit the membership examination or undergo membership by assessment of performance. These examinations are not mandatory. The RCGP presently has around 18 000 members.

Quality control systems

The National Health Service in England is responsible to the Parliamentary Secretary of State for Health. An Executive develops and implements policy through eight regional offices and 100 health authorities, the latter having a strategic role with responsibility for improving the overall health of the population and for reducing health inequalities. Recent years have seen a substantial move towards the implementation of evidence-based practice with a National Institute for Clinical Excellence deciding which treatments should be made available to the population. Audit and feedback are important components of general practice, particularly in relation to prescribing activity. All general practitioners receive individualized feedback on their prescribing activity in the preceding 3 months on a cyclical basis.

Clinical governance can be defined as 'a framework through which NHS organizations are accountable for continuously improving the quality of their services and safeguarding high standards of care by creating an environment in which excellence in clinical care will flourish'.[4] The process aims to develop a culture of quality, and is the responsibility of health authorities and primary care groups and trusts in conjunction with local primary health care teams. Individual quality measures are proposed from time to time—the Government has recently indicated its intention that all patients should be able to see a general practitioner within 48 h of requesting an appointment. Considerable work has been undertaken in recent years regarding the assessment of general practitioners' performance, and a wide range of measures are proposed in this regard.[5]

Policy developments

A publicly financed and comprehensive health care system such as the NHS is subject to substantial political influences, and the years since 1989 have seen radical reforms of the NHS, first through the development of the internal market and the introduction of general practitioner fundholding, and later through removal of the market principle and its replacement with new overarching primary care structures bringing together providers of health and (ultimately) social care. From an early experimental status, primary care based purchasing became a central element of the NHS during the 1990s. Although initially opposed by the British Medical Association, many doctors eventually opted in to the system of fundholding, which by 1997 covered around 50 per cent of the population. The Labour Government of 1997 abolished general practice fundholding on the grounds of inequity and unacceptably high transaction costs, whilst retaining an emphasis on the 'primary care led NHS'.

Primary Care Trusts

Establishment of these central components of delivering primary care was announced in a government white paper in 1997.[6] Primary Care Trusts will be the main agents in the Government's drive towards a more integrated health service. NHS policy involves shifting the balance of power within the NHS towards primary care, and it is anticipated that these primary care organizations will ultimately receive and control around 75 per cent of the total NHS budget. The PCT Board has widespread primary health care representation, including general practitioners, and lay representation. Internal structures allow for representation of the professional groupings within the primary care community. The Chief Executive's team oversees delivery of Board policy.

Primary Care Trusts are responsible for assessing local health needs and (increasingly) for the commissioning of health services for their population of patients. It is anticipated that these organizations will have an increasing role in delivering and co-ordinating local health and social care services in conjunction with hospital and social care organizations. Primary Care Trusts are presently responsible for the administration and delivery of primary care to populations of around 100–200 000 people.

Other primary care initiatives

Primary care in the United Kingdom is based on a model in which general practice and general practitioners play a central role. General practitioners now operate as part of a multi-disciplinary primary health care team involving input and support from practice management and administrative staff, practice nurses, nurse practitioners, health visitors, and close liaison with a wide range of other community-based health care professionals such as pharmacists, optometrists, community mental health teams including community psychiatric nurses, and addiction teams.

The Netherlands

The Netherlands has a strong primary care orientation in its health care system and a high score on international health indicators.[1] Of 7763 general practitioners, 42 per cent of general practitioners currently work in solo practice. There is one full-time equivalent general practitioner for every 2483 inhabitants, but 39 per cent of general practitioners now work part-time. Demographic characteristics of general practitioners are changing rapidly—currently only 21 per cent are younger than 40 (women 43 per cent, men 13 per cent). Women comprise 63 per cent of general practitioner trainees. Among general practitioners looking for a practice, 86 per cent prefer a part-time job and only 8 per cent prefer a single-handed practice.(7)

About two-thirds of the Dutch population have health care insurance in the social insurance system, while one-third have private insurance. Both systems include the same mandatory basic coverage, but individuals may also add private insurance. A national tax-based health insurance system covers major risks such as long-term treatment, long-term care, and psychiatric care. Privately insured patients pay the general practitioner a fee for service, while the general practitioner is reimbursed by a capitation fee for patients covered by social insurance.

The average patient list per full-time general practitioner is 2350 patients. General practitioners play a central role in the health care system, treating the majority of ailments and caring for more than 90 per cent of health care problems presented in their practice. General practitioners function as gate-keepers for other medical specialists and hospital admissions.

It takes 6 years of basic medical training to become fully qualified in medicine. Three additional years of vocational training are required for registration as a general practitioner. Revalidation of Dutch general practitioners occurs every 5 years and requires the doctor to be working as a general practitioner and to earn at least 40 CME credit points (hours) per year. General practice is well established as an academic discipline. Dutch general practitioner investigators contribute on a large scale to the publication of research in international journals.

Quality improvement (QI) is a cornerstone of general practice in the Netherlands. The Dutch College of General Practitioners has set up a comprehensive quality system. The policy of quality improvement is based on the principles of the quality cycle (Box 2).(8)

Since the 1980s, peer groups have met throughout the country on a regular basis. Over 75 clinical practice guidelines have been developed. A translation in English can be seen on the website of the College (http://www.artsennet.nl/nhg). Each guideline provides guidance for the diagnosis and treatment of one medical topic. Guidelines are developed by working groups of volunteer general practitioners, supported by the staff of the Dutch College. New guidelines are being produced and existing guidelines are being updated on a regular basis. The Dutch College promotes the following basic principles:(9)

- the natural course of a disease is of major importance;
- education advice is preferred over medication;
- the use of new drugs has to be considered carefully and to be recommended, new drugs must be proven to have clear advantages over currently well-known drugs;
- treatment in general practice is preferable when treatment by general practitioners and medical specialists is equivalent.

Adoption of clinical guidelines is voluntary. The average rate of implementation is 70 per cent; specific programmes have raised this to 80 per cent in some areas. A comprehensive programme enhances implementation of the guidelines. The programme includes dissemination, assessment procedures, educational products for both general practitioners and supporting staff, support materials focusing on the different organizational aspects of care, telephone cards for practice assistants, patient information leaflets and letters, an electronic prescription system, and interdisciplinary guidelines.

Box 2 Dutch College of General Practitioners quality cycle

1. Formulate what is meant by good quality care in general practice.
2. Choose goals suitable for quality improvement, in accordance with existing practice guidelines, if possible.
3. Collect data and evaluate the care provided.
4. Organize activities for quality improvement.
5. Evaluate and adjust these activities as necessary.

Practice assessment, a 1-day peer visitation, has also become an established part of the quality system. Practice assessment is obligatory for the funding of a nurse practitioner in general practice.

Future goals for the quality programme include involvement of patients in the development of guidelines and cooperation with medical specialists. In collaboration with scientific organizations of specialists, the Dutch College tries to obtain consensus about the treatment and the approach of the specialist and that of the general practitioner. Specialists and general practitioners can use this consensus for local arrangements and cooperation.

Dutch general practice is not 'an island in Europe'. In 1977, the Dutch College organized the Leeuwenhorst conference, at which a European definition of general practice was formulated and thereafter influenced the development of general practice in Europe for decades. In 2002, the Dutch College hosted a WONCA Europe conference (see Chapter 2.13) at Noordwijk, to formulate definitions for the core content of general practice and the core competences of a general practice in a changing society.

Dutch general practice is also an 'export product'. General practitioners from the Netherlands are involved in supporting the development of general practice in Romania, Poland, Greece, the former Soviet republics, China, Costa Rica, and elsewhere. Based on comprehensive research into health systems in eight countries, the quality system of the Dutch College of General Practitioners (together with the government of Switzerland) was awarded the Bertelsmann prize 2000.(10) The award was given for the comprehensiveness of the system and its influence on health care in the Netherlands.

As in every country, changes in society have an influence on general practice in the Netherlands. In many European countries, demographic changes such as ageing and immigration are now taking place. A strong growth in part-time work, a higher rate of general practitioners quitting their jobs, and less enthusiasm for work in health care in general are some reasons for serious potential manpower problems in the years to come. Remuneration of general practitioners is also an issue. A tendency to individualization and consumerism in society stimulates discussions about listed patients and the gate-keeper system.

A new vision of the future of general practice in the Netherlands has been examined in a nationwide discussion among general practitioners. General practitioners have restated their central role in health care, as the place of first contact and with responsibility for continuity of care. More and more single-handed practices will evolve to group practices, tasks will be delegated to supporting staff, and cooperation with other health care workers will grow.

Germany

The German health care system provides care for its 82 million population covering 356 978 km^2 with a structure in which public health and primary and secondary ambulatory care are only loosely distinguished from hospital-based in-patient care. A rapid growth in health care expenditure ended in 1977, with the introduction of the Health Insurance Cost Containment Act. Funding of the health care system has been administered through 453 statutory sickness funds (covering 72 million people) and 52 private health insurance companies (covering 7 million people).

Primary and secondary ambulatory health care is provided by office-based physicians who have responsibility for financing of premises, equipment, and personnel. The majority of such physicians (75 per cent) are solo practitioners. Ambulatory physicians cover all specialties, with a small percentage having admission rights to hospital (e.g. in isolated rural areas)—the remainder transferring responsibility for care during in-patient episodes to hospital-based physicians.

Germany has no gate-keeping system—patients are free to select a sickness-fund-affiliated doctor of their choice. Family practitioners are general practitioners and physicians without specialization. Despite Federal

Government policies and other attempts in recent years, the number of general practitioners has reduced relative to the numbers of office-based specialists, being less than 40 per cent in 1998.

Education and training

Germany has 36 medical schools and a 6-year undergraduate course providing 9500 medical graduates per annum. Curricular reform is ongoing. Undergraduate assessment focuses around four central examinations. Recent years have seen an increasing move towards primary care based education, more bedside teaching, introduction of problem-solving curricula, and integration of basic sciences with clinical teaching.

Secondary professional training involves the specialization of all doctors after graduation, with general practice being recognized as a distinct specialty. The rather weak position of general practice and primary care within the health care system has coincided with the reduction in perceived status of general practice and (since 1999) a move towards increasing support of general practice training by sickness funds and private insurers. Continuing professional development is voluntary and self-regulated by health care professionals. There is a recognition that future and existing health care professionals require to be better qualified in primary care, health promotion, rehabilitation care, and in interdisciplinary cooperation.

Funding issues

Ambulatory physicians receive funding in three steps:

1. Sickness funds make total payments to physician associations for the remuneration of affiliated doctors. Such payments are capitation based.
2. Physician associations disburse total payments amongst affiliated members according to a uniform value scale and additional regulations—the uniform value scale covering all approved medical procedures and services.
3. Office-based physicians invoice their associations on a quarterly basis.

The current average income for an ambulatory physician is 150 000 DM, this also being the average income for a general practitioner, whilst for an ENT ambulatory specialist, average income is around 250 000 DM.

Health care reforms

The major objective of recent reforms has been cost containment, with the introduction of budgets, introduction of reference pricing, and restrictions on the supply of high-cost technology equipment. Other objectives do however exist, including health for all. Although health promotion activities were legally abolished in 1996, the principle continues through the introduction of health care targets that differ between social funds.

At present, general practice and primary care is relatively weakly represented within the German health care system.[(1)] The absence of a gate-keeping role is an issue under review. Current funding structures tend to support ambiguity in policy regarding gate-keeping—although German sickness funds claim to support the principle, their models of health care tend to reinforce the gate-keeping role of the fund and resource allocation, rather than primary care practitioners and clinical need.

Belgium

The Kingdom of Belgium covers 30 528 km^2, and has a population of 10 170 226 (1997). The low-lying terrain accommodates one of the most densely populated, heavily industrialized nations in Europe, with emphases on trade and industry, with some traditional industries (lace making and diamond cutting) persisting. Belgium has three official languages—Flemish, French, and German.

Belgium, along with France, Germany, and the United States, has an unregulated system of primary care whereby national policies do not influence the location of physician practice. There is virtually universal coverage with over a half of health care costs funded by employer/employee contributions. General practice training is strong, and most general practitioners operate from solo practices. Primary care physicians are reimbursed on a fee-for-service fee, with the level being negotiated directly with patients who are then partially reimbursed (except for those on low incomes where there is exemption from payment). In contrast with the United Kingdom there is no patient list system—patients may select to consult any general practitioner or specialist at their own discretion. Home visits are an integral part of the system—in 1997, 25 276 297 visits were made by patients to doctors, and 21 513 465 visits made by doctors to patients at home. The free choice of first doctor to contact leads to patients 'shopping around' for care and to over-consumption of medical care and consequent increases in health care expenditure. There are presently plans to introduce a general medical file for each patient that will allow for the collation of information on patients in one place, and in developing patients' loyalty towards one particular general practitioner.

Training

In 1995, there were 3060 medical students at various stages of undergraduate training in Belgium. The undergraduate course is of 7 years and incorporates a year of practical, hospital-based training. To be able to practice, doctors require postgraduate accreditation, with specialist training courses lasting between 4 and 6 years. In 1997, of the 39 240 doctors in Belgium (of which 35 757 were general practitioners and 3483 specialists), 28.7 per cent were female—a significant increase from only 12 per cent in 1977.[(11)]

Spain

Substantial health reforms followed the introduction of new legislation ('Ley General de Sanidad', *General Health Law*) in 1986 consequent on the Alma-Ata recommendations. Although publicly funded universal coverage of health care has operated in Spain for many years, the reform of the system introduced a very different primary care scenario, with the establishment of a primary care oriented health care system. Currently, the whole population (40 million) benefits from a centrally funded health care system based on tax revenues, with decentralization of planning, and devolution of health care budgets to 17 local government bodies.

Like the United Kingdom, Spain has universal coverage and open access to primary care. Primary care providers are salaried employees of health authorities, operating from health centres that are owned by these bodies. The location of health centres is based on the geographical distribution of the population. Such centres provide a wide range of primary care health services to around 15 000 to 25 000 individuals, this figure being dependant on whether the setting of the centre is urban, semi-urban, or rural. Health centres offer curative and preventive services, as well as rehabilitation and palliative care. Infrequently, and only in rural areas, family physicians may work in solo practice. Group practices usually have between five and 10 family physicians.

The nurse has a central role in primary care delivery, health authorities employing nurses in equal numbers to work with family physicians. Nurses have the main responsibility for the management of chronic problems, preventive activities, and for the home care services. Administrative staff and social workers are also key professionals contributing to care provided at the health centres.

Training for Family Medicine in Spain was established when the new speciality of Family and Community Medicine was recognized in 1978. Unlike other specialities, there had been no postgraduate training programme for primary care prior to that time.

The establishment of a 3-year training programme in 1978, along with other health reforms, saw major changes in the situation. The postgraduate training programme for family medicine in Spain is a common programme for the whole country requiring accreditation of teaching primary health care centres and tutors on the programme. Health authorities also established a theoretical and practical training programme for practising general practitioners who had not previously undergone postgraduate training. Currently, around 2000 of 4000 graduating students from undergraduate programmes enter the postgraduate training system for family medicine. Half of the training takes place in primary care settings and half in hospital settings, including emergency care. As in other European countries and following a European Directive in 1995, completion of training for family medicine is compulsory prior to providing services as a family doctor. Although the training programme has improved the situation considerably, the possibility of extending the course to a period of four years of training is currently being explored.

Training is coordinated through 'Family Medicine Training Units' established by health authorities to oversee the programme. There are about 90 such units in Spain, each with their own training structure and personnel, including support staff for research purposes.

Although the postgraduate structure of family medicine is now well established in Spain, very little has changed in the exposure of undergraduates to primary care. Indeed, there are no departments of family medicine at any of the 19 undergraduate medical schools in Spain (although some have loosely affiliated departments of family medicine or primary care associated indirectly through internal medicine or public health). This situation is under review, with an increasing number of undergraduate primary care attachments being offered, and increasing opportunity for the development of academic careers in a number of medical schools.

In recent years, increasing postgraduate training opportunities for Spanish family doctors has led to increased competition for posts in primary care. A recognition of the standard of Spanish training, and internal workforce pressures has resulted in some European countries (mainly United Kingdom, Ireland, Sweden, and Portugal) offering employment opportunities for Spanish family doctors.

An important third component of primary care development in Spain in recent years was the establishment of the Spanish Society of Family and Community Medicine (semFYC) in 1983. Although membership was initially restricted to trained family doctors, this has now been extended to all family doctors and residents in the training programme.

Among the main achievements of semFYC is the establishment of the preventive and health promotion programme. This programme involves the organization and opportunistic integration of preventive health activities in primary care. The programme has been adopted by many Spanish health authorities, with around 25 per cent of the population benefiting from the arrangements. Other activities of semFYC include the publication of practice guidelines, and the establishment of an accreditation system for continuing medical education activities. An international committee ensures the representation of the organization at the European Society of General Practice–Family Medicine, WONCA, as well as the representation of the organization in various European networks.

France

General practice in France is well established, and there is a long tradition of general practitioners working for the public health system in small practices, usually as solo practitioners. GPs in the health care system in France do not have a gate-keeping role,[12] and individuals may change their general practitioner as frequently as they wish. Practices are unequally distributed throughout the population, and there is no system of patient lists assigned to individual doctors. People may choose the general practitioner they wish to manage any episode of illness. Reimbursement to the doctor from public authorities is based on a common honorarium. Although the number of vocationally trained general practitioners has been low in France, there has been a substantial increase in recent years. Several medical schools in France now have training programmes for family medicine, established since the application of the European directive in 1995.

At least some of this improvement is attributed to the CNGE, the scientific organization of teachers of general practice in France. This organization has been crucial in promoting better standards of training in family medicine, and in publicizing the recent changes in family medicine in France. The journal of the organization, *Exercer*, is an important reference point for all French general practitioners who are involved in teaching and training.

The SFMG is a scientific association of general practitioners that has been of major importance to French general practitioners in recent years, particularly in relation to their continuing medical educational activities. This organization publishes *La Revue du Practicien*, a journal which acts as the main reference resource for continuing medical education of general practitioners in France.

Portugal

Portugal has a rather similar health system to the one previously described for Spain. Like Spain, Portugal has achieved important progress in family medicine in recent years. Family doctors are mostly vocationally trained, delivering primary care from dedicated centres and working together with other professional and administrative staff. Primary care providers are salaried practitioners providing a comprehensive range of curative and preventative health care activities. The Portuguese population is dispersed, and there is a need for family doctors to work in rural health centres. In areas close to Spain, some Spanish family doctors are taking the opportunity to work in Portugal. The APMCG is the scientific association of family doctors in Portugal; this organization has been active in recent years in promoting Portuguese family medicine within the international community. The APMCG has also promoted the attendance of Portuguese family doctors at many recent international conferences.

Italy

Italian general practitioners are independent practitioners within the health care system. They tend to operate as solo practitioners, although in Italy (unlike neighbouring France), family doctors have a gate-keeping role in relation to other health services. Italy has a long history of general practice, claiming to have one of the highest populations of general practitioners in Europe, especially within urban areas. There is, however, no tradition of postgraduate training for family medicine, although the European Directive of 1995 also saw the introduction of a 2-year training programme for general practitioners, which is compulsory for doctors providing care within the public system.

Italian family medicine is represented by a number of associations. The SIMG, the Italian Society of General Practitioners, is a scientific and trade-union organization associated to UEMO, which represents most general practitioners. The Italian Academy of Family Medicine has been responsible in recent years for promoting the training of Italian family physicians. SIMiFaC is the Italian Society of Family and Community Medicine, an organization that has worked hard in recent years to gain recognition, and to disseminate the idea of the need for a broad-based approach in primary care, taking account of the prevailing social environment. Finally, CeReMe is the research organization responsible for collaborating with WONCA in reporting on Italian primary care.

Greece

The health system in Greece was reorganized in the late 1970s following the Alma-Ata recommendations. This reorganization saw the establishment of primary health care delivery services that have been modified over the years to account for the political and administrative structures prevailing in Greece. The basic unit of health administration is the district, this planning unit being the focus for all elements of health care delivery.

Greek general practitioners provide care from primary health care centres, and work alongside other professional groups. The service is publicly funded, with general practitioners being salaried employees. Recent years have seen advances in training for family medicine. The comprehensive 4-year postgraduate training programme is now popular with graduating students from the universities. The University of Crete was one of the first universities in Greece to have an academic general practice focus in a department of social medicine. The Greek Association of General Practitioners (ELEGIA) is the organization responsible for the international representation of Greek general practitioners.

Conclusion

It is of importance to emphasize the significant efforts made in recent years by WONCA (see Chapter 2.13) and the World Health Organization, which have contributed to improvements in primary health care systems in many of the above-mentioned countries. The situation throughout all of the countries of west and southern Europe cannot be described in detail in the present chapter and interested readers are referred to the websites and documentation of some of the previously mentioned organizations[13–15] as important sources for more comprehensive descriptions of the primary care systems within these countries.

References

1. **Starfield, B.** *Primary Care. Balancing Health Needs, Services, and Technology.* New York: Oxford University Press, 1998.
2. **Royal College of General Practitioners.** *Information Fact Sheet 3: Workload.* London: Royal College of General Practitioners. RCGP Information fact sheets, 1999.
3. **General Medical Council Education Committee.** *Tomorrow's Doctors: Recommendations on Undergraduate Medical Education.* London: GMC, 1993.
4. **Department of Health.** *A First Class Service.* London: HMSO, 1998.
5. **Campbell, S.M., Roland, M.O., Quayle, J.A., Buetow, S.A., and Shekelle, P.G.** (1998). Quality indicators for general practice: which ones can general practitioners and health authority managers agree are important and how useful are they? *Journal of Public Health Medicine* **20** (4), 414–21.
6. **Department of Health**. *The New NHS, Modern, Dependable.* London: HMSO, 1997.
7. **Keneens, R. and Hingstman, L.** *Cijfers uit de registratie van huisartsen, Peiling.* Utrecht: Nivel, 2001.
8. **Grol, R.** *Kwalitieitsbevordering voor en door husartsen.* Utrecht: Nederlands Huisartsen Genootschap, 1995.
9. **Thomas, S., Geijer, R.M.M., Laan, J.R., and Wiersma, T.J.** *NHG—Standaarden voor de huisarts II.* Utrecht: Nederlands Huisartsen Genootschap, 1996.
10. **Bocken, J., Butzlaff, M., and Esche, A.**, ed. *Reforming the Health Sector: Results of International Research.* Gutersloh: Bertelsmann Foundation Publishers, 2001.
11. **European Observatory on Healthcare Systems Series: Healthcare Systems in Transition**—Belgium. WHO Regional Office in Europe, 2000.
12. **Boerma, W. and Fleming, D.M.** *The Role of General Practice in Primary Health Care.* Geneva: WHO Europe, 1998.
13. **World Health Organization. Regional Office for Europe.** *Framework for Professional and Administrative Development of General Practice/Family Medicine in Europe.* Geneva: WHO Europe, 1998.
14. **World Health Organization. Division of Development of Human Resources for Health.** *Making Medical Practice and Education More Relevant to People's Needs. The Contribution of the Family Doctor.* Ontario, Canada: WHO WONCA, 1994.
15. **Saltman, R.B. and Figueras, J.**, ed. *European Health Care Reform. Analysis of Current Strategies.* Geneva: WHO Europe, 1997.

2.7 Primary care and general practice in Europe: Central and East

Adam Windak and Peter van Hasselt

Introduction

Until the end of the 1980s, countries of Central and Eastern Europe were strongly influenced politically by the Soviet Union and its socialist economy. Health care in the region was a public responsibility. Organization, management, and delivery of care were undertaken by the state authorities. Financing and administration were strongly centralized and bureaucratic. Primary health care (PHC) was provided exclusively by clinical specialists or under-qualified recent graduates. General practice, well known before the World War II, had been nearly completely abolished.

In this chapter, we will describe the changes in the field of PHC, especially in family medicine/general practice, in those Eastern and Central European countries previously part of or under the influence of the Soviet Union, located north of the former Yugoslavian Republic. The second section will describe the situation during Soviet period. The third section will present the international collaboration for change. The next four sections describe the development of specific training in family medicine, the establishment of departments in universities, professional organizations and structures for quality improvement. The final two sections are concerned with the status at the beginning of the twenty-first century and future plans for family medicine in Central and Eastern European countries.

Health care in Central and Eastern Europe

After World War II, the Siemaszko model, developed in the 1920s in the Soviet Union, was imposed on all the countries concerned. The main features of the model were:

- nearly all inhabitants were entitled to free health care;
- health care was financed by the state, out of general taxation;
- finances were regulated by central and regional state administrations;
- finance was allocated according to the needs of existing or planned infrastructure rather than patient needs;
- financing was based on fixed indicators, mostly the number of Full Time Equivalents of personnel instead of health care needs of the population;
- there were little or no contributions by patients to funds, except for medicines;
- the scope of services was poorly defined but in practice determined by public investments instead of health care needs of the population;
- health care was delivered exclusively by public service providers;
- patients were allocated to local or regional providers according to their place of residence;
- there was a shortage of highly specialized and advanced techniques;
- informal payments were widespread to obtain better access or higher quality services.

Under the Siemaszko model, several clinical specialists provided primary care (usually internal medicine specialists, paediatricians, and gynaecologists). In the larger cities they were employed by large polyclinics, otherwise by rural health centres.

In rural areas, PHC was usually limited to the services of 'district physicians', internists, paediatricians, or newly qualified and unspecialized

Table 1 Per capita health care expenditure in US$ PPP (adjusted for purchasing power parity) and as a percentage of GDP in selected European countries in 1997 (or latest available)

Country	Health care expenditure per capita in US$ PPP	Health care expenditure as a percentage of GDP
EU countries		
Germany	2364	10.7
Denmark	2042	8.0
Netherlands	1933	8.3
EU average	1771	8.5
United Kingdom	1391	6.8
Greece	1196	8.6
Spain	1183	7.4
Portugal	1148	7.9
CEE countries		
Czech Republic	943	7.2
Hungary	642	6.5
Poland	386	5.2
Russian Federation	47[a]	2.2[b]
Ukraine	10[c]	3.5

[a] 1993.

[b] 1995.

[c] 1994.

Source: WHO Regional Office for Europe Health for All database.

doctors. In theory, patients would consult one of them first—for other clinical specialists they needed to be referred. In practice, however, patients had easy or even unlimited access to most outpatient clinical specialists.

District physicians were not properly trained for the job. Those doctors working in primary health care designated as clinical specialists had the same training as those working in hospitals. Physicians had little or no understanding of the complexity of the patients' problems. Indeed they did little more than treat uncomplicated infections or issue medical certificates. Consequently, they referred over 50 per cent of their cases to clinical specialist outpatient or hospital services, requiring a high number of hospital beds.

As a result, they needed a large number of doctors, especially in the former Soviet Union countries. For instance, at the end of the 1990s in the Russian Federation there were 4.2 doctors per 1000 inhabitants compared to 1.6 and 2.5 in the United Kingdom and the Netherlands, respectively, countries with a family doctor/general practitioner model.

Consequently, it was common to find low quality care, low patients' satisfaction, rising costs, and medical staff dissatisfied with their working conditions and salaries.

After the collapse of communism at the beginning of the 1990s in most countries, health care reform started. Emphasis was on the development of insurance-based financing, decentralization of the organization of health care, and maybe most important of all, the re-introduction of family medicine as a new speciality.

Health care expenditure in all the countries of the region is far lower than in Western Europe. (Table 1)—presenting a great obstacle to reform.

International collaboration

At the beginning of the 1990s, new democratic governments in Central and Eastern Europe were forced to seek more cost-effective health care services, able to meet society's expectations.

Since the Alma Ata conference, WHO has promoted the role of PHC.(1) The Regional WHO Office for Europe discussed with governments of the region potential development of PHC. Several meetings were organized, including one in Perugia, Italy, in 1991, which framed the future development of general practice in Europe.(2,3) This policy line was confirmed by several later meetings and documents.(4,5)

PHC reform towards the general practice/family medicine model was approved by decision makers in all the countries of the region. Furthermore, PHC was seen as a core of the reformed health care systems. Such a profound re-orientation of this sector required fundamental changes in the structures and attitudes of patients, medical staff, health care administrators, and decision makers.

This complex process needed external support, both know-how and finance. In many countries, these were provided by the PHARE programme, funded by the European Commission.(6) Between 1990 and 1993, over 90 million US$ was made available for health care reform in Central Europe.(7)

Courses for future trainers of new family doctors were organized. English-speaking, motivated candidates from Central and Eastern countries were selected for training in Western universities to learn the principles of the discipline. After they returned, they were expected to develop and conduct training courses for their colleagues in their native languages. In fact, they also became early leaders and advocates of family medicine.

A second intervention was foreseen—support for establishing university departments of family medicine including model practices to serve future training.

This scenario was repeated in many countries.(8–10) At that early stage international contacts and external support helped to transfer necessary knowledge to initiate the process of change and provided technical support to establish the basic framework, essential for further development.

Collaboration continued through numerous bilateral or multilateral educational and research projects and the work of WONCA and its network organizations, the European Academy of Teachers in General Practice (EURACT), European Working Party on Quality in Family Practice (EQuiP), and European General Practice Research Workshop (EGPRW).

Specific training in family medicine

Training of physicians for PHC based on family medicine was one of the most difficult challenges. Future family doctors were expected to have much broader knowledge and skills than the specialists formerly working in PHC. New attitudes were needed to change from a disease-centred to a patient-oriented approach. Profound changes were also needed in teaching style. Predominant teacher-oriented methods like lectures and seminars had to be replaced by learner-centred methods and active learning. Postgraduate education necessitated to be moved out of hospitals and into the community. Teachers experienced in PHC were needed in place of clinical specialists. Such profound changes necessitated a gradual, step by step strategy. At the beginning of the 1990s nearly all governments in the region recognized family medicine as an independent medical discipline and specialty. Training of first trainers usually took place abroad, as described above.

The new training programmes included two types of training. Since 1993, in nearly all countries, re-training programmes in family medicine have been established for specialists working in PHC wishing to become family doctors. At the same time modern, residency-based programmes for young physicians graduating from medical schools have been initiated. Retraining programmes were designed to allow physicians to acquire necessary knowledge, skills and attitudes without losing contact with daily practice and patients.

Residency-based programmes, lasting from 2 years in Ukraine to 4 years in Poland, were established.

Model practices were new and important places for training, although hospitals and university departments were still involved in the process.

The target numbers of physicians to be trained in different countries varied. In Estonia, 800 family doctors were needed to serve the whole population, while in Poland roughly 20 000 were needed.(6,11) At the end of the twentieth century, some countries (Estonia, Hungary) were close to the target number of family doctors, while others (Bulgaria, Ukraine, Russia) were still in the initial phase.[10–14]

Family medicine as an academic discipline

Establishing university departments of family medicine is crucial for the development of the discipline. They are needed as centres of excellence, teaching undergraduates and postgraduates, and conducting research and quality assurance projects. Their existence is essential for the emergence of family medicine as a recognized discipline within medicine and particularly among academics, who are influential opinion makers. So, the creation of university departments became an important part of the action plan in many countries. Training of staff, renovation of facilities and purchase of equipment were planned as part of family medicine projects.

In Lithuania, Latvia, Estonia, Poland, Hungary, Slovakia, and the Czech Republic, nearly all university medical schools now have departments or chairs of family medicine. In Ukraine and in Romania, nearly half of all medical schools have a department or chair in 1999.[10] There are several departments in Russia.[15]

Gradually, they have developed a full range of academic activities. Originally created to provide vocational training, they quickly introduced undergraduate programmes. Nowadays family medicine is taught within basic medical education programmes in all departments of undergraduate medical schools of the region. The length, content, and methods of the programmes vary. However, nearly all medical students have some exposure to the discipline during undergraduate education.

Departments are usually chaired not by family doctors, but by sympathetic clinical specialists, who hold the necessary degrees to occupy posts and to be allowed to teach within the academic hierarchy.

Research and other scientific work is also conducted by these departments. Scientific papers, written by GPs from Central and Eastern Europe are published in professional and scientific journals all over the world. Many are written in collaboration with more experienced co-authors from Western Europe. Departments are more and more frequently involved in international research networks, especially the EGPRW.[16] GPs from the region actively participate in international conferences and congresses.

Professional organizations

Professional development of family doctors can be supported by colleges, scientific associations, and other organizations, bringing together physicians, nurses, allied health professionals, and sympathizers. Such organizations have now been established in all countries of Central and Eastern Europe.

Colleges usually limit their membership exclusively to licensed family doctors. The overall role of such colleges is to strengthen the development of the discipline and to promote family medicine. Colleges oversee standards of practice. In many countries colleges are also involved in the development of family medicine teaching, especially postgraduate training.

In some countries, these responsibilities are shared with scientific associations, which promote the discipline through research and education. Sometimes the functions overlap. Colleges and associations hold regular national, scientific and educational meetings frequently. Local conferences on particular themes are organized more.

There are larger scale initiatives. Estonia, Latvia, Lithuania, and Poland collaborate as the Baltic group of countries.

Many of the organizations in the region regularly publish newsletters and educational or scientific journals.

At the 2001 WONCA World Council Meeting in South Africa, there were colleges and associations from Czech Republic, Estonia, Lithuania, Poland, Romania, and Ukraine represented as full members, and more will join.

Quality improvement systems

The Siemaszko health care model typically involved a traditional, repressive approach to quality with external control and a system of punishments. By contrast, the modern approach is based on the quality cycle and on continuous improvement. Such approaches are becoming more popular[17] and knowledge about them is shared through the colleges' activities and journal publications. The Czech Republic, Estonia, Hungary, Lithuania, and Poland are represented in EQuiP—the branch of WONCA Europe, responsible for quality development—and more are joining.

In Poland, Czech Republic, and Hungary, guidelines on the management of selected health problems or diseases have been published. There have been systematic efforts to produce reliable and valid guidelines for family doctors in Latvia and Estonia. In Poland, there is now regular training for tutors of peer review groups. These developments are continuing.

Unfortunately decision makers still have limited understanding of the techniques of modern quality improvement. They still prefer traditional, external, and repressive quality control. But the momentum of developments within the profession must soon begin to influence decision makers.

Overview of the position of general practice at the beginning of the twenty-first century

The sections above described a decade of changes in primary health care in Central and Eastern Europe. Reform has re-established the discipline of family practice. However, as the discipline has continued to develop in the rest of the world, especially in North and West Europe, it is very difficult for Central and Eastern European countries to catch up. These countries are still struggling with numerous problems and harmonious development is jeopardized by unstable political situations and frequent changes of decision makers.

There are differences between countries. In Slovakia, Hungary, and Czech Republic although general practice is a formally recognized discipline, taught at the universities, the old fashioned division between physicians treating children and adults has been preserved.[12,18] In several countries, for instance, Estonia and Latvia, family doctors are not 'gate keepers' and have to compete with other specialists.[11] In most countries, patients still have free access to specialists without referral for some specialities such as gynaecology and dermatology.

In Russia, Ukraine, Bulgaria, and Romania, there are still limited numbers of trained family doctors and the old style of polyclinics still predominates. Little progress has been made in Belarus, where primary health care is still provided by specialists, employed by state polyclinics.

Implementation of family medicine in Central and Eastern Europe is seen as a part of health care reform. It is not an absolute priority for decision makers. It is rather a tool for more effective use of resources and increasing the quality of care. Emphasis is often put on privatization and (re)establishment of independent practices, contracting directly with new insurance companies.[6,18]

Future plans for developments

Most of the countries of Central and Eastern Europe are on their way towards modern primary health care, based on general/family practice. There are significant differences in the amount of reform. In all countries the discipline needs systematic development, and in particular:

- explaining and advocating the principles of the discipline to the general public, academic leaders, and decision makers;
- completion of retraining programmes for clinical specialists already working in PHC;

- establishment of departments or chairs of family medicine at all medical faculties in universities;
- establishment of effective undergraduate and postgraduate training programmes;
- clarification of the role of the GP within the health care system, emphasizing teamwork, 'gate-keeping,' and the use of patient lists;
- promotion of modern quality improvements methods.

These goals can be achieved if medical leaders, patients, and decision makers work closely with the international family medicine community.

References

1. **Primary Health Care.** Report of the International Conference on Primary Health Care, 6–12 September 1978, Alma Ata, USSR. Geneva: World Health Organization, 1978.
2. **Evans, P.R.** (1994). Medicine in Europe: the changing scene in general practice in Europe. *British Medical Journal* **308**, 645–8.
3. **The contribution of family doctors/general practitioners to health for all report on a WHO working group**, Perugia, Italy, 22–25 May 1991. Report of the Working Group on the Contribution of Family Doctors/General Practitioners to Health for All 1991, Perugia, Italy.
4. **Making medical practice and education more relevant to people's needs: the contribution of the family doctor.** A working paper for the World Health Organization and the World Organization of Family Doctors. From the joint WHO-WONCA Conference in Ontario, Canada, 6–8 November, 1994.
5. **WHO—Europe Region Declaration** (1996). Ljubljana charter on reforming health care. *British Medical Journal* **312**, 1664–5.
6. **Windak, A.** (1998). The return of old family doctors in the new Europe. *European Journal of General Practice* **4**, 168–70.
7. **Richard, T.** (1995). Challenge is thrown to Europe's GPs. *British Medical Journal* **311**, 1043.
8. **Whitehouse, C.R.** (2000). The development of family medicine training in Poland—a decade of European cooperation. *European Journal of General Practice* **6**, 23–6.
9. **Toon, P.D., Southgate, L.J., Gubachev, Y., Kossovoi, A., and Simbirtsev, S.** (1998). In the steps of Peter the Great—building links between London and St Petersburg. *European Journal of General Practice* **4**, 37–8.
10. **Gibbs, T., Mulka, O., Zaremba, E., and Lysenko, G.** (1999). Ukrainian general practitioners; the next steps. *European Journal of General Practice* **5**, 72–4.
11. **Lember, M.** (1996). Revaluation of general practice/family medicine in the Estonian health care system. *European Journal of General Practice* **2**, 72–4.
12. **Jack, B., Nagy, Z., and Varga, Z.** (1997). Health care reform in Central and Eastern Europe. Family Medicine in Hungary. *European Journal of General Practice* **3**, 152–8.
13. **Goranov, M.N. and Balaskova, M.I.** (1998). General Pactice in Bulgaria. *European Journal of General Practice* **4**, 37–8.
14. **Jogerst, G.J., Lenoch, S., and Ely, J.W.** (1998). Russian family practice training program: a single step on a long journey. *Family Medicine* **30**, 372–7.
15. **Vinkour, V.** (1998). Training general practitioners in St Petersburg. In Education and debate. *British Medical Journal* **317**, 741–4.
16. **Thomas, P., Griffiths, F., Kai, J., and O'Dwyer, A.** (2001). Networks for research in primary health care. *British Medical Journal* **322**, 588–90.
17. **Windak, A., Tomasik, T., and Kryj-Radziszewska, E.** (1998). The Polish experience of quality improvement in primary care. *The Joint Commission Journal on Quality Improvement* **24**, 232–9.
18. **Jurgova, E.** (1998). The transposition of Slovak health care system and its influence on primary care services. *European Journal of General Practice* **4**, 34–6.

2.8 General practice in Europe: Scandinavia

Frede Olesen

This chapter describes general practice in Scandinavia, which covers four North European countries each with 4–9 million inhabitants, that is, Denmark, Norway, Sweden, and Finland (Table 1), as well as Iceland (285 000 inhabitants), Greenland (55 000 inhabitants), and the Faeroe islands (45 000 inhabitants), the last two of which are self-governing Danish dominions. The chapter aims to give an overall impression of the GP's role and function in the Scandinavian health care models without providing detailed descriptions and statistics from individual Scandinavian countries.

The description will focus on the models in Denmark, Norway, Sweden, and Finland. The health care system in Iceland is quite similar to that of the other Scandinavian countries, especially the Swedish, and is influenced by the large size of the country compared with the low number of inhabitants.

All the Scandinavian countries have a long tradition of a firmly established primary health care system and a strong GP sector. Their health care systems are publicly financed through state and county taxes and are organized by national and county authorities. Patient co-payment is minimal. Both the primary and the secondary health care sectors are headed by the same regional and national political and administrative bodies. This has advantages and disadvantages:

- All citizens have health insurance and enjoy equal access to care for equal needs independently of their social position and ability to pay.
- The health care system benefits from a strong political and professional interest in coordinating the different sectors.
- Politicians have a keen wish, springing from considerations of costs, to keep as many health care tasks as possible within the primary sector.
- All Scandinavian countries seek to secure an even distribution of the number of GPs per 1000 inhabitants throughout the countries. Rural areas, for example, in Northern Scandinavia, may seek to have more GPs per 1000 inhabitants due to the great distances (vacancies may be a hindrance to achieving this goal).
- Commercial competition between GPs and between GPs and other specialists or hospitals is almost non-existent. This situation favours a health care system driven solely by people's medical needs.
- The private insurance-paid part of the health care system is small, less than 5 per cent in all countries.
- The very high level of public funding and the lack of economic incentives may, however, be instrumental in creating long waiting lists and bottleneck problems, compromising the feeling of a smooth, seamless health care system.
- Another disadvantage may lie in patients' ability only to exercise indirect influence on health care planning through national and local elections and the ordinary political channels.

Table 1 Number of inhabitants, physicians, and GPs in Finland, Norway, Sweden, and Denmark

	Number of inhabitants	Inhabitants per physician	Number of GPs	Inhabitants per GP
Finland	5 180 000	330	1954	2650
Norway	4 500 000	280	2308	1950
Sweden	8 880 000	320	5324	1670
Denmark	5 330 000	310	4359	1225

Source: Nordic Medical Facts, Swedish Medical Association, Stockholm, 2001.

Public health insurance

All the Scandinavian countries have a public, tax-paid health insurance system. In Norway, Sweden, Iceland, and Finland, the GPs are employed by regional health care authorities. Danish GPs are contractors to the public health insurance and are, therefore, funding their own clinics and covering all costs, including payroll and running costs. Payment of Danish GPs is based on a mixed fee-for-service (70 per cent) and capitation (30 per cent) system. All contacts are paid by the public, whereas there is a small co-payment from patients in the other Scandinavian countries. Doctors in the other Nordic countries are typically paid a fixed salary, but recent years have seen a shift towards different combinations of fee-for-service and fixed salary. In Finland, for example, less than 40 per cent of the GPs are on fixed salaries; the rest receive a combination of fee-for-service, capitation, and salary. The co-payment from patients in Norway, Sweden, Iceland, and Finland is small, typically equivalent to the income earned in 1–2 h by a blue-collar worker and with reduction for chronically ill or financially non-privileged patients.

In Scandinavia, public health insurance is subject to political governance, and incentives are plenty to coordinate hospitals and primary care and to explicitly describe task distribution between primary health care and hospital care (see also chapter about 'Generalists in Hospitals').

Scandinavian GPs are generally trained to a level that puts them at par in terms of specialization with other specialists within the health care system and their income usually matches that of other specialists, depriving physicians of financial or educational incentives to choose one specialty over another.

Gate keeping and list patients

In all the Scandinavian countries, GPs assume an important role as gate keepers to hospital care even if Sweden and Iceland maintain open walk-in hospital clinics, especially in many big cities, besides the GP pathway to health care. All the countries have open accident and emergency services in the big cities.

For decades, Denmark has had a list–patient system, and more than 97 per cent of the population has joined a list and have their own GP (less than 3 per cent have chosen not to be on a list and have to pay a small amount of the GP bill themselves). In recent years, Norway, Sweden, and Finland have taken different initiatives to establish list–patient systems, but these reforms have not yet been fully implemented, partly due to political resistance and partly due to a perceived reduced freedom for patients to choose care givers. In Finland, 60 per cent of the population is listed now, especially in the big cities. Non-listed patients in big cities, therefore, enjoy a free choice of GP, whereas geography for practical purposes enforces a list–patient system in rural areas even if it is not formally implemented. Scandinavian patients signing up on a doctor's list usually do so within a GP setting where the GP is working alone in a single-handed practice or together with other GPs, for example, in a health care centre.

Organization of general practice work

Besides favouring list–patient systems, all countries have taken initiatives to stimulate coordination of care between hospitals and primary health care (see also chapter about 'Generalists in Hospitals'). Icelandic specialists have been less interested in cooperating with the GPs and least committed to gate keeping, but some quarrels between specialists and GPs over the last two decades have now been settled, and Iceland now follows the general Scandinavian trend.

Scandinavian GPs mainly work on the basis of face-to-face contacts with their patients. Their duties in relation to the community, public health care, groups of people, and other non-GP partners are few. Finland, however, has quite strong traditions for GPs taking responsibility for public health. In Denmark, a few non-GP specialists are also working in primary health care, but patients should normally be referred to them through the gate-keeping system; so from a functional point of view these specialists are part of the secondary health care system. Access to eye specialists and ENT specialists is, however, for historical reasons free. In all other Scandinavian countries there are specialists from other disciplines in primary health care. This is especially the case in the big cities.

All the Scandinavian countries have a strong municipality-led home care sector run mainly by nurses. Its aim is to coordinate preventive and curative care for elderly, chronically diseased, and disabled patients. Scandinavian GPs are typically part of an informally run primary health care team that cooperates with this home care sector.

The GPs' clinical work varies among the countries as Finland and Sweden have a strong tradition for fairly large health centres with about 3–10 GPs, whereas clinics in Norway, Iceland, and Denmark remain smaller (two to four GPs), and about one-third of all GPs in Denmark are still single-handed practices. Norway and Iceland also have many single-handed practices, especially in the many sparsely populated rural areas.

The amount of auxiliary staff is smallest in Denmark with 0.5–1 staff member per GP whereas the bigger Swedish and Finnish health centres typically have several nurses and other professionals in the team.

GP services include telephone advice, consultations, and home visits in all the Scandinavian countries. Denmark operates the most well-developed telephone consultation service, and almost all GPs set aside 1 h per day solely for telephone consultation purposes. Some 3–4 per cent of all face-to-face contacts in Denmark are home visits. These figures are somewhat smaller in Norway, and home visits are rare in Sweden and especially in Finland. A typical Danish GP sees 18–20 patients per day and (s)he is in indirect contact, mainly by telephone, with a similar number of patients. These figures are smaller in the other countries.

Scandinavian GPs typically work from 8 AM to 4–5 PM, 5 days a week, that is, around 40 h per week. All the countries have automatic out-of-hours service rota systems. These systems are most well-organized in Denmark, Finland, and Sweden. In Norway, however, the small number of GPs in the large, less densely populated areas makes it necessary to run rota systems with around two to four GPs.

Formally, preventive care is part of Danish GPs' services. They are primarily responsible for preventive child care, they are playing a major role in preventive maternity care, and they are performing all the child immunizations. In Sweden, preventive maternity care and child care are to some extent undertaken by special clinics staffed by nurses and midwives. The Nordic GPs participate in a few other preventive tasks in relation to individual patients, for example, Pap smear screening.

Academic institutions, academic development, and research

All the Scandinavian countries have a rather long tradition for academic university institutions and there are now GP chairs at all the universities. Moreover, several university-based or county-based research units for general practice have been established, lending further strength to the case for evidence-based teaching and training in primary care. The links between research and continuous medical education (CME) activities have traditionally been rather weak in the Scandinavian countries because CME activities have been confined to medical associations and colleges whereas research has been pursued at the universities. However, this gap is now closing and research, teaching, and quality management are now becoming better integrated.

Education and vocational training

The Scandinavian colleges for general practice are generally influential, and there is only one college per country. They have a long tradition for influencing health care planning and for cooperation with the medical associations of which there is also only one per country.

The duration of the medical study is $5\frac{1}{2}$–6 years. All countries have mandatory pregraduate courses in primary health care and general practice including a 2–8-week stay in a general practice setting. All Scandinavian universities have, in one way or another, a final examination involving GP functions.

All countries have mandatory postgraduate training for all doctors. Such training typically lasts around 18 months and includes a period of usually 6 months in general practice.

Physicians who want to become GPs within the public health insurance system must be trained to the level of being a specialist in general practice, and all the countries formally recognize general practice as a medical specialty. The training required to become a specialist in general practice lasts $3\frac{1}{2}$–5 years, varying from country to country. Approximately half of the time or a little less must be supervised clinical training in general practice. Hospital training takes place in different clinical departments, and theoretical courses in the functioning as a GP are mandatory. The duration of these courses is in the range of 200–400 h.

Only Finland has a formal specialist general practice examination and doctors without an examination get paid less. For years, Sweden has had a voluntary specialist examination, whereas there is no formal specialist examination in Denmark and Norway.

Scandinavian family medicine is closely coordinated and enjoys a solid academic standing owing, among others, to the biannual Scandinavian congresses in family medicine, which have been held now for more than 20 years, and to a joint periodical for GPs, the *Scandinavian Journal of Primary Health Care.*

Continuous medical education and quality assurance

Continuous medical education has been driven by a mix of independent education initiatives and initiatives taken by pharmaceutical companies in all the countries. The independent CME has typically been arranged by the medical associations or the colleges and, to some extent, by the health care regions.

None of the countries have mandatory CME. However, both quantitative and qualitative aspects of CME for GPs are receiving much attention both from the public and the public health insurance. There is, generally, a clear tendency in all the Scandinavian countries towards

- Creating publicly and professionally steered CME activities.
- Creating balanced CME schemes to avoid dominance by the interests of the pharmaceutical industry. This effort also involves growing public regulation of industrial sponsoring of CME for GPs.
- Creating multidisciplinary CME as part of the regional activities in cooperation between hospitals, the social sector, and GPs within the region.
- Creating group-based, self-steered CME for small groups of 8–20 GPs with the aim of obtaining maximum activation of participants.
- Creating a liaison between research, CME, and quality development in a system giving priority to evidence-based teaching and evaluation of performance according to well-defined quality indicators.
- Creating regional guidelines followed up by active local CME and formal monitoring of performance within quality assurance protocols.
- Individual monitoring and registration of each GP's CME activities as a tool to ensure appropriate CME for all.
- Creating economic and other incentives for participating in CME activities. Norway has introduced a system with CME points. GPs who do not collect a sufficient number of points over a period of 5 years have deductions in their income from the health insurance.
- Augmenting the number of quality assurance activities. Norway has been setting aside substantial funds for stimulation of quality assurance activities for years. Such funds have also existed in Denmark, Sweden, and Finland, at least for the last 5–10 years.
- A more spirited discussion of the feasibility and the need for a recertification initiative as recertification is not mandatory in any of the Scandinavian countries.

Scandinavia, like the rest of Europe, has given high priority to quality development initiatives. This has been reflected in both the structure and the practical activities and in the creation of different quality networks, including networks within the Scandinavian countries. A few should be mentioned:

- In the 1980s, an audit system was created at the University of Odense, Denmark (Audit Project Odense, APO). The initiative started as a simple practice activity analysis where a few GP groups met and discussed their practice activities. This initiative has developed into a more comprehensive quality assurance process including all the phases of the quality assurance circle. This system has been implemented in all the Scandinavian countries.
- The advent of information technology has given a quality boost to communication in all Scandinavian countries, especially in Denmark where national standards govern all electronic general practice communication and where some 80 per cent of the communication from practices is now electronic.
- Finland has a strong tradition of developing electronically based decision aids and operates a very comprehensive evidence-based system where GPs can get information on clinical problems. This system is now becoming increasingly web-based.
- All countries have different systems for developing national guidelines and for the transformation of national guidelines into regional action plans.

Final remarks

The Scandinavian ambition to create a seamless, comprehensive health care system is firmly rooted in a strong political wish for such a system with the GP as its cornerstone. This political goodwill has been parallelled by a tradition in the Scandinavian medical associations for a strong professional development of all medical disciplines including the discipline of general practice. The Scandinavian health care systems are, therefore, overall enjoying a very privileged position. There is a strong wish for more GPs in Sweden, and there are a few vacancies in GP positions in all countries, especially in the rural areas, mainly the very northern parts of all the countries. All the Scandinavian countries are, to different degrees, facing the threat of poor recruitment due to heavy workload and professional isolation in general practice. Ongoing initiatives to integrate all medical professions in a comprehensive health care scheme may ameliorate this threat, and the educational systems have increased their intake in recent years.

Acknowledgements

I would like to thank Pertti Soveri, Finland, Anders Håkansson, Sweden, and Knut Holtedahl, Norway, for ideas and critical comments on the manuscript.

Further reading

Boerma, G.W., de Jong, F.A.J.M., and Mulder, P.H. *Health Care and General Practice Across Europe.* Utrecht: NIVEL, 1993.

Gérvas, J., Pérez Fernández, M., and Starfield, B.H. (1997). Primary care, financing and gatekeeping in Western Europe. *Family Practice* **11**, 307–17.

Håkansson, A., Kvamme, O., Magnússon, S., Norén, I., Olesgaard, P., and Winell, K. (1996). Trends and traditions in Nordic family medicine. *Almän Medicin* **18** (Suppl.), 4–8.

Websites of the Scandinavian Ministries of Health

Denmark (Ministry of the Interior and Health): http://www.denmark.dk/
Norway (Ministry of Health): http://www.norge.no/
Sweden (Ministry of Health and Social Affairs): http://www.sweden.se/
Finland (Ministry of Social Affairs and Health): http://www.finland.fi/
Iceland (Ministry of Health & Social Security): http://www.iceland.org/

2.9 Primary care and general practice in India

Anan S. Raghunath and A.S. Ramanujam

Introduction

India is a vast country and with a population of around 1027 million, is the second most populous country in the world after China. Although 742 million live in rural areas, nearly 80 per cent of the health facilities, both public and private, are concentrated in the urban areas.[1,2] India also has a highly multicultural, multiethnic, and multireligious society. With increasing capitalism and westernization, there is a widening gap between the rich and poor and the dimensions of health care provision, access and understanding are complex and influenced by a multiplicity of factors.

The general health of the population as reflected in the infant mortality rates (IMRs) have significantly improved with time over the last 20 years (Fig. 1).[1]

Much of this progress has been made against diseases such as diarrhoea and acute respiratory infections, where there have been global initiatives and national programmes.[3] However, over the last 5 years, the official IMR has hardly changed suggesting that much greater investment in safer motherhood and neonatal programmes is required.[4]

Background

The terms primary health care and general practice are not synonymous in the context of health care systems in India. Primary health care refers mainly to governmental organizations providing preventive services. General practice, more popularly known as private practice in India, is the source that the rich and poor access when they become ill (Table 1).

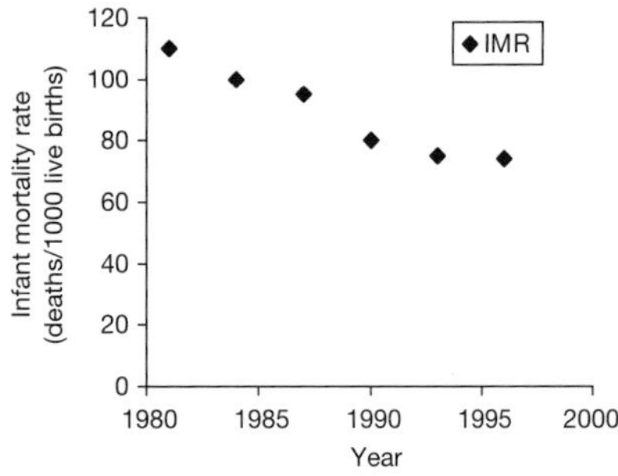

Fig. 1 Trend over time (IMR).

Table 1 Primary health care and general practice in India

Primary health care	General practice
Government, non-government (e.g. voluntary agencies)	Private
Mainly preventive	Mainly curative
Has an organizational structure	No clear structure
Available in cities, towns, and villages	Mainly concentrated in cities and towns
Every individual can access	Those who can afford
Provided by a team of health care professionals	Medical practitioners
Consistent quality	Variable quality
Non-profit making	Profit making

In India, primary health care delivery and medical education are largely governmental functions. India cannot afford a national health service. However, it has a national health policy based on the primary health care approach, with emphasis on rural health in order to achieve the World Health Organization's goal of Health for All by 2000.[5,6] A variety of services are available from the Indian government, the not-for-profit sector, and the for-profit sector (which includes modern allopathic and traditional practitioners, and local healers). Although the private sector provides about 80 per cent of health care in India, the government is the primary source of preventive services such as immunization and family planning. Overall, government spending on health represents only 5 per cent of the gross domestic product.[7] In addition to general health services provided to all people, public sector services to meet the specific health and nutritional needs of Indian women and children are provided through the family welfare programme and integrated child development programme.[4,8]

General practice (private medical practice)

Systems

In India, when the term general practice is used it usually refers to private medical practice by qualified allopathic medical practitioners. Private medical practice, however, is also allowed under government legislation to be carried out by other qualified medical practitioners (Box 1).

Figures on the total number of private health practitioners in India are difficult to obtain but there are possibly more than 400 000 doctors possessing recognized medical qualifications and registered with the medical councils of India.[9]

Organization and service provision (Box 2)

There is no structured organization of private medical care in India. Private allopathic medical practitioners tend to be concentrated in cities and towns. This is related to the concentration of medical colleges providing undergraduate and postgraduate training being mainly located in major cities. As a result there is grossly disproportionate distribution of private medical

Box 1 Who are private medical practitioners?

Allopathic
Basic (MBBS)
Specialists (MD, MS, MRCP, FRCS)
Super specialists (DM in cardiology, cardiothoracic surgery and others)

Non-allopathic
Homeopaths
Other indigenous systems

Unregistered
Quacks

Box 2 Organization of private medical care

- Single-handed practitioner
- Polyclinics
- Nursing homes
- Private hospitals

care across the country. Private medical practice is also being increasingly undertaken from polyclinics that provide for various private specialist services under one roof. Private nursing homes and hospitals have become increasingly popular amongst many that can afford them for conditions requiring in-patient treatment ranging from management of pneumonia and heart attack to major surgical procedures such as brain and heart surgery.

Access to private health care and roles of private practitioners

Private medical practice in most cities and towns provides the first point of contact for the majority of people, rich and poor alike. Many doctors will set up a single-handed private practice in a rented or owned accommodation following completion of their medical training. Since most medical colleges are located in major cities, qualifying doctors tend to aggregate around cities and towns. Private medical practice is also undertaken by non-allopathic doctors, many of whom will practice mixed type medicine incorporating their own indigenous training with self-learnt but not accredited allopathic approach. Private pharmacists not uncommonly provide the first point of contact and under a system that has no clear channels of prescribing regulation are able to prescribe and advise on a range of medical conditions from the common cold to malaria and gastrointestinal infections.

Private practitioners cater essentially to acute medical problems and tend to provide a flexible and friendly service. Apart from those (perhaps between 10 and 20 per cent) verging on extreme poverty lines, most people are willing to access private practitioners. Although there is no clear system of record keeping and continuity of care, many will see the same private practitioner, having established a good doctor–patient relationship.[10] Fees charged per contact are variable and practitioners tend to use their discretion depending on their knowledge of the patients' financial situation.

Private practitioners deal with a range of medical conditions depending on their training, expertise, and experience. The majority of acute and chronic ailments are managed by general or specialist private practitioners (Boxes 3 and 4).

Box 3 Examples of common conditions treated by a general private practitioner

Acute	*Chronic*
Gastroenteritis	Pulmonary tuberculosis
'Fever'	Hypertension
Malaria	Arthritis
Asthma attacks	Angina
Rash in a child	Headaches
Jaundice	

Box 4 Examples of specialist private practice

Acute or chronic medical	*Acute or chronic/elective surgical*
Chest pains/heart attack	Appendix removal
Breathlessness	Abscess drainage
Fits in a child	Gall bladder surgery
Diabetes	Major cardiac/bowel surgery
Heavy periods	
Depression/schizophrenia	
Referrals from general practitioners	

Prescribing

There are few data available in the area of prescribing by health professionals in private practice in India. There may be huge variations in the patterns of prescribing between practitioners for similar health and illness conditions. There also appears to be wide differences in the prescribing behaviour of urban and rural allopathic practitioners with urban practitioners prescribing in a more prolific manner.[11] Antibiotics, vitamins, non-steroidal anti-inflammatory drugs, and respiratory drugs are the most commonly prescribed medications.

The concept of holistic medicine in the context of Indian society, culture, and religion is alien to the mainstream public. This means that health is seen as freedom from medical illness and the ability to earn a livelihood. Psychological and social problems are rarely brought to or addressed during a routine consultation with a private practitioner. There is, however, with increasing westernization, especially in affluent and middle class Indian societies, a greater realization as well as acceptance of psychological health problems. This has therefore led to private specialist psychiatrists providing both outpatient and inpatient services, mainly based in cities like Delhi and Mumbai. Specialist private practitioners (Box 4) tend to be more expensive and are therefore for those who can afford to pay. Private insurance companies are increasingly entering the health care market in India and there is debate about public private partnerships to provide comprehensive health care.

Rural versus urban medical care

An example of rural versus urban medical care is illustrated in Box 5.

Clinical governance and quality assurance

Until recently, there has been no formal performance evaluation or ongoing educational requirement for private practitioners in India.[12] Dangerous and negligent practitioners have thrived as well as, their honest and

Box 5 A hypothetical case scenario of rural versus urban medical care

Gita, a 16-year-old daughter of a labourer has burning urine, weight loss, and nausea for several weeks.

Her management is dependent on several factors; her place of living (remote hilly area, village, town, or city), access to health care facilities, family dynamics and resources, health beliefs and attitudes to health care systems, ideas concerns and expectations of Gita and her family. Gita may, for instance, be pregnant but ashamed to divulge this information since she may not yet be married. Gita may also be harbouring tuberculosis. Her mother may take Gita to a local 'village doctor' or 'healer' who may prescribe 'home made' medications or even an injection unaware of her pregnancy status. Gita may end up being admitted to a local hospital several miles away in a critical condition and be diagnosed to have tetanus presumably following the injection with a dirty needle given by the healer.

If Gita lived in a city like Delhi, she may be taken to see a pharmacist, private qualified, unqualified, or unregistered medical practitioner or to an outpatient clinic of a large city hospital. The outcome to Gita's health will vary depending on the ethical, financial resources, and relationship considerations between health care provider, Gita, and her family.

Equally, if Gita had come from an affluent family and or has connections with the medical fraternity, she would have been quickly and extensively investigated. Her care in this situation would be the same or even better than the best of medical centres in the United Kingdom or the United States.

responsible colleagues. The public for a variety of reasons did not contemplate taking legal action against the medical profession. But this attitude may be changing.[13,14] There have also been political moves towards regulating the medical profession; for instance, in Delhi post-graduate activities are beginning to happen, though the content and seriousness of such sessions are open to criticism and debate.

Primary health care

Systems, structure, and organization

The public health sector in India is organized to provide services ranging from the delivery of primary health care to a relatively small population in a village through to training of doctors and providing advanced medical and surgical care in large specialist and teaching hospitals (Fig. 2, Box 6). Within the public health sector, health care is also provided through the state, central health insurance schemes, and non-governmental organizations.[15]

Total infrastructure[15]

- Village health guides 323 000
- Trained birth attendants 660 996
- Sub-centres 137 027
- Primary health centres 23 266
- Community health centres 2 962

Health problems and major elements of primary health care in India

Communicable diseases, nutrition and environmental, sanitation, and population problems are the major health concerns of India. Therefore, the strategies to tackle these problems are concentrated in the following areas:

- education concerning prevailing health problems and methods of preventing and controlling them;
- promotion of food supply and proper nutrition;
- an adequate supply of safe water and basic sanitation;
- maternal and child health care, including family planning;
- immunization against major infectious diseases;
- prevention and control of locally endemic diseases;
- appropriate treatment of common diseases and injuries;
- provision of essential drugs.

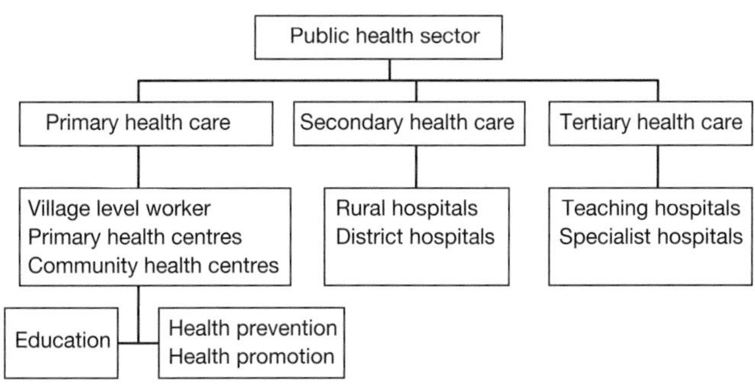

Fig. 2 Flow chart of Indian Health Service (government).

Box 6 Health systems organizations in India

Central
Overall responsibility and strategic planning, resource allocation

State
Prioritizing local needs

Peripheral
Rural development
Programmes for health promotion
Programmes for disease reduction
Multidisciplinary key workers

Major public health issues and diseases[7,16]

The figures cited in Table 2 may vary depending on the source. Official immunization coverage statistics reported by the national government seem to vastly exceed more detailed immunization surveys collected by WHO. For example, in 1996, the Indian government reported 89 per cent coverage for DPT3 at 1 year, whereas the WHO expanded programme of immunization surveys produced estimates of 47 per cent.

Current health programmes in India[8]

Current health programmes in India are illustrated in Box 7.

Description of some important ongoing health programmes

The integrated child development services (ICDS) programme

The aim of the ICDS programme is to improve the nutritional and health status of pregnant and lactating women and of children under 6, and to enable mothers to look after their children's health and nutritional needs. Services such as supplemental food for children, pre-school programmes, and nutrition and education programmes for women are provided by female workers at village health centres.[4,17]

Directly observed short course treatment for tuberculosis (DOTS)

An estimated 500 000 people die from tuberculosis in India every year, more than 1000 every day and one every minute. A WHO study has reported that India is one of the hot zones for the deadly multi-drug resistant tuberculosis (MDR-TB). When the disease is resistant to treatment with commonly used drugs like isoniazid and rifampicin, it is categorized as MDR-TB. Of the estimated 14 million tuberculosis cases in India, 3.5 million are sputum positive. Although the DOTS strategy represents the most important public health breakthrough of the decade, in terms of lives that will be saved, India is lagging behind even neighbouring Bangladesh in implementing DOTS.[18]

The national programme for control of blindness in India (NPCB)

There are today more than 13 million blind persons in India; 80 per cent or more than 10 million of these blind persons suffer from blindness due to cataract. Since its inception in 1976, NPCB is fully centrally sponsored. Around 450 District Blindness Control Societies have now been established to facilitate eye care activities, mainly by organizing eye camps, collaborating with non-governmental organizations and private practitioners and handling funds. Since 1994, NPCB has received a World Bank loan of 118 million US dollars over 5 years for programme implementation in seven major states. With this assistance, the programme has increased considerably in funding and complexity. Only recently has a corresponding increase in capacity in the form of staffing and space been initiated.[19]

Table 2 Major public health issues and diseases

Health/disease	India	China	England and Wales
Mortality			
Infant mortality rate (deaths/ 1000 live births)	65–70	41	5.63
Maternal mortality rate (deaths/100 000 live births)	440	60	7.4
Nutrition			
Wasting (% wt/ht ≤2Z scores)	15.5	2.2	Nearer to 0
Stunting (% ht/age ≤2Z scores)	47	9	Insignificant
Iron deficiency anaemia	Highly prevalent due to inadequate reserves at birth, poor dietary intake and feeding practices, and hookworm and other infections	Similar reasons but prevalence decreasing	Uncommon and causes are mostly related to blood loss and malabsorption
Iodine deficiency	2.2 million people are cretins	37% people live in high-risk areas	Virtually non-existent
% children exclusively breast fed (0–3 months)	51	64	10–20
Tuberculosis			
Notified cases (per 100 000 population)	115	36	4.38 amongst white and 121 in ethnic
Total estimated cases	818 209	636 066	5658
Malaria			
Number of cases	2 666 057	33 382	44 cases (in inner London)
Immunization			
BCG	80%	85%	95–100%
DPT3	78%	85%	>90%
Measles	60%	85%	Recent downtrend (85–90%)
Polio	78%	90%	>90%
Reproductive health			
Total fertility rate	3.1	1.8	1.76
% of antenatal care coverage	62	79	Nearly 100
Contraception prevalence	41%	83%	85–95%
HIV/AIDS			
Estimated numbers living HIV/AIDS	3 500 000	500 000	13 670 (1996)

Box 7 Current health programmes in India

- National malaria eradication
- National filaria control
- National immunization
- Control of tuberculosis
- Leprosy eradication
- Control of sexually transmitted diseases
- AIDS control
- Blindness control
- Goitre control
- Control of diarrhoeal diseases
- Guinea worm eradication
- Kala-Azar control

Conclusions

Most people in India, rich and poor alike, seek the help of private practitioners (allopathic or traditional) for their day-to-day health problems. Primary health care services, such as immunization and disease control programmes, are largely provided through governmental organizations. There are centres of medical excellence in India that match the best in Western Europe and North America, but are available to only a tiny minority who can afford to pay.

With increasing westernization and changing public expectation, health professionals in general, and private practitioners in particular, will have to demonstrate competence, accountability, and value for money.(20) It is therefore vital that before the government imposes regulations that may lack understanding and clarity, private practitioners establish self-regulation through professional guidelines, clinical protocols, ethical principles, voluntary and/or compulsory monitoring systems, and a local and national register of practising private practitioners.(12)

References

1. **Office of the Registrar General, India.** (1998). *SRS Bulletin* **32** (3). Available for download from http://www.censusindia.net/
2. **Apte, N.K. and Kerkar, P.G.** (1994). Health care delivery system and surgical education in India. *World Journal of Surgery* **18** (5), 687–90.
3. **Bhutta, Z.A.** (2000). Why has so little changed in maternal and child health in south Asia? *British Medical Journal* **321**, 809–12.
4. **Costello, A.** (1999). Is India ready for the integrated management of childhood illness strategy? *Indian Pediatrics* **36**, 759–62.

5. **World Health Organization** (1988). From Alma-Ata to the year 2000: reflections at the midpoint. Available for download from the WHO website.
6. **Declaration of Alma-Ata.** International Conference on Primary Health Care, USSR, 6–12 September, 1978. Available for download from http://www.who.dk/policy/almaata.htm.
7. **World Health Organization** (1998). Emergency and humanitarian action health intelligence network for advanced planning v. 1.5: baseline statistics for India. Available for download from http://www.who.int/disasters/stats/baseline.cfm?countryID=24.
8. **Voluntary Health Associations of India.** National health programmes. In *State of India's Health* (compilation of articles), pp. 61–62, 1993. New Delhi: Voluntary Health Association of India.
9. **Health Information of India.** Central Bureau of Health Intelligence, Directorate General of Health Services, Ministry of Health and Family Welfare, 1995/96, p. 99.
10. **Kumar, A.** (1997). Families regarded the general practitioner as their primary care giver. *Indian Journal of Pediatrics* **64** (6), 745.
11. **Srishyla, M.V., Rani, M.A., Venkataraman, B.V., and Andrade, C.** (1995). A comparative study of prescribing pattern at different levels of health care delivery system in Bangalore district. *Indian Journal of Physiology and Pharmacology* **39** (3), 247–51.
12. **Thomas, M.** (1991). Continuing medical education as a strategy for improving general practice—experiences from Vellore. *Family Practice* **8** (3), 243–6.
13. **Bhat, R.** (1996). Regulation of the private health sector in India. *International Journal of Health Planning and Management* **11** (3), 253–74.
14. **Bhat, R.** (1996). Regulating the private health care sector: the case of the Indian Consumer Protection Act. *Health Policy and Planning* **11** (3), 265–79.
15. **Park, K.** *Text Book of Preventive and Social Medicine.* Jabalpur, India: Banarsidas Bhanot, 2000, pp. 621–5.
16. **Gwatkin, D.R., Rustein, S., Johnson, K., Pande, R.P., and Wagstaff, A.** (2000). Socio-economic differences in health, nutrition and population in India. For the HNP/Poverty Thematic Group of the World Bank. Available for download from http://www.worldbank.org/poverty/health/data/india/india.pdf.
17. **Shah, D. and Sachdev, H.P.S.** (1999). Evaluation of the WHO/UNICEF algorithm for integrated management of childhood illness between the age of two months to five years. *Indian Pediatrics* **36**, 767–78.
18. **The World Bank Group and Health Sector Development and Disease Control in India** (1999). Available for download from http://www.worldbank.org/tuberculosis (contact: gchopra@worldbank.org).
19. **The Blindness Problem in India.** 1996-11—The Setting. Available for download from http://www.um.dk/danida/evalueringsrapporter/1996-11/1996-11.3.asp, 1996.
20. **Bhat, R.** (1999). Characteristics of private medical practice in India: a provider perspective. *Health Policy and Planning* **4** (1), 26–37.

2.10 Primary care and general practice in Pakistan

M. Jawad Hashim

Introduction

Primary medical care needs in Pakistan are served by private practitioners including generalists and specialty-trained physicians, government-employed physicians, community health workers, and traditional healers. Primary health care faces the challenges of inappropriate training, lack of consumer protection, and a tertiary care orientation of health care services.

Primary care providers deliver cost-conscious, culturally sensitive care but work virtually without any regulation or continuing education. Private practitioners work on a fee-for-service basis with competition from non-physicians providing primary care. Studies have revealed inappropriate prescribing for common conditions such as watery diarrhoea and upper respiratory infections, indicating a need for improvement in primary care medical education.

Health indicators

Pakistan's last census in 1998 enumerated a total population of 130 million with an average growth rate of 2.6 per cent. Estimated life expectancy at birth for both males and females was 63 years. Most of the population resides in rural areas although larger cities have experienced high rates of urban migration. Karachi, the largest city, had a population of 9.2 million in 1998, a dramatic increase from 5.2 million in 1981. Average household size is 6.8 persons.[1] Household health care expenses account for 4.6 per cent of total expenditure and this proportion is greater in rural and lower socio-economic class families.[1]

Health indicators in Pakistan have shown a positive trend with improvements in life expectancy and infant mortality rate. However, the overall health of the population remains poor compared to countries with comparable economic status. This has been attributed to a low literacy rate, lack of clean water and sanitation, and neglect of the health care sector at the government level.

Structure of health care

Health care services in Pakistan have evolved from traditional medicine with a rich legacy to 'a highly inequitable, western-oriented curative model, which certainly does not fulfil the requirements of a very great majority of the people'.[2] A rapidly growing population, health transition to non-communicable diseases, poverty, and sociopolitical upheavals further strain these services.

The private sector provides the majority of health care while the public sector serves as a safety net for the poor. The private sector itself is varied, ranging from untrained providers working in rural areas to sophisticated technology-intensive hospitals in the larger cities. There are no direct reimbursements to private practitioners by the government as in the Medicare/Medicaid programmes in the United States.

The private sector operates in a fee-for-service mode; competition and financial returns affect the quality of services provided. Providers are sensitive to the health care needs in the cultural and financial context of the patients. Health care consumers are usually at a disadvantage in judging quality, appropriateness of services, or fee structures. Lack of accreditation and regulation makes quality assessment and assurance even more difficult.

Government clinics and hospitals provide essential health care services for those who cannot afford private sector fees—this includes families in the lower and lower-middle socioeconomic classes and government employees. The public sector, operated by provincial health ministries, is limited by centralized control, resource wastage, and poor quality of care. Although direct fees charged are minimal, families end up paying out-of-pocket significantly for 'covered' items such as medicines and surgical supplies.[3] Due to the overwhelming demand for public-sector health care, additional cost-shifting occurs in subtle ways such as long waiting lines that force patients to seek care elsewhere. Rationing of services also occurs with the exclusion of under-served groups to the benefit of 'entitled' classes such as higher-rank government and military officials, and family contacts of health care providers.

Primary care services

Primary care services are rendered by a variety of providers: allopathic physicians, *hakims* (traditional physicians dispensing herbal medicines), homeopathic physicians, faith healers, pharmacy dispensers in independent clinical practice, and drugstore attendants (see Fig. 1).

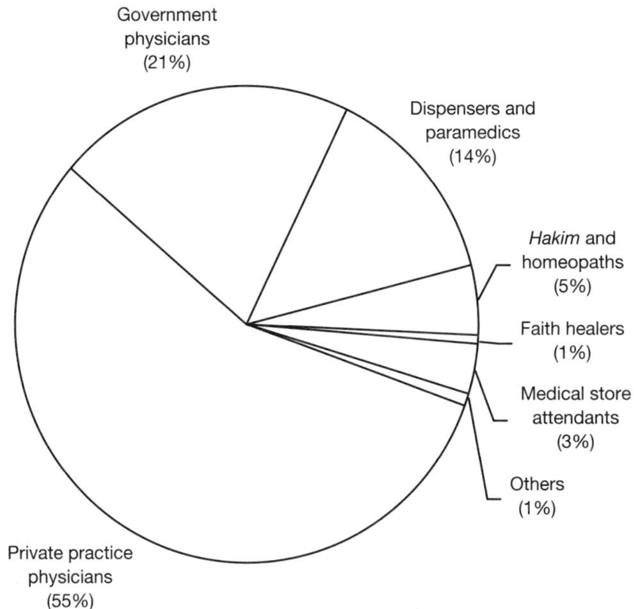

Fig. 1 Healthcare providers contacted for a recent illness by adult males in a national survey.

The private sector provides the majority of first-contact care in urban and rural areas, independent of distance to a public health care facility.[4] This preference is most likely due to public perception of lack of quality of care, long waiting lines, and erratic availability of staff, medical supplies, and medicines at government clinics. Doctors and dispensers at these clinics usually supplement their incomes with private practice, which creates a conflict of interest in treating patients at the government centers.

Prescription writing is not limited to registered physicians (despite the efforts of the Pakistan Medical Association and the Pakistan Medical and Dental Council), resulting in a wide range of primary care providers in terms of qualifications and quality of care. Intense competition results in downward pressure on fees charged with compensatory reduction in quality of care parameters: time per patient encounter, level of clinical sophistication of services provided, and referrals to other providers. There is virtually no documentation of care and medical records are usually not maintained. Clinically inappropriate practices such as prescribing unnecessary injections, systemic steroids, antibiotics, and strong antidiarrhoeal drugs, also become more prevalent to 'satisfy patient preferences'.[5,6]

Unfortunately, the level of training and the fees charged do not seem to correlate with better health care or improved outcomes. Specialty-trained physicians such as paediatricians and obstetrician–gynaecologists also show inappropriate prescribing for common primary care conditions.[7] Restriction of prescription writing to registered doctors is unlikely to bring about a major improvement in quality of primary care.

Training for primary care

Primary care training is improving at most medical colleges—with certain private medical schools leading with new Family Medicine departments. Primary care is included in the Community Medicine curriculum but taught without involvement of primary care clinics. Medical students learn to extrapolate 'primary care' from inpatient wards of teaching hospitals and outpatient specialty clinics. The majority of medical graduates practice primary medical care without any further training (only about 10 000 of the 63 000 registered physicians reported specialty training to the Pakistan Medical and Dental Council in March 2001).

The role of postgraduate training in Family Medicine residency programmes remains unclear—academic teaching and research in primary care are potential roles for advanced trainees in Family Medicine. The Aga Khan University, which initiated the first Family Medicine residency programme, has developed a postgraduate curriculum that includes inpatient training, longitudinal outpatient experience, and community involvement.[8]

The College of Physicians and Surgeons of Pakistan, a public body that conducts specialty-certification examinations, has introduced a Diploma in Family Medicine[9] as well as full specialty certification in Family Medicine. The demand for and future impact of these on primary care in Pakistan is uncertain. Market demands call for a 'specialist' label and the pressure to specialize remains high. Public understanding of the difference between family physicians and generalists remains limited.

Factors limiting improvement of primary care

Financial disincentives to training, lack of continuing medical education (CME), unethical drug detailing, and inappropriate training contribute to poor quality of primary care. The time spent in practice since medical college graduation has been shown to correlate with worsening prescribing patterns, perhaps indicating a need for CME.[10]

As general practice in Pakistan remains fairly unregulated, market factors tend to dominate its distribution and quality of services. Health care consumers are unable to make informed choices about selecting primary care providers. Low earnings, the absence of a career path, and lack of professional recognition and influence at medical institutions add to the frustrations of primary care physicians.

The Primary Health Care model promoted by the World Health Organization appears to hold the greatest promise for sustainable and affordable primary health care. Unfortunately, it remains difficult to implement beyond small-scale pilot projects. Health care insurance has the potential to escalate medical costs, making it unaffordable to the majority of the population.

Future directions

The scope for improvement in clinical practice of primary care remains great. Targets for cost-effective interventions to improve rational drug prescribing have been identified at the medical college level, and in postgraduate training programmes as well as CME for practising physicians.

Direct enforcement of licensure and CME for practising physicians will probably be difficult and innovative approaches to encourage public and professional demand for quality care and CME certification are needed. 'Social marketing' has been used in contraception-promoting programmes that use direct-to-consumer marketing techniques to creating public awareness and demand for these services. Social marketing may be useful in promoting primary care CME certification in Pakistan.

Development of primary care curricula that are evidence-based on local research and socially appropriate should be a priority. A concerted national effort to improve primary health care is needed in Pakistan with participation of medical colleges, professional interest groups, government health departments, and informed public representatives. Integrated work among these groups and across the provinces will help ensure consistency, resource-sharing, and appropriate primary care practices. Such integration will allow improved collaboration with the family physician as a focal point in local Primary Health Care, referrals and pre-hospital care, and community leadership in health promotion.

References

1. **Federal Bureau of Statistics.** *Household Integrated Economic Survey, 1998–99.* Islamabad: Government of Pakistan, 2001.
2. **Zaidi, A.** *Issues in Pakistan's Economy.* Karachi: Oxford University Press, 1999.
3. **Kadir, M.M., Khan, A., Sadruddin, S., and Luby, S.P.** (2000). Out-of-pocket expenses borne by the users of obstetric services at government hospitals in Karachi, Pakistan. *Journal of the Pakistan Medical Association* **50** (12), 412–15.

4. **NoorAli, R., Luby, S., and Rahbar, M.H.** (1999). Does use of a government service depend on distance from the health facility? *Health Policy and Planning* **14** (2), 191–7.
5. **Iqbal, I., Pervez, S., and Baig, S.** (1997). Management of children with acute respiratory infections (ARI) by general practitioners in Multan—an observational study. *Journal of the Pakistan Medical Association* **47** (1), 24–8.
6. **Ahmad, S.R. and Bhutta, Z.A.** (1990). A survey of paediatric prescribing and dispensing in Karachi. *Journal of the Pakistan Medical Association* **40** (6), 126–30.
7. **Nizami, S.Q., Khan, I.A., and Bhutta, Z.A.** (1997). Paediatric prescribing in Karachi. *Journal of the Pakistan Medical Association* **47** (1), 29–32.
8. **Haq, C.L., Qureshi, A.F., Zuberi, R.W., Inam, S.N., and Bryant, J.H.** (1992). Family medicine postgraduate training in Pakistan. *Journal of the Pakistan Medical Association* **42** (3), 69–73.
9. **Zuberi, R.W., Jafarey, N.A., Qureshi, A.F., and Elahi, F.** (1993). The diploma in family medicine examination; a scientific exercise. *Journal of the Pakistan Medical Association* **43** (10), 217–20.
10. **Choudhry, A.J. and Mubasher, M.** (1997). Factors influencing the prescribing patterns in acute watery diarrhoea. *Journal of the Pakistan Medical Association* **47** (1), 32–5.

2.11 Primary care and general practice in the Middle East

Howard Tandeter and Pesach Shvartzman

Background

Countries in the Middle East are quite different one from the other, with different social structures, cultural background, and government types. The development of health services is greatly influenced by these differences. Since most of the countries of this region gained independence only about 50 years ago, health services are still not well established (in comparison to the United States and Europe) and are still developing. This chapter presents available information about the development of primary care in this region. Table 1 presents comparative data between six countries.

Israel

Israel has a well-developed primary care system with clinics located in the community, all around the country (urban, suburban, and rural). About 97 per cent of the population has medical coverage through a National Health Insurance, and they can choose one of four Health Maintenance Organizations as their health services' provider. Twenty per cent of physicians in Israel work in the primary care setting. At present, training (a formal residency programme or postgraduate course) is not a prerequisite to become a primary care physician, and only about 750 of the 5000 or so doctors delivering primary care services in this country are specialists, board certified in family medicine.

The first official residency training programme was initiated in 1977. Today, four medical schools offer residency programs (Ben-Gurion University, Tel-Aviv University, the Technion in Haifa, and the Hebrew University in Jerusalem). After 1 year of internship, residents enter a national 4-year programme composed of hospital and community rotations. Hospital rotations include a year in internal medicine, 6 months in paediatrics, 3 in psychiatry, and 6 in elective rotations (two 3-month rotations chosen from a list of sub-specialties such as ENT, dermatology, ophthalmology, gynaecology, surgery, orthopaedics, and emergency medicine). Community rotations are performed in approved teaching practices, with 9 months under direct supervision of an instructor, followed by 12 months of independent work (not under direct supervision), in what will become the definitive practice of this doctor after certification. In addition, residents participate in a weekly course over six semesters in which they discuss the theoretical background of their work and learn communication skills. Evaluation consists of two examinations—a multiple-choice examination 24 months into their residency, and a final oral examination—for the Board of Family Medicine mandatory examinations—about different areas of knowledge (clinical cases, family presentation, and practice organization). These programmes produce about 60 board certified physicians per year.

Family medicine is a well-acknowledged discipline in this country and it is now recognized by the National Scientific Council as base for sub-specialization in geriatrics, infectious diseases, and emergency medicine.

Lebanon

The American University of Beirut established the first department of family medicine in 1979 and initiated a family practice residency programme in the same year. The curriculum was structured following the guidelines of the American Academy of Family Physicians. This 3-year residency programme is similar to the American programme. Recently, the final year was re-structured into modules of 3 months each: occupational medicine, geriatrics, mental health, and electives. Residents pass through the four modules while continuing patient care under supervision in different primary care settings. The programme has produced between three and six family physicians per year, from which two-thirds have remained in

Table 1 Comparative health system information between countries in the Middle East

	Population (millions)	Physician/ 100 000 population	Total (±) number of physicians	Number of primary care physicians	Medical schools with residencies in Family Medicine
Israel	6.5	385	25 000	5000	4
Lebanon	4.3	210	9 000	NDA	2
Syria	16.1	144	23 000	NDA	NDA
Jordan	5.2	166	8 600	NDA	NDA
Saudi Arabia	21.1	166	35 000	4000	3
Egypt	69.8	202	141 000	NDA	NDA

NDA: no data available.

Lebanon, while the rest have migrated to the USA or work in other Arab countries.

In 1995, Saint Joseph University, Beirut started a residency programme in Family Medicine and both programmes cooperate to improve their role in the community. Satellite clinics were initiated in order to provide comprehensive care to the target population.

Although the graduates of these residency programmes have won quick acceptance and esteem by the community because of the high quality of medicine they provide, the number of family medicine specialists remains minimal in this country, and training is not a prerequisite to become a primary care provider.

Jordan

The Royal Medical Services established the first training programme in family medicine in 1983. The Ministry of Health, the University of Jordan, and the Jordan University of Science and Technology followed, and the Jordan Medical Board established an end-of-training assessment. General practice was then recognized as a separate specialty, but the committee on family medicine was staffed by trained family practitioners only in 1993. Today, Jordan has training programmes in general practice with a 3-year hospital residency component, and a fourth year of supervised training in a health centre. The number of trained general practitioners has increased considerably in the past two decades but still fails to meet the existing population needs in primary health care. Training is not a prerequisite to become a primary care physician. Private and public primary health care facilities have increased considerably in the last two decades and spread throughout the Kingdom. Standards vary considerably from one facility to another even within the public sector. General practice is not well recognized, and patients refer themselves directly to specialists instead of to primary care physicians.

Saudi Arabia

About 11.5 per cent of the physicians in this country work in primary health care centres. The government of Saudi Arabia has developed a comprehensive, cost-effective primary health care system. The first merger of family medicine with community medicine to form a single department took place at the College of Medicine, King Faisal University (KFU) in 1980. King Saud University (KSU) followed in 1982 and in 1985 the King Abdul Aziz University (KAU) followed suit with the Abha branch of KAU in 1986. In 1981, KFU invited international and regional experts in family and community medicine to develop a postgraduate training programme relevant to family physicians in order to produce competent clinicians. A 2-year masters and diploma programme in primary health care was started by KSU in 1983 and from 1995 KFU offered a diploma in family and community medicine. There are two other vocational training programmes in primary health care, one developed by the Ministry of Health in conjunction with the Royal College of General Practitioners in the United Kingdom and locally recognized by KSU (12 months), and the other developed at the military hospital in Riyadh in conjunction with RCGP-UK in which candidates become eligible to sit for membership of the RCGP (3 years). The Arab Board has a final examination at the end of the 3 years of training, while all the others have end-of-course examinations.

Egypt

Each year, around 4000 medical students graduate from 14 medical schools, and obtain licensure by completing a 1-year internship in Medicine and Surgery. Female physicians go into 1 year of urban practice, while male physicians complete their military obligations by practising in the army. Physicians may then select specialty or general practice. Around 20 per cent of graduates go on to a 2-year training programme in a specialty, to obtain a Masters degree to practice as specialists. Of these specialists, a small number go on to obtain a Doctorate in that specialty, and to follow an academic career. The remaining 80 per cent of graduates go directly into urban, suburban, rural, or military practice without further training. There is no requirement for continuing education or certification by the Egyptian Medical licensing board, once a physician is in practice. At present, there is no formal training in Egypt of newly qualified physicians to prepare them for family medicine, to meet the diverse health care needs of the population.

The Family Medicine faculty at the University of California, Irvine offers a programme to train 30 selected physicians from Egypt to become educators in Family Medicine. These physicians are expected to start their own training programmes in teaching hospitals and clinics all around Egypt, under the Public Health sector of the government. These programmes will seed other training centres to disseminate this education to the entire general physician work force, thereby raising the standard of health care for the country.

Historically, the Egyptian health care system emphasized inpatient, institutional care. Efforts are now being made to shift this emphasis toward outpatient, high-quality primary health care. Alexandria was chosen as the site for a pilot project. The lessons from this pilot are expected to be used for expansion to two other areas. Eventually, the programme will be extended to the whole country.

Conclusion

Family medicine is not developing symmetrically in all Middle East countries. In order to develop a strong community-oriented system, recognizing family medicine as a separate discipline and creating academic departments are just the first steps. Political issues within the medical community and education of the population are important factors. Countries should institute a common, national policy that recognizes family medicine (and not hospitals) as the port of entry to the health system. Israel and Saudi Arabia are well developed in this sense. In Jordan, family practice is still not well recognized, and in Lebanon and Egypt it looks more like a local effort from some Universities than a real policy shift. However, since the whole world is moving into a primary care (mainly family medicine) based system, is to be expected that all the countries in the region, sooner or later, will move in this direction.

Acknowledgements

The authors wish to thank Dr Robert Erasmus for his contribution in the writing of the section about family medicine in Saudi Arabia.

Further reading

Aitken, A.M., Sibai, M.H., and Tramimi, T.M. (1988). The King Faisal University fellowship training programme in family and community medicine. *Family Practice* **4**, 253–9.

Albar, A.A. (1999). Twenty years of family medicine education in Saudi Arabia. *Eastern Mediterranean Health Journal* **5** (3), 589–96.

Fabb, W.E. Curricular plan for family medicine. *Proceedings of WONCA/MESAR International Teachers' Training of Family Medicine Education.* Bangladesh, WONCA/MESAR, 1996, pp. 18–21.

Polliack, M.R. (1983). Vocational training for family practice in Israel. *Israel Journal of Medical Science* **19** (8), 783–6.

Tandeter, H. (1995). The family practice residency program in Israel. *Family Medicine* **27**, 610–11.

The Family and Community Medicine Curriculum Document, 2nd edn. Riyadh: King Faisal University Press, 1985.

Weingarten, M.A. and Lederer, J. (1995). The development of family medicine in Israel. *Family Medicine* **27** (9), 599–604.

WHO Estimates of Health Personnel. Physicians, nurses, midwives, dentists and pharmacists (around 1998).

Material found in the Internet written by Professor Mustafa Khogali, Chairman, Department of Family Medicine, American University of Beirut, 2002.

Material found in the Internet written by Dr Mazen M. Al-Bashir, Jordan Center for Family Medicine, Amman, Jordan, 2002.

2.12 Primary care and general practice in North America

Daniel J. Ostergaard, Norman B. Kahn, Jr., and Darrell Henderson

Introduction to the region

General practice has a long and honoured history in both the United States and Canada. Before World War II, the general practitioner was the predominant source of medical care and the major access point to the health care systems in each county. After World War II, great advances in medicine occurred and subspecialties assumed a greater role in health care, especially in the United States. By 2000, fewer than 16 000 general practitioners remained in the United States, compared to an estimated 72 000 family physicians. The number of active civilian family physicians and general practitioners in the US specialty mixis approximately 13 per cent of all active civilian MDs for whom a specialty is known. Approximately 35 per cent of office-based physicians in the United States are considered primary care physicians when one includes general internists and general paediatricians.[1] The proportion of family physicians in the Canadian specialty mix exceeds 50 per cent, due in part to official policies to ensure access to a family physician for all Canadians.[2]

During the 1960s, health planners, medical leaders, and government officials realized that the production of a variety of specialists in North America was advancing; yet people had less access to a competent general practitioner. In the late 1960s and early 1970s, general practice underwent a series of educational and structural changes to emerge as the specialty of family practice.[3,4]

In North America, a general practitioner is now a physician who did not complete formal training in any specialty and is ineligible for specialty certification in family practice or any other discipline. In most states in the United States, such physicians may obtain a license to practice. For newly trained physicians in Canada, general practice is no longer an option. One must complete a 2-year family practice residency and obtain initial certification from the College of Family Physicians of Canada (CFPC), although some provinces have exceptions for practice only within that province.

By the 1980s, general practitioners in the United States and Canada could be active members of the American Academy of Family Physicians (AAFP) or the CFPC only after completing an accredited family practice residency. General practitioners not trained in family practice residencies become fewer each year.

Primary health services are delivered almost entirely by family physicians in Canada. These services are often delivered using a multidisciplinary approach, and with the inclusion of non-physician health care providers as part of the health care team. Family physicians deliver a substantial portion, but not all, of primary care health care services in the United States. Other providers of care share the provision of primary care services in the United States to some degree. Family physicians in the United States are the primary care leaders in a pluralistic health care delivery system that also includes physicians in general internal medicine, general paediatrics, nurse practitioners, and physician's assistants. Family physicians often utilize non-physicians as part of a team approach to practice.[5]

The physician discipline of osteopathic medicine is unique to the United States. Students in colleges of osteopathic medicine leading to the degree of doctor of osteopathy (DO) currently receive medical education similar to students in schools of medicine leading to the degree of medical doctor (MD). In addition to the usual course of medical study, colleges of osteopathic medicine also teach osteopathic manipulation therapy, a technique of musculoskeletal manipulative therapy pioneered by Andrew Still, MD, in the late nineteenth century. This special training and activity forms the basis of the current distinction between doctors of osteopathy and doctors of medicine. As of 2000, there were 48 000 osteopathic physicians in the United States, of which 24 000 were family physicians.[6]

Medical education and family practice

The 125 medical schools in the United States accept approximately 16 500 students each year. The 19 American Osteopathic Association (AOA) accredited colleges of osteopathic medicine accept approximately 2500 students each year. Nearly all matriculants into medical schools in the United States have a college degree, and some have advanced degrees in a variety of fields.

Academic departments of family medicine exist in 113 of the 125 medical and all 19 colleges of osteopathic medicine in the United States. In contrast, all 125 US medical schools have academic departments of internal medicine, paediatrics, obstetrics/gynaecology, psychiatry, and surgery. Academic departments and curricula of family medicine are found in all Canadian medical schools. In 1993, family medicine achieved parity with the other five major disciplines in the curricula of US medical schools. Medical school accreditation language reads, 'clinical education programs involving patients should include disciplines such as family medicine, internal medicine, obstetrics/gynecology, paediatrics, psychiatry and surgery'.[7] All US medical schools have required educational experiences in the other five major medical specialties, but approximately 20 do not yet require educational experiences in family medicine. As a result, graduates of medical schools with both departments and required curricula in family medicine are more than twice as likely to enter careers in family practice as graduates of schools without departments and required curricula in family medicine.[8]

Postgraduate training and professional development

The 16 medical schools in Canada each have family practice residencies, which are closely affiliated. After 4 years of medical school, successful graduates from US medical schools enter residency training in one of the 24 specialties recognized by the American Board of Medical Specialties. Approximately 10–17 per cent of graduates enter residencies in family practice.[9] Family practice residencies in US medical schools are of 3 years duration. Of all 1969 through 1993 graduates of Accreditation Council on Graduate Medical Education (ACGME) accredited US family practice residencies, 91 per cent identified themselves as practising family physicians in January 1994.[10]

In the United States, medical school graduates can deliver primary care services as generalists in internal medicine or paediatrics. Some who do so enter internal medicine or paediatric residencies and do not subspecialize, and others retain some element of primary care services delivery in combination with their subspecialty. Graduates of colleges of osteopathic medicine in the United States enter 3 years of family practice residency programmes accredited by the AOA. In Canada, approximately half of the graduates of Canadian medical colleges enter 2 years of family practice residency programmes accredited by the CFPC.

Successful completion of a residency programme in family practice, internal medicine, or paediatrics qualifies the graduate to take a specialty certifying examination in one of those three specialties. A similar situation applies to DOs in the United States.

Accreditation and professional organizations

Medical schools in the United States and Canada that offer the MD degree are accredited by the Liaison Committee on Medical Education, which is a voluntary private accreditation agency with rigorous standards for medical education.[7] Colleges of osteopathic medicine are accredited by the AOA using similar standards as those for medical education.

The ACGME accredits family practice residencies in the United States upon recommendation of its specialty-specific Residency Review Committee for Family Practice. The ACGME has residency review committees in all major specialties. Canadian family practice residency programmes are accredited by the CFPC, while the Royal College of Physicians and Surgeons of Canada accredits programmes in all other medical specialties. All residency programmes in all specialties in osteopathic medicine, including family medicine, are accredited by the AOA.

As of July 2002, there were 466 ACGME accredited family practice residencies in the United States. In these residencies, there were 10 130 total residents divided approximately equally among the 3 years of training. Family practice residency programmes produced 67 297 graduates since 1 January, 1970.[11] The AOA accredits 111 osteopathic family practice residencies in the United States.[12] Each of the 16 Canadian medical schools has several family practice residency units.

The major specialty societies in the United States are the AAFP, the American Academy of Pediatrics, and the American College of Physicians–American Society of Internal Medicine. Although each of these specialty societies works closely with the American Medical Association (AMA) and provide delegates to the AMA House of Delegates, all three specialty societies are independent of the AMA.

There are several other family practice organizations in the United States that represent various academic constituencies, some of which also have Canadian members.

The American College of Osteopathic Family Physicians (ACOFP) is the largest specialty association affiliated with the AOA. The ACOFP sets the standards for and inspects the osteopathic family practice residencies, which are accredited by the AOA.

In Canada, the CFPC is structured somewhat differently than its sister organizations in the United States. The CFPC is the professional association of family physicians, the entity that accredits family practice residencies, and certifies individual physicians as specialists in family practice. By contrast, in the United States the functions of residency accreditation and individual physician certification as specialists in family practice are the responsibility of separate organizations. Much as there are several family practice organizations in the United States, the specialties of internal medicine and paediatrics also have additional organizations that represent special interests of those physician populations, including the Society of General Internal Medicine and the Ambulatory Pediatric Association.

Continuing education and quality improvement

To be board certified in family practice in the United States, one must be a graduate of an ACGME accredited family practice residency programme, possess a full and unrestricted license to practice medicine in one or more states, and pass a cognitive examination offered by the American Board of Family Practice (ABFP). Created in 1969, the ABFP was the first of the US certifying boards to require periodic recertification by all certificants. Board-certified family physicians in the United States must accrue 300 h of continuing medical education in a 6-year period in order to be eligible to take the recertification examination.[13] Certification in family practice is valid for a 7-year period, hence, family physicians recertify in the sixth or seventh year of their certification period. Recertification includes a cognitive examination and office record review. Practicing family physicians may designate focused areas of concentration for the cognitive examination, while the other part is a broad examination covering all of family practice.

In Canada, certification in family medicine is granted to eligible candidates following successful completion of the Certification Examination in Family Medicine. All active certificants must participate in the CFPC's MAINPRO programme (maintenance of certification). MAINPRO is the CFPC programme that governs the continuing medical educational requirements of its members. It is possible to be a member of the college without being a certificant. In order to maintain membership in the CFPC, all active members, including certificants, are required to obtain a minimum of 250 maintenance of membership study credits per 5-year cycle. Certificants are also required to accumulate 24 maintenance of certification credits within the 250 study credits in a 5-year cycle.[14]

In 2000, the AAFP began a quality improvement programme that combines continuing medical education and practice-based assessment, intervention, and evaluation. The AAFP and ABFP are moving from recertification to the concept of continuous maintenance of certification, as occurs in Canada. Maintenance of certification would include licensure and credentialing, cognitive examination, practice performance evaluation, and lifelong learning/self-assessment.

Practice arrangements: government and private enterprise

Following World War II, payment for physician services in the United States evolved from direct payments by patients to physicians to indemnity health insurance, pre-paid capitation, and managed care. The US government became the largest payer of health care services in 1966 with the passage of Medicare (care of the elderly) and Medicaid (care of the poor) government insurance programmes. Capitated health maintenance organizations (advance payments based on the number of enrollees) emerged to capture a significant portion of the health care market in the 1990s. Large private insurers and payers of health care now offer a combination of indemnity insurance (fee-for-service), health maintenance organizations (capitation), and hybrid preferred provider organizations (discounted fee-for-service), all of which constitute 'managed care'.

In Canada, by contrast, the provincial governments directly reimburse physicians for services rendered. Prices are set through negotiation between physician groups and provincial governments.

Key policy developments

While Canada has both federal and provincial workforce policies to maintain a system of approximately 50 per cent family physicians, the United States has no such proactive federal physician workforce policy. Approximately half the states subsidize the training of family physicians or reimburse part of all of educational loans for graduates of family practice programmes as an inducement to practice in the state.

In the United States, only family physicians are distributed geographically in the same proportion as the population. Approximately 20 per cent of the population of the United States lived outside metropolitan areas (metropolitan statistical areas, MSAs) in 1997,[15] and 21 per cent of non-Federal M.D. family physicians actively providing patient care practised in non-MSA counties, compared to approximately 8 per cent of general internists and 7 per cent general paediatricians.[16]

More than half (52.4 per cent) of active AAFP members engage in direct patient care practice in partnerships or groups with other family physicians. Approximately 20 per cent were in solo practice,[9] compared with 25 per cent of Canadian family physicians.[17]

Because the United States does not have health care coverage for all, there are many primary care health personnel shortage areas, defined as fewer than one primary care physician per 3500 population. Family physicians are the dominant providers in such shortage areas. In 1995, 784 of 3082 counties in the United States were wholly designated as primary care health personnel shortage areas, but an additional 1332 (58.0 per cent) of the remaining 2298 counties would become primary care health personnel shortage areas if not for the family physicians in those counties.[18]

Many states have attempted to provide health personnel for their shortage areas through expanded licensure and scope of practice legislation for nurse practitioners. However, while approximately one-fourth of primary care office-based physicians use physician assistants and/or nurse practitioners for an average of 11 per cent of visits.[19]

Specific primary care initiatives

The United States and Canada have special government programmes that provide care for rural and indigent people who otherwise would not have access to medical care. These programmes are largely primary care based with the major contribution offered by family physicians and significant assistance by physician's assistants and nurse practitioners. Other primary care physicians offer additional services in these areas including contributions by obstetricians/gynaecologists and other specialists. In the United States, the Indian Health Service of the United States Public Health Service (USPHS) provides services specifically for Native Americans. Another programme of the USPHS is the National Health Service Corps, which provides medical services to a variety of physician shortage areas with the major emphasis of its services being primary care.

The Canadian Institutes of Health Research (CIHR) has councils to support research in special needs of specific Canadian populations. Included under CIHR's umbrella are Institutes for Aboriginal Peoples' Health, Ageing, Gender and Health, and Human Development, Child and Youth Health.

For family practice residents who desire to establish a practice in physician shortage areas in rural North America, both United States and Canadian family practice residencies are often tailored to provide specific experience and training for service in those areas. Family practice residencies in the United States can utilize a series of specific curricular suggestions provided by the AAFP. Canada has a specific rural track of 6 months duration, which provides additional rural exposure to meet rural health care needs. A resident may also choose a third year of advanced skills training for rural practice. Family practice residents in both countries are well trained to provide health care services to female patients, and there is no specialty specific to the primary care needs of women.

Overview of the current position of family practice

Family physicians in North America provide the full range of patient services to all ages in the population.

In 1999, 22.5 per cent of all ambulatory office visits in the United States were to family physicians (see Table 1).[9] Family physicians received more office visits than paediatricians, general internists, or obstetricians/gynaecologists. Office visits by females of age 18–64 were made more often to family physicians than to general internists or obstetricians/gynaecologists (see Table 2).[9] Essential hypertension was the most frequent principal diagnosis of all ambulatory visits to family physicians, followed by acute upper respiratory infections of multiple or unspecified sites, general medical examinations, diabetes mellitus, chronic sinusitis, and health supervision of infants or children.[9]

According to data from the CFPC's JANUS project of 2001, half or more of Canadian family physicians offer medical services in chronic disease management, mental health care, palliative care, and sports medicine. At least nine of 10 Canadian family physicians offer blood pressure screening, Pap smears, obtaining histories of tobacco use and smoking cessation counseling/interventions, immunization for the elderly, mammography for women aged 50–69, and clinical breast examinations for women aged 50–69.[17]

Table 1 Distribution of office visits by physician specialty and professional identity, United States, 1999

	Office visits			
	Number of visits (in thousands)			
	Doctor of medicine	Doctor of osteopathy	Total visits	Percentage of total
All visits	709 071	47 663	756 734	100.0
Physician specialty				
Family physicians and general practice	140 003	30 568	170 571	22.5
General internal medicine	133 624	1 983	135 607	17.9
Paediatrics (includes all subspecialties)	71 187	2 858	74 045	9.8
Obstetrics and gynaecology (includes subspecialties)	57 998	1 520	59 518	7.9
Ophthalmology	51 165	a	51 165	6.8
Orthopaedic surgery	38 925	1 591	40 516	5.4
Dermatology	30 797	1 907	32 704	4.3
Psychiatry	21 791	a	22 346	3.0
General surgery	20 127	1 047	21 174	2.8
Urology	17 415	a	17 415	2.3
Cardiovascular diseases	16 574	a	16 566	2.2
Otolaryngology	16 254	a	16 369	2.2
Neurology	8 298	a	8 298	1.1
All other specialties	84 941	5 499	90 440	12.0

a The estimate is too small to be reliable.

Source: US Department of Health and Human Services, Public Health Service, Centers for Disease Control and Prevention, National Center for Health Statistics, 1999 data, unpublished.

Table 2 Office visits by sex and age of patients to all physicians and selected specialties (including doctors of osteopathy): United States, 1999

	Office visits (no. in thousands)				
Patient age (years)	**All physicians**	**GFP**	**PD**[a]	**GIM**[b]	**OBG**[c]
Total	756 734	170 571	74 045	135 607	59 518
Under 3 years	44 506	6 589	31 290	1 973	d
3–17 years	91 121	21 034	40 141	3 356	1 351
18–44 years	227 005	59 838	1 868	33 469	42 738
45–64 years	201 911	47 793	d	44 008	11 342
65 years and over	192 190	35 316	d	52 801	3 922
Female, total	445 566	97 532	35 242	78 822	59 518
Under 3 years	21 227	3 641	14 386	1 115	d
3–17 years	44 589	10 577	19 206	1 910	1 351
18–44 years	147 036	35 510	1 103	17 852	42 738
45–64 years	119 424	27 204	d	24 883	11 342
65 years and over	113 290	20 600	d	33 062	3 922

[a] General paediatrics and paediatric subspecialties.

[b] General internal medicine.

[c] OBG and subspecialties.

d The estimate is too small to be reliable.

Source: US Department of Health and Human Services, Public Health Service, Centers for Disease Control and Prevention, National Center for Health Statistics, 1999 data, unpublished.

Table 3 Types of patient care in family physicians'[a] hospital practices, May 2000

Privilege	Percentage
Obstetrical delivery	22.4
Attend at caesarean delivery	29.8
Newborn care	61.7
Dilatation and curettage	11.8
Tubal ligation	5.3
Surgery	
Assisting	25.9
Minor	36.4
Coronary care unit	47.8
Intensive care unit	51.4
Emergency room	57.8
Psychiatry	36.7
Interpret EKGs	36.0
Flexible sigmoidoscopy	29.0

[a] Includes only active member respondents of the American Academy of Family Physicians.

Source: American Academy of Family Physicians Practice Profile Survey I, May 2000.

Most family physicians in North America include hospital care of patients in their routine clinical practice. In 2000, 86 per cent of active members of the AAFP in direct patient care had hospital admission privileges.[(9)] Twenty-two per cent of active members of the AAFP included hospital deliveries in their obstetrical care[(9)] (Table 3).

The CFPC's JANUS project of 2001 found that 35 per cent of Canadian family physicians practice in hospital inpatient units and 25 per cent practice in emergency departments.[(17)]

Future plans for family practice development

Family practice is a well established specialty in North America. It has grown into a very strong contributor to primary care in both the United States and Canada over the past several years. In both countries, more family physicians are needed to adequately meet the primary care needs of the entire population. The CFPC's *Prescription for Renewal—2000* proposes the establishment of family practice networks throughout Canada. Family physicians would be encouraged to form linkages with one another, nurse practitioners, nurses, midwives, and other health care professionals to work in interdisciplinary, integrated teams.[(20)]

In the United States, the AAFP and its sister organizations of family practice have embarked on a project entitled 'The Future of Family Medicine' scheduled for completion in 2003. This project is designed to transform and renew family practice to meet the needs of people in a changing health care environment.

References

1. **Division of Survey and Data Resources, Department of Physician Practice and Communications Information.** *Physician Characteristics and Distribution in the US*, 2002–2003 edn. Chicago IL: American Medical Association, 2002.
2. **National Information: Southam Medical Data Base.** In *Canadian Institute for Health Information*, 2001 (http://www.cihi.ca/facts/natsmdb.shtml).
3. **Ad Hoc Committee on Education for Family Practice.** *Meeting the Challenge of Family Practice.* Chicago IL: American Medical Association, 1966.
4. **Citizens Commission on Graduate Medical Education.** *The Graduate Education of Physicians.* Chicago IL: American Medical Association, 1966.
5. **Non-Physician Providers** (NPPs). In *AAFP: AAFP Policies on Health Issues*, 2000 (http://www/aafp.org/policy/issues.html).
6. **American Osteopathic Association.** AOA Fact Sheet. *The DO*, 12–15 January, 2001.
7. **Liaison Committee on Medical Education.** *Functions and Structure of a Medical School.* Chicago IL: American Medical Association, 2001.

8. **Pugno, P.A.** et al. (2001). Entry of US medical school graduates into family practice residencies: 2000–2001 and three year summary. *Family Medicine* **33**, 585–93.
9. **American Academy of Family Physicians.** *Facts About Family Practice*, 2002 (http://www.aafp.org/facts).
10. **Kahn, N.B. Jr.** et al. (1996). Specialty practice of family practice residency graduates, 1969 through 1993: a national study. *Journal of the American Medical Association* **275**, 713–15.
11. **Family Practice Residency Programs.** *Reprint 150.* Leawood KS: AAFP, 2002.
12 **American College of Osteopathic Family Physicians.** *ACOFP Fact Sheet.* Arlington Heights IL: ACOFP, 2001.
13. **American Board of Family Practice.** *Recertification Candidate Information Booklet.* Lexington KY: ABFP, 2001.
14. **MAINPRO.** *The College of Family Physicians of Canada*, November 2001 (http://www/cfpc/ca/cme/mainpro/mainpro.htm).
15. Population estimates for metropolitan areas and components, annual time series April 1, 1990 to July 1, 1999. In *Population Estimates Program, Population Division, US Census Bureau* (http://eire.census.gov/popest/archives/metro/ma99–03a.txt).
16. **The Robert Graham Center.** *The Effect of Accredited Rural Training Tracks on Physician Placement.* Washington DC: American Academy of Family Physicians, 1999.
17. **The College of Family Physicians of Canada.** *Initial Data Release of the 2001 National Family Physician Workforce Survey: The Janus Project*, 2001.
18. **Fryer, G.E.** et al. (2001). The United States relies on family physicians unlike any other specialty. *American Family Physician* **63**, 1669.
19. **Hooker, R.S. and McCaig, L.F.** (2001). Use of physician assistants and nurse practitioners in primary care, 1995–1999. *Health Affairs* **20** (4), 231–8.
20. **Primary Care and Family Medicine in Canada: a Prescription for Renewal.** *The College of Family Physicians of Canada*, October 2000 (http://www.cfpc.ca/communications/prescription.asp).

2.13 International organizations

Chris van Weel and Wes E. Fabb

Introduction

International contact and cooperation has been a feature of general practice/family medicine since the early days of the founding of national professional and academic organizations. At the heart of it were family doctors who questioned the effectiveness of their own professional setting and looked for other experiences. This is a pattern that is still a powerful driving force behind primary care development and most of these contacts remain informal. Formalization of contacts facilitates the organization of conferences and journal publications—the traditional modes of international contacts—and more recently websites.

In line with the natural development of primary care, initially the emphasis of international exchanges has been to compare and exchange experience with the professional role of general practice and family medicine in health care. From that followed the agenda of the generic professional development of general practice which features teaching, training, quality assurance, and research. The systematic in-depth exploration of clinical and methodological parts of the profession followed after this and primary care organizations that have their mission here are a fairly recent development.

Primary care has always fostered close links to other disciplines and other medical organizations often attract a significant input from GPs. In some cases, GPs played a leading role in their founding—for example, the International Epidemiological Association. These links fall outside the brief of this chapter.

When considering professional organizations and networking, the core characteristic of primary care should be kept in mind: integration of care, cure, and diagnosis for a variety of health problems. Rather than splitting the field there is a strong drive towards gathering organizations under one umbrella and this has been, in particular, the position of the World Organization of Family Doctors, WONCA. As this is a dynamic process, organizations that are outside WONCA at one time may have joined the umbrella at another. For that reason this chapter focuses in particular on WONCA, but will start with a short overview of other organizations. Because it involves parts of the world where 'family physician' and 'family medicine' are the terms used for what in Europe is referred to as 'general practitioner' and 'general practice' in this chapter, the two are considered synonymous.

Science and politics

Most organizations of GPs contribute to the development of the content of the profession and are therefore 'academic' in their mission. Primary care in its professional functioning is a direct product of the health care system and this reflects the medico-political frame of the profession. As national political powers take precedence over medico-political issues, national organizations are usually the most appropriate for this. The obvious exception is Europe, where the EU presents more and more an agenda that involves the medical profession and where there are EU-wide directives for minimally required professional training for entry into general practice.

The Union Europeainne de Medicin Omnipracticien (UEMO) unites the medico-political organizations of the EU member countries, the candidate member countries and important non-EU countries like Switzerland, Norway, and Iceland. Its leading role is in producing the directives for training for general practice, the recognition of diplomas and the free movement of doctors, in legislation related to the medico-ethical aspects of general practice, and in regulations that address quality of care and consumer protection. UEMO functions through the direct involvement of the boards of its member organizations, which enhances the implementation of its decisions. These meetings take place at least twice a year and additional meetings are organized for a broader audience—some together with WONCA-Europe. In fact, the UEMO mission touches directly on the 'academic' development of general practice and the roles of WONCA and UEMO are to a considerable degree complimentary.

Academic general practice organizations

North American Primary Care Research Group (NAPCRG)

North American Primary Care Research Group (napcrg.org) is the leading North American research organization of general practice. Membership is based on individual subscription. Although it was in its origins centred on Canada and the United States, membership is open to anyone who feels related to its mission. In particular, from Europe there is a substantial following. Its annual conferenced are organized in the United States and Canada. NAPCRG has contributed to full breadth of general practice research development and capacity building but has in the past decades contributed to the establishment of (sentinel and research) practices networks, mental health research, and the development of qualitative methodology to evaluate health of indigenous populations.

Society of Teachers of Family Medicine (STFM)

The Society of Teachers of Family Medicine (stfm.org) is a large academic organization, dedicated to improving health through education, research, patient care, and advocacy. It was founded in 1967 and now has a membership of more than 5000 teachers of family medicine. Its principal goals are to promote excellence and innovation in family medicine education, to foster a scholarly approach to clinical practice and teaching, to promote members' interests and skills in appraising, applying, and conducting research in family medicine, and to assure education in the fundamentals of family medicine to all physicians. The Society supports collaboration within the discipline of family medicine and has a particular focus on promoting educational models which address the needs of families and communities, with an emphasis on under served populations. *Family Medicine*, a scholarly journal featuring clinical and educational research articles, is published monthly and STFM sponsors annual conferences in North America.

European networks EURACT, EQUIP, EGPRW

The European Academy of Teachers of General Practice (EURACT, euract.org) functioned for a long time as a stand-alone organization for GPs involved in teaching and training, before it became a co-founder of WONCA-Europe in 1995. The European Association for Quality in Family Practice (EQUIP, www.equip.ch) had established itself as an important resource group for European primary care innovation when it supported the initiative of founding WONCA-Europe. The European General Practitioners Research Workshop (EGPRW, www.synapse.net.mt/egprw) had a long tradition as a forum for GPs with a research interest when it joined as a founding organization in 1995 WONCA-Europe. All three groups continue to organize regular meetings in their own domain but have now integrated as a network in WONCA-Europe.

Iberoamerican Confederation of Family Medicine

An influential organization in Latin America is the Iberoamerican Confederation of Family Medicine (CIMF, cimf.net). Centred in Buenos Aires, it brings together the national general practice organizations of Latin America and fosters close ties with Spain and Portugal. It has played a major role in the development of general practice in Central and South America. It has encouraged medical schools to include departments of family medicine, and has facilitated the development of national colleges throughout the region. It has its own organizational structure with an annual conference. As mentioned above, CIMF has in 2002 become part of the WONCA organization, and a sixth WONCA region, Latin America, will be created.

General practice clinical groups

In the last decade, a number of general practice groups have been founded to explore in greater details the role of primary care and the primary care physician in particular clinical area. These groups have grown out of a recognition of the distinctive contribution made by primary care to the management of a range of disorders, of the need to undertake epidemiological, interventional, and health services research in the primary care setting, to provide evidence-based education for general practitioners and to collaborate with specialist colleagues in secondary care in the management of many of these conditions.

Primary Care Society of Gastroenterology (PCSG) and European Society for Primary Care Gastroenterology (ESPCG)

The Primary Care Society of Gastroenterology (www.pcsg.org.uk) was founded in the United Kingdom in 1985, bringing together general practitioners with a special interest and expertise in gastrointestinal problems. Its European counterpart, the European Society of Primary Care Gastroenterology (ESPCG, gp-gastro@med.uu.nl), was founded in 1995, and has a membership drawn from over 20 European countries. It has been involved in the production of clinical guidelines on topics such as the management of *Helicobacter pylori* infection and the early detection of colorectal cancer. Both societies publish a journal, *Gastroenterology in Perspective* from the United Kingdom and *Eurogut* in Europe, and both contribute to international conferences, including the British Society of Gastroenterology, the American Gastroenterology Association and WONCA, have had a significant impact on the relationship between primary and secondary care in clinical care and research in gastroenterology, and have been used as models for the development of similar clinical groups.

European Primary Care Cardiovascular Society

The European Primary Care Cardiovascular Society (EPCCS) focuses on the diagnosis, treatment, and prevention of cardiovascular disease in primary care, in order to improve the quality of care for patients in general practice. It has links to WONCA as well as to cardiology meetings in Europe and North America.

International Primary Care Respiratory Group

The International Primary Care Respiratory Group (IPCRG) has its origins in a WONCA meeting held in Dublin in 1998. Asthma and COPD are its main themes of work, but respiratory infections also feature. Membership is open for everyone interested in these topics. Symposia at WONCA are mirrored by similar events at European and North American respiratory conferences. IPCRG organizes a stand-alone conference every 2 years.

World Organization of Family Doctors

The largest international organization in primary care, and the most representative of the world's family doctors, is the World Organization of Family Doctors (WONCA). Its motto is *World Family Doctors. Caring for People.*

WONCA was founded in 1972 in Melbourne, Australia as the 'World Organization of National Colleges, Academies, and Academic Associations of General Practitioners/Family Physicians'—thus the acronym WONCA, the first letter of the first five words. Later, the short name was adopted. It is governed by a representative Council and an Executive. Its Secretariat is currently in Singapore.

WONCA's mission

The mission of the organization is to improve the quality of life of the peoples of the world through defining and promoting its values, and by fostering high standards of care in general practice/family medicine. It does this by championing personal, comprehensive, and continuing care for the individual in the context of the family and the community; encouraging and supporting the development of academic organizations of general practitioners/family physicians; providing a forum for the exchange of knowledge and information between member organizations and between general practitioners/family physicians; and representing the policies and the educational, research and service provision activities of general practitioners/family physicians to other world organizations and forums concerned with health and medical care.

This global scientific mission to promote and improve primary medical care, family medicine, or general practice brings together academic national organizations ('colleges'). At present 65 national colleges from 58 countries are currently members of WONCA, representing over 150 000 family doctors world-wide. As a result of a recent agreement with the Latin American organization, ICFM, there will soon be the addition of a number of colleges from Central and South America.

WONCA contributes to the improvement of the health of individuals around the world, and works through primary health care to achieve this. The prime objective is the development of primary health care for everyone around the world. The availability of general practice/family medicine contributes substantially to effective and efficient (cost-effective) health care. The provision of general practice/family medicine in the local community contributes to the accessibility of health care for all, and to equity. Another objective of WONCA is to pursue excellence in primary care in order to guarantee general practice/family medicine services of the highest standards. Tools to achieve this include teaching, training, research, and development.

Medical teaching must address illness and disease *in* the community in order to be able to enhance clinical competence that is relevant to physicians working there. This requires a medical curriculum with teaching based on community-oriented primary care, which emphasizes prevention, early diagnosis, family-oriented care, continuity of care medical interventions, and patients' perceived health/quality of life.

Entry into general practice/family medicine should be conditional upon *specialist training* in the primary care setting. Only through working under these conditions can future primary care physicians be prepared for their task. The teaching hospital can provide future general practitioners/family physicians with important knowledge and skills, and experience in that setting can be highly relevant for practice in primary care. However, the clinical experience the hospital can offer is in itself dramatically incomplete for primary care practice.

Treatment of illness and disease must be based on scientific evidence. For general practice/family medicine this implies that it is based on *research* that analyses the natural history of illness and diagnostic and therapeutic outcomes *in* the primary care setting. Innovative approaches must be *developed* in, built upon, and tested in the community settings where it is to be practised.

From mission to implementation

In order to achieve its objectives, WONCA applies a number of strategies. The most important is that general practice/family medicine is put into practice everywhere patients are cared for—in other words, in the communities where physicians are working. As national organizations are in a better position to provide this than is a world body, WONCA pursues its mission through its member organizations.

Member organizations

The availability of an academic organization of general practice/family medicine in every country in the world is essential. Where there is none, this usually signals the need for primary care development. An important task for WONCA in the past decades has been the facilitation of the growth of national academic organizations. This process is now well advanced in Europe and North America, has come a long way in Asia-Pacific, is showing encouraging results in Middle East, South Asia, and Latin America, but has only just started in Africa. To promote the development of national initiatives, regional support can be vital. Therefore, an important WONCA strategy is the development of its regions.

WONCA regions

The problem in the regions is that where the need is highest, the going is toughest. Currently the process of regionalization is well underway. The regions with many member organizations (Europe and Asia-Pacific) have recently developed a solid regional structure and have demonstrated the ability for concerted action and the provision of a general practice/family medicine platform for regional needs and demands. The development of WONCA regions in Africa and the Middle East and South Asia will be a strong stimulating factor for the development of primary care there.

Conferences

The organization of conferences is a traditional method of bringing together general practitioners/family physicians. Every 3 years, WONCA organizes a world conference, hosted by one of its member organizations. In fact, the founding of WONCA as an organization followed a number of world conferences of family medicine in the 1960s. As a forum for research, development, and training/teaching, WONCA conferences are important and are attracting an increasing number of participants. However, the impact of an occasional world conference on the actual state of affairs in primary care is limited. Since the regional structure allows a more targeted networking of primary care experience, there are increasing numbers of large- and small-scale regional conferences organized under the WONCA banner.

Working parties and special interest groups

WONCA facilitates the regular meeting of groups devoted to aspects of health care. The most important sustained contribution has come from the WONCA International Classification Committee. Over a period of 25 years, this group has developed a primary care-specific classification of diseases (the International Classification of Health Problems in Primary Care)[1] and later an integrated classification of signs, symptoms, diseases and procedures, the International Classification of Primary Care.[2] Through the work of this group, WONCA stimulated the analysis of the content of general practice/family medicine with reference to terms, criteria, and concepts fundamental to primary care.

Other working groups include Research, which has worked on the measurement of functional status;[3] Quality Assurance;[4] Informatics; Health Behaviour Change, Women in Family Medicine and Care of the Elderly. Of particular importance has been the work of two working parties. The rural doctors' initiative has drawn attention to the special needs of populations and their practitioners who live in isolated circumstances.[5] Through the involvement of the working party on Rural Practice the general practice/family medicine focus has been preserved. The working party on Smoking Cessation is enabling WONCA to play a leading role in combating smoking related diseases.

Recently, within WONCA a number of groups have organized themselves with a special clinical focus: general practitioners/family physicians with particular expertise in gastroenterology, cardiovascular diseases, and respiratory illness.

Invitational meetings, policy documents, and site visits

Another way in which WONCA has contributed to the development of primary care has been the publication of policy documents on key issues. Input into the documents has been based on invitational meetings of experts and circulation of the resultant document. Targeted site visits provided a means of follow-up. The most impressive examples in this respect have been:

- The work on primary care in China. After developing documentation relevant for the developmental status of China,[6] WONCA was able to play a leading role in China's health care reform. A number of visits of international experts were made, during a period when foreign influence was difficult to establish.
- Documentation of the role of the general practitioner/family physician and the consequent needs for medical education and specialty training,[7] which followed a World Health Organization/WONCA invitational conference in London, Ontario, in 1994. This document has subsequently played a major role in health care reform in Central and Eastern Europe, and has had an influence on ministries of health, medical schools, and medical curricula around the world.
- In 1997, another WHO/WONCA conference organized by the Royal College of General Practitioners reviewed the implications of physicians' funding on the performance of health care systems. Given the central role of the general practitioner/family physician, issues such as access, capitation, competition, and fee-for-service have a direct impact on the outcome of care.
- A policy document on research in primary care is currently in preparation.

WONCA website

WONCA is in the process of expanding its website with the inclusion of a wide range of educational material. It aims to become a major resource for medical education, research, and public information, particularly in developing countries.

Cooperation with other global organizations

In pursuing its objectives, WONCA works with partners. For special projects there is an important role for funding bodies like the Kellogg Foundation. WONCA has developed close links with the World Health Organization, and in an effort to foster primary care around the world has published *Improving Health Systems: The Contribution of Family Medicine—A Guidebook.* Two of the policy documents mentioned above were developed with WHO. WONCA supports WHO's *Towards Unity for Health* initiative that proposes to bring together public health and clinical medicine.

Cooperation takes place on a regional level as well as on a global level. In Europe, WONCA and WHO have joined in the development of primary care in Central and Eastern countries, in particular the former Soviet republics. A significant sign of the impact of this has been that in Europe general practice/family medicine is regarded the key factor in primary care.[(8)]

Membership: colleges, individuals, and university departments

As stated, national academic organizations of general practice/family medicine are the constituent members of WONCA. In addition, WONCA is open for individual membership. Individual membership allows for personal benefits in participation in WONCA activities and is particularly attractive for academic leaders of the discipline of general practice/family medicine.

Recently, the importance of university departments of general practice/family medicine in the work of WONCA has been recognized, and in the near future it will be possible for university departments to join—again qualifying for special benefits.

A case in depth: WONCA-Europe

Societas Internationalis Medicinae Generalis (1959–1995)

The position of WONCA in Europe warrants extra attention. The linkage of Europe into WONCA proved to be a strong element in the development of WONCA. In Europe, the Societas Internationalis Medicinae Generalis (SIMG) was founded in 1959 in Vienna. SIMG included individual general practitioners in Europe, though later colleges also could join. The emphasis of SIMG was on Central and Eastern Europe, with German the main language for a long time. A major achievement of SIMG was to bring together general practitioners, leaders from West and East, in a period when the Iron Curtain still cast its large shadow over the continent. Annual conferences in Austria provided ground where both sides could meet. In that respect, the personal membership basis was of fundamental importance and personal relations were established that paid off long after the curtain had come down. Membership grew in the 1980s and 1990s leading to an increase in the SIMG conferences from one to two. In addition to the 'Austrian' one, a Spring meeting was held in other countries. With the opening of the East, the basis of SIMG started to change and in 1995 SIMG merged into the European region of WONCA. This spurred WONCA to change its constitution into an organization with more emphasis on regional structures.

European networks

General practice in Europe has always been characterized by the free flow of ideas and experience between countries. General practice was faced with the implications of specialty training and general practice undergraduate teaching. A gathering of leaders formed the Leeuwenhorst group in 1974, which a few years later turned into the European Academy of Teachers of General Practice, EURACT, where individuals involved in teaching and training met regularly. Researchers established their network to present and discuss studies: the European General Practice Research Workshop (EGPRW), which provides a structure where the training of researchers is combined with the exchange of original research findings. In the 1990s, the issue of quality of care appeared on the health care agenda and this resulted in the foundation of EQuiP as the network of quality assurance experts.

Networks and WONCA-Europe

When SIMG and WONCA merged, the networks were involved and designated the position of expert groups within the European-WONCA region. They maintained their function as a forum for individuals with a special interest and a leading role in the development of general practice/family medicine. Since 1995, a network of experts on prevention (EUROPREV), and a network of general practitioners working in rural and remote areas (EURIPA), have been established and included within WONCA-Europe.

Primary care organizations can be identified from the primary care internet guide (www.uib.no/isf/guide/family.htm).

References

1. **WONCA.** *ICHPPC-2-defined: International Classification of Health Problems in Primary Care* 3rd edn. Oxford: Oxford University Press, 1983.
2. **Lamberts, H. and Wood, M.**, ed. *ICPC: International Classification of Primary Care.* Oxford: Oxford University Press, 1987.
3. **Van Weel, C., König-Zahn, C., Touw-Otten, F.J.M.M., van Duijn, N., and Meyboom-de Jong, B.** *Measuring Functional Health with the COOP/WONCA Charts—A Manual.* Groningen: Northern Centre for Health Care Research, 1995.
4. **Makela, M., Booth, B., and Roberts, R.**, ed. *Family Doctors' Journey to Quality.* Helsinki: STAKES National Research and Development Centre for Welfare and Health, 2001.
5. **Strasser, R.** *Policy on Training for Rural Practice.* Melbourne: WONCA, 2000.
6. **Almagor, G.**, et al. *Medical Education and the Development of General Practice/Family Medicine in China.* Report of the WONCA Task Force, December 20, 1992–January 9, 1993. Hong Kong: WONCA, 1993.
7. **Brown, S.** *Physician Funding and Health Care Systems—An International Perspective.* London: The Royal College of General Practitioners, 1999.
8. **World Health Organization (WHO) and World Organization of Family Doctors (WONCA).** *Making Medical Practice and Education more Relevant to People's Needs: The Contribution of the Family Doctor.* Hong Kong: WONCA, 1994.

3

Reasons for consultation

3 Reasons for consultation

3.1 Use of health services

Sally Wyke

The majority of health care is undertaken at home without recourse to professional advice. People perceive, evaluate, and manage symptoms of illness using evidence based on their own experience together with information gleaned from a range of sources (such as family and friends, magazines, and television programmes).

By far the most important factor that influences whether formal health services are consulted is the severity of the illness experience. Nevertheless, a range of cultural, social, environmental, and health service factors also influence service use. Cultural values such as stoicism, self-reliance, or being unwilling to acknowledge psychological distress also influence service use. These values may vary by age, sex, where people live, and by ethnicity and this variation may result in variation in use of services between groups.

The presence of social support can influence use of services in a range of ways, both increasing and decreasing the likelihood of consultation with formal primary care services. For example, talking to family and friends about worrying symptoms may either increase the likelihood of consultation (where friends feel it is better 'safe than sorry') or decrease the likelihood of consultation (where just talking is enough to reduce the burden of worry and 'normalize' the experience). The expectation of benefit from a consultation is also an important factor that influences service use, but expectations are modified by experience. For example, the expectation that a child's cough will get better with treatment by antibiotic is likely to increase if consultations consistently result in prescription, but to decrease if it is explained that antibiotics are unlikely to help. All of these factors are dealt with in more detail in the following chapters in this section.

An important context for any consideration of use of health services is the health system experienced by people in different countries. Different health systems lead to differences in the way in which primary medical care is used. The most important difference between health systems is the way in which they are financed; the underlying norms and values of the broader society and macro-economic resources available to countries influence this in turn.[1] For example, most Western European countries, Australia, Canada, and New Zealand are committed to the principles of universal access to health care for all citizens, and to sustainable financing of health care. Health systems in these countries are financed either through universal taxation or through social insurance, with some co-payment for services by patients in some countries. In the United States of America, on the other hand, there is no historical commitment to universal access to health care, and the health system is funded through mainly privately accountable insurers. Countries in Central and Eastern Europe, in the Commonwealth of Independent Countries, and in the developing world, often face such difficult macro-economic pressures that even with a collective commitment to universal access to care, it is rarely achievable.

Another difference in health systems that influences use of primary medical care is the extent to which citizens have a choice of provider, and direct access to specialist physicians. Citizens of the United States of America experience maximum choice, having direct access to either family or specialist physicians. In Australia, New Zealand, and many countries in the European Union (except Belgium, Luxembourg, Germany, and France),[2] citizens must consult primary medical practitioners who then refer to specialist physicians as appropriate.

Bearing in mind these key contextual influences, this chapter examines differences in the use of primary medical care services, first by populations in a range of different countries and second by different population groups. Finally, the chapter introduces the issue of access to primary care, and explores some of its potential influence on use of services.

The data used in this chapter rely on the conduct of periodic community-based surveys of health and use of health services and on the systematic collection and collation of routine contacts between patients and primary care practitioners. Inevitably, these are much more common in the developed world, where resources are more plentiful. The chapter therefore relies heavily on data collected in the European Union (especially the United Kingdom), in the United States of America and in New Zealand.

An international perspective

Table 1 compares both likelihood of having consulted a GP at least once in the previous 12 months, and mean consultation rates with GPs, between countries of the European Union in 1996. The data are drawn from a community survey (the European Community Household Panel (ECHP)), reported by Koolmand and Van Doorslaer.[3]

Variation in both these measures are high. For example, Austrians have nearly 2.5 times the mean annual consultation rate than Greeks. Figures on the probability of at least one contact with a GP in the previous 12 months in Europe are comparable with those from New Zealand and Australia. In New Zealand in 1996/97, 79.1 per cent of adults visited a GP at least once in the last year,[4] compared to 82 per cent of Australians in 1999/2000.[5]

Data from the United States of America are not directly comparable. As US citizens have direct access to specialist providers, the biannual National Health Interview Study does not distinguish between primary medical care and other physician contacts. Table 2 shows the proportion of the civilian population who had contact with physicians in emergency department, doctors' offices, or at home in 1998 by age.[6] Eighty-four per cent of the adult population had at least one contact with a physician in the last year.

The mean number of visits to a GP or specialist doctor in the European Union in 1996 was 6.2,[3] which is broadly comparable to the 6.5 visits made by adult Australians in 1998–1999.[7]

Table 1 Contact with general practitioners, EU countries, 1996[a]

Country	Probability of at least one contact with a GP in previous 12 months (%)	Mean number of GP visit in previous 12 months
EU–12[b]	74.7	4.2
Austria	89.3	5.4
Belgium	84.7	5.2
Germany	77.4	5.1
Denmark	74.5	3.1
Spain	65.2	3.7
Greece	52.5	2.2
Italy	76.1	4.5
Ireland	70.4	3.7
Luxembourg	81.7	3.3
Netherlands	71.6	2.9
Portugal	71.3	3.6
United Kingdom	77.9	3.8

[a] Rates are standardized to impose similar age–gender distributions for all countries.

[b] The French survey does not ask these questions and Sweden does not take part in the ECHP.

Table 2 Health care visits to doctors' offices, emergency departments, and home visits within the past 12 months by age, USA, 1998

Age	Number of health care visits			
	None	1–3 visits	4–9 visits	10 or more visits
All persons	15.9	46.8	23.8	13.5
Under 18 years	11.7	54.4	25.6	8.2
18–44 years	21.6	47.7	18.6	12.2
45–64 years	15.9	43.6	24.3	16.2
65+ years	7.3	34.1	35.3	23.4

Differences between population groups

There are large differences in rates of health services utilization between population groups. In health systems that aspire to universal access to primary medical care, such as the United Kingdom, much of this variation is explained by morbidity differences between social groups. In other health systems, financial access to care is an important influence on use.

Age

Table 2 shows the U-shaped distribution of health services utilization with age in the United States. This distribution is confirmed across the developed world. For example, the UK Fourth National Study of Morbidity in General Practice[(8)] shows the annual general practice consultation rates in 1991–1992 for ages 0–4, 16–44, and over 74 were, respectively, 5.5, 2.2, and 6.4 for males and 5.3, 4.6, and 7.1 for females. These patterns are confirmed in a more recent UK community survey,[(9)] and in New Zealand,[(4)] where the proportions of 0–4, 25–44, and over 75 year olds with at least one consultation in the past year was, respectively, 88, 68, and 95 per cent for males and 92, 90, and 95 per cent for females. The differences are likely to reflect greater risk of morbidity amongst the young and old, and increased attendance for preventive health services such as immunization amongst the young.

Sex

As the figures from the UK National Morbidity Study[(8)] and the New Zealand National Health Survey[(4)] show, in general women consult more than men, particularly between the age of 16 and 64. The conditions for which this difference is most evident include genitourinary disease, mental disorders, diseases of the blood and blood-forming organs, symptoms, signs, and ill-defined conditions, and for reasons classified as supplementary (reproductive care, screening). Because of these data, it is often assumed that women have a greater propensity to consult than men for any condition. However, analyses that examine women's and men's response to particular symptoms of ill health[(10)] and to underlying conditions[(11)] challenge this assumption. They find that women are no more likely than men to consult a doctor once a symptom or condition is experienced, except for symptoms and conditions of mental health.

Ethnicity

Patterns of health service utilization between different ethnic groups are complex, vary between countries, and defy simple explanation. In addition, ethnicity and race are conceptualized differently in countries with different histories of migration. This makes cross-national comparisons impossible. Here, we consider data from the United Kingdom, New Zealand, and from United States of America.

In the UK Fourth National Morbidity Study[(8)] people who described themselves as black were no more likely to have consulted a GP in the past 12 months for any reason as any other group. Adults who described themselves as originating in the Indian sub-continent were more likely to have consulted for serious illness. For example, adjusted odds ratios of people from Indian sub-continent consulting for serious conditions at ages 16–44 and 45–64 were, respectively, 1.5 and 2.1 for women, and 1.5 and 1.4 for men. This pattern is likely to reflect the increased risk of cardiovascular disease and diabetes in this group.

In the New Zealand Health Survey,[(4)] similar proportions of adults in European, Maori, and Pacific ethnic groups had visited a GP at least once during the year. However, Maori people were more likely to have had six or more visits to a GP than any other group (Maori 18.9 per cent, Pacific people 16.3 per cent, European 15 per cent, other ethnic groups 8.9 per cent). These patterns reflect greater health needs amongst Maori people, although Pacific people are also more likely to have higher health needs than European people, which might suggest some discrepancy between health needs and use of GP services in Pacific people.

Table 3 shows age-adjusted rates of health care visits in the United States of America in 1998, by race and Hispanic origin, and poverty status. Large differences in use of services are apparent between both ethnic and racial groups, and between people at or near poverty and the more affluent. Differences between groups in the proportion of people with no health care visits are likely to be explained by differential access to health insurance, and financial barriers to health care. On the other hand, differences between groups with 10 or more visits are likely to be explained by higher rates of morbidity amongst poor people.

Socio-economic status

People who are socio-economically disadvantaged have higher rates of ill health than those who are more affluent,[(3,4,6,8)] and this tends to result in higher consultation rates. For example, in the United Kingdom one measure of socio-economic status is occupational social class. People are distinguished on the basis of the usual or last occupation of the 'head of household' into five groups. Analysis of the Fourth National Morbidity Study[(8)] shows that people in occupational social classes IV and V (semi-skilled and unskilled) were more likely than those in social classes I and II (professional and managerial) to consult a doctor: for any illness (odds ratios 1.2 males, 1.2 females); for any serious illness (odds ratios 1.5 males, 1.4 females); and for mental disorder (odd ratios 1.8 males, 1.6 females). Most of the excess is due to morbidity differences. Table 3 shows that even

Table 3 Health care visits to doctor's offices, emergency departments, and home visits in the past 12 months, USA, 1998, by race and Hispanic origin, and poverty status

Race and Hispanic origin, and poverty status	Number of health care visits			
	None	1–3 visits	4–9 visits	10 or more visits
White, non-Hispanic				
Poor	17.0	38.2	24.0	20.7
Near poor	17.1	41.7	23.2	18.0
Non-poor	12.8	48.1	25.7	13.4
Black, non-Hispanic				
Poor	18.0	37.9	25.1	19.1
Near poor	20.7	41.6	22.5	15.2
Non-poor	13.9	51.0	24.6	10.5
Hispanic				
Poor	30.8	36.6	17.5	15.1
Near poor	26.3	42.4	20.4	11.0
Non-poor	17.1	51.4	22.0	9.5

in a non-universal health care system such as the United States of America, poor people are most likely to be highest users of services across all race and ethnic groups because of greater burden of ill health.

Access to care

Access to care is an important factor influencing the decision to consult a primary medical practitioner. Here we distinguish between three forms of access: financial access, organizational access, and geographical access.

Financial access

As we have seen, financial barriers to care are particularly important in non-universal systems of health care such as in the United States of America and children can be particularly vulnerable. In the 1994–1995 National Health Interview Study,[12] children from higher-income families were more likely to have health insurance coverage than those in lower-income families. Over 20 per cent of poor and near-poor children had no health insurance whereas 9 per cent of middle-income children and 4 per cent of high-income children were uninsured. These differences were reflected in less use of health care for low-income children with poor uninsured children particularly unlikely to have seen a doctor: nearly 25 per cent of poor uninsured had not seen a doctor in the last 12 months compared to 8 per cent of poor children with insurance. Financial barriers mean that when poor children do consult, it is more likely to be in an emergency room than planned care.[12]

In universal health systems that nevertheless demand some co-payment for services from patients, such as in New Zealand, lack of money can be suggested as a reason for not consulting a doctor when care was felt to have been needed. The New Zealand National Health Survey asked if respondents had not visited a GP when they felt they had needed to, as a measure of unmet need. Of those who felt they had unmet health needs, nearly half identified cost as their main reason for not consulting.[4]

In the European Union, however, there is little evidence of financial barriers to use of GP services in the face of similar need. Koolmand and Van Doorslaer[3] ask the question 'to what extent do groups of people with equal needs receive equal treatment, irrespective of their income?' (p. 5). Using data from the EUHP they test whether, after having taken need for care into account across quintiles of the income distribution, mean use of GP services is still systematically related to income.

Table 4 shows that for the European Union as a whole there is no general pattern to suggest there are financial barriers to primary medical care across the income groups. In only two countries (Austria and Portugal) were higher-income groups more likely to have higher rates of GP use given equal need.

Table 4 Mean number of GP visits in last 12 months in top and bottom quintile of the income distribution (standardized for age, sex, and morbidity), EU countries, 1996

Country	Income quintiles (Q)		Q1/Q5	Q1–Q5
	Bottom 20%(Q1)	Top 20%(Q5)		
EU–12	4.3	4.0	1.08	0.3
Austria	5.1	5.8	0.88	−0.7
Belgium	5.3	5.1	1.05	0.2
Germany	5.0	4.7	1.07	0.3
Denmark	2.9	2.8	1.03	0.1
Spain	4.0	3.4	1.17	0.6
Greece	2.2	2.1	1.03	0.1
Italy	4.6	4.2	1.08	0.4
Ireland	4.1	3.5	1.17	0.6
Luxembourg	3.3	3.0	1.11	0.3
Netherlands	2.8	2.8	1.00	0.0
Portugal	3.2	3.7	0.88	−0.5
United Kingdom	4.0	3.6	1.12	0.4

Organizational access

The way in which primary medical care is organized can act as a barrier to use of care. Not being able to get an appointment acts as a particularly irksome barrier to patients. For example, in the New Zealand Health Survey,[4] nearly 20 per cent of people who felt that they had not consulted a doctor in the last year when they needed to, said that they had not done so because they could not get an appointment soon enough at a time that suited them. The 1998 National Survey of NHS patients, England[13] showed that nearly 20 per cent of respondents felt that they should have been able to have their last appointment with their GP sooner, and 25 per cent had had to wait 4 or more days for an appointment.

Geographical access

Distance from a health facility is negatively associated with using health services. These issues may be particularly acute in some remote and rural areas. The UK's Fourth National Morbidity Survey showed that even when other factors such as socio-economic status are taken into account people living in rural areas were 10 per cent less likely to consult a doctor than those living in urban areas. Distance from the practice was also a general deterrent to consultation, whether in rural or urban areas. The deterrent effect of distance was less for more serious illness.[8]

Summary

Between 50 and 80 per cent of citizens of the developed world consult a primary medical practitioner at least once in every 12 months. Nevertheless, there is substantial variation between countries in average health service utilization, which is mostly explained by differences in the extent to which health systems seek to achieve universal access to care, health care financing, and the level of co-payment for care expected from patients. However, cultural differences in response to illness should not be ignored and later chapters cover this in some detail. Difference in rates of health service utilization between social groups are largely explained by differences in need for care, particularly in countries with universal access to care. Financial, organizational, and geographical barriers to care can interact with other factors to reduce the likelihood of appropriate consultation.

References

1. **Figueras, J., Saltman, R.B., and Sakellarides, C.** (1998). Introduction. In *Critical Challenges for Health Care Reform in Europe* (ed. R.B. Saltman, J. Figueras, and C. Sakellarides), pp. 1–19. Buckingham: Open University Press.
2. **Mossialos, E. and Le Grand, J.** (1999). Cost containment in the EU: an overview. In *Health Care and Cost Containment in the European Union* (ed. E. Mossialos and J. Le Grand), pp. 1–154. Aldershot: Ashgate.
3. **Koolmand, X. and Van Doorslaer, E.** *Inequalities in Self-Reported Health and Utilisation of Health Care in European Union Countries.* Ecuity II, Project Working Paper #2. Erasmus University, Department of Health Policy and Management, 2001.
4. **Ministry of Health.** *Taking the Pulse. The 1996/97 New Zealand Health Survey.* Wellington, New Zealand: Ministry of Health, 1999.
5. **Britt, H.** et al. *General Practice Activity in Australia 2000–01.* Canberra: Australian Institute of Health and Welfare (General Practice Series No. 8), 2001.
6. **National Center for Health Statistics.** *Health, United States, 2000. With Adolescent Health Chartbook.* Hyattsville MD: National Center for Health Statistics, 2000.
7. **Australian Institute of Health and Welfare.** *Australia's Health 2000: The Seventh Biennial Health Report of the Australian Institute of Health and Welfare.* Canberra: Australian Institute for Health and Welfare, 2000.
8. **Royal College of General Practitioners, the Office of Population Censuses and Surveys, and the Department of Health.** *Morbidity Statistics from General Practice. Fourth National Study 1991–92* Series MB5 No. 3. London: HMSO, 1995.
9. **Office for National Statistics Social Survey Division.** *Living in Britain. Results from the 1998 General Household Survey.* London: The Stationary Office, 2000.
10. **Wyke, S., Hunt, K., and Ford, G.** (1998). Gender differences in consulting a general practitioners for common symptoms of minor illness. *Social Science and Medicine* **46**, 901–6.
11. **Hunt, K.** et al. (1991). Are women more ready to consult than men? Gender differences in family practitioners consultation for common chronic conditions. *Journal of Health Services Research and Policy* **44**, 96–100.
12. **Pamuk, E.** et al. (1998). *Socioeconomic Status and Health Chartbook. Health, United States, 1998.* Hyattsville MD: Center for Health Statistics, 1998.
13. **Airey, C.** et al. *National Surveys of NHS Patients. General Practice 1998.* London: National Center for Social Research, 1999.

3.2 Illness behaviour

Eloy H. van de Lisdonk

Introduction

Illness behaviour is a term used to describe what people do when they are ill. Doctors are familiar with a variety of illness behaviours. They observe the illness behaviour during history taking and when formulating a treatment programme. As an area of scientific study, illness behaviour is elucidated in particular by scientists from the fields of psychology and sociology. This chapter is inspired both by the experiences of doctors and their studies into illness behaviour, and by theories and studies from psychology and sociology.

The chapter has seven sections. First, some definitions are given. Second, the development of illness behaviour is summarized. Third, Parsons' model of the sick role is described. Fourth, some remarks are made regarding methods of measuring illness behaviour. Fifth, the appropriateness of illness behaviour is considered. Sixth, figures on the various forms of illness behaviour and differences between people in applying these forms are discussed. Seventh, explanations are sought for differences in medical consumption.

Definition

Falling ill is a common experience for everyone. The process of becoming ill includes questions like: why am I sick?; what is it?; what can be done?; what can I do myself? The latter question refers to what is called 'illness behaviour' (Box 1). Illness behaviour is diverse, and may even look capricious. It varies much between people. For a common cold one individual may continue with his daily routine as normally as possible, another may stay at home simply sleeping a few extra hours, and a third may consult a pharmacist or doctor or both. This is the case probably not because the common colds are so different, but because of the subjective aspects of both illness and the inclination to react. Illness is defined by Cassell as 'what the patient feels when he goes to the doctor,' illustrating this subjective aspect.[(2)] Hence, it is not surprising that illness behaviour is not easily predictable from the complaints or illness itself. For individuals, however, illness behaviour does not change so much. Rather it seems that consulting seldom or often is connected more to the person than to his/her state of health.

Behaviour, connected to specific actions (or omission of actions), is defined according to the thesaurus of PsycInfo (www.psycinfo.com) as: 'adaptive or non-adaptive behaviour exhibited by an individual during the course of an illness or dysfunction'. Other definitions also include process variables preceding the behaviour. Variables important to understanding behaviour include psychological phenomena as cognition and emotions.[(3)] In this chapter, a combination of two aspects is meant when speaking of illness behaviour: the cognition and emotions associated with feeling ill, and the actions one decides to take after the assessment of the cognition and emotions. Helman, moreover, stresses the social context proposing: 'illness is the subjective response of the patient, and of those around him, to his being unwell; particularly how he, and they, interpret the origin and significance of this event; how it affects his behaviour, and his relationship with other people; and the various steps he takes to remedy the situation'.[(4)] Consulting friends and family is an important aspect of illness behaviour, but can be seen as part of the actions.

Therefore, illness behaviour in the comprehensive definition of Mechanic, means dynamic behaviour over the course of time. For instance, after continuing as prior to the illness, an individual may decide to remain at home after a few days, and another few days later he or she may decide to consult a doctor. Changes in the illness behaviour are related to various factors, including deterioration in the health status, recovery time, and the patient's expectations of the course of the illness. As reactions to illness seem to vary with certain characteristics of an individual, it is probably fruitful to study illness behaviour as learned behaviour. This topic is addressed in the next section.

Box 1 Illness behaviour

The ways in which given symptoms may be differentially perceived, evaluated, and acted (or not acted) upon by different kinds of people.[(1)]

The development of illness behaviour

Behaviour develops during the different stages of a person's life cycle. It is believed that the basis for illness behaviour is laid down in the early years. What is going on when small children show disturbed health? It is the caregivers who become alarmed. They can be alarmed by the child's changes in bodily appearance and bodily functions. Crying, refusing the bottle, and exanthemas, for example, attract the caregiver's attention to the health of the child. The caregiver assumes physical (pain, constipation), emotional (fear) symptoms, or changes in the interpersonal relations ('did you miss mum?'). One can hypothesize, that the caregiver's interpretation of the observed bodily appearance and bodily functions reflects his or her own experiences. Thus, some caregivers will show great confidence in nature's ability to heal. They will console the child and monitor the child's condition. Other caregivers react differently. They will be alarmed, not so much by the objective condition of the child but by their own thoughts. The young child feels and sees the confidence of the former caregiver and the fear of the latter. As a consequence, the child learns to react with confidence or fear. This simplified scenario exemplifies the intergenerational patterns of illness behaviour that are seen and reported by doctors.[5]

The role of the family, the mother in particular, in the shaping of attitudes, beliefs, and illness behaviour is important.[6,7] Illness behaviour as learned behaviour is part of the socialization process. Norms, attitudes, and beliefs learned early in life do not change greatly nor easily once they are stabilized in the young adult. The literature even suggests a certain rigidity of illness behaviour pointing out intergenerational family patterns for presented morbidity and frequency of consultation.[8,9] Furthermore, attitudes and health beliefs, which are significant items in understanding illness behaviour, have been shown to be strongly correlated between children and their parents. This is consistent with the concept of 'family scripts'. These scripts contain among others, the rules on how to behave.[10]

It is clear that illness behaviour develops in a process of social learning. Influences of culture and social class are dominant in this process. Among others it is the cultural influences that lead to differences in symptom-experience, symptom-interpretation, naming of the symptoms, and, ultimately, illness behaviour.[11,12] It seems that in our world, despite the enormous possibilities of transport and the amount and accessibility of information, cultural aspects, including religious aspects, of health and illness are still understudied.

The sick role

Parsons' vision of the social aspects of being ill found wide recognition. By defining patients' and doctors' roles, the rules of the health care arena were also defined. Parsons' concept of the sick role (Box 2) was based on a functionalist view of society, which was seen as a system characterized by norms and rules that helped citizens to live their lives in harmony. Sickness was seen as deviance from the normal state, that is, a state of full health and functioning, needed to contribute to the development of society. Deviant behaviour was seen as threatening to the status quo, requiring rules for its containment. In this context, the concept of the sick role was formulated.

In the years to follow, major criticisms of this concept were formulated, pointing in particular to the complexity of patient–doctor interactions (see also Chapter 5.4). Two other points can be made:

1. The concept of the sick role lacks an empirical base. In practice, patients are often neither as passive nor as adherent to doctors' advice as the model suggests. Rather, patients often want to be involved in decision-making processes, ask for information, are eager to know what they can do themselves, and negotiate with doctors details of regimens, duration of stay, and control frequency. They want a personal doctor, who adapts his protocols and standards to the very private needs and wants of the patient. This creates pressure for doctors who have to be objective and make decisions based on clinical evidence.
2. The concept of the sick role does not fit very well to patients with chronic diseases. In established chronic diseases cure is not an option. Management is centred around symptom control, and the preservation of quality of life and functional status. Most of the time the chronically ill remain at home, with a great deal of self-management. Often they are only partly free of normal obligations, do not consider their status as undesirable, cannot get entirely well, and as a consequence stop seeking medical help. Parsons acknowledged these critics, and showed that chronically ill go in and out of the sick role, depending on periods of aggravation and complications of their disease.[14]

Box 2 Rights and responsibilities of the sick role[13]

The patient:

- is free of the normal obligations of work and school
- is not responsible for being ill
- has the obligation to get well as soon as possible
- has the obligation to seek medical help

The doctor:

- should be clinically highly competent
- should be emotionally neutral and objective
- is given access to normally intimate areas

Measuring illness behaviour

In 1961, Mechanic obtained data from respondents (mother–child pairs), teachers, and school reports. Mothers were interviewed (about their psychological state and health attitudes among other things), and daily illness diaries were completed. In 1977, a follow-up study among the children from the 1961 study was performed.[15] Mechanic showed that illness behaviour could be studied objectively. However, analysing data on illness behaviour is not easy, partly because there is no accepted classification of illness behaviours. The most commonly used methods of assessment of illness behaviour are interviews, checklists (open ended or checklists with symptoms), and health diaries, each with its own advantages and disadvantages.[16,17]

In the history of measuring illness behaviour, diary studies have evolved. The oldest diaries (1938–1975) allowed for entries about restriction of daily activities on the one hand and medical, pharmacological or nursing treatments on the other. In the 1970s, two new categories were incorporated: consultations with lay people and self-care. The former concept of lay referral was introduced by Freidson.[18] The interest in self-care reflects recognition of the increasing emancipation of patients as expressed in inquiries for more information, democratic decision making and respect for autonomy. Between 1980 and 2000, the four main categories of illness behaviour found in diaries are:

- consultations of lay people;
- non-medical self-care;
- medical self-care;
- seeking professional care.

The researcher's interests determine what information is gathered on these main themes. By using words indicating actual behaviour, conceptual misunderstanding can be avoided.

Appropriateness of illness behaviour

The appropriateness of illness behaviour will be considered for each of the four categories mentioned above.

Consultation of lay people

Seeking information is a basic component of illness behaviour. Information can be acquired from other people and from impersonal sources (books, newspapers, magazines, television, Internet). Elliot-Binns concluded that impersonal sources of information more often resulted in harmful advice than personal sources, and amounted to 18 per cent of the advice resulting in excessive anxiety, incorrect treatment, and delay before seeing a doctor.[19]

Advice in books and on the Internet often end with the recommendation to consult a doctor if you are not sure. How often this recommendation actually prompts people to consult, and whether this advice driven consultation behaviour is adequate, is not known.

Non-medical self-care

Research into this field faces many difficulties. What exactly was the health complaint? What remedy was chosen? How and how long the remedy was used? What outcome parameters are useful for evaluation? What is a representative sample to be studied? And which cultural factors have to be studied as well? These questions are explored further in Chapter 3.5.

Medical self-care

Medical self-care can usually be classified as harmless. In the 1970s, it was found that about half the people consulting a doctor had attempted self-treatment, and that most remedies were relevant, probably with an indifferent outcome. About 1 per cent of the medications used proved to be potentially harmful.[20] Reports of harmful self-medication with alternative drugs and herbs have been published[21,22] (see Chapter 3.5).

Seeking professional care

In theory, reasons for encounter can be adequate or not. But, who should judge these ratings of adequacy, and which criteria can be followed? In individual cases it can usually be understood why patients consult, but it is very difficult to indicate which signs, symptoms and conditions ought to prompt the patient to consult (perhaps with the exception of acute traumatic conditions and a few alarm symptoms).[23,24] Hannay found that about 9 per cent of the consultations he studied were for non-serious physical symptoms ('trivia').[25]

It can be concluded that scientific information on the appropriateness of illness behaviour is lacking, whether 'appropriateness' is defined from the point of view of the patient or the doctor. Even more limited is the knowledge of factors associated with the appropriateness of illness behaviour.

Self-care and professional care

This section concerns the demarcation between consulting and not consulting, and elaborates on three forms of illness behaviour: non-medical self-care, medical self-care, and seeking professional care.

Studies of illness behaviour show that most illnesses are acted upon without consulting professional health workers. It all began with the so-called Peckham experiment: '. . . routine medical examination was offered to a group of people between the years 1935 and 1939. Ninety per cent were subsequently classified as having some identifiable disorder or disease, although less than a tenth of these had previously been receiving medical attention'.[26] Since the early 1960s, the term 'clinical iceberg' or 'iceberg phenomenon' has become the familiar term to describe this robust finding (Box 3).[27,28]

Most of the time people seem to be satisfied by doing nothing or using some form of self-care for complaints and problems. In only about 10–20 per cent of the reported complaint episodes is a doctor consulted. As episodes have a mean duration of about 3–4 days, the consultation behaviour takes place in about 3–5 per cent of the reported complaint days.

Box 3 The iceberg of morbidity, a global picture[25,29–31]

- In a period of 1 week respondents report a mean of one to two complaints about their bodily health.
- In a month most reported are: musculo-skeletal problems, headaches, common colds and other respiratory problems, and gastrointestinal problems.
- Episodes have a mean duration of 3–4 days; in case of muscle pain the mean duration is 8 days, in case of headaches 3 days, for common cold 5 days and for abdominal pain 3 days.
- In a period of 1 year about 15 per cent of the respondents did not report any complaint, 70 per cent regularly, and 15 per cent reported complaints approximately daily.

In children, a consultation-rate was found of 11 per cent of all complaint days.[32]

Non-medical self-care

Non-medical self-care includes various activities, such as staying in bed, activities in and around the house like gardening, and social visits. Freer found that in almost all medical problems at least one non-medical self-care action was reported, and in half of these actions the presence of at least one other person was required.[33] That was not the case when respondents reported doing nothing as a response to their complaints. The figures for 'doing nothing' differ greatly. Wadsworth mentioned that 19 per cent of the respondents reported that no action was taken for complaints.[34] Van de Lisdonk, asking 277 respondents to report their behaviour during each complaint day, found that the category 'doing nothing' included 27 per cent of all reported actions.[35] Wilkinson et al., interviewing 340 patients over the age of 15 years with one or more complaints in the last 14 days, found that 37 per cent of these people did not take any action as response to their complaints.[36]

Medical self-care

Regarding medical self-care in particular, self-medication is studied widely. Wadsworth mentioned that two-thirds of the medication taken by respondents in the last 14 days, was not medically prescribed (interview, 14 days, $n = 2153$).[34] Hannay found that about one-third of the 1344 respondents (interview, previous 14 days) were taking non-prescribed medications.[25] Van de Lisdonk found that in 33 per cent of the reported episodes the respondents used medicines of which two-thirds was not medically prescribed. In 20 per cent of the complaint days self-medication was used.[35] Dahlquist reports non-prescribed medication use on 34 per cent of the symptom days.[37] Wilkinson found that 28 per cent used over-the-counter (OTC) medication.[36] See Chapter 3.5 for further discussion of this issue.

Seeking professional care

The results of several studies investigating the occurrence of symptoms, and the extent to which they lead to consultations with doctors, are given in Table 1. These studies confirm the finding that health disturbance is a common occurrence and that only a minority of the patients experiencing symptoms consult a doctor. The differences in the findings may be explained by the variables studied: the country in which the research was conducted, and the characteristics of that country's health care system; patient selections and response rates; differences in content of the diaries used; the time period of reporting; instructions given to respondents; method and unit of analysis; and outcome measures. These and other variables have not been studied in depth to explain differences in self-care.

Table 1 Frequencies of perceived complaints and consultations with doctors

Authors	Country	Number, sex, and age	Instrument	Period	Prevalence of complaints	Prevalence of consultation
White et al., 1961[27]	England, USA	≥16 years	Interview	1 month	75% ≥1 episode of ill-health	25/100/month
Folmer, 1968[38]	Norway	Practice population 20–75 years old	Questionnaire Registration GP	Complaints regularly present 1 year	Mean: 6 for men and 8 for women 50% ≥1 episode of ill-health	10% of perceived complaints presented to GP
van der Velden, 1971[39]	Netherlands	424, female, 20–55 years old	Checklist 87 symptoms	'Lately'	3 complaints per respondent	18% of perceived complaints presented to GP
Rhogmann and Haggerty, 1972[40]	USA	512 families, 1081 adults, 1466 children, 71 316 person-days	Diary	28 days	Adults: 22% days with complaint Children: 14% days with complaint	Adults: 6% of days with symptoms Children: 7% of days with symptoms
Banks et al., 1975[41]	England	198, women, 20–44 years old	Diary	4 weeks	Mean of 10 symptom days, 6.2 episodes	1 consultation per 37 symptom episodes
Freer, 1980[33]	Ontario, Canada	26, women, 34–44 years old	Diary	4 weeks	A new medical problem every 2 days, a new non-medical problem every 4–5 days	10% of respondents consulted a doctor
Hannay, 1979[25]	Scotland	1344 all ages, men and women	Interview using a checklist of 44 symptoms	2 weeks	68% of respondents reported ≥1 physical symptom, 51% ≥1 mental symptom	34% of physical symptoms, 17% of mental symptoms
Scambler et al., 1981[42]	England	79, women, 16–44 years	Diary	6 weeks	32% of all days with symptoms	6% of days with symptoms
van de Lisdonk, 1985[35]	Netherlands	277 persons, >15 years	Diary	4 weeks	86% of resp. ≥1 complaint, 33% of days with symptoms	20% of respondents, 10% of episodes, 2.4% of days with symptoms
Verbrugge and Ascione, 1987[43]	USA	243 men, 346 women	Diary	6 weeks	Men 31%, women 43% days with symptoms	5% of days with symptoms
Dahlquist et al., 1987[37]	Sweden	185 young families	Diary	4 weeks	27% of individual days a health problem	10% of days with symptoms

Probably, factors contributing to variation in patients' consulting behaviour can help to formulate hypotheses in this field.

Differences in patients' consulting behaviour

Probably the most important factor related to differences in patients' consulting behaviour concerns the perception of physical complaints. It is obvious that not everyone with complaints asks for help, even if the complaints are serious (as perceived by either patients or doctors). Hannay found that 23 per cent of his respondents ($n = 1344$) had at least one medical symptom for which they did not seek professional or formal advice although they said that either the pain or disability was severe, or the symptom was serious.[25] In a Dutch study, Huygen found that 12 per cent of the respondents ($n = 631$) experiencing potentially serious symptoms according to doctors, did not consult.

In case of minor symptoms, the tendency to consult a doctor is linked to the structure of the health care system (see Chapter 3.1), to demographic factors (of patient, doctor, and practice) and to cognitive, affective, and cultural factors (dominant factors among others in the patient–doctor communication). Gender, age, and socio-economic status are related to consultation behaviour: more women than men, more old than young, and more people in lower than in higher socio-economic groups consult. The number of patients on a doctor's list and the practice organization (single-handed or group practice) are not particularly important issues in this respect. Geography also contributes: people in inner-cities consult more often than in rural areas. These findings, of course, also depend on the availability of resources. Studies comparing frequent attenders and non-attenders (Box 4) show that cognitive, affective, and cultural factors all

Box 4 Characteristics of non-attenders

- People who seldom consult a doctor are not distinguishable by any particular characteristics.
- There is no remarkable illness behaviour that could explain why people do not consult a doctor.
- People who seldom consult differ from those who consult frequently in their beliefs and ideas, such as: caring about health problems; beliefs concerning personal health; beliefs concerning GPs; their confidence in GPs; perceived obstacles in visiting a GP.

Based on a Dutch literature review from H. Beukema-Siebenga[46–50] affect the tendency to consult doctors. Personality is probably not an important contributing factor, and the role of psychological distress is unclear.[44]

On the other hand, health beliefs do seem to play an important role. The Health Belief Model is based on the assumption that, whether a person acts upon perceived health disturbances, depends upon; (a) the value placed on a certain goal (i.e. the desire to avoid illness); and (b) the belief that the specific action will achieve that goal (see the next Chapter 3.3).[45] In the literature, the main question is whether the few dimensions of the Health Belief Model can predict the great variety of outcomes that occur in different social settings, and for individuals with different sickness biographies. For doctors, the Health Belief Model is of great practical importance as it contains factors that permit intervention, something that cannot be said of the demographic factors mentioned above.

Research into differences in consultation rates is still more complicated in people with chronic diseases. Such research refers to three different aspects: (i) the chronic condition itself, and the medical need to monitor and control the condition and its sequelae; (ii) the disabilities and handicaps accompanying the chronic condition, which require the individual patient and his or her social environment to cope, and to seek affirmation from others, paramedical help and psycho-social support; and (iii) all concurrent illnesses and worries about one's health (related or not to the chronic disease) that also bring people without a chronic condition to a doctor.

Discussion

Illness behaviour is an intriguing issue. To understand this particular form of behaviour, somatic, psychological, and social dimensions have to be considered. There is no comprehensive theory, but various aspects have been researched. In practice, doctors can gain a better understanding of illness behaviour by asking themselves: why does this patient consult me now, and for what reason? Elucidating each part of this question at the beginning of the consultation will help to direct the search for an answer to the patient's concerns. Systematic research on patients' answers to this question can be of great value for understanding illness behaviour.

References

1. **Mechanic, D.** (1962). The concept of illness behavior. *Journal of Chronic Diseases* **15**, 189–94.
2. **Cassell, E.J.** *The Healer's Art: A New Approach to the Doctor–Patient Relationship.* New York: Lippincott, 1976.
3. **Ajzen, I. and Fischbein, M.** *Understanding Attitudes and Predicting Social Behavior.* Englewood Cliffs NJ: Prentice Hall, 1980.
4. **Helman, C.G.** *Culture, Health and Illness* 2nd edn. London: Wright, 1990.
5. **Huygen, F.J.A.** *Family Medicine. The Medical Life History of Families.* London: The Royal College of General Practitioners, 1990. First published by Dekker & van de Vegt, Nijmegen, The Netherlands, 1978.
6. **Litman, T.J.** (1974). The family as a basic unit in health and medical care: a social behavorial overview. *Social Science & Medicine* **8**, 495–519.
7. **Broderick, C.B.** (1993). The Socialization process—Chapter 8. *Understanding Family Process* pp. 212–43. Newbury Park: Sage Publications.
8. **Schor, E., Starfield, B., Stidley, C., and Hankin, J.** (1987). Family health. Utilization and effects of family membership. *Medical Care* **25**, 616–26.
9. **Huygen, F.J.A.** (1988). Longitudinal studies of family units. *Journal of the Royal College of General Practitioners* **38**, 168–70.
10. **Byng-Hall, J.** (1988). Scripts and legends in families and family therapy. *Family Practice* **27**, 167–79.
11. **Zborowski, M.** (1952). Cultural components in responses to pain. *Journal of Social Issues* **8**, 16–30.
12. **Payer, L.** *Medicine and Culture.* New York: Henry Holt, 1988.
13. **Parsons, T.** *The social system.* New York: Free Press, 1951.
14. **Parsons, T.** (1975). The sick role and the role of the physician reconsidered. *Millbank Memorial Fund Quaterly* **53**, 257–78.
15. **Mechanic, D.** (1980). The experience and reporting of common physical complaints. *Journal of Health and Social Behavior* **21**, 146–55.
16. **Verbrugge, L.M.** (1980). Health diaries. *Medical Care* **18**, 73–95.
17. **Kooiker, S.E.** (1995). Exploring the iceberg of morbidity: a comparison of different survey methods for assessing the occurence of everyday illness. *Social Science & Medicine* **41**, 317–32.
18. **Freidson, E.** *Profession of Medicine.* New York: Dodd, Mead and Company, 1970.
19. **Elliot-Binns, C.P.** (1986). An analysis of lay medicine: fifteen years later. *Journal of the Royal College of General Practitioners* **36**, 542–4.
20. **Eliot-Binns, C.P.** (1973). An analysis of lay medicine. *Journal of the Royal College of General Practitioners* **23**, 255–64.
21. **Angell, M. and Kassirer, J.P.** (1998). Alternative medicine—the risk of untested and unregulated remedies. *New England Journal of Medicine* **339**, 839–41.
22. **Kessler, D.A.** (2000). Cancer and herbs. *New England Journal of Medicine* **342**, 1742–3.
23. **Kalimo, E. and Sievers, K.** (1968). The need for medical care; estimation on the basis of interview data. *Medical Care* **6**, 1–2.
24. **Cough, H.G.** (1977). Doctor's estimates of the percentage of patients whose problem do not require medical attention. *Medical Care* **11**, 380–4.
25. **Hannay, D.R.** *The Symptom Iceberg.* London: Routledge & Kegan Paul, 1979.
26. **Pearse, I. and Cocker, L.** *The Peckham Experiment.* London: George Allen and Unwin, 1943. Cited in: Williamson, J.D. and Danaher, K. *Self-care in Health.* London: Croom Helm, 1978, p. 35.
27. **White, K.L., Williams, T.F., and Greenberg, B.G.** (1961). The ecology of medical care. *New England Journal of Medicine* **265**, 885–92.
28. **Last, J.M.** (1963). The iceberg: completing the clinical picture in general practice. *Lancet* **ii**, 28–31.
29. **Bentzen, N., Christiansen, T., and Pedersen, K.M.** *The Danish Health Study.* Occasional paper no. 3. Department of Economics, Odense University, Odense, 1988.
30. **Navig, B., Nessioy, I., Brougaard, D., and Rutle, O.** (1995). Musculosceletal symptoms in a local community. *European Journal of General Practice* **1**, 25–8.
31. **Musil, C.M., Ahn, S., Haug, M., Warner, C., Morris, D., and Duffy, E.** (1998). Health problems and health activities among community dwelling older adults: results of a health diary study. *Applied Nursing Research* **11**, 138–47.
32. **Cunningham-Burley, S. and Irvine, S.** (1987). 'And have you done something so far?' An examination of lay treatment of children's symptoms. *British Medical Journal* **295**, 700–2.
33. **Freer, C.B.** (1980). Self-care: a health diary study. *Medical Care* **18**, 853–61.
34. **Wadsworth, M.E.J., Blaney, R., and Butterfield, W.J.H.** *Health and Sickness: The Choice of Treatment.* London: Tavistock Press, 1971.
35. **van de Lisdonk, E.H.** (1989). Perceived and presented morbidity in general practice. *Scandinavian Journal of Primary Health Care* **7**, 73–6.
36. **Wilkinson, I.F., Darby, D.N., and Mant, A.** (1987). Self-care and self-medication. *Medical Care* **25**, 965–78.
37. **Dahlquist, G., Sterky, G., Ivarsson, J.-I., Tengvald, K., and Wall, S.** (1987). Health problems and care in young families—load of illness and patterns of illness behavior. *Scandinavian Journal of Primary Health Care* **5**, 79–86.
38. **Folmer, H.R.** Huisart en ijsberg. Thesis, University of Utrecht, Utrecht. (Dutch, summary in English), 1968.
39. **van der Velden, H.G.M.** Huisvrouw, huisarts, huisgezin. Thesis, Dekker & van de Vegt, Nijmegen (Dutch, summary in English), 1971.
40. **Rhogmann, K.J. and Haggerty, R.J.** (1972). The diary as a research instrument in the study of health and illness behavior. *Medical Care* **10**, 143–63.
41. **Banks, M.H., Beresford, D.C., and Morrell, D.C.** (1975) Factors influencing demand for primary care in women aged 20–44 years; a preliminary report. *International Journal of Epidemiology* **4**, 189–95.
42. **Scambler, A., Scambler, G., and Craig, D.** (1981). Kinship and friendship networks and women's demand for primary care. *Journal of the Royal College of General Practitioners* **31**, 746–50.

43. **Verbrugge, L.M. and Ascione, F.J.** (1987). Exploring the iceberg. Common symptoms and how people care for them. *Medical Care* **25**, 539–69.
44. **Schrire, S.** (1986). Frequent attenders—a review. *Family Practice* **3**, 272–5.
45. **Jantz, N.K. and Becker, M.H.** (1984). The Health Belief Model: a decade later. *Health Education Quaterly* **11**, 1–47.
46. **Kessel, N. and Shepherd, M.** (1965). The health and attitude of people who seldom consult a doctor. *Medical Care* **3**, 6–10.
47. **Baker, C.D.** (1976). Non-attenders in general practice. *Journal of the Royal College of General Practitioners* **26**, 404–9.
48. **Mackay, H.A.F.** The occasional patient; a ten year study of patients who consult a doctor infrequently. Thesis, Dundee University, Dundee, 1986.
49. **Anderson, J.A.D., Buck, C., Danaher, K., and Fry, J.** (1977). Users and non-users of doctors—implications for self-care. *Journal of the Royal College of General Practitioners* **27**, 155–9.
50. **Corney, R. and Murray, J.** (1988). The characteristics of high and low attenders at two general practices. *Social Psychiatry and Psychiatric Epidemiology* **23**, 39–48.

3.3 Health beliefs

Natalie O'Dea and Deborah C. Saltman

In this chapter, health beliefs are explored through several perspectives. First, health and illness will be defined. These definitions will then be incorporated into a historical overview of theoretical models of health and illness. Psychological models that aim to describe and predict health behaviour are described, followed by empirical models deriving from sociology and anthropology. Some models focus on health, whereas others have a focus on illness. The order in which the models are described reflects the developing body of knowledge about health beliefs and how they were developed to address criticisms made of earlier models.

Definitions of health and illness

Traditionally, health and illness have been defined in relation to each other. That is, health is the absence of illness and vice versa. More contemporary definitions of health have broadened this view. For example, the World Health Organization (WHO) defines health as 'a state of full physical, psychic and social well-being and not the mere absence of disease'.[1] This definition has also been incorporated into lay thinking. The Australian Pocket Oxford Dictionary defines health as 'a state of being well in body or mind; a person's mental or physical condition; or soundness, especially financial or moral'.[2]

Webster defines health as a response to change and subsequent adaptation.[3] Through this definition, he argues that life is a trajectory, which incorporates development and ageing. Health is a resource for everyday life. A person's health determines how well they are able to function emotionally and physically in society. Diseases are, therefore, no more than artefacts along the way.

In contrast, the definition of illness is medically based as 'a disease or state of being ill'.[2] Illness, by reference to processes inside the individual body, defines the reason that a body reacts to some disorder, temporary or permanent, for example, the invasion of the body by a virus or germ.[4] Sociologists and anthropologists, however, distinguish between illness and disease, using the former to refer to the subjective experience of ill-health and the latter to refer to the categories of biomedicine.

Personalistic and naturalistic conceptions of illness

Foster and Anderson suggested that the models describing illness can be conceptualized in one of two ways: personalistic or naturalistic.[5] The difference between the two systems is in the way they apportion causation. Murdock later extended the personalistic concept and labelled it supernatural.[6]

The personalistic concept attributes causation of illness to a purposive intervention by an entity. This agent may be an ancestor, a ghost, a witch, another individual, or a deity. Illness is a misfortune linked to cosmological activity that impacts on human beings. The act of aggression instigated by one of these agents is not arbitrary; rather, it has a cause and a purpose that requires a skilled shaman or diviner to identify. The fundamental principles of treatment are to identify the source of the problem and restore cosmic balance and health.

One of the earliest examples of the personalistic concept comes from Greek medicine of the Cretan–Mycenean period. As was common in many ancient civilizations, virtually all gods could cause illness. For example, Apollo and his sister Artemis could shoot arrows that would bring on illness, deterioration, and old age. Some gods could deliver health. For example, Chiron, the half-brother of Zeus, was the patron of healing.

The supernatural concept coined by Murdock is an extension of the personalistic concept. Causation may be attributed to fate, foreboding sensations (dreams, sights, sounds, mystical crimes, and retributions), issues of the soul and spirit, sorcery, or witchcraft. The most predominant supernatural causes of illness are aggressive spirits, sorcery, taboo, and retribution. The aim of the healer is to exorcize the supernatural destructive force and restore balance and health.

Throughout history there have been many models based on the supernatural concept. In Mayan culture, for example, causation arose inevitably from the other world. Illness represented a loss of balance between unfavourable and favourable influences. In order to fight illness, the Mayans used a blend of magic, religion, and science. However, magic and religion were more important in curing illness than science. The priests (hemenes) were responsible for curing the magical elements of causation whereas the technical or surgical procedures were delegated to people of lower status (hechiceros).

In contrast, the naturalistic causation of illness, as the name implies, attributes disease causation to natural or impersonal factors such as extremes of heat or cold, strong emotions such as fear or anger, infective agents, deterioration of the body, and accidents. In each of these cases there is an observable relationship between the causes and their specific effects.

An example of a naturalistic concept is ancient Chinese medicine. In China, health was determined by the interaction between the yin (passive, dark, cold, moist, negative, feminine) and the yang (active, light, dry, warm, positive, masculine). The ultimate principle of the universe, tao, was determined by the proportions of yin and yang in any individual. However, forces beyond one's control, such as the wind, could upset the yin/yang balance.

Another example is from Greece, where the philosopher-scientists who followed after Asclepios also adhered to a naturalistic approach to illness. Four elements, each with their own unique characteristics, were the basis of all substances: water (wet), earth (dry), fire (hot), and air (cold). The number four became significant to health, and the four qualities later went on to form the four humors.

Hippocrates, perhaps the greatest of the philosopher-scientists in medicine, developed the system linking illness to the four basic humors: blood (which was warm and moist), phlegm (which was cold and moist), yellow bile (which was warm and dry), and black bile (which was cold and dry). When all these humors were balanced, the body was in health. An excess or deficiency of one or more caused illness. Any disease had three stages. The first stage was a change in humoral proportions caused by external factors. The second stage was the body's reaction to this change, usually through fever. The final stage was the discharge of the excess humor or death.

The Hippocratic belief about medicine was that nature, not the physician, cured disease. Hippocrates clearly believed that objective observation

Table 1 Typology of ethnomedical models of health and illness

Feature	Personalistic	Naturalistic
Causation	Active agent	Loss of equilibrium
Nature of illness	Misfortune	Unrelated to misfortune
Supernatural elements	Religion/magic related to illness	Unrelated to illness/magic
Responsibility	Beyond patient	With patient
Prevention	Active	Passive by avoidance
Cultures	Tribal	Western

rather than adherence to supernatural doctrines was the key feature in defining illness. Patients were seen as victims of natural causes who deserved rational methods of care. The role of the healer in this model is to work with the patient to restore balance.

Foster and Anderson argued that both naturalistic and personalistic/supernatural systems are used concurrently to explain illness and treat problems. Whilst causation in both models is attributed differently, the principles of rectification are similar—to restore balance in an individual. This combined concept of causation is in keeping with the more traditional definitions that place health and illness on a single continuum for an individual. Health is the optimum end of the spectrum and anything less is viewed as ill.

The possibility that a total shift to the health end of the spectrum may not be possible, as is the case in patients who have chronic illnesses, is not part of the naturalistic and personalistic/supernatural framework. The unilinear focus on the capacity of an individual to achieve health also excludes public, societal, and cultural perspectives. In addition, collective notions such as contagion and prevention of epidemics are not incorporated.

Many of the newer models encompass a more holistic view of multiple problems to include societal and cultural causation.

In an attempt to integrate culture into naturalistic and personalistic models of health and illness, Foster superimposed a cross-cultural typology.[7] The key features of this framework are summarized in Table 1, which has been adapted from Foster.[7]

Theoretical models of health and illness

Recent theorists have attempted to specifically include health in models, instead of just focusing on illness. Highlighting the differences between health and illness, Tamm outlined six models.[8] Three of these models focus on health; religious, humanistic, and transpersonal. The other three have illness as their central tenet; biomedical, psychosomatic, and existential.

The religious model

This model is one of the oldest models to be described in writing. Health is perceived as 'the correct way of living', not just the absence of disease. Religious aspects are more significant than biological, psychological, or social dimensions. When there is harmony with nature, other individuals and most importantly, with the gods, there is a state of health. In keeping with the naturalistic/personalistic framework, the concept of illness in this model is a result of disharmony. Healing and, therefore, health are related to restoring the correct cosmic balance. In the model, illness is thought to affect the whole person, even though it may manifest itself in a particular part of the body.

The healer is often both a religious leader and a doctor, who in the healing process, diagnoses the disease, communicates with the spiritual world, carries out religious rites, and administers medication thereby restoring the sick person to the correct level of harmony and health.

The biomedical model

In this model, the mind and body are viewed as two distinct entities. The mind is associated with abstract and systematic thinking, governed by rationality and logic. Unlike the mind, the body is considered to be like a machine that can be studied scientifically. The concept of health and illness is naturalistic. Illness affects a person from without; for example, bacteria and viruses enter a body and cause illness. Illness is conceptualized as a pathological or mechanical dysfunction within an individual. The curing of diseases is the responsibility of the doctor, not gods, priests, or other sacred figures. In this model, using both mind and body, a person possesses strong powers of self-healing and the doctor's role is to help them find expression through these powers. Medication and surgical intervention are tools to assist the individual cure themselves and health is defined as the absence of illness.

The psychosomatic model

Developed in the 1930s, this model links the mind and the body in causation of illness. There are no somatic diseases without emotional and/or social antecedents, and no emotional illnesses without somatic symptoms. Illness involves both the body and the mind. These two aspects are so interrelated that they cannot be separated from each other. Illness develops through an interplay between physical and mental factors using a feedback loop mechanism. In the same way, recovery from disease is thought to be through positive attitudes and stress-reducing techniques that help the mind/body system. Reattainment of balance is the ultimate goal to achieve good health. Curing illness is thought to be the responsibility of the individual, with help sought from people such as medical personnel, friends, workmates, and family.

The existential model

Developed in the mid-1940s, the emphasis of this health model is subjectivity. The individual's concrete experience of reality defines health and illness. Central to this model is the belief that individuals can choose how to exist. For example, if individuals choose to be fit, they are choosing health. Conversely, a person can choose to be ill, through inactivity. The responsibility of the doctor or therapist is not necessarily to cure, but to help the patient attain a better understanding of themselves, and thereby a functioning life.

The humanistic model

This model, developed in the 1950s, links health and illness. The humanistic model views individuals as psychological and biological organisms in interaction with their social environment. It is the first model that describes health as a process, not a condition. It focuses on subjective thought processes, rather than objective and quantifiable facts. There is also scope in this model for individuals to be supported by others through societal measures for promoting health, such as parks and childcare centres. As health is a process, the individual is capable of taking responsibility for their own health. Maslow and Mahrer describe a healthy person as one who is striving for self-actualization and living an authentic life.[9,10] An ill person is someone whose internal relationships are disintegrative and whose inside is confused and negative.

The transpersonal model

First described in the mid-1960s, this model extends the concepts aired in the humanistic, existential, and religious models. Both health and illness are related to the supernatural. An individual is in a state of health and well-being when they transcend the spiritual–body dualism they are used to perceiving in existence and reach a stage of uniform consciousness. Insight and mindfulness are the primary healthy factors.

Consciousness and the experience of dualism create human suffering and disease. Agitation, worry, and anxiety are the central features of mental illnesses. Rectification of health problems occurs through reaching altered states of consciousness by meditating. In this way an individual can attain cosmic consciousness. Through different meditative techniques, an individual successively and gradually can assume their consciousness, become infused with physic energy, and develop powers necessary for self-healing. The healer in this model assists the person to develop the appropriate meditative technique.

Whilst these models described by Tamm represent varying approaches to health and illness, each of them deals specifically with one aspect of health or illness and says very little about the other. Several other empirically based models describe a more complex interplay of health and illness.

Psychological models

Psychological models focus on the extent to which health behaviours can be predicted by health beliefs.

The health belief model

Originating in 1952, the health belief model (HBM) is based on the theories of Kurt Lewin. Lewin postulated that the world of the perceiver determines what an individual will and will not do. This model expands on Lewin's theory and provides a link between attitudes and behaviour. The HBM is the first model that attempts to predict behaviour rather than just describe it. The model presents a systematic method that can be used to describe and predict preventive behaviour.[11] It seeks to explain why people participate in preventive activities and screening programmes.

The underlying principle is that positive and negative influences in an individual's world affect their behaviour. If the objective is to avoid a particular illness, then an individual must feel personally vulnerable or susceptible to the illness, the illness must be potentially serious to the individual, and the person must be able to reduce the threat by a specific action. To effect a particular preventive or health promotive action, an individual must be triggered by a stimulus either from within or without that is greater than any perceived barrier to action.

There are five key descriptors that define the HBM:

Perceived susceptibility, which is a person's subjective perception of the risk of contracting an illness. There are widespread individual differences in perception of susceptibility. At one extreme there is denial. At the other extreme there is high level of belief that an illness will be contracted. In the middle, there is a moderate level of belief in which the individual admits that there is a statistical possibility of contracting an illness.

Perceived severity, which refers to an individual's beliefs about the effects of a given illness on their well-being. The effects may be emotional, financial, interpersonal, or a precursor to more serious illness.

Perceived benefits, or a person's beliefs about the benefits that may be accrued by taking a preventive action. The greater a person's belief that the preventive strategies they will undertake are likely to reduce the threat of illness, the more likely they are to act.

Perceived barriers, which refers to a person's beliefs about the potential negative consequences that may result from taking a particular preventive action. Potential barriers include: inconvenience, expense, pain, upset, and unpleasantness. These barriers would diminish the likelihood of a person undertaking a preventive action.

Cues to action, are the events that either bodily or environmentally motivate a person to take action. These cues are a combination of the effects of perceived susceptibility, seriousness, and the benefits (minus the barriers).

In recent revisions, the HBM has been expanded to include more depth in the predictive elements by focussing on motivation. An individual's motivation to undertake health behaviour can be defined by three principles: individual perceptions, modifying behaviours, and the likelihood of action. Individual perceptions are the factors that affect the way a person views their health or illness. Each person ascribes certain levels of importance, susceptibility, and severity in relation to their health problems.

Many mechanisms modify individual perceptions. They can be internal, such as perceived threat, a person's general health values and beliefs, or external, such as demographic variables. After all these variables have been considered, it is the likelihood of taking a preventive action that is the final determinant of whether a patient will actually undertake a preventive activity.

Although generally accepted as a comprehensive and contemporary model of health beliefs, the HBM has a number of limitations. Its main emphasis is on the individual and their responses. The influence of moods and habits of an individual are not incorporated in the model. Also external factors such as societal attitudes, the environment, and the economic context are not included. Also, whilst the model proposes behavioural modification it provides no measure of any modifying factors.

The protection motivation theory

In 1977, Bandura added a self-efficacy component to the HBM.[12] The 'self-efficacy model' outlines an individual's belief in their ability to successfully execute the behaviour required to produce desired outcomes. The 'protection motivation theory' was developed as an expansion of the HBM that included self-efficacy as well as response effectiveness, that is, whether the proposed change is thought to be effective in improving health.[13] However, like the HBM, the 'self-efficacy model' and 'protection motivation theory' are restricted to self and self-beliefs and do not take into account external factors such as culture, gender, and class.

The theory of reasoned action

The 'theory of reasoned action' was first introduced by Fishbein in 1980.[14] It is an example of a social cognition model, so called because it includes the individual's representation of their social world.[15] The underlying principle in this model is the connection between rational thought and action. Intention is a function of the attitude of an individual towards performing a behaviour and how a person judges what is normal for any situation. The intention to act is a reasoned thought that is followed by a behaviour. 'Reasoned action' looks at personal beliefs and also adds a social component, by looking at what society views as normal.

The intention to perform an action, and the relationship of the intention to an action, are described through four variables:[16]

Behaviour, which is comprised of action, target, context, and time. For example, implementing an action, such as a youth suicide prevention risk strategy, may include providing a toll-free helpline for homeless youth (target) to ring (action) when (time) they are feeling depressed, angry, or just want to talk to someone (context).

Intention, or a person's intent to perform a behaviour, is the best predictor that a particular behaviour will occur. Intention is also influenced by attitudes and societal norms.

Attitude, which describe a person's positive or negative attitude towards performing a behaviour.

Norms, which are a person's perceptions of other people's opinions about a defined behaviour. Normative beliefs are also influenced by a person's willingness to conform to those views.

The theory of planned behaviour

The 'theory of reasoned action' was further developed by Ajzen and colleagues, who proposed the theory of planned behaviour (TPB).[17] The TPB proposed that behavioural intentions are the outcomes of three sets of beliefs: attitudes towards a behaviour, including evaluation of that behaviour and beliefs about its outcome; subjective norm, referring to perceived pressure to behave in a certain way and the individual's motivation to comply with this pressure; and perceived behavioural control.

As with other behavioural models, one of the limitations of the 'theory of reasoned action' is that it focuses on intent rather than actual behaviour. The relationship between intent and action is often only postulated or predicted. Assessing the efficacy of models is therefore quite complex.

The health action process approach

The health action process approach (HAPA) was developed by Schwarzer[18] in order to include a temporal element in models of health beliefs, and to bridge the gap between intentions and behaviour. The HAPA includes a motivation stage and an action stage. The motivation stage includes three components: self-efficacy; outcome expectancies including effects on other people; and threat appraisal, which incorporates perceptions of severity and susceptibility. The action stage consists of cognitive, situational, and behavioural factors.

Whilst the more recent models include a societal component, at best they acknowledge that a particular action by an individual is determined in part by their view of society and expectations on them. Incorporation of other demographic and cultural components into behavioural models seldom occurs.

Sociological studies of lay beliefs about health and illness

Sociologists and anthropologists have carried out empirical studies of lay models of health and illness. These have shown that lay models, even those of uneducated people, are often complex and sophisticated.[19] Through the study of lay health beliefs, sociologists have come to appreciate the extent to which people's ideas and practices are socially embedded. These beliefs are shaped by people's situation in the social structure, their cultural context, personal biography, and social identity.

Blaxter's interview-based study of working-class grandmothers in Aberdeen identified a range of causes of disease and the diseases attributed to each cause.[19] These included infection and the environment; heredity and familial tendencies; stress, strain, and psychological explanation; disease which is secondary to trauma and surgery; behaviour and the constraints of poverty; individual susceptibility; the ageing process; and diseases without cause such as cancer and tuberculosis. Causes were often seen as multiple, and the women distinguished between causal agents and precipitating factors. Blaxter concluded that while lay models of the causes of illness might be scientifically wrong in their details, they may not be unscientific in principle.

Cornwell[20] conducted an ethnographic study in a working class area of London. She distinguished between public and private accounts of health and illness. Public accounts tended to be given in response to formal questions, and were dominated by questions of acceptability and legitimacy. Private accounts consisted of stories based on personal experiences. In the public accounts, health and illness were morally problematic: good health was presented as morally worthy and illness as discreditable. The moral prescription for a healthy life was cheerful stoicism characterized by a refusal to worry, complain, or be morbid.

Cornwell identified three categories of health problem: 'normal illness', 'real illness', and 'health problems not seen as illness'. Normal illnesses included childhood illnesses and infectious illnesses in adults that are not severe such as common respiratory diseases and infections of the kidneys or tonsils. Real illnesses included major disabling and life-threatening diseases such as cancer or heart disease. These diseases were thought real due to their severity, poor prognosis, and effect on people's lives. Health problems not seen as illness were problems associated with the natural processes of ageing and the reproductive cycle. These problems were not seen as amenable to medical treatment. In all cases, if the legitimacy of an illness could be established, the moral implications of having it disappeared. If the person was unable to establish the legitimacy of their illness, for example, when their problem fell into the third category, the moral status of the condition remained problematic. The onus to prove that one was not responsible for one's condition was much greater in these cases. In the private accounts of health and illness, these moral considerations were less apparent. Instead, people's experiences of illness were placed in the context of the conditions of their employment and the demands of their work; their position in the sexual division of labour; and their previous experience of health and medical services.

The Health and Lifestyle Survey, based on interviews with over 9000 respondents in the United Kingdom, aimed to build on the findings of these smaller in-depth studies using a larger representative sample.[21] Respondents were asked to describe someone they knew who was very healthy as well how they felt when they were healthy. The responses were grouped into 10 categories: negative answers when respondents had very little to say; health as 'not-ill'; health as absence of disease or health despite disease; health as a reserve; health as healthy behaviour; physical fitness; energy and vitality; health as social relationships; as ability to function; and health as psycho-social well-being. The Health and Lifestyle Survey thus confirmed the complexity of lay concepts of health and illness, and allowed for comparisons according to age and gender. The tendency to mention these concepts varied over the life course, with younger men, for example, talking of physical strength and fitness, and older people talking in terms of function. There were also clear gender differences, women of all ages giving more expansive answers than men. Women of higher social class or higher educational qualifications expressed many-dimensional concepts. Many women but few men included social relationships in their definition of health. For these respondents, health was not a unitary concept, but included several dimensions.

There are two aspects of the WHO definition of health,[1] which are relevant to lay models. The first aspect is the focus on well-being as a criterion for health. The second aspect is the incorporation of mental and social components into the definition. Rodwin identifies four other features that define lay models: the perspective of the patient as a consumer, the uneasy tension between market forces in health and patient perspectives, the reinforcement of the subservient patient role, and the medicalization of patient's lives.[22]

Current reviews of consumer literature about health describe an increasing dissonance between the differing ways that consumers, health care providers, and health theorists see health.[23] The notion of the individual as a consumer, not a patient, predominates in the consumer model of health. For example, consumers in one North American study identified self-concept, fitness, and role performance as the strongest indicators of health not the absence of illness.[24]

Conclusion

Ideas about health and illness vary according to a person's position in the health arena, whether they are a consumer, patient, nurse, government minister, doctor, or psychologist. Interpretation of health and illness is also consequent upon an individual's age, outlook on life, current state of health, and societal approaches. Views do not fit neatly into one model or another—they are usually a compilation of aspects of several models. The relevance for practitioners is that they need to understand lay models of health and illness if they wish to engage with patients' own understandings of their health problems.

References

1. **World Health Organization (WHO).** *Preamble to the WHO Constitution*, 1948.
2. **The Australian Pocket Oxford Dictionary,** 4th edn. Melbourne: Oxford University Press, 1999.
3. **Webster, I.** (1998). *Choices in Health in the Tasks of Medicine: An Ideology of Care* (ed. P. Baume). Sydney: Maclennan + Petty.
4. **Davis, A. and George, J.** *States of Health and Illness in Australia* 3rd edn. Sydney: Addison Wesley Longman, 1998.
5. **Foster, G.M. and Anderson, B.M.** (1978). *States of Health and Illness in Australia* 3rd edn. (ed. A. Davis and J. George). Sydney: Addison Wesley Longman.
6. **Murdock** (1980). *States of Health and Illness in Australia* 3rd edn. (ed. A. Davis and J. George). Sydney: Addison Wesley Longman.

7. Foster, G.M. (1998). Disease etiologies in non-Western medical systems. As cited by Soudemire, A. In *Human Behaviour* 3rd edn. Philadelphia PA: Lippincott Williams & Wilkins, 1998.
8. Tamm, M.E. (1993). Models of health and disease. *British Journal of Medical Psychology* **66**, 213–28.
9. Maslow, A. *Towards a Psychology of Being.* Toronto: Van Nordstrands, 1962.
10. Mahrer, A. *Experiencing. A Humanistic Theory of Psychology and Psychiatry.* New York: Brunner/Mazel, 1978.
11. Health Belief Model. University of South Florida, November 2001 (http://hsc.usf.edu/kmbrown/Health_BeliefModel_Overview.htm).
12. Bandura, A. (1977). Self-efficacy: toward a unifying theory of behavioral change. *Psychological Review* **84** (2), 191–215.
13. Rogers, R.W. (1983). Cognitive and physiological processes in fear appels and attitude change: a revised theory of protection motivation. In *Social Psychology: A Source Book* (ed. J.R. Cacioppo and R.E. Petty), pp. 153–76. New York: Guildford Press.
14. Fishbein, M. (1980). A theory of reasoned action: some applications and implications. *Nebraska Symposium on Motivation* **27**, 65–116.
15. Ogden, J. *Health Psychology: A Textbook* 2nd edn. Buckingham: Open University Press, 2000.
16. Ajzen, I. and Fishbein, M. *Understanding Attitudes and Predicting Social Behaviour.* New Jersey: Prentice-Hall, 1980.
17. Ajzen, I. (1985). From intention to actions: a theory of planned behaviour. In *Action-control: From Cognition to Behavior* (ed. J. Kuhl and J. Beckman), pp. 11–39. Heidelberg: Springer.
18. Schwarzer, R. (1992). Self efficacy in the adoption and maintenance of health behaviors: theoretical approaches and a new model. In *Self Efficacy: Thought Control of Action* (ed. R. Schwarzer), pp. 217–43. Washington DC: Hemisphere.
19. Blaxter, M. (1983). The causes of disease: women talking. *Social Science and Medicine* **17**, 59–69.
20. Cornwell, J. *Hard Earned Lives: Accounts of Health and Illness from East London.* London: Tavistock Publications, 1984.
21. Blaxter, M. *Health and Lifestyles.* London: Tavistock/Routledge, 1990.
22. Rodwin, M.A. (1994). Patient accountability and quality of care: lessons from medical consumerism and patients' rights, women's health and disability movements. *American Journal of Law and Medicine* **XX**, 147–67.
23. Saltman, D.C. (1997). Feminism and the health care movement. In *Contemporary Australian Feminism* 2nd edn. (ed. K. Pritchard-Hughesd), pp. 216–41. Melbourne: Longman.
24. Kenney, J.W. (1992). The consumer's views of health. *Journal of Advanced Nursing* **17** (7), 829–94.

3.4 Medicine and the media

Angela Coulter

Introduction

Health is of prime importance to most people in the world, so it is no surprise that the mass media reflect this interest by devoting a considerable amount of attention to stories about health risks, new treatments, patients' concerns, and the politics of health care. Medical and health features are very popular and can be found in every newspaper and on most broadcasting schedules. In responding to public interest in these issues, journalists, producers, and editors play an important part in shaping public expectations.

Health professionals are often wary of the media's role, perceiving it as presenting an exaggerated and distorted view of the realities of health care. The tendency to simplify and sensationalize to grab the reader's, viewer's, or listener's attention is viewed with suspicion by health professionals trained in a more cautious scientific tradition. Many clinicians resent the fact that they may have to deal with raised expectations or inappropriate demands resulting from the media 'getting it wrong once again'. But how often do the media get it wrong and why does this happen? What are the sources of, and influences on, media coverage of health issues? What impact does media presentation of these stories have on public expectations and on consultation patterns?

This chapter reviews the evidence and argues that an understanding of media influence is essential for those working in primary care, not only because they may have to deal with its ill-effects, but also because the mass media has a positive role to play in increasing public understanding of health and disease.

Coverage of health and illness in the mass media

First, we must clarify the scope of the chapter. The definition of mass media that we will adopt here encompasses communications targeted at a broad population, that is media which provide information at low cost or free to the user. So this includes newspapers (both broadsheets, which aim to cover issues in some depth, and mass-circulation tabloids aimed at a more popular audience), television programmes (including news, documentaries, and drama), radio programmes, and magazines. Excluded from this definition are books, specialist journals, and targeted communications aimed at specific audiences, for example, health education leaflets or patient information booklets about specific diseases or treatments.

Logically, this definition should also exclude the Internet. Despite their growing importance as a medium for communicating about health and illness, health websites rely on being sought out by people looking for information on specific topics and hence have more in common with books than with newspapers or television programmes. However, patients are increasingly turning to the Internet for explanation and second opinion, and primary care professionals need to be aware of what they are finding there. We are starting to see a convergence of technologies as uptake of digital television becomes more widespread. Interactive digital television already encompasses e-mail and Internet access and it will soon become commonplace to use the television for information, education, and personal research as well as for entertainment. Television programmes about health topics offer viewers the chance to access further information via Internet links, now accessible via the family TV set. Before too long, the Internet will have become a central part of the mass media.

Journalists, TV producers, and editors are obliged to be selective in their choice of topics. Their choices, or news values, are governed largely by their knowledge of their readership or audience and their interests. This knowledge also influences the way in which the information is presented. Writing in 1988 about medical news stories in British radio and television programmes, Karpf[1] distinguished seven types of story which featured regularly:

- *the breakthrough* (scientific discoveries leading to potential new treatments);
- *the disaster* (health consequences of earthquakes, fires, explosions, or accidents);
- *the ethical controversy* (e.g. surrogate mothers, test-tube babies);
- *the scandal* (e.g. deaths from prescribed drugs, violence by psychiatric patients);
- *the strike* (health service dispute or political debate);
- *the epidemic* (its course and treatment);
- *the official report or speech* (government or medical) (ref. 1, pp. 28–9).

The amount of attention given to each of these categories of news stories is likely to vary over time and from country to country, depending on factors such as the extent of political interest in health care issues. For example, in Britain the emphasis on strikes and staff disputes gave way in the 1990s to a concern with access and waiting times, hospital closures, and health care rationing. Nevertheless, the list effectively captures the range of issues covered as news items by much of the mass media.

Media interpretations of health news

News items often provide a peg for features which aim to explore the issues in more depth or to develop a particular angle. The facts are analysed and interpreted by journalists to make them appeal to their audiences. Karpf[1] distinguished four main types of story, or interpretative frameworks, into which, she argued, most media news and documentary features could be fitted: the medical approach, the consumer approach, the look-after-yourself approach, and the environmental approach. These four frameworks continue to provide a valid means of classifying most newspaper and television coverage of health and disease. Quotes from the British broadsheet newspaper, the *Sunday Times*, have been used below to illustrate the different approaches or genres.

The medical approach

> A spice used in curries might help treat bowel cancer, according to the UK pharmaceutical company Phytopharm. Turmeric is believed to inhibit the production of an inflammation-related enzyme found in abnormally high levels in certain cancers. Phytopharm's turmeric-based product, P54, has been used in a study of 15 patients with advanced colon cancer at the Leicester Royal Infirmary NHS Trust.
>
> (*Sunday Times*, 28 January 2001)

The medical approach celebrates medical advances, with stories about new developments in scientific knowledge and medical technology leading to the prospect of curative breakthroughs and life-saving treatments. Generally optimistic and uncritical in tone, these stories promote the idea of scientific progress successfully conquering disease. Doctors and scientists are the heroes in this battle (military metaphors are common) and they are frequently interviewed and quoted. Much news and features coverage is triggered by press releases issued by organizations wanting publicity for specific purposes. Stories publicizing medical breakthroughs are often initiated by pharmaceutical companies or research funding bodies keen to promote public approval for their efforts. Such stories encourage the view that continued investment in research and development of new treatments is essential for progress to be maintained.

The consumer approach

> A damning report into the scandal of 3500 retained organs stored from dead babies at Liverpool's Alder Hey hospital will attack failures in management systems as well as criticising a number of senior doctors and administrators. The long-awaited report will also condemn the prevailing culture among doctors who believe it is acceptable to keep dead children's body parts without the knowledge of their parents.
>
> (*Sunday Times*, 28 January 2001)

The consumer approach tends to side with the patient rather than the doctor, highlighting treatment disasters, unintended side-effects, and victims of medical mishaps. Stories about doctors' errors reflect growing awareness that medical interventions can sometimes cause more harm than benefit. Doctors in this type of story (and occasionally nurses and other health professionals) are often portrayed as arrogant and out-of-touch. Despite evidence that errors and adverse events are usually the result of system failures rather than the actions of rogue individuals, journalists prefer to identify particular villains who can be named and shamed. Drawing on press releases from consumer groups, political parties, health care providers, official enquiries, and government sources, the consumer approach brings medical care firmly into the political arena.

The look-after-yourself approach

> You may think the gym is the healthiest place you can spend time on a regular basis, but it's also where you will encounter all sorts of nasty bugs. Gyms and health clubs are, after all, unnaturally intimate—where else do you undress, sweat a lot and shower in close proximity to a load of strangers? But before you use it as an excuse not to exercise regularly, there are some simple measures you can take to reduce your chances of picking up any bugs while you are there.
>
> (*Sunday Times*, 21 January 2001)

The patient or lay person is also at the heart of the look-after-yourself approach, but in this case in an active role rather than as passive victim. Influenced by health promotion campaigns, these features aim to satisfy the public's appetite for information on how they can involve themselves actively in keeping healthy. The focus is on individual behaviour and lifestyle change, on healthy diets and exercise, and on self-help. Women's magazines tend to favour this approach, publishing articles about diseases, treatments and prevention, intended to satisfy their readers' desire to understand issues affecting their health. Complementary therapies are often featured alongside orthodox ones, but on the whole these advice columns celebrate rather than challenge medical wisdom.

The environmental approach

> Have you ever stayed awake at night worrying about invisible rays zapping you in your sleep? Have you considered the toaster, television or electric heater to be a threat to your health? What about the risks involved in having a cool glass of water on a summer's day? All of the above may sound like the stuff of sci-fi novels, but invisible rays do ooze from floors in the form of radon, a colourless, odourless gas produced by decaying uranium-238 in the ground.
>
> (*Sunday Times*, 28 January 2001)

The environmental approach is also concerned with health promotion and disease causation, but at a population rather than an individual level. Stories in this genre focus on health risks beyond the control of the individual. Often instigated by environmental pressure groups, documentaries and feature articles use investigative techniques to uncover previously unknown health risks and expose scandals. Targets include government departments, industry, in particular the pharmaceutical, food, tobacco, and agri-chemical industries, and politicians who are seen as failing to protect public health. Also in this group are stories which focus on health inequalities and socio-economic causes of ill-health, in which the individual is portrayed at the mercy of government economic and social policies, the victim of external circumstances rather than the agent of their own destiny.

Shaping the agenda

The categorization into four genres is an over-simplification of course and many media stories are hybrids drawing on two or more of these approaches (ref. 1, p. 9). Nevertheless, it provides a useful illustration of the way in which the media shapes the agenda and draws particular issues to public attention. Our illustrative quotes demonstrate that each of the four types of story could be found within two consecutive issues of a single Sunday paper.

The broadsheets' appetite for health stories is increasing, presumably because their market research supports its popularity among readers. Radio programmes cover a similar set of issues, often in more depth. Readers of tabloid newspapers tend to be presented with a more restricted diet of stories, but each of the four genres can be found in these as well. Tabloids tend to place greatest emphasis on stories that focus on individuals, both as victims of the health system (the consumer approach) and as interested participants in their own health and health care (the look-after-yourself approach).[2]

In selecting what to write about and what to publish, journalists and editors are influenced by the characteristics of the newspaper or television channel, the source of the story and the availability of specialist expertise, competition from other types of story or feature, interest from other media outlets, and their intuition and views on 'newsworthiness'. Much news is 'manufactured', in the sense that it is generated by organizations and interests external to the news media to suit a particular purpose. Journalists do not usually reproduce press releases uncritically or without looking for alternative interpretations of a particular story, but the news agenda tends to be shaped by those who have a vested interest in influencing public opinion. The views of large institutions, both statutory or public bodies and commercial corporations, tend to dominate, particularly in the United States.[3] In the health arena these can include industrial or commercial interests, political interests, professional and patient groups, and those with an interest in promoting public health.[4]

News is not produced in a vacuum. It is shaped by the cultural and economic context of the society that consumes it. The media can stimulate public debate or present a one-sided view. The informed consumer of news stories needs to be aware of the biases inherent in the selection and presentation of material. An independent press and broadcasting industry and a diversity of news media reflecting different views, coupled with interested but not uncritical readers, listeners and viewers, are essential to a healthy democracy.

Impact of the mass media on attitudes to health and health care

Apart from those with a professional medical training, most people derive most of their information about health and disease from the media. This supplements and influences the effects of our own experiences of ill-health and helps to shape our attitudes to the nature and effects of illness experienced by other people. It may also affect our attitudes to health professionals and the way in which we evaluate, and act upon, medical advice. Understanding the way in which the media shapes beliefs and attitudes is therefore important for understanding the context in which patients consult health professionals, the factors which prompt them to do so, and their willingness to accept the advice or treatment offered.

Television drama and features programmes have entertainment as their primary aim, but information is often an important by-product. Drama series or 'soaps' deal with a variety of social issues and themes relating to health and disease are common. For example, the popular soap *Brookside* has dealt with teenage pregnancy, domestic violence, HIV/AIDS, and mental illness. Medical care settings have provided the backdrop for a number of popular drama series. Television series like *ER*, *Casualty*, and *Peak Practice* provide viewers with behind-the-scenes pictures of health care, which help to shape expectations of real-life health professionals and institutions. Although many such programmes strive for realism, the requirements of drama, including programme length and narrative pace, ensure that the picture they present is a distorted one.[5] In American medical soaps, doctors are usually heroes working in high-tech palaces, patients mostly suffer traumatic acute illnesses which are quickly resolved, and participants manage to juggle stressful workloads and dramatic love-lives, apparently with impunity.

The dramatization of social issues in fictional series can contribute to the stigmatization of particular social groups. Concerned about negative media images of mental illness, the Glasgow Media Group studied the impact of both fictional and non-fictional stories on public attitudes. Stories about mentally ill people causing harm to others predominated. Two-thirds of media references to mental health related to violence and these negative images tended to receive headline treatment while more positive items were relegated to problem pages or health advice columns.[6] Portrayals of mentally ill people in drama series focused on weird and sometimes dangerous behaviour. These stories undoubtedly contributed to people's fear of mental illness and reinforced negative attitudes, but the research illustrated the complexity of the way in which media messages are selectively assimilated and mediated by people's personal experience. Those who had direct experience of mental illness, either because they or their relatives or friends were sufferers, were more likely to reject the dominant media accounts. Those without such experience often treated the issue as taboo, neither discussing nor evaluating what they saw, despite their absorption with the story line and characters.[7]

Reporting science

The distinction between the information and entertainment functions of the media is not as clear cut as it may at first appear. As well as informing their readers, listeners or viewers, news journalists also hope to entertain them. This can result in dramatization of stories which begin life as dry articles in scientific journals. Sometimes, the media sensationalize topics in such a way as to distort perceptions of their prevalence or importance. One such example occurred in 1994, when European papers were full of stories about 'the killer bacteria' necrotizing fasciitis.[8,9] This was not a new bacterium and it was still rare. There was no evidence that it was increasing in prevalence. Indeed there was nothing particularly new about the story, but it coincided with public interest in alarming tropical diseases ('the Ebola epidemic' was the subject of a bestselling book, *The Hot Zone* by Richard Preston, which was published in 1994) and the spread of AIDS had renewed public concern about infectious diseases. The 'killer bacteria' story fitted with the general mood of growing alarm about hitherto unrecognized disease risks. A few cases of necrotizing fasciitis were identified by enterprising journalists, leading to sensationalist headlines and lurid newspaper accounts of the victims' suffering, and the story spread rapidly throughout the European media. The newspapers continued to spread alarm about 'killer bacteria' for several weeks until specialist correspondents finally published more balanced articles and interest in the story subsided.

The popularity of the 'killer bacteria' story was the result of a particular congruence of events, including a bestselling book. The journalists who picked up the story and passed it on were seizing an opportunity to compete for column inches and air time against other sensational news stories. No one deliberately set out to mislead the public, but the effect was to seriously overstate a minimal risk to public health.

Quality of information about medical treatments

Journalists have occasionally been guilty of credulousness in the face of unscrupulous people peddling quack remedies. Uncritical reporting of claims of a miracle cancer cure 'invented' by Luigi Di Bella, an 85-year-old physician from Modena in Italy, exposed the vulnerability of ill people to hopes of a cure, no matter how scientifically dubious. Di Bella's claims, which were not substantiated by published evidence, were widely reported in the Italian media, giving rise to more than 50 television interviews and about 300 newspaper articles. Despite the advice of oncologists and the Minister of Health, patients tended to view the media reports optimistically, leading to a campaign for free provision of Di Bella's therapy to all cancer patients who wanted it. In a survey at the height of the publicity campaign, 1120 patients attending 13 medical oncology centres in various regions of Italy were asked for their views on the Di Bella therapy. The results revealed considerable confusion among cancer patients despite the scepticism of their doctors: 42 per cent of patients judged the Di Bella therapy effective, 1 per cent said it was ineffective, and 57 per cent said they were unsure.[10] The media presented Di Bella as a misunderstood person persecuted by the leaders of official medicine. The fact that a substantial proportion of the Italian public preferred to believe this version of events was evidence of a considerable level of disillusion with the products of orthodox medicine.

Prompted by concern that patients may get hold of unreliable information, a number of studies have evaluated the quality of news stories about new medical treatments,[11] health advice columns in newspapers,[12] and health websites.[13] These have revealed cause for concern about accuracy and balance, although it would be wrong to assume that people follow such advice blindly or uncritically.[14] Faced with a plethora of often conflicting information sources, most people show themselves capable of sorting out which to trust and which to act upon when given the opportunity to make their own choices.[15]

There is, nevertheless, a case for public education in critical appraisal of health information, to help them sort out the wheat from the chaff. On the whole, efforts to help lay people evaluate the quality of health information have been restricted to the provision of specific patient information materials about diseases and treatments. Various checklists have been published to assist patients and information providers to judge the reliability of health information in written and electronic form,[16–18] but none of these was designed to help the casual newspaper reader or television viewer.

Influence of the media on use of health services

People depend on the mass media for most of their information about the world beyond their immediate experience. The media respond to the public's thirst for information about health and medical care. In doing so, they may either inform or mislead. The media help to shape attitudes and expectations, but what impact do they have on people's use of health services?

Evidence on the impact of media stories on health behaviour presents a complex picture. Stories that provoke alarm can cause people to take action, sometimes with adverse consequences. For example, press coverage of research linking oral contraceptive use with an increased risk of venous thromboembolism led some women to cease taking effective contraceptives, resulting in an increase in the numbers seeking abortion.[19] Parental concern about adverse publicity surrounding childhood vaccinations for pertussis in the 1970s and MMR in the 1990s resulted in reduced immunization rates and an increase in the incidence of serious childhood illnesses.[20] In both cases, media reports of research studies had failed to emphasize the cautious nature of the researchers' conclusions, focusing instead on raising alarm about the implied risks.

Direct-to-consumer advertising of pharmaceutical products is allowed in the United States but officially outlawed in Europe. Nevertheless, the drug companies have shown themselves adept at getting publicity for their products by encouraging features stories, some of which have had a profound effect on demand. The publication in 1990 of a prominent article about Prozac in the international news magazine *Newsweek*, resulted in widespread publicity in many European news media and a dramatic increase in sales of the drug.[21] Similarly, the anti-impotence drug Viagra became a news sensation throughout the world. This type of free publicity is not necessarily benign. It carries the risk that it can increase demand for inappropriate medical interventions, potentially causing harm to patients and increasing pressure on scarce health resources.[22]

There is, however, evidence that the mass media can have a positive effect on health behaviour, and many health education campaigns have incorporated media publicity as a key component. For example, well-designed media campaigns succeeded in achieving small reductions in the number of young people who take up smoking.[23] In the Netherlands, a mass media campaign on the use of folic acid to reduce the risk of foetal neural tube defects increased awareness and use of folic acid among pregnant women.[24] Following extensive media publicity about excessive and rising hysterectomy rates in Canton Ticino in Switzerland in 1984, the rates dropped by 33 per cent.[25] A British campaign to reduce the stigma associated with depression employed newspaper and magazine articles, radio and television programmes, leading to significant positive changes in attitudes.[26] A systematic review of the effects of mass media interventions on health services utilization identified 17 studies, 14 of which evaluated formal campaigns and three looked at media coverage of health-related issues.[27] All but one concluded that mass media coverage was effective in promoting beneficial change, including uptake of immunization and cancer screening, education about HIV risk, and reducing delay in admission to hospital for patients with suspected myocardial infarction.

Response to health scares

Stories about salmonella in eggs and chickens, BSE in cattle and genetically modified food sources have also had dramatic effects on consumer behaviour, demonstrating the lengths people will go to avoid externally imposed, and hard-to-quantify potential risks to their health. They also illustrate the increasing scepticism with which the public views reassurances from scientists and public health experts. Attempts to persuade people that the risks from these health hazards are small, and indeed much smaller than those most people face with equanimity every day, such as driving a car or crossing a busy road on foot, do not have the same direct effect.[28] Scientists often complain of difficulties in persuading the media, and through them the public, to take a more balanced view of risk and probability.

The very different perspectives of medical scientists and journalists lead to tensions, which can get in the way of providing clear, usable information to the public.[21] Science proceeds slowly and tentatively, becoming more reliable as studies are criticized, peer-reviewed, re-tested and replicated. News, on the other hand, must be seen to be dramatic, fresh and controversial, the more bizarre the better. Consensus is boring to the journalist, who is trained to seek out conflict and debate. Fast publication of emerging results is preferred to the slow time-frame of most academic publications. Journalists aim to produce colourful, readable copy which cuts to the essence of a story, while scientists are trained to write in a dense and cautious style, omitting no potentially relevant detail or qualification. Journalists use personal stories and case studies to illustrate important events while scientists eschew these in favour of statistics and regularities.

The gulf between these two perspectives often manifests itself as a struggle for control over the dissemination of information, but mutual suspicion is overlaid with a recognition that both sides need each other.[29] Most scientists seek media publicity. It helps to generate research funds, it improves the circulation and hence the impact factor of the academic journals which publish the original research, and it can also help to further academic careers.[30] For journalists, the peer-reviewed journals provide an endless source of stories to fill their columns and programmes and they depend on academic experts for background information and comment.[31] Recognition of reciprocal benefits from the relationship between scientists and journalists has led to greater sophistication on the part of medical scientists and research funding bodies in the management of media messages. This in turn has caused some journalists to probe more critically into the sources of the stories they are fed.[21] For those concerned about public information, this should be a positive development as mutual misunderstanding cannot, by definition, be illuminating.

Implications for primary care

Patients seeking medical help bring their expectations, knowledge, attitudes, and beliefs with them to the consultation. These are the product of direct personal experience, the influence of significant others, and people's knowledge of the world gained through formal education and the mass media. As we have seen, the influences of the media can be both malign and benign. There are good and bad journalists, just as there are good and bad doctors. It is incumbent on doctors to help their patients to understand their health state and how to cope with, treat, and prevent illness. The primary care professional who wishes to understand the factors influencing patients' understanding of illness and expectations of health care cannot ignore or dismiss the influence of the mass media. Those who consult them may have been prompted to come by something they read in the newspaper or saw on the television. Advice from health professionals is usually well received, but it will be mediated by the patient's beliefs and opinions which in turn may be partly shaped by the media. Ensuring that journalists have access to reliable information about health, disease, and the medical system, and assisting them in their task of reproducing a range of opinions is an important activity for those concerned with public health.

References

1. **Karpf, A.** *Doctoring the Media: The Reporting of Health and Medicine.* London: Routledge, 1988.
2. **Entwistle, V. and Hancock-Beaulieu, M.** (1992). Health and medical coverage in the UK national press. *Public Understanding of Science* **1**, 367–82.
3. **Priest, S.H.** *A Grain of Truth: The Media, the Public and Biotechnology*, Maryland: Rowman and Littlefield, 2001, pp. 7–16.
4. **Entwistle, V.A. and Sheldon, T.A.** (1999). The picture of health? Media coverage of the health service. In *Social Policy, the Media and Misrepresentation* (ed. B. Franklin), pp. 118–34. London: Routledge.
5. **Turow, J.** (1996). Television entertainment and the US health-care debate. *Lancet* **347**, 1240–3.
6. **Philo, G., McLaughlin, G., and Henderson, L.** (1996). Media content. In *Media and Mental Distress* (ed. G. Philo) Chap 4, pp. 45–81. Harlow: Addison Wesley Longman.
7. **Philo, G.** (1996). The media and public belief. In *Media and Mental Distress* (ed. G. Philo), pp. 82–104. Harlow: Addison Wesley Longman.
8. **De Semir, V.** (1996). What is newsworthy? *Lancet* **347**, 1063–6.
9. **Radford, T.** (1996). Influence and power of the media. *Lancet* **347**, 1533–5.
10. **Passalacqua, R.** et al. (1999). Patients' opinions, feelings, and attitudes after a campaign to promote the Di Bella therapy. *Lancet* **353**, 1310–14.
11. **Moynihan, R.** et al. (2000). Coverage by the news media of the benefits and risks of medications. *New England Journal of Medicine* **342**, 1645–50.
12. **Molnar, F.J.** et al. (1999). Assessing the quality of newspaper medical advice columns for elderly readers. *Canadian Medical Association Journal* **161**, 393–5.
13. **Impicciatore, P.** et al. (1997). Reliability of health information for the public on the world wide web: systematic survey of advice on managing fever in children at home. *British Medical Journal* **314**, 1875–9.
14. **Entwistle, V.** (1999). Who's afraid of the newspaper advice column? *Canadian Medical Association Journal* **161**, 397–8.
15. **Turney, J.** (1996). Public understanding of science. *Lancet* **347**, 1087–90.
16. **Coulter, A., Entwistle, V., and Gilbert, D.** *Informing Patients.* London: King's Fund, 1998.
17. **Jadad, A.R. and Gagliardi, A.** (1998). Rating health information on the internet: navigating to knowledge or Babel? *Journal of the American Medical Association* **279**, 611–14.
18. **Charnock, D.** et al. (1999). DISCERN: an instrument for judging the quality of written consumer health information on treatment choices. *Journal of Epidemiology and Community Health* **53**, 105–11.
19. **Drife, J.O.** (2001). The third generation pill controversy ('continued'). *British Medical Journal* **323**, 119–20.
20. **Nicoll, A., Elliman, D., and Ross, E.** (1998). MMR vaccination and autism 1998: Deja-vu—pertussis and brain damage 1974? *British Medical Journal* **316**, 715–16.
21. **Nelkin, D.** (1996). An uneasy relationship: the tensions between medicine and the media. *Lancet* **347**, 1600–3.
22. **Medawar, C.** (2000). Prescription drugs: direct advertising? *International Journal of Risk & Safety in Medicine* **13**, 81–6.
23. **Sowden, A.J. and Arblaster, L.** (2001). Mass media interventions for preventing smoking in young people (Cochrane Review). In *The Cochrane Library* Issue 1. Oxford: Update Software.
24. **De Walle, H.E.K.** et al. (1999). Effect of mass media campaign to reduce socioeconomic differences in women's awareness and behaviour concerning use of folic acid: cross sectional study. *British Medical Journal* **319**, 291–2.
25. **Domenighetti, G.** et al. (1988). Effect of information campaign by the mass media on hysterectomy rates. *Lancet* **2**, 1470–3.
26. **Paykel, E.S., Hart, D., and Priest, R.G.** (1998). Changes in public attitudes to depression during the Defeat Depression campaign. *British Journal of Psychiatry* **173**, 519–22.
27. **Grilli, R.** et al. (2001). Mass media interventions: effects on health services utilisation (Cochrane Review). In *The Cochrane Library* Issue 1. Oxford: Update Software.
28. **Mohanna, K. and Chambers, R.** *Risk Matters in Healthcare: Communicating, Explaining and Managing Risk.* Abingdon: Radcliffe Medical Press, 2001, pp. 3–9.
29. **Deary, I.J., Whiteman, M.C., and Fowkes, F.G.R.** (1998). Medical research and the popular media. *Lancet* **351**, 1726–7.
30. **Wilkes, M.S. and Kravitz, R.L.** (1992). Medical researchers and the media: attitudes toward public dissemination of research. *Journal of the American Medical Association* **268**, 999–1003.
31. **Entwistle, V.** (1995). Reporting research in medical journals and newspapers. *British Medical Journal* **310**, 920–3.

3.5 Self-care and self-medication

Alison Blenkinsopp and Christine Bond

Self-care and self-medication

In this chapter, we will consider the scope of self-care and self-medication (see Box 1 for definitions) and the contexts of minor illness and chronic conditions. Self-medication, the availability of medicines over-the-counter (OTC), and the potential benefits and drawbacks are described. The roles of health professionals in supporting self-care are explored.

Choices: what people do when they feel ill

As van de Lisdonk has noted in Chapter 3.2, people make their own decisions and choices about what to do when they feel ill and may undertake a number of actions including:

- consulting with lay people;
- undertaking non-medical self-care (including lifestyle changes and 'home remedies');
- undertaking medical self-care (including self-medication);
- seeking professional care.

Lay advice networks are extensively used instead of or prior to other actions. We would add another action to van de Lisdonk's list, that of information and resource-seeking, including use of the Internet. Seeking professional care might involve 'supported self-care' such as advice from a pharmacist or nurse, formal consultation with a physician, other health professional, or complementary therapy practitioner. Kate Thomas (Chapter 3.6) notes the 'Family' and 'Folk' sources of advice and information to support self-care. Consultations with care providers may take place face to face, by telephone, or electronically.

Box 1 Definitions

Self-care describes the actions that an individual takes to maintain good health or respond to illness. Although the term self-care is often used in relation to minor ailments it applies across a spectrum of ill-health through to chronic diseases.

Self-medication describes treatment that is initiated and managed by the individual rather than prescribed by a health professional. While the term is generally used in relation to minor ailments it can also apply to intermittent and chronic conditions.

As pressures have increased worldwide on health care budgets, one response has been to encourage more self-care as a way of managing demand for health care services. Limiting access to physicians through triaging is becoming more widely used and in the future it is likely that nurses and community pharmacists (those working in retail pharmacies) will become the health professionals most involved in managing minor illness. In the United States and, more recently, the United Kingdom, this has included nurse-led telephone triage. Evaluation has shown that such systems do not increase clinical risk and that patient satisfaction with the service is high. Other recent developments in the UK National Health Service have included an open access website with algorithms providing decision support and information about conditions and treatment (see www.nhsdirect.nhs.uk). The same material has been used as the basis for a book distributed free of charge through medical practices and community pharmacies to encourage self-care. The NHS is also experimenting with schemes to divert minor ailments away from medical consultations by providing treatment through community pharmacies.[1] Patient follow-up showed that pharmacy consultations substituted for those with the GP and there was no evidence of additional GP consultations nor of adverse health effects. Patients were satisfied with the service and 40 per cent chose it instead of an appointment with their doctor.[1] It has been suggested that physicians should recommend the use of OTC treatments to their patients as a way of changing future behaviour. While physicians have been cautious about such recommendations, research suggests that they are increasing[2] and are acceptable to patients.[3] There has been an overall increase in the level of approval among GPs for the provision of a wider range of medications by community pharmacists.[4]

Self-care for minor illness

Research has identified symptoms and conditions for which the public regularly treat themselves, as indicated in Table 1.

Experience of symptoms of minor illness, such as the above examples, may trigger both non-medication and medication-related behaviours. Some non-medication behaviours, for example, hot water bottles for stomach ache, are based on adages and are not evidence based. Their apparent effectiveness runs counter to the current rationale for evidence-based clinical practice. Indeed, some of the homely remedies may even be counter to current clinical advice, such as warmly wrapping up a child with a fever. A review of information on the world wide web about the management of fever in young children found the content and accuracy of sites variable.[5]

Taking medication is a common initial response to symptoms of minor illness. It will often be self-medication, which includes the following and may or may not be associated with professional advice:

- using a medicine already available at home (prescribed or over the counter);
- purchasing a new medicine from a pharmacy or non-pharmacy outlet.

Table 2 provides information on the proportions of people behaving in these various ways, including those seeking professional advice.

For children, the ailment most likely to be left untreated is a digestive ailment, and sensory ailments are the most likely to be treated. For adults, women are more likely to self-treat than men. Thinning hair and bruising are the adult symptoms least likely to be treated, and skin conditions and indigestion the most likely. Symptoms of minor ailments were less likely to result in a visit to the doctor than 10 years ago, and this is particularly marked for pain, a symptom for which new OTC products have become available during this period. Individual decisions about what, if any, action to take, are influenced by a myriad of factors including social setting, health beliefs, prior experience, and possible available treatments (see Chapter 3.2 for a further discussion of the supporting literature).

There are 'expert' and 'novice' users of self-medication. The former group would include those with previous successful experience of the particular symptoms and treatment. The latter would include new symptoms and newly available treatments. 'Expert' users are less likely to seek professional advice while 'novice' users may seek advice from a pharmacist or nurse. While a relatively small percentage of people consult the pharmacist about an episode of minor illness, the numbers involved are large, with an average of about 10 people seeking advice about symptoms in each community pharmacy every day,[6] for symptoms which may range from pain to skin disease, and from travel advice to homeopathy. Table 3 shows the top five presenting categories of such symptoms.

Thus, community pharmacies undoubtedly see many initial presentations of illness and are a key gateway for triage and referral to other sources of advice. Criteria have been identified to assess the appropriateness of advice-giving by community pharmacists and their staff.[7] However, concerns have been expressed about the quality of advice provided by community pharmacists and their staff to pharmacy customers.[8,9] Community pharmacists and their staff have to supervise the sales of such products reliably according to the OTC licensing restrictions, and some surveys indicate

Table 1 Everyday ailments for which people in the UK report treating themselves rather than seeking a consultation with a doctor[a] ($n = 2000$)

Ailment	% of people reporting ailment
Headache	80
Athlete's foot	79
Dandruff	73
Heartburn	62
Migraine	62
Period pain	61
Colds	60
Coughs	56
Mouth ulcers	51
Acid stomach	50

[a] *PRISM (Progressive Research in Self-Medication) 94*. London: Readers' Digest, 1994.

Table 2 Responses to minor ailments experienced in the past 2 weeks by adults ($n = 9032$) and children ($n = 646$) in the UK[a]

Response	% children	% adults
Saw doctor or dentist	8	10
Saw another health professional	3	4
Used a prescription medicine already in the house	11	14
Used an OTC medicine	27	27
Used a home remedy	7	9
Did not use anything	37	46

[a] British Market Research Bureau. *Everyday Health Care. A Consumer Study of Self-Medication in Great Britain*. London: BMRB, 1997.

Table 3 Top five categories of symptoms presented in pharmacies in the UK

Symptom	%
Respiratory	52
Skin	24
ENT	9
Gastrointestinal	9
Eye	6

that these may not always be adhered to. A professional response to this has been the introduction of mandatory supervision protocols covering the OTC sales of medicines[10] and a requirement that all medicines counter staff should hold a minimum qualification.[11] Pharmacists themselves have also expressed a need for educational initiatives in this area.[12]

Guidelines in community pharmacy

Following on from clinical practice in other areas, particularly medicine, guidelines for OTC counselling in different therapeutic areas have become increasingly available in the United Kingdom and other countries. These are already widely distributed to community pharmacists, produced by academic groups and the industry, and disseminated through professional journals, mailings, and educational events. The best of such guidelines are evidence based and developed by multidisciplinary groups.[13] Information includes not only how to treat the presenting symptoms but also supports the differential diagnosis of symptoms, and provides guidance on symptoms of significant or serious disease that need referral on to another practitioner or even an urgent referral to hospital. Unfortunately, the mere publication of clinical guidelines is unlikely to change clinical behaviour without further dissemination and implementation activities. A recent UK evaluation of a community pharmacy guideline shows that, in fact, pharmacists probably already have the knowledge covered by the guidelines and that failure always to apply the rigid requirements of the OTC license[14] may be due to other factors. These may include professional judgement, patient pressure, and doctor recommendations. In response to a perceived conflict between guideline content, patient preference, and their own professional experience, pharmacists may, however, pragmatically decide on a different management strategy.[15]

There is little published research about pharmacists' decision-making processes in selecting OTC product recommendations. Studies with community pharmacists in Australia indicate that perceived clinical effectiveness, personal and customer experience, manufacturer support, and commercial factors all play a part. Concern has been expressed that pharmacists and their assistants in developing countries recommend 'prescription' medicines for OTC use (e.g. antibiotics for diarrhoea or cough) and there is evidence that this occurs.[16,17] There is undoubtedly variation in the extent to which the law relating to medicines is enforced or not in different countries as well as in the extent to which pharmacists adhere to guidelines.

Self-care for chronic conditions

Self-care is not only restricted to minor self-limiting conditions. There is increasing recognition of people's capacity to self-manage chronic conditions following initial diagnosis and stabilization. This is sometimes referred to as the 'Expert Patient' movement.[18,19] There is good evidence that lay-led self-management training programmes, where patients learn from other patients, can produce health benefits and reduce medical consultations.[20,21] Although many patients currently need to access their treatment through a physician due to the 'Prescription only' status of many of the medicines used, research shows that substantial numbers of patients also self-regulate this treatment, largely without discussion with a health professional.[22] The move towards the concept of 'concordance', where patient and health professional negotiate and agree upon a treatment plan, will underpin self-management. Health professionals need to change to adopt a greater sharing of power with the patient (see Chapter 7.5).

People may also undertake self-care for chronic conditions through self-medication with an OTC product. Research into people's management of chronic pain demonstrates parallel use of prescribed and OTC medicines. A study of purchasers of OTC ibuprofen showed that one-fourth of respondents were in the 'chronic pain' category and were either solely self-medicating or self-medicating concurrently with their prescribed medications.[23] Some of the concurrent self-medication duplicated the prescribed treatment, raising questions about GPs' awareness of the use of OTC medication, safety, the GP's role in developing rapport with the patients, and monitoring long-term medication for efficacy in controlling pain.

Access to treatments: medicines available over the counter

Each country has a system to control the availability of medicines with a basic division between those medicines that can only be prescribed by a physician and those that can be purchased OTC. In general, OTC treatments tend to be for acute self-limiting conditions.

There are differences of detail between countries. For example, in the United Kingdom over the counter medicines have one of two legal classifications: Pharmacy medicine (P) or General Sales List (GSL). The former can only be sold from registered pharmacies and under the supervision of a pharmacist. The latter can be sold from pharmacy and non-pharmacy outlets. In the United States, however, for example, there is no 'Pharmacy only' category so that if a medicine is not restricted to prescription it can be purchased anywhere. However, because of the frequent location of pharmacies within major retail outlets, in practice a pharmacist will be readily available to provide advice if requested to do so, if not actually being aware of every sale. Australia has an additional sub-category of pharmacy only medicines that requires the pharmacist's personal involvement in all sales of the designated medicines. The higher level of control compares with the more general requirement that P only be sold from pharmacies, overseen by a pharmacist who need not be directly involved in each transaction.

Prescription only medicines (POMs) may be deregulated to OTC status providing certain criteria are met, primarily on the basis of patient safety. The legal status of medicines is, therefore, constantly under review to protect safety yet maintain accessibility. Recent high-profile deregulations in the United Kingdom include emergency hormonal contraception, and conversely the return to prescription control of the non-sedating antihistamines, terfenadine, and astemizole.

Criteria for switching from POM to P

Before a medicine can be switched from POM to P, Governments must be satisfied that it would be safe to allow it to be supplied without a prescription. This move to switch medicines is happening worldwide as governments seek to reduce drug budgets and increase individual responsibility for health. The principles of deregulation have been supported by the World Health Organization, based on a study of self-medication in Europe,[24] which concluded that there should be 'a framework of orderly development, including reforms in professional education and practice'. In Europe, a decision was made that 'no medicine should remain POM unless necessary for reasons of safety'. In 1992, this became European Community directive for medicines classification 92/26/CEE and the basis on which further medicines have been deregulated (see Table 4).

Despite common principles for deregulation, availability of medicines varies from country to country, even within Europe, demonstrating the difficulty of interpreting the guidance in practice (see Table 5 for selected examples). A further influencing factor is the support of the manufacturer of the medicine, which is usually a prerequisite for switching since data on efficacy and safety are required. While pharmaceutical companies are generally the instigators of POM to P switches, several have joined together in the United States to oppose a proposal that non-sedating antihistamines should become OTC medicines.[25] This is a noteworthy development because the same manufacturers previously promoted the switch of these

Table 4 European community directive for medicines classification 92/26/CEE

Medicines should only be 'prescription only medicines' if:

- Dangerous if used other than under medical supervision
- Frequently used incorrectly
- New and needs further investigation
- Normally injected

Table 5 International availability of selected medicines

	Australia	Belgium	New Zealand	Portugal	Singapore	UK	USA
Chloramphenicol (topical eye)	POM	OTC	POM	OTC	POM	POM	POM
Famotidine	OTC	POM	OTC	POM	OTC	OTC	OTC
Fluconazole (oral)	POM	POM	POM	POM	POM	OTC	POM
Levonorgestrel	POM	POM	POM	POM	POM	OTC	POM
Prochlorperazine	OTC	NA	OTC	NA	POM	OTC	POM
Salbutamol	Inhaler OTC	POM	Inhaler OTC	POM	Oral OTC	POM	POM

Source: www.aesgp.be/ingredients OTC Ingredient Classification Tables.

NA = medicine not available in that country.

Table 6 Differences in dose and licensed indications between selected 'prescription only' and 'pharmacy' products in the UK

Drug	POM product, dose, and indications	P product, dose, and indications	Key differences
Ranitidine	Zantac 150 and 300 mg tablets, 300–600 mg daily. Treatment and prevention of peptic ulcer; reflux oesophagitis	Zantac 75, 75 mg dose, followed by second 75 mg if no effect after 1 h. Maximum four tablets per day. Treatment of heartburn and indigestion. Prevention of these symptoms when food and drink-related. Maximum 2 weeks use	OTC dose substantially lower than POM dose; different indications
Hydrocortisone (topical)	0.5 and 1% strengths. For use in mild inflammatory skin disorders, unlimited treatment period	1% strength for allergic contact dermatitis, irritant dermatitis, insect bite reactions, mild to moderate eczema. Maximum 1 week use. Contra-indicated for use on face, ano-genital region, broken skin, children under 10	Indications restricted

Source: British National Formulary 42. September 2001. British Medical Association and Royal Pharmaceutical Society of Great Britain.

medicines in a number of other countries where they have now been available OTC for several years.

Where a medicine is reclassified to allow OTC sale there may be differences from its POM usage in the indications for use and dosage (see Table 6). The package labelling states the licensed OTC dose and maximum dose and the indications for use.

The implications for health professionals are the need to:

- Ask patients about any previous self-medication, including the dose of drug, frequency, and duration of use.
- Make an assessment of whether a different treatment might be needed, or a stronger dose of the same drug.
- Be aware of the licensed indications for OTC treatments when making any recommendation to purchase a medicine.
- Be aware that the same ingredients may be licensed for one indication, or patient group by one proprietary brand, and not another. Examples of such anomalies include Nicotine Replacement Therapies, ibuprofen paediatric syrup, and vaginal imidazoles.

Systematic enquiry about previous treatments used should be incorporated into all health professionals' practice[26] and research indicates this will require a change in practice.[27,28] There may also be tensions between a patient who wishes to determine his/her own treatment, which may not be endorsed by the regulations, and based possibly on the basis of valid experience, and the health care professional with a responsibility to ensure that to the best of their ability the conditions of the OTC license are being adhered to. This has led both to allegations of professional paternalism that are seen to run counter to the philosophy of self-care[29] and conversely of professional negligence.

A current example of such tension in the United Kingdom is in the recent availability OTC of 'emergency hormonal contraception'. The rationale for this switch was to increase access to emergency contraception and reduce the numbers of unwanted pregnancies. The OTC sale is restricted to women over the age of 16. Pharmacists have the unenviable task of deciding how to implement this policy. They want, on the one hand, to meet clients' needs and not to deter legitimate purchasers but also not wanting to upset parents and the public by apparently 'liberal' behaviour.

Unlike medical consultations, those in community pharmacies do not usually involve the keeping of patient-specific records for OTC medicines. Sharing of information with other health professionals about purchasers of medicines would require patient consent, an issue that is yet to be addressed in this context. Pharmacists are bound by their professional ethical code to maintain patient confidentiality.

Benefits and drawbacks of self-medication with OTC medicines

As pressure on health care resources has increased throughout the world there has been a renewed emphasis on self-care and self-medication as a means of both increasing patient empowerment and limiting demand for state health care systems. Brass has summarized the potential benefits and areas of concern arising from reclassification of medicines for OTC use[30] and these are relevant to a wider discussion about self-medication (Table 7).

Safety of OTC medicines

An important consequence of increased self-medication is that the use of such medicines is outside the formal systems of prescribing and monitoring of treatment. While there is no evidence to date of major public health problems arising from OTC treatment, research has shown that some people may be at risk. For example, small percentages of people in the United Kingdom buying ibuprofen OTC[23] reported having current or previous peptic ulcer, or were taking doses higher than the maximum OTC level (1200 mg total dose in 24 h). Some were even exceeding the maximum prescribed dose of the drug. The study demonstrated the potential for collection of pharmaco-vigilance data on specific OTC medicines through

Table 7 Self-medication: potential benefits and areas of concern

Potential benefits	Areas of concern
Increased public access to effective medicines	Risks associated with side-effects and interactions with other medication Public health risks, e.g. increase in antimicrobial resistance Lack of pharmaco-epidemiology data on OTC medicines use and adverse effects
Decreased frequency of visits to physicians, hence possible reduced staff costs to third-party payers	Inaccurate self-diagnosis Delayed or sub-optimal treatment of serious conditions
Increased patient autonomy/empowerment	Diminished role of physicians in supervision of care (perceived loss of control)
Enhanced patient education	Risks associated with inappropriate use where package/labelling instructions not followed
Reduced medication costs for third-party payers	Redistribution of medication costs with increased cost to consumers Inequity of access
Increased patient awareness of effective treatments	Patient demand for new treatments from prescribers

Source: Adapted from Brass, E.P. (2001). Changing the status of drugs from prescription to over the counter availability. *New England Journal of Medicine* **345**, 810–16.

pharmacies. In a UK study of paracetamol use, 4 per cent of purchasers were at risk of overdose, and 13 per cent appeared to experience side-effects or were using it in contraindicated circumstances. Almost two-thirds (61 per cent) were on other concurrent medication.

It has recently been proposed that community pharmacists should record their sales of OTC medicines and should be required to report suspected adverse reactions to treatment.[31] Community pharmacists are included in national reporting schemes for adverse reactions in some countries, for example Australia and the United Kingdom. These schemes are voluntary and under-reporting is recognized as a problem. More active monitoring of OTC medicines by pharmacists poses a number of important challenges. First, there is no culture of identifying and documenting individual patients' use of OTC medicines and nothing is known about what the public's response might be. The relative informality and anonymity of the pharmacy setting has generally been seen as a benefit of self-medication and there is evidence that at least some consumers are less than happy when asked questions on the purchase of an OTC medicine.[32] An additional and larger potential problem is that the availability of OTC medicines from non-pharmacy outlets would make recording incomplete.

Misuse (or abuse or overuse) of OTC medicines is a relatively under-researched area but is known to occur. In a Scottish survey of community pharmacists, 70 per cent said they believed OTC products were being misused, including antihistamine containing sleep aids, codeine preparations, cough medicines, stimulant cold remedies, and laxatives.[33] Pharmacists reported reasons for their suspicions as being unexpected increased turnover, individual excessive requests, and suspicious appearance. Professional concerns mean that they tried to manage the situation by suggestions to visit a doctor if symptoms did not improve, keeping a record of sales, refusing sales, and not stocking certain products. Nonetheless, they are frustrated by their lack of control over the situation as if people really want to purchase something they can always try elsewhere. These findings have been confirmed by other surveys, which also concluded that pharmacists feel that the issue should be addressed in a structured way with national guidelines on management.[34] Conversely, recent research on codeine-containing analgesics in Finland did not support the view that widening access to medicines liable to misuse would increase usage.[35]

Finally, it is unclear whether the sorts of overuse and misuse reported above are intentional or unintentional. Do some people believe that any medicine available without a prescription is safe, and perhaps treat the same drug on prescription with more respect? Whilst all OTC medicines come with clear patient information leaflets, detailing likely side-effects and contraindications, there are concerns that these are not read, or that the presentation of the information is hard for the lay reader to interpret. Further consideration must be given to these leaflets to ensure that they are realistic in presenting associated risks whilst encouraging appropriate usage. Whilst many pharmacy sales of OTC preparations are supported by informed advice, the increasing availability of drugs from non-health care outlets means that leaflets will increasingly become the main source of information for those wishing to self-medicate.

Supported self-care

The future for self-care of chronic conditions lies in developing scenarios where health professionals are accessed by patients when their advice and support is needed. Further reclassification of medicines will support this by widening access to treatments previously available only on prescription. The implementation of prescribing by non-medical health professionals is well advanced in some countries, with nurses and pharmacists playing a key role. Future deregulation of medicines is likely to include treatments for chronic conditions where self-care is an option for patients following an initial diagnosis by an authorizing health professional. Applications have already been made in the United States (unsuccessfully so far) to the FDA for the deregulation of the proton pump inhibitor omeprazole[36] and also for lovastatin and pravastatin in lipid-regulating treatment.[37] In 2001, it seems unlikely that any move of statins to OTC status will occur in the near future. Nevertheless, the principle of widening access to medicines for chronic use would enable patients to take greater control of the management of their condition.

The challenge for health professionals will be to develop concordant consultation styles that support, rather than try to control, patients' self-care and to recognize that patients' support needs will change over time and according to context.[20]

References

1. **Hassell, K., Whittington, Z., Cantrill, J., Bates, F., Rogers, A., and Noyce, P.** (2001). Managing demand: transfer of management of self limiting conditions from general practice to community pharmacies. *British Medical Journal* **323**, 146–7.
2. **Proprietary Association of Great Britain**, Annual report, London, 1997.
3. **Bradley, C.P., Riaz, A., Tobias, R.S., Kenkre, J.E., and Dassu, D.Y.** (1998). Patient attitudes to over the counter drugs and possible professional responses to self-medication. *Family Practice* **15**, 44–50.
4. **Erwin, J., Britten, N., and Jones, R.** (1996). General practitioners' views on over the counter sales by community pharmacists. *British Medical Journal* **31**, 617–18.
5. **Impicciatore, P., Pandolfini, C., Casella, N., and Bonati, M.** (1997). Reliability of health information for the public on the world wide web: systematic survey of advice on managing fever in children at home. *British Medical Journal* **314**, 1875–7.
6. **Bissell, P., Ward, P.R., and Noyce, P.R.** (2000). Appropriateness measurement: application to advice-giving in community pharmacies. *Social Science and Medicine* **51**, 343–59.
7. **Smith, F.J. and Salkind, M.R.** (1990). Presentation of clinical symptoms to community pharmacists in London. *Journal of Social and Administrative Pharmacy* **7**, 221–4.

8. **Goodburn, E., Mattosinho, S., Mongi, P., and Waterston, A.** (1991). Management of childhood diarrhoea by pharmacists and parents: is Britain lagging behind the Third World? *British Medical Journal* **302**, 440–3.
9. **Krska, J., Greenwood, R., and Howitt, E.P.** (1994). Audit of advice provided in response to symptoms. *Pharmaceutical Journal* **252**, 93–6.
10. **Sharpe, S.E., Norris, G.W., Ibbitt, M.L., Staton, T.J., and Riley, J.S.** (1994). Protocols: getting started. *Pharmaceutical Journal* **253**, 804.
11. **Evans, D. and Moclair, A.** (1994). Vocational qualifications for pharmacy support staff. *Pharmaceutical Journal* **252**, 631.
12. **Scottish Department Executive** (1992). Report on the council meeting of the Royal Pharmaceutical Society. *Pharmaceutical Journal* **248**, 219.
13. **Watson, M.C., Grimshaw, J.M., Bond, C.M., Mollison, J., and Ludbrook, A.** (2001). Oral versus intra-vaginal imidazole and triazole anti-fungal treatment of uncomplicated vulvovaginal candidiasis (thrush): a systematic review. *Cochrane Library of Systematic Reviews.*
14. **Watson, M.C., Bond, C.M., Grimshaw, J.M., Mollison, J., and Ludbrook, A.** (2001). Educational strategies to promote evidence based community pharmacy practice: a cluster randomised controlled trial. *International Journal of Pharmacy Practice* **9** (Suppl.), R12.
15. **Seston, E.M., Nicolson, M., Hassell, K., Cantrill, J.A., and Noyce, P.R.** (2001). Community pharmacy management of acute diarrhoea in adults. *International Journal of Pharmacy Practice* **9**, 1–8.
16. **Chue, N.T., Larsson, M., Falkenberg, T., Do, N.T., Binh, N.T., and Tomson, G.B.** (2001). Management of childhood acute respiratory infections at private pharmacies in Vietnam. *Annals of Pharmacotherapy* **35**, 1283–8.
17. **Ross-Degnan, D., Soumerai, S.B., Goel, P.K., Bates, J., Makhulo, J., Dondi, N., Sutoto, A.D., Ferraz-Tabor, L., and Hogan, R.** (1996). The impact of face-to-face educational outreach on diarrhoea treatment in pharmacies. *Health Policy and Planning* **11**, 308–18.
18. **Department of Health.** *The Expert Patient. A New Approach to Chronic Disease.* London, 2001.
19. **Carter, J.** (2001). The expert patient. *British Medical Journal* **323**, 3.
20. **Lorig, K.R., Ritter, P., Stewart, A.L., Sobel, D.S., Brown, B.W. Jr, Bandura, A., Gonzalez, V.M., Laurent, D.D., and Holman, H.R.** (2001). Chronic disease self-management program: 2-year health status and health care utilization outcomes. *Medical Care* **39**, 1217–23.
21. **Thorne, S.E. and Paterson, B.L.** (2001). Health care professional support for self-care management in chronic illness: insights from diabetes research. *Patient Education and Counselling* **42**, 81–90.
22. **Grime, J., Pollock, K., and Blenkinsopp, A.** (2001). Proton pump inhibitors: perspectives of patients and their GPs. *British Journal of General Practice* **51** (470), 703–11.
23. **Sinclair, H.K., Bond, C.M., and Hannaford, P.C.** (2000). Over the counter ibuprofen: how and why is it used? *International Journal of Pharmacy Practice* **8**, 121–7.
24. **Levin, L.S.** (1988). Self medication in Europe: some perspectives on the role of the pharmacist. In *The Role and Function of the Pharmacist in Europe* (ed. I. Lund and G. Dukes). Report of a WHO Working Group. Groningen: Styx Publications.
25. **Charatan, F.** (2001). US manufacturers resist moves to sell drugs over the counter. *British Medical Journal* **322**, 1270.
26. **Lowe, N.K. and Ryan-Wenger, N.M.** (1999). Over the counter medications and self-care. *Nurse Practitioner* **24**, 34–44.
27. **Bradley, C.P., Kenkre, J., Tobias, R., Dassu, D., and Riaz, A.** (1996). GPs' rate of recommending over the counter drugs varies. *British Medical Journal* **313**, 115–16.
28. **Pal, B.** (1996). GPs lack awareness of non-steroidal anti-inflammatory drugs available over the counter. *British Medical Journal* **313**, 116.
29. **Brazier, M. and Prayle, D.** (1998). Supply of medicines: paternalism, autonomy and reality. *Journal of Medical Ethics* **24**, 93–8.
30. **Brass, E.P.** (2001). Changing the status of drugs from prescription to over the counter availability. *New England Journal of Medicine* **345**, 810–16.
31. **Clark, D., Layton, D., and Shakir., S.A.W.** (2001). Monitoring the safety of over the counter drugs. *British Medical Journal* **323**, 706–7.
32. **Morris, C.J., Cantrill, J.A., and Weiss, M.C.** (1997). One simple question should be enough: consumers' perceptions of pharmacy protocols. *International Journal of Pharmacy Practice* **5**, 64–71.
33. **Bond, C.M., Matheson, C.M., and Hickey, F.** *Community Pharmacists' Involvement with Drug Misusers: A National Survey of Pharmacists' Attitudes and Practice.* Report to the Scottish Office, 1997.
34. **MacFadyen, L., Eadie, D., and McGowan, T.** (2001). Community pharmacists' experience of over-the-counter medicine misuse in Scotland. *Journal of the Royal Society for the Promotion of Health* **121**, 185.
35. **Almarsdottir, A.B. and Grimsson, A.** (2000). Over the counter codeine use in Iceland: the impact of increased access. *Scandinavian Journal of Public Health* **28**, 270–4.
36. **Gottlieb, S.** (2000). FDA panel advises against omeprazole as over the counter drug. *British Medical Journal* **321**, 1099.
37. **Gottlieb, S.** (2000). FDA says statin cannot be sold 'over the counter'. *British Medical Journal* **321**, 198.

3.6 Alternative sources of advice: traditional and complementary medicine

Kate Thomas

Professional, family, and folk medicine

Most health care takes place outside the formal health care system. Many episodes of minor morbidity resolve with no care, self-care, or care within the family, sometimes with recourse to over the counter purchases of supporting pharmaceuticals (see Chapter 3.5).[1,2] The choice not to seek professional care will vary according to perceptions of the seriousness of the problem, ease of access to the health care system, and health beliefs, all of which shape behavioural responses to an illness episode. Still other types of care will be sought from carers working outside the formal health care system. Recognizing this, the anthropologist Kleinman proposed the existence of three sectors of health care: 'professional', 'family', and 'folk'. The third sector 'folk medicine' describes all the alternative sources of care available within a society that are delivered outside the formal health system and beyond the family. A patient's pathway through these three sectors may entail exclusive use of one, sequential use of each, or the simultaneous use of two or more sectors of care.[3]

Traditional or complementary?

Systems of medicine embedded in historically identifiable and culturally specific beliefs about the nature of ill health that predate Western scientific medical thinking, are frequently described as 'traditional medicine' (e.g. Chinese medicine or Ayurvedic medicine).[4] In contrast, therapies and modalities that have emerged more recently in parallel to scientific medicine are usually described as 'alternative' or 'complementary', depending on their degree of divergence from Western medical diagnosis and the extent to which they are seen to support conventional treatment regimes.

In Western societies today, the 'folk' sector embraces traditional and complementary medicine. For simplicity's sake, the use of the term 'CAM' (complementary and alternative medicine) has been coined to embrace both approaches, and will be used in this chapter.

In the most commonly used operational definition of CAM, it comprises those health-related practices that are not taught in medical schools or generally available in mainstream medicine.[5–7] These boundaries are clearly relaxing however, and the United States Office of Alternative Medicine has offered a more durable definition:

> [CAM is] A broad domain of healing resources that encompasses all health systems, modalities and practices and their accompanying theories and beliefs, other than those intrinsic to the politically dominant health system of a particular society or culture in a given historical period. CAM includes all such practices and ideas self-defined by their users as preventing or treating illness or promoting well-being. Boundaries within CAM and between the CAM domain and the domain of the dominant system are not always sharp or fixed.[8]

Classifications and shared characteristics of CAM

Broad definitions are very useful to help us understand the position of CAM in a society. However, they are less useful for understanding the content of CAM and its contextualized role within health care. Attempts have therefore been made to classify the individual modalities that are thought to comprise CAM based either on the character of the therapies, or on their relationship to mainstream care (Fig. 1).

However, CAM practice is also distinguished from conventional medicine by its philosophy, or shared alternative belief system, comprising distinctive views of the body, health, and the cause of illness[11] (Fig. 2). The extent to which elements of this philosophy are shared by patients, and its contribution to understanding why patients are using CAM, are discussed below.

Access to CAM

CAM is accessed by patients in hospital as well as community settings, through consultations with CAM practitioners, and via over-the-counter purchases of alternative remedies and products for self-medication. In the United States and Canada, insurance coverage offers only limited access to CAM. In the United Kingdom, 90 per cent of all reported CAM visits are conducted in the private sector and paid for out-of pocket, despite access to a national health care system that delivers treatment free at the point of delivery.[16]

Most patients seek care from a CAM practitioner who is not qualified as a medical doctor. Freedom to practice and the regulation of titles in CAM vary considerably between countries.[17] In the United Kingdom, the number of CAM practitioners exceeds the number of primary care physicians.[18] Some overlap exists between the two systems however, as patients may be referred to CAM care by a physician, or receive care from a physician who is also trained in a CAM modality. In 1995, 40 per cent of UK primary care practices offered access to CAM via referral, provision, or treatment.[19]

Is CAM primary care?

Direct access, generalist care, longitudinal care, and delivery in a community setting are identified as four key attributes of primary care.[20] Few data exist to support or refute the existence of longitudinal care in CAM. Most practitioner-delivered CAM care is accessed directly by patient self-referral in a community setting (albeit a private one). Generalist care is seen as a defining characteristic of alternative systems of medicine such as acupuncture or homeopathy. Other modalities are more often perceived as specialist services (e.g. osteopathy and chiropractic), and still others would define their role as 'supplementary' to medicine.

Pathways to care—professional and lay networks

Surveys of CAM users have shown that by far the most common pathway to CAM treatment reported is a recommendation by a family member, friend, or colleague.[21,22]

Therapeutic similarity[9]

- 'ethnic medical systems' (e.g. traditional Chinese medicine, Ayurvedic medicine)
- 'non-allopathic medicinal systems (e.g. homeopathy, herbal medicine)
- manual therapies (e.g. chiropractic, osteopathy, therapeutic massage)
- 'mind–body' therapies (e.g. hypnotherapy, psychic healing, Reiki)
- 'nature cure therapies' (e.g. anthroposophical medicine, naturopathy)

Integrative potential (acceptability, evidence-base, and degree of potential for integration into mainstream care)[10]

- modalities with some scientific evidence of efficacy (acupuncture, chiropractic, homeopathy, herbal medicine, and osteopathy)
- modalities perceived to be working in a supportive capacity alongside conventional medicine, and not offering independent diagnosis (e.g. massage, aromatherapy, reflexology, hypnotherapy, and yoga)
- traditional systems of medicine that are perceived to be backed by historical practice only (e.g. Ayurvedic and traditional Chinese medicine), and recent diagnostic modalities with little supportive evidence (such as iridology and kinesiology)

Fig. 1 Classifications of CAM.

Mode of action

- supporting self-healing processes in order to improve wellness and treat disease
- an individualized approach to diagnosis and treatment
- working with, not against, symptoms to uncover underlying historical and constitutional causes of ill health

Healing intent

- a 'holistic' understanding of health as the interrelationship of physical, mental, emotional, and spiritual well-being
- attention to intangible healing energies
- 'vitalism'or life force in the body and in the environment
- a focus on achieving and maintaining individual optimum wellness, or 'salutogenesis'

Fig. 2 Characteristics of a CAM general belief system.[9,12,13]

The decision to seek help for a health problem occurs in a social context. 'Lay consultations' with friends and family help to define, clarify, and legitimize a concern as a 'health problem', and through such discussions a decision is reached about appropriate action. Such 'lay referral networks' may be extensive or limited, and the health beliefs which underlie them may be more or less congruent with those shaping the delivery of mainstream health care. The relationship between lay referral networks and CAM has been explored empirically in a Canadian population using a social network approach. While the networks described were embedded in strong ties to immediate family, and all featured professional or mainstream sources of advice, people reporting larger, looser, and more diverse networks, with greater participation of friends, were more likely to access CAM.[23,24]

Using this model, we can speculate that the diffusion of the use of CAM will accelerate as 'early adopters' influence choices in their immediate networks, and sources of personal recommendation expand, supported by wider cultural acceptance and the messages available via the mass media.[25] Patients appear to make pragmatic choices regarding the types of problem that they take to CAM practitioners and the point at which they choose to do so. Thus, for most users, CAM is a supplement rather than a substitute for conventional care.[26]

Levels of CAM use

Levels of CAM use recorded in Western industrialized societies appear to transcend differences between health care delivery systems. Estimates of the level of CAM use are always a product of the definition of CAM used in the survey;[27] however, population-based national surveys have repeatedly demonstrated significant levels of use in Australia, United Kingdom, Canada, and United States. These estimates range from 13 to 20 per cent for practitioner visits in the past year, and from 30 to 40 per cent for use that includes self-medication with purchased CAM remedies and dietary products.[6,15,16,28] Despite common perceptions that use is increasing in these countries, longitudinal data demonstrating trends over time are only available for the United States.

Characteristics of CAM users

The profile of CAM users in Western countries shows greater use in the middle age groups, amongst women compared to men, and by people with greater educational attainment, higher incomes and professional or non-manual occupations.[6,15,16,28,29] Surveys have shown a mixed picture with regard to race/ethnicity and use of CAM, primarily because the population-wide samples and survey tools are not adequate to the task of unravelling behavioural patterns in small sub-groups.[30] Compared to primary medical care, children and the elderly are under-represented amongst CAM users.

The caricature of the CAM user as female, middle aged, and college educated with disposable income has served to fuel some of the 'lifestyle' explanations of CAM use. However, it also disguises some facts about CAM use. Most importantly, while CAM use may be more common in particular sections of the population, a level of CAM use is apparent across all social groups. For example, 8 per cent of people aged 65 and over were found to have made a visit to a CAM practitioner in the United Kingdom in 1998.[16]

How CAM is used

People using CAM report poorer health status than the general population. The clinical profile of users does not support the contention that CAM use can be dismissed as an outlet for the 'worried well'. In particular, they report high levels of chronic pain, back problems, muscle sprains and strains, arthritis, allergies, fatigue, addictive problems, depression or anxiety, and headaches. Musculoskeletal problems (particularly back and neck pain) dominate the clinical reasons for consulting CAM practitioners in Canada, Australia, United Kingdom, and United States.[6,15,26] This would seem to explain the predominance of visits to manipulative and bodywork therapists found in surveys. However, musculoskeletal problems also form a large part of the workload of other therapists.[31,32] Recent longitudinal data from Canada suggests that this profile may be changing over time, with patients seeking help for more varied problems and consulting a wider range of practitioners.[20] High levels of CAM use have been reported in surveys of specific patient groups including rheumatology patients, patients with chronic digestive disorders and some groups of cancer patients.

Finally, a significant minority of patients report no specific health problem at the time of use. These patients cite enhanced wellness, relaxation, or health maintenance as their main reason for using various CAM therapies. This group forms a substantial proportion of patients visiting some of the bodywork therapies, such as aromatherapy and reflexology.[16]

Reported satisfaction with CAM

Patient satisfaction is generally regarded as an accepted measure of heath care quality in primary care. Studies evaluating the provision of CAM have found high levels of reported satisfaction with care, especially in the domains of communication and access to care.[33,34] High levels of overall satisfaction with CAM care have also been reported by consumer surveys in the United Kingdom and the United States. However, questions about overall satisfaction with care in mainstream medicine also tend to elicit positive responses.

Studies that have compared patient satisfaction with orthodox primary care and CAM care suggest that CAM users are more satisfied with the quality of the interpersonal care that they received; but differences were less obvious with respect to perceived efficacy.[35,36] However, studies of patients who use CAM following a diagnosis of cancer, show that satisfaction with CAM therapies can be high, even without the hope for anticancer effect.[37] More research is needed to understand the role of patient expectations in the context of CAM care.

Perceived risks of CAM care

The public perception of CAM is often one of minimal intervention and 'natural remedies'.[7,13] The dangers of an uncritical belief in the benign properties of CAM to the exclusion of any possible harmful effects have been highlighted by a number of commentators who stress a number of potential problems, including contaminants in unregulated herbal medicines, possible interactions with conventional treatment, and the risks of unregulated providers of CAM.[38] Recent UK research has shown that acupuncture is a safe procedure when conducted by appropriately trained practitioners.[39,40] Similar evidence is needed about safety in other therapies.

Reasons for seeking CAM care

A number of theories have been developed to explain the rising interest in, and use of CAM therapies. Some involve 'pull' factors, drawing patients towards CAM use; others focus on the factors that are perceived to be pushing people away from mainstream care. Some are speculative; others have a sounder base in theory or empirical evidence (Fig. 3). Six of the most popular explanations are discussed in turn.

Flight from science

The phrase 'flight from science' in relation to CAM use and users first appeared in *British Medical Journal* editorial in 1983.[41] 'Flight from science' encapsulates the idea that patients' use of CAM is an indication of a false fear, or ignorance, of the domain of empirical science. If patients and the public had a better understanding of scientific medicine and what it had achieved, they would not fall back on credulous faith, risk false hope, waste

Evidence-based 'pull' factors

- pragmatism; desire for symptom reduction
- belief in the effectiveness of CAM
- lifestyle choice; congruence with values and principles of CAM; especially a 'holistic' approach to health (mind, body, and spirit)
- desire for increased well-being
- opportunity to take active part in own treatment and care and gain greater control and choice
- perceived natural and/or non-invasive nature of treatments

Other possibilities

- search for a satisfactory therapeutic relationship (especially for continuing CAM use)
- explanations offered by CAM 'makes sense'
- desire for a more person-centred approach to care approach
- accessibility of CAM
- affordability of CAM

Evidence-based 'push' factors

- pragmatism; perceived lack of effective conventional treatment for a particular problem
- dissatisfaction with conventional medicine;
  - poor prior experience with conventional medicine
  - experience of poor communication with doctors in relation to specific health problems
- concern about unpleasant side-effects of conventional care

Other possibilities

- flight from science; rejection of science/ gullibility and naivety
- dissatisfaction with medical care in general
- high costs of orthodox care (USA)
- affluence
- being a member of the 'worried well'

Fig. 3 Motivations for using CAM.

their money, or worse still, turn their backs on mainstream medicine and what it has to offer. A similar argument was developed and strongly upheld in the first of two British Medical Association reports on CAM.(42,43) This explanation is less commonly put forward today. The ascendancy of an evidence-based medicine culture has highlighted the need for empirical evidence of efficacy in all areas of medicine, and created a slightly more even playing field with regard to claims to the scientifically robust demonstration of effectiveness (or the lack of it).

The adequacy of this explanation is also challenged when the epidemiological evidence shows that the strongest socio-demographic predictor of CAM use is receipt of higher education. Furthermore, the majority of CAM users do not appear to have rejected orthodox medicine, rather they are willing to make use of both systems of care at different points in their lives, guided by choices that are mediated by the context and history of a particular health problem.

A lifestyle choice

A less patronizing and more sophisticated view of the cultural implications of CAM use is found in the literature describing this behaviour as a lifestyle choice linked to sympathy with the principles underlying CAM and their compatibility with patients' values, worldviews, and beliefs about the meaning of health and illness.(7,31) A recent study operationalized this hypothesized 'philosophical congruence' in a US population study. Astin found that a 'holistic philosophy of health' (mind, body, and spirit) predicted CAM use in this sample, as did membership of a group described as 'cultural creatives': people who expressed a commitment to environmentalism, feminism, and personal growth psychology.(7) Similar findings regarding a positive valuation of CAM philosophy and principles have been reported in studies of Canadian and UK populations.(13,31)

This explanation sits well with models of CAM diffusion that identify value congruence as a key mechanism by which people seek advice, and take action in response to particular symptoms and health concerns. It can be thought of as a 'pull' factor propelling people towards the use of CAM.

Dissatisfaction with orthodox care

Chief amongst the 'push' factors offered to explain the reasons for CAM use is that of dissatisfaction with mainstream care. The logic is clear: if people are not getting their needs met, they will seek help elsewhere. Four major elements of dissatisfaction are discussed in the literature: ineffectiveness of orthodox care; poor communication with doctors; a perceived lack of control or choice in mainstream care; and the perceived dangers and adverse side-effects of some orthodox treatments. Asked to score reasons for seeking CAM care, the statement 'Because orthodox treatment was not effective for my particular problem' was strongly endorsed by patients using acupuncture, osteopathy, or homeopathy.(31)

Communication with doctors may be particularly problematic for patients experiencing ill-defined and functionally debilitating conditions. Lacking an orthodox diagnosis, patients may be left without a satisfactory explanation of their symptoms, or a sense of legitimacy regarding their condition; the reported experience of chronic fatigue syndrome patients illustrates the impact of this lack of recognition well. This explanation of CAM use fits well with the profile of CAM users. Older and less well-educated patients have been shown to be more deferential to doctors, and these groups are less likely to use CAM. Being less deferential may be expressed as a desire for more choice and control in health care.

The profile of patients using CAM includes a large proportion of patients with chronic, non-life-threatening conditions. For some of these patients, control of the process from the vantage point of their own experience and expertise, may be paramount and lead them to seek new treatments and alternative ways of reducing the negative impact of illness on their lives. For other patients, poor experiences of orthodox care, and concerns about adverse side-effects of orthodox treatments may propel them to look elsewhere for help.

Studies have shown that dissatisfaction with orthodox care makes a significant contribution to predicting CAM use only when measured in terms of specific negative experiences. Reported 'general dissatisfaction' with conventional medicine is not a good predictor of use.(7,31) General dissatisfaction with orthodox medicine and distrust of doctors may however predict CAM use for the small minority of patients reporting a primary reliance on CAM for their health care.(7)

Active well-being and health maintenance

A significant minority of CAM users report no current health problem, estimates suggest an overall figure of 10 per cent, but this will vary according to the therapy used. Patients are more likely to use bodywork therapies, especially massage, aromatherapy, and reflexology, for general well-being and relaxation. Chiropractic and osteopathy use may involve regular but infrequent 'maintenance treatments' designed to aid the patient in keeping an achieved level of wellness. The line between health care and well-being enhancement is not always easy to draw and CAM use may have an important role to play in current debates concerning the appropriate boundaries of 'health need' or 'medical necessity'. These patterns of use illustrate the fourth reason put forward to explain the popularity of CAM; namely the support it can offer patients wishing to take a more active part in maintaining their health.

Qualitative research suggests that CAM use is perceived as a valuable support mechanism for people wishing to take greater responsibility for their health, and quantitative studies in the United Kingdom and Canada demonstrate that this is a strongly endorsed reason for using CAM, as well as showing that CAM patients are more likely to engage in health promoting behaviours such as regular exercise, monitoring their diet and taking vitamin supplements than matched patients of family GPs.(13,31) Not surprisingly perhaps, social theorists have begun to link CAM use to a growing 'fitness culture' emerging in North America and Western Europe.(44)

Pragmatism and anticipated symptom relief

All studies that have set out to explore the reasons why people turn to CAM have reported that the single most influential factor is the need for symptom relief, coupled with a belief in the potential effectiveness of CAM. This is unlikely to be expressed as a blanket endorsement of the efficacy of all CAM modalities for every problem, but rather as a considered choice, made in the context of a particular existing health problem.(26,45,46)

Decisions about appropriate care will be made in the context of what conventional care is perceived to offer for the problem in question. Survey literature that shows patients are using a 'mixed economy' of health care, supports the hypothesis that CAM use is based less on blind faith, and more on a 'pragmatic' approach to identifying and assessing the full range of options available, and making a decision in the light of the accessibility and affordability of the alternatives.

In addition to a positive belief in the effectiveness of CAM for a given problem, a more general health optimism has been identified, characterized as the belief that health can always be improved.(35) To the extent that this belief overlaps with basic CAM philosophy, it is likely to fuel dissatisfaction and encourage help seeking elsewhere, especially if the message from orthodox medicine is one that emphasises the intractability of a chronic condition. A healing philosophy that is positive about the capacity for everyone to gain some benefit from restoring balance and enhancing well-being, makes CAM an attractive option under such circumstances. However, a pragmatic orientation to care suggests that those patients who do not get the expected benefits from CAM, will soon move on to find another source of care.(21)

The search for a satisfactory therapeutic relationship

The final reason for CAM use considered here is the counterbalance to the consumerist orientation suggested above. Whilst CAM patients may appear to be displaying the principles of rational consumerism in their choice of medical encounter, the affective aspects of health care, including patients' needs to gain support in the face of uncertainty and fear, may be equally important in determining behaviour and satisfaction with care received.(47–49)

Three key elements of a good therapeutic relationship are commonly discussed in relation to CAM: holistic care, empathetic listening, and partnership. Holistic care, defined as care that attends to the body, the emotions and the spirit, is not exclusive to CAM. Elements of holistic care, such as paying close attention to the person with the illness rather than the illness itself, will be present in all medical encounters to a greater or lesser degree. Nor is it a uniform expectation within CAM. Some modalities and practitioners will offer care which is much more 'holistic' than others. However, the potential of CAM care to attend to the whole person is greatly enhanced by a common approach to diagnosis and treatment. This usually requires divergent sources of information, obtained by eliciting a detailed personal history that skilfully takes on board the physical, emotional, spiritual, and practical elements of a patient's experiences.

Opportunities to tell their story, and be treated as a whole person are valued by many CAM patients, as is the opportunity CAM affords to make sense of illness experiences.(31,46) Both of these require a degree of empathetic listening on the part of the practitioner. Again, such skills are not exclusive to CAM, but studies comparing patients' experiences suggest that patients who used CAM rated GPs listening skills lower than matched patients who had not.(35)

CAM consultations have been characterized as following a 'partnership' model, with acknowledged expertise on both sides, and a high degree of shared information and shared decision-making.(21) CAM patients have reported a more equal relationship with their CAM practitioner and this fits with the evidence suggesting that some patients report using CAM to find a way of gaining more involvement and control over their health.(21,31)

As a reason for choosing CAM, the search for a satisfactory therapeutic relationship may exist alongside more pragmatic and problem-oriented reasons for seeking care. However, it is important to remember that CAM patients will always consist of two distinct groups; those seeking help for the first time, and those continuing or returning for further care. The choices made by these two groups will be based on different experiences and most likely governed by different expectations of the therapeutic relationship.(22,31,46) As the pool of patients exposed to CAM continues to grow, so will the likelihood of being a returning patient. In order to understand why people are using CAM, it will become increasingly important to distinguish between these two behaviours. Longitudinal studies are required to explore these questions further.

Conclusions

Searching for a simple explanatory model for the reasons why people use CAM is like seeking the Holy Grail. CAM users reflect the diversity of the wider populations in which they are embedded. Multiple regression techniques may uncover the relative importance of the factors tested, but they also serve to disguise the diversity of users described in survey after survey. Middle-aged people may use CAM more often, but children and the elderly are also users. Higher social class, income, and education may be related to higher levels of use, but people with little education and low incomes also use CAM. Economic considerations will be context specific, and depend on the cost to patients of access to mainstream care. Ultimately, the evidence points to the dominant reason for seeking help from CAM being the same as that propelling people to seek any health care—a problem that they perceive cannot be managed by self-care alone. How this happens is always an expression of 'lifestyle', social networks, and the cultural norms within which people operate and make decisions on a day-to-day basis.

CAM use shows no signs of abating. Primary care must decide whether to adopt a 'laissez faire' stance and allow the present parallel care system to continue, or to encourage and facilitate further integration of the 'folk' and professional or mainstream sectors. At the very least, the benefits of increased integration will include greater integrity of GP care, with patients and their doctors openly sharing information about the range of treatments being accessed by patients at any particular time. However, the real challenge for primary care lies in its assessment of the potential contribution of CAM to health care as a whole, whether viewed in terms of the specific therapeutic tools on offer, or the lessons which might be (re)learned about the intrinsic value of the therapeutic relationship. True integration will entail changes in both systems of care, carrying with it both the promise of positive transformation and the risks of uncertainty and change.(12,33,50)

References

1. **Hannay, D.** (1980). The 'iceberg' of illness and 'trivial' consultations. *Journal of the Royal College of General Practitioners* **30**, 551–4.

2. **Wadsworth, M., Butterfield, W., and Blaney, R.** *Health and Sickness: The Choice of Treatment.* London: Tavistock, 1977.
3. **Kleinman, A.** *Patients and Healers in the Context of Culture.* Berkley CA: University of California Press, 1985.
4. **World Health Organization.** The Promotion of Traditional Medicine. Technical Report Series No. 622, Geneva, 1978.
5. **Ernst, E.** (2000). The role of complementary and alternative medicine. *British Medical Journal* **321**, 1133–5.
6. **Eisenberg, D., Davis, R., Ettner, S., Appel, S., Wilkey, S., Von Rompay, M., and Kessler, R.** (1998). Trends in alternative medicine use in the United States, 1990–1997. *Journal of the American Medical Association* **280** (18), 1569–75.
7. **Astin, J.** (1998). Why patients use alternative medicine. *Journal of the American Medical Association* **279** (19), 1548–53.
8. **Office of Alternative Medicine, NIH Committee on Definition and Description** (1997). Defining and describing complementary and alternative medicine. *Alternative Therapies in Health and Medicine* **3** (2), 49–57.
9. **Fulder, S.** (1998). Basic concepts of alternative medicine and their impact on our views of health. *Journal of Alternative and Complementary Medicine* **4** (2), 147–58.
10. **House of Lords Select Committee on Science and Technology.** *Complementary and Alternative Medicine.* London: The Stationary Office, 2000.
11. **O'Connor, B.** (2000). Conceptions of the body in CAM. In *Complementary Medicine: Challenge and Change* (ed. M. Kelner and B. Wellman). Amsterdam: Harwood Academic Publishers.
12. **Jonas, W.** (1998). Alternative medicine—learning from the past, examining the present, advancing the future. *Journal of the American Medical Association* **280** (18), 1616–18.
13. **Kelner, M. and Wellman, B.** (1997). Health care and consumer choices: medical and alternative therapies. *Social Science and Medicine* **45** (2), 203–12.
14. **Pelletier, K.** et al. (1997). Current trends in the integration and reimbursement of complementary and alternative medicine bymanaged care, insurance carriers, and hospital providers. *American Journal of Health Promotion* **12**, 112–22.
15. **Millar, W.J.** (1997). The use of alternative health care practitioners by Canadians. *Canadian Journal of Public Health* **88**, 154–8.
16. **Thomas, K.J., Nicholl, J., and Coleman, P.** (2001). Use and expenditure on complementary medicine in England—a population-based survey. *Complementary Therapies in Medicine* **9** (1), 1–11.
17. **Saks, M.** (2000). Professionalization, politics and CAM. In *Complementary and Alterative Medicine: Challenge and Change* (ed. M. Kelner and B. Wellman). Amsterdam: Harwood Academic Press.
18. **Mills, S. and Peacock, W.** Professional Organization of Complementary and Alternative Medicine in the United Kingdom. Report to the Department of Health. University of Exeter, 1997.
19. **Thomas, K.J., Fall, M., and Nicholl, J.** (2001). Access to complementary medicine via general practice. *British Journal of General Practice* **51**, 25–30.
20. **Steiner, A., Godber, E., and Robinson, R.** (1998). What is primary care? *Journal of Health Services Research and Policy* **3** (2), 127–8.
21. **Kelner, M.** (2000). The therapeutic relationship under fire. In *Complementary Medicine: Challenge and Change* (ed. M. Kelner and B. Wellman). Amsterdam: Harwood Academic Publishers.
22. **Thomas, K.J., Carr, J., Westlake, L., and Williams, B.** The Utilisation of Alternative Health Care Systems in Relation to Orthodox Medicine. Report to Nuffield Provincial Hospitals Trust, 1990.
23. **Freidson, E.** *The Profession of Medicine.* New York: Dodd Mead and Co, 1970.
24. **Wellman, B.** (2000). Partners in illness: who helps when you are sick? In *Complementary Medicine: Challenge and Change* (ed. M. Kelner and B. Wellman). Amsterdam: Harwood Academic Publishers.
25. **Valente, T.** (2000). Social networks and mass media: the diffusion of CAM. In *Complementary Medicine: Challenge and Change* (ed. M. Kelner and B. Wellman). Amsterdam: Harwood Academic Publishers.
26. **Thomas, K.J., Carr, J., Westlake, L., and Williams, B.T.** (1991). Use of non-orthodox health care in Great Britain. *British Medical Journal* **302**, 207–10.
27. **Harris, P. and Rees, R.** (2000). The prevalence of complementary and alternative medicine use among the general population: a systematic review of the literature. *Complementary Therapies in Medicine* **8** (2), 88–96.
28. **MacLennan, A.H., Wilson, D.H., and Taylor, A.W.** (1996). Prevalence and costs of alternative medicine in Australia. *Lancet* **347**, 569–73.
29. **Blais, R., Maiga, A., and Aboubacar, A.** (1997). How different are users and non users of alternative medicine? *Canadian Journal of Public Health* **88**, 159–62.
30. **Wooton, J. and Sparber, A.** (2001). Surveys of complementary and alternative medicine: Part 1. General trends and demographic groups. *Journal of Alternative and Complementary Medicine* **7** (2), 195–208.
31. **Vincent, C. and Furnham, A.** (1996). Why do patients turn to complementary medicine? An empirical study. *British Journal of Clinical Psychology* **35**, 37–48.
32. **Wadlow, G. and Peringer, E.** (1996). Retrospective survey of patients of practitioners of traditional Chinese acupuncture in the UK. *Complementary Therapies in Medicine* **4** (1), 1–7.
33. **Luff, D. and Thomas, K.J.** (2000). Getting somewhere, feeling cared for: Patient perspectives on complementary therapies in the NHS. *Complementary Therapies in Medicine* **8** (4), 253–9.
34. **Goldstein, M. and Glik, D.** (1998). Use of and satisfaction with homeopathy in a patient population. *Alternative Therapies* **4** (2), 60–5.
35. **Furnham, A. and Forey, J.** (1994). The attitudes, behaviours and beliefs of patients of conventional versus complementary (alternative) medicine. *Journal of Clinical Psychology* **50** (3), 458–69.
36. **Pincus, T., Vogel, S., Savage, R., and Newman, S.** (2000). Patients' satisfaction with osteopathic and GP management of low back pain in the same surgery. *Complementary Therapies in Medicine* **8** (3), 180–6.
37. **Downer, S.M., Cody, M.M., McCluskey, P., Wilson, P.D., Arnott, S.J., Lister, T.A., and Slevin, M.L.** (1994). Pursuit and practice of complementary therapies by cancer patients receiving conventional treatment. *British Medical Journal* **309**, 86–9.
38. **Ernst, E.** (2001). Safety issues in complementary medicine. In *The Desktop Guide to Complementary and Alternative Medicine; an Evidence-Based approach* (ed. E. Ernst). Edinburgh: Mosby/Churchill Livingstone.
39. **MacPherson, H., Thomas, K.J., Walters, S., and Fitter, M.** (2001). The York acupuncture safety study: prospective survey of 34,000 treatments by traditional acupuncturists. *British Medical Journal* **323**, 4886–7.
40. **White, A., Hayhoe, S., Hart, A., and Ernst, E.** (2001). Adverse events following acupuncture: prospective survey of 32,000 consultations with doctors and physiotherapists. *British Medical Journal* **323**, 4885–6.
41. **Smith, T.** (1983). Alternative medicine. *British Medical Journal* **287**, 307–8 (editorial).
42. **British Medical Association.** *Alternative Therapy: Report of the Board of Science and Education.* London: BMA, 1986.
43. **British Medical Association.** *Complementary Medicine. New Approaches to Good Practice.* Oxford: Oxford University Press, 1993.
44. **Goldstein, M.** (2000). The culture of fitness and the growth of CAM. In *Complementary Medicine: Challenge and Change* (ed. M. Kelner and B. Wellman). Amsterdam: Harwood Academic Publishers.
45. **Cassidy, C.** (1998). Chinese medicine users in the United States. Part II: preferred aspects of care. *The Journal of Alternative and Complementary Medicine* **4**, 189–202.
46. **Sharma, U.** *Complementary Medicine Today: Practitioners and Patients.* London and New York: Tavistock/Routledge, 1992.
47. **Lupton, D.** (1997). Consumerism, reflexivity and the medical encounter. *Social Science and Medicine* **45** (3), 373–81.
48. **Mitchell, A. and Cormack, M.** *The Therapeutic Relationship in Complementary Health Care.* Edinburgh: Churchill Livingstone, 1998.
49. **Paterson, C. and Britten, N.** (2000). In pursuit of patient-centred outcomes: a qualitative evaluation of the Measure Yourself Medical Outcome Profile. *Journal of Health Services Research and Policy* **5**, 27–36.
50. **Paterson, C.** (2000). Primary Health Care transformed: complementary and orthodox medicine complementing each other. *Complementary Therapies in Medicine* **8** (1), 47–9.

3.7 Patients' expectations of treatment

Michel Wensing

Introduction

Many patients have specific expectations of primary medical care. An international study showed that patients expect to have enough time in the consultation with the care provider to talk about their health problem; to get adequate information and effective treatment; and that services for emergency health should be well organized.(1) Some patients may not have specific expectations, but only general ideas. A qualitative study suggested that their expectations may develop over time, as they get more experienced in primary medical care.(2) This chapter describes patients' expectations of primary medical care in more detail and discusses their relevance for care providers.

Knowing patients' expectations is important for a number of reasons. Firstly, it is an ethical imperative that health care meets patients' needs and preferences as much as possible, which implies that patients' expectations should be taken into account in the design and delivery of services. Secondly, effective treatment is based on adequate insight into patients' expectations of health care. For instance, a patient with low back pain who wants to know whether she has serious damage in her back is not effectively helped by advice to keep active. Thirdly, specific expectations can influence patients' health behaviour and effective use of treatment. For instance, patients may have hearing problems, but if they do not expect benefits from a hearing aid they will probably decide not to seek health care or use a hearing aid. So patients' expectations can directly influence functional health status and other outcomes of health care. Fourthly, in a competitive market patients' expectations are important because they influence the choice between different care providers. Fifthly, learning about patients' expectations can be educational for care providers, because it helps them to clarify their own expectations and to set priorities for learning and improvement.

Terminology is confusing in this area. This chapter focuses entirely on *normative expectations*, which are defined as patients' opinions about what should happen, either because it is desirable in itself or because it is related to specific values or objectives. *Descriptive expectations*, on the other hand, are ideas about what will actually happen, regardless of whether this is desired or not ('background expectations').(3) *Priorities* are normative expectations that are most important within a larger set of expectations. Patients' expectations can refer to the interaction with the care provider ('interaction expectations') or to the actions performed by the care provider ('action expectations').(3)

Expectations can be distinguished from other ideas and attitudes with respect to health care, such as: *experiences* which are perceptions of actual events or situations in health care; *satisfaction with care*, which is an evaluation of health care in terms of poor or excellent, for which expectations may be a frame of reference; *preferences*, which are opinions about what is the favourable alternative out of two or more alternatives, for instance, different treatment options, in a specific choice (Box 1).

Expectations can be held by individuals not seeking health care, although they may seek health information outside the health care setting; by patients or consumers, individuals who are actually seeking and using medical care; and by groups or organizations of patients, who have developed ideas and opinions about health care through discussions amongst themselves. These three groups do not necessarily have the same expectations, particularly if it is taken into account that time and money are limited. For instance, specific patients may prefer an expensive treatment, while citizens may prioritize preventive services for larger numbers of people. This chapter focuses on patients who seek primary medical care.

The remaining part of this chapter contains three sections. The first section describes patients' overall expectations of primary medical care; the second section focuses on patients' expectations of specific consultations; and the third section deals with patients' expectations of specific treatments. Each section also describes how well primary care physicians assess patients' expectations and how patients' expectations influence treatment provided in primary medical care. Where possible the chapter is based on research evidence. This chapter describes general trends in patients' expectations of primary medical care, but the reader should remember that individual patients may deviate from these overall trends. Patients' expectations vary across different patients, but also (within the same patient) across different health problems and different moments in time.

Box 1 Patients' expectations, health-related quality of life, and satisfaction with care(4)

Although measures of health-related quality of life (HRQL) are widely used, it is unclear whether individual patients conceptualize their health in the theoretical models used for HRQL. In particular, the source of items in the measures may reflect expert opinions rather than patients' own expectations. Patient expectations have been linked with satisfaction, but there is little empirical evidence for the theoretical models. Expectations may be tentative in nature and partly emerge from the consultation process itself. Expectations were explored in a qualitative interview study with 33 cardiac inpatients. The results were used to develop a questionnaire for assessing patients' expectations that was given to 400 cardiac patients. This study showed that the content of patients' expectations showed some overlap with the domains of the SF-36, a generic HRQL measure, but that patients seemed to adopt a broader approach to their health. For instance, patients emphasized aspects of the prognosis, such as knowing what will happen to their condition and chances of surviving. The authors conclude that the concept of patients' expectations differs from HRQL and from patient satisfaction with care.

Patients' overall expectations of primary medical care

A systematic review of the literature covering the period 1966 until 1995 provided 57 studies on patients' overall expectations of primary medical care.(5) This review focused on surveys with heterogenous patient samples in different primary care settings. Some studies included patients consulting the GP, while others included individuals independent of their visits to primary care. Box 2 reports on the importance rank order of patients' expectations, based on 19 studies that provided sufficient detailed information to categorize specific items into a pre-defined list of aspects of general practice.

The highest prioritized expectation proved to be 'humanity', that is, respect and personal interest for the patient as an individual. Highly prioritized were also 'professional competence' and 'adequate involvement in decisions'. The overall picture is that patients gave a very high priority to aspects of their communication with the care provider as well as the professional competence of the care provider, and (less strongly) effective treatment. They also prioritized the provision of specific services, such as preventives services, availability/accessibility, particularly availability in case of emergencies, and (less strongly) continuity of care. Patients did not prioritize organizational aspects: these aspects were less important than other aspects of care. Nevertheless, some of the aspects could be crucial for specific subgroups of patients, for instance, the care providers' support for his or her relatives is probably important for patients with chronic illness.

An international survey study of patients' priorities in general practice confirmed the results of this literature review.(1) This study focused on patients visiting the GP. Eight countries participated (Denmark, Germany,

Box 2 Overall rank order of patients' priorities[5] (based on 19 studies; percentage of studies with item in highest quartile)

1. Respect and personal interest for the patient as an individual (humanity) (86%).
2. Availability and adequate use of clinical knowledge and skills (competence) (64%).
3. Adequate involvement in decisions about treatment (63%).
4. Time for patient care (60%).
5. Other aspects of availability/accessibility, e.g. emergency care (60%).
6. Adequate provision of all relevant information (58%).
7. Exploring patients' needs and wishes with regard to treatment (57%).
8. Other aspects of relation/communication (57%).
9. Availability of special services, e.g. preventive screening and vaccination (57%).
10. Attention for the negative consequences of treatment for patients (50%).
11. Continuity over time (50%).
12. Effectiveness of treatment: improvement of patients' health status (33%).
13. Other aspects of medical care (33%).
14. Stimulating patients' self-management (33%).
15. Attention for patients' coping and psycho-social problems (counselling) (29%).
16. Short waiting time before a care provider can be consulted (25%).
17. Other aspects of information/support (20%).

Box 3 Top 10 priorities of patients in Europe[1] ($n = 3540$ patients from eight countries; range of percentages very/most important)

1. During the consultation a GP should have enough time to listen, talk, and explain to me (85–93%).
2. A GP should be able to provide quick service in case of emergencies (87–94%).
3. A GP should guarantuee the confidentiality of information about all his/her patients (77–88%).
4. A GP should tell me all I want to know about my illness (69–89%).
5. A GP should make me feel free to tell him or her about my problems (68–89%).
6. It should be possible to make an appointment with a GP at short notice (69–86%).
7. A GP should go to courses regularly to learn about recent medical developments (70–84%).
8. A GP should not only cure diseases, but also offer services to prevent disease (64–86%).
9. A GP should critically evaluate the usefulness of medicine and advice (66–79%).
10. A GP should explain the purpose of tests and treatment in detail (61–79%).

Israel, Netherlands, Norway, Portugal, Sweden, and United Kingdom) and the response rate was 55 per cent. Box 3 shows the 10 items that were most important for patients out of a list of 38 aspects. Highly prioritized were enough time in the consultation, availability in case of emergencies, and confidentiality of patient information. What is new compared to the literature is that patients highly prioritized the confidentiality of patient information and the possibility to make an appointment at short notice. A relatively low ranking was given to aspects such as waiting time before the consultation, GPs helping patients to deal with emotional problems, convenient facilities in the practice, concern about costs of medical treatment, written information on surgery hours, and phone numbers of the practice.

Do GPs and patients have different priorities, and are GPs well informed about the patients' priorities? A study in the Netherlands explored aspects of general practice prioritized differently by GPs and patients.[6] The study included a patient sample and two independent samples of GPs, each several hundreds of individuals. There was a high correlation between the priorities of patients and doctors, and doctors were also able to estimate the priorities of patients reasonably well. However, some differences were found as well. Patients gave, for instance, a higher rating than GPs to the provision of information on illness, getting an appointment within short notice, seeing the same GP at each visit, a GP who is willing to check health status regularly, and a GP who is easy to speak on the phone. GPs, on the other hand, gave a higher priority than patients to written information on practice organization, good cooperation between GP and staff, making visits to seriously ill patients, and a GP coordinating different types of care.

GPs proved to underestimate the value that patients attach to discussing the need for and usefulness of investigations, referrals, and medications, and to GPs going to courses regularly. So, professional competence and critical assessment of medical procedures were more important for patients than GPs thought. On the other hand, GPs overestimated the priority given by patients to showing a personal interest in patients' lives and to making home visits when patients are seriously ill. Personal attention may be important for specific sub-groups of patients, but not for the total patient population seen in primary care. Although GPs can estimate patients' expectations reasonably well, they should take into account that many patients expect the GP to be professionally competent and less focused on psycho-social issues than they might think patients expect.

Patients' expectations of consultations

This section focuses on expectations of individuals who seek primary medical care. Patients visit the GP if they think that the health problem threatens their health status and normal activities; it is not, or no longer, possible to cope with the problem alone; (primary) medical care can solve or reduce the problem; and the risks and costs of health care are acceptable.[7] These individuals primarily expect effective treatment. Another reason to visit the GP is a need for more or better information on the health problem and its treatment. A further reason is the advice to seek health care provided by family members, friends, mass media, or care providers. Such external triggers may result in less specific expectations of primary medical care (Box 4).

Box 4 Reasons to visit a GP[8]

A British study based on 500 consecutive patients showed that 33% consulted the doctor because the symptoms became worse, 30% came because the doctor had told them to come back, 27% visited the GP because the symptoms were interfering with their life, and 26% of the patients came because their own treatment did not work. Other reasons were: being worried about serious disease (14%), somebody had told them to go to the doctor (11%), a need for a specific explanation (11%), and need for a certificate (6%). There was considerable variation in the reasons for consulting a care provider, and many patients had more than one reason.

Most patients come to the consultation with a specific agenda. A content analysis of written agenda forms provided by 819 patients who consulted 46 GPs in the United Kingdom showed that patients typically brought one or two health problems (mean = 1.6, standard deviation = 1.0) and one or two symptoms (mean = 1.8, standard deviation = 1.0).[9] Most patients had a specific request, such as an explanation (which was expected by 69 per cent of the patients), a prescription (55 per cent), an investigation (44 per cent), an official certificate or a letter (15 per cent). As the percentages show, many patients had more than one request. This study did not address consultations that had been initiated by the doctor, for instance, to deliver preventive services.

Another British study among 824 patients who completed a pre-consultation questionnaire shows that many patients wanted a patient-centred approach, which implies good communication, partnership and health promotion (Box 5).[10] Only 14 per cent very strongly wanted full examination (54 per cent wanted this to some extent) and 5 per cent very strongly wanted a prescription (25 per cent to some extent). A desire for a prescription was positively associated with desire for good communication (odds ratio = 1.20), partnership (OR = 1.46), and health promotion (OR = 1.61). So patients' expectations of patient centredness may even be higher in patient populations with stronger preferences for a prescription.

A survey by Salmon and colleagues[11] distinguished between patients seeking global explanation, detailed information, medical treatment, or support. Strikingly, these expectations were almost unrelated to patients' physical symptoms (a list of 25 specific symptoms such as headache, sleeping problems, and dizziness). So, patients' physical and mental symptoms should be distinguished from expectations of the consultation with the care provider. The only clear predictor of patients' expectations was psychological distress, which was correlated to a higher desire for support. So, a primary care provider who knows patients' health problem and symptoms does not automatically know patients' expectations of care.

Several studies have shown that many patients desire information, regardless of what specific treatment is provided. Focus groups with patients identified a range of underlying reasons for expecting information: to understand what is wrong, to get a realistic idea of prognosis, to make the most of consultations, to understand the processes and likely outcomes of possible tests and treatments, to assist in self-care, to learn about available services and sources of help, to provide reassurance and help to cope, to help others to understand, to legitimize seeking help and their concerns, to learn how to prevent further illness, to identify further information and self-help groups, and to identify the 'best' health care providers.[12] The number of items on which patients desire information can be so high that the information should be spread over different consultations or it should be given outside the consultation.

Do patients want to be involved in decision-making in the consultation? The research literature suggests that patients' desire for information is stronger than their desire to be involved in decision-making.[13] It has been suggested that patients dislike the uncertainty of doctors related to shared decision-making.[14] Much of the research in the field of decision-making, however, used hypothetical questions and scenarios that may not truly reflect patients' views when they are actually taking part in a consultation. It is also unclear to what extent research findings from secondary care can be transferred to primary care.[15]

The study by Salmon and colleagues showed that doctors were able to detect patients' desire for support to some extent, but that they were insensitive to other expectations such as detailed information or medical treatment. Doctors recognized patients' distress, but not their need for information or effective treatment. Patients and doctors may also have different perceptions of patients' functional, psychological, and social factors related to the health problem. For instance, GPs were frequently unaware of functional disability, social factors, anxiety, and depression in their patients with osteoarthritis.[16] In the great majority of these cases, the GP was the only health professional involved. This implies that a primary care provider should explicitly address patients' expectations of the consultation.

Doctors' ideas of patients' expectations are an important predictor of the decisions in a consultation. For instance, doctor's perceptions of patients' expectations was a strong predictor of the decision to prescribe in a survey study in general practice.[17] In a British study with 544 patients consulting 15 GPs, the odds ratio of receiving a prescription was 2.34 if the patient hoped for it, but 7.04 if the doctor thought that the patient wanted a prescription. The writing of prescriptions was also associated with the doctor's sense of feeling pressured and to patients' ethnicity. If the GPs thought that the patient wanted a prescription, patients received it in 89 per cent of the cases. Other studies have shown similar findings (see Box 6). These studies suggest that a care provider should be careful with interpreting patients' expectations, because a wrong perception of patients' expectations can lead to inappropriate decisions.

Box 5 **Patients' expectations shortly before the consultation[10] (824 patients; percentage 'very strongly agree')**

1. Clearly explain what the problem is (45%).
2. Be friendly and approachable (42%).
3. Find out how serious my problem is (40%).
4. Clearly explain what should be done (40%).
5. Listen to everything I have to say about my problem (34%).
6. To feel really understood (34%).
7. Be interested in how the problem affects my life (29%).
8. Understand my main reason for coming (28%).
9. Deal with my worries about the problem (27%).
10. Discuss and agree with me what the problem is (27%).
11. Discuss and agree with me on treatmeent (27%).
12. Be interested in what I think the problem is (26%).
13. Be interested in what I want to know (24%).
14. Give advice on how to reduce the risk of future illness (24%).
15. Give advice on how to stay healthy in future (23%).
16. Give advice on what I can do (23%).
17. Be interested in what I want done (23%).
18. Be interested in what treatment I want (22%).
19. Understand my emotional needs (17%).
20. Examine me fully (14%).
21. Prescription (5%).

Box 6 **Patients' expectations and prescribing in general practice[18]**

A sample of 22 GPs in Australia recruited 336 patients with a newly diagnosed medical condition. About half of these patients received a prescription. The study compared patients' expectations and doctors' judgements of patients' expectations of receiving a prescription. When the patient did not expect a medication the practitioner's judgements of the patient's expectation agreed in 80% of cases and when the patient did expect a medication the practitioner's judgement agreed in 65% of cases. The doctors were more likely to ascribe an expectation of prescription to women than to men. After controlling for the presenting condition, patients who expected medication were nearly three times more likely to receive medication (OR = 2.9). A GP who thought that the patient expected medication was 10 times more likely to prescribe it (OR = 10.1). So, the strongest predictor of medication prescribing was not the patients' actual expectations but the practitioners' judgements of these expectations.

Patients' expectations of specific treatments

Treatment options in primary medical care include advice, medication, counselling, and referral to another care provider. Test ordering, preventive screening, and monitoring of chronic illness are also options. Patients' expectations of specific treatment options are embedded in 'lay theories' of a health problem. These are more or less consistent sets of ideas about the diagnosis, causes, prognosis, and treatment of the health problem. This section describes patients' expectations of specific options for treatment.

Test ordering

Diagnostic information is highly valued by many patients. Pregnant women who received prenatal care at a Health Maintenance Organization were prepared to pay considerable amounts of money for ultrasound while they knew it had no consequences for the medical treatment.(19) Many patients seem to value medical information related to their body for its own sake. Some patients explicitly request diagnostic tests, although health care professionals do not think they are necessary. For instance, a small study in which patients with acute upper gastrointestinal bleeding and primary care physicians considered alternative diagnostic strategies, using a formal decision-making process, showed that 92 per cent of these patients expected a gastrointestinal endoscopy against 52 per cent of the doctors.(20) These patients thought that diagnostic testing could prevent complications and identify the cause of the bleeding. The physicians did not necessarily wish to know the cause of the problem, because this knowledge did not influence their clinical treatment.

Advice

As was described in the previous section, many patients desire information regardless of what treatment is provided. In some cases advice is the only treatment provided, for instance, as part of a 'wait and see' approach. Patients (and doctors) may oppose this approach, because they perceive it as 'doing nothing'. If specific tools are used for providing advice, such as written information, illustrations and models, and computer output, this approach may be acceptable for more patients.

Medication

A qualitative study among 30 general practice patients revealed that patients had a range of positive and negative views on medication.(21) Drugs were seen as one of the benefits of modern medicine. Some medicines, such as penicillin, were accepted because they have been used for a long time. Individuals with positive views usually took their medication according to instructions. On the other hand, drugs were also seen by many as unnatural to the body, addictive and potentially damaging, for instance, because they reduce the body's ability to combat infection naturally. Some individuals felt that drugs dealt with the symptoms and not the cause of the disease. Some said they would not take medication if they could avoid it or if it was not really necessary. They would not start with the first symptom of discomfort or they would only use medication if the symptoms interfered with their performance at work. Previous experience of side-effects was also associated with negative views of drugs. Those with negative orientations or mixed views said they did not always take their medication as prescribed (Box 7).

Referral

Patients' expectations of referral are particularly relevant if formal permission from a primary care professional is needed to see the other health care professional. Some patients do not want to be referred, which can lead to potentially dangerous delays for treatment. For instance, older patients with stable angina feared hospitals, operations, and medical tests.(23) Another study among patients who had attended a hospital suggested that delays in referral and treatment in general practice were often associated with chronic health problems (such as persistent back pain), stigmatizing conditions (such as mental illness and alcohol dependency), and problems thought to be of psychological or social origin.(24)

Other patients expect to be referred. This may indicate a lack of trust in the competence and resources of the primary medical care provider or a strong belief in the competence and resources of the health professional the individual wants to be referred to. For instance, patients may value the expertise of the medical specialist and his extensive possibilities for performing diagnostic tests (e.g. X-rays in case of sprained ankle). Providing information on the diagnostic and therapeutic skills of primary care physicians and creating opportunities for patients to get positive experiences with primary care may change such expectations.

Box 7 Prescribing antibiotics for acute lower respiratory tract illness(22)

GPs recruited 787 adult patients who consulted with an acute lower respiratory illneess, defined as new cough and at least one other symptom, including sputum production, dyspnoea, wheeze, or chest pain for which there was no obvious explanation. Most patients thought that their problem was caused by infection (87%). Most patients wanted antibiotics (72%) and had expected to be prescribed them in this consultation (72%). One-fifth explicitly asked for antibiotics (19%). Of the patients who thought their symptoms were caused by an infection 90% considered antibiotics would help compared to 49% who did not think that they had an infection. Of the patients who wanted antibiotics 90% expected to be prescribed them compared with 17% who had not wanted them. The GPs said that of the patients who received antibiotics only one-fifth absolutely needed them (20%) and about a one-fifth did not need them (22%). The GPs also said that non-clinical factors influenced their decision to prescribe antibiotics in 44% of the cases. Most often mentioned were patients' expectations, social factors for the patient, and the GP's expectation that the patient would otherwise return.

Prevention

Activities to prevent health problems are highly valued by patients,(1) but patients' expectations may, on the other hand, prevent a healthy life-style. In one study, smokers had 'already made their own evaluation about smoking, did not believe doctors' words could influence their smoking, believed that quitting was down to the individual, and felt that doctors who took the opportunity to talk about smoking should focus on the individual patient'.(25) The smokers anticipated that they would be given antismoking advice by the doctor; and this realization influenced the health care seeking behaviour of some of them. The authors concluded that doctor–patient relationships can be damaged if doctors routinely advise all smokers to quit.

A qualitative study on immunization of babies suggested that mothers prefer the general practice over health centres for immunization of babies.(26) GPs were seen as more like to explore worries and to offer explanations. 'Mothers valued highly those immunising health professionals who engaged their baby, touched, spoke to or induced a smile from their baby, encouraged them to cuddle their baby in the immediate aftermath and whose demeanour seemed to acknowledge the emotional pain they, the mothers, were experiencing'.(26)

Disease monitoring

Most patients with chronic illness receive long-term primary medical care. A qualitative study with asthma patients suggested that some patients wished to be seen regularly in the clinic and others wished to attend only when needing help.(27) The majority of these patients were in favour of asthma care aiming to teach people to manage their asthma for themselves. Some of the patients who wished to manage their asthma actively also wished to be seen in the clinic regularly, because it gave them the confidence to take responsibility for their asthma the rest of the time. Some patients thought that a specialized asthma nurse knows more about asthma than a doctor, but several people had reservations about seeing the nurse, especially when the asthma was more severe.

On the other hand, patients with mild to moderate asthma may not regard it as a chronic disease that needs regular monitoring and therapeutic adjustments.[28] These patients prefer 'to manage asthma as an intermittent acute disorder, and they are uncomfortable with a guided self-management plan that reinforces asthma as a chronic, ongoing disease needing monitoring and managing'. They emphasized that they knew their body best and knew best what drugs worked for them. These attitudes may explain poor attendence of asthma clinics and adherence to self-management plans among these patients. GPs were ambivalent about self-management plans, but nurses thought that ongoing patient education and monitoring was crucial for these patients.

Conclusions

Most patients expect primary medical care to meet high standards of professional competence; they want appropriate information about their health problem and its treatment; and they desire patient-centred communication. Organizational aspects tend to be less important, but primary medical care should be sufficiently available and accessible, particularly in case of emergencies. Individual patients may have specific expectations that differ from these overall trends. For instance, patients with chronic illness may value specific aspects higher. On the other hand, groups and organizations of patients and consumers at local and national levels may emphasize other aspects, because their ideas are influenced by each other.[29]

Patients' expectations are important, because these influence their behaviour and, in many situations, the care providers' decisions. Primary care providers can reasonably estimate patients' expectations, but they can have misconceptions. The care provider should, therefore, explore explicitly patients' expectations and the patient should express his or her expectations clearly. Discrepancies between patients' expectations of care and professional standards should be solved by finding a balance between being responsive to patients' needs and convincing patients about the need to adhere to professional standards.

Acknowledgement

I thank Richard Grol, Hans Peter Jung, and the editors of this section for their comments on earlier versions of the chapter.

References

1. **Grol, R., Wensing, M., Mainz, J., Ferreira, P., Hearnshaw, H., Hjortdahl, P., Olesen, F., Ribacke, M., Spenser, T., and Szécsényi, J.** (1999). Patients' priorities with respect to general practice care: an international comparison. *Family Practice* **16**, 4–11.
2. **Fitzpatrick, A. and Hopkins, A.** (1983). Problems in the conceptual framework of patient satisfaction: an empirical exploration. *Sociology of Health and Illness* **3**, 297–311.
3. **Stimson, G. and Webb, B.** *Going to See the Doctor: The Consultation Process in General Practice.* London and Boston: Routledge and Kegan Paul, 1975.
4. **Staniszewska, S.** (1999). Patient expectations and health-related quality of life. *Health Expectations* **2**, 93–104.
5. **Wensing, M., Jung, H.P., Mainz, J., Olesen, F., and Grol, R.** (1998). Which aspects of general practice care are important for patients? A systematic literature review. *Social Science and Medicine* **47**, 1573–88.
6. **Jung, H.P., Wensing, M., and Grol, R.** (1997). What makes a good general practitioner: do patients and doctors have different views? *British Journal of General Practice* **47**, 805–9.
7. **Van de Kar, A.** et al. (1992). Why do patients consult the general practitioner? Determinants of their decision. *British Journal of General Practice* **42**, 313–16.
8. **Martin, E., Russell, D., Goodwin, S., Chapman, R., North, M., and Sheridan, P.** (1991). Why patients consult and what happens when they do. *British Medical Journal* **303**, 289–92.
9. **McKinley, R.K. and Middleton, J.F.** (1999). What do patients want from doctors? Content analysis of written patient agendas for the consultation. *British Journal of General Practice* **49**, 796–800.
10. **Little, P., Everitt, H., Williamson, I., Warner, G., Moore, M., Gould, C., Ferrier, K., and Payne, S.** (2001). Preferences of patients for patient centred approach to consultation in primary care: observational study. *British Medical Journal* **322**, 1–7.
11. **Salmon, P., Sharma, N., Valori, R., and Bellenger, N.** (1994). Patients' intentions in primary care: relationship to physical and psychological symptoms, and their perceptions by general practitioners. *Social Science and Medicine* **38**, 585–92.
12. **Coulter, A., Entwistle, V., and Gilbert, D.** (1999). Sharing decisions with patients: is the information good enough? *British Medical Journal* **318**, 318–22.
13. **Guagdagnoli, E. and Ward, P.** (1998). Patient participation in decision-making. *Social Science and Medicine* **47**, 329–39.
14. **Logan, R.L. and Scott, P.J.** (1996). Uncertainty in clinical practice: implications for quality and cost of health care. *Lancet* **347**, 595–8.
15. **Elwyn, G., Edwards, A., and Kinnersley, P.** (1999). Shared decision-making in primary care: the neglected second half of the consultation. *British Journal of General Practice* **49**, 477–82.
16. **Memel, D.S., Kirwan, J.R., Sharp, D., and Hehir, M.** (2000). General practitioners miss disability and anxiety as well as depression in their patients with osteoarthritis. *British Journal of General Practice* **50**, 645–8.
17. **Britten, N. and Ukoumunne, O.** (1997). The influence of patients' hopes of receiving a prescription on doctors' perceptions and the decision to prescribe: a questionnaire study. *British Medical Journal* **315**, 1506–10.
18. **Cockburn, J. and Pit, S.** (1997). Prescribing behaviour in clinical practice: patients' expectations and doctors' perceptions of patients' expectations—a questionnaire study. *British Medical Journal* **315**, 520–3.
19. **Berwick, D.M. and Weinstein, M.C.** (1985). What do patients value? Willingness to pay for ultrasound in normal pregnancy. *Medical Care* **23**, 881–93.
20. **Dolan, J.G., Bordley, D.R., and Miller, H.** (1993). Diagnostic strategies in the management of acute upper gastrointestinal bleeding: patient and physician preferences. *Journal of General Internal Medicine* **8**, 525–9.
21. **Britten, N.** (1994). Patients' ideas about medicines: a qualitative study in a general practice population. *British Journal of General Practice* **44**, 465–8.
22. **MacFarlane, J., Holmes, W., MacFarlane, R., and Britten, N.** (1997). Influence of patients' expectations on antibiotic management of acute lower respiratory tract illness in general practice: questionnaire study. *British Medical Journal* **315**, 1211–14.
23. **Gardner, K. and Chapple, A.** (1999). Barriers to referral in patients with angina: qualitative study. *British Medical Journal* **319**, 418–21.
24. **Preston, C., Cheater, F., Baker, R., and Hearnshaw, H.** (1999). Left in limbo: patients' views on care across the primary/secondary interface. *Quality in Health Care* **8**, 16–21.
25. **Butler, C.C., Pill, R., and Stott, N.C.H.** (1998). Qualitative study of patients' perceptions of doctors' advice to quit smoking: implications for opportunistic promotion. *British Medical Journal* **316**, 1878–81.
26. **Harrington, P.M., Woodman, C., and Shannon, W.F.** (2000). Low immunisation uptake: is the process the problem? *Journal of Epidemiology and Community Health* **54**, 394–400.
27. **Paterson, C. and Britten, N.** (2000). Organising primary health care for people with asthma: the patient's perspective. *British Journal of General Practice* **50**, 299–303.
28. **Jones, A., Pill, R., and Adams, S.** (2000). Qualitative study of views of health professonals and patients on guided self management plans for asthma. *British Medical Journal* **321**, 1507–10.
29. **Williamson, C.** (2000). Consumer and professional standards: working towards consensus. *Quality in Health Care* **9**, 190–4.

4

Descriptive epidemiology

4 Descriptive epidemiology

4.1 The iceberg of illness

Ruut A. de Melker

Introduction

Although general practitioners (GPs) are supposed to have a complete overview of medical histories of their practice populations, this is untrue. Most illnesses are *not* presented to the GP. And how should we know whether all chronic diseases are completely detected and registered? Several studies show that in a period of 14 days to 2 months, 65–95 per cent of respondents experience one or more symptoms.[1–6] Ten to 20 per cent of all these illnesses are presented to the GP.[3,5] As on average 1 or 2 days a week respondents have complaints about their health, it is clear that health does not mean total physical, mental, and social well-being.[7]

In this chapter we will present definitions and describe measurement problems in health surveys, total and hidden illnesses and diseases. We will discuss changes in the iceberg over time and between (sub)cultures, including differences between families. Finally, the consequences of the iceberg phenomenon will be discussed.

Definitions and concepts

Health is defined by the World Health Organization (WHO) as 'a state of complete physical, mental and social well-being and not as merely the absence of disease or infirmity'.[1,8] Other definitions underline the dynamic aspect of health and the capacity of the individual or group to cope with all living circumstances.[8] The *metaphor of 'the iceberg' of morbidity* represents the presented morbidity as the '*tip of the iceberg*' as a fraction of total morbidity in a population, including the reservoir of hidden morbidity: *the 'iceberg under water'* (see Fig. 1).[1,5,6,8,9] The *submerged portion of the iceberg*, the 'hidden' morbidity below the water surface, comprises diseases not medically attended, medically attended but not accurately diagnosed, and diagnoses not reported to GPs.[8] The iceberg metaphor relates not only to objective morbidity ('disease') but also to subjective experiences ('illness'). *Disease* is a physiological/psychological dysfunction and *illness* is a subjective state of the person who feels aware of not being well.[1,8] So the words disease and illness are not synonymous.

Can we compare findings of different studies?

Reliable measurement of health status and illnesses is difficult. Self-reports of various aspects of health have been widely used in health surveys. Surveys are more efficient for getting data from large samples than for instance

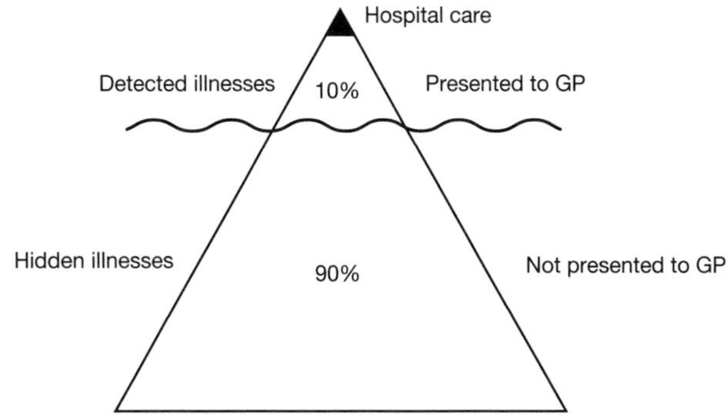

Fig. 1 The iceberg of illnesses above and below the water surface.

examinations by physicians. However, data from surveys register only symptoms and do not classify diseases according to doctors' criteria. Some researchers ask for experiences, either 'ever' or in a specified period, of common symptoms or conditions such as asthma, headache, migraine and so on.[10] Other researchers ask for reports of experiences of acute or chronic illnesses and for the name of this condition afterwards.[10] Survey health interviews and health diaries often lead to different results.[11] Checklists are sensitive to psychological distress and not limited to physical illness alone. Open-ended questions prevent biased responses, but result in fewer symptoms recorded. Health diaries with open-ended questions 'produce' more symptoms, but take more effort complete, requiring motivated respondents. Comparisons among more than 1000 volunteers of reported symptoms and seriousness of colds, with assessments by a trained clinical observer, showed extremely high correlations for all ages, occupation and marital status. Men were significantly more likely than women to over-rate their symptoms in comparison with the clinical observer.[11]

Exploring the iceberg of illnesses

High frequency of symptoms in populations

Although most repondents report in health surveys at least some complaints, still most of them asses themselves as 'healthy'.[3,7] In a large interview survey in Glasgow, United Kingdom, nearly 90 per cent of responding adults and children reported at least one physical symptom in a 2-week period with a mean of more than four per person, maximum 25. Only 14 per cent had no illnesses at all during this period.[2] In an American study, 31 per cent of men had symptoms in a 6 weeks registration compared to 43 per cent of females.[6] In a Dutch study, respondents reported 1 day with symptoms every 3–4 days. Half of them reported less than 7 days with symptoms and one out of seven reported no symptoms during a 4-week period.[5] There are large differences between respondents according to age, sex, and culture.[2,3,5,12] Elderly people and females experience more symptoms than

Table 1 The top 10 symptoms in two health surveys

Symptom	Prevalence (%)
A. (Hannay)[2] $n = 1344$ (symptoms of chronic diseases included; mental, social, behavioural problems *not* included)	
1. Stuffy/runny nose	27
2. Cough now or past 2 weeks	21
3. More tired than usual	20
4. Headache	17
5. Bunions, corns, callosities	14
6. Phlegm now or during past 2 weeks	13
7. Rash or irritation	13
8. Shortness of breath when hurrying on level ground or walking up slight hill	12
9. Usually cough first thing on getting up	12
10. Varicose veins	11
B. (van de Lisdonk)[5] $n = 277$ (mental symptoms included, symptoms of chronic diseases *not* included)	
1. Fibrositis	45
2. Headache	34
3. Common cold	24
4. Abdominal pain	18
5. Menstrual pain	10
6. Tiredness	8
7. Small injuries	8
8. Nervous disorders	7
9. Dermatitis	4
10. Vomiting and/or diarrhoea	4

younger subjects and males.[5–7] A study in a very elderly cohort showed a high prevalence of reported physical symptoms, which increased with age. Still 70 per cent of respondents rated their health as 'good' or 'very good'.[7] In a Dutch study, 5 per cent reported no complaints during 2 weeks, nearly a third 1–3, half 4–10, and 20 per cent more than 10 complaints. Parents reported more symptoms than their children and mothers more than fathers.[3]

Common symptoms well known to GPs

In the survey in Glasgow, respiratory symptoms—rhinorrhoea and cough—tiredness and headache were the most common symptoms (Table 1A). Half of adults had one or more mental symptoms in a 2-week period, for example, anxiety, depression, paranoid ideas (not in table). A quarter of children showed behavioural symptoms, for example, developmental, school problems (not in table). Almost a quarter of adults had at least one social problem, such as unemployment, financial problems (not in table).[2] In a smaller Dutch study, fibrositis, headache, common cold, and abdominal pain were the most common complaints (Table 1B).[5] In the UK study, data were collected with a coded questionnaire during home interviews. Mental problems were classified separately and not included in the table.[2] In the Dutch survey, data were collected with day-to-day reporting avoiding daily registration of complaints of chronic diseases. These complaints were registered with a checklist separately and in contrast to the British study, not included in the table. On the other hand, in the Dutch study, psycho-social problems were, contrary to the British one, included in the daily registration printed in the table.[5] This explains why the list of top 10 illnesses in the Dutch study does not contain complaints of chronic diseases like phlegm and shortness of breath and the UK one, no mental problems. However, complaints such as the common cold (rhinorrhoea and cough), headache and tiredness are on the top 10 list in both studies.[2,5] In most studies, respiratory and muscoskeletal problems are most commonly reported.[2,5,6]

Exploring the iceberg of diseases

The iceberg of *diseases* below the water surface consists of sub-clinical and undiagnosed diseases such as diabetes, glaucoma, and tuberculosis as shown by Last.[1] A prevalence of sub-clinical coeliac disease of more than

Table 2 Estimated prevalences presented, total, and 'hidden' chronic diseases in the Netherlands, numbers (% presented/total morbidity)

Disease	Presented	Total	'Hidden'	Presented/ total (%)
Contact eczema	109.100	745.700	636.600	15
Depression	78.900	484.200	405.300	16
Dementia	32.600	162.400	129.800	20
Age-related macula degeneration	19.100	58.600	39.500	33
Hearing loss	498.100	1384.400	886.300	36
M Parkinson	23.500	44.500	21.000	53
Rheumatoid arthritis	80.700	145.400	64.700	56
Diabetes	268.300	442.300	174.000	61
Heart failure	93.500	147.100	53.600	64
Arthrosis	403.000	548.400	145.400	73
Apoplexia	83.900	100.200	16.300	84

Source: National Institute for Public Health and the Environment, Bilthoven, the Netherlands.[18]

three per 1000 was found after screening more than 3000 students aged 11–15 years.[13] Cases of invasive group A streptococcal infection seem to reflect the tip of the iceberg with regard to the burden of colonization of a specific invasive streptococcal clone in the community.[14] In a study among 15-year-olds the self-reported rate of psychiatric morbidity was seven times greater than that suggested by their medical records.[15] Hidden cases of bulimia nervosa are relatively common in general practice.[16] The elderly seem to be a risk group for 'hidden' morbidity. In a recent British study, patients under 75 years of age with stable angina pectoris patients felt old, had low expectations of treatment and knew little about new developments in treatment of angina.[17] In a Dutch governmental paper, the iceberg of 'hidden' diseases was estimated by comparing results of morbidity studies in health care with population based studies.[18] Prevalences of nearly all chronic conditions are one to two times higher in population-based studies compared to registrations of presented cases in general practice and hospitals. Mental disturbances are 3–15 times more frequent in populations compared to registrations of presented morbidity, for anxiety even 40 times (Table 2). These estimations should be interpreted carefully, because different sources have been used with complex classification problems. Fifty six per cent of men and 49 per cent of women reported 'no diseases' at all. For chronic diseases these percentages were higher: 71 and 69 per cent, respectively. These values were 60 per cent for England and 77 per cent for Sweden.[18] There are several explanations for this hidden part of the iceberg of diseases. Firstly, many persons (even with serious complaints) do not ask for professional help. People with certain mental problems can bypass the GP and present these to institutions with free access. Clinicians will often use more strict diagnostic criteria than epidemiologists in population-based studies. Finally physicians can mis-diagnose symptoms, because the clinical picture is not (yet) clear or is non-specific.[18] The iceberg below the water surface is relatively large for contact eczema, depression, dementia, age-related macular degeneration, and hearing problems.

The iceberg and the GP

As most illnesses are *not* presented to the GP, professional health care is confronted with a small and selected part of total morbidity. In the Glasgow study, a quarter of all physical symptoms were presented to professionals, while 17 per cent of mental and half of social symptoms were.[2] This may reflect the non-acceptance of mental problems. About 10 per cent of physical, mental, and social symptoms are presented to lay and informal care. Behavioural symptoms lead in 20 per cent to lay care.

For GPs it is very important to know that self-care is most important. Several studies show that on average 10–20 per cent of all experienced symptoms only are presented to the GP.[3,5,9] Although self-reliance in their own capacity to cope with daily illnesses seems well developed, some symptoms lead more often to professional care than others. In a Dutch study the proportion of cases presented to GPs were higher for trauma, skin, and psychological problems, and of abdominal and lower respiratory tract symptoms lower than average (10 per cent). Twenty per cent of respondents consulted their GP during the 4-week study: mothers more than fathers and children less than their parents (Table 3).[5] In an American study, medical care was sought for only 3 per cent of musculoskeletal and respiratory symptoms.[6]

Are GPs aware of 'hidden' serious symptoms?

It is a misunderstanding to think that 'hidden' illnesses represent non-serious symptoms. A Dutch study shows that the greatest portion of these serious symptoms are never seen by any physician (Table 4).[3] This study was carried out in a stable general practice population in the Netherlands, a country with a listing system and well-defined practice population. However, during the years after this study these serious symptoms never came to light. In another study doctors expressed a greater need for treatment than patients. This difference was greater for non-serious than for serious symptoms.[19] In the Glasgow survey, the degree of incongruous 'referral', defined as either failure to consult with symptoms assessed by patients themselves as 'serious' or consulting for symptoms assessed as 'minor', was estimated. All symptoms were graded for pain, disability, seriousness, and duration, with patients' or parents' own assessment. For each subject, a severity score was calculated. Twenty-six per cent of respondents with physical, mental, or behavioural symptoms did not seek professional help for serious symptoms. On the other hand, 11 per cent sought professional help for minor symptoms. Failure to consult for serious symptoms was significantly associated with neuroticism, poor past and present health, increasing age, and female sex. Consultation for minor symptoms was associated with a greater number of present illnesses, divorce/separation, increasing age, female sex, few years in present residence, poor experience with doctors, difficulties to contact doctors, and number of hospital stays.[2]

Table 3 Presented symptoms to GPs, percentages of total complaints of participating repondents and their family members

Traumata	17
Skin symptoms	16
Psychological	13
Musculoskeletal	11
Upper respiratory tract	9
Circular tract	7
Urogenital tract	7
Digestive tract	3
Lower respiratory tract	1

n = 580 complaints; on average 10% of complaints were presented.

n = 277 respondents; on average 20% of respondents, of participating mothers 25, of fathers 16, of daughters 12, and of sons 3% were presented.

Source: van de Lisdonk.[5]

Table 4 'The iceberg below the water surface' of more or less serious symptoms, percentages of respondents with certain symptoms and percentages of symptoms not presented to GPs; (n = 631 respondents)

Symptom	Respondents with symptom (%)	'Hidden' (%)
Pain on chest	6	90
Short of breath	6	85
Heart palpitation	5	86
Hoarseness	5	92
Wheezing	3	84
Swallowing problems	4	88
Lumps, swollen glands	2	85
Weight loss	3	84
Abnormal loss blood	2	75
Micturition problems	3	90
Haematuria	<1	50

Source: Huygen et al.[3]

Key points

- Although GPs encounter nearly all listed patients in 3 years, they see just the tip of an iceberg of illnesses and diseases.
- About 80–90 per cent of illnesses are hidden 'below the water surface'.
- Even a lot of serious complaints are not presented to the GP, although these mostly show a self-limiting course.
- The iceberg of diseases under the water surface contains undetected chronic diseases varying from a high degree of undetected mental problems, hearing loss, coeliac disease to a lower number of cases with diabetes mellitus and epilepsy.

Does the GP knows best?

For physicians it can be difficult to accept that their medical construction of clinical reality, based on pathology, is only one of many possible constructions.[3,9] The meaning and interpretation of a symptom is an individual one and relates to three personal factors. Firstly, the extent to which these are perceived as threatening, disruptive, and painful. Secondly, the familiarity and the perceived personal responsibility for their occurence. Finally, how embarrassing the symptoms are.[20] Although results of health surveys suggest women's morbidity and need for medical care to be higher than men's, this is relative. In one study, 40 per cent of the higher overall female morbidity were gynaecological–obstetric diagnoses. One-fifth of the overall sex differences accounted for psychosomatic symptoms.[21] Another study did not support the widely suggested explanation for gender differences in consulting GPs that perceived symptoms by women are more frequently presented than those of men.[22]

The changing pattern of the iceberg of illnesses

The dynamic pattern of illness and disease

The iceberg is a dynamic pattern of illnesses and diseases depending on time, country, culture, and sub-culture. Scientific knowledge increases and interpretations change. So opinions of physicans and expectations of patients will change over time, especially in response to the Internet and the media. In the past a child's earache was accepted as a self-limiting *illness* belonging to normal life. It was treated with reassurance and simple medication. Nowadays it is a highly over-treated *disease.*[23,24] (Sub)culture is the most important determinant for a persons' interpretation of his/her illness and expectations of the physician.[12,23] For instance, the duration of illnesses depends mainly on cultural factors in different countries.[12] Medical treatment differs all over the world. Dutch doctors prescribe antibiotics in about 20 per cent of cases of acute otitis media, in contrast with nearly 100 per cent in most other countries.[24] In Germany, low blood pressure is treated as a disease; in the United States, it is rewarded with reduced insurance rates.[23] Medicine itself is a sub-culture with its own set of unstated assumptions and expectations.[9] A patient entering this medical sub-culture is like a traveller visiting a foreign country.[9]

GPs' specialty: the family

The most important sub-culture relating to the iceberg phenomenon is *the family*. The sense of well-being and the number of symptoms experienced are significantly correlated between family members. The same is true for readiness to seek medical help. Huygen found strong inter-relationships of frequency of illnesses between parents and children. These associations tended to be stable over the years.[25] The family is an *epidemiological unit*, because of shared living conditions such as housing, environment, and hygiene. Moreover, it is a *social unit*, because of shared illness and help-seeking behaviour and self-care activities. Although most respondents showed in surveys much self-reliance for common diseases, there are clear differences between families in the need for professional care for these mostly self-limiting diseases.[3,5,25] The tip of the iceberg is greater for smaller families and mothers showing neurotic instability. The same is true for children with neurotic parents.[25] Finally, the iceberg relates to specific circumstances and life events.[9] So the iceberg 'above the water surface', is for some families far greater than for others. Family medicine means that the family is the unit of thinking, diagnosing, and management.

Key points

- Family medicine means that the family is the unit of thinking, diagnosing, and management.
- The family sharing common pathogenic factors is an epidemiological unit: there are strong inter-relationships of frequency of illness between family members.
- The family is a social unit: there are strong inter-relationships of illness behaviour between parents and children.

More attention for the iceberg phenomenon in medical research

The iceberg phenomenon has major consequences for evidence-based medicine and makes clear that the development of more dynamic definitions is a major scientific challenge. These should underline the great importance of adequate coping mechanisms. Health could be defined as 'the optimal dynamic balance of all capacities to cope with life problems, illnesses and diseases'.[8] Medical research should focus more on the iceberg below the water surface. What is the natural course of the illnesses never seen by doctors? Do these ilnesses differ from those seen in health care? Are people themselves better 'doctors' than the professional ones? So the importance of the self-limiting course of most illnesses seems to be highly underestimated by the medical world. The effectiveness of self-care activities needs to be given more attention in medical research.

Changing focus of health care policy

The need for a shift in medical thinking

There is a need for a shift in medical thinking. On the level of *public health*, medical policy should focus more on health education to improve self-care of self-limiting common diseases. Most common illnesses need no medication or intervention. Professional care can be even dangerous, because of side-effects, somatization, and medicalization.[3,9,25] On the other hand, more systematic attention should be paid to early detection, treatment, and control of those individuals at risk for certain chronic diseases, for which detection has been proven to be cost-effective. On the level of *primary and hospital care* doctors should be aware of the consequences of the iceberg phenomenon. As an example: as GPs see during an outbreak only the tip of the iceberg of invasive group A streptococcal infections, they should be aware of the circulation of virulent clones in their practice populations. The high number of asymptomatic carriers are a major threat for those at high risk for invasive bacteria such as the elderly and other patient groups.[14] So the focus of care should be populations and families at risk instead of only individuals presenting symptoms. As a consequence, people should be well informed. In modern times this should be possible with the help of information communication technology.

Are patients well informed nowadays?

Nowadays people are often misinformed by the media, that only show the triumphs of medicine (see Chapter 3.4). Information about the limitations of medicine is not 'sensational news'. The impressive development of medical knowledge and technology has led to a new belief of limitless progress of medicine solving all health disturbances and life problems.[26] Results of research are however unpredictable. Most successes were a matter of 'trial and error', luck, and positive surprises after a lot of negative surprises. No one can predict new successes and further progress is bounded by limitations of research.[26]

Early detection of chronic diseases: should we do it?

Wilson and Junger formulated 10 criteria to determine the need for screening programmes.[9,27] The disease in question should be a serious health problem, treatment in an early phase should be effective and acceptable, screening tests should be sensitive and specific and the screening procedure cost-effective. In most cases, these criteria are difficult to fulfil.[9] For some chronic diseases, for instance depression and hearing loss, the iceberg under water seems relatively large. However, various studies showed that the spectrum of depression in general practice differs from that in psychiatric practice. A much larger proportion of patients in general practice have mild depression and one can doubt whether treatment is always necessary.[9] One can expect that undetected cases show at least the same mild course as those diagnosed in general practice.

Key points

- The iceberg phenomenon shows that the focus of medical thinking should be changed from patients presenting symptoms to populations and families at risk.
- In general, it is not worthwhile to bring all hidden chronic diseases above the water surface.
- Specific criteria can inform the GP which cases should be detected, for instance risk factors for heart diseases, heart failure, and coeliac disease.
- Health education is an important activity to improve and stimulate self-care for common self-limiting diseases.

One can doubt if it is effective to detect more hearing problems knowing treatment with hearing aids is only effective in selected serious cases. It seems more appropiate to focus on specific information and health education for those at risk, as for instance the elderly. On the other hand, some chronic diseases seem to meet the criteria mentioned above. In a study in more than 3000 students, screening for coeliac disease was feasible and involved only slight discomfort to the population. The number of detected cases was more than three per 1000 and an effective and simple intervention is available: gluten-free diet.[13] European studies suggest that there is an increasing epidemic of heart failure. Most cases are asymptomatic, but treatment with angiotensin-converting enzyme inhibitors has been found effective in randomized trials.[28]

Early detection of chronic diseases: how should we do it?

Early detection does not necessarily mean large-scale screening programmes; case-finding may be a good alternative. Case-finding is the active and specific detection of certain diseases during contacts with patients unrelated to the presented complaints.[9] The method is cheap, easy to perform, and more cost-effective compared to screening programmes.

Case-finding in general practice: simple and effective

Case-finding is the method of choice in general practice, because GPs are confronted with about three-quarters of their practice population in 1 year and nearly all patients in 3 years.[9,25] Case-finding is most effective and efficient when it focuses on specific risk groups and risk profiles based on registration data, as for instance familial disease and lifestyle factors such as smoking.[9] For example, in a 55-year-old obese manager, smoking cigarettes and with a family history of coronary diseases and presenting a skin disease, the GP measures the blood pressure, determines weight and height, and carries out tests for diabetes mellitus and cholesterol levels. Surveillance of risk groups by GPs is closely interwoven with curative care (see Chapter 5.2).

Key points

- Case-finding and surveillance of risk groups is most appropiate in general practice.
- Each contact with a patient could be used to identify unknown risk factors and diseases.
- The lesson of the iceberg phenomenon is that GPs should look far beyond presented cases to work effectively and efficiently.

The consequences and management of detected cases can be discussed by the GP with his or her patients without any complex administrative procedures. Information can be given in line with past medical history, living conditions, and other family factors. This has the great advantage of a lower chance for medicalization and somatization, compared to screening programmes. So the lesson of the iceberg phenomenon is that GPs, in general, can work effectively and efficiently with surveillance of risk groups and looking beyond presented symptoms.

Health education: the most effective intervention for GPs?

Families with high consumption of health care for common illnesses should be approached as risk groups in an attempt to improve self-reliance by explanation, health education, and support. Self-reliance relates to insight into possibilities of self-care and support systems of family members and others.[5] High consumers are at risk for the life problems such as divorce and unemployment.[25] Low consumers, such as the elderly, adolescents, and people with poor health, are at risk for under-reporting serious diseases.[2] Health education is not only a task for GPs, but even more for health visitors, practice nurses, other health personnel, and the media.

References

1. **Last, J.M.** (1963). The iceberg: 'completing the clinical picture in general practice'. *Lancet* **II**, 28–31.
2. **Hannay, D.R.** *The Symptom Iceberg: A Study of Community Health.* London: Routledge & Kegan Paul, 1979.
3. **Huygen, F.J.A., Van den Hoogen, H., and Neefs, W.J.** (1983). Gezondheid en ziekte; een onderzoek van gezinnen. (Health and disease; a study of families.) *Nederlands Tijdschrift Geneeskunde* **127**, 1612–19.
4. **Folmer, H.R.** *Huisarts en ijsberg.* (General Practitioner and iceberg). Thesis, University of Utrecht, Avanti, Zaltbommel 1968 (Summary in English).
5. **van de Lisdonk, E.H.** (1989). Perceived and presented morbidity in general practice. *Scandinavian Journal of Primary Health Care* **7**, 73–8.
6. **Verbrugge, L.M. and Ascione, F.J.** (1987). Exploring the iceberg: common symptoms and how people care for them. *Medical Care* **25**, 539–69.
7. **Dening, T.R.** et al. (1998). Changes in self-rating health, disability and contact with services in a very elderly cohort: a 6-year follow-up study. *Age and Ageing* **27**, 23–33.
8. **Last, J.M.**, ed. *A Dictionary of Epidemiology.* Oxford: Oxford University Press, 1988.
9. **McWhinney, I.R.** *A Textbook of Family Medicine.* Oxford: Oxford University Press, 1989.
10. **Maccintyre, S. and Pritchard, C.** (1989). Comparisons between the self-asessed and observer-assessed presence and severity of colds. *Social Science and Medicine* **29**, 1243–89.
11. **Kooiker, S.E.** (1995). Exploring the iceberg of morbidity: a comparison of different survey methods for assessing the occurence of everyday illness. *Social Science and Medicine*, **41**, 317–32.
12. **De Melker, R.A., Touw-Otten, F.W.M.M., and Kuyvenhoven, M.M.** (1997). Transcultral differences in illness behaviour and clinical outcome: an underestimated aspect of general practice. *Family Practice*, **14**, 472–7.
13. **Catassi, C.** et al. (1994). Coeliac disease in the year 2000: exploring the iceberg. *Lancet* **343**, 200–3.
14. **Cockerill, F.R.** et al. (1997). An outbreak of invasive group A streptococcal disease associated with high carriage rates of the invasive clone among school-aged children. *Journal of the American Medical Association* **277**, 38–43.
15. **Potts, Y., Gillies, M.L., and Wood, S.F.** (2001). Lack of mental wellbeing in 15-year-olds: an undisclosed iceberg? *Family Practice* **18**, 95–100.
16. **Whitehouse, A.M.** et al. (1992). Prevalence of eating disorders in three Cambridge general practices: hidden and conspicuous morbidity. *British Journal of General Practice* **42**, 57–60.
17. **Gardner, K. and Chapple, A.** (1999). Barriers to referral in patients with angina: qualitative study. *British Medical Journal* **319**, 418–21.
18. **Maas, I.A.M., Gijsen, R., Lobbezoo, I.E., and Poos, M.J.J.C.** *Volksgezondheid (Health) 1997. De gezondheidstoestand: een actualisering. (Health Status: an Actualisation).* Bilthoven: National Institute for Public Health and the Environment, 1997.
19. **Peay, M.Y. and Peay, E.R.** (1998). The evaluation of medical symptoms by patients and doctors. *Journal of Behaviour Medicine* **21**, 57–81.
20. **Jones, R.A.** et al. (1981). On the perceived meaning of symptoms. *Medical Care* **19**, 710–17.
21. **Gijsbers van Wijk, C.M.T.** et al. (1992). Male and female morbidity in general practice: the nature of sex differences. *Social Science and Medicine* **35**, 665–78.
22. **Wyke, S., Hunt, K., and Ford, G.** (1998). Gender differences in consulting a general practitioner for common symptoms of minor illness. *Social Science and Medicine* **46**, 901–6.
23. **Payer, L.** *Medicine and Culture.* New York: Penguin Books, 1989.
24. **Froom, J.** et al. (1997). Antimicrobials for acute otitis media? A review from the International Primary Care Network. *British Medical Journal* **315**, 89–102.
25. **Huygen, F.J.A.** *Family Medicine: The Medical Lifehistory of Families.* Nijmegen: Dekker & Van de Vegt, 1978.

26. **Le Fanu, J.** *The Rise and Fall of Modern Medicine.* London: Little, Brown and Company, 1999.

27. **Wilson, J.H.G. and Junger, G.** Principles and practice of screening for disease. Public Health paper no. 34. Geneva: World Health Organization, 1968.

28. **Hoes, A.W., Mosterd, A., and Grobbee, D.E.** (1998). An epidemic of heart failure? Recent evidence from Europe. *European Heart Journal* (Suppl. L) L2–8.

4.2 Physical and mental illness

François G. Schellevis

Introduction

In Chapter 4.1, it has been shown that everyone from time to time perceives symptoms from his or her body or mind, but that people—fortunately for doctors and for the health care system—present only a small proportion of these symptoms to a doctor. This chapter is concerned with the profile of symptoms, illnesses, and diseases (further referred to as 'morbidity') presented to primary care doctors. It is important to acknowledge that morbidity presented to primary care doctors is only a small part of all morbidity perceived by people in the community.

In the first section the profile of morbidity presented to primary care doctors will be discussed and the relation between the position of the primary doctor in the health care system and the profile of morbidity presented to him will be explained. It will be shown that this is a core element in justifying the existence of primary care medicine as a separate medical discipline in its own. In the second section the diagnostic process of primary care doctors will be dealt with, including the relevance of making a medical diagnosis and the validity of diagnoses. The third section provides an overview of sources of information about the profile of morbidity presented to primary care doctors. In the fourth section information will be given about the frequency and nature of physical and mental illness presented to primary medical care. In the last section attention will be paid to the translation of this epidemiological information to daily patient care, including the occurrence of rare diseases and the occurrence of more than one disease in the same patient. Finally, the information provided in this chapter will be summarized in a number of key messages.

Morbidity profile

Introduction

The broad definition of health of the World Health Organization (WHO), 'Health is a state of physical, mental and social well-being,' reflects very well the variety of health problems that is presented to primary care doctors. In this section, the variety of health problems will be discussed first. Secondly, the relation between the position of the primary care doctor in the health care system with the profile of morbidity presented to him will be explained.

The variety of health problems

The WHO definition of health includes three dimensions of well-being. Primary care doctors are familiar with the entanglement of these three dimensions in the health problems presented to them. Patients may present their symptoms as a merely physical problem, but the primary care doctor will be alert to recognize the psychological and social dimensions of the physical problem. The same holds true for presented problems of a predominantly psychological or social nature. In the last decades, the frequency of psychological and social problems or physical problems with important psycho-social dimensions presented to primary care doctors has been varying.[1] The recognition of these different dimensions is not only necessary to make the right diagnosis but also to assess the health problem in the context of the patient. Such a comprehensive approach is important in view of preventing medicalization.[2] Focusing exclusively on the physical aspects of the presented health problem without paying attention to the psychological context bears the risk for unnecessary medical interference. However, overestimation of the psycho-social aspects could lead to undetected physical diseases. Especially in primary care, where a defined medical diagnosis often cannot be made (see next section), a doctor needs specific skills and attitude for paying balanced attention to both physical and psycho-social aspects.

The health care system and the profile of morbidity presented to primary medical care

In most countries, the primary care doctor is the first medical professional to be consulted within the health care system by people when they perceive a health problem. Usually, the primary care doctor is freely accessible. In countries with a so-called gate-keeper system (e.g. in the United Kingdom and the Netherlands), the primary care doctor is also the only medical professional with free access and in such systems access to secondary specialist care is only possible via the primary care doctor. The free accessibility of primary care strongly determines the profile of symptoms, illnesses, and diseases presented in primary care. When access to secondary specialist care is restricted it can be expected that the profile of morbidity presented to primary medical care reflects the profile of symptoms perceived by people in the community. However, the profile of presented morbidity also depends on the health care seeking behaviour of people—and this varies largely because people differ in:

- perceiving signs and symptoms that might threaten their health;
- (the perception of) the seriousness of these signs and symptoms;
- their inclination to seek professional medical help;
- the sensitivity for opinions of family and friends whether they should consult a doctor or not.

In addition, these determinants of health care seeking behaviour vary with the nature of the signs and symptoms.

Therefore, the profile of morbidity presented to primary care doctors is primarily a result of a complex process that takes place before the patient decides to see a doctor (sometimes referred to as the 'pre-medical phase') and secondarily a result of the position of the primary care doctor in the health care system (see Section 3 on reasons for consultation).

However, this profile is very different from the profile of morbidity seen by medical specialists in hospitals or ambulatory specialist care settings.[3] This is best illustrated by countries where the primary care doctor has a gate-keeper role in the health care system. In these countries, the vast majority (up to 90 per cent or more) of the health problems presented to them is managed by primary care doctors. The small proportion of health problems for which people are referred to medical specialists represents a highly selective part of the morbidity spectrum, for example, complex diagnostic situations requiring specific diagnostic techniques, diseases which cannot be managed by primary care doctors for technical or complexity reasons, and acute diseases requiring urgent specialist intervention. The recognition of this difference in morbidity profile between primary care and secondary or specialist care is essential and has been the basis of the emancipation of primary medical care throughout the world. It has major implications for basic medical education, vocational training of future primary care doctors, and continuous medical education. Traditionally, the medical curriculum is dominated by medical specialists

for use of these classification systems include registration and classification at 'the highest true level of understanding' referring to the nature of diagnostic certainty in primary care. Finally, it should be emphasized that, although a diagnosis may consist of a symptom, the diagnosis always reflects the doctor's assessment and not the opinion of the patient.

Frequency and nature of physical and mental illness

Introduction

In this section, information will be presented about the incidence and prevalence of diseases presented to primary care doctors. The information originates from the Dutch National Survey of General Practice, which includes nationally representative data of 1987–8 for the Netherlands[9] and from the fourth National Morbidity Survey in General Practice carried out in the United Kingdom.[10] It can be assumed that the morbidity profile is globally the same in most European countries, especially when looking at the ranking of the diseases in frequency order, rather than the exact numbers. In case differences between countries occur, these can usually be explained by differences in help-seeking behaviour and cultural differences rather than 'real' differences in the frequency of diseases in the population.[11]

Incidence of diseases

In Table 1, an impression is given of the distribution of incident morbidity presented to primary doctors in the Netherlands according to the different organ systems.

Table 1 shows a number of important aspects:

- among the diseases presented, respiratory, musculoskeletal, and skin diseases are by far the most frequently affected organ systems;
- the frequency of diseases is high;
- the morbidity includes physical as well as pyschological and social health problems.

A much more detailed insight into the morbidity of primary care is provided by the 20 most frequently presented incident diseases (Table 2).

This list of most frequent 'new' episodes of diseases presented to primary care doctors demonstrates that 'common diseases' are the core business of primary care doctors. It also shows a number of diagnoses that are formulated at the level of a symptom (e.g. myalgia, cough). As explained before, this is an characteristic element of diagnoses made by primary care doctors. The diagnostic label of 'no diagnosis' is used in those cases where no pathological sign or symptom could be traced by the doctor. The predominance of diseases of the respiratory tract, the musculoskeletal system, and the skin as shown in Table 1 is confirmed in Table 2.

Prevalence of diseases

Tables 3 and 4 provide information about prevalent diseases as measured in the United Kingdom in 1991–2.[10] In Table 3, the prevalence rates per ICD chapter are shown.

Table 3 shows high prevalence rates in the ICD chapters XVI and XVIII; this illustrates that the ICD is less appropriate for classifying morbidity in primary medical care. Diseases of the respiratory system, the nervous system, and the musculoskeletal system are the most prevalent conditions. Although the structure of the ICPC and ICD classifications does not allow direct comparisons, important similarities become visible compared to the incident diseases (Table 1) when ranked according to frequency. Diseases of the respiratory system, the musculoskeletal system, and the skin are among the most frequent incident and prevalent diseases.

In Table 4, the most prevalent diseases are showed in more detail.

Table 1 Morbidity according to ICPC chapter (incidence per 1000 per year)

ICPC chapter	Incidence per 1000 per year
A General and unspecified	134.4
B Blood	16.0
D Digestive	147.6
F Eye	62.8
H Ear	102.0
K Circulatory	67.2
L Musculoskeletal	324.4
N Neurological	40.0
P Psychological	90.4
R Respiratory	338.0
S Skin	259.2
T Endocrine/metabolic/nutrition	19.6
U Urology	57.6
W Pregnancy/family planning	51.2
X Female genital	64.8
Y Male genital	14.0
Z Social	28.0

Source: ref. 9.

Table 2 Twenty diseases (ICPC codes) with the highest frequency (incidence per 1000 per year)

Diseases (ICPC codes)	Incidence per 1000 per year
Upper respiratory tract infection (R74)	123.2
Myalgia (L18)	57.6
Cystitis (U71)	46.4
No disease (A97)	43.2
Acute bronchitis (R78)	38.8
Cough (R05)	36.4
Sinusitis (R75)	34.8
Cerumen (H81)	33.2
Eczema (S88)	29.6
Acute otitis media (H71)	26.8
Infection of digestive tract (D73)	26.4
Lumbago (L03)	26.4
Influenza (R80)	24.8
Acute tonsillitis (R76)	24.0
Other viral disease (A77)	23.6
Dermatomycosis (S74)	23.2
Allergic conjunctivitis (F71)	21.6
Warts (S03)	20.0
Tendinitis/synovitis (L93/L99)	17.2
Irritable bowel syndrome (D93)	16.0

Source: ref. 9.

Table 3 Morbidity according to ICD chapter (1-year period prevalence per 1000)

ICD chapter		Prevalence per 1000
I	Infectious and parasitic diseases	139.9
II	Neoplasms	23.9
III	Endocrine, nutritional and, metabolic diseases and immunity disorders	37.7
IV	Diseases of blood and blood-forming organs	9.7
V	Mental disorders	72.8
VI	Diseases of the nervous system and sense organs	173.2
VII	Diseases of the circulatory system	93.1
VIII	Diseases of the respiratory system	307.0
IX	Diseases of the digestive system	86.6
X	Diseases of the genitourinary system	113.3
XI	Complications of pregnancy, childbirth, and the puerperium	10.8
XII	Diseases of the skin and subcutaneous tissue	145.5
XIII	Diseases of the muculoskeletal system and connective tissue	152.1
XIV	Congenital anomalies	5.3
XV	Certain conditions originating in perinatal period	1.3
XVI	Symptoms, signs and ill-defined conditions	151.0
XVII	Injury and poisoning	139.0
XVIII	Supplementary classification of factors influencing health status and contact with health services	334.8

Source: ref. 10.

Table 4 Twenty diseases (ICD codes) with the highest frequency, excluding preventive services (1-year period prevalence per 1000)

Diseases (ICD codes)	Prevalence per 1000
Acute upper respiratory infections (465)	77.2
Contraceptive management (V25)	72.8
Acute bronchitis and bronchiolitis (466)	71.9
Asthma (493)	42.5
Disorders of conjunctiva (372)	41.5
Essential hypertension (401)	41.2
Acute pharyngitis (462)	40.9
Disorders of external ear (380)	40.9
Acute tonsillitis (463)	40.7
Ill-defined intestinal infections (009)	39.4
Other and unspecified disorders of back (724)	37.2
Symptoms involving respiratory system (786)	36.6
Non-suppurative otitis media and Eustachian tube disorders (381)	34.6
Neurotic disorders (300)	34.4
Common cold (460)	32.0
Osteoarthrosis and allied disorders (715)	31.5
Candidiasis (112)	31.3
Atopic dermatitis (691)	30.3
Certain adverse effects not elsewhere classified (995)	29.4
Allergic rhinitis (477)	28.3

Source: ref. 10.

There are similarities and differences with the list of diseases in Table 2. Of course, among the most prevalent diseases are also the most frequent incident diseases, as can be understood from the definition of prevalence. However, a number of other diseases and health problems are listed among the most prevalent diseases, including diseases of the cardiovascular system (hypertension) and psychological health problems (neurotic disorders). Another difference with the diseases listed in Table 2 is that the prevalent diseases in Table 4 include more exact medical diagnoses and less symptom diagnoses.

The lists of diseases in Tables 2 and 4 represent an important part of the morbidity profile presented to the primary care doctor and describe which health problems he deals with in daily practice.

Rare diseases and multimorbidity

Introduction

In this section, attention will be paid to two other aspects of the morbidity presented to primary care doctors that cannot be read from the incidence and prevalence figures: rare diseases and multimorbidity.

Rare diseases in primary care

From Tables 1–4, one could draw a false conclusion that primary care doctors only deal with frequent and common diseases. Although these diseases represent the majority of daily work, and take up most time, the primary care doctor will always be alert about the possible existence of an unexpected symptom that may point towards the existence of a rare (and often serious) disease. Besides the management of so many common diseases and frequent chronic diseases, this alertness and attitude of sound suspicion is a basic element of primary medical care. The Bayesian mathematical model (provides some basis for rational evaluation, but the 'feeling' of the doctor is equally important. This dealing with uncertainty has to be learned in daily practice and grows with experience over the years. Finding a balance between suspicion and comfort (usually taking place via the trial-and-error path) implies balancing between the unnecessary use of diagnostic examinations (resulting sometimes in false-positive findings) and diagnostic delay (which may have bad prognostic consequences). In this respect, the work of primary care doctors differs from the work of specialized colleagues. Where a primary care doctor starts his diagnostic reasoning from 'the patient is healthy unless there are signs and symptoms of a disease', the medical specialist will focus on the exclusion of all possible diseases with a range of diagnostic tools. Or expressed otherwise: a primary care doctor will justify his diagnostic examinations by his 'working hypothesis' or diagnosis, and a medical specialist will justify his diagnosis by his diagnostic examinations.[6]

Multimorbidity

Another aspect that is not reflected in the incidence or prevalence figures is the existence of more than one disease in the same patient at the same time, usually referred to as 'co-morbidity' or 'multimorbidity'.[12,13] In many countries the primary care doctor is a 'generalist' and is the 'best' doctor to keep the overview of all health problems existing in the same patient. This includes keeping a complete medical record of the patient, but also, for example, an oversight of prescribed drugs, contra-indications, and interactions. Patients with multimorbidity, often elderly, are a vulnerable group among the practice population and deserve special attention. In daily practice, a primary care doctor will be familiar with multimorbidity, but when only looking at descriptive epidemiological information from primary medical care, this phenomenon remains unseen.

Within the scope of physical and mental illness, multimorbidity also reflects the combination of physical and mental illness in the same patient. While it is generally accepted that people with chronic, somatic diseases are at higher risk for a serious psychiatric disorder, such as a major depression;[14] the reverse has been much less studied. The association between physical and mental illness can be explained by several mechanisms:

- a common biological substrate;
- stress as a common cause;
- as a consequence of the deterioration due to chronic somatic diseases.

This relationship underlines the need for primary doctors to pay attention to possible psycho-social problems accompanying physical illness.

Paying attention to multimorbidity in older patients, and especially the combination of chronic physical diseases and serious psychiatric disease, is an important feature of the work of the primary care doctor.

Key points

- *The profile of morbidity presented to primary care doctors is unique and justifies primary care medicine being a separate discipline on its own.*
  The free accessibility of the primary care doctor strongly determines which health problems are presented. In health care systems where the primary care doctor acts as a gate keeper for specialized health care, there are major differences between the profiles of morbidity presented to primary care doctors and to secondary care medical specialists.
- *Most incident health problems presented to primary care doctors are self-limiting common diseases.*
  Balancing between sound suspicion for the existence of a rare disease and feeling comfortable in observing the natural course of a health problem is an important skill for a primary care doctor.
- *In primary medical care, the prognosis of a health problem is often more important than the exact medical diagnosis.*
  For appropriate management of a health problem presented to a primary care doctor it is usually not necessary to establish an exact medical diagnosis. Knowledge about the probability of the occurrence of symptoms and diseases in the adhering population is essential for assessing the probability of a disease. A 'working hypothesis' guiding further diagnostic or therapeutic interventions is usually sufficient, together with information about the time course of a health problem.
- *Primary care doctors are alert to rare diseases and multimorbidity.*
  Although primary care doctors do not focus on excluding rare diseases in case of presentation of symptoms that may refer to such a disease, a sound alertness for this is an important skill that has to be developed, mainly by experience.

References

1. **Verhaak, P.F.M., van de Lisdonk, E.H., Bor, J.H.J, and Hutschemaekers, G.J.M.** (2000). GPs' referrals to mental health care during the past 25 years. *British Journal of General Practice* **50**, 307–8.
2. **Grol, R.P.T.M.** *To Heal or to Harm. The Prevention of Somatic Fixation in General Practice.* Exeter: The Royal College of General Practitioners, 1988.
3. **Hodgkin, K.** *Towards Earlier Diagnosis in Primary Care* 4th edn. New York: Churchill Livingstone, 1978.
4. **Fry, J.** *Common Diseases* 4th edn. Lancaster: MTP Press Ltd, 1985.
5. **Huygen, F.** *Family Medicine.* Nijmegen: Dekker en Van de Vegt, 1978.
6. **van der Velden, H.G.M.** (1983). Diagnosis or prognosis (in Dutch, with English summary). *Huisarts & Wetenschap* **26**, 125–8, 148.
7. **Wulff, H.R.** *Rational Diagnosis and Treatment.* Oxford: Blackwell Scientific Publications, 1976.
8. **Schellevis, F.G., van de Lisdonk, E.H., van der Velden, J., van Eijk, J.Th.M., and van Weel, C.** (1993). Validity of diagnoses of chronic diseases in general practice. The application of diagnostic criteria. *Journal of Clinical Epidemiology* **46**, 461–8.
9. **van der Velden, J., de Bakker, D.H., Claessens, A.A.M.C., and Schellevis, F.G.** *Dutch National Survey of General Practice. Morbidity in General Practice.* Utrecht: Netherlands Institute for Health Services Research (Nivel), 1992.
10. **McCormick, A., Fleming, D., and Charlton, J.** *Morbidity Statistics from General Practice. Fourth National Study 1991–1992. Office of Population Censuses and Surveys Series MB5 no. 3.* London: Her Majesty Stationary Office, 1995.
11. **Payer, L.** *Medicine and Culture.* New York: Henry Holt and Company, Inc., 1988.
12. **Schellevis, F.G., van der Velden, J., van de Lisdonk, E.H., van Eijk, J.Th.M., and van Weel, C.** (1993). Comorbidity of chronic diseases in general practice. *Journal of Clinical Epidemiology* **46**, 469–73.
13. **van den Akker, M., Buntinx, F., Metsemakers, J.F.M., Roos, S., and Knottnerus, J.A.** (1998). Multimorbidity in general practice: prevalence, incidence, and determinants of co-occurring chronic and recurrent diseases. *Journal of Clinical Epidemiology* **51**, 367–75.
14. **Wells, K.B., Golding, J.M., and Burnam, M.A.** (1988). Psychiatric disorder in a sample of the general population with and without chronic medical conditions. *American Journal of Psychiatry* **145**, 976–81.

4.3 Classification and the domain of family practice

Inge M. Okkes and Henk Lamberts

Summary and scope of this chapter

Several systems are available for *documentation* in family practice; however, only one family practice *classification* exists that is designed to describe the domain, and to allow the collection of aggregated data on morbidity in family practice. The International Classification of Primary Care (ICPC)-2 caters for the coding of reasons for encounter, diagnoses and interventions in an episode of care structure, and allows, for more clinical detail, the use of ICD-10 as a nomenclature. It was designed to meet family physicians' needs both in practice and in research. Its prime purpose is not documentation; rather, it aims at hierarchically ordering the family practice domain in order to better understand its content. While a clinical terminology aims at being as specific, detailed, and comprehensive as possible, the aim of ICPC as a family practice classification is to bring about an effective reduction, based on the frequency distribution of reasons for encounter and diagnoses in family practice.

Within this perspective, we illustrate and discuss the relation of ICPC with other classifications, nomenclatures, and terminologies. Also, we illustrate the usefulness of ICPC by presenting aggregated data on probabilities based on the relations between reasons for encounter and diagnoses, and data from an international comparative study.

It is stressed that family doctors who, for documentation purposes in electronic patient records, use Controlled Medical Vocabularies such as the Clinical Terms-Version-3 or the Systematized Nomenclature of Medicine-Clinical Terms (SNOMED-CT), still may have access to the diagnostic mode of ICPC as the ordering principle of their domain, since reliable mapping of these systems' diagnostic terms to the International Statistical Classification of Diseases and Related Health Problems (ICD-10) exists.

Over the years, discussions on the potential value and practical usefulness of classification systems in medicine at large, and in family practice in particular, often have been difficult, because of conflicting vested interests of national or international organizations, and because a different use of terms sometimes led to incommensurability. We aim to prevent at least some potential confusion by adding a glossary of terms used in this chapter.

Introduction

Science requires ordering by a taxonomy or classification. The first attempt at a disease classification dates from 1662, when Graunt prepared the *London Bill of Mortality*, listing 83 causes of death. In the following centuries, many classifications for causes of deaths, and increasingly, also for diseases have been developed. By far the most widely used is the ICD, now in its 10th revision (ICD-10).[1,2] Basically, each of its 21 chapters deals with a medical specialty (e.g. dermatology, gynaecology, neurology). In its successive revisions, ICD has grown in size, largely under the influence of (sub-) specialists and epidemiologists who wanted 'their' field to be described in the greatest detail possible; ICD-10 contains well over 12 000 three or four digit diagnostic rubrics. However, as White put it, in trying to accommodate everyone, it pleases few.[3]

This is especially true for family practice.[3,4] As opposed to most medical specialists, family doctors deal with literally all diseases, symptoms, feelings of unease and fear, and psychological, social and daily life problems; the frequency distribution in family practice, however, is skewed towards common problems. Consequently, a *disease* classification such as ICD that, in addition to its lack of focus on the context of family practice, does not cater for this frequency distribution, cannot adequately characterize daily family practice. As early as 1972 it was acknowledged that international family practice required its own ordering principle, tailored to fit its domain.[5–7] In the following decades, WONCA (the World Organization of Family Doctors) developed the ICPC (described in detail in Box 1), that allows the classification and coding of three core elements of each encounter: the patient's *reason for encounter*, the physician's *diagnosis*, and the (diagnostic and therapeutic) *interventions*, organized in an *episode of care* structure.[4,8,9]

Figure 1 summarizes the essential terms related to documentation and classification in the family practice context used in this chapter (see also Appendix).[4,8,10–15] A patient visits a family doctor, who asks the patient for his/her reasons for encounter, and identifies, after history taking and/or examination, the medical objects involved. A medical vocabulary provides the terminology to conceptualize medical objects with a term. Terms refer to health problems, structured with a nomenclature that allows an optimal description. The classification provides classes and codes for the core elements of episodes of care (reasons for encounter, diagnoses, and interventions), allowing the arrangement into classes given the domain's boundaries, and the systematic inclusion of episode data in a patient record.[4,16] The related issues of registration, medical record keeping, and record linkage are covered in Chapter 10.2.

Clinical terminology versus classification

A Clinical Terminology or Controlled Medical Vocabulary is a structured list of all terms for use by health care professionals, describing the care and treatment of patients, covering a wide range of areas: diseases, operations, treatments, special investigations, appliances, drugs, occupations, administrative items, etc.[17] A clinical terminology, as a consequence, contains several hundred thousands of terms of which diagnostic terms are only a small proportion. A very comprehensive terminology will be the SNOMED-CT, currently under development, meant to replace Clinical Terms Version 3

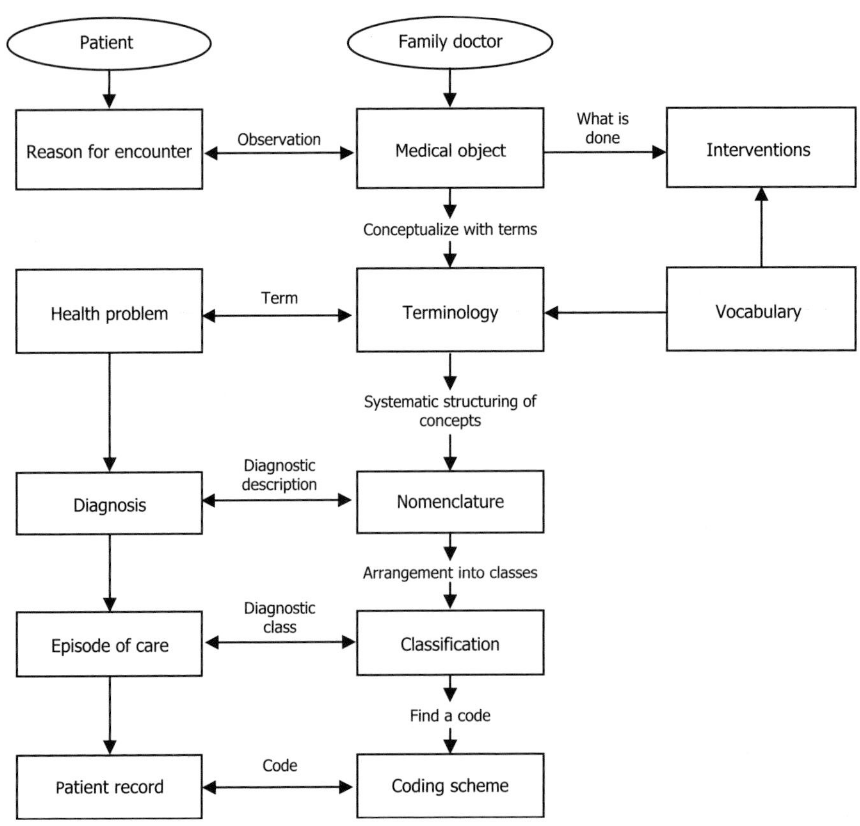

Fig. 1 Terms related to documentation and classification in the family practice context.

Box 1 The International Classification of Primary Care (ICPC)

ICPC is designed to order the domain of family practice, providing codes for the description of the content of encounters in an episode of care structure. The *content of encounters* entails three core elements: the patient's reason(s) for encounter, the doctor's diagnosis, and the intervention(s). Family doctors manage their patients' problems over time. Sometimes a problem is over and done with in one encounter, but sometimes it takes (far) more encounters. Since diagnoses may change over time (e.g. from URTI to bronchitis, or pneumonia), it is essential to link data belonging to one problem. Therefore at the heart of ICPC data is the framework of the *episode of care*: a health problem from its first presentation by the patient to a health care provider until the completion of the last encounter for it. An episode of care encompasses all contact elements related to that health problem (see Fig. a).

Fig. a Core elements for coding encounters in an episode of care structure with ICPC

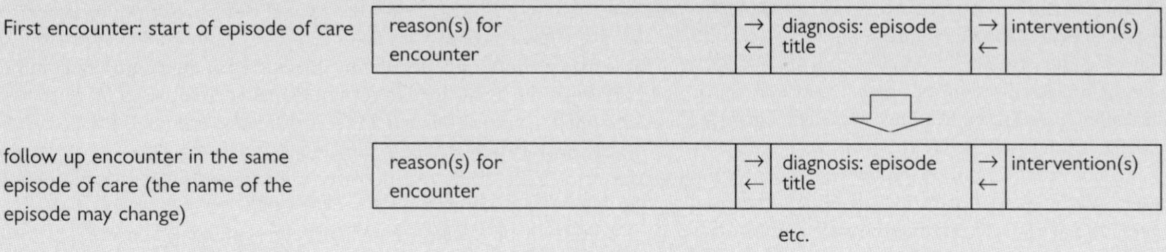

First encounter: start of episode of care	reason(s) for encounter	→ ←	diagnosis: episode title	→ ←	intervention(s)
follow up encounter in the same episode of care (the name of the episode may change)	reason(s) for encounter	→ ←	diagnosis: episode title	→ ←	intervention(s)

etc.

ICPC is a biaxial classification system. Seventeen chapters with an alpha code referring to a body system/problem area form one axis; seven components (rubrics with a two-digit numeric code) form the second. An ICPC code consists of an alpha for the chapter, and of a two digit numeric code for the rubric within the chapter and component structure (Fig. b).

Fig. b ICPC structure: 17 chapters, 7 components

Chapters⇒ Components⇓	A	B	D	F	H	K	L	N	P	R	S	T	U	W	X	Y	Z
1. Symptoms and complaints																	
2. Diagnostic, screening, preventive																	
3. Medication, treatment, procedures																	
4. Test results																	
5. Administrative																	
6. Referrals and other reasons for encounter																	
7. Diseases																	

Chapters:

A: General and unspecified
B: Blood, blood-forming organs and immune mechanism
D: Digestive
F: Eye
H: Ear
K: Circulatory
L: Musculoskeletal
N: Neurological
P: Psychological
R: Respiratory
S: Skin
T: Endocrine, metabolic, and nutritional
U: Urological
W: Pregnancy, child-bearing, family planning
X: Female genital
Y: Male genital
Z: Social problems

ICPC reflects the characteristic distribution of reasons for encounter, diagnoses, and interventions in family practice. All frequent reasons for encounter, diagnoses, and interventions (roughly: occurring at least once per 1000 patients per year) are included as a separate code; less frequent diagnoses/ reasons for encounter are, therefore, relatively often included in a 'ragbag' rubric: a miscellaneous collection of symptoms and complaints, of interventions or of diseases not classified elsewhere (the last codes of all components). As opposed to disease classifications, ICPC caters for the classification of the typical questions patients bring to family doctors, that is, not only symptoms, complaints and diseases, but also social and daily life problems, fears, and requests for advice, medication, examination, or referral etc. In order to provide the necessary additional clinical detail, ICPC has been mapped to ICD-9(-CM), and to ICD-10.

For coding *reasons for encounter*, all rubrics from all components may be used; a reason for encounter may be:

1. a symptom or complaint (component 1): e.g. I have a cough: R05, I'm feeling so low (P03);
2. a request for an intervention (components 2–6): e.g. I need a new prescription for my asthma (R50), I would like you to check my blood pressure (K31);
3. a disease (component 7): e.g. I am here for my diabetes (T90).

For coding a *diagnosis*, all rubrics from components 1 and 7 may be used, which include all diagnostic categories. If needed, additional diagnostic detail can be derived from ICD-10; e.g., by coding: ICPC-2 code K72, cardiovascular neoplasm, together with ICD-10 code C45.2, mesothelioma of pericardium.

For coding an *intervention*, all codes from components 2, 3, 5 and 6 may be used: examination of ear (H31), suture of skin (S54), referral to a cardiologist (K67).

ICPC has significant mnemonic quality that facilitates its routine use by doctors. Rubrics within components are as much the same as possible throughout the chapters, e.g. the first code in component 1 (symptoms/complaints) mostly refers to 'pain': H01: ear pain, D01: abdominal pain, N01: headache. Components 2–6 are entirely identical per chapter: e.g. D50 is medication for an episode of care in chapter D(igestive), S50 medication in chapter S(kin).

ICPC was first published in 1987; the second edition ICPC-2 was published in 1998, followed by a (corrected) electronic version: ICPC-2-E. ICPC-2-E contains a full mapping to ICD-10, and for relevant rubrics, inclusion and exclusion criteria, synonyms and 'consider' (indicating other codes that might be considered). ICPC has been translated in the following languages: Afrikaans, Basque, Chinese, Danish, Dutch, German, Finnish, French, Greek, Hebrew, Hungarian, Italian, Japanese, Norwegian, Polish, Portuguese, Romanian, Russian, Spanish, and Swedish; more are under development.

(CTV-3 or Read Codes) and SNOMED-RT in electronic patient records (EPRs).[18–22] CTV-3 is made available and updated by the British National Health Service Information Authority; it is a hierarchical system in which the Read codes characterize the concepts, to which several terms with a term identifier may be added as synonyms. SNOMED was first published in 1975 by the College of American Pathologists: a concept based reference terminology that allows the coding of clinical concepts with clear relationships between terms and concepts. SNOMED-CT will be a joint effort of both organizations.[23]

A clinical terminology is no classification: in order to retrieve aggregated data for epidemiological use, a classification is needed. Therefore, for CTV-3 and SNOMED-CT, ICD-10 is designated to summarize the documented diagnostic data, in the form of, for example, incidences and prevalences of diseases.[23] Reliable cross-maps to ICD-10 are, therefore, essential, but do only provide diagnostic terms; for areas such as treatments, investigations, occupations, drugs, appliances, other mappings are required. The Unified Medical Language System (UMLS) of the National Library of Medicine in the United States, contains a metathesaurus offering a wide perspective on the terms included in many systems.[24,25] Galen provides a terminology server that systematically orders all terms in a specific domain.[26]

Coding diagnoses

ICPC was designed to meet family physicians' needs both in practice and in research. Its prime purpose is not documentation; rather, it aims at hierarchically ordering the family practice domain in order to better understand its content (Box 1). While a clinical terminology aims at being as specific, detailed, and big as possible, the aim of ICPC as a family practice classification is to bring about an effective reduction, based on the frequency distribution of reasons for encounter and diagnoses in family practice.[4,8,9] The diagnostic classes of ICPC allow the establishment of an episode of care database on the basis of reasons for encounter and episodes of care with a high prevalence in family practice, and big enough to allow adequate retrievals. The classes in ICPC were primarily selected because they are common in family practice (rule of thumb: at least one episode of care per 1000 patients per year). Empirical data available at that time supported this rule of thumb, because reported error rates in family practice data bases practically prohibited to rely on the quality of (multipractice) sampling frames when studying a 'low prevalent' disease (<1 case per 2000 patient years).[4,10] In the future, however, it might be feasible to rely on clinical data on rare diseases from high quality electronic patient records with a long observation period. Once this is sufficiently supported by empirical data, the number of classes of ICPC could well be extended.[5,11–13]

Right now, however, it is evident that ICPC does not cater for the diagnostic specificity needed for coding clinical data in patient records in family practice (where, of course, also very rare diseases occur).[27–33] Therefore, ICPC can use ICD-10 as a nomenclature, with a vocabulary in the form of a thesaurus with well over 80 000 diagnostic terms, based on the alphabetic index of ICD-10.[8,9] A prototype of such a thesaurus was recently developed in the Netherlands;[34] since all included terms are double coded with ICPC-2 and ICD-10, semi-automated coding is available to a family doctor who works with an electronic patient record that allows picking the correct diagnostic description from this thesaurus.[9,35] This is illustrated in Table 1 with the one-to-one mapping of the multilanguage ICPC class 'T85- hyperthyroidism/thyrotoxicosis' to the three digit ICD-10 class E05 with the same title. The four-digit ICD-10 classes E05.1–9, represented in English, French, Spanish, and Dutch, allow the family doctor to describe the patient's condition in much more clinical detail. The use of the alphabetical index of ICD-10 as a terminology in the four languages is illustrated by the terms for E05.0 'thyrotoxicosis with diffuse goitre': clinical terms such as Basedow's disease, exophtalmic goitre, Graves', Flajani's, and Perry's disease become readily available.[34]

Coding reasons for encounter

Reason for encounter codes are, as yet, not widely used in routine documentation in EPRs. ICPC contains over 200 codes for symptoms and complaints for use in the reason for encounter mode.[4,8,9] These codes appear to greatly enhance the clinical reliability and relevance of patient documentation, and play a major role in estimating probabilities for diagnoses in standard sex/age groups.[36] In principle, codes for diagnoses, symptoms, and complaints from another system could also be used to code reasons for encounter. However, only ICPC provides codes for reasons for encounter in the form of a patient request (for a prescription, an advice, an X-ray). This type of reasons for encounter has proved to play an important role in explaining variation in the distribution of interventions: family doctors are generally inclined to grant their patients' requests.[37] There is only one other classification system for reasons for encounter: the Reason for Visit Classification (RVC) in the United States;[38] because it is the predecessor of ICPC in its reason for encounter mode, the mapping between both is quite straightforward.

In this chapter, we do not discuss the potential of controlled medical vocabularies for future inclusion in an EPR through natural language dictation by family doctors without data entry on a keyboard. In family practice, the dictum that 'doctors dictate and will continue to dictate' and that 'nurses write and will continue to write' appears to apply neither now nor in the near future.[39] In some medical (sub and super) specialties, the details to be documented are, by their nature, relatively suitable for dictation, because of, for example, the usually rather fixed order of standardized events to be documented, and the relatively small size of the domain (e.g. obductions, X-ray reports). In our perspective, however, family doctors will for good reasons continue to, themselves, enter data in a structured format. They know they often deal with fuzzy data in a fuzzy health care world, where only a limited amount of hard clinical information is available.[40] A substantial proportion of the medical history of family practice patients is not, already before the encounter, 'out there', ready to be documented, but is, to a large extent, constituted during the communication between doctor and patient.[35,41,42] This is at the same time a major incentive to consequently identify, classify, and code the patients' reasons for encounter.[33,42]

Summary

Although other systems may well be able to document the detail of what goes on in family practice, it is by now widely acknowledged that only data on reasons for encounter, diagnoses, and interventions ordered with the limited number of selected and meaningful classes of ICPC, in an episode of care structure over time, will add to knowledge about morbidity patterns in family practice.[27,43–47] This perspective will be further elaborated in the following paragraphs.

Practical use of ICPC

Relation with other systems

Recent progress in the development of electronic patient records and of mapping structures on the diagnostic level may now allow family doctors to use ICPC together with other—often mandatory—diagnostic systems that are used for administrative, reimbursement, or policy purposes. In principle, it is possible to comply with coding requirements for the use of ICD-9-CM, ICD-10(-CM), Clinical Terms Version-3 (CTV-3), and SNOMED-CT, and have, at the same time, access to ICPC in its diagnostic mode as a part of the organizing principle of international family practice, for retrieval purposes, to structure patient data in episodes of care, and to use family practice decision support systems (e.g. guidelines for prescribing and the selection of tests, epidemiological data, protocols, etc.).[8,9,12,47–49]

We illustrate this using a famous case history by Weed in 1968 (Fig. 2).[50,51] In Table 2, we have listed the episodes of care from this history in an episode or problem list, with ICPC-2 and ICD-10 codes, as well as with CTV-3 Read codes, together with the term identifiers, thus providing access to the underlying coding structure in the three systems. We tried to formulate each problem at its most realistic level of specification. Additional detail about important events, and other characteristics of the episodes of care in this individual patient are included in the diagnostic label of the

Table 1 The mapping between ICPC-2 class T85 hyperthyroidism/thyrotoxicosis (labels in various languages) with ICD-10 on the 3- and 4-digit level, and the available ICD-10 terms in English, French, Spanish, and Dutch

ICPC-2 code	ICPC-2 label	ICD-10 codes	ICD-10 labels (English)	ICD-10 labels (French)	ICD-10 labels (Spanish)	ICD-10 labels (Dutch)
T85	**Hyperthyroidism/thyrotoxicosis**	E05	Thyrotoxicosis (hyperthyroidism)	Thyréotoxicose (hyperthyroïdie)	Tirotoxicosis (hipertiroidismo)	Thyrotoxicose (hyperthyroïdie)
	Hypertyreose/tyreotoksikose (Danish)	E05.0	Thyrotoxicosis with diffuse goitre	Thyréotoxicose avec goitre diffuse	Tirotoxicosis con bocio difuso	Thyrotoxicose met diffuse struma
	Hyperthyreoidie/thyreotoxicose (Dutch)	E05.1	Thyrotoxicosis with toxic single thyroid nodule	Thyréotoxicose avec nodule thyroïdien simple	Tirotoxicosis con nódulo solitario tiroideo tóxico	Thyrotoxicose met solitaire toxische schildkliermodus
	Hyperthyroïdie/thyréotoxicose (French)	E05.2	Thyrotoxicosis with toxic multinodular goitre	Thyréotoxicose avec goitre multinodulare toxique	Tirotoxicosis con bocio multinodular tóxico	Thyrotoxicose met toxische multinodulaire struma
	Hyperthyreose/Thyreotoxikose (German)	E05.3	Thyrotoxicosis from ectopic thyroid tissue	Thyréotoxicose due à des nodules thyroïdiens ectopiques	Tirotoxicosis por tejido tiroideo ectópico	Thyrotoxicose door ectopisch schildklierweefsel
	Ipertiroidismo/tireotossicosi (Italian)	E05.4	Thyrotoxicosis factitia	Thyréotoxicose factice	Tirotoxicosis facticia	Thyrotoxicosis factitia
	Hipertiroidismo/tireotoxicose (Portuguese)	E05.5	Thyroid crisis or storm	Crise aiguë thyréotoxique	Crisis o tormenta tirotóxica	Thyrotoxische crisis of storm
	Hipertiroidismo/tirotoxicosis (Spanish)	E05.8	Other thyrotoxicosis	Autres thyréotoxicoses	Otras tirotoxicosis	Overige gespecificeerde vormen van thyrotoxicose
		E05.9	Thyrotoxicosis, unspecified	Thyréotoxicoses	Tirotoxicosis	Thyrotoxicose
			Terms referring to E05.0 in the alphabetical index of ICD-10 (English)	**Terms referring to E05.0 in the alphabetical index of ICD-10 (French)**	**Terms referring to E05.0 in the alphabetical index of ICD-10 (Spanish)**	**Terms referring to E05.0 in the alphabetical index of ICD-10 (Dutch)**
			Basedow's disease	Basedow	Basedow; enfermedad	Basedow
			Exophthalmic; goitre	Flajani	Bocio; exoftálmico	Exoftalmie; struma
			Flajani's disease	Goitre; adénomateux; exophtalmique	Bocio; hipertiroidismo	Flajani
			Goitre; exophthalmic	Goitre; exophtalmique	Bocio; tirotoxicosis	Graves
			Goitre; hyperthyroidism	Goitre; hyperthyroïdie	Bocio; tóxico	Hyperthyroïdie; struma
			Goitre; thyrotoxicosis	Goitre; thyréotoxicose	Enfermedad; Basedow	Parry
			Goitre; toxic	Goitre; toxique	Enfermedad; Flajani	Struma; exoftalmie
			Graves' disease	Goitre; toxique, diffus	Enfermedad; Graves	Struma; hyperthyroïdie
			Hyperthyroidism; goitre	Graves	Enfermedad; Parry	Struma; thyrotoxicose
			Parry's disease	Hyperthyroïdie; goitre	Hipertiroidismo; bocio	Toxisch; struma
			Thyrotoxicosis; goitre	Parry	Tirotoxicosis; bocio	
			Toxic; goitre	Thyréotoxicose; goitre	Tóxico; bocio	
				Toxique; goitre		
				Toxique; goitre; diffus		

PROBLEM LIST

6/17 #1 Rheumatic Heart Disease
- a. Mitral insufficiency
- b. Atrial fibrillation
- c. Compensated congestive failure TTB
- d. Cardiac catheterization
- e. Successful cardioversion

#2 Presumed SBE
#3 Mild diabetes mellitus—adult onset
#4 Repeated pulmonary embolism
#5 Post. Inferior Vena Cava Ligation
#6 Allergic dermatitis
9/3 #7 Arthralgia
9/8 #8 Family problems

8/5—CARDIOLOGY
TEMP—36.6 WEIGHT 73.6 kg

#1 *RHD:*
Sx—excellent exercise tolerance—does housework, taking walks etc. no SOB
Obj—wt up again 4 lbs P 100 reg. c rare PVC BP 150/90 chest few rales @ (l.) base that do not clear c cough; cor.—unchanged
Rx—unchanged—see flow sheet
Plans—in view of excellent clinical response and exercise tolerance I am not concerned about rates but will continue to watch
a. Quinidine 0/200 q2h#300
continue other meds

#5 *Post IVC Ligation:*
Sx—o
Obj—leg swelling continues to be a problem esp. during the hot weather
Rx—unchanged
Plan—1. Naqua up to 0/002 QD
2. Coumadin 0/005 QD
3. protime today
RTC 3 mos.

9/8
#1 *Arthralgias*—see EW note 9-3-66
SX—continues @ about same intensity but more concentrated in r arm (cath. done in that arm)
Obj—ASO neg. RH factor—not significantly up
Repeat sed. rate—films of shoulders, elbows, wrists
Rx—symptoms exacerbated by ASA—some relief by heat
Plan—1. uric acid, serum glob, LE prep
2. observe

#8 *Family Problems:*
pt. has been upset lately by husband's constant admonitions not to over-do herself and his general over protective attitude. Today was very upset, depressed and crying—it is now obvious that more fundamental conflicts exist in this marriage. Husband drinks, is jealous of attention she gives the children, etc.
Plan—have asked her to have husband call me and will get a greater feel for the situation starting with the part of the conflict revolving around her medical condition.

9/23
Was pelvic (& pap) done during adm? if not, suggest having these done.

#1 *RHD:*
Sx—continued excellent exercise tolerance
Obj—wt up 2 kg; B 160/70;P 100 reg; chest-clear;
cor—as above
Rx—Digitalis 0/100 QD, Quinidine 0/200 qid

#5 *Post IVC Ligation:*
(R) leg now back to normal s oedema but (L) leg now swells even more and often does not go down @ night—becomes heavy and cumbersome
Rx—Naqua seems to help but not taking QD
Plan—1. Naqua QD
2. refer to peripheral vasc. clinic
3. D/C Coumadin

#7 *Arthralgia:*
Sx—comes and goes but essentially about the same overall. A.M. had stiffness seems to be her biggest complaint
Obj— joint films → osteoarthrosis changes in elbows and hands
Rx— o—heat, rest, ASA
Plan—continue above

#8 *Family Problem:*
marked improvement p she mentioned to husband that I wanted to talk c him. He has not called but has been much improved in his attitude toward her and the children.

List of problems and associated clinic notes on a patient being seen in a busy outpatient department of a large urban hospital. This list is a permanent part of the record, and new problems are added as they appear such as the arthralgia and family problems in the particular case. The latter is an example of a good physician who did not limit himself to the strictly medical or organic questions. (Note that all problems are not necessarily dealt with on each visit; the extent of the thought and care given to each situation is clearly defined.)

Fig. 2 Weed's famous case history.[50]

Table 2 Problem list of Johanna Weed (28-10-1947), in practice since 15-4-1996; office encounter September 23, 2001, 16:43

	ICPC-2	ICD-10	Read code	Term ID	Problem	First encounter	Last encounter
1	K71	I05.1	G111.	Y204t	Rheumatic mitral insufficiency (1987) catheterized (1995)	<15-04-1996	23-09-2001
2	K78	I48	G5730	Y20AP	Atrial fibrillation (1992) with cardio-version (3x; last 1998)	<15-04-1996	23-09-2001
3	K77	I500	XEOV8	Y20C6	Congestive heart failure with nocturnal asthma cardiale (1993)	<15-04-1996	23-09-2001
4	K70	I330	G5101	Y2041	Presumed subacute bacterial endocarditis (1995); penicillin prophylaxis	<15-04-1996	18-03-2000
5	T90	E11.9	XaEL8	Yaemw	Non-insulin dependent diabetes without complications; diet controlled	11-08-1996	02-07-2001
6	K93	I26.9	G401	Y20DV	Pulmonary embolism (repeated) without cor pulmonale	02-12-1996	14-05-1999
7	K99	I87.9	G8y21	Y20N2	Vena cava inferior syndrome after ligation in 1997	08-02-1998	23-09-2001
8	S88	L23.2	M1281	YMAsO	Contact dermatitis both axillae, rollerball deodorant	11-09-2000	14-06-2001
9	L91	M15.0	XE1Gm	YMJbx	Osteoarthrosis both elbows/wrists/hands	11-09-2000	23-09-2001
10	ZIZ	Z63.0	XEOP7	Y7DkW	Strained relation with husband (drinking, jealous)	08-09-2001	23-09-2001

episode. Standard labels in a nomenclature or classification are adequate for retrieval and for research purposes, but are, evidently, often insufficient to describe the clinical situation of an individual patient. The dates of the start and the last encounter of the episode are included in the list; four episodes already existed at the time this patient first came to the practice. For retrieval purposes, the mapping of ICPC to the other systems result in compatibility, in the direction from highly detailed towards the diagnostic classes of ICPC. Tables 3 and 4 show part of the relations between the different systems for rheumatic heart disease and pulmonary embolism, respectively, illustrating the systems' different levels of granularity and specificity. Also, it becomes evident that however detailed a vocabulary, it will always need the addition of individual detail to the (readymade) terms.

In Table 5, the two encounters for the episode 'Vena cava inferior syndrome' from Weed's case history are documented and classified according to the ICPC-2 structure; in doing so, we had to adapt some of the patient information. The core elements of encounters—reasons for encounter, diagnoses, and interventions, including prescriptions—are coded with ICPC-2 and the ICPC drug code.[52] The column 'findings/free text' shows that a personalized narrative will almost always be needed.[53,54]

In order to illustrate the potential of double coding of clinical terms with ICD-10 as a nomenclature and ICPC as a classification system, we studied patient data for a group of very rare diseases in family practice. Two notoriously difficult ICPC 'ragbags' with rare malignancies were selected (D77: malignant digestive neoplasm other/unspecified, and R85: malignant respiratory neoplasm other), together also dealing with the crossing of the respiratory and the gastrointestinal tracts. From a 5-year database, collected within the framework of the Transition Project, with *Transhis* as an EPR (1995–99, approximately 19 000 listed patients with approximately 45 000 episodes of care), all episodes of care with either of these codes were identified ($n = 30$). Additional clinical information was extracted from the active database, or—in case a patient had died—from the inactive database, in order to establish the reliability of the diagnosis (Table 6). All episodes of care proved to be correctly included in the two ragbag codes. The two cases of carcinoid of the appendix were incorrectly included in ICPC rubric D77, in conformity with an error in the ICPC–ICD-10 mapping at that time. In ICPC-2, this neoplasm of uncertain behaviour has been included in D78.[8,9,27] It may be concluded that the use of ICPC as a classification with ICD-10 as a nomenclature (within a high quality EPR) allows the collection of reliable data on episodes of care with a prevalence as small as approximately 0.1 per 1000 listed patients; this also supports the feasibility of the thesaurus for routine double coding. However, it is also clear that the establishment and the upkeep of mappings requires much attention.

Table 3 Part of the mapping between ICPC code K71 (rheumatic fever/heart disease), ICD-10 (4-digit), and ICD-9-CM

ICD-9-CM code	ICD-9-CM label	ICD-10 code	ICD-10 label	ICPC-2 code	ICPC-2 label
398.0	Rheumatic myocarditis	I09.0	Rheumatic myocarditis	K71	Rheumatic fever/heart disease
397.0	Triscuspid valve disease	I07.1	Triscuspid insufficiency	K71	Rheumatic fever/heart disease
395.1	Rheumatic aortic insufficiency	I06.1	Rheumatic aortic insufficiency	K71	Rheumatic fever/heart disease
391.9	Acute rheumatic heart disease NOS	I01.9	Acute rheumatic heart disease unspecified	K71	Rheumatic fever/heart disease
391.9	Acute rheumatic heart disease NOS	I01.8	Other acute rheumatic heart disease unspecified	K71	Rheumatic fever/heart disease
392.0	Rheumatic chorea with heart involvement	I02.0	Rheumatic chorea with heart involvement	K71	Rheumatic fever/heart disease
392.9	Rheumatic chorea NOS	I02.9	Rheumatic chorea without heart involvement	K71	Rheumatic fever/heart disease
393.0	Chronic rheumatic pericarditis	I09.2	Chronic rheumatic pericarditis	K71	Rheumatic fever/heart disease
391.8	Acute rheumatic heart disease NEC	I01.8	Other acute rheumatic heart disease	K71	Rheumatic fever/heart disease
394.1	Rheumatic mitral insufficiency	I05.1	Rheumatic mitral insufficiency	K71	Rheumatic fever/heart disease
395.2	Rheumatic aortic stenosis with insufficiency	I06.2	Rheumatic aortic stenosis with insufficiency	K71	Rheumatic fever/heart disease
395.0	Rheumatic aortic stenosis	I06.0	Rheumatic aortic stenosis	K71	Rheumatic fever/heart disease

Table 4 Part of the mapping of Read codes and terms with ICD-10 for pulmonary embolism

Read code	Term identifier	Term[60]	ICD-10 code	ICD-10 label
G40.	Y20DC	Acute pulmonary heart disease	I260	Pulmonary embolism with mention of acute cor pulmonale
G400.	Y20DD	Acute cor pulmonale	I260	Pulmonary embolism with mention of acute cor pulmonale
G401.	YE0Qj	(Pulmonary embolus) or (pulmonary infarction)	I269	Pulmonary embolism without mention of acute cor pulmonale
G401.	Y20Dj	Pulmonary infarction	I269	Pulmonary embolism without mention of acute cor pulmonale
G401.	Y20DX	Pulmonary embolus	I269	Pulmonary embolism without mention of acute cor pulmonale
G401.	YMK5e	Infarction—pulmonary	I269	Pulmonary embolism without mention of acute cor pulmonale
G401.	Y20DV	Pulmonary embolism	I269	Pulmonary embolism without mention of acute cor pulmonale
G4010.	Yacwm	Postoperative pulmonary embolus	I269	Pulmonary embolism without mention of acute cor pulmonale
G402.	Y20Dj	Pulmonary infarction	I269	Pulmonary embolism without mention of acute cor pulmonale
G402.	Y20Dj	Pulmonary infarction	I260	Pulmonary embolism with mention of acute cor pulmonale
G402.	YMH3U	Pulmonary infarct	I260	Pulmonary embolism with mention of acute cor pulmonale
G402.	YMH3U	Pulmonary infarct	I269	Pulmonary embolism without mention of acute cor pulmonale

Table 5 Two encounters for episode K99—Vena cava inferior syndrome (after ligation 1998)

	Reason for encounter	History	Intervention	Medication	Findings, free text
8-5-2001	K07 swollen ankles	T07 weight gain	K31 partial examination K34 prothrombin time K50 medication	Furosemide =ICPC drug K20 =ATC C03CA01 Acenocoumaroli =ICPC drug B00 =ATC B01AA07	73.6 kg + 2 kg Both sides pitting oedema, L > R, during hot weather Disposition 3 months
23-9-2001	L14 leg symptoms/complaints K31 request examination K61 request test result		K31 partial examination K50 medication K67 referral vascular surgeon	Furosemide =ICPC drug K20 =ATC C03CA01 Acenocoumaroli =ICPC drug B00 =ATC B01AA07	Oedema R gone, L worse. Heavy, cumbersome feeling legs, swelling also during night Does not comply with Furosemide although it helps Pothr. time: 12 s Will talk with vascular surgeon before she sees him Disposition: return after seeing vascular surgeon

Table 6 The content of two 'difficult' ICPC ragbag rubrics: R85-malignant respiratory neoplasms, other, and D77-malignant digestive neoplasms, other/NOS; based on 30 patients

ICPC code	Localization of malignant neoplasm	ICD-10 code
R85 (*n* =7)	Larynx (*n* = 4)	C32
	Tonsil (*n*= 2)	C09
	Mesothelioma pleurae (*n* = 1)	C45.0
D77 (*n* = 23)	Lip (*n* = 5)	C00
	Gall bladder (*n* = 5)	C23
	Oesophagus (*n* = 4)	C15
	Small intestines (*n* = 3)	C17
	Carcinoid appendix (*n* = 2)	D37.3[a]
	Tongue base (*n* = 1)	C01
	Floor mouth (*n* = 1)	C04
	Parotitis (*n* = 1)	C07
	Other salivary gland (*n* = 1)	C08

[a] Erroneous, but 'correct' at the time.

Describing the domain of family practice

The relations between reasons for encounter and diagnoses, together with the diagnostic and therapeutic interventions, at the start and during follow up of episodes of care over time ('transitions') form the basis of knowledge about morbidity patterns in family practice.[4,16,39,45–47,55] At the heart of the use of ICPC is the establishment of prior and posterior probabilities for important diseases in family practice when patients present with a specific symptom or complaint.[40] Tables 7 and 8 present epidemiological data from the Transition Project (1985–2000, 185 016 patient years, collected by 56 Dutch family doctors). Table 7 shows the distribution of episodes of care starting with the reason for encounter R02 shortness of breath ($n = 5093$) in the form of probabilities, per 1000 reasons for encounter with 95 per cent confidence intervals, for seven standard age groups. The 'mirror' table (Table 8) presents, in a similar way, the reasons for encounter presented at the start of 7670 episodes of R78, acute bronchitis, per 1000 episodes of care. Cells with 5 or less observations were excluded in both tables, and the resulting distributions support the rule of thumb that diseases with a prevalence in family practice of less than 1 per 1000 will hardly ever—even in a large database as this one—reach the sufficient clinical significance required for generic research in family practice.[35,39,54] Age differences are responsible for considerable variation, and reflect characteristic differences in the clinical perspective of these reasons for encounter and diagnoses in the context of family practice. Evidently, this type of data has great potential value for family practice as an academic discipline, and for family physicians in that it can support their medical decision making.

In order to prove the utility of ICPC for comparative studies, Table 9 presents the most common symptoms and complaints at the start of episodes of care per 1000 patients per year from an international comparative study in the Netherlands, Japan, Poland, and the United States (the NAMCS data from the United States coded with RVC and ICD-9-CM have been mapped to ICPC).[39,56] Only 35 groups of symptoms/complaints covered the top-30s in all databases, at the same time including 45–60 per cent of all symptom/complaint reasons for encounter. In Table 10, the most frequent face-to-face encounters per episode of care per 1000 patients per year is given for the four countries, showing an overall very high number of face-to-face encounters per episode in Japan. The proportion of all encounters per 1000 patients per year covered by the top 30 for each country was 70–75 per cent. These tables support that aggregated ICPC data are suitable for use in comparative national studies into the content of family practice.

Discussion

Generally, the world becomes increasingly complex; however, with regard to classifications and nomenclatures in family practice, the world has become less complicated. The long-standing feud in the field of family practice classification between the 'lumpers' (who want to give precedence to the main classes of ICPC) and the 'splitters' (who prefer a system with the highest granularity) has become less relevant. Family practice as an academic discipline has a well-defined clinical domain, characterized by reasons for encounter, diagnoses, and interventions classified and coded with ICPC-2 in an episode of care structure.

This principle now can also be accepted in an operational form by family doctors working with EPRs based on the (mandatory) use of other systems such as ICD-9-CM, ICD-10(-CM), CTV-3 (and in the future SNOMED-CT), because of the reliable mapping structures with ICPC. This only applies to the diagnostic terminology; the available mapping structures, however, can greatly enhance continuity of care and the exchange of information on episodes of care between FPs and specialists. In the same vein, the American Psychiatric Association has developed the Diagnostic and Statistical Manual of Mental Disorders (now in its fourth edition: DSM-IV), for the characterization of the domain of psychiatry, at the same time maintaining a good comparability with the chapter on mental disorders in ICD-10.[57,58]

For classifying and coding reasons for encounter, ICPC has a unique approach, so far unlike any other system. However, ICPC offers only a very basic classification of interventions in family practice, and depending on the national situation, additional classifications of procedures should be considered for inclusion.[59] The ICPC drug code, directly derived from ATC (the Anatomical Therapeutical Chemical Classification Index), is a

Table 7 Final diagnoses of episodes of care starting with the reason for encounter R02, shortness of breath/dyspnoea ($n = 5093$), per 1000 reasons for encounter

Rank	ICPC Code	Label	Total	0–4	5–14	15–24	25–44	45–64	65–74	75+
1	R78	Acute bronchitis/bronchiolitis	254 ± 12	316 ± 37	279 ± 51	181 ± 45	248 ± 28	244 ± 28	282 ± 31	230 ± 23
2	R02	Shortness of breath/dyspnoea	118 ± 9	51 ± 18	101 ± 34	98 ± 34	108 ± 20	166 ± 24	130 ± 23	126 ± 18
3	R96	Asthma	93 ± 8	155 ± 29	248 ± 49	199 ± 46	124 ± 21	74 ± 17	44 ± 14	24 ± 8
4	K77	Heart failure	73 ± 7	—	—	—	—	30 ± 11	113 ± 22	198 ± 22
5	R98	Hyperventilation	72 ± 7	—	47 ± 24	181 ± 45	124 ± 21	106 ± 20	54 ± 16	34 ± 10
6	R74	URI (head cold)	62 ± 7	162 ± 30	87 ± 32	59 ± 27	83 ± 18	33 ± 12	31 ± 12	34 ± 10
7	R81	Pneumonia	39 ± 5	32 ± 14	—	—	31 ± 11	26 ± 10	38 ± 13	70 ± 14
8	R77	Acute laryngitis/tracheitis	38 ± 5	164 ± 30	77 ± 30	—	26 ± 10	25 ± 10	10 ± 7	12 ± 6
9	R95	Emphysema/COPD	22 ± 4	—	—	—	6 ± 5	24 ± 10	52 ± 15	31 ± 9
10	R05	Cough	16 ± 3	10 ± 8	—	—	28 ± 10	30 ± 11	8 ± 6	9 ± 5
11	K76	Ischaemic heart disease	16 ± 3	—	—	—	—	14 ± 8	26 ± 11	34 ± 10
12	A97	No disease	14 ± 3	19 ± 11	20 ± 16	—	13 ± 7	16 ± 8	10 ± 7	14 ± 6
13	R75	Sinusitis acute/chronic	14 ± 3	—	—	35 ± 21	28 ± 10	19 ± 9	9 ± 6	—
14	A77	Other viral diseases NOS	11 ± 3	25 ± 13	—	—	12 ± 7	11 ± 7	8 ± 6	6 ± 4
15	R91	Chronic bronchitis/bronchiectasis	8 ± 3	—	—	—	—	11 ± 7	19 ± 9	11 ± 6
16	L04	Chest symptoms/complaints	8 ± 3	—	—	—	16 ± 8	10 ± 6	8 ± 6	6 ± 4
17	K78	Atrial fibrillation/flutter	8 ± 2	—	—	—	—	7 ± 5	21 ± 10	13 ± 6
18	A04	General weakness/tiredness	7 ± 2	—	—	—	10 ± 6	9 ± 6	—	8 ± 5
19	A85	Adverse effect medical agent in proper dose	7 ± 2	—	—	—	—	12 ± 7	14 ± 8	9 ± 5
20	R99	Other disease respiratory system	6 ± 2	—	—	—	13 ± 7	7 ± 5	—	6 ± 4
		Total	5093	592	298	287	939	911	795	1271

Table 8 Reasons for encounter presented at the start of episodes of R78, acute bronchitis ($n \pm 7670$), per 1000 episodes of care

Rank	ICPC code	Label	Total	0–4	5–14	15–24	25–44	45–64	65–74	75+
1	R05	Cough	694 ± 10	698 ± 24	773 ± 31	730 ± 46	681 ± 25	715 ± 23	693 ± 27	628 ± 27
2	R02	Shortness of breath/dyspnoea	169 ± 8	130 ± 17	122 ± 25	142 ± 36	174 ± 20	155 ± 19	194 ± 23	232 ± 23
3	A03	Fever	154 ± 8	293 ± 24	214 ± 31	107 ± 32	117 ± 17	100 ± 16	109 ± 18	121 ± 18
4	R74	URI (head cold)	49 ± 5	56 ± 12	52 ± 17	82 ± 28	72 ± 14	56 ± 12	26 ± 9	21 ± 8
5	R03	Wheezing	46 ± 5	101 ± 16	31 ± 13	52 ± 23	42 ± 11	30 ± 9	19 ± 8	34 ± 10
6	A04	General weakness/tiredness	34 ± 4	28 ± 8	43 ± 15	41 ± 20	28 ± 9	29 ± 9	26 ± 9	51 ± 12
7	R78	Acute bronchitis/bronchiolitis	33 ± 4	15 ± 6	15 ± 9	27 ± 17	40 ± 11	50 ± 11	46 ± 12	29 ± 9
8	R25	Abnormal sputum/phlegm	30 ± 4	8 ± 5	—	49 ± 22	40 ± 10	44 ± 11	33 ± 10	32 ± 10
9	*31[a]	Request partial med. exam/health evaluation	24 ± 3	27 ± 8	21 ± 11	—	26 ± 9	23 ± 8	17 ± 8	32 ± 10
10	*50[a]	Request medication/prescription/injection	23 ± 13	11 ± 5	12 ± 8	19 ± 14	27 ± 9	38 ± 10	26 ± 9	23 ± 8
11	R21	Symptoms/complaints throat	16 ± 3	—	24 ± 11	38 ± 20	34 ± 10	17 ± 7	9 ± 5	6 ± 4
12	R01	Pain attributed to respiratory system	14 ± 3	—	9 ± 7	—	36 ± 10	16 ± 7	12 ± 6	10 ± 6
13	R07	Sneezing/nasal congestion	8 ± 2	11 ± 5	—	—	7 ± 4	10 ± 5	8 ± 5	—
14	N01	Headache	6 ± 2	—	9 ± 7	—	10 ± 5	6 ± 4	5 ± 4	5 ± 4
15	D10	Vomiting	5 ± 2	17 ± 7	—	—	—	—	—	—
16	R80	Influenza (proven) without pneumonia	5 ± 2	—	—	—	7 ± 5	8 ± 5	10 ± 6	—
17	*64[a]	Provider initiated episode new/ongoing	5 ± 2	4 ± 3	—	—	—	—	8 ± 5	10 ± 5
18	L04	Chest symptoms/complaints	5 ± 2	—	—	—	7 ± 5	6 ± 4	7 ± 5	5 ± 4
19	R04	Other breathing problems	4 ± 1	5 ± 4	—	—	—	4 ± 3	5 ± 4	6 ± 4
20	R27	Fear of other respiratory disease	4 ± 1	—	—	—	7 ± 4	6 ± 4	—	—
		Total	10 645	2103	967	517	1906	1975	1510	1667

[a] Numerical ICPC code without indication of chapter; e.g. *50 means all requests for medication.

Table 9 Most frequent (groups of) reasons for encounter in the form of a symptom/complaint per 1000 patients per year, standardized for the 1996 sex/age distribution of the US population, based on top 30 of the Netherlands, Japan, Poland, and NAMCS (between brackets, percentages dealt with by a family physician in the United States). Italicized figures indicate highest rates

ICPC codes	Symptom/complaint	The Netherlands	Japan	Poland	NAMCS (% family physician)
R05/R07	Cough/sneezing/nasal congestion	163	292	*684*	295 (41)
R21/R22/R23	Throat/voice/tonsil symptoms/complaints	66	81	*250*	102 (33)
A02/A03	Fever/chills	71	*158*	155	99 (29)
L02/L03/L05	Low back/back/flank symptoms/complaints	88	28	64	*135* (51)
D01/D06	Abdominal pain	*77*	34	76	42 (34)
A04	Tiredness	*76*	21	35	60 (26)
R02/R03	Shortness of breath/wheezing	*73*	9	14	59 (27)
S06/S07	Redness skin	*72*	52	42	64 (31)
N01	Headache	46	49	39	*68* (40)
H01	Earache	47	12	24	*59* (33)
L15	Knee symptoms/complaints	45	20	28	*55* (12)
P03	Feeling depressed	16	a	8	*53* (16)
S04	Localized swelling skin	*53*	14	19	28 (56)
L14	Leg/thigh symptoms/complaints	38	11	14	*51* (25)
K01/K02/L04	Heart/chest pain/tightness	48	15	*49*	42 (34)
D09/D10	Nausea/vomiting	34	*49*	24	42 (37)
F05/F07	Vision problems	8	2	38	*48* (8)
P01	Feeling anxious/nervous/tense	26	1	14	*47* (17)
U01/U02/U03	Urination symptoms/complaints	22	3	*47*	37 (25)
L01	Neck symptoms/complaints	36	16	18	*44* (48)
L08	Shoulder symptoms/complaints	*42*	12	16	40 (52)
S03	Warts	*40*	1	4	12 (27)
D11	Diarrhoea	20	*38*	21	28 (36)
S02	Pruritus	*37*	19	25	25 (29)
L12	Hand/finger symptoms/complaints	27	12	14	*36* (21)
D02/D03	Stomach pain/heartburn	28	25	33	*34* (33)
L17	Foot/toe symptoms/complaints	*34*	10	19	22 (17)
N17	Vertigo	29	14	17	*32* (34)
H02	Hearing complaints	*29*	2	15	12 (15)
R09	Sinus symptoms/complaints	24	2	14	*29* (47)
H13	Plugged feeling ear	*22*	1	10	12 (36)
P06	Sleeping disturbance	18	6	9	*20* (25)
S18	Laceration	*18*	17	14	10 (46)
D19/D20	Mouth/tongue/teeth symptoms/complaints	15	*15*	12	2 (51)
S12	Insect bite	3	*11*	2	3 (42)
	Total top 30s	1491	1052	1867	1747
	All symptom/complaint reasons for encounter per 1000 patients per year	3362	1923	3375	2598 (31)

a Less than 0.5 per 1000 patients per year.

good example of this.[52] A major decision with regard to the documentation of interventions is whether family doctors will primarily take on the responsibility to classify and code the interventions for which they are, themselves, responsible, or whether they wish to document and code all interventions that their patients face in their national health care system. Controlled medical vocabularies contain large numbers of entries focusing on interventions, laboratory tests, disposition, administrative procedures, occupations, drugs, and a variety of other health-related subject fields. The CTV-3 is a good example of this; its large terminology contains well over 300 000 terms, but only 87 000 of these have a direct link with ICD-10, and, consequently, a mapping to ICPC.

A caveat should be put in with regard to the potential utility of medical vocabularies used through their mapping to ICD-10. Their content is 'Anglo-Saxon', and their utility in countries other than the United Kingdom

Table 10 Diagnoses in the most frequent direct encounters per episode (group) per 1000 patients per year, standardized for the 1996 sex/age distribution of the US population and based on top 30s of the Netherlands, Japan, Poland, and NAMCS (between brackets, percentages dealt with by a family physician in the United States). Italicized figures indicate highest rates

ICPC codes	Diagnosis	The Netherlands	Japan	Poland	NAMCS (% family physician)
K86/K87	Hypertension	181	*619*	153	203 (38)
A97/A98	Prevention/no disease	171	42	*538*	254 (44)
A77/A78/R05/R07/R21/R74/R77/R80	All URTI	165	509	*511*	198 (46)
R72/R76/R90	Tonsillitis/strep throat	26	30	*274*	26 (33)
L95	Osteoporosis	9	*234*	27	9 (39)
L02/L03/L05/L84/L86	Back pain/ischiatica	92	*186*	24	67 (45)
D84/D90	Disease of oesophagus/hernia	16	*161*	3	25 (36)
R78	Acute bronchitis	58	32	*144*	67 (47)
D85/D86	Duodenal/peptic ulcer	5	*136*	12	11 (34)
T90	Diabetes	63	*128*	81	99 (39)
R96	Asthma	51	*125*	15	52 (25)
L89/L90/L91	Arthritis	24	*122*	28	55 (43)
L01/N02/L83	Neck symptoms/complaints, cervical syndrome	43	*120*	36	21 (42)
D87	Gastritis	20	*117*	22	9 (40)
S86/S87/S88	Dermatitis	85	*115*	52	41 (21)
	All musculoskeletal trauma	*93*	55	18	20 (45)
W78/W84/W90/W92	Pregnancy	68	a	18	*90* (8)
P06	Sleeping disturbance	40	*90*	8	6 (51)
T93	Lipid metabolism disorder	28	*89*	41	23 (34)
R75	Sinusitis	37	20	54	*85* (41)
K89/K90	TIA/CVA	19	*82*	5	13 (27)
H71/H72	Otitis media	38	14	15	*81* (23)
P76/P03	Depression/depressed feeling	78	34	13	*79* (27)
K74/K75/K76	Ischaemic heart disease	38	*79*	28	66 (21)
S18	Laceration/cut	27	*78*	20	11 (41)
D12	Constipation	26	*78*	20	8 (39)
B80	Iron deficiency anaemia	15	*67*	7	17 (33)
D11/D73	Diarrhoea/gastro-enteritis	27	*63*	27	25 (35)
	Malignancy	42	28	10	*52* (11)
R97	Hay fever	23	40	14	*50* (28)
T80/T81/T85	Thyroid disorders	10	27	*50*	4 (26)
K77	Cardiac insufficiency	24	*48*	14	23 (31)
U71	Cystitis	35	13	*47*	5 (49)
L08/L92	Shoulder symptom/complaint/syndrome	*46*	29	5	16 (42)
D72	Viral hepatitis	1	*46*	2	2 (–)
S03	Warts	*45*	4	5	15 (31)
F92	Cataract	3	*43*	10	40 (3)
N01/N89	Headache/migraine	32	*43*	18	36 (36)
W11	Oral contraception	*41*	a	8	12 (25)
P01/P74	Feeling anxious/anxiety disorder	*40*	38	8	26 (30)
S74	Dermatophytosis	40	36	10	13 (21)
A04	Tiredness	*40*	15	16	14 (50)
X14/X16/X72/X84/X85	All vaginitis	*39*	a	8	23 (27)
H81	Earwax	*39*	2	12	12 (29)
T82/T83	Overweight/obesity	10	1	8	*36* (42)
R91/R95	COPD/emphysema	32	*35*	6	29 (32)
T92	Gout	5	*35*	2	6 (38)
R81	Pneumonia	16	18	*34*	14 (31)
S96	Acne	11	2	8	*27* (10)
A85	Side-effects of medication	*24*	8	4	5 (38)
Y85	Benign prostatic hypertrophy	6	*22*	11	21 (24)
D06	Localized abdominal pain	*20*	11	18	5 (38)
D22	Worms	2	1	*18*	2 (–)
	Total top 30s	2169	3970	2530	2159
	All face-to-face encounters p1000 ppy	2785	5330	3936	2955 (26)

a Less than 0.5 per patient per year.

and the United States is, especially in family practice, not certain.[60] International Classification of Primary Care is available in close to 20 languages, and because the mapping between ICPC-2 and ICD-10 is alphanumeric, it is, in principle, to be expected that a multilanguage use can easily be established. The application of ICPC, however, as the organization principle of international family practice, based on a mapping with national diagnostic terminologies/nomenclatures (ICD-9 or -10) requires explicit testing.[8,27,60]

The increasing availability of EPRs in family practice allows to shift the focus from the classification predicaments in the Anglo-Saxon world towards the multilanguage and multicultural aspects of family practice. For the international family practice community it now becomes increasingly possible to focus on one of the original goals of ICPC: to empirically characterize the clinical content of family practice under very different language and national health care conditions in international comparative studies. That is the royal route to elucidating what is generic for the family practice discipline, and what is, to some extent, the result of local or national conditions.

Appendix: glossary of terms

Note: this glossary is based on the WONCA International Glossary for Family Practice, and on the *Dictionary of Epidemiology* 4th edn. In addition, several definitions have been added from other sources. In case no international agreement existed, the authors decided which definitions to include.

Axis

Direction or reference within a classification system. ICPC is biaxial: one axis represents 17 body systems/problem areas (chapters), and the other seven components.

Classification of diseases

Arrangement of diseases with common characteristics into groups or classes. The usefulness depends on the user's objectives.

Classification system

Arrangement of all concepts in a domain into groups/classes according to established criteria. Prerequisites for a classification are:

1. naturalness: the classes correspond to the nature of the thing being classified;
2. exhaustiveness: every member of the group will fit into one (and only one) class;
3. usefulness: the classification is practical;
4. simplicity: the subclasses are not excessive;
5. constructability: the set of classes can be constructed by a demonstrable procedure.

Classify

To aggregate concepts from a domain into groups/classes for a purpose.

Code

Fixed sequence of numerical and/or alphabetical characters, serving to designate an object, a concept, or a term. In many coding systems (e.g. ICPC and ICD), codes are *significant*: they describe the position of the concept in a hierarchy. Other systems use *non-significant* codes that are context-free and not related to the concept's meaning.

Compatibility

Ability to exist together in harmony. Classifications are compatible when they are inter-related in an established and consistent manner through mapping/linkage.

Comparability

Quality or state of being equivalent or similar. Classifications are comparable when, and in so far as their rubrics allow mapping/linkage of identical concepts.

Concept

Unit of knowledge created by a unique combination of characteristics.

Contact

See Encounter.

Diagnostic categories

Family practice uses three diagnostic categories:

1. *pathological/pathophysiological diagnoses* with a proven pathological/ pathophysiological substrate and/or aetiology (e.g.: carcinoma, hypertension);
2. *symptom diagnoses* label a patient's symptom or complaint as the diagnosis (e.g.: diarrhoea, tiredness);
3. *nosological diagnoses* (synonym: *syndrome)* label the diagnosis as a symptom complex based on consensus between physicians, without (as yet) a proven pathological or pathophysiological basis or aetiology (e.g.: migraine, depressive disorder).

Diagnostic criteria

Symptoms and complaints, together with the objective signs and test results that are essential for labelling a health problem with a specific diagnosis.

Diagnosis

Formal statement of the provider's understanding of the patient's health problem, representing the formal establishment of an episode of care.

Diagnostic and statistical manual (DSM)

Manual (developed by the American Psychiatric Association) that aims at systematizing and standardizing definitions of mental disorders, listing all psychiatric diagnoses with their criteria. Latest edition: DMS-IV, 1994.

Disease

Physiological or psychological dysfunction. To be distinguished from *illness* (the subjective state of not feeling well), and from *sickness* (state of social dysfunction, i.e. the role an individual assumes when feeling ill).

Domain

Field of special knowledge; its borders are defined from a purpose-related point of view.

Encounter

Professional interchange between a patient and (a) member(s) of a health care team. One or more episodes of care may be dealt with at an encounter. An encounter may be direct (face to face) or indirect (telephone call, letter, through a third party, or administrative).

Episode of care

A health problem from its first presentation by the patient to a health care provider until the completion of the last encounter for it. It encompasses all contact elements related to that health problem; its name (diagnosis) may change over time.

Health problem

Health concern of a patient as determined by the health care provider. Problems should be recorded at the highest level of specificity possible.

1. *new problem:* the first presentation of a problem;
2. *continuing problem:* a previously assessed problem requiring ongoing care (follow-up).

Incommensurability

See Paradigm.

International Classification of Primary Care (ICPC) (1st edn., 1987; 2nd edn., 1998; electronic edn., 2000)

The official classification of the World Organization of Family Doctors (WONCA) (see Box 1).

International Statistical Classification of Diseases and Related Health Problems (ICD)

Classification of health and health related concepts, classifying diseases, symptoms, other reasons for encounter, and external causes of injury; developed by WHO, now in its 10th revision: ICD-10 (1992) ICD-10 has 21 chapters and now uses alphanumeric codes in order to provide a larger coding frame than previously, leaving room for future expansion. Some chapters are aetiologic (e.g. *Infective and Parasitic Conditions*), others relate to body systems (e.g. *Circulatory System*), and some to classes of a condition (e.g. *Neoplasms, Injury*). This heterogeneity of categories reflects prevailing uncertainties about causes of disease.

International Classification of Health Problems in Primary Care (ICHPPC)

Predecessor of ICPC. Produced by the WONCA Classification Committee in 1975, revised as ICHPPC-2 (1979), and as ICHPPC-2-Defined (1983) with inclusion criteria to reduce miscoding and coding variability. Structured in the same way as ICD-9.

ICPC-Drug classification

ICPC classification of drugs (1993); compatible with the Anatomical Therapeutic Chemical Classification Index (ATC), but following ICPC's chapter structure in that classes were selected according to their relevance for family practice.

IC-PROCESS-PC

International Classification of Process in Primary Care, produced by the WONCA Classification Committee (1986) to classify and code the diagnostic and therapeutic elements in the process in primary care.

Intervention

See Process.

Linkage/mapping

Establishment of a relation between the representation of a concept in one system to the most similar representation in another system.

Mode

A way a classification may be used. ICPC can classify: (a) reasons for encounter; (b) diagnoses; and (c) interventions. Comprehensive use includes the simultaneous use of all three modes.

Modification, diagnostic

Revision of a diagnosis in the course of an episode of care.

Morbidity

Collective term for all health problems of an individual patient, a group of patients or a practice population during a defined period of time.

Narrative

Free text part in a medical record.

Nomenclature

A terminology that is systematically structured according to pre-established rules.

NOS

Not otherwise specified: the term to be coded cannot be classified to a more specific rubric.

Nosology

Classification of diseases into groups with explicit criteria, based on agreement as to the boundaries of the groups.

Object

Anything perceivable or conceivable.

Paradigm

Typical example, pattern of thought, conceptualization, overall way of regarding phenomena of a group of scientists. A paradigm may dictate what explanation will be acceptable, but paradigms may change. *Incommensurability* exists when two paradigms are in conflict.

Process (intervention)

What is done for the management of a reason for encounter and/or a health issue by a health care provider.

Ragbag

Miscellaneous collection of symptoms and complaints, of interventions or of diseases not classified elsewhere.

Read-codes (Clinical Terms Version 3, CTV-3)

The terminology used by the NHS for health service in the United Kingdom, including a wide range of objects.

Reason for encounter

The statement of the reason(s) why a person enters the health care system, representing that person's demand for care. The coded/documented reason for encounter should be recognized by the patient as an acceptable description of her/his demand for care.

Rubric

Medical phrase for designating/identifying a class in a coding system.

SNOMED (Systematized Nomenclature of Medicine)

Multi-axial systematized nomenclature developed by the College of American Pathologists. It is a concept-based reference terminology that allows coding of clinical concepts with clear relationships between terms and concepts.

Symptom

Any subjective evidence of a health problem, as perceived by the patient, for example, cough, pain, and tiredness.

Terminology

List of terms referring to the concepts in a particular domain.

Term

Verbal designation of a concept in a specific subject field.

Thesaurus

Systematic set of professionally used words, including terms and jargon, in which each word is represented with possible synonyms, and related words designating broader or narrower concepts. A thesaurus may serve as a dictionary or as a translation from jargon to terminology.

Transition

Process of change during episodes of care developing over time through health care.

Unified Medical Language System (UMLS)

Unified Medical Language System: a Controlled Medical Vocabulary, developed by the National Library of Medicine (United States) as a knowledge source with references to classifications (including ICPC-2 and ICD-10), and terminologies such as SNOMED and CTV-3.

Vocabulary

Terminological dictionary containing the designations from one or more specific subject fields. A 'Controlled Medical Vocabulary' contains the terminology of related subject fields in medicine: diseases, reasons for encounter, external causes, health interventions, preventive measures, microbial causes, morphology, environmental factors, living conditions, body functions, etc.

References

1. **International Classification of Diseases.** Manual of the International Statistical Classification of Diseases, Injuries and Causes of Death. Ninth revision, ICD-9. Geneva: World Health Organization, 1977.
2. **International Classification of Diseases.** Manual of the International Statistical Classification of Diseases, Injuries and Causes of Death. Tenth revision, ICD-10. Geneva: World Health Organization, 1993.
3. **White, K.L.** (1987). Historical preface. In *ICPC. International Classification of Primary Care* (ed. H. Lamberts and M. Wood), pp. 11–14. Oxford: Oxford University Press.
4. **Lamberts, H. and Wood, M.**, ed. *ICPC. International Classification of Primary Care.* Oxford: Oxford University Press, 1987.
5. **ICHPPC.** *International Classification of Health Problems in Primary Care.* Chicago IL: American Hospital Association, 1975.
6. **ICHPPC-2.** *International Classification of Health Problems in Primary Care* 2nd edn. Oxford: Oxford University Press, 1979.
7. **ICHPPC-2-Defined.** *International Classification of Health Problems in Primary Care* 3rd edn. Oxford: Oxford University Press, 1983.
8. **ICPC-2.** *International Classification of Primary Care* 2nd edn. Oxford: Oxford University Press, 1998.
9. **Okkes, I.M., Jamoulle, M., Lamberts, H., and Bentzen, N.** (2000). ICPC-2-E: the electronic version of ICPC-2. Differences from the printed version and the consequences. *Family Practice* **17**, 101–6.
10. **Bentzen, N.**, ed. (1995). An international glossary for general/family practice. *Family Practice* **12**, 341–69.
11. **Last, J.M.**, ed. *A Dictionary of Epidemiology* 4th edn. Oxford: Oxford University Press, 2001.
12. **Health Informatics—Vocabulary on Terminological Systems.** ISO/TC 215/WG 3 N 000, 2000-10-21 ISO/WD nnn-n. ISO/TC 215/WG3.
13. **Ingenerf, J. and Giere, W.** (1998). Concept-oriented standardization and statistics-oriented classification: continuing the classification versus nomenclature controversy. *Methods of Information in Medicine* **37**, 527–39.
14. **Rector, A.L.** (1998). Clinical terminology: why is it so hard? *Methods of Information in Medicine* **38**, 239–52.
15. **De Keizer, N.F., Abu-Hanna, A., and Zwetsloot-Schonk, J.H.M.** (2000). Understanding terminological systems I: terminology and typology. *Methods of Information in Medicine* **39**, 16–21.
16. **Lamberts, H. and Hofmans-Okkes, I.M.** (1996). Episode of care: a core concept in family practice. *Journal of Family Practice* **42**, 161–7.
17. **Cimino, J.J.** (1998). Desiderata for controlled medical vocabularies in the twenty-first century. *Methods of Information in Medicine* **37**, 394–403.
18. **Smith, N., Wilson, A., and Weekes, T.** (1995). Use of Read codes in development of a standard data set. *British Medical Journal* **311**, 313–15.
19. **Cimino, J.J.** (1996). Review paper: Coding systems in health care. *Methods of Information in Medicine* **35**, 273–84.
20. **Côté, R.A., Rothwell, D.J., Palotay, J.L., Becket, R.S., and Brochu, L.**, ed. *The Systematized Nomenclature of Medicine SNOMED International.* Northfield IL: College of American Pathologists, 1993.
21. **NHS Centre for Coding and Classification.** *Read Codes, Version 3.* London: NHS Management Executive, Department for Health, 1994.
22. **Rothwell, D.** (1995). SNOMED-based knowledge representation. *Method Information in Medicine* **34**, 209–13.
23. **NHS Website:** http://www.nhsia.nhs.uk/terms/pages/faq.asp.
24. **Lindberg, D., Humphreys, B., and McGray, A.** (1993). The Unified Medical Language System. *Method of Information Medicine* **34**, 281–91.
25. **Unified Medical Language System (UMLS) Knowledge Sources,** 12th edn. Hyattsville: US Department of Health and Humans Services, National Institutes of Health, National Library of Medicine, 2001.
26. **Rector, A., Solomon, W., Nowlan, W., Rush, T., Zanstra, P., and Claassen, W.** (1995). A terminology server for medical language and medical information systems. *Methods of Information in Medicine* **34**, 147–57.
27. **Lamberts, H., Wood, M., and Hofmans-Okkes, I.**, ed. *The International Classification of Primary Care in the European Community, with a Multi-language Layer.* Oxford: Oxford University Press, 1993.
28. **Britt, H.** (1997). A new coding tool for computerised clinical systems in primary care: ICPC Plus. *Australian Family Physician* **26**, S79–82.
29. **Lamberts, H. and Hofmans-Okkes, I.M.** (1997). Sense and specificity in computer based patient records in general practice. The ICPC-ICD-10 conversion structure as the Holy Grail. *Australian Family Physician* **26**, S57–9.
30. **Bernstein, R.M., Hollingworth, G.R., and Viner, G.S.** ENCODE-FM (Electronic Nomenclature and Classification of Disorders and Encounters for Family Medicine), Version 2.1, May 1997. Ottawa: Insite-Family Medicine, 1997.
31. **Virtanen, M., Liukko, M., Hartikainen, K., and Lorensen, F.** *Handbook of Diagnostic Classification for Primary Care.* First draft for expert use. Kuntaliito: STAKES, 1996.
32. **Lorentzen, E.F.** (1996). International Classification of Primary Care converted to ICD-10. In *Medical Informatica in Europe 1996* (ed. J. Brendel et al.), pp. 188–92. Amsterdam: IOS Press.
33. **Hofmans-Okkes, I.M. and Lamberts, H.** (1996). The International Classification of Primary Care (ICPC): new applications in research and computer-based patient records in family practice. *Family Practice* **13**, 294–302.
34. **Becker, H.W., Van Boven, C., Oskam, S.K., Okkes, I.M., Hirs, W., and Lamberts, H.** ICPC-2-NL/ICD-10-NL Thesaurus. CD-ROM. Amsterdam: Project Dutch College of General Practitioners/Family Doctors and the Academic Medical Centre/University of Amsterdam on Adaptation of ICPC, Integration and Implementation of ICD-10(-CM), 2001.
35. **Lamberts, H. and Hofmans-Okkes, I.** (1996). The generic patient record: an alliance between patient documentation and medical informatics. *Methods of Information Medicine* **35**, 5–7.
36. **Okkes, I.M., Oskam, S.K., and Lamberts, H.** (2002). The probability of specific diagnoses for patients presenting with common symptoms to Dutch family physicians. *Journal of Family Practice* **51**, 31–6.
37. **Hofmans-Okkes, I.M.** (1993). An international study into the concept and the validity of the 'reason for encounter'. In *The International Classification*

of Primary Care in the European Community, with a multi-language layer* (ed. H. Lamberts, M. Wood, and Halman-okkes), pp. 34–42. Oxford: Oxford University Press.

38. **Patients' Reasons for Visiting Physicians: National Ambulatory Medical Care Survey United Sates, 1977–8.** DHHS Publication 82-1717. Hyattsville: US Department of Health and Human Services, 1981.
39. **Rector, A.** (2001). AIM; a personal view of where I have been and where we might be going. *Artificial Intelligence in Medicine* **23**, 111–27.
40. **Sadegh-Zadeh, K.** (2001). The fuzzy revolution: goodbye to the Aristotelian Weltanschauung. *Artificial Intelligence in Medicine* **21**, 1–25.
41. **Lamberts, H.** (1996). Generic research in general practice. *European Journal of General Practice* **2**, 129–31.
42. **Okkes, I.M., Polderman, G.O., Fryer, G.E., Yamada, T., Bujak, M., Oskam, S.K., Green, L.A., and Lamberts, H.** (2002). The role of family practice in different health care systems. A comparison of reasons for encounter, diagnoses and interventions in primary care populations in the Netherlands, Japan, Poland and the US. *Journal of Family Practice* **52**, 72.
43. **Mennerat, F. and Jamoulle, M.** Updated ICPC Bibliography http://www.ulb.ac.be/esp/wicc/icpc_ref.html
44. **Grimsmo, A., Hagman, E., Falkø, E., Matthiesen, L., and Njalsson, T.** (2001). Patients, diagnoses and processes in general practice in the Nordic countries. An attempt to make data from computerised medical records available for comparable statistics. *Scandinavian Journal of Primary Health Care* **19**, 76–82.
45. **Klinkman, M.S. and Green, L.A.** (1995). Using ICPC in a computer-based primary care information system. *Family Medicine* **27**, 449–56.
46. **Brage, S., Bentsen, B.G., Bjerkedal, T., Nygård, J.F., and Tellnes, G.** (1996). ICPC as a standard classification in Norway. *Family Practice* **13**, 391–6.
47. **Donaldson, M.S., Yordy, K.D., Lohr, K.N., and Vanselow, N.A.** *Primary Care. America's Health in a New Era.* Washington DC: Institute of Medicine, National Academy Press, 1996.
48. **Iggulden, P.** *Towards an 'Episode of Care' Approach: A Project Briefing.* Winchester GB: NHS Information Authority, 2000.
49. **Baegan, E., Øystein, N., and Grimsmo, A.** (2001). Ranking of information in the computerized problem-oriented patient record. In *Medinfo 2001* (ed. V. Patel et al.), pp. 594–9. Amsterdam: IOS Press.
50. **Weed, L.L.** (1968). Medical records that guide and teach. *New England Journal of Medicine* **278**, 593–9.
51. **Weed, L.L.** (1968). Medical records that guide and teach. Concluded. *New England Journal of Medicine* **278**, 652–7.
52. **De Maeseneer, J.** (1993). The ICPC classification of drugs. In *The International Classification of Primary Care in the European Community* (ed. H. Lamberts, M. Wood, and I.M. Hofmans-Okkes), pp. 163–70. Oxford: Oxford University Press.
53. **Kay, S. and Purves, I.N.** (1996). Medical records and other stories: a narratological framework. *Methods of Information in Medicine* **35**, 72–87.
54. **Tange, H.J., Schouten, H.C., Kester, A.D.M., and Hasman, A.** (1998). The granularity of medical narratives and its effect on the speed and completeness of information retrieval. *Journal of the American Medical Information Association* **5**, 571–82.
55. **Okkes, I.M., Groen, A., Oskam, S.K., and Lamberts, H.** (2001). Advantages of long observation in episode-oriented electronic patient records in family practice. *Methods of Information in Medicine* **40**, 229–35.
56. **Commission on Professional and Hospital Activities.** *International Classification of Diseases,* 9th Revision, with Clinical Modifications (ICD-9-CM). Ann Arbor, 1978.
57. **Lamberts, H., Magruder, K., Kathol, R.G., Pincus, H.A., and Okkes, I.M.** (1998). The classification of mental disorders in primary care: a guide through a difficult terrain. *International Journal of Psychiatry in Medicine* **28**, 159–76.
58. **American Psychiatric Association Committee on Nomenclature and Statistics.** *Diagnostic and Statistical Manual of Mental Disorders* 4th edn. (DSM-IV). Washington DC: American Psychiatric Association, 1994.
59. **IC-Process-PC.** *International Classification of Process in Primary Care.* Oxford: Oxford University Press, 1986.
60. **Berg, M.** (1998). Medical work and the computer-based patient record: a sociological perspective. *Methods of Information in Medicine* **37**, 294–301.

4.4 Age and gender

Willem Jan van der Veen and Betty Meyboom-de Jong

Introduction

Like the traveller who uses a map to follow a certain route to reach his destination, a GP uses a set of patient characteristics to arrive at a certain diagnosis. Age and gender are important coordinates of the GPs mental map, aiding in the task of making sense of the verbal and non-verbal appearance of the patient, identifying underlying pathological processes, assessing the prognosis for the patient, and choosing an appropriate course of action. Some medical conditions are more frequently, or even exclusively, seen in men, whereas other conditions are more frequently brought to the attention of the GP by female patients. Gender—as a variable encompassing the biological aspects of sex together with its social, cultural, and political dimensions—matters in many primary care situations, as it affects the type of conditions seen by GPs and the way patients disclose their problems. Age as a variable functions in roughly the same way as gender, in providing the GP with cues to structure the contact with the patient in terms of past events, the present condition, and possible outcomes in the future. Many disorders are closely related to certain ages and stages in life or to a transition from one stage to another. Their severity may, moreover, be related to the age at onset. Age is, moreover, a marker of the patient's birth generation, which may affect help-seeking behaviour, ways of communicating, and use of medical services. In short, age represents a stage in the medical, sociocultural, and relational biography of a patient.

This micro-perspective on primary care can be complemented with an epidemiologic, population-based macro-perspective. The amount and type of care demanded by a general practice population is strongly affected by its age and sex distribution. General practices with relatively young populations do have other patterns of care compared to those focusing on elderly populations with an over-representation of women. The age and sex distribution of a general practice population is determined by its increments (birth, entry into practice) and decrements (departure, death). Whereas the sex ratio at the lower ages is likely to be slightly in favour of men (as there is a slight excess of men over women at birth), women tend to become more numerous from about age 60 onward as a result of a lower male life expectancy. The amount or volume of care demanded and provided is partly a function of the size and distribution of the underlying population being served by a general practice and partly affected by the relative frequencies of the health problems for which advice and assistance are being sought over the age and sex groups. To make a comparison for descriptive epidemiologic purposes, standardization by age and sex serves to distinguish between the effect of different population sizes and the effect of different prevalences of health problems.

Before causal hypotheses can be raised and tested, new descriptive studies may serve to provide an adequate map of this study area.(1) In this chapter, we aim to provide such a map by bringing together these two connected perspectives on the role of age and gender in primary care and presenting some empirical findings on the subject. The micro-perspective on primary care has a focus on the types of problems presented by patients, the management of patient trajectories, and the amount of care demanded and provided. The epidemiologic approach, on the other hand, has a focus on the underlying processes that help to explain why events occur as they do in general practice and why they occur with particular intensities, patterns, and frequencies.

In our attempt to treat this vast subject in a compact manner, we use several theoretical insights that together serve to consider age and gender as the markers of an unfolding (medical) lifecourse. Age reflects the stage a patient has reached within his or her lifecourse. With the structuring of health data by age, it may become visible that patients go through distinct sequences and that there is a certain commonality in human life throughout time. Gender points to the heterogeneity in the experience of this unfolding lifecourse and in the way medical problems arising from particular lifecourse stages are brought to the attention of a GP. Women are biologically different from men and thereby encounter different problems. The organization of their lifecourse in time may also differ, in terms of leaving the parental home, sexuality, reproductive experiences, family formation and dissolution, adoption of health-damaging behaviours, education and work, and growing older. The unfolding lifecourses of women and men can be seen as a set of careers developing in sequences or side by side, such as the reproductive career, family career, and work career. The combination of these careers and the transitions from one stage to the other may be experienced and coped with differently by women and men, resulting in different demand for care patterns across gender.

Apart from a theoretical exploration, we aim to illustrate several key features of the role of age and gender with empirical data taken from the morbidity and medication Registration Network Groningen (RNG).(2) The database of the RNG is based on the electronic patient files of 16 GPs in the north of the Netherlands with a total of about 30 000 patients on their lists. The GPs are working in three single-handed practices and one group-practice in the University town of Groningen and in two group-practices in the smaller towns of Hoogezand-Sappemeer and Hoogeveen. Data refer to the 3-year period 1998–2000. We realize that every dataset covering a relatively small local or regional population carries with it all the peculiarities of local policies, habits, and health care structures. Nevertheless, we believe that our findings bear relevance to other primary care contexts as well. With a dataset like the one used here, the underlying epidemiology of a population broken down by age and gender can be described, as the Dutch GP is often the first medical resource person being contacted for diagnosis, treatment, medication, and referral.

Theoretical perspectives

The events occurring in general practice and their distributions by age and gender have their own underlying epidemiology. This section serves to introduce several concepts and perspectives from the literature to enhance our understanding about the types of health problems encountered by men and women during their lifecourse and their underlying forces.

The epidemiologic transition

Omran defined three stages in the epidemiologic transition that eventually led to the mortality and morbidity regimes and patterns of today's low-mortality countries and the certainty of life for most of their citizens.(3) The first stage, the 'age of pestilence and famine', is characterized by fluctuations in death rates resulting from epidemics, famines, and war. Most deaths were attributed to infectious diseases, malnutrition, and maternity complications. High infant and child mortality kept life expectancy at low levels. Moreover, women who survived infancy and childhood continued to face high risks because of the complications associated with pregnancy and delivery. The second stage, called the 'age of receding pandemics', was characterized by a smoothing out of the peaks and troughs of mortality, and a redistribution of deaths from early life to advanced ages. The most favourable effects on survival were concentrated among infants, children, and women of childbearing age.(4) The third stage, called the 'age of degenerative and man-made diseases', emerged in the first half of the twentieth century but became manifest mostly after World War II, with chronic diseases underlying most deaths at higher ages. This stage was initially considered a plateau phase in our epidemiologic history where an equilibrium of mortality was achieved and theoretical limits to mortality declines were approached.(4) With the arrival of this stage a shift from acutely fatal infectious disease to chronic degenerative diseases had been completed. Several epidemiologic changes thereafter gave rise to further extensions of the epidemiologic transition theory and to new approaches in the study of risk factors, chronic disease, and ageing.

Life's risks

In spite of rapid economic progress in many post-war low-mortality countries there were several 'epidemics' of chronic disease among adult males, including a rise in mortality due to cardiovascular disease. In the Netherlands, for instance, the epidemic of cardiovascular disease originated in urban centres where adverse lifestyle habits were picked up first, and gradually spread out to more peripheral regions.(5) In many countries, similar regional diffusions of lifestyles took place, resulting in increases in cardiovascular mortality, and in a few countries reduction in male life expectancy. It became apparent that diseases can be man-made, and that affluence may have its price in terms of increases in diseases resulting from adverse lifestyle habits or from new environmental hazards emerging in modern society and still with us today.

Several approaches came to the fore to account for the new and largely unanticipated dimensions of mass disease.(6) One of these perspectives was concerned with society as the first cause of mass disease. There were sufficient grounds for believing that the new modern societies brought new man-made hazards as well as a sharpening of epidemiologic differences along the lines of socio-economic status, ethnicity, and also gender. Other commentators emphasized the individual's will and moral responsibility and they saw personal lifestyle as underlying the leading causes of death.(6) This perspective was adhered to by those who believed that health is attainable by everyone through the adoption of a healthy lifestyle and the avoidance of adverse environmental factors. This found widespread support when studies appeared on the associations between lifestyle-related behaviour (with an initial emphasis on cigarette smoking) and chronic diseases such as cancer and cardiovascular disease. Rogers and Hackenberg interpreted chronic disease epidemiology primarily from a 'risk factor perspective', and proposed an extension of the epidemiologic transition theory with a new 'hybristic stage'.(7) This stage was characterized by the dominance of diseases and injuries having their roots in personal behaviour and lifestyle.

With a risk factor perspective, the gender differences in health can be understood to a certain extent. The extensive literature on the subject points at the uptake of health-damaging behaviour, particularly among men, which expresses itself in elevated risks for men of accidental injuries, coronary heart disease, (lung) cancer, liver cirrhosis, and premature death. Prevention in primary care of conditions and events like these would rest on advices to stop smoking, avoid chronic alcohol abuse, reduce fat consumption, manage stress, and performing physical exercise on a regular basis. A central tenet in the risk factor paradigm is that health problems are not inevitable and that epidemiologic differences by gender can be reduced through the promotion of healthy lifestyles. Lawlor et al. found that the geographical variations in the sex ratio for coronary heart disease were associated with environmental factors like the mean per capita fat consumption and thus concluded that these gender differences were not inevitable.(8) Gender differences may become smaller when men adopt more healthy lifestyles or, instead, when women follow them in adopting health-damaging behaviours. The rising female mortality due to lung cancer is an example of such a trend.(9)

The focus on lifestyle factors underlies the theory of successful ageing as put forward, for example, by Rowe and Kahn.(10) Successful ageing does not refer to prosperity, but to a complex made up of low risks of disease and disease-related disability, high mental and physical function, and active engagement with life. In a Swedish study of living conditions with 12 675 persons followed from 1982 until 1991, attendance at cultural events, reading books, making music, or singing in a choir contributed to a longer life after controlling for gender, age, socio-economic status, long-lasting disease, smoking, and physical exercise.(11) Maintaining close relationships with others and remaining involved in meaningful and purposeful activities are also important for well-being. Individual lifestyle came to be regarded as an important factor affecting how we age.

Age(ing) and health

The plateau phase during which risk factor epidemiology emerged proved to be short-lived, as mortality started to fall again after the 'epidemics' of cardiovascular disease among men in many low-mortality countries had faded out around the 1970s. Olshansky and Ault reserved another separate name for this new (fourth) stage in the epidemiologic transition that was set in motion around that time: the 'age of delayed degenerative diseases'.[4] This stage was characterized by reductions in cardiovascular disease that were largely unanticipated. One aspect that was new in the appraisal of these reductions was the possible existence of processes of delay and postponement of death due to chronic disease. To a certain extent the interest in risk factors made way for an increased focus on time, ageing, disease origins and evolvement, and years of life lived in good health.

In the post-war societies with their ageing populations, several theories were formulated on ageing and senescence. According to Kirkwood, organisms have developed several physiological defence, maintenance, and repair mechanisms that work sufficiently to ensure reproductive success, that is, 'evolutionary fitness'.[12] Once the reproductive stage and the period of parental care have passed, the body is disposable. In line with this theory, Olshansky and Carnes suggested that extended survival beyond the ages required for successful reproduction should be associated with a never-ending and progressively more difficult battle against the disorders of old age.[13] When diseases and disorders of old age are successfully postponed, the law of diminishing returns predicts that new or infrequently observed diseases will reveal themselves. The emergence of competing causes of death would put a halt to further rises in life expectancy. Manton et al. argued, however, that much higher life expectancies could be reached if important changes in health-related behaviour could be accomplished.[14] They emphasized the synergism of senescence and exogenous factors, where medical intervention and risk factor modification may modify chronic disease processes in terms of their incidence and progression.

The consequences of increased survival were discussed in terms of the quality and the functional status of the years added to life. Nusselder distinguished between the 'expansion-of-morbidity hypothesis', the 'compression-of-morbidity hypothesis' and the 'dynamic-equilibrium hypothesis'.[15] In an article called *The failures of success*, Gruenberg suggested that a prolongation of life had become within reach for most persons as a result of medical progress and a retreat of several important risk factors, but that the quality of these added years was questionable.[16] Mortality reductions were believed to produce an increase in years lived with morbidity and disability. As the lethal sequelae of degenerative conditions were reduced due to medical interventions, the lives of the chronically ill were prolonged, and the population was pushed into the oldest-old ages where degenerative diseases are extremely prevalent.[15] In short, mortality reductions gave people more time to be ill.[17] Bonneux et al. suggested that postponed acute mortality (e.g. due to myocardial infarction) was traded off for increased chronic morbidity due to heart failure among the elderly.[18] In particular, women may expect to spend more years with chronic morbidity, disability, and dependency on long-term care than men, suggesting that the advantage to women in terms of their life expectancy is a disadvantage in terms of their healthy life expectancy.[19] However, Fries proposed, a 'compression of morbidity'.[20] If a morbid period, defined from the onset of chronic infirmity until death, can be postponed and life expectancy is relatively constant, then morbidity will be compressed into a shorter period of time. An intermediate position was taken by Manton who suggested a dynamic equilibrium between life expectancy increases, slowing down in the rate of progression of chronic diseases, medical intervention, and lifestyle change.[21] In line with this perspective, Robine et al. showed that an increase in the number of years lived with disability may ensue from increases in life expectancy but that these years are not years of severe morbid states.[22] The life expectancy increases among women occurred in parallel with a stagnation in disability-free life expectancy where the disabilities were generally of a mild or moderate kind.

Another approach to the understanding of (chronic) diseases, arising from a discontent with risk factor epidemiology and a poor precision of the temporal dimensions of disease processes was put forward by a research group in Southampton led by David Barker.[23,24] The so-called 'Barker hypothesis', elaborated in many journals and several books, asserts that chronic diseases at the adult stages of life may have their origin in the foetal stage through nutritional programming. This hypothesis was built on associations between infant mortality by geographic area in the past and adult mortality in the same area at present and on data of a particular cohort in the United Kingdom (the so-called 'Hertfordshire studies'). The Hertfordshire studies established a close association between the presence or absence of ischaemic heart disease among the study subjects and their birth weight as obtained from their obstetric records. Barker contended that the environment encountered during foetal and infant life programmes children from socio-economically unfavourable circumstances to an elevated risk of cardiovascular disease in adult life.[24] Early life factors thereby could have influenced the disease and mortality patterns in the population as we observe them currently and face them in primary care. Moreover, the context within which human beings procreate today shape the disease patterns in the future: 'the seeds of inequalities in health in the next century are being sown today—in inner cities and other communities where adverse influences impair the growth, nutrition and health of mothers and their infants'.[24] In the shift from the 'lifestyle paradigm' to the 'early life experience paradigm' the focus was redirected to other health problems than ischaemic heart disease alone, including artherosclerosis, hypertension, breast cancer, and diabetes.[25]

Integration

What we experience today in a setting of primary care is the result of shifts, transitions, behaviours, accumulation of risks, and survival in the lives of individual patients in the past within their immediate contexts. Kuh and Ben-Shlomo developed a lifecourse approach to chronic disease epidemiology which integrates Barker's hypotheses on the role of time and critical periods in human development with the perspectives developed in risk factor epidemiology on human behaviour and lifestyle.[26] Their approach is characterized by a focus on the interaction of social and biological processes and the effects such interactions have on present disease risks. It incorporates various contextual variables (including genetic, biological, and social levels) and emphasizes a temporal level of analysis and the interactions between past and current life experiences. The human lifecourse is an evolving structure that generates health problems that have to do with changes and transitions, conflicts between several dimensions of life, accumulation of risk, and selective survival.

Empirical findings

The morbidity in a modern society is, paradoxically, the sum of diseases not being prevented and the mortality that has actually been prevented.[27] Whereas the epidemiologic transition is about the emergence of chronic disease and their changing lethality, primary medical care is still dealing with an array of health problems such as infections that were more lethal in the past but are manageable nowadays. We use data from the RNG to capture these health problems and their distributions by age and gender.[2]

The complaints and diagnoses are electronically recorded using the International Classification of Primary Care (ICPC) within a medical journal and a linked list of episodes-of-care.[28] The data on prescribed medication include an ICPC-based indication and a reference to the type of medication with the Anatomical Therapeutic Chemical (ATC) classification.[29] The denominator representing the population at risk is calculated using the number of person-years lived within the 3-year period mentioned above on account of the patients' entry and exit dates.

The distributions of health problems by age and gender are presented over the 3-year period, 1998–2000. We speak in the same terms as Gijsbers van Wijk et al. did where they defined health problems as 'all diseases, symptoms and reasons for consultation that are dealt with by general practitioners'.[30] Distributions are first considered for gender, thereafter for the different age groups. The measures presented in the tables are based on two types of calculations. Prevalences are defined as the number of persons with at least once a particular ICPC code within the study period, divided by the number of person-years lived during the study period. Average numbers are calculated as the number of different events (for instance, a contact coded with a particular ICPC code) divided by the number of patients having had at least one code during the study period.

The obvious shortcoming of using these registration data is that they only pertain to those conditions that were brought to the attention of the GP and stored with timed ICPC codes in the GP's databases. Differences in biological risks, acquired risks, illness behaviour, health reporting behaviour, and prior health care utilization generate gender differences in reported health problems, but with our data we cannot disentangle the risks, experiences, and events leading to consultation.[31] A common finding is that, once symptoms are experienced and recognized, there are no gender differences in seeking help from GPs. Verbrugge and Ascione reported a great commonality in how men and women react to common bothersome problems.[32] Focusing on common symptoms of minor illness, Wyke et al. concluded that, with the exception of consulting for headaches and for skin rash or problems in a young cohort, gender differences in consulting arise from differences in the reported experience of symptoms.[33]

Population dynamics

The population size and distribution in terms of age and gender have an autonomous influence on the amount and patterns of care in general practice. The population size may fluctuate as a result of changing birth and death rates and as a result of entry into practice and departure. Whereas fertility and mortality have the strongest impact on the size of large national populations, local factors and policies determining entry into and exit from practice are likely to have a strong influence on smaller general practice populations. It, moreover, matters whether a general practice is situated in a rural peripheral region or in a commercial or educational urban centre. Table 1 shows the age and gender distribution of the population of the RNG at the start of the period 1998–2000 and the distributions of the patients moving in, departing, and dying. Table 1 exemplifies that entries are mostly concentrated at birth and the younger ages and that departures are somewhat differently distributed. It is interesting to note that there is a peak in the entries in the age group 15–24 years because students start to live and study in the town. There is a peak in the departures in the age group 25–34 years, consisting mainly of former students moving out again after having completed their studies and building up their lives somewhere else. The well-known difference in longevity between men and women is reflected in the last column of Table 1. The result of the different age profiles of mortality by gender is a predominance of women in the elderly population. Table 2 presents data on the causes of death for a subset of the patients who died in the study period. These data reinforce the idea that the lifecourses of men and women end in a different manner and with a different pace. Acute myocardial infarction and lung cancer represent the two main processes leading to gender differences in longevity. Women are more likely to die at later ages as a result of a complex array of conditions (as exemplified by 'general deterioration') or heart failure.

Table 1 Population dynamics of the RNG practices; 1998–2000, by age groups and gender, in numbers of patients

Age group (years)	Population, 1998		Entries, 1998–2000		All exits, 1998–2000		Deaths, 1998–2000	
	M	F	M	F	M	F	M	F
0–4	935	801	791	670	193	158	1	4
5–14	1647	1585	213	248	187	188	2	
15–24	1857	2063	806	1173	341	515	1	
25–34	2983	3094	858	691	707	835	3	3
35–44	2565	2524	456	317	359	336	9	11
45–54	2042	1871	263	222	205	207	26	20
55–64	1018	1061	125	123	107	105	32	25
65–74	749	997	86	114	104	125	60	47
75–84	439	775	45	81	139	168	108	102
85+	157	292	37	52	75	157	53	108

Reported health problems

An important facet of primary care involves the management of health problems arising from the female reproductive cycle, sexuality, and the regulation of fertility matters. Health problems may stem, for example, from menstrual and menopausal irregularities (in terms of frequency, pain, timing, etc.), hormonal change, and sexually transmitted diseases. The regulation of fertility matters may involve the avoidance of pregnancy through contraceptives, the management of pregnancy, the treatment of subfertility or infertility, and male sterilization. Table 3 reveals that the prevalences of most health problems in the gynaecological and reproductive ICPC chapters 'X' and 'W' are far higher than those in chapter 'Y' on male genital problems. Several conditions and female matters for which the GP is consulted have a high prevalence, indicating that a considerable part of the total demand for care relates to reproductive and female genital matters, including Pap-smears, menopausal and menstrual problems, family planning, candidiasis, and pregnancy.

It is well known that there is excess morbidity among women.[34] Even after removing reproductive and gynaecological problems and standardizing for age women frequent their GP more often than men. Table 4 shows male/female ratios for prevalent health problems with either a female or male predominance. There is a relative over-representation of women with regard to problems like urinary infections, headache, and feelings of depression, patterns which confirm what was already known from the literature. There are only a few health problems with a predominance of men. Table 4 shows that there is an over-representation of men for inguinal hernia, foreign body in the eye, and several chronic diseases (ischaemic heart disease, lung cancer). The higher male prevalence for external injuries is reflected in the figures for lacerations and cuts. The well-known over-representation of male children and adolescents with attention-deficit

Table 2 Deaths in the RNG population, 1998–2000, by gender and cause of death ($n = 594$)

ICPC code	Description	Gender	*n*	% of deaths	Median age at death
A05	General deterioration	M	22	7.6	84
		F	38	12.5	88
A20	Euthanasia request/discussion	M	0	0.0	
		F	7	2.3	84
K75	Acute myocardial infarction	M	53	18.3	73
		F	35	11.5	82
K77	Heart failure	M	17	5.9	77
		F	21	6.9	90
K90	Stroke/cerebrovascular accident	M	20	6.9	81
		F	30	9.9	82
R84	Malignant neoplasm bronchus/lung	M	22	7.6	69
		F	8	2.6	68
X76	Malignant neoplasm breast	M	0	0.0	
		F	12	3.9	67
	All other	M	156	53.8	75
		F	153	50.3	78
	Total	M	290	100.0	75
		F	304	100.0	80

Table 3 Prevalences of selected health problems from the gender-specific ICPC chapters, RNG population, 1998–2000

ICPC code	Meaning	Male prevalence	Female prevalence
X	*Female genital system*		
X37	Pap-smears		76.3
X72	Urogenital candidiasis proven		24.1
X14	Vaginal discharge		20.0
X11	Menopausal symptoms/complaints		16.2
X07	Menstruation irregular/frequent		11.2
X02	Menstrual pain		9.8
X06	Menstruation excessive		8.9
X08	Intermenstrual bleeding		8.9
X16	Symptoms/complaints vulva		8.8
X19	Lump/mass breast		8.6
W	*Pregnancy/delivery/puerperium*		
W11	Family planning/oral contraceptives		107.1
W78	Pregnancy confirmed		21.7
W10	Morning after pill		8.7
W12	Family planning/IUD		5.3
W14	Family planning/other		4.8
W15	Complaints of infertility		4.0
W01	Question of pregnancy		3.6
W02	Fear of being pregnant		3.5
Y	*Male genital system*		
Y13	Family planning/sterilization	6.4	
Y04	Other symptoms/complaints of penis	5.4	
Y85	Benign prostate hypertrophy	4.7	
Y75	Balanitis	3.6	
Y73	Prostatitis/seminal vesiculitis	3.6	
Y07	Symptoms/complaints potency	3.6	

Note: prevalences are calculated as the number of patients with at least one contact because of the specified ICPC code per 1000 person-years lived within the period 1998–2000.

Table 4 Sex ratios and prevalences of selected health problems with female or male predominance, RNG population, 1998–2000

ICPC code	Meaning	Male prevalence	Female prevalence	Sex ratio M:F
U71	Cystitis/other urinary infection	10.9	64.7	0.2
B80	Iron deficiency anaemia	4.6	18.7	0.3
K07	Swollen ankles/oedema	4.8	15.9	0.3
D06	Other localized abdominal pain	15.2	35.2	0.4
S82	Nevus/mole	7.2	16.4	0.4
P03	Feeling depressed	6.2	15.8	0.4
N01	Headache	10.8	21.8	0.5
N17	Vertigo/dizziness	9.8	20.4	0.5
A85	Adverse effect medical agent	9.0	19.8	0.5
P18	Medication abuse	8.5	17.9	0.5
L13	Hip symptoms/complaints	7.3	14.9	0.5
D89	Inguinal hernia	3.9	0.5	8.1
F76	Foreign body in eye	6.4	1.1	5.6
P21	Overactive child/ hyperkinetic syndrome	2.5	0.6	4.5
P19	Drug abuse	1.8	0.7	2.7
K76	Other/chronic ischaemic disease	8.9	3.4	2.6
P15	Chronic alcohol abuse	3.4	1.4	2.4
R84	Malignant neoplasm bronchus/lung	1.2	0.5	2.4
T92	Gout	3.2	1.4	2.3
K75	Acute myocard infarct	5.5	2.5	2.2
S18	Laceration/cut	24.4	13.5	1.8
K01	Pain attributed to heart	5.6	3.1	1.8

Note: prevalences are calculated as the number of patients with at least one contact because of the specified ICPC code per 1000 person-years lived within the period 1998–2000.

hyperactivity-disorder (ADHD) is revealed by our findings for ICPC code P21.

Several studies have pointed out that women are more likely to consult for neurological, psychological, and social problems than men, suggesting that there are gendered health responses to the vicissitudes of life.[34,35] Arising from a complex interplay between biological sensitivity, hormonal change, and social demands, women may increasingly come to their GP for tiredness, headache, feeling depressed, and depression itself. This pattern is confirmed by Table 5, which shows sex ratios and prevalences for several of these problems from ICPC chapters 'N', 'P', and 'Z'. The relative over-representation of women holds true for the symptoms and complaints in these chapters, but also for the diseases and diagnoses including depressive disorders. These problems are likely to be of a more chronic and severe character for which medication is being prescribed more often. The only exception in this selection of relatively prevalent problems is chronic alcohol abuse, which is 2.4 times more prevalent in men.

From the results on gender presented above, it is not clear whether health problems are experienced more frequently by women because of biological, psychological, or social differences between the sexes or arises from differences in the age distributions of their respective populations. These results, moreover, do not reveal how this differential epidemiology is built up over the lifecourse for the selected ICPC codes. Table 6 provides some insight into the relative prevalences of selected health problems in four different age groups (0–14 years for infants and children; 15–44 years for adolescents and the reproductive stage; 45–64 years as an intermediate stage after reproduction and before retirement; and 65 years and over). The multiplication factors serve to make an easy comparison between the age groups and between men and women. They reflect the number of times the overall

Table 5 Sex ratios and prevalences of selected health problems from ICPC chapters 'N', 'P', and 'Z', RNG population, 1998–2000

ICPC code	Meaning	Male prevalence	Female prevalence	Sex ratio M:F
N	*Neurological system*			
N01	Headache	10.8	21.8	0.5
N02	Tension headache	5.1	12.1	0.4
P	*Mental/psychological disorders*			
P01	Feeling anxious/nervous/ tense	14.4	27.8	0.5
P02	Acute stress	8.3	14.0	0.6
P03	Feeling depressed	6.2	15.8	0.4
P04	Feeling/behaving irritable	1.7	1.7	1.0
P06	Disturbances of sleep/insomnia	13.0	24.6	0.5
P15	Chronic alcohol abuse	3.4	1.4	2.4
P74	Anxiety disorder/anxiety state	2.0	4.1	0.5
P75	Hysterical/hypochondriacal disease	0.8	1.9	0.4
P76	Depressive disorder	9.8	16.7	0.6
P77	Suicide attempt	0.6	0.8	0.7
Z	*Social problems*			
Z12	Relation problem partners	3.9	7.8	0.5
Z13	Problem with behaviour partner	0.9	2.9	0.3
Z21	Problem behaviour parents/ other family	0.8	2.5	0.3

Note: prevalences are calculated as the number of patients with at least one contact because of the specified ICPC code per 1000 person-years lived within the period 1998–2000.

Table 6 Overall and relative prevalences of selected health problems, by age groups, gender, and ICPC code, RNG population, 1998–2000

ICPC code	Meaning	Prevalence	Gender	Index figures (years)			
				0–14	15–44	45–64	65+
A03	Fever	9	M	4.2	0.3	0.4	1.1
			F	3.6	0.3	0.5	0.6
A04	General weakness/tiredness	35	M	0.6	0.6	0.7	1.2
			F	0.8	1.4	1.0	2.0
H71	Acute otitis media/myringitis	18	M	4.5	0.3	0.3	0.2
			F	3.7	0.4	0.4	0.4
K75	Acute myocardial infarction	4	M	0.0	0.1	2.3	9.5
			F	0.0	0.0	0.6	4.1
K86	Uncomplicated hypertension	29	M	0.0	0.2	1.6	3.8
			F	0.0	0.3	2.0	5.5
K90	Stroke/cerebrovascular accident	5	M	0.0	0.1	1.0	7.5
			F	0.0	0.1	0.9	7.1
N01	Headache	16	M	0.5	0.6	0.8	0.9
			F	0.9	1.5	1.4	1.4
P03	Feeling depressed	11	M	0.1	0.6	0.7	1.1
			F	0.0	1.6	1.6	2.3
P06	Disturbances of sleep/insomnia	19	M	0.2	0.4	0.9	2.8
			F	0.1	0.7	1.8	4.4
P76	Depressive disorder	13	M	0.0	0.9	1.0	0.9
			F	0.0	1.4	1.6	2.0
R05	Cough	45	M	1.5	0.5	1.0	1.5
			F	1.5	0.8	1.3	1.9
R74	Upper respiratory infection	52	M	1.7	0.7	0.8	1.1
			F	1.7	1.0	0.9	1.2
R78	Acute bronchitis/bronchiolitis	39	M	1.5	0.4	1.0	2.6
			F	1.1	0.7	1.2	2.4
R84	Malignant neoplasm bronchus/lung	1	M	0.2	0.0	2.0	11.2
			F	0.0	0.0	1.4	2.6
R96	Asthma	33	M	1.9	0.7	0.6	1.8
			F	1.1	0.9	1.1	1.5
S18	Laceration/cut	19	M	2.2	1.2	0.9	1.0
			F	1.3	0.6	0.7	0.8
T90	Diabetes mellitus	18	M	0.1	0.3	1.6	4.3
			F	0.0	0.2	1.6	5.5
U71	Cystitis/other urinary infection	39	M	0.1	0.1	0.3	1.5
			F	0.9	1.6	1.6	3.5

Note: overall prevalences are calculated as the number of patients with at least one contact because of the specified ICPC code per 1000 person-years lived within the period 1998–2000; the index figures reflect the number of times the overall prevalence should be multiplied to arrive at the prevalence by age group and gender.

prevalence for both sexes combined should be multiplied in order to arrive at the prevalence for the particular population by age group and gender. The female prevalence of headache in the age group 15–44 years is thus 1.5 times 16. This equals 24 patients per 1000 person-years lived in the 3-year study period.

Table 6 shows that most health problems with a high prevalence among infants and children do not have a particular gender bias, except for fever, acute otitis, asthma, acute bronchitis, lacerations, and cuts with higher prevalences among boys. Whereas there is a clear increase in numbers and frequencies of women needing GP consultations and medication when the reproductive cycle starts, men apparently have a different story. For them a relative reduction in their contacts with a GP may occur after reaching adulthood, and from data of the RNG (not shown here) it appears that there is a concentration of patients not having contact with their GPs in the group of adolescent and young grown-up men. This is consistent with other results published for the Netherlands and the United Kingdom.[36–38] As compared to women, their reproductive change and development apparently do not lead to the same amount of problems for which consultations are being sought. Moreover, fertility matters and contraceptive behaviour are still predominantly female matters and the contraceptive pill is the most frequently prescribed medication in many general practices. In the male lifecourse, different rhythms and patterns may be discerned that are less determined by fertility cycles but more affected by changes in their educational, working, and relational careers. More importantly perhaps, the consequences of adverse lifestyles including smoking, alcohol consumption, and excessive stress may accumulate and become manifest in an intermediate stage between ages 45 and 65, as revealed by the sharp increases in myocardial infarction and lung cancer. The stage of old age is the domain of surviving women again, where they may develop co-morbidities, their functional status declines, and they tend to use different types of medication in combination.

Table 7 Average number of different health problems per patient, by ICPC categories, age groups, and gender, RNG population, 1998–2000

Age group (years)	All symptoms, complaints, diseases, and diagnoses		All, except chapters W, X, and Y		All symptoms and complaints, except chapters W, X, and Y		All diagnoses and diseases, except chapters W, X, and Y	
	M	F	M	F	M	F	M	F
0–14	4.9	5.0	4.8	4.9	2.2	2.3	2.5	2.6
15–44	4.5	7.3	4.4	5.6	2.2	2.9	2.1	2.7
45–64	6.6	9.1	6.4	8.3	3.1	4.3	3.3	4.0
65+	10.4	12.3	10.1	12.1	4.2	5.8	5.9	6.3

Table 8 Average number of all and different prescriptions per patient, by age groups and gender, RNG population, 1998–2000

Age group years	Average number of prescriptions per patient		Average number of different prescriptions per patient	
	M	F	M	F
0–4	8.3	7.8	3.2	3.1
5–14	7.8	7.1	2.6	2.8
15–24	6.2	12.7	2.5	3.9
25–34	10.4	15.1	2.9	4.2
35–44	13.5	20.8	3.3	4.6
45–54	22.2	32.7	4.1	5.5
55–64	35.8	48.4	5.2	6.4
65–74	55.9	64.3	7.1	7.7
75–84	63.8	78.9	8.1	9.0
85+	65.6	92.6	8.3	9.5
All	19.8	27.9	3.8	5.0

Note: the first two columns pertain to all prescriptions; the last two columns pertain to different prescriptions only; prescriptions are different when they differ on the ATC three-digit level.

Co-morbidity and polypharmacy

Thus far the ICPC codes were evaluated on their patterns by age and gender. The data and prevalences presented were person-based, that is, based on counts of patients having had at least once the ICPC code of interest within the 3-year period. This only gives partial insight into patterns of demand for care, because there is likely to be a clustering of health problems within individual patients themselves that also tends to increase with advancing age.[39] Table 7 presents the average number of different ICPC codes being registered for the study population. Only the codes with numbers 1–29 (symptoms and complaints) and 70–99 (diagnoses and diseases) are selected, with the exception of code A97 ('no disease'). Table 7 reveals that there is an increase in the average number of different ICPC codes per patient by advancing age, with the notable exception of men in the age group 15–44 years. The variety of different ICPC codes is larger for women than for men, even after removing the health problems from chapters 'W', 'X', and 'Y'. The patterns for symptoms and complaints versus diagnoses and diseases are somewhat different in the sense that the gender bias in the oldest age category is stronger for the first category of problems compared to the second category. This probably confirms the findings in the literature that there is a less sharp gender difference when the serious health problems are concerned.[38]

The prescription of medical drugs is a common event in general practice and the patterns found will reflect the distribution and patterns of their underlying health problems. Table 8 shows that the average number of prescriptions rises with advancing age and that women have on average more prescriptions than men.

The sharpening of gender differences at the start of the female reproductive cycle is also visible here, as there is a decline in the average number of prescriptions for men but an increase for women due in part to the contraceptive pill. The effects of age and gender become reinforced when only counting the different prescriptions per patient. With these data and other results from the RNG registration, we conclude that medical drugs are more frequently prescribed to female patients, that prescription itself is slightly less common among the intermediate age groups and men, and that the number of different medical drugs prescribed per patient correlates positively with female sex and advancing age.[2]

Evaluation

The task of the GP has been described as the management of patient trajectories.[40] In the treatment of our subject we have come close to this view by arranging our data using the concept of the human lifecourse while acknowledging the heterogeneity of patient trajectories by gender. With a theoretical and descriptive approach to the subject we aimed to integrate two interrelated perspectives: the micro-perspective of the GP whose first interest may concern the amounts, types, and patterns of care he has to provide, and the macro-perspective of the epidemiologist focusing on population distributions and relative frequencies of various health problems.

There are important differences between the medical biographies of men and women. The first stage of life is not qualitatively and quantitatively different (except for asthma with a predominance of boys) but in the stage thereafter there is a clear widening of experiences with primary care by gender. Among adolescent and grown-up men there is a clear downfall in the volume of care demanded (as revealed by prevalences and different ICPC codes per patient), whereas among women there is an increase for reproductive, gynaecological, psychological, and social matters. It is the stage of the reproductive cycle where the excess morbidity among women clearly starts to build up. In that stage, men probably accumulate certain risks for which they do not immediately seek a GP's consultation but which later in life become manifest as chronic diseases. After their initial contacts with a GP in their early life years, related to infectious diseases and to lacerations and cuts, they tend to frequent their GP less frequently when growing up. This sharp differential morbidity is softened somewhat during the intermediate age range 45–64 years, where men enter a stage with elevated risks of acute myocardial infarction, bronchitis, lung cancer, diabetes mellitus, and mortality.

The distribution of events in primary care by gender arises from a set of underlying epidemiologic forces. There is a growing difference in male and female population numbers over the lifecourse, resulting in a predominance of women at the older ages. Women experience more health problems at the various stages of their lives than men for which they seek advice, consultation, care, or therapy. In addition, their variety of different health problems (co-morbidity) and medication prescriptions (polypharmacy) is larger than in the male population. Each facet of the human lifecourse brings forth its own patterns of health problems and demand for care.

The differences in the epidemiology of health problems by age and gender can only be mitigated in primary care to a certain extent. The risk factor approach to gender differences tells us that part of the excess mortality among men can be reduced through the promotion of healthy life styles. Women nevertheless face several health problems that are not related so much to their risk profiles but to their own (reproductive) biology and—not in the least—their enhanced longevity. Theories on ageing, co-morbidity, competing causes of death, and quality of life tell us that the prevention of risk factors and mortality may allow other chronic disease processes and disabling conditions to become manifest. The experience that has been built up with the epidemiology of elderly women may provide us with an idea about what the future would hold for men should they adopt more healthy lifestyles.

Summary

The variables gender and age provide the GP with cues to structure the contact with the patient in terms of past events, the present condition, and possible outcomes in the future. This micro-perspective on primary care can be complemented with an epidemiologic, population-based macro-perspective. In this chapter, we aimed to bring together these two connected perspectives based on several theoretical insights from the literature and some empirical findings on the subject. The empirical data are taken from the morbidity and medication Registration Network Groningen, based on the electronic patient files of 16 GPs with about 30 000 patients on their lists, refering to 1998–2000.

Theoretical insights are introduced to portray our primary care experiences of today as the result of life course transitions, behaviours, accumulation of risks and survival in the lives of individual patients in the past within their immediate contexts.

In the medical biographies of men and women, there are important differences. The first stage of life is not qualitatively and quantitatively different (except for asthma and ADHD with a predominance of boys) but in the stage thereafter there is a clear widening of experiences with primary care by gender. Among adolescent and grown-up men there is a clear reduction in the volume of care demanded (as revealed by prevalences and different ICPC codes per patient), whereas among women there is an increase for reproductive, gynaecological, psychological, and social matters. It is the stage of the reproductive cycle where the excess morbidity among women clearly starts to build up. In that stage, men probably accumulate certain risks for which they do not immediately seek a GP's consultation but which later in life become manifest as chronic diseases. After their initial contacts with a GP in their early life years, related to infectious diseases and to lacerations and cuts, they tend to frequent their GP less frequently when growing up. This sharp differential morbidity is softened somewhat during the intermediate age range 45–64, where men enter a stage with elevated risks of acute myocardial infarction, bronchitis, lung cancer, diabetes mellitus, and mortality.

Key points

- Most health problems with a high prevalence among infants and children do not have a particular gender bias, except for fever, acute otitis, asthma, acute bronchitis, lacerations and cuts with higher prevalences among boys.
- From early adulthood, women present an excess morbidity compared to men, not only referring to reproductive and gynaecological problems, but also to several psycho-social problems. The only psycho-social problem with male dominance is chronic alcohol abuse.
- With advancing age, there is an increase in the average number of different ICPC codes per patient and the variety of different ICPC codes is larger for women than for men, even after removing the health problems from gynaecological and childbearing problems. The prescription of medical drugs reflects the distribution and patterns of their underlying health problems.

References

1. **Malterud, K. and Okkes, I.** (1998). Gender differences in general practice consultations: methodological challenges in epidemiological research. *Family Practice* **15**, 404–10.
2. **Van der Werf, G.T.H., Smith, R.J.A., Stewart, R.E., and Meyboom-de Jong, B.** *Spiegel op de huisarts.* Groningen: Universiteitsdrukkerij Groningen, 1998.
3. **Omran, A.R.** (1971). The epidemiologic transition. A theory of the epidemiology of population change. *Milbank Memorial Fund Quarterly* **49**, 509–38.
4. **Olshansky, S.J. and Ault, A.B.** (1986). The fourth stage of the epidemiologic transition: the age of delayed degenerative diseases. *Milbank Memorial Fund Quarterly* **64**, 355–91.
5. **Mackenbach, J.P., Looman, C.W.N., and Kunst, A.E.** (1989). Geographic variation in the onset of decline of male ischemic heart disease mortality in the Netherlands. *American Journal of Public Health* **79**, 1621–7.
6. **Kunitz, S.J.** (1987). Explanations and ideologies of mortality patterns. *Population and Development Review* **13**, 379–408.
7. **Rogers, R. and Hackenberg, R.** (1987). Extending epidemiologic transition theory: a new stage. *Social Biology* **34**, 234–43.
8. **Lawlor, D.A., Ebrahim, S., and Davey Smith, G.** (2001). Sex matters: secular and geographical trends in sex differences in coronary heart disease mortality. *British Medical Journal* **323**, 541–5.
9. **Levi, F.** et al. (1992). Trends in cancer mortality sex ratios in Europe 1950–1989. *World Health Statistics Quarterly* **45**, 117–64.
10. **Rowe, J.L. and Kahn, R.L.** *Succesful Aging.* New York: Random House, 1999.
11. **Bygren, L.O., Konlaan, B., and Iohansson, S.E.** (1996). Attendance at cultural events, reading books or periodicals, and making music or singing in a choir as determinants for survival: Swedish interview survey of living conditions. *British Medical Journal* **313**, 1577–80.
12. **Kirkwood, T.B.L.** (1977). Evolution of aging. *Nature* **270**, 301–4.
13. **Olshansky, S.J. and Carnes, B.A.** (1996). Prospect for extended survival: a critical review of the biological evidence. In *Health and Mortality Among Elderly Populations* (ed. G. Caselli and A.D. Lopez). Oxford: Clarendon Press.
14. **Manton, K.G., Stallard, E., and Tolley, H.D.** (1991). Limits to human life expectancy: evidence, prospects, and implications. *Population and Development Review* **17**, 603–37.
15. **Nusselder, W.** *Compression or Expansion of Morbidity? A Life-table Approach.* Amsterdam: Thela Thesis, 1998.
16. **Gruenberg, E.M.** (1977). The failures of success. *Milbank Memorial Fund Quarterly* **55**, 3–24.
17. **Porter, R.** *The Greatest Benefit to Mankind. A Medical History of Humanity from Antiquity to the Present.* London: Fontana, 1997.
18. **Bonneux, L., Barendrecht, J.J., Meeter, K., Bonsel, G.J., and van der Maas, P.J.** (1994). Estimating clinical morbidity due to ischemic heart disease and congestive heart failure: the future rise of heart failure. *American Journal of Public Health* **84**, 20–8.
19. **Van Den Bos, G.A.M.** (1995). The burden of chronic diseases in terms of disability, use of health care and healthy life expectancies. *European Journal of Public Health* **5**, 29–34.
20. **Fries, J.F.** (1980). Aging, natural death, and the compression of morbidity. *New England Journal of Medicine* **303**, 208–32.
21. **Manton, K.G.** (1982). Changing concepts of morbidity and mortality in the elderly population. *Milbank Memorial Fund Quarterly* **60**, 183–244.
22. **Robine, J.M., Mathers, C., and Brouard, N.** (1996). Trends and differentials in disability-free life expectancy: concepts, methods, and findings. In *Health and Mortality Among Elderly Populations* (ed. G. Caselli and A.D. Lopez). Oxford: Clarendon Press.
23. **Barker, D.J.P.**, ed. *Fetal and Infant Origins of Adult Disease.* London: BMJ Publishing Group, 1992.
24. **Barker, D.J.P.**, ed. *Mothers, Babies, and Disease in Later Life.* London: BMJ Publishing Group, 1994.
25. **Robinson, R.J.** (1992). Is the child father of the man? Controversy about the early origins of cardiovascular disease. *British Medical Journal* **304**, 789–90.
26. **Kuh, D. and Ben-Shlomo, Y.** *A Life Course Approach to Chronic Disease Epidemiology.* Oxford: Oxford University Press, 1977.

27. **Barendrecht, J. and Bonneux, L.** Degenerative disease in an aging population; models and conjectures. Dissertation, Erasmus University, Rotterdam, 1998.
28. **Lamberts, H. and Wood, M.** *International Classification of Primary Care.* Oxford: Oxford University Press, 1987.
29. **WHO Collaborating Centre for Drug Statistics Methodology.** *ATC Index with DDS.* Norway: WHO, 1999.
30. **Gijsbers van Wijk, C.M.T., Kolk, A.M., van den Bosch, W.J.H.M., and van den Hoogen, H.J.M.** (1995). Male and female health problems in general practice: the differential impact of social position and social roles. *Social Science and Medicine* **40**, 597–611.
31. **Verbrugge, L.M.** (1989). The twain meet: empirical explanations of sex differences in health and mortality. *Journal of Health and Social Behavior* **30**, 282–304.
32. **Verbrugge, L.M. and Ascione, F.J.** (1987). Exploring the iceberg. Common symptoms and how people deal with them. *Medical Care* **25**, 539–69.
33. **Wyke, S., Hunt, K., and Ford, G.** (1998). Gender differences in consulting a general practitioner for common symptoms of minor illness. *Social Science and Medicine* **46**, 901–6.
34. **McDonough, P. and Walters, V.** (2001). Gender and health: reassessing patterns and explanations. *Social Science and Medicine* **52**, 547–59.
35. **Macintyre, S., Hunt, K., and Sweeting, H.** (1996). Gender differences in health: are things really as simple as they seem? *Social Science and Medicine* **42**, 617–24.
36. **Lamberts, H.** *In het huis van de huisarts. Verslag van het transitieproject.* Lelystad, Meditekst, 1994.
37. **McCormick, A., Fleming, D., and Charlton, J.** *Morbidity Statistics from General Practice, Fourth National Study 1991–1992.* London: HMSO, 1995.
38. **Mant, D. and Silagy, C.** (1998). The epidemiology of men's health. In *Men's Health* (ed. T. O'Dowd and D. Jewell). Oxford: Oxford University Press.
39. **Van den Akker, M., Buntinx, F., Metsemakers, J.F.M., Roos, S., and Knottnerus, J.A.** (1998). Multimorbidity in general practice: prevalence, incidence, and determinants of co-occurring chronic and recurrent diseases. *Journal of Clinical Epidemiology* **51**, 367–75.
40. **Berg, M., Goorman, E., Harterink, P., and Plass, S.** *De nacht schreef rood. Informatisering van zorgpraktijken.* Den Haag: Rathenau Instituut, 1998, studie 37.

4.5 Socio-economic differences in health

Sara Willems and Jan de Maeseneer

Introduction

The discussion of socio-economic health differences starts from the concept of social stratification, which layers society into bottom, representing the less-favoured members of society, and top, representing the most favoured. The term 'socio-economical health differences' indicates the systematic differences in health between people with a lower position in the social stratification on the one hand and people with a higher position on the other hand.

This chapter includes five parts. The first part gives an overview of the historical context of research on unhealthy inequalities. In the second part, some methodological and conceptual problems in measuring socio-economic health differences are presented. In the third part, we go deeper into the present status of health inequalities research and look at its epidemiology. Part four explores the social differences in the utilization of health care services and the way family doctors deal with poor patients in their practice. Finally, in the fifth part, we report on possibilities to tackle health inequalities and reflect on the consequences of socio-economic health differences for the organization of the health care system.

History

A classic topic within today's public health research concerns socio-economical health differences. When in the nineteenth century in a number of European cities committed doctors and citizens established the Sanitary Movement, interest in this topic arose. This movement's goal was to tackle the major problems of public health at that time. Extensive attention was paid to different mortality and morbidity rates between the rich and the poor.(1)

One of the oldest known studies in this area concerns the mortality in Geneva in the seventeenth century. Using ecclesiastical registers the life-course of a large sample of the population of Geneva was reconstructed. The profession of the individuals also being registered, it was possible to analyse mortality by social class and to provide evidence for the existence of socio-economic health differences. Studies about other large cities in Europe, performed on data from the eighteenth century, equally show explicit discrepancies between social classes(1) (Table 1).

Equal accessibility to the health care system for all citizens being an important objective of the welfare state, some believed that the implementation of this welfare system in the 1960s and 1970s would be able to at least decrease the problem of socio-economic health differences. Though measures taken in this spirit led to a stronger increase in the use of health services by lower-income groups than the average increase for the total population, health differences did not disappear.

In 1977, the Secretary of State for Social Services of the Labour government in the United Kingdom appointed a Research Working Group to assess the national and international evidence on health inequalities and so draw conclusions for policy. The report concluded that the poorer health experience of lower occupational groups applied to all stages of life. Moreover, if mortality rates of professional workers and members of their families had been applied to partly skilled and unskilled manual workers and the members of their families during 1970–2, 74 000 lives of people aged under 75 would not have been lost.(2)

Mainly because of the publication of the Black Report in the United Kingdom, renewed attention to socio-economic health differences arose and new studies and intervention programmes were designed.(1)

The World Health Organization (WHO) put emphasis on 'equity in health' too, referring to a situation in which everyone has equal chances to reach his/her maximal potential health, rather than everyone having the same health status. In 1984, the member states of the Regional Bureau for Europe of the WHO recognized the importance of focused attention for socio-economic health differences. The first target in the 'Health for all by the year 2000' declaration states: 'By the year 2000, the differences in health status between countries and between groups within countries should be reduced by at least 25 per cent, by improving the level of health of disadvantaged nations and groups.' Hence, the monitoring of the differences in health status between different geographical areas and socio-economic groups within each country should be strengthened, priority should be given to the implementation of measures to reduce differences in health status, the basic prerequisites for health, such as food, housing, and education, should be available for all, the living and working environments supporting health and adequate health care should be more accessible and disadvantaged nations should obtain 'special assistance and attention'.(3) The newer 'Health 21' programme equally considers socio-economic health inequalities a major issue.(4)

Table 1 Health life expectancy in a number of European cities in the seventeenth and eighteenth centuries

City	Period	Mean age at death (in years)			Ratio higher class/ lower class (in %)
		Higher class	Middle class	Lower class	
Berlin	1710–99	29.8	24.3	20.3	147
Geneva	17th century	35.9	24.7	18.3	196
Rouen	18th century	32.5	33.0	24.5	133
Trier	1770–1800	41.0	—	36.5	112
Neuruppin[a]	1732–1830	33.2	28.6	28.9	115
Durlach[a]	1751–1800	53.1	58.2	40.1	132
Spandau	1720–1869	58.5	56.5	54.0	108

[a] Only adults.

Source: Schulz H. (1991). Social differences in mortality in the eighteenth century; an analysis of Berlin church registers. *International Review of Social History* **36**, 232–329.

Methodological and conceptual problems

As stated above, in the last decades a huge amount of research has been done concerning the differences in health between society's higher and lower socio-economic classes. Based on this literature, the relation between socio-economic status, on the one hand, and physical and mental health, on the other hand, has been established. Still, methodological and conceptual problems hamper the comparison, generalization, and interpretation of these—sometimes contradictory—findings.

Health inequalities versus inequities

In this chapter, the term 'socio-economic health differences' is used to describe the systematic differences in health between people from different layers of the social stratification. This definition does not imply any value judgment about the fairness of these health differences. Hence, the terms 'inequalities in health' and 'inequities in health' can be used. The strict definition of 'inequalities in health' refers to a broad range of differences in both health experience and health status between countries, regions, and socio-economic groups. Most inequalities are not biologically inevitable but reflect population differences in circumstances and behaviour that are in the broadest sense socially determined. Likewise, 'health inequities' are inequalities that can be avoided and are henceforth unfair and unjust.

Despite these formal definitions, health inequalities and inequities are not understood worldwide in the same way, which complicates interpreting research results. For example, in literature from industrialized countries such as the United Kingdom, the term 'inequalities in health' is used to refer to differences in health status between regions and population subgroups that are regarded as inequitable. In reality, the term 'inequities' is mainly applied to unfair and unjust differences in access to health services between regions and population subgroups within a country.

In western European countries, in which access to health services is relatively universal and not strongly dependent on socio-economic circumstances or geography, much of the research on inequalities in health has been focused on the mechanisms that generate socio-economic gradients in illness, health, and mortality. From this perspective, inequalities in health are mainly a function of the aetiology of disease, and the policy solutions that arise concern primary prevention. In low- and middle-income countries, by contrast, people working on inequities in health tend to see the problem as one of trying to ensure more equitable provision of health care.[(5)]

Measuring inequalities and socio-economic status

Individual or household income, educational level, and occupational social class are the main principles to define one's socio-economic status. In some research, however, proxy variables such as being the owner of a house, possessing a car, etc. are used.[(6)] Since there is no universal consensus about how to measure these variables, making valid comparisons of health inequalities between socio-economic groups becomes more problematic. Despite these difficulties, research has nevertheless established real international variations in the magnitude of socio-economic differences in health status and mortality for specific diseases. Thus, it is clear that socio-economic variation is not a fixed and inevitable feature of society.[(7)] Further, since lower-income countries do not always have disposal of the necessary infrastructure to collect relevant data, comparison between countries also turns out to be difficult. Even in the higher-income countries the available data often do not allow the measurement of the distribution of health status within the country.[(5)]

Finally, difficulties in the measurement of inequalities in health are compounded by yet another problem. The less-favoured groups are not always represented in clinical research (e.g. RCTs). Moreover, when they are included in the research population, it still remains unclear in which way the results can be applied to these population groups.

Explanatory models: selection or causation?

The relation between health and socio-economic status has been documented above. Different hypotheses exist about the causality in this relationship and about the explanatory mechanisms. In this section, we give a short overview of the most common frames of reference.

The artefact hypothesis states that the observed differences in health between the socio-economic classes are explained by artefacts in the research. An example of this is the nominator/denominator bias that arises when different sources provide data for the nominator on the one hand and for the denominator on the other. Because of different definitions used by the two sources, the nominator and the denominator are measured in a different way and the result can be biased. For example, when comparing the healthy life expectancy in two countries, based on the national health surveys, the definition used to determine the healthy life expectancy in the one country can vary from the definition used in the other. Still, the amount of evidence for socio-economic health differences delivered by studies with a high methodological quality, avoiding this artefact bias, is growing. Nevertheless, one should heed this hypothesis' warning and be careful in interpreting research results.[(1)]

The social selection theory asserts that one's health status strongly determines one's life chances, which implies that health 'selects' people into different strata. In this theory, social mobility (moving within the social strata) is an expression of selection through health. The hypothesis of genetic predisposition stands close to the social selection hypothesis by stating that one's place in the social stratification is determined by one's genetic predisposition. Some evidence has been published to confirm these theories, though all socio-economic health differences cannot be explained.[(1)]

According to the social causation theory, one's socio-economic status determines one's health through intermediate factors. Socio-economic health differences occur when the quality of these intermediate factors are unevenly distributed between the different socio-economic classes. Four groups of intermediate factors can be identified. The group of behavioural factors and lifestyle include eating habits, smoking, risk behaviour, the use of health services, etc. Housing and working conditions, individual income are structural factors.

Psychological factors include stressors (e.g. life events), coping-style, psycho-social stress, social network, etc. Finally, the group of intermediate factors are related to the early years of life such as the living conditions in childhood, health status as a child, etc.[1,8,9] Though many determinants are identified, the relative impact of these determinants on health and the joint impact of determinants on health remain unclear.

In this context we refer to the work done by Wilkinson on the impact of relative versus absolute material standards. In most explanatory models for socio-economic differences in health, the direct impact of absolute material standards such as bad housing, poor diets, inadequate heating, ... is implicated, though material conditions do not adequately explain health inequalities in western countries. In richer countries, wellbeing is more closely related to relative income than to absolute income. A low relative material standard affects health through the psychosocial effects of its emotional and social meaning. Social dominance, inequality, autonomy and the quality of social relations have an important impact on psychosocial wellbeing and are among the most powerful explanations for the patterns of population health in rich countries. The distinction between the direct effects of material conditions such as malnutrition and bad housing on health and the psychosocially mediated health effects of relative deprivation has important implications for policy.[10,11]

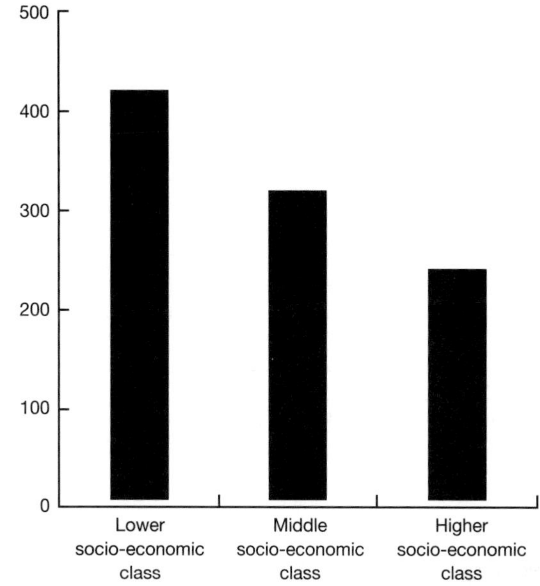

Fig. 1 New cases of morbidity per 1000 patients per year, per social class (1971–1988). *Source:* van de Lisdonk, E.H. et al. (ed.). *Diseases in the Family Medicine Practice.* Utrecht: Wetenschappelijke uitgeverij Bunge, 1990.

Epidemiology

Socio-economic inequalities in health

Notwithstanding increased attention paid to socio-economic health inequalities and the measures taken by governments, mortality and morbidity inequalities between lower and higher socio-economic classes can still be observed nowadays, even in western, industrialized countries. Despite marked health improvements of the overall population, literature shows higher mortality rates for most diseases and for major causes of death for the socio-economically disadvantaged.[12,13] Scientific evidence indicates that less-educated people are more likely to be affected by disabling back pain than educated people.[14]

High-income inequality in a country also confers an increased risk of poor mental health,[15] coronary heart disease,[16,17] and smoking-related cancers.[15] In the study of Power et al., the prevalence of subjects who reported poor health increased with declining social class at age 33: from 8.5 per cent in classes I and II to 17.7 per cent in classes IV and V among men, and from 9.4 per cent to 18.8 per cent among women.[18] An analysis of the registered morbidity in three representative primary care practices in the Netherlands during the period 1971–88 concludes that between the three defined social classes (lower social class, middle class, and higher class, based on profession) large differences can be noted. In the lower social class, more new cases of morbidity per year are registered than in the higher class (Fig. 1). When looking at the seriousness of the disease, the same pattern can be found. For example, hypertension is diagnosed three times more often in the lower social class than in the higher social class (Fig. 2).[19]

This inequality exists for both males and females at every stage of the life-course.[11,20] Already in the early stages of life inequalities in health appear. So, literature reports that the hospitalization rate for inner-city infants is much greater than that for suburban infants in the United States. A substantial portion of the difference, namely that attributable to mandatory admissions, reflects higher rates of serious illness. Dissimilarities attributable to discretionary admissions may reflect higher rates of serious illness to some extent, but also appear to reflect less-effective health services to a substantial degree.[21] When looking at inequalities after the age of retirement, relative differences in mortality between low and high employment grades are less than before retirement, partly because the background incidence for all subgroups extends with age. The absolute differences in mortality between less- and more-advantaged groups, however, increase at older ages.[22]

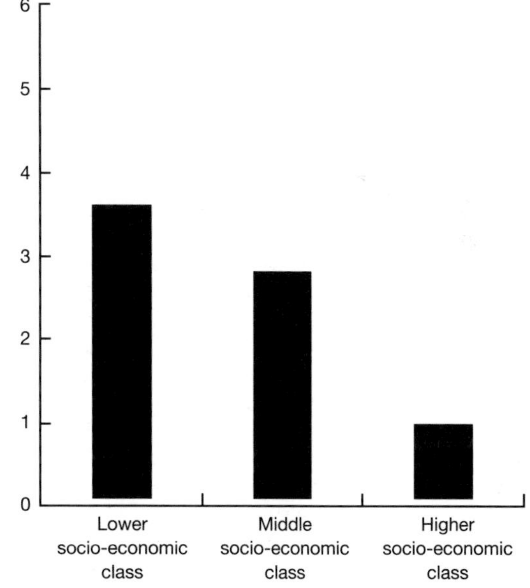

Fig. 2 New cases of hypertension per 1000 patients per year, per social class (1971–1988). *Source:* van de Lisdonk, E.H. et al. (ed.). *Diseases in the Family Medicine Practice.* Utrecht: Wetenschappelijke uitgeverij Bunge, 1990.

In relation to health inequalities, the high concentration of smoking among more-disadvantaged social groups is reflected in the distribution of smoking-related deaths in the early 1980s. It is shown that a man with an unskilled manual occupation (e.g. cleaners, unskilled labourers) is more than four times as likely to die of lung cancer than a person with a professional occupation (e.g. doctors, accountants, lawyers) and twice as likely to die from coronary heart disease.[23]

There is also growing evidence that mortality inequalities have widened in western countries over time. These increasing disparities appear to be due to faster declines in mortality among those of higher socio-economic status. In some countries, on the other hand, there is evidence of an actual increase in mortality rates for some conditions among the most disadvantaged.[20,24–26] For example, in Scotland relative deprivation increased between the 1981 and 1991 censuses and was mirrored by a worsening of relative death rates. Changes in relative mortality were explained by differences in the decline in death rates according to the affluence of an area; among men the decline in deprived areas was only about half that in affluent areas and among women it was only about one-third.[25]

Further, literature substantiates an unprecedented widening of income differences during the 1980s and a growth of relative poverty in Britain, as in several other developed countries. Official figures of incomes after taxes and benefits, adjusted for household size, show that at the start of the decade the incomes of the richest 20 per cent of the population were four times as large as those of the poorest 20 per cent. By 1991, they were almost six times as large. Moreover, in the late 1980s not only was the most rapid part of this unprecedented widening of income differences seen, but also a cessation in the long-term fall in national mortality rates among men and women aged 15–44.[27]

An important set of studies looking at changes in social inequalities over time are the Whitehall studies. The Whitehall I study of British civil servants started in 1967, and showed a steep inverse association between social classes, as assessed by grade of employment, and mortality from a wide range of diseases. Between 1985 and 1988, the Whitehall II study analysed the degree and causes of the social gradient in morbidity in a new cohort of 10 314 civil servants (6900 men, 3414 women) aged 35–55. In the 20 years separating the two studies there was no decrease in social class difference in morbidity: an inverse association between employment grade and prevalence of angina, electrocardiographic evidence of ischaemia, and symptoms of chronic bronchitis was found. Self-perceived health status and symptoms were worse for people with lower-status jobs. There were clear employment-grade differences in health-risk behaviours, including smoking, diet, and exercise, in economic circumstances, in possible effects of early-life environment as reflected by height, in social circumstances at work (e.g. monotonous work characterized by low job control and low satisfaction), and in social supports.[28,29]

The WHO Health Report 2000 indicates that health differences occur between people from different socio-economic classes within the same country as well as between countries. When looking at life expectancy at birth (in years) large differences can be noted, differing from 74.7 years for males and 79.7 years for females in the United Kingdom to 33.2 years for males and 35.4 years for females in Sierra Leone. Differences in the average level of population health are even larger. This is reported in terms of disability-adjusted life expectancy (DALE) at birth, most easily understood as the expectation of life lived in full health, and differs between countries from 69.7 years for males and 73.7 years for females in the United Kingdom to 25.8 years for males and 26.0 years for females in Sierra Leone (Table 2).

Concerning Europe, the inequalities in life expectancy are increasing. In 1970, male life expectancy at age 15 was 56 years in countries that now form the European Union, 55 in the communist countries of central and eastern Europe (excluding the Soviet Union), and 52 in the Soviet Union. In 1997, male life expectancy increased to 60 in the countries that now form the European Union and decreased to 54 in the former communist countries of central and eastern Europe (excluding the former Soviet Union), and to 48 in Russia. The relative disadvantage for women was similar, though the absolute differences were smaller. Mortality changes after 1989 in eastern Europe were correlated with changes in gross domestic products and alterations in income inequalities. There was a life expectancy gap of 6 years between eastern and western Europe in the mid-1990s. Of these 6 years, 0.9 years were due to differences in infant mortality. The biggest contribution to the gap was in middle age. Cardiovascular disease accounted for more than half of the 6-year gap, and external causes of death accounted for another fifth.[20,30]

Socio-economic differences in the use of primary health care services

Differences in health care utilization by socio-economic status and gender have been reported by a number of researchers. Most studies conclude that people with low socio-economic status make more use of health care facilities, especially primary care consultations, than people with higher socio-economic status.[31–33] For this more frequent use of primary health care, a variety of reasons are mentioned.

First of all there is an association between socio-economic status and health locus of control. This term refers to the way people perceive the events related to their health as controllable (internal control), as a coincidence (coincidence oriented) or as controlled by others (mostly by doctors) (external control). The extent of being external control oriented is related to lower socio-economic status. It has been reported that doctor-oriented patients tend to visit the doctor more often. Further, financial aspects could also be significant: people with a lower income might prefer going to their primary practices rather than paying the more expensive specialist a visit.

Finally, and apparently the most important reason, people from a lower socio-economic class tend to be in a worse health condition than people from a higher socio-economic class. This implicates that the former need more health care. However, if the analyses of the health care utilization are controlled for the higher morbidity in lower socio-economic groups, these people consume less health care than people from higher socio-economic groups.[33–35]

As a result, the question whether the health care system is available and accessible for all is raised. The availability of good medical care tends to vary inversely with the need for it. This inverse care law operates more completely where medical care is most exposed to market forces, and less so where such exposure is reduced.[36]

Concerning the accessibility of the available health care, various types of barriers have been identified: geographical, financial, cultural, psycho-social barriers, the behaviour of the physicians, administrative barriers, and health care system related barriers (see Chapter 3.1).

In the following section we look closer at this latter possible barrier.

How do family doctors deal with poverty?

According to the theoretical framework of Fishbein and Azjen (theory of reasoned action), behaviour is determined by cognition, attitude, and

Table 2 Life expectancy at birth (in years) and disability-adjusted life expectancy (DALE) (in years) for males and females

Country	Males				Females			
	Life expectancy at birth	Uncertainty interval	DALE at birth	Uncertainty interval	Life expectancy at birth	Uncertainty interval	DALE at birth	Uncertainty interval
United Kingdom	74.7	74.4–75.0	69.7	69.4–70.1	79.7	79.4–80.0	73.7	73.5–74.4
USA	73.8	73.0–74.6	67.5	67.0–68.1	79.7	79.4–80.0	72.6	72.2–73.3
Peru	65.6	64.6–66.6	58.0	56.9–59.0	74.1	73.1–75.0	60.8	59.6–62.0
South Africa	47.3	45.4–49.0	38.6	37.7–39.5	49.7	47.7–51.8	41.0	39.9–42.1
Sierra Leone	33.2	30.7–35.2	25.8	24.5–26.8	35.4	33.0–37.5	26.0	24.8–27.1

Source: WHO Health Report 2000, 206 pp. Available from URL: http://www.who.int/whr/2000/en/report.htm.

intentions. Following this theory, the way family physicians deal with poor patients in their everyday practice is determined by the information and the perception they hold of the poor and of poverty, by their attitude towards poverty and poor people, and by their intentions to be responsive to these problems. Research findings on this topic have shown that among others a major barrier to health care for the homeless are indeed the family physicians themselves, more specifically their training, their perceptions of homeless people, and their consultation style. Investigation also suggests that the beliefs and attitudes of GPs concerning the issue of homelessness can lead to a medical- or a social-oriented behaviour. The choice of the GP to adopt a purely medical approach to the patient's problem may form a barrier to primary care for homeless people.[37] A qualitative, unpublished study concluded that the participating family physicians, all involved in primary health care for the poor and the underserved, identify three concepts in their definition of poverty: socio-economic aspects, psychological and personality characteristics, and socio-cultural concepts. Family physicians adopt different types of approaches to deal with deprived patients: adaptation of the doctor–patient communication, lowering of the financial threshold, referral to specialists and other health care professionals. These results illustrate the importance of the function of an accessible family physician operating at the crossroad between society and the health care system. They point out the need for specific attention towards the poor and underserved, as well as the need for adequate training and health care organization in order to meet these objectives.[37]

Tackling inequalities in health

Reviews of evaluated interventions tackling inequalities in health reveal four main policy levels for action: strengthening individuals, strengthening communities, improving access to essential facilities and services, and encouraging macro-economic and cultural change.[22]

At the first level, policy responses are aimed at strengthening individuals in disadvantaged circumstances and employing person-based strategies. These policies are based on the premise that building up knowlegde, motivation, and/or competence of skills, enables one to alter behaviour in relation to personal risk-factors, or to cope better with the stress imposed by external health hazards from other layers of influence. This approach is refered to as the 'empowerment' model of health promotion. Although these policies may be expected to have a direct impact on health (e.g. being succesful in reducing smoking rates among people in poor socio-economic circumstances), very often the potential effect will be more indirect (e.g. health services for people who are unemployed do not reduce the unemployment rate, but may ameliorate the worst health effects of unemployment and prevent further damage).

The second policy level concerns strengthening communities. Here, the model of community oriented primary care (COPC model) may contribute to reduce unhealthy social inequalities (see Chapter 1.4). The focus of COPC is not only on the curative and the preventive efforts at the level of the individual patient, but also enhances a 'community diagnosis'. This approach starts from a primary health care facility, is targeted at a well-defined population, and develops a systematic intervention towards the most important health problems of the population. The COPC model comprises four steps: definition of the target population, detection of the most important health problems, development of intervention programmes, and evaluation and monitoring. Different information sources are used: experiences of the own practice (as family physician, nurse, social worker, etc.) and secondary analyses of health-related data (about unemployment, migration, vulnerable groups in society, etc.). In some cases new data are collected, both quantitatively and qualitatively (e.g. focus groups). All this information contributes to the 'community diagnosis' in which the relation between social class and health condition is an important focus. Intervention programmes are defined starting from clear objectives, realistic timing, adequate methods and, most important of all, participation of the target group during the whole process.[38] In a community health centre in a deprived area of Ghent (Belgium), for example, family physicians and nurses observed young children in a poor physical condition. They suspected that the children spent too much time in front of the television. This was the starting point of a COPC action. A survey in the neighbourhood revealed that on average the children in that community took two times less physical exercise during a week than an average child in the country, and that they spent twice as long in front of the television. In a discussion with the children and their parents and teachers, it became clear that the lack of safe playgrounds in the neighbourhood was a major problem. Action was undertaken in order to improve possibilities for physical activities and different playgrounds were created and activities (with a high participation rate) were organized during the holidays. Since the police reported a decrease in minor street crime during that period, it can be concluded that this intervention had a positive effect, not only on the physical level, but also on the psycho-social level.[39]

The COPC approach recognizes the importance of social cohesion, as well as the need to create the conditions in deprived neighbourhoods for community dynamics to work.[38]

The third policy level focuses on improving access to essential facilities and services. These policies tackle the physical and psycho-social conditions in which people live and work, including clean water, sanitation, adequate housing, safe and fullfilling employment, safe and nutritious food supplies, essential health care, education services, and welfare in times of need. Most such improvements require multisectoral action. Within the health care system, specific actions in order to decrease psycho-social and financial barriers can be undertaken. For example, family physicians should be accessable without financial cost to the patient. Hindering the accessibility of the most cost-effective level of the health care system obviously lacks all logic. Taking all financing systems into account, capitation and salary-system theoretically guarantee financial accessibility of health care for the poor and the underserved.

Physicians have a special responsibility for the use of financial resources for health care: a cost-effective, evidence-based approach will enable the largest part of the population to have access to high quality of care.[40]

The fourth and final policy level is aimed at encouraging macro-economic or cultural changes to reduce poverty and the wider adverse effects of inequality on society. These include macro-economic and labour market policies, the encouragement of cultural values promoting equal opportunities, and environmental hazards control on a national and international scale. These policies tend to span several factors and work across the population as a whole.[23] Some policies, however, are not primarily introduced for health reasons, let alone with the aim of reducing inequalities in health. In this way they are not monitored for health outcomes. Family physicians, operating at the crossroads between society and the health care system, have a privileged position to discover and document unhealthy inequalities and to signal health consequences of bad social circumstances. Some family physicians will even consider it their duty to put social inequalities on the political agenda. The personal views of the doctor and the political context will determine which responsibility the family physician assumes. Eventually, it is clear that social health inequality is a socio-political problem. Fighting poverty on a worldwide scale will be most effective.

Key points

Health inequalities can be tackled by four approaches

- Helping individuals change their behaviour to cope better with health risks
- Helping communities to take effective social action
- Improving access to essential facilities and services
- Encouraging macro-economic and cultural change to reduce poverty

References

1. **Mackenbach, J.P.** *Unhealthy Differences. About Social Stratification and Health in The Netherlands.* Assen: Van Gorcum, 1994.
2. **Department of Health and Social Security.** *Inequalities in Health: The Black Report.* Harmondsworth: Penguin, 1982.
3. **WHO Regional Office for Europe.** *Targets for Health for All. The Health Policy for Europe.* Summary of the updated edition. Copenhagen: WHO, 1991.
4. **WHO Regional Office for Europe.** *Health 21—Health for All in the 21st Century: An Introduction.* Copenhagen: WHO, 1998.
5. **WHO Health Report 2000,** 206 pp. Available from URL: http://www.who.int/whr/2000/en/report.htm.
6. **Kunst, Z.E. and Mackenbach, J.P.,** ed. *Measuring Socio-economic Inequalities in Health.* Copenhagen: WHO Regional Office, 1994.
7. **Leon, D.A. and Walt, G.** (2001). Recent advances: international perspectives on health inequalities and policy. *British Medical Journal* **322**, 591–4.
8. **Marmot, M. and Wilkinson, R.G.,** ed. *Social Determinants of Health.* New York: Oxford University Press, 1999.
9. **Power, C.** (1994). Health and social inequality in Europe. *British Medical Journal* **308**, 1153–6.
10. **Marmot, M. and Wilkinson, G.W.** (2001). Psychosocial and material pathways in the relation between income and health: a response to Lynch et al. *British Medical Journal* **322**, 1233–6.
11. **Wilkinson, G.W.** (1997). Socioeconomic determinants of health: health inequalities: relative or absolute material standards? *British Medical Journal* **22: 314** (7080), 591–5.
12. **Turrell, G. and Mathers, C.** (2001). Socio-economic inequalities in all-cause and specific-cause mortality in Australia: 1985–1987 and 1995–1997. *International Journal of Epidemiology* **30**, 231–9.
13. **Gornick, M.E., Eggers, P.W., and Reilly, T.W.** (1996). Effects of race and income on mortality and use of services among Medicare beneficiaries. *New England Journal of Medicine* **335**, 791–9.
14. **Dionne, C.E.** et al. (2001). Formal education and back pain: a review. *Journal of Epidemiology and Community Health* **55**, 455–68.
15. **Kahn, R.S.** et al. (2000). State income inequality, household income, and maternal mental and physical health: cross sectional national survey. *British Medical Journal* **321**, 1311–15.
16. **Davey Smith, G.** et al. (1996). Socio-economic differentials in mortality risk among men screened for the multiple risk factor intervention trial. 1. White men. *American Journal of Public Health* **86**, 486–96.
17. **Davey Smith, G.** et al. (1998). Individual social class, area-based deprivation, cardiovascular disease risk factors, and mortality: the Renfrew and Paisley study. *Journal of Epidemiology and Community Health* **52**, 399–405.
18. **Power, C., Matthews, S., and Manor, O.** (1996). Inequalities in self rated health in the 1958 birth cohort: lifetime social circumstances or social mobility? *British Medical Journal* **313**, 449–53.
19. **van de Lisdonk, E.H.** et al., ed. *Diseases in the Family Medicine Practice.* Utrecht: Wetenschappelijke uitgeverij Bunge, 1999.
20. **Lynch, J.** et al. (2001). Income inequality, the psychosocial environment, and health: comparisons of wealthy nations. *The Lancet* **358**, 194–200.
21. **McConnochie, K.M., Roghmann, K.J., and Liptak, G.S.** (1997). Socio-economic variation in discretionary and mandatory hospitalization of infants: an ecologic analysis. *Pediatrics* **99**, 774–84.
22. **Marmot, M.G. and Shipley, M.J.** (1996). Do socio-economic differences in mortality persist after retirement? 25 Year follow up of civil servants from the first Whitehall study. *British Medical Journal* **313**, 1177–80.
23. **Townsend, J.,** ed. (1995). The burden of smoking. In *Tackling Inequalities in Health* (ed. M. Benzeval, K. Judge, and M. Whitehead), pp. 82–94. London: King's Fund.
24. **Pappas, G.** et al. (1993). The increasing disparity in mortality between socio-economic groups in the United States, 1960 and 1986. *New England Journal of Medicine* **329**, 103–9.
25. **McLoone, P. and Boddy, F.A.** (1994). Deprivation and mortality in Scotland, 1981 and 1991. *British Medical Journal* **309**, 1465–70.
26. **Phillimore, P., Beattie, A., and Townsend, P.** (1994). Widening inequality of health in northern England, 1981–91. *British Medical Journal* **308**, 1125–8.
27. **Wilkinson, R.G.** (1994). Divided we fall. *British Medical Journal* **308**, 1113–14.
28. **Marmot, M.G.** et al. (1991). Health inequalities among British civil servants: the Whitehall II study. *Lancet* **337** (8754), 1387–9.
29. **North, F.** et al. (1993). Explaining socio-economic differences in sickness absence: the Whitehall II study. *British Medical Journal* **306**, 361–6.
30. **Marmot, M. and Boba, M.** (2000). International comparators and poverty and health in Europe. *British Medical Journal* **321**, 1124–8.
31. **De Prins, L.F., Peersman, W.P., and De Maeseneer, J.M.** (1998). Lower educated, more consultations in general practice? A study in Flanders (Belgium). *Huisarts en Wetenschap* **41** (4), 173–8.
32. **Nolan, B.** (1994). General practitioner utilization in Ireland. The role of socio-economic factors. *Social Science and Medicine* **38**, 711–16.
33. **Van der Meer, J., Van Den Bos, J., and Mackenbach, J.** (1996). Socio-economic differences in utilization of health services in a Dutch population: the contribution of health status. *Health Policy* **37**, 1–18.
34. **Saxena, S., Majeed, A., and Jones, M.** (1999). Socio-economic differences in childhood consultation rates in general practice in England and Wales: prospective cohort study. *British Medical Journal* **318**, 642–6.
35. **Cooper, H., Smaje, C., and Arber, S.** (1998). Use of health services by children and young people according to ethnicity and social class: secondary analysis of a national survey. *British Medical Journal* **317**, 1047–57.
36. **Hart, J.T.** (1971). The inverse care law. *The Lancet* **1**, 405–12.
37. **Lester, H. and Bradley, C.** (2001). Barriers to primary healthcare for the homeless. The general practitioner's perspective. *European Journal of General Practice* **7**, 6–12.
38. **Rhyne, R.** et al., ed. *Community-Oriented Primary Care: Health Care for the 21st Century.* Washington DC: American Public Health Association, 1998.
39. **Willems, S., Swinnen, W., and De Maeseneer, J.,** ed. *'Tell me about poverty': Perceptions of Family Physicians.* Unpublished research report, 2001.
40. **Brown, S.,** ed. *Physician Funding and Health Care Systems—An International Perspective.* Cambridge: The Royal College of General Practitioners, 1999.

5

The consultation

5 The consultation

5.1 The patient–doctor relationship

Ann Louise Kinmonth and Moira Stewart

Introduction

The consultation has been elegantly described by Dr James Spence as 'The essential unit of medical practice, the occasion when, in the intimacy of the consulting room or sick room, a person who is ill, or believes himself to be ill, seeks the advice of a doctor whom he trusts'. The consultation is thus seen as the main manifestation of the patient–doctor relationship, and the primary situation in which it is built or destroyed.[1]

The relationship between patient and family doctor can also be seen as an indicator of the current values of a society, and of its evolution over time. The expectations brought to the relationship are moderated not simply by experience of previous consultations, but by a wide range of social and cultural influences within which the consultation takes place. These influences play on doctor and patient alike, although to different effect.

Expert commentaries from sociology[2] and social history[3,4] draw attention to the curious mood of disorientation and uncertainty that beset western medicine at the end of the twentieth century—a loss of confidence in the proper way in which doctors should relate to patients, a deep unhappiness expressed by doctors, accompanied by media articles questioning their power, competence, attitudes, and position in society. Porter[3] concluded that '... for centuries medicine was impotent and thus unproblematic. Today, with "mission accomplished" its triumphs are dissolving in disorientation ... it is losing its way, or having to redefine its goals ...'.

In this essay, we examine the traditions of holistic, person-centred medical practice on the one hand, and of reductionist, disease-centred biomedicine on the other. By tracing their origins, and reviewing the evidence for their strengths and limitations, we reflect on the key elements of a patient–doctor relationship adapted to twenty-first century primary care.

The tasks of medicine

Confusion about the tasks of medicine may contribute to the current disorientation of doctors. The central tasks of medicine have been defined in a variety of ways: enhancement of the public's health, which implies an epidemiological approach;[5] strengthening the ability of the patient to cope, which invokes psychology;[6] or alleviation of suffering, which implies recognition of the individual's predicament and active listening.[7] The dominant, traditional medical model holds that the central tasks are threefold: diagnosis (including explanation), prognosis, and treatment. Not only are the tasks of medicine contested, but so is the nature of the patient–doctor relationship that can best underpin them. The debate stems from issues of deep interest to individuals and society such as 'What is the nature of disease and illness?' 'Do (as Spence implies) intimacy and trust make important contributions to the effective fulfilment of the tasks of medicine?' It can obviously be confusing for both parties if a patient who believes that disease is a tiresome, mechanical derangement, to be identified and fixed, meets a doctor steeped in traditions of whole person medicine, valuing also the meaning of the illness experience. Those holding to the first belief might regard the relationship with a physician as unimportant and embrace substitution of interactive computerized diagnosis for the patient–doctor relationship with satisfaction. Those holding to the second might espouse protection and enhancement of the patient–doctor relationship through longer consultations and continuity of care.

Holistic approaches: the school of Cos

The polarities between these two approaches to medicine can be traced back to ancient Greece and the schools of Cos and Cnidus.[8] The school of Cos was concerned with the whole organism's expression of disease and attempted, by careful observation of the patient, to describe the illness in all its dimensions over time. As Hippocrates describes in 'First Epidemics', attention was paid to 'what was common to every and particular to each case; to the patient, the prescriber and the prescription; to the epidemic constitution generally and in its local mood'.[9] Diagnosis in this school required careful listening to the patient's ideas and accounts of illness, exploration of both the social context and the inner life, and observation of present state. Attention was paid 'to the habits of life and occupation of each patient; to his (sic) speech, conduct, silences, thoughts, sleep, wakefulness and dreams—their content and incidence; to his pickings and scratchings ...'. Diagnosis at the level of the whole organism in its environment led naturally to explanations and management at this level; with attention to a regimen of care, personal lifestyle changes, and environmental modification to support health.

From this holistic approach to medicine can be traced at one end of the spectrum the doctor as advocate, aiming to improve the health of a population, and at the other the rise in understanding of the influence of the doctor–patient relationship on the well-being of the individual.

Population health and advocacy

Work in the area of public health advocacy includes elucidation of the environmental and social determinants of disease from Snow[10] to Brown and Harris[11] building on the importance given to social context in the school of Cos. It leads to definition of the patient–doctor relationship beyond the consultation, and clarifies the position of the doctor in relation to the Government of the day in terms of advocacy for the nation's health. As Cicero said 'The health of the people is the highest law', and the position of doctor as advocate for the people's health is movingly described[12,13] and exemplified in the working lives and advocacy of doctors in deprived areas.[14–17]

The second thread of the school of Cos is the power of the patient–doctor relationship.

The patient–doctor relationship

Among the many individuals who have observed or explored the patient–doctor relationship in the twentieth century, the work of George Engel in the United States, and Michael and Enid Balint's work with the Balint Society, stand out. Both studies sought a deeper understanding of the patients' problems than was offered by biomedical diagnosis alone. Engel advanced the influential idea of a biopsychosocial model of illness that combined the classical biomedical model with the emerging insights of sociology.(18) The Balints drew on psycho-analytic ideas to demonstrate the potential for the process of the consultation to be therapeutic. Their work has strongly influenced medical education with its emphasis on the doctor as the treatment, and the need for doctors to understand themselves if they are to understand their patients in the clinical encounter.

Balint(19) pointed out that listening is a difficult undertaking that must be learned; he wrote, 'The ability to listen is a new skill, necessitating a considerable though limited change in the doctor's personality. While discovering in himself an ability to listen to things in his patient that are barely spoken because the patient himself is only dimly aware of them, the doctor will start listening to the same kind of language in himself' (p. 121). Listening is key to understanding the patient and the presence of a listening doctor can lead to healing; 'Doctors may fail to realize that what a patient wants is something very simple: a recognition of his or her unique suffering or perhaps only our presence at a time of need' (ref. 9, p. 96). This presence can restore the patient's sense of connectedness, a connectedness that may have been broken by physical or emotional suffering.(7,20) The process of recognition requires the patient to be treated as the 'expert' on his or her illness. The patient–practitioner relationship thus becomes more one of partnership than of supplication.(21)

Seminal qualitative studies describe such processes as beginning with the practitioner listening, followed by the patients beginning to trust in the relationship, becoming a more active partner in care, being empowered to mobilize their own resources, and leading finally to healing and health.(22,23)

In summary, then, the great strength of the school of Cos is its potential for influencing advocacy and enablement at the level of both the population and the individual. It encourages us to remember the interaction between the organism and its environment. It points to a patient–doctor relationship based on a deep connection, in which the particulars of each patient are listened to and recognized.

We judge that this school will become increasingly influential as the scientific base of medicine becomes more integrative in approach, stimulated both by the current opportunities to understand more about the development of disease processes (seen as the result of dynamic mind–body and environmental–gene interactions) and by the rising social expectation of partnership in health care.

Reductionist approaches: the school of Cnidus

In contrast to the emphasis on the organism in its environment in understanding the manifestations and management of disease, the school of Cnidus in Ancient Greece was concerned primarily with diseases as abstract entities and their effects on organs rather than organisms. The disease was seen as an entity independent of the patient. Thus, while in diagnosis the Coans attempted a full description of the patient's state, with an emphasis on understanding, the Cnidians attempted to classify the disease, independent of the patient's illness experience, as an abstract proposition in accordance with a taxonomy that emphasized prediction and prognosis. In treatment, while the Coans managed each patient individually and symptomatically with a view to assisting nature in restoring the functional unity of the organism, the Cnidians employed a specific remedy for each named disease.

The power of prediction

The great potential of the school of Cnidus was that of explanation of cause, prediction of course, and rational development of specific remedy. It could not, however, begin to exploit this potential until methods became available to make rational taxonomies of disease. Sydenham—'the English Hippocrates'—(1624–89) made some progress by developing the study of the natural history of disease and correlating clinical categories with their course and outcome. Using careful observation of the patient, he was remarkable in his success in differentiating many of the common infectious diseases.

However, the major step forward did not come until the nineteenth century when the French School of Clinical Pathologists began to link the signs of disease found on physical examination with the post-mortem appearances of the body organs. The powerful classification of disease based on morbid anatomy forms the basis of the clinical method still in general use in specialist and generalist practice today. It has greatly influenced the patient–doctor relationship.

As Armstrong has put it, 'the core task of medicine became not the elucidation of what the patient said but what the doctor saw in the depths of the body'.(24) Foucault has famously defined how the patient's body becomes subject to a 'medical gaze' in the context of the clinic where an array of instruments allowed new ways of 'seeing' the disease within.(25) This new clinical method came to dominate the education of doctors, providing the student with a conceptual structure within which to formulate a diagnosis based on underlying pathology.

This approach tended to downplay public health strategies. It neglected the growing burden of chronic conditions where patients undertake the daily care of their condition and distracted attention from the management of illnesses without pathological diagnosis such as chronic fatigue or widespread pain, and the presentations of anxiety and depression, which form such an important part of medical care.

The rise of counting and accountability

The tradition of classifying and counting includes the development of tools to assess the cost-effectiveness of treatments summed across individual consultations which has also strongly influenced the patient–doctor relationship. At the beginning of the twentieth century, clinical competence in doctors and effectiveness of medicine was broadly taken as given. By the 1970s this position was in question. Evidence suggested that relatively little of the long-term health of populations was directly due to biomedicine, that many commonly used interventions were not beneficial when evaluated, that medical errors were more common than expected, and that doctors varied widely in their use of procedures (independent of case mix).(26) The spate of evidence-based protocols and guidelines that ensued has provided much of the current base for discussions of doctor substitution in health care. Practitioners have been seen simply as a means to implement guidelines and, the doctor–patient relationship mistrusted as a shield to hide incompetence rather than trusted as the bedrock for effective practice. New drugs and technologies are now reviewed by national organizations for safety and cost-effectiveness before acceptance into practice. In most countries, the management of rationing has been introduced into the patient–doctor relationship along with the potential for further erosion of trust as the patient wonders if the doctor is an advocate for him or her or for the State.

Quantitative studies of patient–doctor relationship

An important example of the coming together of the holistic and reductionist traditions is in the application of analytical methodology from epidemiology to studies of the patient–doctor relationship. Despite considerable limitations in terms of definitions of the interventions and measures, power, study quality, and length of follow-up, studies demonstrate that processes in the consultation contribute significantly to what patients think and do as reflected in their satisfaction, their recall and understanding of information, and their responsiveness to advice.(27) Patients also prefer doctors who communicate well, especially those who are seen as approachable and able to explain clearly what the problem is and what should be done.(28) Characteristics of the interaction between patient and practitioner also influence outcome, predicting resolution of symptoms in general,(29,30) headache,[31] sore throat,[32] and anxiety and distress.[33] However, few trials in this area are yet available with objective health outcomes.

Building on a 1995 review by Stewart,[34] our more recent systematic review of 35 intervention trials has found that most interventions significantly improved patient–doctor communication measures (22/30) while slightly more than half of the interventions improved physical symptoms, anxiety, depression, well-being, or functional status/quality of life where these were measured (14/25).[35] The evaluated interventions targeted all stages of the patient–doctor interaction, the most frequently evaluated approaches encouraging patient participation in the consultation (19/30). Six trials measured health outcomes objectively among patients with diabetes, hypertension, or mixed presentations.[36–41] Only two of these trials showed a significant positive effect on blood glucose in one case and on blood pressure in the other.[36,37]

Moving from evidence to practice

Despite this evidence that the nature of the patient–doctor relationship can affect process and outcome of medical care, it has had relatively little impact on medical policy or practice. This may be, in part, because of the lack of rigour of some of the evidence, a weakness in the theoretical underpinnings of the interventions evaluated, and the lack of data on the mechanisms by which they may be achieving their ends. However, there may also be a resistance to patient-centred practice because of the perceptions of time pressure under which medicine is increasingly practiced. There is in fact little evidence that patient-centred medicine is more time consuming than disease-centred practice.[35] However, modern medicine puts daunting pressures on doctors to be both efficient and accurate in diagnosis and treatment of disease, pressures arguably arising from the Cnidian worldview. In this context, consideration of Coan attitudes to the individual and their social context, which further embrace complexity and uncertainty, may feel overwhelming.

Solutions to this complexity have largely been more compatible with the biomedical than the holistic approach to practice. They include larger practice teams, and extended computer use that are associated with a reduction in personal continuity of care, implying 'team' rather than 'personal' loyalty and an increasing dependence on the medical record as the only purveyor of the patient–practitioner relationship over time. This may assist systematic monitoring and accountability rather than the development of therapeutic alliances; it leads medical practice towards quality assured packages to which patients have rights, and away from a partnership between patient and doctor built on trust.

Partnership and trust

Trust in doctors implies a range of confidences; for example, confidence in the safety of committing patients' bodies to medical care, confidence in doctors' commitment to patients' best interests, confidence in doctors' technical competence, and humanity.

The depersonalization of medical care, with loss of continuity, conflicts of interest associated with its commercialization, and the growth of managed care, alongside media attention to medical uncertainty and error, all challenge trust.[42,43] Studies across countries repeatedly demonstrate widespread problems with communication and respect for patients' wishes in primary and secondary care.[44–46]

Concerns about erosion of trust find practical responses at institutional and individual levels. At the institutional level regulatory frameworks for medical practice are being reviewed across the world in line with societal expectations. Such frameworks make transparent both rights and obligations and aim to protect both patients and their doctors.[47] Similarly, clinical institutions are taking measures to help restore trust; for example, eliciting patients' views on care, providing more information to them, and teaching staff communication skills.[42] Paradoxically, these attempts to shore up trust can erode it further. Thus, the wholly admirable aim of increasing information has resulted in the public having to confront the risks and uncertainty that limit medical practice, and which were less explicit under the traditional paternalistic medical model (when ironically there was less to offer). This can increase the work needed at the individual level to construct trust, on both sides, not as the blind faith of the past, but as the basis of a working partnership between patient and doctor.

Doctors and patients might benefit from an explicit new contract that admitted the strengths and limitations of biomedicine and led to a more honest relationship.[4,48] However, patients will still benefit from flexibility. For example, they may be best served on occasion by a temporary dependence on the doctor[49] or by being allowed to hope when hope is not strictly warranted by the stage of disease alone.[29]

What next? A patient-centred clinical method

In spite of the many pressures that continue to keep the schools of Cos and Cnidus in opposing corners, there are others that are pushing forward their integration. An integrated model accepts a wide range of causes of illness and disease, psychological, social, and physiological. It combines respect for the biomedical clinical method with a parallel respect for the individual's particular predicament in making diagnosis both of the disease and of the illness. It realizes the power of the therapeutic alliance in framing the way the presenting problem is seen and in motivating action or adaptation. It thus integrates the rational with the experiential in effective practice.

The clinical method to support this integration is already well developed and taught in some medical schools. It is called the Patient-centered Clinical Method and comprises six interacting components.[50] The first three components encompass the process between patient and doctor. The second three focus more on the context within which patient and doctor interact. Inherent in the clinical method is the notion that power is shared between the patient and the doctor, that doctors will connect at an emotional level with patients, and that there is a need for physician self-knowledge.

The first component of the patient-centred clinical method is the assessment of the two conceptualizations of ill health: the biomedical concept of disease and the holistic concept of illness. In addition to assessing the disease process by history and physical examination, the physician actively seeks to enter into the patient's world to *understand his or her particular experience of illness* (patients' feelings, ideas, function, and expectations).

The second component is the integration of the concepts of disease and illness with an *understanding of the whole person*: the patient's unique personality, life story, and the context (environment) in which he or she lives.

The mutual task of *finding common ground* between doctor and patient is the third component of the method and focuses on three key areas: (a) defining the problem, (b) establishing the goals of management, and (c) identifying the roles to be assumed by doctor and patient. Mutual discussion encourages the patients to participate as fully as they desire in the process.

The fourth component highlights the potential of each visit as an opportunity for (relevant) discussion about *prevention and health promotion.* The fifth component emphasizes that each consultation should be used to build on the *patient–physician relationship*, using empathy to support enablement and healing.

The sixth component requires that, throughout the process, the physician be *realistic* about time, and availability of resources, including the personal resources of emotional and physical energy.

The key message of the patient-centred clinical method is the integration of the biomedical knowledge (of disease) with the personal knowledge (of the patient's illness experience), seen within the patient's and doctor's environment (context).

Research

Need for quantitative and qualitative methods

The evidence base of the new clinical method comes from a range of quantitative and qualitative research. Traditionally, biomedicine has depended on the former, and holistic medicine on the latter. In our view, both are impoverished by this boundary.

There is a pressing need to value qualitative research on patient–doctor relationships equally with quantitative research that evaluates the effectiveness of efforts to improve patient–doctor relationships. Qualitative components can illuminate the 'black box' of an unspecified intervention, and promote deep reflection, while quantitative components can answer specific questions about effectiveness and costs.

Developing and evaluating new interventions

Our systematic reviews of trials of patient–practitioner interaction demonstrated how few rigorous trials of well-defined interventions have been reported. The reviews identified a range of promising approaches to improving patient–practitioner interaction in a cost-effective manner, which have yet to be fully evaluated. These include simple techniques to encourage patients to ask questions in the medical interview, or to tell practitioners what their concerns are. They include teaching practitioners how to explore their patients' ideas, concerns and expectations, provide clear information about the disease and its treatment and incorporate both into problem-framing and shared plans. They also include attention to emotion in the consultation.

These interventions require careful specification and their evaluation requires attention to appropriate measures of process and outcome, as well as study design.(51)

A multidisciplinary research agenda

There is a wide cross-disciplinary research agenda relating to the patient–doctor relationship that reaches well beyond the use of clinical trials. It spans ethics, sociology, history, law, and economics, as well as the more traditional medical disciplines, psychology, and neuroscience. We expect it to address such questions as the mechanisms of effect of the so-called 'non-specific' factors in health care, the meaning of trust, the effects of accountability and transparency in medicine on hope, optimism, and health, and the true cost-effectiveness of applications of the patient-centred method in long-term studies with disease and patient-centred outcomes among defined patient groups.

Conclusion

There is a moral responsibility on us to retain humanity in medical practice. There is an evidence base to support particular attributes of the consultation in improving the processes of care. To develop this work further and apply it more widely is clearly challenging. We believe that the challenge must be addressed if we are to achieve a patient–practitioner relationship fit for twenty-first century primary medical care that integrates the best of the traditions of Cos and Cnidus.

Acknowlegement

We thank John Benson and Ian McWhinney for their thoughtful comments.

References

1. **Spence, J.C.** *The Purpose and Practice of Medicine: Selections from the Writings of Sir James Spence.* London: Oxford University Press, 1960.
2. **Fox, R.** (2000). Medical uncertainty revisited. In *The Handbook of Social Studies in Health and Medicine* (ed. G.L. Albrecht, R. Fitzpatrick, and S.C. Scrimshaw), pp. 409–25. Newbury Park: Sage Publications.
3. **Porter, R.** *The Greatest Benefit to Mankind: A Medical History of Humanity* 1st edn. New York: W.W. Norton, 1998.
4. **Smith, R.** (2001). Why are doctors so unhappy? *British Medical Journal* **322**, 1073–4.
5. **White, K.** *The Task of Medicine: Dialogue at Wickenburg.* Menlo Park CA: Henry J. Kaiser Family Foundation, 1988.
6. **Folkman, S. and Lazarus, R.S.** (1988). The relationship between coping and emotion: implications for theory and research. *Social Science and Medicine* **26**, 309–17.
7. **Cassell, E.J.** *The Nature of Suffering and Goals of Medicine.* New York: Oxford University Press, 1991.
8. **Crookshank, F.G.** (1926). The theory of diagnosis. *Lancet* **1**, 939.
9. **McWhinney, I.R.** *A Textbook of Family Medicine.* Oxford: Oxford University Press, 1997.
10. **Snow, J.** *Snow on Cholera* cited in Pickles, W.N. Epidemiology in Country Practice: bibliography p II. Bristol: John Wright and Sons Ltd. London: Simpkin Marshall Ltd, 1939 (reissued 1949). London and New York, 1936.
11. **Brown, G. and Harris, T.** *Social Origins of Depression: A Study of Psychiatric Disorder in Women.* London: Tavistock Publications, 1978.
12. **Cronin, A.J.** *The Citadel.* New York and Boston: Little Brown and Co, 1983.
13. **Coles, R.**, ed. *The Doctor Stories.* New York NY: New Directions, 1984.
14. **Tudor-Hart, J.** *A New Kind of Doctor.* London: Merlin Press, 1988.
15. **Heath, I.** *The Mystery of General Practice.* London: Nuffield Provincial Hospitals Trust, 1995.
16. **Macaulay, A.C.** et al. (1998). Participatory research with native community of Kahnawake creates innovative Code of Research Ethics. *Canadian Journal of Public Health* **89**, 105–8.
17. **Masi, R. and Disman, M.** (1994). Health care and seniors: ethnic, racial and cultural dimensions. *Canadian Family Physician* **40**, 498–504.
18. **Engel, G.** (1977). The need for a new medical model. A challenge for biomedicine. *Science* **196**, 129–34.
19. **Balint, M.** *The Doctor, his Patient and the Illness.* London: Pitman, 1964.
20. **Suchman, A.L. and Matthews, D.A.** (1988). What makes the patient–doctor relationship therapeutic? Exploring the connexional dimension of medical care. *Annals of Internal Medicine* **108**, 125–30.
21. **Tuckett, D.** et al. *Meetings Between Experts: An Approach to Sharing Ideas in the Consultation.* London: Tavistock, 1985.
22. **Seifert, M.H., Jr.** (1992). Qualitative designs for assessing interventions in primary care: examples from medical practice. In *Assessing Interventions: Traditional and Innovative Methods* (ed. F. Tudiver, M.J. Bass, E.V. Dunn, P. Norton, and M.A. Stewart). Newbury Park: Sage Publications.
23. **McWilliam, C.L.** et al. (1997). Creating empowering meaning: an interactive process of promoting health with chronically ill older Canadians. *Health Promotion International* **12**, 111–23.
24. **Armstrong, D.** (1984). The patients' view. *Social Science and Medicine* **18**, 737–44.
25. **Foucault, M.** *The Birth of the Clinic: An Archaeology of Medical Perception.* New York: Vintage, 1975.
26. **Light, D.** (2000). The sociological character of health care markets. In *The Handbook of Social Studies in Health and Medicine* (ed. G.L. Albrecht, R. Fitzpatrick, and S.C. Scrimshaw). Thousand Oaks CA: Sage.
27. **Starfield, B.** *Primary Care: Balancing Health Needs, Services and Technology.* New York: Oxford University Press, 1998.
28. **Little, P.** et al. (2001). Preferences of patients for patient-centred approach to consultation in primary care: observational study. *British Medical Journal* **322**, 468–72.
29. **Little, P.** et al. (2001). Observational study of effects of patient-centredness and positive approach on outcomes of general practice consultations. *British Medical Journal* **323**, 908–11.
30. **Stewart, M.** et al. (2000). The impact of patient-centered care on outcomes. *Journal of Family Practice* **49**, 796–804.
31. **Headache Study Group** (1986). Predictors of outcome in headache patients presenting to family physicians—a one year prospective study. *HEADACHE Journal* **26**, 285–94.
32. **Little, P.** et al. (1999). Clinical and psychosocial predictors of illness duration from randomised controlled trial of prescribing strategies for sore throat. *British Medical Journal* **319**, 736–7.
33. **Roter, D.** et al. (1995). Improving physicians' interviewing skills and reducing patients' emotional distress: a randomized clinical trial. *Archives of Internal Medicine* **155**, 1877–84.

34. **Stewart, M.A.** (1995). Effective physician–patient communication and health outcomes: a review. *Canadian Medical Association Journal* **152**, 1423–33.
35. **Kinmonth, A.L.** Systematic review. Orlando, 2000.
36. **Greenfield, S.** et al. (1988). Patients' participation in medical care: effects on blood sugar control and quality of life in diabetes. *Journal of General Internal Medicine* **3**, 448–57.
37. **Kaplan, R. and Ganiats, T.G.** (1989). Trade offs in treatment alternatives for non-insulin-dependent diabetes mellitus. *Journal of General Internal Medicine* **4**, 167–71.
38. **Meland, E., Laerum, E., and Ulvik, R.** (1997). Effectiveness of two preventive interventions for coronary heart disease in primary care. *Scandinavian Journal of Primary Health Care* **15**, 57–64.
39. **Kinmonth, A.L.** et al. (1998). Randomised controlled trial of patient-centred care of diabetes in general practice: impact on current well-being and future disease risk. *British Medical Journal* **317**, 1202–8.
40. **Pill, R.** et al. (1998). A randomized controlled trial of an intervention designed to improve the care given in general practice to Type II diabetic patients: patient outcomes and professional ability to change behaviour. *Family Practice* **15**, 229–35.
41. **Reuben, D.B.** et al. (1999). A randomized clinical trial of outpatient comprehensive geriatric assessment coupled with an intervention to increase adherence to recommendations. *Journal of the American Geriatric Society* **47**, 269–76.
42. **Mechanic, D.** (1996). Changing medical organisation and the erosion of trust. *Milbank-Quarterly* **74**, 171–89.
43. **Kearley, K., Freeman, G., and Heath, A.** (2001). An exploration of the value of the personal doctor–patient relationship in general practice. *British Journal of General Practice* **51**, 712–18.
44. **Compas Inc. Multi-Audience Research.** Muddled mandate: ambivalence, conflict, frustration, and other plaints of public opinion on healthcare policy. Interview Schedule, 2001.
45. **Coulter, A. and Cleary, P.D.** (2001). Patients' experiences with hospital care in five countries. *Health Affairs (Millwood)* **20**, 244–52.
46. **Grol, R.** et al. (2000). Patients in Europe evaluate general practice care: an international comparison. *British Journal of General Practice* **50**, 882–7.
47. **Irvine, D.** (2001). Doctors in the UK: their new professionalism and its regulatory framework. *Lancet* **358**, 1807–10.
48. **Hart, J.** (2001). Unhappiness will be defeated when doctors accept full social responsibility. *British Medical Journal* **322**, 1363–4.
49. **Thomas, K.** (1974). Temporarily dependent patient in general practice. *British Medical Journal* **1**, 626.
50. **Stewart, M.** et al. *Patient-centered Medicine: Transforming the Clinical Method.* Thousand Oaks: Sage Publications, 1995.
51. **Campbell, M.** et al. (2000). Framework for design and evaluation of complex interventions to improve health. *British Medical Journal* **321**, 694–6.

5.2 Consultation tasks

Nigel C.H. Stott

Background

Something as complex as the consultation in clinical medicine requires a number of tasks to be performed within the domains of:

- skills (competences);
- knowledge (which is the basis of clinical reasoning);
- attitudes (that enable an effective clinical process);
- values (that inform individual integrity, probity and purpose);
- performance (disciplined and appropriate application);
- clinical experience that informs the other five domains.

Excellence in clinical consultation technique requires all of these attributes at a high level of function. Dysfunctional consultations are likely to occur when a clinician is seriously deficient in one or more of these domains. Every clinical practitioner needs to develop in all six domains from the undergraduate stage onwards. However, the content of each domain is far from static. Research constantly modifies the knowledge in each domain and changing social attitudes move the boundary of what is acceptable in different age, gender, and need groups.

External issues also have a potential impact on the quality of clinical consultations: peer pressure, organizational factors, and political factors can help or hinder the consultation process but they are not an excuse for sloppy consultations. Quality improvement in general practice depends on achieving some agreement about the tasks and standards that need to be measured to demonstrate improvement. However, despite years of research, there are persisting concerns about the diversity of systems and standards of primary care on the world scene.(1) For example, Grol et al.(2) surveyed 21 countries in Europe plus United States, Canada, Australia, New Zealand, and Hong Kong. Most were using traditional morbidity data or chart audit as markers of quality in 1995. Only two or three countries were using trained observers, self-recording or audiotape to test quality in the consultation in a systematic way. However, the authors were encouraged by a distinct improvement in attitude over the previous 5 years towards the introduction of innovative and transparent measures for quality improvement in general practice/family medicine.

The basic licensing of doctors to work as general practitioners/family physicians was shown to depend mainly on completion of vocational training schemes (22 out of 26 countries), and re-certification schemes were poorly developed.(2) Traditional CME points systems are now regarded as unsatisfactory indicators of competence or performance. It is in this context that the United Kingdom provides an interesting case study.

The General Medical Council (GMC) of the United Kingdom has transformed its approach to the regulation of medical practitioners during the 1990s. The GMC used to focus on major negative events in a doctor's behaviour when finding serious professional misconduct. The publication by the GMC of 'Good Medical Practice'(3) changed this scene by shifting the emphasis to a set of positive standards that were regarded by many people as being aspirations when first published. These have evolved into a set of 57 professional standards that now need to be met by all doctors who provide patient care, teach students, work with colleagues, conduct research, or have any professional financial/commercial dealings. 'The Duties of a Doctor' (Table 1) underpin the 57 standards and they resonate with many of the consultation tasks that are described in detail below.

By 2004 a quinquennial revalidation for all practising doctors should replace the old CME points system with a personal learning portfolio. The process of revalidation will reflect attention to all the standards spelled out in 'Good Medical Practice'.

The clinical consultation lies at the hub of most medical practice because this is where doctor meets the patient, and this is where primary clinical decisions are taken which initiate advice, investigation, treatment, or referral, often with important implications for patient, family, health service staff, and the economy.

Corporate (population) health promotion and prevention involves a separate set of tasks that are not addressed in this chapter. It is the individual consultation that we focus on here. Yet in primary care issues to do with family and small populations do overlap with care of individuals. The tasks described will therefore include elements that reflect this overlap. A high proportion of people consult every year, particularly among women and children and this level of contact provides many opportunities for clinicians to be proactive as well as responsive in their day to day work.

Table 1 The duties of a doctor registered with the General Medical Council[3]

Patients must be able to trust doctors with their lives and well-being. To justify that trust, we as a profession have a duty to maintain a good standard of practice and care and to show respect for human life. In particular as a doctor you must:

- make the care of your patient your first concern;
- treat every patient politely and considerately;
- respect patients' dignity and privacy;
- listen to patients and respect their views;
- give patients information in a way they can understand;
- respect the right of patients to be fully involved in decisions about their care;
- keep your professional knowledge and skills up to date;
- recognize the limits of your professional competence;
- be honest and trustworthy;
- respect and protect confidential information;
- make sure that your personal beliefs do not prejudice your patients' care;
- act quickly to protect patients from risk if you have good reason to believe that you or a colleague may not be fit to practice;
- avoid abusing your position as a doctor; and
- work with colleagues in the ways that best serve patients' interests.

In all these matters you must never discriminate unfairly against your patients or colleagues. And you must always be prepared to justify your actions to them.

Art or science? The pull between patient and population priorities is complicated by another tension that exists between 'rational analysis' underpinning scientific endeavour and the expression of emotion/intuition, values and spirituality that underpin most motivation and inductive, aesthetic, artistic, and literary achievement.[4] All these dimensions are important aspects of being fully human and they are manifested in clinical consultations. To 'feel understood' is essential to a good relationship, and the pursuit of this primary goal encourages the development of humanity and compassion in medical practice.[5,6]

The unfortunate separation in learning environments of 'science' from 'art' was brought into relief in 1956 by C.P. Snow[7] and the debate about these two cultures has continued ever since. Danger arises when the two sides cannot or will not communicate. The modern emphasis on evidence based medicine should bring the two together if clinical experience, patients' values and the best evidence are integrated.[8–10] But evidence narrowly defined can become a vehicle for intellectual hubris. So, clinicians need to be vigilant as they bring the dimensions together in their daily tasks.

The 'Grand Round' and 'chart round' and 'case conference' are all examples of corporate clinical events that major on rational evidence, often without the patient/family being present. Issues of intuition, emotion, and spiritual values are easily sidelined in such a context.

Multiprofessional health care should encourage the meeting of different mindsets and the modern clinician has a special responsibility to be a protector of the humanity in corporate clinical events where the individual can become too easily lost among the issues. She/he should ensure that the six domains described in the first paragraph are not side-lined and that the 'Duties of a Doctor' (Table 1) are always remembered.

The tasks

Process and management tasks are components of all consultations but the weight of each will vary according to the problem presented to the clinician. For this reason most consultation analysts fudge the difference between art and science and then amalgamate them in a variety of ways. In this section the tasks will be reduced to a manageable number of sets. An overview of key published work will then follow. This approach is possible because there is substantial agreement between analysts about the content of consultation tasks but some divergence about the sub-divisions and the presentation of content.

The first task in every consultation is for the patient to feel valued and recognized as a person. This is good manners and good clinical practice because it reveals that the clinician is aware of the disadvantage that most patients feel when they consult an expert about a problem. Anything less than a gracious and respectful consultation is to abuse a position of authority. Patients who are too ill to respond to the clinician are so vulnerable that they merit particular care in showing respect at every encounter. The few patients who are habitually offensive or difficult in clinical encounters may be anticipating being handled in a high handed way, and many will respond well to explicit and consistent respect for them as persons.

The second set of tasks lie in clarifying the *reason(s) for the consultation* so both clinician and patient understand the agenda(s). This is what Tuckett has called 'meeting between experts'[11] because the patient is the expert in describing his/her own problems, but she/he may be ill understood. The doctor is an expert in clarifying and re-framing the patient's problems into a format that raises therapeutic possibilities. This process involves the doctor in a set of competences that are a complex mixture of active listening (history taking skills) and direct observation (clinical skills) and self-knowledge (insight). The undergraduate first learns these skills as a logical sequential process.[12] The graduate should learn to integrate the three into a coherent and efficient whole without loss of respect for the person, or loss of a disciplined scientific process. There is always the risk that either scientific reductionism or intuitive insight will dominate and distort the effectiveness of the consultation. This is less likely to occur if the doctor checks back regularly to ensure that she/he has elucidated the essential components:

- The nature, history and evolution of the problem(s).
- Patient concerns, ideas, doubts, fears that relate to each problem.
- The impact of each problem on lifestyle/function of the patient.
- The likely cause(s) of each problem.
- An appropriately comprehensive approach to examination of systems.
- Agreed priority ordering of the problems and goals for treatment.

Some analysts break this set of tasks down into a large number of separate components[13] and this is helpful for scientific analysis, but it is unhelpful if the student needs an easy-to-recall framework.

The third set of tasks relates to achieving a *shared understanding* of each problem with the patient (and family if this is appropriate).[13,14] Any management plan that is agreed can then be seen as appropriate to both doctor and patient. The skills involved in these interactions and the tools needed to support major clinical decisions are still relatively underdeveloped in clinical practice. Indeed they are both being subjected to on-going programmes of research (see Chapter 5.5). The behavioural objectives underlying this work can be summarized in a series of questions for our convenience, but even these are in a state of experimental flux:

- How to involve patient and family in their own care appropriately?
- How to achieve concordance over clinical management?
- How to optimize the therapeutic success of every encounter?
- How will the illness experience influence future use of services?
- How to help clinicians to remain humble and honest about what they do not know?

The fourth set of tasks involves the clinician considering any *on-going clinical problems or risk factors* that merit evaluation. By implication this often means that the patient has not raised the issues spontaneously and that the clinician has a comprehensive clinical record that reveals each problem and when it was last reviewed. Sometimes the clinician will have observed a new problem of which the patient seems unaware. Obvious examples are suspected hypothyroidism, unexplained bruise, a suspicious mole, hidden depression, or anxiety.

In each situation the time available, the organization of the practice, and the persona of the patient will influence the sequence of what happens next.

This task may need to be sensitively re-scheduled to a more appropriate time but it cannot be abandoned completely in modern primary care. Attention to task four is usually facilitated by good records and continuity of care.

The fifth set of tasks involves consideration of *primary preventive issues* or interventions of relevance to health promotion. Every person has a set of well-proven benefits that can come from primary prevention but not every person is willing or ready to make the behavioural changes or to agree to the clinical interventions that will produce these benefits. The task for the doctor is to clarify what is desirable and appropriate under the circumstances of the consultation. Like the fourth task, the doctor will be greatly helped by good clinical records that reveal what has been achieved and what remains to be achieved when the patient is ready. Guidelines that reflect good clinical practice may facilitate the process, and an understanding of the psychology of readiness to change is an essential set of knowledge and skills (elaborated in Chapters 5.1, 5.3–5.5). In an ideal world, the patients carry their own comprehensive record and are enabled through skilled interaction to be fully and appropriately involved in the choices. Unfortunately, the world is far from ideal and patients may try to shop from one doctor to the next until they get what they want. Clinical records can be too brief and superficial, time for consultation can be tight and 'patient lists' non-existent. In these circumstances the professionalism of the clinician is severely tested because the context in which she/he works actually militates against high quality primary care. The clinician's role may broaden to draw the shortcomings of the system to the attention of management, funding body, or politician.

It must be emphasized that the five sets of tasks do not carry equal priority. The first three are critical to every consultation. The fourth and fifth are only essential when the time and context is appropriate.

Underpinning the consultation tasks

A 'model' is a precise but simplified representation of a complex system. It can be used to portray form or function and can sometimes be used in training. The clinical consultation is a very complex system that has been heavily influenced by the traditional medical case-history method. It is usually reductionist and focused on the pursuit of accurate diagnosis.

In primary care, the clinical agenda may be focused onto an important diagnostic problem and the reductionist traditional model becomes relevant and helpful. But, much more commonly, the presenting problem is either undifferentiated or straightforward and the agenda is wide and person-focused rather than disease-focused. The patient with problems in an evolving lifecycle and changing context is much more challenging to professionals than the patient with a disease at one point of time.

Many analysts and researchers have contributed to the construction of models to help students understand the consultation in primary care or to analyze consultations. The models are not rigid or unresponsive to change, but each one has influenced thinking and research in the discipline. All of them have been influenced to some extent by the seminal work by a working party of the UK Royal College of General Practitioners that formulated a job description for the future general practitioner and used imaginative educational objectives as the starting point for vocational training programmes in 1972.[15]

In the United States, Engel also challenged the prevailing reductionist hospital model,[16] and his work influenced the emergence of the school of Patient Centred Medicine.[13,17] This important clinical method is detailed in Chapter 5.1. In Europe, the Leeuenhorst Working party published their formative statement on the work of the general practitioner in 1977.[18]

It is interesting that during the 1990s there was a reaffirmation of the fundamental purpose of the consultation but there have been two attempts to achieve fresh social constructions of that purpose. Hart argues that patients are not consumers of health care but co-producers of health in partnership with doctors.[19] Heath describes a different kind of partnership. She places the family doctor/general practitioner at the interface between illness and disease, there to witness and interpret the patient's experiences through honest reflection and empathy.[20]

Many nurses could claim that both these views simply bring the analysis full circle to where nurses have seen their roles as articulated by Newman and Young as early as 1972.[21] Modern primary care is of course a multiprofessional activity and the doctor has no monopoly over consulting. Furthermore, a greater 'community orientation' may compete with individual care. It is likely that during the next decade there should be more research on the primary care consultation in the context of a modern evolving scene. The relative strengths of doctors, nurse practitioners, and nurses can then be appropriately harnessed in a skill-mix that most benefits patients.[22] It would, however, be a retrograde step if well-established and tested international principles of primary care that are already inherent in the various consultation models become lost in this process.[23,24]

Models that have informed the understanding of consultation tasks are:

(a) Six phases in the consultation (Byrne and Long, 1976).[25]

(b) Exceptional potential in each consultation (Stott and Davis, 1979).[26]

(c) Seven tasks for the consultation (Pendleton et al., 1984).[27]

(d) Five checkpoints model (Neighbour, 1987).[28]

(e) The patient-centred clinical method (McWhinney, 1989).[17]

(a) *Byrne and Long first described six phases in the consultation* after their detailed empirical study of nearly 2000 tape-recorded consultations from more than 100 general practitioners. This yielded a classification of the sequence of events in consultations:

- the doctor establishes a relationship with the patient;
- the doctor attempts to discover the reason for patient's attendance;
- the doctor conducts a verbal and/or physical examination;
- the doctor, or the doctor and the patient, or the patient (alone) considers the condition;
- the doctor, and occasionally the patient, details further investigation or treatment;
- the consultation is terminated, usually by the doctor.

Each of these phases is focused primarily on the presenting problem(s) and the nature of the interaction between doctor and patient. At the time of the study this was a remarkable analysis of this most confidential aspect of a general practitioner's work. It was also remarkable for the evidence it provided of how the fourth phase (sharing information) was often limited to information giving. Unsurprisingly, incomplete collection of accurate information in phase-2 was often associated with dysfunctional consultations. Another startling discovery was that only 25 per cent of the general practitioners studied in the early 1970s had the open and flexible consulting styles that enable patient's full expression of their problems and participation in the consultation. The rest of the doctors studied had quite tightly controlled interview styles and timings that limited patient participation in the consultation. These important findings threw down the gauntlet to the educational and research teams and powerfully influenced the next decade of professional research and development.

(b) *The exceptional potential in each primary care consultation* is portrayed by Stott and Davis in a simple 2×2 open diagram designed to be an aide memoir to reveal what may be achieved (rather than what must be achieved) in each consultation (see Fig. 1).

The framework in Fig. 1 was built with three prior assumptions that arose partly from the work of Byrne and Long and partly from other data on consultation skills:

- the professional should be skilled at exchanging information with patients in primary care;
- the professional should be able to make patients feel that their needs are being taken seriously;
- the professional has adequate diagnostic and therapeutic skill to deal with the diversity of problems encountered in primary care.

A. Management of presenting problems	B. Modification of help seeking behaviour
C. Management of continuing problems	D. Opportunistic health promotion

Fig. 1 The exceptional potential in each primary care consultation.

- To define the reason for the patient's attendance, including:
  - the nature and history of the problem;
  - the aetiology;
  - the patient's ideas, concerns and expectations;
  - the effects of the problems.
- To consider other problems:
  - continuing problems;
  - at-risk factors.
- With the patient, to choose an appropriate action for each problem.
- To achieve a shared understanding of the problems with the patient.
- To involve the patient in the management and encourage him to accept appropriate responsibility.
- To use time and resources appropriately:
  - in the consultation;
  - in the long-term.
- To establish or maintain a relationship with the patient which helps to achieve the other tasks.

Fig. 2 Seven tasks for the consultation.

Figure 1 was described by the authors as 'an aide memoir' and also as the 'surface anatomy of primary care'.[29] It was an early practical attempt to encourage general practitioners to broaden their consultation approach. They were being encouraged to adopt new health care responsibilities that could be addressed in and through their many clinical encounters with patients. This wider view was also consistent with the emerging international agenda for primary care where the consultation hub becomes surrounded by a number of supporting services and structures to deliver modern primary care. It prioritizes clinical tasks but it does not address detailed consultation skills or behaviours.

(c) *Seven tasks for the consultation* were defined by Pendleton et al. in their book on the consultation (see Fig. 2). The tasks were devised primarily to inform postgraduate teaching and learning, particularly when analysing videotaped consultations. The first five tasks are separate statements of what a doctor needs to achieve in the consultation. The final two are general observations about use of time and resources and about building trust. The publication of these tasks coincided with enormous interest in the use of the video recording of consultations for training. Generations of doctors were brought up on this particular form of consultation analysis.

(d) *The five checkpoints model* of Neighbour approaches the consultation in a way that is complementary to the others described here. It starts from the young doctor's dilemma of wanting to apply all the tasks and skills but feeling overwhelmed by the possibilities. Neighbour tries to address this prioritization dilemma by encouraging the learner to imagine that they have two heads: the 'Organizer head' is rational and intellectual and the 'Responder head' is intuitive, naïve, and spontaneous. Either head may be talking to the patient at any one point in time but the doctor must become aware that the non-talking head may well be whispering distracting or contradictory thoughts internally while the external dialogue is progressing.

This imagery replicates standard psychotherapeutic teaching in which the therapist must grow to recognize his/her own inner intuitive observations as well as the intellectual/logical observations. When there is a perceived mismatch between the two in a therapeutic dialogue a critical point is looming. Much of the skill in psychotherapy is built around learning how to use these nodal points in the therapeutic dialogue to help a patient

- *Connecting:* which involves establishing and maintaining a relationship with the patient;
- *Summarizing:* involves telling the patient what you have found;
- *Handing over:* is involving the patient in management decisions;
- *Safety netting:* is ensuring that important things are not omitted;
- *House-keeping:* is ensuring that the doctor's needs are addressed.

Fig. 3 The five checkpoints model.

release or expose inner tensions and fears. Patients who grow to be sensitive to the same duality often become much less stressed and anxious because they have discovered a legitimate reason for the feelings that had previously overwhelmed them. The verbal and non-verbal languages people speak often reflect the same duality.

Neighbour encourages the learner to view the consultation as a therapeutic journey in which the success is not in the destination but in the journey itself. He weaves the continuing doctor–patient relationship into an evolving and constantly changing set of interactions with each patient. Each consultation is then just one nodal point along the road of life. This approach has the great merit of taking away the self-imposed stress of trying to deliver a tranche of tasks and skills at every consultation. It also introduces the learner to simple psychotherapeutic techniques.

The 'five checkpoints' were devised as an extension of the analogy with a motor journey (see Fig. 3). They are key places 'to make for' in any one consultation.

Neighbour is frank about the extensive overlap with the models described above and with behavioural studies of consultation behaviour. But he feels that his approach can help young doctors to prioritize their efforts in consultations. Also that the doctor has needs that must not be forgotten in the pressure to deliver so many tasks. Neighbour separates consultation behaviours from the tasks associated with the consultation. His book is a very comprehensive manual of options laid out under the broad checkpoint categories.

(e) *The patient-centred clinical method* is an analysis of consultation tasks with clear descriptions of the behaviours or methods required for its implementation (see Chapter 5.1). The Canadian group responsible for this work has collaborated with others from several countries to produce laudable precision in this area.[13,17] The principles that underlie patient-centred styles are, however, espoused by many of the reflective physicians already cited and by others around the world.[30–34]

Conclusions

Students of medicine must understand the six domains outlined in the opening paragraph of this chapter. Approaches to the consultation in family medicine have a common core that is encapsulated in the five sets of tasks described earlier. A model is just a convenient map on which to place the results of learning, analysis and experience. Each task/phase/behaviour model described has contributed to the development of a disciplined approach to consulting in primary care. From the patient's viewpoint, there should be reassurance in the knowledge that primary care clinicians are working towards common themes and common priorities. An increasing emphasis is placed on enabling the patient/family to be as much involved in their health care and health promotion as they wish to be.

References

1. **Boerma, W.G.W., Van Der Zee, J., and Fleming, D.M.** (1997). Service profiles of general practitioners in Europe. *British Journal of General Practice* **47**, 481–6.
2. **Grol, R., Baker, R., Roberts, R., and Booth, B.** (1997). Systems for quality improvement in general practice. A survey of 26 countries. *European Journal of General Practice* **3**, 65–8.

3. **General Medical Council.** *Good Medical Practice.* London: GMC, 2001 (updated regularly since 1995).
4. **Downie, R.S.,** ed. *The Healing Arts. An Oxford Illustrated Anthology.* Oxford: Oxford University Press, 2000.
5. **Balint, M.** *The doctor, His Patient and the Illness* 2nd edn. London: Pitman, 1964.
6. **Engel, G.L.** (1977). The need for a new medical model: a challenge for biomedicine. *Science* **196,** 126–36.
7. **Snow, C.P.** *The Two Cultures and a Second Look.* Cambridge: Cambridge University Press, 1964.
8. **Silagy, C. and Haines, A.,** ed. *Evidence-based Practice in Primary Care.* London: BMJ Books, 2001.
9. **Bensing, J.** (2000). Bridging the gap. The separate worlds of evidence-based medicine and patient-centred medicine. *Patient Education and Counseling* **39,** 17–25.
10. **Edwards, A. and Elwyn, G.,** ed. *Evidence-based Patient Choice.* Oxford: Oxford University Press, 2001.
11. **Tuckett, D., Boulton, M., Olson, C., and Williams, A.** *Meetings between Experts.* London: Tavistock, 1985.
12. **Fraser, R.,** ed. *Clinical Method. A General Practice Approach* 3rd edn. Oxford: Butterworth-Heinemann, 1999.
13. **Stewart, M., Brown, J.B., Weston, W.W., McWhinney, I.R., McWilliam, C.L., and Freeman, T.R.** *Patient-Centred Medicine. Transforming the Clinical Method.* Thousand Oaks: Sage Publications, 1995.
14. **Middleton, J.F. and McKinley, R.K.** (2000). What kind of partnership in the consultation? *British Journal of General Practice* **50,** 268–9.
15. **Royal College of General Practitioners** (1972). *The Future General Practitioner: Learning and Teaching.* London: British Medical Journal.
16. **Engel, G.L.** (1977). The need for a new medical model: a challenge for biomedicine. *Science* **196,** 126–36.
17. **McWhinney, I.** (1989). The need for a transformed clinical method. In *Communicating with Medical Patients* (ed. M. Stewart and D. Roter), pp. 25–40. Newbury Park: Sage Publications.
18. **Leeuwenhorst Working Party** (1977). The work of the general practitioner. Statement by a working party appointed by the Second European Conference on the teaching of general practice. *Journal of the Royal College of General Practitioners* **27,** 117.
19. **Hart, J.T.** *Feasible Socialism.* London: Socialist Health Association, 1994.
20. **Heath, I.** *The Mystery of General Practice.* London: Nuffield Provincial Hospital Trust, 1995.
21. **Newman, B. and Young, R.J.** (1972). A model for teaching total person approach to patient problems. *Nursing Research* **21,** 264–9.
22. **Richards, G. and Maynard, A.** *Fewer doctors? More nurses? A review of the knowledge base of doctor–nurse substitution.* Discussion Paper 135, Centre for Health Economics, University of York, 1995.
23. **Starfield, B.** (1994). Is primary care essential? *Lancet* **344,** 1129–33.
24. **Starfield, B.** (2001). New paradigms for quality in primary care. *British Journal of General Practice* **51,** 303–10.
25. **Byrne, P.S. and Long, B.E.L.** *Doctors Talking to Patients.* London: HMSO, 1976.
26. **Stott, N.C.H. and Davis, R.H.** (1979). The exceptional potential in each primary care consultation. *Journal of the Royal College of General Practitioners* **29,** 201–5.
27. **Pendleton, D., Schofield, T., Tate, P., and Havelock, P.** *The Consultation: An Approach to Teaching and Learning.* Oxford: Oxford University Press, 1984.
28. **Neighbour, R.** *The Inner Consultation.* Lancaster: MTP Press, 1987.
29. **Stott, N.C.H.** *Primary Health Care: Bridging the Gap between Theory and Practice.* Berlin: Springer-Verlag, 1983.
30. **World Health Organisation** (1980). *Primary Health Care.* Joint Report by WHO and UNICEF: International Conference on Primary Health Care at Alma Ata\in 1978. *Health for All Series No.1. WHO. Geneva.*
31. **Henbest, R.J. and Fehrsen, G.S.** (1992). Patient-centredness: is it applicable outside the West? Its measurement and effect on outcomes. *Family Practice* **9** (3), 311–17.
32. **Novack, D.H., Suchman, W.C., Epstein, R.M., Najberg, E., and Kaplan, C.** (1997). Calibrating the physician. Personal awareness and effective patient care. *Journal of American Medical Association* **278** (6), 502–9.
33. **Lipkin, M., Lazare, A., and Putnam, S.** *The Medical Interview.* New York: Springer-Verlag, 1995.
34. **Usherwood, T.** *Understanding the Consultation.* Buckingham/Philadelphia: Open University, 1999.

5.3 Communication skills

Theo Schofield

Other chapters in this book have defined patient-centred consulting and considered the evidence that supports it. They have also described the tasks that need to be achieved in a patient-centred consultation. These include:

- understanding the patients and their problems;
- sharing understanding about the problem and its management;
- making decisions about management with the patient;
- enabling the patient to make decisions about and manage their care;
- using time appropriately;
- establishing and maintaining an effective relationship.

These tasks are central to the work of doctors in primary care and much of the research and writing about communications skills has focused on the medical interview. However, the tasks and skills are shared by nurses and other health professionals and the chapter is intended to be relevant to all those who work in primary care. This chapter will describe the skills and strategies that can be used to conduct an effective patient-centred consultation.

Understanding the patients and their problems

The first task in a consultation or medical interview is to understand the reason for the patient's attendance.(1) This includes his/her problem; its nature, history, possible causes, and its effects. It also involves understanding the persons and their perspective; their personal and social circumstances; their ideas about health and their problem; their concerns about the problem; and their expectations for information, involvement, and care. Achieving these tasks requires skills in opening, listening to, exploring, and summarizing the patient's story.

The opening gambit

Doctors employ a variety of opening gambits such as 'How are you today', 'What can I do for you today' or just saying nothing and allowing the patient to start talking. It is essential that the opening gambit does not direct the patient, or close off new problems by making assumptions about why they are there, for example, by saying 'Are your new tablets helping your arthritis'.

Listening to the opening statement

Most patients come to the consultation prepared to tell their story to their doctor, and hope to have the opportunity to express their ideas about their problem, concerns for what it may mean, and expectations of what they would like to be done. Beckman and Frankel(2) in their classic study of medical interviews found that doctors frequently interrupted these opening statements, after a mean time of only 18 seconds. If they were interrupted, the majority of patients did not complete their statement and did not express their concerns at any time during the interview. In contrast, doctors who were trained to allow the patients to complete their opening statement found that it rarely lasted more than 2 min, and that the patients were much more likely to state their main complaint and to express their concerns.

Listening to the patient's opening statement without interruption is not, however, a passive process. It involves communicating interest and encouragement to continue by non-verbal behaviour such as maintaining eye contact, adopting an open posture, facial expressions of interest, and by avoiding expressions of disinterest such as looking at the notes. Verbal expressions such as 'go on', 'I see', 'Yes' also convey interest.

The most difficult skill during this phase of the consultation is to hear, remember, and to interpret the verbal and non-verbal communications from the patients while they are telling their story. If the patients tell their full story there may well be a considerable amount of information to retain and interpret. As the patients are presenting a set of symptoms of 'disorganized illness', the doctor can be ordering them in his or her head into a history of the presenting complaint. These symptoms may include salient features that trigger hypotheses about the nature of the problem that will require further testing. Hearing the whole story avoids the risk of a premature closure or an inappropriate hypothesis.

The patients may also make statements about their concerns or fears, or they may be conveying their anxieties non-verbally. This may provide cues to the patients' problems, particularly if there is any dissonance between their verbal and non-verbal communications.

The reasons for Beckman and Frankel's finding that doctors interrupt so quickly may be explained by medical teaching that every symptom requires clarification and qualification; it may be because of the difficulty of retaining all the information that is presented and the need to establish control by starting to ask questions; or it may be in the mistaken belief that interruptions save time. Having the patient's whole agenda early in the consultation enables the available time to be used more appropriately.

To illustrate the importance of avoiding interruptions, imagine a patient who starts by saying:

> Three or four months ago I was having slight discomfort in my chest which I thought was indigestion, but in the last month it has become more pressing and I have started thinking about what happened to my father and have become rather worried about it.

Having heard the whole story the doctor is left with a partial history of chest pain, and an indication that this man has a significant family history. The doctor can start to think that this may be of oesophageal or cardiac origin and that these hypotheses require further exploration. The doctor also has a verbal cue that he is anxious, and this may also be reinforced by the non-verbal communication in the way that the story was told. Imagine what would have happened if the doctor had interrupted after the word 'indigestion' to ask what he meant by indigestion and whether it occurred before or after meals, or, if after the mention of pressing chest pain, the doctor asked whether it was related to exertion or radiated to the neck. Important clues to the diagnosis and cues to the patient's concerns would have been lost.

Exploration

After the introductory phase of the consultation strategic choices have to be made. If the patient has presented a number of separate or only loosely linked problems, the choice is which one is a priority for this consultation. This choice can be openly negotiated with the patient. If, on the other hand, the patient presents cues to a number of different aspects of a single problem, all of which require exploration, the doctor still needs to choose where to start. Medical training would give priority to exploring serious physical disease such as the causes of chest pain in our imaginary patient. However, the doctor could choose to acknowledge the patient's anxiety and to establish that the patient's father in fact died from carcinoma of the oesophagus and that that was his main fear. This would not deflect the doctor from going on to explore the causes of chest pain but it would mean that a partnership had been built by addressing the patient's concerns, and that the exploration and subsequent explanations would also meet those concerns.

Having made the strategic decision about which topics are a priority, a range of questioning techniques and other skills can be used to explore it. Questions can be totally *open* such as:

> How are you feeling in yourself.

Such questions are most appropriate to encourage the patients to tell their stories in their own words, and during the phase when hypotheses are still being generated rather than tested.

The mainstay of the exploratory phase is the *open focused* question. Examples are:

> Tell me more about your chest pain.
> Have you noticed anything that brings it on?
> What thoughts have been going through your mind?
> What is your worst fear?

These questions clearly indicate to the patients the information being sought but encourages them to answer in their own words.

Other approaches to exploring ideas or concerns may include more explicit legitimization of the topic, for example, 'I am interested in hearing what you think yourself' or the use of an empathic statement such as 'I can understand that it might be worrying for you' followed by attentive silence. The use of *silence* can be very powerful. It gives the patients space to formulate their thoughts and to choose what they want to say or reveal. It can, however, put pressure on a patient and the doctor needs to be prepared to break it either by a supportive statement such as 'This must be difficult for you' or by moving on to another topic.

During this exploratory phase, there can be a sequence from fairly open questions to focused questions to closed questions, which was first described by Goldberg as the 'Open–Closed Cone'.[3] It may well be that at the end of open and focus questions there are still pieces of necessary information that have not been mentioned and these can be gathered by closed questions, for example, 'Does the pain go down your arm or up into your neck'. However, these questions come from the doctor's agenda and the doctor needs to be aware that by using them he or she is taking control of the content of the consultation at that point.

Apart from questioning there are two other important sources of information available to the doctor. The first is the patients' non-verbal communication, for example, demeanour, eye contact, tone of voice, posture, movement, and physical appearance. These may all give cues to their mental state, for example, anxiety or depression, to their social situation, and to the way that they relate to other people. It may be that the doctor may choose to pick up a non-verbal cue and explore it verbally, for example, 'it seems to me you're anxious about this, am I right' or 'You don't seem your usual self today'.

The other source of information is the feelings that the patient engenders in the doctor. There is a grain of truth in the aphorism, 'patients who make me feel anxious have anxiety, patients who make me feel depressed are depressed, and patients who make me feel confused are psychotic'. Also, patients may seek to transfer their feelings and expectations onto their doctor. An awareness of this, and of the feelings that it engenders, may give the doctor insight into the patients' relationship, not only with their doctor, but also with other people in their lives.

Summarizing

At the end of this process of exploration the doctor should be developing pictures of the patients and their problems. A strategy that many doctors find valuable at this stage is to check with the patient that this understanding is correct by some statement which starts with a phrase such as 'Have I got this right' or 'so in summary'. This enables the doctor to pause for thought, to clarify the problem, and to check that all the necessary information has been obtained. For the patients it conveys the fact that the doctor has listened and understood their problems. It gives them the opportunity to correct or to add to what has been said, and it is also an opportunity for the patient to introduce any other problems that they wish to be included in the consultation. It also provides a transition to the next task in the consultation, which is to share understanding about the problem and management options.

Sharing understanding

Ensuring that patients understand the nature of their problem, its possible causes, the options for management, and the opportunities for prevention are a fundamental task in the consultation. This understanding will enable the patients to make informed choices, increase their involvement in their own care, and use health care appropriately in the future.

Sharing understanding is also therapeutic, as it reduces uncertainty, helps to meet concerns, and can re-frame or change the meaning of the illness to the patient. For example, a patient suffering from headaches who is uncertain about what is wrong and is fearful that he/she may have a serious physical disorder can be helped to understand the relationship between stress and headaches. The reduction in uncertainty and concern may in itself relieve the headaches, and also gives the patient the opportunity to consider how best to manage stress rather than focus on symptomatic relief for headaches.[(4)]

Ley studied the relationship between giving information to the patient in the consultation and subsequent satisfaction and compliance.[(5)] He argued that patients remembering what information they had been given was a prerequisite for using that information, and that recall could be improved by a number of techniques including:

- simple messages given with short words, in short sentences, and avoiding jargon;
- explicit categorization, for example, statements such as 'I am first going to explain what I think the problem is and then the ways in which it can be managed';
- repetition;
- using specific rather than general statements.

He also advocated the use of drawings and diagrams and written material to back up the explanation.

Tuckett et al.[(6)] in their book *Meeting Between Experts*, described sharing information more as a two-way process in which the doctor was an expert on diseases and their treatments, and the patients experts in their own problems and experiences. They described the concept of the 'reactive explanation' in which the content and language of the explanations given by the doctor matched the individual patient's ideas, explanatory models, and language. To be able to give such an explanation requires the doctor to have established the patients' ideas and what their explanatory models of health and illness are. They found a high level of recall and understanding of the important messages that were given by doctors (73 per cent) and that the commonest explanation for lack of understanding was when the doctor was using an explanatory model that was very different from that of the patient.

Simple examples of effective reactive explanations would be asking questions such as 'What have you been told already' or 'What do you understand by ... ' and when the patient says 'I caught a chill' starting an explanation with 'The way you catch a chill is ...' rather than 'You have got a virus infection'. In their sample of consultations, Tuckett et al. found that reactive explanations were uncommon, largely because the doctors had not established the patient's ideas beforehand.

Sharing understanding becomes more difficult the greater the distance between the culture of the doctor and the culture of the patient. Culture is not just an issue of ethnic origin but includes a wide variety of factors including age, gender, and socio-economic status. The wider the gap the greater the danger of losing sight of the individual and stereotyping the patient.[(7)]

Whilst doctors and other health professionals remain a very important source of information for patients, there is a growing variety of other sources, for example, the media, health books, and the Internet (see Chapter 3.4). The challenge for doctors is not to see this as a threat to their authority but as an opportunity to work with better informed patients who are more able to participate in decisions and in their care. This may involve establishing what information the patients have obtained and how they have interpreted it, and reacting appropriately to those ideas. It may also involve helping the patients access reliable sources of good-quality information. Doctors and nurses may need to use a series of consultations, rather than an individual consultation, to share understanding and come to decisions about management.[(8)]

Making decisions about management

The majority of consultations include making decisions about the management of the patient's problem. Management can involve investigations, medication, referral, other procedures, therapy, self-help, and lifestyle change, and always the option of doing nothing. However, until recently this was a relatively neglected part of the consultation.[(9)] The central issues are how decisions are made and who makes them (see Section 6).

The treatment decision-making process can be conceived as having two components. The first is information about the treatment options, their benefits, and their risks, with this information being increasingly evidence based. The second being the patients' preferences and values and the weight that they place on different outcomes (utilities). The rational decision would be to opt for the most desirable, most likely option (expected utility).

The second issue is who makes the decision. Charles et al.[(10)] described three possible models. The first is *paternalistic*. In this model, the doctor makes the decision and gives the patient just sufficient information required to implement or 'comply' with that decision. However, it is possible to be both paternalistic and patient-centred if the patient requests the doctor to make the decision. If the doctor is to do this and base the decision both on his/her own understanding of the evidence and on the patient's views and preferences, this model requires the doctor to have elicited what those views and preferences are.[(11)] This converts the decision from being 'the best treatment for arthritis' to 'the best treatment for you'.

At the other extreme is the *informed patient choice* model in which the doctor provides information about treatment options, and the patients make their own decision. This requires the doctor to provide the information in a way that enables patient choice and is not aiming to persuade the patient to adopt a particular line of action. This model is based on a respect for the patient's autonomy and has also been described as evidence-based patient choice.[(12,13)]

The third model occupying the middle ground is *shared decision making* (see Chapter 5.5). Despite some reservations about feasibility, this model has attracted support from patients and professionals,[(14)] and patient partnership is part of the policy agenda in the United Kingdom.[(15)]

Enabling patients to implement decisions

Decisions, whether they are to take medication or to change lifestyle, may or may not be adhered to by the patient after the consultation. The literature on patient adherence and trials of methods to improve it has recently been reviewed.[(16)] The authors concluded that

> If measures are to be taken to improve compliance, these should primarily be based on a closer understanding of the patient's experience of their illness and medication, rather than the perceptions and expectations of health care professionals.

These measures include understanding the patient's capacities and circumstances so that the actions that are agreed are appropriate to that person, and maximize the involvement of the patient in his/her own care.

In their review of the placebo effect, Crow et al.[(17)] reviewed the evidence that shows that patients' expectations about the effectiveness of their treatment and their beliefs that they could carry out the actions necessary for successful management of a disease or coping with the treatment (self-efficacy) are related to positive health outcomes. These outcomes included improvements in both symptoms and disease status such as blood pressure or diabetic control. Self-efficacy is a person's belief about his/her ability to achieve specific goals, for example, losing weight, and can be enhanced by giving information, involving people in decisions, and specific skills training.[18]

Time management

In Chapter 5.6, Belle Brown reviews the evidence about the length and the outcome of consultations and concludes that 'while longer consultations do on the whole lead to better outcomes for patients, some physicians are able to achieve these outcomes without spending more time'. This section will consider some of the ways that time in the consultation can be used effectively.

A number of the patient-centred strategies already described have built-in economies of time. Establishing the reason for the patients' attendance and their expectations means that the consultation can be focused on meeting those expectations. Establishing the patient's ideas and concerns means that any explanation and information can be directed at meeting those concerns. Summarizing and checking at each stage in the consultations allows the doctor to maintain a structure to the interview and to signal the transition from one stage to the next. Allowing the patient to make an opening statement without interruption minimizes the risk that 'hidden agendas' will be produced later.

Time management is not just about how to bring a consultation to a close, though this is a very important phase of the consultation. Patients are well aware that time in the consultation is limited and if they have been in control of the early part of the consultation they may well initiate closure themselves. Closure by the doctor may include a concluding summary, checking that no important issues remain, and contracting for the next steps for both the patient and doctor. Neighbour[19] described the process of 'safety netting', explaining what the patient should do if things do not go according to plan or any unexpected events occur. This means that patients are taking responsibility for their own care but are being given very clear criteria on which to base their decisions. Examples of safety netting would include statements such as 'If you get a rash with the tablets stop them and come and see me again'. This helps to preserve the doctor–patient relationship and is also a very important part of risk management (the advice should also be written in the notes!).

Time can also be managed between one consultation and the next. This interval can be used for the patient to obtain information from other sources. The patient can take time to consider decisions and choices before they are finally made, and this process of decision-making can be assisted by decision aids.[20] Time can be used as an investigation to gain more information from the way that a problem evolves and it is also an opportunity for patients to do emotional work, reframing, and reconsidering their problems in the light of new insights that they have gained in the consultation.

Consultations can be seen as part of a cycle of care[21] in which patients develop their understanding of health and their problems, become more enabled to cope with and manage these problems themselves, and learn to use future consultations more appropriately.

Developing and maintaining the doctor–patient relationship

By describing what is to be achieved in a consultation, one can then define the characteristics of an effective relationship between doctor and patient. These include:

- the doctor is interested in the whole person and not just their disease;
- the patients are able to tell their story in their own words without interruption;
- the patients' ideas and opinions are sought and respected;
- the patients' desire for information and for involvement are responded to;
- decisions are shared between the doctor and patient.

Initiating a consultation

Building a relationship starts with the first impressions and these can be made more positive by such simple social skills as greeting the patient by name, introducing oneself, standing up and shaking hands, and giving the patient one's undivided attention. This attention can be conveyed verbally, and non-verbally by eye contact, posture, and being relaxed. Neighbour[19] describes the process of housekeeping, clearing one's mind of the previous consultation and other thoughts so that the impression of being relaxed and attentive to the patient is a genuine one.

Personal qualities

Rogers[22] described the personal qualities necessary for an effective interpersonal relationship as warmth, genuineness, and unconditional positive regard. A doctor needs to posses these qualities and be able to communicate them to his/her patients. It is perhaps easier to consider how this is done by thinking of the opposite behaviour: coldness, failing to interact with and respond to the other person; artificiality when statements are made that are not meant, and when there is a discrepancy between verbal statements and non-verbal behaviour; and judgmental non-acceptance of the patients, their ideas, or their lifestyle. These qualities are difficult to learn, and to a large extent they depend on the doctor's own confidence, inner comfort, and recognition and acceptance of their own imperfections.

Empathy

Empathy involves being able to identify and understand patients' thoughts and feelings and to see the world as they see it. It also involves being able to express that understanding to the patient by such statements as 'I can understand your worries about what this might mean'. Expressions of empathy are a powerful way of building a relationship between the doctor and patient, 'My doctor understands me', and in themselves can be very therapeutic. Empathy is different from sympathy, which is about the doctor's own feelings 'feeling sorry for the patient' and expressions of sympathy run the risk of creating a distance between the doctor and the patient.

Trust

Trust can be defined as the patient's belief that the doctor would always act in the patient's best interests.[23] It can also include trusting the doctor to be competent, tell the truth, and maintain confidences. Within a trusting relationship people can disclose their personal problems and concerns and accept information and advice. Trust can be undermined if the patient feels that the doctor's advice is based on constrained resources or other external pressures, or on the possibility of personal gain, for example, fees or target payments. Patients would also like to be able to trust their doctor to be there for them when he or she is needed. The changes in the pattern of care in practices may make this very difficult at times.

Therapeutic aspects of the relationship

Balint coined the phrase 'The Drug Doctor' to describe the importance of the doctor–patient relationship in improving patients' health.[24] Illnesses have physical, psychological, and social components. They may be the physical manifestations of social or psychological distress, or the psychological and social reactions to some physical disease. Whatever the cause there is potential to improve the patients' illness experience by increasing the patients' understanding and reducing uncertainty, helping the patients to develop new strategies to tackle their feelings, their relationships, and often their guilt, and by offering hope, encouragement, and support. This is what personal doctoring is all about.

Conclusions

Consultations take place in the context of a health care system, a legal and professional framework, and of society as a whole. All these are changing rapidly and are influencing the nature of the interaction between doctors and patients.

Some of these changes are to be welcomed: the expectations of patients for information and involvement in their care; the increased range of effective management, particularly for chronic diseases; the availability of information and evidence-based reviews to both doctors and patients; computerization of the medical record and the development of records shared with the patient; and the development of teamwork in health care.

Other changes in health care and society are less welcome: changes in working practices that lead to reduced continuity of care and personal doctoring; the undervaluing of public services leading to low morale and difficulties with recruitment and retention; the undermining of trust in professional competence; and frequent recourse to complaint, litigation, and even violence when patients are dissatisfied.

Our response must be to adapt to change, to attempt to influence change, but also to adhere to what doctors and patients believe to be of value, patient-centred consultations that meet the needs of the whole person, and in which information and decisions are shared.

References

1. **Pendleton, D., Schofield, T., Tate, P., and Havelock, P.** *The Consultation: An Approach to Learning and Teaching.* Oxford: Oxford University Press, 1984.
2. **Beckman, H.B. and Frankel, R.M.** (1984). The effect of physician behavior on the collection of data. *Annals of Internal Medicine* **101**, 692–6.
3. **Goldberg, D.P.** et al. (1980). Training family doctors to recognise psychiatric illness with increased accuracy. *Lancet* **2**, 521–3.
4. **Fitzpatrick, R.M., Hopkins, A.P., and Harvard Watts, O.** (1983). Social dimensions of healing: a longitudinal study of outcomes of medical management of headaches. *Social Science and Medicine* **17** (8), 501–10.
5. **Ley, P.** *Communicating with Patients.* London: Chapman and Hall, 1988.
6. **Tuckett, D., Boulton, M., Olson, C., and Williams, A.** *Meetings Between Experts: An Approach to Sharing Medical Ideas in Medical Consultations.* London: Tavistock, 1985.
7. **Kai, J.** (2000). Cross cultural communication. *Medicine* **28**, 36–8.
8. **Holmes-Rovner, M.** et al. (2001). Patient choice modules for summaries of clinical effectiveness: a proposal. *British Medical Journal* **322**, 664–7.
9. **Elwyn, G.J., Edwards, A., and Kinnersley, P.** (1999). Shared decision-making in primary care: the neglected second half of the consultation. *British Journal of General Practice* **49**, 477–82.
10. **Charles, C., Whelan, T., and Gafni, A.** (1999). What do we mean by partnership in making decisions about treatment? *British Medical Journal* **319**, 780–2.
11. **Gafni, A., Charles, C., and Whelan, T.** (1998). The physician–patient encounter: the physician as a perfect agent for the patient versus the informed treatment decision-making model. *Social Science and Medicine* **47** (3), 347–54.
12. **Hope, T.** *Evidence-based Patient Choice.* London: Kings Fund, 1996.
13. **Edwards, A. and Elwyn, G.J.** *Evidence-based Patient Choice: Inevitable or Impossible?* Oxford: Oxford University Press, 2001.
14. **Coulter, A.** (1997). Partnerships with patients: The pros and cons of shared clinical decision-making. *Journal of Health Service Research Policy* **2**, 112–21.
15. **NHS Executive.** *Patient Partnership: Building a Collaborative Strategy.* Leeds: NHS Executive, 1996.
16. **Vermeire, E.** et al. (2001). Patient adherence to treatment: three decades of research. A comprehensive review. *Journal of Clinical Pharmacology and Therapeutics* **26**, 331–42.
17. **Crow, R.** et al. (1999). The role of expectancies in the placebo effect and their use in the delivery of health care: a systematic review. *Health Technology Assessment* **3** (3), 1–96.
18. **Bandura, A.** (1977). Self-efficacy: toward a unifying theory of behavioural change. *Psychology Review* **84**, 191–215.
19. **Neighbour, R.** *The Inner Consultation: How to Develop an Effective and Intuitive Consulting Style.* Lancaster: Kluwer Academic, 1987.
20. **O'Connor, A.M.** et al. (1999). Decision aids for patients facing health treatment or screening decisions: systematic review. *British Medical Journal* **319**, 731–4.
21. **Pendleton, D.** (1983). Doctor–patient communication: a review. In *Doctor–Patient Communication* (ed. D. Pendleton and J. Hasler). London: Academic Press.
22. **Rogers, C.R.** *On Becoming a Person.* London: Constable, 1967.
23. **Fugelli, P.** (2001). James Mackenzie Lecture. Trust—in general practice. *British Journal of General Practice* **51**, 575–9.
24. **Balint, M.** *The Doctor, His Patient and the Illness.* London: Tavistock, 1957.

5.4 Doctors' perceptions of their patients

Louise M. Millward and Michael P. Kelly

Introduction

The perceptions that medical staff have of their patients have received much attention in the medical, nursing, sociological, and more recently, medico-legal literature. Specifically, it is argued that doctors find a sizeable minority of patients 'difficult', and that they negatively label such patients. The capacity for patients to exasperate, defeat, and overwhelm their doctors has been widely reported.(1) It is easy to understand how, when faced with exasperation, defeat and a sense of being overwhelmed, doctors respond with negative evaluations. However, as naturally human as this type of behaviour may seem to be, the fact that it is doctors who are doing it is discordant with widely held expectations about what ought to be appropriate doctor behaviour. It seems to run counter to the privileged position doctors enjoy, and to undermine the trust, which is such an important part of the doctor patient relationship. The doctor's capacity to heal, and to reach out to people when they are sick and at their most vulnerable, is special. The access which doctors are allowed to the most private parts of a patient's physical and emotional world, depends in large part on the doctor–patient relationship being qualitatively different from other kinds of human contact. Surely we expect more of our doctors? Surely they should be above stereotyping and venality? The almost sacred and certainly unique and special nature of the relationship seems to be at risk. It is this kind of concern that has fuelled discussions of this issue.

The discussion has also been driven by a sense that things have changed. Undoubtedly, the nature of health care and its delivery has altered in recent years. Communication between doctors and patients and compliance with medical advice appear to be different to how they used to be. The ethos that the doctor knows best and accompanying unquestioning acceptance of the expert advice by its recipients, has been replaced by skepticism about the advice, and indeed the right to give it. Of course, in the past there was always doubt about medical knowledge among some sections of society, and the ideal of a paternalistic doctor and a submissive patient was perhaps a figment of popular and sociological imagination. Nevertheless, many commentators have noted that the nature of the relationship seems to have changed in subtle ways and as part of an analysis of these changes, the kinds of perceptions that doctors develop of their patients have been scrutinized.(2,3)

In part the change in the nature of the doctor–patient relationship may be attributed to a range of much broader changes in contemporary society.

Amongst other things this has involved a loss of legitimacy of a range of social institutions, from the police and the church, to the monarchy and including medicine.[4] Within health care, a number of very specific phenomena provide the backdrop against which the doctor–patient relationship is now acted out and which simply did not exist, or were remote from normal experience, in an earlier age. Such things include consumerism, patient advocacy, willingness to resort to litigation, health service management which values patient satisfaction, health promotion strategies which encourage people to take greater responsibility for their own health, and the growth in alternative and complementary medicine. Patients now have access to much more medical knowledge. With increasing prevalence of long-term chronic illnesses under medical management and an ageing population, doctors have to deal with more 'expert' patients and relatives. All of this renders the relationship between doctors and their patients intrinsically more difficult than it was once thought to have been.

Doctors' perceptions of patients

'Difficult' patients

The terms 'difficult' and 'heartsink' patients are widely used.[1,5–13] Coupled with patients who cause 'trouble' for their doctors, these concepts serve as a primary focus of investigation in identifying how and why doctors may perceive patients in different ways. Over 25 years ago, Stimson[14] found that of a cohort of 453 general practitioners, 94 per cent readily interpreted and identified patients in terms of the 'trouble' they caused. Groves[15] later produced typologies of the 'hateful patient', Gerrard and Riddell[5] outlined characteristics of the 'difficult patient' and with specific reference to general practice, O'Dowd[1] used the term 'heartsink patient'. It has been estimated that British general practitioners have an average of six 'heartsink patients' per practitioner.[6] These figures appear conservative compared to the United States where primary care physicians have defined almost one of every six patients seen as 'difficult'.[7]

Work on 'good' and 'bad' patients, and patients negatively stereotyped by doctors and nurses,[16,17] also contributes to an understanding of why some therapeutic encounters may be problematic. Several characteristics have been associated with 'difficult', 'heartsink', and 'troublesome' patients. However, the evidence is equivocal. In some cases this is a methodological artefact; that is, different concepts, measures, and epistemologies generate contradictory results. In some studies, however, inconsistency arises from a failure to acknowledge the dynamics produced by the situation and interaction that may arise between doctors and their patients.

Patient characteristics

In order to assess the ways in which patients might be characterized by doctors, a literature search was conducted using a range of relevant terms (e.g. 'Doctor/s', 'General Practitioner/s', 'Patient/s', 'Negative', 'Attitudes', 'Heartsink'). Some of the key studies of patient labelling generated by this strategy appear in Table 1, along with a range of labels that have been used to characterize 'difficult' patients.

The results detailed in Table 1 reveal first, that 'difficult' patients and labelling processes continue to cause concern. Second, the findings of current studies tend to show very similar results to those conducted over 25 years ago.[14] Third, the ways in which patients are characterized are not theoretically uniform. In some cases stereotypes are generated by demographic criteria (e.g. gender, social class). In others, they relate to medical factors (e.g. mental health, alcohol/drug misuse), behavioural factors (e.g. frequent attenders, demanding), and/or value judgements (e.g. dissatisfied, inadequate), or to a combination of these.

It is important to note that whilst the terms 'difficult', 'heartsink', and 'troublesome' are associated with types of patients who frequent primary care and beyond, their status is defined with reference to patients who are not perceived to create problems for practitioners. Very few studies

Table 1 Characteristics associated with 'difficult' patients

Reference	Characteristic(s) of 'difficult' patients
Gerrard and Riddell (1988)[5]	Attend frequently. Demanding. Dependent. Cause despair, anger, frustration, and helplessness
Groves (1978)[15]	Hateful. Dependent clingers. Entitled demanders. Manipulative help-rejecters. Self-destructive deniers. Masochistic. Reap secondary gains. Display self-murderous behaviour
Hahn et al. (1996)[7]	Use services more. Frustrating. Difficult to communicate with. Time-consuming. Dissatisfied. Self-destructive. Have functional impairment. Have mental disorders (e.g. mulitsomatoform disorder; panic disorder; dysthymia; generalized anxiety; major depressive disorder; probable alcohol use/dependence). Cause doctors to feel manipulated
John et al. (1987)[8]	Female. Older. Divorced. Widowed. Have more acute problems, chronic problems, medical tests and examinations, referrals and visits. Have thick charts
Mathers and Gask (1995)[11]	Manipulative. Able to abuse and manipulate those helping them
Mathers et al. (1995)[6]	Attend frequently. Hypochondriac. Difficult to communicate with. Have multiple symptoms/psychiatric problems. Cause angry helplessness
Najman et al. (1982)[17]	Vulgar. Garrulous. Know-it-alls. Alcohol/drug abusers. Those who lack hygiene, are unemployed/on welfare/are deviant. Those with sexually transmitted diseases or seeking vaccinations or blood pressure checks
O'Dowd (1988)[1]	Attend frequently. Demanding. Have endless complaints. Dissatisfied. Exasperate, defeat, overwhelm doctors. Cause distress, puzzlement, frustration, disappointment, and clinical insecurity
Schwenk et al. (1989)[9]	Female. Have vague, difficult to describe, undifferentiated medical problems. Have an abrasive behavioural style. Unable to contribute to definition of problem. Cause frustration, unmet expectations, and dissatisfaction
Sharpe (1994)[10]	Attend frequently. Distressed. Lower satisfaction. Psychological and psycho-social factors. Medically unexplained symptoms, coexisting social problems and severe untreatable illness. Are more adversely affected by their illness. Are more likely to misunderstand or disagree with the explanation and treatment offered
Smith (1995)[12]	Display abnormal illness behaviour, somatize, or suffer from a personality disorder
Stimson (1975)[14]	Female. Demanding. Hypochondriac. Time-consuming. Uncooperative. Neurotic. Ungrateful. Malingerers. Workshy. Lonely. Unsettled. Inadequate. Insecure. Pseudo-sophisticated. Nouveau riche. Geriatric. Lack common sense. Have inadequate personalities and low intelligence. Reside in unhygienic conditions. Have trivial/vague complaints, psychiatric illness, psychological symptoms. Unable to judge when to consult. Do not follow advice. Critical of doctors. Not trusting of doctors. Unable to cope

highlight this point. One exception is Stimson.[14] Stimson found that patients who caused least 'trouble' for general practitioners were those who could judge when to consult, were undemanding, did not take time, described problems clearly, were healthy, presented with specific symptoms of an organic/physical nature, were easy to diagnose and manage, could be treated, had medical rather than social problems, wanted to get better and got well, acknowledged the limits of the doctor's skill, accepted the judgement of the doctor, had confidence in the doctor, followed advice, were grateful, cooperative, intelligent, had common sense, could cope, were happy, settled, adequate, working, and had good homes. Patients who deviated from these criteria were more likely to be perceived as 'troublesome' (see also May and Kelly,[18] Millward,[19] and Stockwell[20]).

Doctor characteristics

Literature relating to doctors' characteristics and their links to their behaviour in labelling patients, is notable for its relative absence. The majority of work in this area tends to reflect 'situational' rather than 'demographic' or 'personal' features of doctors. Mathers et al.[6] examined whether characteristics of British general practitioners were associated with numbers of 'heartsink' patients reported. Their results found associations between greater perceived workload, lower job satisfaction, lack of communication/ counselling skills or training, lack of appropriate postgraduate training, and the volume of these patients reported. Unsupported professional needs,[1] hurried working conditions,[1] perceived workload,[6] and job satisfaction,[6] have also been associated with the experience of 'difficult' and 'heartsink' patients.

Doctors' behaviours have frequently been defined as the *response* to 'difficult' and 'heartsink' patients rather than causal factors in the way the interaction develops. As Gerrard and Riddell[5] remarked, 'We have been taught that these feelings often originate in the patient' and O'Dowd[1] suggested that ' "Heartsink" more clearly refers to the doctor's emotions which are triggered by certain patients'. Akin to patient characteristics this is an important point because, as mentioned above, doctors' perceptions of patients may not necessarily reflect patients' own interpretations of their behaviour. Also, these interpretations may not necessarily designate anything inherent in the patients themselves as they are rather meanings which doctors ascribe.

The therapeutic encounter

A number of studies attempt to understand why the encounter between some patients and their doctors may be problematic. The explanations offered have included an inadequate understanding of patients by doctors,[1] counter-transference whereby negative feelings are stimulated in the doctor,[12,15] and doctor and patient personalities coupled with demographic and medical care outcomes.[8] Lack of time and resources have been suggested as confounding the situation.[6,13] The majority of studies of 'difficult' and 'heartsink' patients suggest that problems in the doctor–patient relationship are associated with the limited focus of medicine. Specifically, this concerns the distinction between physical/organic/disease states and psycho-social criteria. It has been suggested that patients may be influenced by particular cultural norms that frame medical encounters as being properly concerned with organic disease. Within such a worldview, personal and social problems are given a biological form. The problem is that this may lead doctors to deny the medical legitimacy of such patients.[13] Comparisons of the responses of 'difficult to help' hospital patients and their doctors, suggest that commonly patients *believe* in an organic cause of their symptoms and hope for a cure, whereas some doctors will focus on psycho-social criteria in intractable cases and in certain circumstances therefore provide supportive rather than curative care.[10] This situation is seen to generate uncertainty. Butler and Evans[13] argued that 'heartsink' is a symptom of tension within the philosophical foundations of general practice and that 'GPs are supposed to be able to accommodate all problems including social, psychological, and spiritual, but their biomedical focused training makes this difficult'. This work suggests that, 'the defining characteristic of the heartsink patient is a negative response from a clinician to the presentation of personal, social, or spiritual suffering in "clinical" terms'.[13] Najman et al.[17] suggest that whilst doctors' stereotypes of patients may relate to therapeutic dilemmas, they also relate to negative sanctions of deviant behaviour in relation to the sick role and prevailing societal values.

Remedies

Problematic doctor–patient relationships are medically, socially, financially, and legally detrimental.[9] Over the years, many authors have offered solutions and remedies (for earlier work see Kelly and May[16]). In respect of patients these include providing brief psychiatric intervention.[8] In respect of doctors the list is longer and different, and remedies tend to reflect current fashion in education and psychotherapy. A good example of this genre is Blalock and Devellis[21] who present four strategies to decrease stereotyping and/or its effects: being attentive to cultural factors; increasing active involvement of the patient; encouraging patient self-disclosure of factors that may dispel stereotypes, and being attentive to information provided by patients. Other remedies include: having a greater understanding of patients;[1,5] recognizing difficult to help patients and reviewing them;[10] recognizing doctors' own responses to patients and seeing these as targets of intervention;[12] adopting a reflexive response that considers the roles of both the doctor and the patient, the framework of the relationship and the relationship between biological and social knowledge;[13] improving communication skills and developing better interviewing, patient rapport, and medical solving skills;[9] increasing counselling/communication training and stress management techniques[6] and making more use of specialist support services.[10] On a management level, models, including coping strategies, have been suggested.[11] Organizational recommendations include a reduction in workload and strategies to increase job satisfaction.[6]

A sociological contribution

While interesting, the strategies outlined above tend to overlook pragmatic, and particularly time constraints in general practice. In contrast, sociological insights offer a number of practical remedies.

In his seminal account of the sick role, Parsons[22] suggested that illness is profoundly relevant to the needs of the social system. In the Parsonian model, illness is synonymous with deviant behaviour. This is because it stops people from performing their normal social activities. This in turn, albeit in a small way in the case of a single episode of illness, undermines the functional basis of society. Because illness is not of course a rare occurrence in the population as a whole, the totality of the morbidity in a society requires a response to manage the interruptions to normal life which illness causes. Advanced societies have generated the sick role and a special group of professionals, doctors, to manage this. Several mechanisms contribute to the successful accomplishment of this goal. These are embedded within the patterning of the roles of patients and doctors and their specific situations within the social structure.

In the 'sick role', patients will be exempt from normal responsibilities, must be willing to accept professional help and to cooperate with it, must desire to get well, and will not be held responsible for the state of affairs in which they find themselves. The reciprocal nature of the doctor–patient relationship means that doctors provide the legitimation for this state of affairs.

Parsons[22] recognized that patients only play the sick role to varying degrees. An exploration of deviations from the sick role provides some interesting insights into the concept of difficult patients. First, Parsons viewed legitimations of sickness by doctors as having a moral connotation that functionally protects against 'malingerers'. Second, he acknowledged that patients might utilize the sick role for the purpose of secondary gain. Third, he remarked, 'One very possible reaction is to attempt to deny illness or various aspects of it, to refuse to "give in" to it. Another may be exaggerated self-pity and whining, a complaining demand for more help than is necessary or feasible, especially for incessant personal attention'.[22] Parsons suggests that the sick role is a self-regulating mechanism because families and carers place very strong pressures upon the sick person to return to 'normal' and in doing so reinforce and validate the doctor's role and that ascribed by the institution of medicine.

Parsons' concept of the sick role has been widely criticized, most notably by Freidson[2,23] and Bloor and Horobin.[24] Tuckett[25] has noted how the Parsonian framework may be impossible to achieve for several reasons. First, the doctor's role is based on clinical experience that is practically, rather than theoretically applied, whereby treatment may include elements of scientific uncertainty, and which, rather than being objective and universalistic, is subjective and particularistic. Second, within this climate the scarcity of resources lead doctors to appraise which patients receive particular interventions. Third, 'interesting cases' may invoke increased medical interest compared to other 'more ordinary cases'. Fourth, numerous value judgements do enter into the encounter as are, for example, exemplified in the terms 'difficult' and 'heartsink' patient.

The point is that complex human encounters such as the doctor–patient relationship involve moral reasoning, in the face of inadequate or contradictory guidelines, extenuating circumstances, or clinical ambiguity.[26] The doctor's role is far more complex than the Parsonian framework acknowledges. As Tuckett[25] noted, the doctor 'frequently has to arbitrate between a single patient's interests and those of all his patients, between one patient and another, between a patient's interests now and in the future, between patient and family, between patient and society or community, between the patient's interests and his own interests, between his own interests as a doctor and his interests in other roles'.

However, although it would be naïve to see the problem of difficult patients as residing in a failure of either doctors or patients to play appropriate Parsonian roles (which most of them will never have heard of anyway) the interesting point is that deviations from the ideal as outlined by Parsons more than half a century ago, still point to the major points of fracture in the relationship, that is, the points where patients are perceived not to have a *real* illness but seek the exemptions from work, where individuals positively seem to enjoy being ill and all the fuss and attention they receive, where they fail to follow the advice of the doctor, and on the other side where the doctor fails to keep appropriate distance and becomes angry, or frustrated by the actions and behaviours of the patient. In fact, it might be argued that many of the theoreticians who have criticized Parsons have missed this point. It is not that the empirical real world somehow does not match the Parsonian theoretical schema, so much as the theoretical schema catches the common sense understanding of what should happen in the doctor–patient relationship, and the deviations from it. In other words, Parsons' roles pick up widely understood cultural norms about appropriate patient and doctor behaviour. As noted above, where the behaviour of patients corresponds to the Parsonian ideal they receive very positive evaluations from their carers.

Further light is shed on this by interactionist sociology which followed in the tradition of writers like Schutz,[27] Mead,[28] and Goffman.[29] Interactionists approach the question of patient labelling as follows.[3,18,19] They do not account for it in terms of moral departures from cultural standards as in the classic Parsonian influenced approaches. Instead, they take the existence of labelling of all kinds as a normal feature of human interaction. They then pose two questions. How is meaning generated in social encounters? (Labelling is but one way in which meaning is generated.) And, what needs do labels fulfil? The argument is that professionals enter encounters with patients with a number of ideas in their minds, about what skills and services they can provide to patients. They have learned these in their professional training and have honed them through practice. Their very sense of who and what they are as an individual, and as a worthwhile and competent professional, is wrapped up in these concepts of themselves as providers of skills and services to others. They also bring with them a range of other ideas and notions that they possess simply because they are members of the human race. These reflect cultural and sub-cultural values to varying degrees, and, very importantly, may never have been reflected upon in the kind of sustained intellectual way that their professional practice will have been.

Patients bring with them likewise, whatever component of cultural values that reflects their position in the social structure. However, many, if not most, will also bring some degree of concern, worry, anxiety about some aspect of their body or their emotional life. Unlike the doctor they, or the vast majority of them, will not have access to a discourse of science or medical taxonomies through which to express their signs and symptoms. It is the doctor's task to try to bring the lay discourse and his/her professional discourse together, and begin arriving at a diagnosis and the provision of treatment. As the interaction unfolds over an individual, or series of consultations, the two discourses may come closer together in a socially shared sense of what is going on. However, they may remain where they are, or indeed they may get further apart. If they come together, a shared sense of the problem will be negotiated. If they remain apart, meaning still has to be generated, but those meanings are neither shared, nor joint. As such they lead to the parties in the interaction having to generate meanings which make sense to them. In schematic terms, the patient in these circumstances may decide that the doctor is no use, unsympathetic, and indeed they may generate highly negative perceptions of the professional. The doctor, on the other hand, may conclude that they are a bad patient, especially if the behaviour the patient engages in indicates that they don't think much of what the doctor is doing for them.

And this is the crux of the matter. At the point that the doctor senses that the patient is not taking seriously what he/she is trying to do for them, then that sense of the doctor *qua* professional is undermined. The central reason for the doctor being in the encounter seems to be attacked by the failure on the part of the patient to take it seriously. As this immediately opens up all kinds of dangerous threats to professional competence, the meanings that are generated flow back to the patient. The patient is identified as bad, difficult and so on, and on whom a range of other negative attributes may be applied, albeit tacitly, which draw on broader cultural values.

In other words, the use of negative labels *and* positive perceptions of patients follow from the problematics of the encounter or encounters. It is the method by which both parties cope with the intrinsic difficulties that arise if they are not able to arrive at a shared account of the interaction through negotiation. Of course, such processes are not confined to doctors and their patients, and similar process will be found in any setting where one party stands ready to provide a service and the other may or may not agree that that is what they want. The interplay is more complex than this schematic outline has suggested and a whole range of idiosyncratic cultural and other assumptions will be brought to bear on particular interactions, but the principle is clear. Research which fails to get at the interactive elements involved will only ever give a partial picture of the issue.

Three rules can be derived from these perspectives: the *awareness* rule, the *avoidance* rule, and the *assumptive* rule. In the *awareness* rule, the doctor needs to be aware that they are playing a part in a broader set of social relationships and that patients bring with them a constellation of broader social factors. Ideal types of encounters that reflect moral and cultural norms sit uneasily with the realities of practical clinical experience. In the *avoidance* rule, the doctor needs to avoid reinforcing disadvantages that the patient may already experience. The doctor should reflect on their powerful position and pause to consider whether their behaviour or actions might exacerbate any disadvantage or inequality.[30] In the *assumptive* rule, the doctor needs to realize that 'problematic' and 'difficult' patients may be a product of doctors and not patients. Doctors should not assume that the dynamics that give rise to 'problematic' and 'difficult' patients are unidimensional. Doctors should acknowledge that what they bring to the interaction is as important in determining how patients come to be perceived, as is what both patients and doctors do or say.[30] These unfold in interaction.

Discussion

There is much evidence to suggest that doctors may perceive certain patients in a negative fashion. Calling on Schutz's work, Stimson[14] remarked that, 'Typifications of other people are especially apparent in those situations where one group of people process another. The processors use typifications of those being processed in order to cope with the problems at hand'. Doctors define who are and who are not 'heartsink' patients[6,13] by reference to patients that are least likely to cause 'trouble'.[14] Differences in numbers of 'heartsink' patients cannot be accounted for by individual characteristics of patients'.[6] Doctors practise medicine from a desire to help people,[9] rarely dislike patients,[10] and one doctor's list of 'difficult' or 'heartsink' patients may not be the same as another's.[5] Doctors' perceptions of certain patients are a situational response to a therapeutic dilemma that concerns the nature of the doctor's role and where, within the doctor patient encounter, that role is not legitimated. It is not simply about patients challenging the doctor's authority, rather it is bound up with challenging the very foundations of the situational role that doctors occupy, and patients' legitimation of that role.

References

1. **O'Dowd, T.C.** (1988). Five years of heartsink patients in general practice. *British Medical Journal* **297**, 528–30.
2. **Friedson, E.** *Professional Dominance: The Social Structure of Medical Care.* Chicago IL: Aldine, 1960.
3. **Jeffery, R.** (1979). Normal rubbish: deviant patients in casualty departments. *Sociology of Health and Illness* **1**, 98–107.
4. **Kelly, M.P. and Field, D.** (1998). Conceptualising chronic illness. In *Sociological Perspectives on Health, Illness and Health Care* (ed. D. Field and S. Taylor), pp. 3–20. Oxford: Blackwell.
5. **Gerrard, T.J. and Riddell, J.D.** (1988). Difficult patients: black holes and secrets. *British Medical Journal* **297**, 530–2.
6. **Mathers, N.J., Jones, N., and Hannay, D.** (1995). Heartsink patients: a study of their general practitioners. *British Journal of General Practice* **45**, 293–6.
7. **Hahn, S.R.** et al. (1996). The difficult patient. *Journal of General Internal Medicine* **11**, 1–8.
8. **John, C.** et al. (1987). Medical care and demographic characteristics of 'difficult' patients. *The Journal of Family Practice* **24** (6), 607–10.
9. **Schwenk, T.L.** et al. (1989). Physician and patient determinants of difficult physician–patient relationships. *The Journal of Family Practice* **28** (1), 59–63.
10. **Sharpe, M.** (1994). Why do doctors find some patients difficult to help? *Quarterly Journal of Medicine* **87**, 187–93.
11. **Mathers, N.J. and Gask, L.** (1995). Surviving the 'heartsink' experience. *Family Practice* **12** (2), 176–83.
12. **Smith, S.** (1995). Dealing with the difficult patient. *Postgraduate Medical Journal* **71**, 653–7.
13. **Butler, C. and Evans, M.** (1999). The 'heartsink' patient revisited. *British Journal of General Practice* **49**, 230–3.
14. **Stimson, G.V.** (1975). General practitioners, 'trouble' and types of patients. In *The Sociology of the National Health Service* (ed. M. Stacey). Sociological Review Monograph, 22.
15. **Groves, J.E.** (1978). Taking care of the hateful patient. *New England Journal of Medicine* **298**, 16.
16. **Kelly, M.P. and May, D.** (1982). Good and bad patients: a review of the literature and a theoretical critique. *Journal of Advanced Nursing* **7**, 147–56.
17. **Najman, J.M., Klein, D., and Munro, C.** (1982). Patient characteristics negatively stereotyped by doctors. *Social Science and Medicine* **16**, 1781–9.
18. **May, D. and Kelly, M.P.** (1982). Chancers, pests and poor wee souls: problems of legitimation in psychiatric nursing. *Sociology of Health and Illness* **4**, 279–301.
19. **Millward, L.M.** Attitudes towards alcoholics: staff patient relationships in the acute hospital setting. Unpublished PhD thesis. King's College, University of London, UK, 2000.
20. **Stockwell, F.** *The Unpopular Patient.* Royal College of Nursing Research Project, Series 1, No. 2. London UK: Royal College of Nursing, 1972.
21. **Blalock, S.J. and Devellis, B.M.** (1986). Stereotyping: the link between theory and practice. *Patient Education and Counselling* **8**, 17–25.
22. **Parsons, T.** *The Social System.* London UK: Routledge & Kegan Paul, 1951.
23. **Freidson, E.** (1975). Dilemmas in the doctor/patient relationship. In *A Sociology of Medical Practice* (ed. C. Cox and A. Mead). London UK: Collier-Macmillan.
24. **Bloor, M.J. and Horobin, G.W.** (1975). Conflict and conflict resolution in doctor/patient interactions. In *A Sociology of Medical Practice* (ed. C. Cox and A. Mead). London UK: Collier-Macmillan.
25. **Tuckett, D.** (1976). Doctors and patients. In *An Introduction to Medical Sociology* (ed. D. Tuckett). London UK: Tavistock Publications.
26. **Green, M.J., Mitchell, G., Stocking, C.B., Cassel, C.K., and Siegler, M.** (1996). Do actions reported by physicians in training conflict with consensus guidelines on ethics? *Archives of Internal Medicine* **156**, 298–304.
27. **Schutz, A.** *The Phenomenology of the Social World.* Translated by G. Walsh and F. Lehnert. Evanston IL: Northwestern University Press, 1967.
28. **Mead, G.H.** *Mind, Self and Society: From the Standpoint of the Social Behaviorist.* Chicago IL: University of Chicago Press, 1934.
29. **Goffman, E.** *Encounters: Two Studies in the Sociology of Interaction.* London UK: Penguin, 1972.
30. **Cochrane, A.L.** *Effectiveness and Efficiency: Random Reflections on Health Services.* London: BMJ and Nuffield Provincial Hospitals Trust, 1972.

5.5 Shared decision-making in clinical practice

Glyn Elwyn, Adrian Edwards, and Melody Rhydderch

Introduction

Shared decision-making has become a term used to describe the process whereby patients participate in decision-making processes about health care issues, typically in consultations,[1] but increasingly by using other media, such as interactive technologies.[2] An innocent concept, you might think. But it belies a fundamental debate between a belief in *rationality* based on the scientific method and the relativist post-modern condition where our world is portrayed as one of multiple perspectives and values. It may be useful to step back and place the method in the wider context of shifting relationships between society and experts, influenced in part by the information revolution.[3,4]

The wider context

The ethical imperative to respect self-determination is clear but it is not the only factor that has led to the interest in shared decision-making. When considering the arrival of modern medical practice, we should visualize the arrival of medical institutions in the late nineteenth century, the period in which Michael Foucault recognized 'the birth of the clinic'.[5] Until then, Western medicine was based largely on patronage and not on institutions and formalized professionals.[6] It was also a time when the contribution of the physical sciences was largely anatomical and medicine was based on beliefs rather than on physiological and biochemical pathways. But as medicine incorporated knowledge from the biosciences, the position of individuals vested with medical training was elevated.[6] Mainstream Western medicine, up until the 1960s, was largely centred on unquestioned professional expertise.[7] It was the clinician's knowledge that dominated the discourse, and decision-making was assumed to be in the professional domain. Recent developments mark the erosion of that assumed position by three factors.

The first is the increasing influence of accountability frameworks. These frameworks primarily focus on cost, quality, and effectiveness. In tax-based services where the payer is the government, the 'freedom of the clinician' is being constrained by a range of techniques that include guidelines, clinical governance, and budgets. Secondly, better informed citizens demand more justification for decisions and are more alert to recent developments, often challenging restrictive policies set by payer-systems. On a more pervasive level, the mass media regularly report new advances. The third factor is the medico-legal pressure on all professionals to share information with patients, and ultimately, the responsibility for decision-making.

In this wider context, it can be seen that the concept of sharing decisions with patients becomes more a necessity than an embellishment. There are debates about the difference between shared decision-making and patient-centredness but these could be summarized by saying that 'patient centredness' is a broad approach that emphasizes in-depth understanding of patients' perspectives and needs.[8] In contrast, 'shared decision-making' examines the core process of medical practice, that of making decisions, and, by using definitions of the principles[1] and skills required of professionals,[9] takes patient participation to new levels of responsibility.

Ethical perspectives

Many commentators think that the priority given to individual choice is problematic[10]—that reifying personal values overlooks our 'social embeddedness' and causes us to lose sight of mutual interdependence.[11] Others suggest that a criticism of 'individualism' should be tempered by a realization that a balance is necessary between societal priorities versus those of individuals. Whether increasing patient participation in decision-making leads to improved health outcomes is also a largely unresolved issue. This uncertainty adds to the intricate ethical debate about the role of rational approaches to decision-making. At the heart of the issue is the tension between ethical principles. As de Haes has stated: 'The ethical principle of autonomy is not necessarily beneficial and may conflict with the principle of beneficence'.[12] Insisting that patients take full responsibility for decision-making is the stance taken by extreme autonomists, who argue that there are only very limited circumstances where others could assume an agency role. Schneider calls this *mandatory autonomy*, where patients are given decisional responsibility, even if they resist.[13] Clinicians recognize the impracticality of this position. It is a position that some patients have also rejected, complaining of 'abandonment' and anxiety.[14] The middle ground, where patients are invited to participate to the level that they prefer or feel able, is equivalent to the ethical position of *optional autonomy*:[13] a method that also recognizes that health professionals have responsibilities to guide and reduce the potential of decisional distress.

Shared decision-making and other proposals—evidence-based patient choice,[4] concordance,[15,16] participatory decision-making[17]—share a common but often unvoiced assumption: that patients are rational decision-makers. This starting position appeals to the ethical principle of veracity and demands that attention be given to the processes of presenting data. But how much detail is required? Many effective interventions have a number of serious side-effects albeit rare. Translating population data into relevant information at the individual level is becoming an important cognitive science.[18,19] Yet, these debates assume that decision-making follows *rational* pathways, whereas it seems that people only demonstrate this quality to very limited degrees.[20]

Does the partial rationality of human decision-making undermine the concept of shared decision-making? Is it more the case that inter-subjective processes, both in consultations and, more importantly, between family and others, are the dominant influences on decisions? Those who agree with Habermas that it is important to achieve as much *rationality* as possible in human affairs will occupy the middle ground: that it is important to make the most of 'truths', albeit grasped from different standpoints, and will agree with this central thesis about the outcomes, which are:

> distinguished by how they [the actors] specify this coordination among the goal directed actions of different participants—as the interlacing of egocentric calculations of utility, as a socially integrating consensus about norms and values ...[21]

Habermas is in effect describing the shared decision-making process by using phrases such as the 'interlacing' of utilities. Judgements on the appropriateness or otherwise of decisions can be largely suspended if we place our trust in a *process* where people act in each other's best interests, and pursue their goals, provided these goals are not grand, distant, or overtly unachievable.[22]

The principles and competences of shared decision-making

This chapter considers the principles and a suggested skill framework for shared decision-making and draws on the following sources: electronic searches of Medline and PubMed using relevant key words, hand search of *Health Expectations* (Blackwell Journal), systematic search for measurement instruments,[23] Oxford SDM Summer School, 2001,[24] Ottowa Health Decision Centre website,[25] Foundation for Informed Medical Decision-making.[26]

What is clearly evident from empirical work is that clinicians rarely involve patients in decisions.[27,28] Medical sociologists have described the physician–patient decision-making process as one that has a high probability of conflict because of the different agendas brought to the encounter and the different types of discourse used to discuss health care concerns.[29,30] Health economists have raised the issue of agency, the term given to the role taken when one person acts on behalf of another. Gafni and colleagues, for instance, viewed the treatment decision-making process as requiring two components—technical information about available treatment alternatives, their benefits and risks, and information about patient preferences and values.[31] Since information is typically in the domain of the clinician and the latter with the patient, some way must be found to bring the two together in the same individual. Health economists recognize that a perfect agency relationship between physician and patient exists in theory only and in practice, the relationship will be influenced by factors such as physician motivation and incentives in the health care system. The best-known recent conceptual framework for treatment decision-making is the one published by Charles and colleagues[1,32] (see Table 1).

Table 1 Conceptual framework for treatment decision-making[a]

Analytical stages	Models	Paternalistic	Shared	Informed
Information exchange	Flow	One way (largely)	Two way	One way (largely)
	Direction	Physician → patient	Physician ⇆ patient	Physician → patient
	Type	Medical	Medical and personal	Medical
	Amount[b]	Minimal legally required	All relevant for decision-making	All relevant for decision-making
Deliberation		Physician alone or with other physicians	Physician and patient (plus potential others)	Physician and patient (plus potential others)
Deciding on treatment to implement		Physicians	Physician and patient	Patient

[a] Illustration for an encounter focusing on the case of a (treating) physician–patient dyad.

[b] Minimum required.

On the basis of this analysis, four shared decision-making principles were put forward:

- shared decision-making involves at least two participants—the doctor and the patient—and often many more (their respective networks of family or professional colleagues);
- both parties (doctors and patients) take steps to participate in the process of treatment decision-making;
- information sharing is a prerequisite to shared decision-making;
- a treatment decision (which may be to do nothing) is made, and both parties agree to the decision.

This framework for treatment decision-making could be easily adapted for other types of decisions, such as screening or the use of diagnostic interventions. But it is not the principles that cause difficulty. Making the transition to a set of agreed practical skills has been more of a challenge, and a task embedded in the wider debate about the development of interpersonal communication skills.

Interpersonal communication skills

The extent to which interpersonal skills can be analysed and taught is a controversial issue. Hartley[33] defines a social skill as a 'process whereby the individual implements a set of goal-directed, interrelated, situationally appropriate social behaviours which are learned and controlled'. Accepting that professionals can develop these skills, facilitating patient involvement in treatment decision-making is only one aspect of a more comprehensive communication process in medical encounters. Some argue that it is not appropriate to isolate components and warn against the reduction of a complex activity into a sequence of defined tasks.[34,35]

But advocates of communication skill development argue that it is easier to isolate and master individual steps before attempting to combine them into accomplished performances.[36] In addition, recent literature in organizational psychology increasingly speaks of evaluating 'competences' and 'competencies'.[35,37] Distinctions are drawn between characteristics that are personal attributes (*competencies*) and skills that task linked (competences). *Competencies*, as defined by Boyatzis, describe inherent aspects of a person such as the ability to sing in tune or draw. *Competencies* are individual characteristics that enable people to add to them, that is, develop *competences*, which are situational and linked to tasks. It is relatively straightforward to deconstruct situation-specific *competences*; it is much harder to deconstruct *competencies*. Learning programmes need to pay attention to both inherent and acquired skills.

Identifying the competences of shared decision-making

Should the skills of shared decision-making be derived from theoretical conceptual frameworks or would it be better to construct a competence framework using empirical methods? Specific techniques for identifying 'competences' have been developed. They include the Critical Incident Technique and the Repertory Grid Analysis, although they have not been used to assess shared decision-making. The methods used to date include interviews and observational studies.[9,38] Elwyn et al. used a key informant method using selected general medical practitioners to provide a bridge between 'theoretical' ideas about the process of involving patients in decision-making and the practical problems met in practice. The method was used to obtain opinions 'grounded' in specific contexts. Six sequential focus groups were held where 'shared decision-making' was debated until a list of competences was agreed.[9] These competences were investigated using further empirical techniques, and modified over time[39–41] (see Box 1),[42] and patient perspectives added.[43] Each competence will be discussed in turn.

Box 1 Shared decision-making competences

- Problem definition
- Portray equipoise
- Portray options
- Check understanding
- Explore ideas, concerns, and expectations about intervention
- Role preference
- Decision-making
- Deferment if necessary
- Review arrangements

Problem definition

Empirical examination of actual practice revealed the importance of achieving well-defined problems.[39] The issue of whether some decisions are easier (or more appropriate) to 'share' with patients needs further elaboration. It is certainly true that where there are prior views about the 'best' outcome, differing views about the appropriateness of using antibiotics for viral illnesses, for example, then it is difficult to 'share' the decision.[41,44] Agreeing agendas is a basic feature of the patient-centred approach but this step takes on added importance in shared decision-making. Problems have specific characteristics that must be delineated in order to achieve solutions or containment. It is not possible to provide information without first having exactly defined the scope and nature of the problem. For example, hormone replacement therapy requires patients to understand the difference between short- and long-term treatment effects. Short-term hormone replacement therapy relieves menopausal symptoms. Long-term treatment has preventative aims, for example, the reduction of osteoporosis risk. These two different aims have to be distinguished for patients. It is only long-term treatment that carries an increased risk of breast cancer. The decision to take hormone replacement therapy is contingent on understanding the relative harms and benefits of using oestrogen, not for a year or two, but continuously over a 10-year period. This may seem blindingly obvious to clinicians but patients may not realize the implications of this distinction. Until patients understand the relevant decisional issues, the latter stages of shared decision-making are superfluous.

Qualitative studies have showed that problem definition is often bypassed, although it lies at the core of shared decision-making. Many patients have no experience of sharing decisions and find it strange to be drawn into such a requirement. This problem structuring approach is also novel for many clinicians and is a skill that needs specific development.

Portray equipoise

An analysis of consultations by clinicians who were aiming to share decisions revealed the existence of phrases that have been described as 'equipoise' statements, a term that describes a position of balance. These statements were identified in the talk of clinicians who wanted to contextualize the *process* of sharing decisions, to emphasize that there was genuine room to discuss patient preferences and values. Equipoise statements are a recognition that there are patient factors within the professional's realm that should influence the decision-making process.

Many medical situations are characterized by uncertain long-term outcomes and by having more than one treatment option. The shared decision-making method facilitates a discussion about these issues, in effect highlighting the uncertain nature of medical knowledge and practice. Patients, in general, find it novel to participate in such discussions. There is, therefore, a need to be explicit that patient values must be fully integrated into the process. To facilitate this step, professionals should orientate patients to the concept of professional *equipoise* so that the options can be legitimately explained and that the overall aim of the communication process is understood. It has been suggested that shared decision-making should only be considered in situations of clear 'equipoise', that is, where there are debates about the most effective intervention. Whilst a valid standpoint, the authors of this chapter regard this position as being too restrictive. Treatment 'standards' or 'guidelines' may well exist but each individual has a unique psychological and social context to consider, factors that are not considered by the available evidence base: this in effect allows the condition of equipoise to be relevant in a much wider set of circumstances.

Portray options

Choice cannot be exercised without the presence of valid options and it is recognized that the range of options provided by the clinician will determine the scope of discussions.(45) It is also known that patients find the option of 'doing nothing' very difficult to accept. This problem may be avoided by using a more positive term such as 'watchful waiting'. It is also important to explore the options that patients may consider relevant. Choices are often presented from a biomedical menu with little time spent exploring what other strategies may be pertinent.

Studies have demonstrated that it is preferable to provide an outline of options first, before providing detailed information.(9) In other words, clinicians may find it more effective to state that 'for this particular problem, there are three possible options, A, B, or C', a process known as *option listing*. This allows patients to contextualize decisions. The use of decision aids also helps patients assimilate information.(2) Unless detailed information is conveyed appropriately, it is unreasonable to expect patients to become involved in decisions. Asking patients to make choices without adequate information is like asking people to place bets without knowing the odds. It is becoming feasible for a clinician to have a 'basket', so to speak, of data formats, graphs, bar charts, tables, and so on, which can be used to illustrate the concepts of relative and absolute risks.(46) The practicality of this type of information exchange is increasing as online decision aids become available.

Check understanding and conduct an exploration of ideas, concerns, and expectations about the intervention

Checking that patients have understood information is a well-described element of effective communication. Kurtz and colleagues advocate the method of 'chunking and checking'.(36) Exploring patient ideas, concerns, and expectations (in this context pre-conceived notions and fears about interventions, not diagnoses) are a familiar part of the patient-centred method. These techniques ensure that professionals stay in touch with patient perceptions as they become involved in decisions.

Role preference

There is a large literature that has explored patient views about their preferred role in decision-making.(17,47) The work can be summarized by stating that the majority of studies have asked patients to consider their 'preference' either in a hypothetical situation or shortly before engaging in a decision-making process. These methods are not ideal. One of the main difficulties is that an individual's preferred participation in decisions is unlikely to be stable and will change with time, and with the nature and severity of the problems faced. This is made more problematic by the fact that it is only when individuals have understood the scope and the nature of issues facing them that decisions about whether to participate can be taken.(9) Individuals may retract from the responsibility of taking difficult decisions if faced with post-decision regret or guilt.(13) It is also likely that there is a 'learning' or experiential component to such preferences and that a positive experience of the process may well lead to higher future preferences for involvement.

It has been argued that it is important to assess role preference in decision-making processes at the start of consultations.(38) But it may be difficult for patients to understand the relevance of such a question. Clinicians found it difficult at first to evaluate patient role preference and often met with puzzlement.(9) Patients assumed that by communicating with clinicians they were *implicitly* taking active roles in decision-making. Insisting on *explicit* role clarity was regarded unnecessary. This step can be conceptualized as a meta-communication (communication about the process of communication) and is a difficult leap. Nevertheless, the clinicians wanted the step retained as a means of alerting professionals to the need to monitor patient acceptance. Clinicians regarded implicit engagement in the decision-making process as a reasonable proxy for explicitly negotiated role preference *provided* they remained sensitive to signs of discomfort or reluctance.

Decision-making and possible deferment

It has been demonstrated that, irrespective of the total consultation duration, clinicians initiate the decision-making part of the interaction when 80 per cent of the total time has elapsed,(39) that is, decision-making talk seems to act as a closure cue to both parties. It follows, therefore, that the initiation of decision talk should be carefully planned and initiated only after the other stages of the shared decision-making process have been completed. In the absence of an urgent need to make decisions (which is unusual), practitioners should advise patients to deliberate and discuss options with a range of other people. In other words, deferment and reflection should be encouraged and patients advised to explore the implications of decisions with relatives and others.

Review arrangements

The need to review patients is particularly relevant for the shared decision-making method. The process may have generated uncertainty or unwelcome responsibility. Clinicians should ensure that patients do not perceive reviews as an implied criticism of either patient adherence or clinician judgement but as a necessary part of a longitudinal process of decision-making.

Other frameworks for patient participation in decisions

The focus of the 'patient-centred' method was on information gathering and understanding the patient's perspective on the illness experience. The method was not fully developed to cover the decision-making process and it is becoming clear from empirical work that patient-centredness and shared decision-making can be distinguished.(48) It is only in the late 1990s that in-depth attention was given to patient participation in clinical decisions. Towle listed eight *competencies* for shared decision-making: 'skills and attitudes that represent the instructional intents of a programme, stated as specific goals'.(38) Dowell and Dowie have also proposed a consultation method named as a 'concordant therapeutic alliance' that draws on the concept of achieving 'concordance' about taking medication (an agreement between the patient and the clinician)—an alternative and less coercive term than the notion of 'compliance'.(15,16) Further evaluations are awaited.

Measurement of shared decision-making

Is not surprising to find that there is a dearth of valid and reliable measures for shared decision-making. A systematic search did not find an instrument that adequately covered the theoretical and empirically derived framework

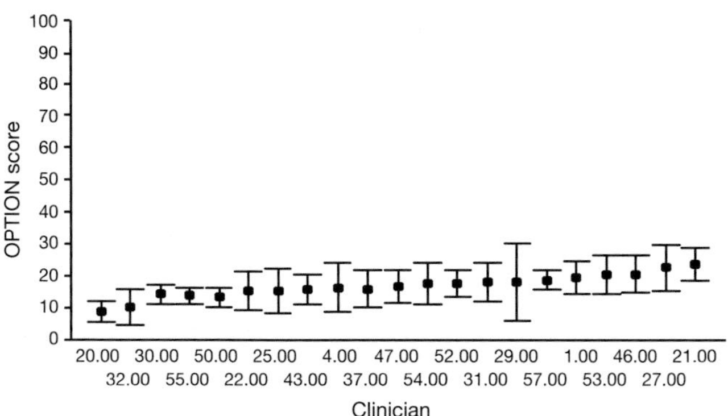

Fig. 1 Patient involvement scores in routine general practice consultations. (Mean option scores (0–100), 95 per cent confidence intervals.)

of shared decision-making.(23) As a response to this gap, an instrument named OPTION (Observing Patient Involvement) has been developed. The scale was developed on the basis of a series of qualitative and quantitative studies,(42) and consists of a 12-item scale that was specifically designed to assess the extent to which clinicians involve patients in decisions, irrespective of the type of problems presented. The degree of patient involvement achieved by recruited general practitioners during routine consultation in service settings is shown in Fig. 1.(49) It has since been shown that these relatively low levels can be significantly improved by skill development interventions.(42)

Future challenges

There is a growing realization that shared decision-making cannot be contained in single episodes. The method describes a complex, longitudinal process that requires a detailed understanding of risks and benefits. It is also clear that the current structure of medical practice is not well suited to these tasks and that communication skills on their own cannot satisfy the information demands. Care is required not to force decision-making on the unwilling(50) or the unable and attention given to the emotional support that is needed when patients are ill, anxious, or lack the willingness, for whatever reason, to engage in rational models of decision-making.(13,51) But as medicine moves towards an anticipatory model—screening, predicting, and preventing problems *before* they occur—clinicians will have to deal with *consumers* not *patients*, and paternalism will no longer satisfy an increasingly well-informed clientele. Clinicians will need fast and accurate portals of information or they will be left behind. The ability to appraise and explain data in order to arrive at shared decisions will become the bedrock of future clinical practice. This chapter has tentatively traced the steps that need to be taken in that direction.

References

1. **Charles, C., Gafni, A., and Whelan, T.** (1997). Shared decision-making in the medical encounter: what does it mean? (Or it takes at least two to tango). *Social Science and Medicine* **44**, 681–92.
2. **O'Connor, A.M., Rostom, A., Fiset, V., Tetroe, J., Entwistle, V., Llewelyn-Thomas, H., Holmes-Rovner, M., Barry, M., and Jones, J.** (1999). Decision aids for patients facing health treatment or screening decisions: systematic review. *British Medical Journal* **319**, 731–4.
3. **Kendall, L.** *The Future Patient.* London: Institute for Public Policy Research, 2001.
4. **Edwards, A. and Elwyn, G., ed.** *Evidence Based Patient Choice: Inevitable or Impossible?* Oxford: Oxford University Press, 2001.
5. **Foucault, M.** *The Birth of the Clinic.* London: Tavistock, 1973.
6. **Johnson, T.J.** *Professions and Power.* London: Macmillan, 1972.
7. **Greaves, D.** *Mystery in Modern Medicine.* Aldershot: Avebury, 1996.
8. **Stewart, M., Brown, J.B., Weston, W.W., McWinney, I.R., McWilliam, C.L., and Freeman, T.R.** *Patient Centred Medicine: Transforming the Clinical Method.* Thousand Oaks CA: Sage Publications, 1995.
9. **Elwyn, G., Edwards, A., Kinnersley, P., and Grol, R.** (2000). Shared decision making and the concept of equipoise: defining the competences of involving patients in healthcare choices. *British Journal of General Practice* **50**, 892–9.
10. **Parker, M.** (2001). The ethics of evidence-based patient choice. *Health Expectations* **4**, 87–91.
11. **Etzioni, A.** *The Spirit of Community.* London: Fontana, 1993.
12. **de Haes, H.C. and Molenaar, S.** (1997). Patient participation and decision control: are patient autonomy and well-being associated? *Medical Decision Making* **17**, 353–4.
13. **Schneider, C.E.** *The Practice of Autonomy: Patients, Doctors, and Medical Decisions.* New York: Oxford University Press, 1998.
14. **Quill, T.E. and Cassel, C.K.** (1995). Nonabandonment: a central obligation for physicians. *Annals of Internal Medicine* **122**, 368–74.
15. **Marinker, M.** (1997). From compliance to concordance: achieving shared goals in medicine taking. *British Medical Journal* **314**, 747–8.
16. **Britten, N.** (2003). Concordance and compliance. In *Oxford Textbook of Primary Medical Care.* Oxford: Oxford University Press.
17. **Guadagnoli, E. and Ward, P.** (1998). Patient participation in decision-making. *Social Science and Medicine* **47** (3), 329–39.
18. **Edwards, A. and Elwyn, G.** (2001). Understanding risk, and lessons for clinical risk communication about treatment preferences. *Quality Health Care* **10** (Suppl.), i9–13.
19. **Edwards, A., Elwyn, G., and Mulley, A.** (2002). Explaining risks: turning numerical data into meaningful pictures. *British Medical Journal* **324**, 827–30.
20. **Evans, J.St.B.T.E., Over, D.E., and Manktelow, K.I.** (1993). Reasoning, decision making and rationality. In *Reasoning and Decision Making* (ed. P.N. Johnson-Laird and E. Shafir). Cambridge: Cambridge University Press.
21. **Habermas, J.** *The Theory of Communicative Action: Reason and Rationalization of Society.* Cambridge: Polity, 1984.
22. **Elwyn, G. and Charles, C.** (2001). Shared decision making: inevitable or impossible? In *Evidence Based Patient Choice* (ed. A. Edwards and G. Elwyn). Oxford: Oxford University Press.
23. **Elwyn, G., Edwards, A., Mowle, S., Wensing, M., Wilkinson, C., Kinnersley, P., and Grol, R.** (2001). Measuring the involvement of patients in shared decision making: a systematic review of instruments. *Patient Education and Counseling* **43**, 5–22.
24. **Abstracts and Programme.** Shared Decision Making Summer School Conference Proceedings. Oxford: St Catherine's College, 2001.
25. **Ottowa Health Decision Centre.** Decision Support Courses, (http://www.lri.ca/programs/ceu/ohdec), University of Ottowa.
26. **Foundation for Informed Medical Decision-Making.** www:healthdialog.com, 2000.
27. **Stevenson, F.A., Barry, C.A., Britten, N., Barber, N., and Bradley, C.P.** (2000). Doctor–patient communication about drugs: the evidence for shared decision making. *Social Science and Medicine* **50**, 829–40.
28. **Campion, P., Foulkes, J., Neighbour, R., and Tate, P.** (2002). Patient-centredness in the MRCGP video examination: analysis of large cohort. *British Medical Journal* **325**, 691–2.
29. **Mishler, E.** *The Discourse of Medicine: Dialectics of Medical Interviews.* Norwood NJ: Ablex, 1984.
30. **Waitzkin, H.** (1985). Information giving in medical care. *Journal of Health and Social Behaviour* **26**, 81.
31. **Gafni, A., Charles, C., and Whelan, T.** (1998). The physician–patient encounter: the physician as a perfect agent for the patient *versus* the informed decision-making model. *Social Science and Medicine* **47**, 347–54.
32. **Charles, C., Gafni, A., and Whelan, T.** (1999). Decision making in the physician–patient encounter: revisiting the shared treatment decision-making model. *Social Science and Medicine* **49**, 651–61.

33. **Hartley, P.** *Interpersonal Communication* 2nd edn. London: Routledge, 1999.
34. **Eraut, M.** *Developing Professional Knowledge and Competence.* London: Falmer Press, 1993.
35. **Barnett, R.** *The Limits of Competence.* Buckingham: Open University Press, 1994.
36. **Kurtz, S., Silverman, J., and Draper, J.** *Teaching and Learning Communication Skills in Medicine.* Abingdon: Radcliffe Medical Press, 1998.
37. **Boyatzis, R.E.** *The Competent Manager. A Model for Effective Performance.* New York: John Wiley and Sons, 1982.
38. **Towle, A. and Godolphin, W.** (1999). Framework for teaching and learning informed shared decision making. *British Medical Journal* **319**, 766–9.
39. **Elwyn, G., Edwards, A., Wensing, M., Hibbs, R., Wilkinson, C., and Grol, R.** (2001). Shared decision-making observed: visual displays of communication sequence and patterns. *Journal of Evaluation in Clinical Practice* **7**, 211–21.
40. **Elwyn, G., Edwards, A., Gwyn, R., and Grol, R.** (1999). Towards a feasible model for shared decision-making: a focus group study with general practice registrars. *British Medical Journal* **319**, 753–7.
41. **Elwyn, G., Gwyn, R., Edwards, A.G.K., and Grol, R.** (1999). Is a 'shared decision' feasible in a consultation for a viral upper respiratory tract infection: assessing the influence of patient expectations for antibiotics using discourse analysis. *Health Expectations* **2**, 105–17.
42. **Elwyn, G.** Shared decision making in clinical practice. PhD thesis, Centre for Quality Care Research, Nijmegen University, Nijmegen, 2001.
43. **Edwards, A., Elwyn, G., and Smith, C.** (2001). Consumers' views of quality: identifying the consultation outcomes of importance to consumers, and their relevance to 'shared decision-making' approaches. *Health Expectations* **4**, 151–61.
44. **Gwyn, R. and Elwyn, G.** (1999). When is a shared decision not (quite) a shared decision? Negotiating preferences in a general practice encounter. *Social Science and Medicine* **49**, 437–47.
45. **Redelmeier, D.A. and Shafir, E.** (1995). Medical decision making in situations that offer multiple alternatives. *Journal of the American Medical Association* **273**, 302–5.
46. **Edwards, A., Elwyn, G., and Gwyn, R.** (1999). General practice registrar responses to the use of different risk communication tools: problems and opportunities. *British Medical Journal* **319**, 749–52.
47. **Benbassat, J., Pilpel, D., and Tidhar, M.** (1998). Patients' preferences for participation in clinical decision-making: a review of published surveys. *Behavioural Medicine* **24**, 81–8.
48. **Wensing, M., Elwyn, G., Edwards, A., Vingerhoets, E., and Grol, R.** (2002). Deconstructing patient centred communication and uncovering shared decision making: an observational study. *BMC Medical Informatics and Decision Making* **2**, 2.
49. **Elwyn, G., Edwards, A., Wensing, M., Hood, K., Atwell, C., and Grol, R.** (2003). Shared decision making: developing the OPTION scale for measuring patient involvement. *Quality and Safety in Health Care* **12**, 87.
50. **McKinstry, B.** (2000). Do patients wish to be involved in decision making in the consultation? A cross sectional survey with video vignettes. *British Medical Journal* **321**, 867–71.
51. **Charles, C., Gafni, A., and Whelan, T.** (2000). How to improve communication between doctors and patients. *British Medical Journal* **320** (7244), 1220–1.

5.6 Time and the consultation

Judith Belle Brown

Introduction

In the twenty-first century time is a precious commodity. In many health care systems in the industrialized world time dictates the quality of care provided to patients. In this chapter, the history of time in relation to the consultation in primary care will be examined. The objective evidence, supported by empirical studies, will demonstrate the relationship of time to patient factors (i.e. satisfaction, age, socio-economic status) and physician factors (i.e. satisfaction, malpractice, practice behaviour). Intricately woven between patient and physician factors are systemic factors (i.e. remuneration, appointment schedules, managed care). As it is difficult to isolate these systemic factors they are examined throughout the chapter. The subjective experience of time, drawn from narratives of both patients and providers and qualitative inquiry, will provide an additional perspective on time and the consultation. Finally, the future role of time and the consultation, as it relates to continuity of care and challenges for future research, will be examined.

Time and the objective evidence

In the last 30 years, as family medicine has become a distinct discipline, considerations on time and the consultation, in particular of the question how much time is enough, have been of interest to primary care physician scholars and researchers. As such, most research about the impact of time on the patient–physician consultation has been conducted in the primary care setting.

The history of time in the consultation

Early studies on time and the consultation were driven by an interest in establishing the optimal consultation length, in order to establish appropriate booking in appointment systems.[1] In addition, initial research was in response to concerns about the brevity of consultations conducted, especially in the United Kingdom, and the subsequent impact on the patient–physician interaction.[2,3] However, methodological issues, for example data collected from a single practice or practice group, and small sample sizes, limited generalizability of early findings.[1,2,4,5] In contrast, a recent study[6] using data from the National Ambulatory Medical Care Survey (NAMCS) of the National Center for Health Statistics in the United States reported on surveys collected from office-based physicians over a 10-year period.[6] The number of patient visits sampled per year ranged from 24 715 to 43 469.[6] Another large data set, collected in the United States, consists of 4454 patient visits with 138 physicians in 84 practices.[7] In this study, research nurses directly observed consecutive patient visits with additional data being gathered from various sources (i.e. chart audit, patient and physician surveys, and ethnographic field notes).[7] These studies demonstrate how research on time and the consultation has become more rigorous and complex in design, reflecting significant advances in the field of inquiry over the last three decades.

How long are consultations in primary care?

The length of the consultation varies around the world—ranging from 5 min or less to over 10 min in the United Kingdom[8] and Hong Kong to as long as 21 min in Sweden.[5] Concern has been voiced that managed care, a reality in the US health care system, has resulted in primary care physicians spending less time with patients.[9] However, recent studies from the United States indicate that the length of time family physicians are spending in consultations has increased.[6,10,11] For example, NAMCS data from 1978 to 1994 showed an increase in consultation length from family physician visits of 2.6 min (13.5–17.1 min).[10] Mechanic et al.[6] also using NAMCS data, found a 2 min increase from 1989 to 1998.

Consultations in Australia are on average 12 min long.[12] In South Africa, Henbest and Fehrsen[13] have documented the mean length of a family practice visit as 11 min. In the United Kingdom, where consultation times have been historically short (i.e. 8.7 min in 1977),[1] Little et al.[14] documented patients' preferences for a patient-centred encounter. Stewart et al.'s[15] research in Canada determined that 9.4 min was a sufficient time frame to achieve a patient-centred consultation.

How do we reconcile these vast ranges in consultation time across the globe? The organization of the health care system, cultural influences, and patient expectations may all serve as influential factors. Yet the question remains—how much time is enough?

How much time is enough?

Roland et al.'s[16] contention that the 'ability to communicate effectively may be largely a function of the time available for the consultation' characterizes the controversy surrounding how much time is enough. There is conflicting literature on the subject of consultation length. On the one hand, studies report that patient–physician interaction (i.e. positive or negative) is not affected by the length of the encounter; while, on the other hand, length of time has been found to impact on the nature and outcome of the patient–physician consultation.

The following studies provide evidence to support the belief that optimal patient–physician interactions do not require in longer office visits. In Marvel et al.'s[17] study, comparing the interviews of exemplary family physicians (physicians who had received postgraduate training in family therapy) versus community family physicians (physicians who had no additional training), there was no difference in the length of the office visits between the two physician groups. Of note, however, was that in the same length of time, the exemplary physicians engaged the patients in more in-depth interactions, including exploration of psycho-social issues and patient collaboration.

Consultations, described by both physicians and patients as being positive, were reported as taking less time than negative consultations.[18] Furthermore, Arborelius and Bremberg[18] found that in the positive consultations more time was devoted to exploring patients' ideas and concerns, which is similar to Marvel et al.'s[17] findings. Greenfield et al.[19] observed that while the total amount of conversation between experimental group patients and their physicians was greater than control group patients, there was no corresponding change in the length of the visit. The intervention (to improve information-seeking skills of the patient) produced a more active interchange, but not a longer visit. Again, this is in concert with Marvel et al.'s[17] findings on enhanced patient collaboration. Henbest and Fehrsen[13] found that consultations, which were the most patient-centred, did not take longer than those that were less patient-centred and stated that the 'frequent assumption that it takes longer to conduct a patient-centered consultation was not supported. Lack of time cannot be legitimately offered as an excuse for not conducting patient-centered consultations' (p. 316).

In contrast, other authors suggest that optimal patient–provider communication requires longer consultations,[1,3,8,20] concluding that there is a trade-off between increasing time and the expectations of the provider, the patient, and the many and varied professional organizations generating clinical practice guidelines. For example, Howie et al.[8] found that significantly higher proportions of favourable responses were shown for long compared with short consultations for 17 of 33 questions asked. The question, 'Did the doctor give you a chance to say what was really on your mind?' was positively associated with length of visit. They concluded that 'The advantages of longer consultations do not simply lie in more services being provided but in a larger proportion of the needs which have been recognized being followed up by the doctor'. (ref. 8, p. 54). Williams and Neal[21] found that when booking appointments were extended from 5 to 10 min patients reported more satisfaction with the consultation, a better understanding of their illness, and improved coping strategies.

In conclusion, the controversy on how much time is enough will continue until there is sufficient research evidence to sway the debate. At present we can only conclude that while longer consultations do on the whole lead to better patient outcomes, some physicians are able to achieve these outcomes without spending more time. These lead us to consider in more detail the various patient factors that influence and are influenced by the length of the consultation.

Patient factors

Patient satisfaction

Patient satisfaction is a frequently used outcome variable in primary care research and is certainly pertinent to the issue of time and the consultation.[22] An association between length of visit, patient volume, and patient satisfaction was found by Zyzanski et al.[23] Lower patient satisfaction was more common among high-volume physicians whose visits were 30 per cent shorter than those of low-volume physicians. Patients reported less follow-up on their problems, less attention to their responses, and less than adequate explanations for their concerns. In addition, high-volume physicians had significantly fewer patients who were up to date on the recommended guidelines for screening, counselling, and immunization. In the discussion the authors suggest that increased efficiency may be at the expense of patient satisfaction, adequate preventive care, and finally may have a negative impact on the patient–provider interaction.

From the same data set, Gross et al.[24] identified two specific patient–provider exchanges that would improve patient satisfaction. First, providers need to allow a brief period of time to 'chat' about topics of a non-medical nature. This, they suggest, may help the patient to connect with the provider. Secondly, sufficient time must be taken when providing patients with feedback on clinical findings.

Patient characteristics

Certain patient characteristics may either increase or decrease the consultation length. There is strong evidence around the globe that elderly patients have longer visits.[1,4,11,25–27] This is not a surprising finding given the co-morbidity of this patient population and the complexity of their problems. Thus, as we face the reality of the aging population, consideration must be given to providing adequate appointment times for this sector of the population. At the other end of the age spectrum are adolescents who are reported to have their family physician spend significantly less time with them than any other age group.[27,28] Teenagers are a potentially vulnerable population who could benefit from time spent on discussions of risk avoidance such as alcohol and drug use and sexual activity.

Studies have established that individuals in lower socio-economic brackets are more likely to experience short consultations.[1,12,29] There is conflicting evidence as to whether non-English-speaking patients in English-speaking countries have shorter consultation lengths. Tocher and Larson[30] found that there was no difference in the length of consultation between English-speaking patients and non-English-speaking patients. In contrast, Rivadeneyra et al.'s[31] study, examining whether primary care physicians used a patient-centred approach with patients accompanied by an interpreter, found that physicians were less patient-centred with non-English-speaking patients. They speculated that one reason for this finding may be the time-consuming process of using an interpreter. One drawback of this study was that they did not specifically measure consultation length. However, their findings suggest that patients requiring the services of an interpreter may need longer visits.

For over two decades researchers have consistently found that patients with psychological difficulties have longer consultations. Westcott,[1] in 1977, reported that patients with a diagnosis of psychoneurosis had significantly longer consultations. In a recent report by Blumenthal et al.,[11] again using the NAMCS data, consultation length for patients with psychosocial problems was significantly longer. The need for longer visits when dealing with patients' psychological concerns also appears to reflect a global trend with similar findings being reported in Sweden,[4] Australia,[29] the United States,[20] and the United Kingdom.[8]

But are disenfranchised populations such as the poor, the elderly, and the psychologically disadvantaged receiving adequate consultation times to address their needs? This raises multiple issues: is the remuneration for caring for these groups of patients insufficient; do primary care physicians lack the necessary skills to address the concerns of these patients, or are the expectations of practice so demanding that the needs of this patient group is negated in the face of other pressing medical demands? Further research will be needed to address these questions.

Physician factors

Physician satisfaction

As early as 1979, Mawardi[32] in the United States reported that family physicians were dissatisfied with the time pressures they experienced in practice. Grol et al.[33] in the Netherlands, documented similar findings 4 years later. In fact, their study indicated that physicians who experienced negative feelings such as being frustrated, tense, and short of time prescribed more and gave less explanation to patients.[33] Thus, spending additional time may result in less physician stress[34] and increased job satisfaction.[35] However, Morrell et al.[22] reported that there was no evidence of less physician stress in consultations of 5, 7.5, or 10 min in length.

One source of stress for primary care physicians is the anxiety related to a malpractice claim. Levinson et al.[36] found that no-claims primary care physicians spent a significantly longer time with patients than primary care physicians involved in claims (18.3 versus 15 min, respectively). Thus, one way to reduce physician stress, at least about the risk of a malpractice claim, may be to spend a few more minutes with patients.

Another source of dissatisfaction for primary care physicians is a lack of adequate remuneration.[37] Martin et al.[26] argue that certain patients, such as those with chronic illnesses, require more time and hence should be reimbursed accordingly. Similarly, patient visits dealing with complex problems, for example, the concerns of the elderly, patients with substance abuse problems, or individuals in psychological distress, are more time consuming, yet no compensation is provided for caring for these patients.[27,29,38]

Physician practice behaviour

But how do physicians use time in the consultation? Beckman and Frankel[39] found that on average physicians interrupt patients 18 s after they begin to speak. They suggest that this early interruption of the patient's story may extend the consultation length as patients may re-introduce unaddressed concerns later in the visit.

Time also impacts on physician practice behaviour within the visit. Longer consultations have been found to include more health promotion activities[8,16,22,40] and prevention strategies.[10,16,41] There is conflicting evidence on the influence of visit length on physician prescribing behavi-our. Some studies[2,33] report that longer consultations result in lower prescription rates while other studies, manipulating the length of the consultation time, have observed no change in the physicians' prescription rate.[22,42]

As communication skills are covered in Chapter 5.3 of this volume, only brief mention will be made of the relationship between time and patient–doctor communication. Clearly, when physicians spend more time with patients they are more likely to discuss psycho-social issues[8,20,42] and to engage patients in an explanation of the problem and the proposed management plan.[16,42] These findings are noteworthy in light of Little et al.'s[14] description of patients' expectations of patient-centred care already discussed.

Thus, we have gone full circle, back to the question of how much time is enough from the perspective of both doctors and patients. While this section has examined patient factors and physician factors separately, what becomes evident is the inextricable link between the needs, expectations, and desires of both patients and doctors in relation to time and the consultation. As Andersson et al.[5] eloquently stated: 'Time is a concept of importance in the search for quality consultation. But time itself is not the quality. The quality is what takes place in a period of time' (p. 67). Thus, what takes place is often a complex, dynamic, and sometimes intimate exchange, between patients and their physicians.

Time and the subjective experience

The aforementioned studies clearly document the evidence regarding the multiple issues in relation to time and the consultation. Yet, beyond this are the real experiences of patients and physicians as described in their narrative accounts. In the last several decades there has been a resurgence in the medical literature of a historical form of story-telling—the narrative which provides a different and richer perspective of both patients' and physicians' experiences.[43,44] As Heath notes, in Greenhalgh and Hurwitz's[44] compilation of narratives:

> Stories can only be told when people have time to talk and time to listen and to hear. The richer the narrative the more time is needed. The magnificent advantage of general practice as a mode of clinical care is its longitudinal dimension and the opportunities this gives both doctor and patients to develop and respond to complex narratives in relatively short instalments but over a sustained period of time. (p. 90)

Borkan et al.'s[43] stories reveal how doctors are also influenced by their relationships with patients, and how time can play an important dimension. The physicians' perspective on the role of time is also revealed in Herman's[25] story of the use of time following his retirement wherein 'time' afforded him the opportunity to understand and respond to patients in a different manner.

In addition to narratives, qualitative studies provide further evidence of the importance of time. McWilliam et al.[45] in their qualitative study of breast cancer survivors' communication challenges in interacting with their physicians, found that time was essential in building relationships and sharing information about present and future care. As one of the study participants described:

> Time was taken . . . to help predict what the procedures were going to be like and how I was going to choose them and in what manner I would choose them. That kind of ten or fifteen-minute introduction to the relationship made a massive difference for me. I wasn't unclothed. I wasn't sitting in some little examining room. I wasn't wondering who was going to walk in the door, how many students were going to be there . . . Those two occasions were very important to me. They set the tone which was easy then for me to sustain. (p. 194–5)

Martin et al.'s[26] qualitative study examining consultation length and chronic illness in general practice found that physicians dominated the encounter (i.e. review of illness and treatment and provision of information). Only in consultations of 20 min and over was the patients' narrative—their unique experience of illness—revealed.

Thus, both narratives and qualitative inquiry provide a different perspective through which we can understand the role of time and the consultation. Future research should be encouraged to use multi-method approaches combining the best of both quantitative and qualitative methodologies.

Time and continuity

A discussion of time in primary care would be lacking if there was no mention of the relationship between time and continuity. The issue of time is embedded in the concept of continuity of care in that continuity is longitudinal, with care being delivered over time, and within the context of a long-term relationship between patient and physician. McWhinney[46] describes continuity as the connection between doctor and patient, describing it as the interpersonal relationship that develops between a patient and physician over time. Similarly, Loxterkamp[47] emphasizes the connection between time and continuity: 'Continuity of care . . . the words themselves emphasize the importance of a connected and unbroken course, of inherent qualities that continue without essential change in the lives of our patients and over the course of our careers'. Continuity of care is fully discussed in Chapter 7.6.

For older patients, in particular, continuity of care and length of the patient–physician relationship are important determinants of health. For example, Weiss and Blustein[48] found that older participants who had an extended relationship with their physicians had a decreased likelihood of hospitalization and lower costs of inpatient and outpatient care. Similarly, Wasson et al.[49] concluded that older patients who had been randomized to receive provider continuity of care had fewer emergency admissions and a shorter average length of stay than those who did not receive continuity of care. Thus, taking time with this population, through a longitudinal relationship, may result in better patient outcomes and reduced costs to the health care system.

The future

There is no debate that health care systems around the globe are at a critical juncture in relation to the issue of time. Still in question are: how much time is enough; which patients require more time; and how to remunerate adequately this expenditure of medical resources.

Future research on time and the consultation faces several methodological challenges. Securing a representative sample may be difficult as physicians agreeing to participate in studies about consultation length may reflect a biased sample. The greatest challenge, however, may be the method used to measure consultation length. Patients' and physicians' self-reports of consultation length may be inaccurate. Physicians may spend considerable time on non-clinical activities such as note-keeping or other administrative activities. Noteworthy is Stange et al.'s[7] finding that the average consultation length they directly observed in primary care was 10 min—6 min shorter than the consultation length of visits provided by physician self-report in the NAMCS data. Therefore, the most accurate measure of consultation length is direct observation of the actual encounter between the patient and physician.[7,12] This can be achieved through various means including direct observation where a third person sits in on the interview or views it through a one-way mirror. Audio- or videotaping the encounter is less intrusive and more amenable to subsequent analysis. However, these methods are more labour-intensive and expensive.

Another important issue in examining the impact of time on the patient–physician consultation is the context of the encounter. Context, in this sense, refers to outpatient versus inpatient care, as well as fee-for-service versus capitated systems. The clinical setting may dictate the amount of time available for the visit. Primary care physicians are in a position to build on the interaction over multiple encounters suggesting that future research needs to examine a series of consultations as well as individual isolated encounters, hence acknowledging the connection between time and continuity.[50]

Time and the consultation remains a controversial issue. More detailed and rigorous studies, using both qualitative and quantitative methods, such as the work by Gross et al.,[24] Zyzanski et al.,[23] and Stange et al.,[7] will contribute to this debate and further our understanding of patients' and physicians' experiences of time and the consultation.

References

1. **Westcott, R.** (1977). The length of consultations in general practice. *Journal of the Royal College of General Practitioners* **27**, 552–5.
2. **Hughes, D.** (1983). Consultation length and outcome in two group general practice. *Journal of the Royal College of General Practitioners* **33**, 143–7.
3. **Hull, F.M. and Hull, F.S.** (1984). Time and the general practitioner: the patient's view. *Journal of the Royal College of General Practitioners* **34**, 71–5.
4. **Andersson, S.O. and Mattsson, B.** (1989). Length of consultations in general practice in Sweden: views of doctors and patients. *Family Practice* **6**, 130–4.
5. **Andersson, S.O., Ferry, S., and Mattsson, B.** (1993). Factors associated with consultation length and characteristics of short and long consultations. *Scandinavian Journal of Primary Health Care* **11**, 61–7.
6. **Mechanic, D., McAlpine, D.D., and Rosenthal, M.** (2001). Are patients' office visits with physicians getting shorter? *New England Journal of Medicine* **344**, 198–204.
7. **Stange, K.C.** et al. (1998). Illuminating the 'black box'. A description of 4454 patient visits to 138 family physicians. *Journal of Family Practice* **46**, 377–89.
8. **Howie, J.G.** et al. (1991). Long to short consultation ratio: a proxy measure of quality of care for general practice. *British Journal of General Practice* **41**, 48–54.
9. **Gordon, G.H., Baker, L., and Levinson, W.** (1995). Physician–patient communication in managed care. *Western Journal of Medicine* **163**, 527–31.
10. **Stafford, R.S.** et al. (1999). Trends in adult visits to primary care physicians in the United States. *Archives of Family Medicine* **8**, 26–32.
11. **Blumenthal, D.** et al. (1999). The duration of ambulatory visits to physicians. *Journal of Family Practice* **48**, 264–71.
12. **Wiggers, J.H. and Sanson-Fisher, R.** (1997). Duration of general practice consultations: association with patient occupational and educational status. *Social Science and Medicine* **44**, 925–34.
13. **Henbest, R.J. and Fehrsen, G.S.** (1992). Patient-centredness: is it applicable outside the west? Its measurement and effect on outcome. *Family Practice* **9**, 311–17.
14. **Little, P.** et al. (2001). Preferences of patients for patient centred approach to consultation in primary care: observational study. *British Medical Journal* **322**, 468–72.
15. **Stewart, M., Brown, J.B., and Weston, W.** (1989). Patient-centred interviewing III: five provocative questions. *Canadian Family Physician* **35**, 159–61.
16. **Roland, M.O.** et al. (1986). The 'five minute' consultation: effect of time constraint on verbal communication. *British Medical Journal* **292**, 874–6.
17. **Marvel, M.K., Doherty, W.J., and Weiner, E.** (1998). Medical interviewing by exemplary family physicians. *Journal of Family Practice* **47**, 343–8.
18. **Arborelius, E. and Bremberg, S.** (1992). What can doctors do to achieve a successful consultation? Videotaped interviews analysed by the 'consultation map' method. *Family Practice* **9**, 61–6.
19. **Greenfield, S.** et al. (1988). Patients' participation in medical care: effects on blood sugar control and quality of life in diabetes. *Journal of General Internal Medicine* **3**, 448–57.
20. **Marvel, M.K.** (1993). Involvement with the psychosocial concerns of patients. Observations of practicing family physicians on a university faculty. *Archives of Family Medicine* **2**, 629–33.
21. **Williams, M. and Neal, R.D.** (1998). Time for a change? The process of lengthening booking intervals in general practice. *British Journal of General Practice* **48**, 1783–6.
22. **Morrell, D.C.** et al. (1986). The 'five minute' consultation: effect of time constraint on clinical content and patient satisfaction. *British Medical Journal* **292**, 870–3.
23. **Zyzanski, S.J.** et al. (1998). Trade-offs in high-volume primary care practice. *Journal of Family Practice* **46**, 397–402.
24. **Gross, D.A.** et al. (1998). Patient satisfaction with time spent with their physician. *Journal of Family Practice* **47**, 133–7.
25. **Herman, J.** (1997). Three unhurried consultations. *Journal of Family Practice* **44**, 313–15.
26. **Martin, C.M.** et al. (1999). Consultation length and chronic illness care in general practice: a qualitative study. *Medical Journal of Australia* **171**, 77–81.
27. **Carr-Hill, R.** et al. (1998). Do minutes count? Consultation lengths in general practice. *Journal of Health Services & Research Policy* **3**, 207–13.

28. **Jacobson, L.D., Wilkinson, C., and Owen, P.A.** (1994). Is the potential of teenage consultations being missed? a study of consultation times in primary care. *Family Practice* **11**, 296–9.
29. **Martin, C.M.** et al. (1997). Characteristics of longer consultations in Australian general practice. *Medical Journal of Australia* **167**, 76–9.
30. **Tocher, T.M. and Larson, E.B.** (1999). Do physicians spend more time with non-English-speaking patients? *Journal of General Internal Medicine* **14**, 303–9.
31. **Rivadeneyra, R.** et al. (2000). Patient centredness in medical encounters requiring an interpreter. *The American Journal of Medicine* **108**, 470–4.
32. **Mawardi, B.H.** (1979). Satisfactions, dissatisfactions, and causes of stress in medical practice. *Journal of the American Medical Association* **241**, 1483–6.
33. **Grol, R.** et al. (1985). Work satisfaction of general practitioners and the quality of patient care. *Family Practice* **2**, 128–35.
34. **Wilson, A.** et al. (1991). Longer booking intervals in general practice: effects on doctors; stress and arousal. *British Journal of General Practice* **41**, 184–7.
35. **Wilson, A.** (1985). Consultation length: general practitioners' attitudes and practices. *British Medical Journal* **290**, 1322–4.
36. **Levinson, W.** et al. (1997). Physician–patient communication. The relationship with malpractice claims among primary care physicians and surgeons. *Journal of the American Medical Aassociation* **277**, 553–9.
37. **Groenewegen, P.P. and Hutten, J.B.** (1991). Workload and job satisfaction among general practitioners: a review of the literature. *Social Science and Medicine* **32**, 1111–19.
38. **Arborelius, E. and Thakker, K.D.** (1995). Why is it so difficult for general practitioners to discuss alcohol with patients? *Family Practice* **12**, 419–22.
39. **Beckman, H.B. and Frankel, R.M.** (1984). The effect of physician behavior on the collection of data. *Annals of Internal Medicine* **101**, 692–6.
40. **Wilson, A.** et al. (1992). Health promotion in the general practice consultation: a minute makes a difference. *British Medical Journal* **304**, 227–30.
41. **Wilson, A.** (1989). Extending appointment length—the effect in one practice. *Journal of the Royal College of General Practitioners* **39**, 24–5.
42. **Ridsdale, L.** et al. (1989). Study of the effect of time availablity on the consultation. *Journal of the Royal College of General Practitioners* **39**, 488–91.
43. **Borkan, J.** et al. *Patients and Doctors. Life Changing Stories from Primary Care.* Madison WI: University of Wisconsin Press, 1999.
44. **Greenhalgh, T. and Hurwitz, B.** *Narrative Based Medicine. Dialogue and Discourse in Clinical Practice.* London: BMJ Books, 1998.
45. **McWilliam, C.L., Brown, J.B., and Stewart, M.** (2000). Breast cancer patients' experiences of patient-doctor communication: a working relationship. *Patient Education & Counseling* **39**, 191–204.
46. **McWhinney, I.** (1982). Continuity of care. *Journal of Family Practice* **15**, 847–8.
47. **Loxterkamp, D.** (1991). Being there: on the place of the family physician. *Journal of American Board of Family Practice* **4**, 354–60.
48. **Weiss, L.J. and Blustein, J.** (1996). Faithful patients: the effect of long-term physician–patient relationships on the cost and use of healthcare by older Americans. *American Journal of Public Health* **86**, 1742–7.
49. **Wasson, J.H., Sauvigne, A.E., and Mogielnicki, R.P.** (1984). Continuity of outpatient medical care in elderly men. A randomized trial. *Journal of the American Medical Association* **252**, 2413–17.
50. **Gray, D.P.** (1998). Forty-seven minutes a year for the patient. *British Journal of General Practice* **48** (437) 1816–17.

5.7 Computers in the consultation

Michael Richard Kidd

Introduction

Welcome to the Computer Age. Advances in information technology and communications are impacting on the traditional ways we deliver service in primary health care. While many of our patients are embracing new technologies, many clinicians are distinctly uncomfortable with the rate of change. Yet, good information management and improved communication offer the opportunity to significantly enhance the quality of care delivered by primary health practitioners around the world.

In this chapter, we will explore how access to a computer in the consultation is changing our knowledge, our skills, and our attitudes as primary health care providers, as well as the impact on our relationship with patients and their changing expectations.

Given the pace of change in this field, it is likely that some of the concepts presented will become outdated in a very short time. Trying to predict future developments in information technology is fraught with peril. If you are reading this chapter in 2005 or beyond, please accept this as an historical discussion and try not to laugh too hard at the outmoded notions that follow.

It is also very difficult to quantify the current clinical usage of computers in consultations. While some clinicians in a number of countries have full electronic medical records and are moving towards embracing the concept of 'The Paperless Practice',[1] others use their computers for one or more of a variety of clinical purposes. These include, among others, word processing reports and referral letters, electronic prescribing and medication management, decision support in chronic disease management, recall and prompting about preventive care interventions, access to electronic information resources, electronic connectivity to pathology and other service providers, and data collection and reporting to meet government requirements or financial imperatives.

Rates of computer use in primary care consultations also vary significantly between countries. While general practitioners in countries such as the United Kingdom, the Netherlands, New Zealand, and the nations of Scandinavia have been early adopters, many colleagues in other parts of the world, and especially the United States of America, are still to adopt clinical computerization in large numbers. Interestingly, there are clinicians in some developing parts of the world who have embraced the use of the computer in the consultation to a greater extent than their peers in some of the most developed nations.

Changes in knowledge and access to information

The breadth of clinical knowledge necessary for safe, competent, and current primary health care delivery is ever expanding. Most clinicians now accept that we cannot carry all the facts we need in our heads. A cultural shift is evident as clinicians seek current information based on the best available evidence, attempt to access current clinical guidelines and treatment protocols, and look for answers to clinical questions arising during the consultation.

It is no coincidence that the culture of Evidence-Based Medicine has emerged at the same time as the Information Technology Revolution and especially at the time when the world's information resources have become available to everybody through the Internet. Computers provide possible solutions to many of the challenges posed by the advocates of evidence-based medicine. They have the potential to assist us in planning the management of our patients, in coordination of their care, in provision of our own continuing education, and in the process of accessing the findings of clinical research. Computer-based assistance has the potential to make us more efficient and effective health care providers if used carefully in the consultation.[2] Information technology has the potential to be the cornerstone of the delivery of evidence-based health care.

As clinical computer use in general practice becomes more widespread, evidence of quality benefits has begun to emerge. This is a slow process and many benefits will not be fully evident until widespread adoption of clinical computerization and electronic connectivity has taken place, and until clinical software reaches a level of maturity in matching the immediate clinical needs and information requirements of primary health care providers. Nevertheless, early systematic reviews of trials of the effects of computer-based clinical decision support systems on physician performance have demonstrated improvements in antibiotic prescribing, drug dosing, preventive care, and other core components of primary medical care in a variety of different clinical settings.[3–7]

The Internet has also arrived at the same time that health consumers are starting to seriously question the traditional doctor–patient relationship and to take a greater role in the management of their own health care needs.[8–10] If general practitioners are to continue to be the trusted cornerstone of health care delivery, they need to start to adapt to the changing expectations of their patients and their use of the Internet to seek knowledge about their health care options.

Soon patients may be able to select their preferred primary health care provider through the use of the Internet. At least one USA site offers a review of doctors in categories such as postgraduate education, accreditation status, and experience.[11] The potential use of such systems appears to be highest among younger people and those who are seeking a new doctor for reasons such as moving city or the development of a new health concern.

Perhaps some patients may believe that they will be able to dispense with their doctors completely and instead consult with an online medical advisor. At the moment, most online doctor services provide only text-based answers to questions posed and paid for by health consumers. However, online teleconsultations across international boundaries may become the norm soon. There may be a demand for doctors with a good teleconsulting manner. Perhaps being photogenic will become more important than clinical competence and qualifications. Eventually, agent-based technology may allow for the use of intelligent Internet-based animated figures, endowed with an individual doctor's personality, quirks, and wisdom, which will dispense sound advice on that doctor's behalf to their patients while the doctor carries out other work or recreational activities.

The idea of teleconsulting is very challenging and already some of the early adopters of this innovative way of working are suffering under a rapidly growing workload that is usually not reimbursed and can lead to increased patient irritation if there are delayed response times to requests.

A wealth of health knowledge is now available through the Internet; however, our patients need to be wary. In the words of the information technology visionary Nicholas Negroponte, 'On the Internet, no-one need know you're a dog'.[12] Anyone can establish a website on a health-related topic and claim to be a local or international expert. The Internet is littered with potentially dangerous sites offering dubious health advice. Cyberquackery is alive and well. And so is cyberchondria with many people using the web as the first step to determine possible causes of their worrying symptoms and seeking cures for as yet undiagnosed health problems.

Many consumer groups, medical organizations, and professional bodies offer Internet portals with links to sites of health information that they have evaluated and believe will be of benefit to their members and other visitors to their own site. There may well be a place for the homepage of an individual general practice to become the portal to useful and validated information on the Internet for the patients who attend that practice. One recent online survey showed that 50 per cent of online users would be interested in using a website operated by their own doctor's office.[13] Indeed, many doctors have started to develop and promote their own websites as a first step in engaging their patients online. But visitors still need to be wary. A few clicks and a patient can leave a validated site and start surfing into questionable territory.

The Internet also provides potential access to information about available health services. This will be particularly valuable to the primary health care provider who is responsible for the referral of patients to other suitable services. Internet-based databases of local health service providers and virtual hospitals can assist doctors to locate suitable and affordable resources for their patients. Such resources can also provide information about waiting lists, readmission rates, wound infection rates, and even allow the development of 'league table' ratings of one health care service or hospital against another.

Changes in skills

The computer era poses a challenge for many existing health care professionals and especially for those who belong to 'The Lost Generation'.[14] This includes those who missed out on learning about information technology as part of their primary, secondary, and tertiary education, and who are as yet unable to retire to escape the anticipated impending technological onslaught in the clinical workplace.

Many clinicians find computers an unnecessary imposition in the workplace and a challenge to their traditional delivery of health care. Clinicians lacking computer literacy may feel threatened by the skills of their younger clinical colleagues, their students, and their own children. At the same time, they may feel they lack the time offered to the retired members of their communities who often show remarkable prowess at surfing the Internet to find their own health-related information and then confront their health care providers with their findings.

Yet, most clinicians hovering between adolescence and senescence now appear to accept that advances in information technology can offer significant potential benefits for the delivery of higher quality health care services. The Internet has made medical information resources easily available to everybody. Like their patients, and the next generation of health care professionals, current clinicians should be poised to reap the benefits of this technology. Clinicians in both developed and developing parts of the world are becoming more comfortable with the use of the Internet at home and with the concept of the use of computer technology in the workplace.

Many general practitioners express feelings of fear and inadequacy when confronted with the possibility of imposed computer use in the consulting room. The implementation of information technology into clinical areas needs to be accompanied by appropriate programmes of staff training. Strategies are needed to educate clinicians about the use of information technology in clinical practice, demonstrating its value, and promoting its benefits. As well as education it is important to remember that most clinicians will also need technical support to allow them to focus on their major priority, the provision of clinical care.

Rapid obsolescence of current technology is another significant concern for many health care workers. However, what is important is perhaps not the actual technology itself but the change in belief that technological advances can improve the quality of aspects of clinical care and a preparedness to attempt to incorporate these changes into daily routine.

Many health care professionals find current education about the use of computers in health care can be dry and not very appealing, especially if the emphasis is on the technology itself, rather than its applications in clinical care. Working through clinical scenarios and identifying the information issues and their personal implications for learners may be a far more effective education strategy.[15] It has been argued that much education about information technology for health care workers requires a three-pronged approach.[16] Clinicians need to learn *about* computers (i.e. their potential applications in health care). They need to learn *through* computers (i.e. how to use the technology to receive their continuing education). Most powerfully, they need to learn *with* computers (i.e. through using this technology as part of their daily work, and through using its features to assist them to identify and meet their educational needs while on the job).

The National Health Service in the United Kingdom has produced recommendations for health informatics training in the education of their clinicians.[17] These recommendations identify common elements across clinical practice relevant to all health care workers and provide advice on education strategies. The eight elements addressed are communication, knowledge management, data quality and management, confidentiality and security, secondary uses of clinical data and information, clinical and service audit, working clinical systems, and telemedicine and telecare. The recommendations also provide a list of 10 basic computing skills that are required by all health care professionals. A more clinically targeted list of essential clinical informatics skills[18] has also been recommended for health care professionals. Together, these recommendations could form the basis for an informatics education curriculum for primary health care clinicians.

There is, however, a danger in thinking that one-off education will provide all the skills that a doctor will require to use information technology in a clinical setting for the rest of her or his career. Ongoing programmes of education, training, and support will be required as technology advances and new software becomes available, and as the demands of patients for protection of the privacy of their health information grows at the same time as potential risks to the security of computer-based data become more apparent.

One of the ways to encourage clinician use of the computer in the consultation is to provide tools which are directly relevant to each doctor–patient interaction and which have instant benefits for clinician and consumer.

Decision support tools to benefit electronic medication management have been used successfully to introduce the computer into the consultation in Australian General Practice. In 1998, less than 10 per cent of Australia's general practitioners were using a computer for clinical applications. By 2001, over 80 per cent were using electronic prescribing.[19] Most Australians now receive a computer-generated prescription from their general practitioner. The decision support software embedded in the computer prescribing software conducts a check when a new medication is being prescribed and alerts the doctor to any potential interactions with the patient's other medications, or contraindications with their other listed health problems. It also provides alerts if the patient may be pregnant or breastfeeding, and ensures that the new medication is not a member of a class of drugs to which the patient is recorded to have known allergies. This is quality use of medicines in action.

In addition, during autumn and winter, Australia's general practitioners have been reminded by their prescribing software of the need to immunize their aged population against influenza each time people over 65, or over 55 for indigenous Australians, have presented to the surgery. This is population health in action and the first of many major initiatives sure to come to improve preventive care intervention rates through general practice.

These are early examples of decision support tools being used to assist doctors in clinical care. The potential for this area to grow is huge. Already some doctors are receiving online pathology and radiology results, using CD-ROM and Internet-based clinical guidelines and education resources on the management of chronic disease, developing individual immunization requirements using electronic travel medicine advice, plotting the vital signs and key pathology findings of individual patients over time. The list goes on and on. As more and more information is entered into the computer on the doctor's desk, there is more potential for decision support tools to be used to assist in improving the quality of care.

Taking computer-based patient information out of the consulting room is another challenge. The potential now exists for sharing personalized health information with health care providers across the rest of a nation's health service. The shared electronic health record will reveal new challenges in data management. Computerized data can be lost just like paper-based data, especially if different aspects of an individual's record are to be stored in a number of separate databases.

General practitioners will require mobile access to information when they are on home visits or attending patients in hospitals or nursing homes. Handheld technology through Personal Digital Assistants (PDAs) is starting to have an impact in health care. Already hospital resident staff are experimenting with the use of PDAs. It will be fascinating to observe how this technology is adapted to the needs of primary health care.

New skills will also be required for dealing with electronic communication with patients. It is becoming apparent that many patients would like to communicate with their doctors online. Many patients would probably be pleased to e-mail their general practitioners in their clinics, particularly in following up the results of pathology and radiology tests or with follow-up questions following a consultation.

This poses additional challenges to the doctor–patient relationship. Just as general practitioners have had to develop a method for handling telephone-based consultations with patients, they will also have to develop ways of handling requests for information received via the Internet. This raises significant issues about the security of personalized health information discussed using e-mail. Until general practitioners are convinced that adequate safeguards are in place they need to be very cautious about such developments.

However, these developments may also revolutionize health care delivery. In the place of discrete episodic visits to the doctor, contact and management advice may be able to be delivered in a continuous and ongoing manner. This could become a very powerful clinical tool when the ability for home monitoring and Internet-based transmission of vital signs and home pathology results is also added. The role of the general practitioner could become even more central in the management of many chronic health care problems. True continuity of care becomes a reality as computer systems allows primary medical care providers to keep track of their patients' clinical care on a daily or even more frequent basis.

General practitioners may soon also start to spam their patients with useful health information and electronic recall reminders. This could represent a method of direct promotion of their clinical services. However, it could also become a way of reminding members of their own patient populations about the need to adopt a healthy lifestyle, and to undertake regular health checks and interventions for preventable conditions, and that their prescription for a continuing medication is about to expire and that it is time for another visit.

The Internet represents a serious challenge to traditional method of clinical care delivery. If general practitioners do not meet their patients' expectations and start to provide Internet-based medical services, others surely will.

Changes in attitudes

Attitudes are changing towards the use of a computer in the consultation. There is growing acceptance of the use of information technology for clinical purposes among many primary health care providers. And there are growing expectations that this technology will be used in primary medical care among patients, policy makers, and health care managers. The information technology industry also sees health care as a very large and important market for their products and ongoing developments.

Health care systems around the world are becoming progressively more consumer-focused. Patients expect their health care providers to have accurate, up-to-date, and accessible medical records. They also require that their personal electronic health information is being protected by high-level privacy and security safeguards.[20] It is essential that primary health care providers pay close attention to privacy issues. If we allow breaches of privacy, we risk losing the great trust that our patients currently have in us. We are a long way from being able to accept a statement like 'Trust me, I'm a computer'.

Patients are also challenging their general practitioners with evolving attitudes towards their own health records. At the moment, many patients desire access to the information their doctors have collected over time and stored in their individual medical records. I can see a time approaching when consumers actually assume total control over their own personalized health information and when we, the providers, will have to seek the permission of our patients to access any aspect of their records, including the information we contributed to the record.

One of the more recent challenges for general practitioners is the patient who presents with information gained from a search of the Internet. This seems to be particularly relevant for people with chronic health problems who may have a degree of dissatisfaction with some aspect of their current health care management. It may surprise some general practitioners to know that many of their patients believe they know more about their chronic health problem than their doctors.

The pharmaceutical industry is, of course, well ahead of many other groups in the use of the Internet for product promotion. The Internet enables the user to cross international boundaries and bypass local laws restricting direct advertising of products to consumers. It is apparent that the Internet will increasingly be used by pharmaceutical companies for delivering direct-to-consumer advertising.

An approach to the person who arrives with information gained from the Internet is to try to determine why this person has really brought this information today. Do not get angry and imagine an implied lack of trust in your judgement or knowledge. Do not get stressed and wonder when you will have the time to absorb scads of computer printouts. Do not feel threatened by your patient's assumption that he or she knows more than you do because, after all, he or she is the expert in their own response to their own health problems. Do try to discover what concerns have led to this fact-finding mission.

Try to adopt an open approach and gather some key information:

> Thank you for sharing this information with me. I'd like to ask what did you find most useful in this article? How do you see this as being relevant to you? Are there any issues that this article raises which you would like to discuss with me? As a result of reading this article, what do you think we should do?

Of course, as clinicians we need to also accept that not all our patients will be comfortable with computers and the use of the Internet. We must be prepared to deal with a wide variety of patients with a wide variety of knowledge and skills and attitudes. This is nothing new in our discipline. As always flexibility in communication is very important in primary health care.

Conclusion

Many concerns remain about the impact of the computer in the consultation. Some doctors are concerned about the impact of computer use on communication with their patients. Many nations are addressing widespread concerns about privacy and confidentiality and levels of patient acceptance. The quality of the software being utilized in some primary care settings has caused concern. The quality and appropriateness of some of the data sources being utilized in decision support software still need to be verified.

This is the beginning of a new era of health care. This is an era of shared responsibility for decision-making, with the health consumer as the rightful centre of attention in the management of their own health concerns, and with access to health information by health care providers and consumers alike. The role of general practitioners is increasingly to assist their patients to interpret what information they have found and to determine how this information applies to them as individuals. The challenge we face as primary medical care providers is to determine how we might use this information together with our patients to provide better health care outcomes for the people who trust us for their health care advice.

Key points

1. Rates of computer use in primary care consultations vary significantly between countries.
2. Computers provide possible solutions to many of the challenges posed by the advocates of evidence-based medicine.
3. The Internet has also arrived at the same time that health consumers are starting to seriously question the traditional doctor–patient relationship and to take a greater role in the management of their own health care needs.
4. Strategies are needed to educate clinicians about the use of information technology in clinical practice, demonstrating its value and promoting its benefits.
5. Many concerns remain about the impact of the computer in the consultation.

Acknowledgement

This paper draws on previous work of the author published in *Australian Family Physician*[10] and the *Medical Journal of Australia.*[14]

References

1. **Ellis, N.** *Going Paperless: A Guide to Computerisation in Primary Care.* Abingdon, Oxon: Radcliffe Medical Press, 2001.
2. **Purves, I.N.** (1996). Facing future challenges in general practice: a clinical method with computer support. *Family Practice* **13** (6), 536–43.
3. **Pestonik, S.L., Classen, D.C., Scott Evans, R., and Burke, J.P.** (1996). Implementing antibiotic practice guidelines through computer-assisted decision support: clinical and financial outcomes. *Annals of Internal Medicine* **124** (10), 884–90.
4. **Sullivan, F. and Mitchell, E.** (1995). Has general practitioner computing made a difference to patient care? A systematic review of published reports. *General Practice* **311**, 848–52.
5. **Balas, E.A., Weingarten, S., Garb, C.T., Blumenthal, D., Boren S.A., and Brown, G.D.** (2000). Improving preventive care by prompting physicians. *Archives of Internal Medicine* **160**, 301–8.
6. **Bates, D.W.** et al. (1999). The impact of computerized physician order entry on medication error prevention. *Journal of the American Medical Informatics Association* **6**, 313–21.
7. **Hunt, D.L., Haynes, R.B., Hanna, S.E., and Smith, K.** (1998). Effects of computer-based clinical decision support systems on physician performance and patient outcomes—a systematic review. *Journal of the American Medical Association* **280**, 1339–46.
8. **Jadad, A.R.** (1999). Promoting partnerships: challenges for the internet age. *British Medical Journal* **319**, 761–4.
9. **Eysenbach, G.** (2000). Consumer health informatics. *British Medical Journal* **320**, 1713–15.
10. **Kidd, M.R.** (2001). General practice on the Internet. *Australian Family Physician* **4**, 359–61.
11. www.healthgrades.com
12. **Negroponte, N.** *Being Digital.* Knopf, 1995.
13. **Pyke, B.** The rise of the Internet health consumer: impacts of the Internet on the doctor–patient relationship (www.cyberdialogue.com/pdfs/white_papers/wp-cch-1999-doctors.pdf).
14. **Kidd, M.R. and McPhee, W.** (1999). The 'lost generation': IT education for healthcare professionals. *Medical Journal of Australia* **171**, 510–11.
15. **Approaches for informatics in postgraduate medical and dental education: an account from four national pilot sites.** National Health Service Education and Training Program in Information Management and Technology for Clinicians, 1997.
16. **Koschmann, T.** (1995). Medical education and computer literacy: learning about, through, and with computers. *Academic Medicine* **70** (9), 818–21.
17. **NHS.** Learning to manage health information. National Health Service Executive, 1999, Bristol, UK (www.enablingpp.exec.nhs.uk).
18. **Coiera, E.** (1998). Medical informatics meets medical education. *Medical Journal of Australia* **168**, 319–20.
19. http://www.gpcg.org/topics/pip.html.
20. **Rigby, M., Forsstrom, J., Roberts, R., and Wyatt, J.** (2001). Information in practice: verifying quality and safety in health informatics services. *British Medical Journal* **323**, 552–6.

Further reading

www.globalfamilydoctor.com (Website of WONCA, The World Organization of Family Doctor, featuring links to many useful resources for primary medical care providers).

www.gpcg.org (Website of the General Practice Computing Group, the peak national organization for primary medical care computing in Australia featuring resources targeted to the needs of general practitioners involved in the computerization of the consultation).

www.imia.org (Website of the International Medical Informatics Association with links to resources which promote informatics in health care and biomedical research).

www.phcsg.org.uk (Website of The Primary Health Care Specialist Group of the British Computer Society with a link to *The Journal of Primary Care Informatics*).

www.amia.org (Website of the American Medical Informatics Association with links to *The Journal of the American Medical Informatics Association*, a peer-reviewed journal published bi-monthly containing articles about all aspects of medical informatics).

6

Diagnosis and decision-making

6 Diagnosis and decision-making

6.1 Undifferentiated illness and uncertainty in diagnosis and management

Geert-Jan Dinant

Introduction

Most patients prefer a doctor who is kind, patient, omniscient, and confident of his or her diagnoses and the information he or she provides. However, such doctors are rare. Being kind and patient can be learned, but knowing everything and always being certain about the right diagnosis and best treatment is practically impossible. The reason is that there is simply too much knowledge and scientific evidence to remember, and that such knowledge and evidence change too fast, while at the same time the available evidence, in particular, regarding diagnosis and management in daily general practice, may be lacking or not applicable.(1) Another reason is that general practitioners are frequently consulted by patients in the early and as yet undifferentiated stages of diseases, who present with complaints that may reflect a great variety of diseases.(2) Thirdly, patients in everyday general practice tend to present with complaints that reflect combinations of organic and psychosomatic origins; some of these combinations of complaints have not been described in the literature and little evidence on effective management is available. As a result, uncertainty is a part of daily life in general practice.

This chapter discusses the nature and content of this uncertainty, and the way in which general practitioners tend to deal with it. Between 'vague' complaints, presented by the patient to the general practitioner, and being uncertain as a doctor, certain aspects of uncertainty can be distinguished: unexplained complaints, ill-defined complaints, ill-defined dieases, uncertain diagnoses, and uncertain management. Each of these aspects is discussed below.

Vague or unexplained?

Complaints that do not allow a diagnostic conclusion are often called 'vague'. In the patient's view, however, complaints are rarely vague. His or her pain or fatigue is real, despite difficulties in expressing their nature or explaining the exact location in the body, or the disabilities they cause in everyday life. It is the doctor's problem that he or she cannot produce an explanation that fits into existing and widely used diagnostic or therapeutic models or categories. Such complaints, therefore, deserve the adjective 'medically unexplained' (hereafter 'unexplained') rather than 'vague'.

Doctors may feel uncomfortable with patients presenting with unexplained complaints. One reason is the risk that unexplained complaints can be the first symptoms of serious or even life-threatening diseases, including malignancies, severe infections, or cardiovascular events, and that, in the doctor's view, early diagnosis might prevent unnecessary, prolonged suffering, or a fatal outcome. It is for these reasons that doctors tend to fear missing the correct diagnosis. Furthermore, telling a patient that 'To my regret, I cannot find the cause of your complaint', seems contrary to how they experience the impact of their work. During their years in medical school, they were trained in detecting and treating diseases rather than in dealing with uncertainty. The result is that they often order laboratory and radiological testing for such patients, despite relatively high probabilities of normal results, or of coincidently finding abnormalities that do not relate to the complaints presented. In the end, this may lead to a cascade of diagnostic interventions and referrals, leaving both the patient and the doctor frustrated and worried.(3–6)

Unexplained or ill-defined?

Unexplained complaints are common in daily general practice, but their exact frequency is not well established (estimates vary from 10 to 20 per cent across all reasons for encounter). It is unclear what kind of complaints other than fatigue, dizziness, and pain are most often seen as unexplained.(7–10) One cause of this frequent occurrence is that it is particularly the general practitioner who sees the early, less-developed stages of diseases. Furthermore, out of a wide variety of complaints presented, only a small proportion predicts the presence of a particular disease, while other complaints have a familial or social background.(11) It has been found in the United States that in 50 per cent of the patients who visited their general practitioner, no somatic origin for the complaint could be established.(12) And in less than 70 per cent of the patients presenting to the general practitioner with (often unexplained) complaints for which, according to the general practitioner, determination of the erythrocyte sedimentation rate (ESR) was indicated, could a diagnosis be established in retrospect 3 months later.(13) It is unclear, however, whether the investigators were really unable to draw a diagnostic conclusion, or whether they simply could not find an accurate definition for their diagnostic findings.

The International Classification of Primary Care (ICPC) tried to solve these diagnostic problems by allowing the classification of individual complaints, for example, headache and fatigue.(14) The Dutch College of General Practitioners went a step further, by publishing the following definition of unexplained complaints: 'Complaints are unexplained when after adequate history taking and physical examination, taking psychological and social circumstances into account, no definite conclusion can be drawn'.(15) The relevant guideline advises general practitioners to refrain from blood tests for at least 4 weeks after the first presentation to the general practitioner of an unexplained complaint. If general practitioners do decide to investigate, they should limit themselves to the following four tests: determination of haemoglobin, blood glucose level, ESR, and thyroid-stimulating hormone. It remains to be determined whether this guideline is sufficiently evidence-based.

Ill-defined complaints or ill-defined diseases?

Most complaints can be fitted into the ICPC classification, whether or not they are explained. But what should we think about so-called ill-defined diseases? In the classical taxonomy, a disease is defined as a set of (closely) related signs or symptoms, with a specific aetiological background, a plausible physiological pathway, a predictable natural history, and the need for a specific therapy. In everyday general practice, however, such diseases are found only in a minority of the patients, for example, in those suffering from more classical and relatively uncommon infectious diseases, like tuberculosis.[16] Symptoms presented are often non-specific, or combinations of symptoms point into more than one diagnostic direction. Heart failure is a typical example of an increasingly common, multi-aetiological condition that requires active and proactive management by the general practitioner, but whose first symptoms are rather non-specific. It becomes even more complicated when several unspecific signs or symptoms are present together in one patient, allowing almost no aetiological or physiological explanation.[17,18] The increasing prevalence of these, often chronic, sets of complaints (or syndromes) has resulted in new diagnostic entities, like the chronic fatigue syndrome, fibromyalgia, irritable bowel syndrome, and repetitive strain injury.[19] Strictly speaking, none of these syndromes are diseases, and the fact that their definitions are no more than descriptive allows the conclusion that they are as yet ill-defined.

Uncertain diagnoses or uncertain management?

Unexplained complaints and ill-defined syndromes together form the group of uncertain diagnoses. More research is needed to improve understanding of the background and management of uncertain diagnoses, taking inter-cultural differences in their presentation and inter-doctor variability in their management into account. Until the results of this research are published, general practitioners will inevitably feel uncomfortable with uncertain diagnoses and tend to do what they can to relieve these feelings. The rationality of this uncertain management is often questionable, in particular, if doctors decide to order 'blindly' additional (laboratory or imaging) tests, whose predictive values are implicitly limited.

Not only the selection of tests, but also the interpretation of test results is a challenge for every general practitioner. Reference values for laboratory tests, for instance, are usually derived from setting borders around the 95 per cent of a non-diseased population in whom the test has been performed. This means that the probability of finding an abnormal test result without clinical significance is implicitly 5 per cent, or 2.5 per cent if a test can only cross the reference values in one direction. If two tests are done, there is a $2 \times 2.5 = 5$ per cent chance of finding at least one such falsely abnormal test result. Furthermore, since the probability that a patient presenting with an unexplained complaint is suffering from an as yet undetectable serious disease is low, a test needs to be normal in nearly all non-diseased people before its abnormal result can be trusted to indicate the presence of the suspected disease.[20,21] Only very few of the tests that are regularly done in general practice are able to discriminate so well. For example, anaemia was found to have a similar frequency in patients who do and those do not complain of fatigue,[22,23] and the ESR is often slightly elevated in patients without an infectious disease.[13]

However, it remains to be seen to what extent abnormal test results in patients presenting with unexplained complaints predict the presence of serious diseases in the long term. More research is needed to find the answer to this question, research that is complicated because it requires large groups of patients and long follow-up periods.[24,25] Such studies should also pay attention to the psychological background of complaints presented. Depression and anxiety disorders may very well be presented to the general practitioner in the guise of complaints that are difficult to explain at first sight, or that worry the patient much more than the doctor.

Uncertain management or uncertain doctors?

Ultimately, it is the doctor who plays the key role in managing uncertainty. Not surprisingly, the number of years in practice is related to the general practitioner's frequency of feeling uneasy or uncertain. Having seen more rare cases helps to detect the next case sooner, and, more importantly, to rule out the presence of a potentially harmful disease. Young doctors try to cope with diagnostic uncertainty by ordering more tests and doing more additional testing, and by more frequently reassessing the patient.[26] But fear of missing a diagnosis, or even fear of court cases, will always be present in the minds of general practitioners.[27–29] The doctor's fears, however, do not always match the patient's feelings.[30] The patient may very well be able to live with the doctor's conclusion that he or she does not (yet) know the diagnosis, or that the complaint presented does not even allow a diagnosis. Furthermore, treating the patient as a partner by taking sufficient time for a proper history-taking, including an exploration of the patient's fears and worries, and a good explanation of the doctor's conclusions, will help the patient to understand the doctor's uncertainty. In addition, general practitioners might use a more problem-solving approach, given that they have had some preliminary training in handling psychological therapy.[31]

Time and the opportunity for continuing care are very powerful diagnostic instruments in the hands of the general practitioner. Two studies have found that, of the patients consulting their general practitioners with non-acute abdominal pain, 68 per cent had recovered 1 year later,[32] while headaches were found to disappear within 4 weeks after presentation.[33] Comparable figures were found in patients who presented with unexplained somatic complaints at an outpatient clinic for internal medicine.[34] The presence of real 'pathology' becomes more manifest over time, because the patients will start to suffer more intensely and experience more related symptoms.[35] Waiting and reassessing the patient are, therefore, good diagnostic instruments, and general practitioners are experts in this approach.[36]

References

1. **Knottnerus, J.A. and Dinant, G.J.** (1997). Medicine-bases evidence, a prerequisite for evidence-based medicine. *British Medical Journal* **315**, 1109–10.
2. **Knottnerus, J.A.** (1991). Medical decision making by general practitioners and specialists. *Family Practice* **8**, 305–7.
3. **Dinant, G.J., Knottnerus, J.A., and Van Wersch, J.W.J.** (1992). Diagnostic impact of the erythrocyte sedimentation rate in general practice: a before–after analysis. *Family Practice* **9**, 28–31.
4. **van Hemert, A.M., Hengeveld, M.W., Bolk, J., Rooymans, H.G.M., and Vandenbroucke, J.P.** (1993). Psychiatric disorders in relation to medical illness among patients of a general medical out-patient clinic. *Psychological Medicine* **23**, 167–73.
5. **Kassirer, J.P.** (1989). Our stubborn request for diagnostic certainty: a cause of excessive testing. *New England Journal of Medicine* **320**, 1489–91.
6. **Putterman, C. and Ben-Chetrit, E.** (1995). Clinical problem solving. Testing, testing, testing. *New England Journal of Medicine* **333**, 1208–11.
7. **Flink, P., Sorensen, L., Engberg, M., Holm, M., and Munk-Jorgensen, P.** (1999). Somatisation in primary care. Prevalence, health care utilization, and general practitioner recognition. *Psychosomatics* **40**, 330–8.
8. **Katon, W.J. and Walker, E.A.** (1998). Medically unexplained symptoms in primary care. *Journal of Clinical Psychiatry* **59**, 15–21.
9. **Kroenke, K. and Mangelsdorff, D.** (1989). Common symptoms in ambulatory care: incidence, evaluation, therapy and outcome. *American Journal of Medicine* **86**, 262–6.
10. **Portegijs, P.J.M.** *Somatization in Frequent Attenders of General Practice; Determinants, Psychiatric Problems, Consequences for Every Day Life and Health Care Utilization.* Maastricht: Maastricht University, 1996.
11. **Firth, J. and Knowlden, S.** (1992). Undifferentiated illness. *Medical Journal of Australia* **156**, 472–6.

12. **Marple, R., Kroenke, K., Lucey, C., Wilder, J., and Lucas, C.** (1997). Concerns and expectations in patients presenting with physical complaints. *Archives of Internal Medicine* **157**, 1482–8.
13. **Dinant, G.J., Knottnerus, J.A., and Van Wersch, J.W.J.** (1991). Discriminating ability of the erythrocyte sedimentation rate: a prospective study in general practice. *British Journal of General Practice* **41**, 365–70.
14. **Lamberts, H. and Wood, M.** *ICPC: International Classification of Primary Care.* Oxford: Oxford University Press, 1987.
15. **Dinant, G.J.** et al. (1994). NHG-Standaard Bloedonderzoek. Huisartsen Wetenschap **37**, 202–11.
16. **McWhinney, I.** (1993). Why we need a new clinical method. *Scandinavian Journal of Primary Health Care* **11**, 3–7.
17. **Malteraud, K.** (1992). Women's undefined disorders—a challenge for clinical communication. *Family Practice* **9**, 299–302.
18. **Crombie, D., Cross, K., and Fleming, D.** (1992). The practice of diagnostic variability in general practice. *Journal of Epidemiology and Community Health* **46**, 447–54.
19. **Kroenke, K., Wood, R.D., Mmangelsdorff, A.D., Meier, N.J., and Powell, J.B.** (1988). Chronic fatigue in primary care: prevalence, patient characteristics and outcome. *Journal of the American Medical Association* **260**, 929–34.
20. **Owen, P.** (1995). Clinical practice and medical research: bridging the divide between the two cultures. *British Journal of General Practice* **45**, 557–60.
21. **Woolf, S.H. and Kamerov, D.B.** (1990). Testing for uncommon conditions: the heroic search for positive test results. *Archives of Internal Medicine* **150**, 2451–8.
22. **Knottnerus, J.A., Knipschild, P.G., Van Wersch, J.W.J., and Sijstermans, A.H.J.** (1986). Unexplained fatigue and hemoglobin, a primary care study. *Canadian Family Physician* **32**, 1601–4.
23. **Kenter, E.G.H. and Okkes, I.M.** Patients with fatigue in general practice; prevalence and treatment. *Nederlands Tijdschrift voor Geneeskunde* **143**, 796–801.
24. **Moran, J.** (2000). A plea for research on the epidemiology of symptoms—the key to earlier diagnosis of colorectal cancer. *European Journal of General Practice* **6**, 40–2.
25. **Summerton, N.** (2000). Diagnosis and general practice. *British Journal of General Practice* **50**, 995–1000.
26. **Calman, N., Hyman, R., and Licht, W.** (1992). Variability in consultation rates and practitioner level of diagnostic certainty. *British Journal of General Practice* **35**, 1.
27. **Gerrity, M.S., DeVillis, R.F., and Earp, J.A.** (1990). Physicians' reactions to uncertainty in patient care. *Medical Care* **28**, 724–36.
28. **Grol, R., Whitfield, M., De Maeseneer, J., and Mokkink, M.** (1990). Attitudes to risk taking in medical decision making among British, Dutch and Belgian general practitioners. *British Journal of General Practice* **40**, 134–6.
29. **Murtagh, J.** (1990). Common problems: a safe diagnostic strategy. *Australian Family Physician* **19**, 733–41.
30. **Williams, S., Weinman, J., Dale, J., and Newman, S.** (1995). Patient expectations: what do primary care patients want from the GP and how far does meeting expectations affect patient satisfaction? *Family Practice* **12**, 193–201.
31. **Wilkinson, P. and Mynors-Wallis, L.** (1994). Problem-solving therapy in the treatment of unexplained physical symptoms in primary care: a preliminary study. *Journal of Psychosomatic Research* **38**, 591–8.
32. **Muris, J., Starmans, R., Fijten, G., Crebolder, H., Krebber, T., and Knottnerus, J.** (1993). Abdominal pain in general practice. *Family Practice* **10**, 387–400.
33. **Lamberts, H. and Hofmans-Okkes, I.M.** (1993). The classification of psychological and social problems in general practice. *Huisarts en Wetenschap* **36**, 5–13.
34. **Speckens, A.E., van Hemert, A.M., Rooijmans, H.G., and Hengeveld, M.W.** (1996). Unexplained physical symptoms: outcome, utilization of medical care and associated factors. *Psychological Medicine* **26**, 745–52.
35. **Krakau, I.** (1991). Severity of illness and diagnoses in a Swedish general practice population. *Family Practice* **8**, 28–31.
36. **Rosser, W.** (1996). Approach to diagnosis by primary care clinicians and specialists: is there a difference? *Journal of Family Practice* **42**, 139–44.

6.2 Clinical diagnosis: hypothetico-deductive reasoning and other theoretical frameworks

Geert-Jan Dinant and Yvonne D. van Leeuwen

Introduction

Over the last two decades, considerable efforts have been made to increase our understanding of the 'black box' of diagnostic reasoning. Nevertheless, reaching a diagnostic conclusion to a certain extent remains a magic process. What medical students experience when they first observe doctors engaged in consultations, seems to them a rather illogical mixture of unrelated questions and random physical examinations. Yet the resulting diagnoses are usually much more accurate than those resulting from the more systematic history-taking and physical examinations done by medical students. This shift from following the books to efficiently finding the correct diagnosis has often been described as a three-step process:

1. generating a list of diagnostic hypotheses, given the problem presented by the patient;
2. imposing a hierarchy on the list, based on the likelihood of each hypothesis;
3. establishing a definite diagnostic conclusion, after excluding the hypotheses one by one.

The first and second steps involve a process of so-called *induction*, whereas the third step can be seen as a process of *deduction*, consisting of logical diagnostic reasoning on the basis of the results of history taking and physical and other (laboratory) examinations.[1,2] This is where the true art of medicine is found: knowledge and experience join forces.

This chapter intends to clarify what kind of information doctors use in establishing a diagnosis. Insight into this process may help them to improve the accuracy and efficiency of their diagnostic work. Moreover, it may facilitate the teaching of medical students on how to establish a diagnosis, and enable doctors to discuss their diagnostic conclusions with peers. The chapter discusses the above mentioned steps in more detail, using clinical examples to clarify the concepts behind them. For a proper understanding of the three phases, it is useful to describe the development of medical expertise first.

Development of medical expertise

Generating medical knowledge and making this knowledge applicable to everyday practice is a process in which four steps can be distinguished. During their first years in medical school, students store fragmented knowledge in their memories.[3] After some time, relationships between findings and diseases become clear, and they find out, for instance, that an elevated glucose level relates to the presence of diabetes. Once the student begins to wonder how insulin shortage relates to glucose levels, the second phase can start.

As a result of the increasing factual knowledge, the so-called 'if–then' type of reasoning gradually starts to develop during the second phase. For instance, *if* the release of insulin is reduced, *then* glucose levels rise, after which the elevated glucose levels result in glucosuria and hence in polyuria and thirst. This process establishes networks of knowledge and relates newly acquired knowledge to familiar networks. The frequent use of these networks leads to concentrated conglomerates of knowledge in the students' and doctors' minds. New cases or problems presented to them by patients will quickly be compared with those that have been committed to memory, and recognizing diagnostic patterns, rather than detailed diagnostic reasoning using basic pathophysiological knowledge, becomes a routine part of the students' and doctors' everyday work.[4,5]

During this third phase, the so-called 'illness scripts' gradually develop.[6] Doctors claim to need no more than a limited number of findings to recognize the presence of a certain disease. When asked to explain their hypotheses, doctors might say things like: 'Because her shoulder pain is combined with vaginal blood loss, she is most likely to have an extra-uterine pregnancy'. While illness scripts can still be traced back to the textbooks, it is only in everyday practice that doctors can become experienced in recognizing less typical presentations of diseases and infrequently found abnormal findings. As a result, their illness scripts become more varied and complex, and doctors become increasingly able to recognize exceptional cases. This process of optimizing the integration of knowledge and experience can be seen as a final and in fact never-ending phase in the development of medical expertise.[7,8]

Generating diagnostic hypotheses

Experienced doctors have no difficulty in listing the main origins of chest pain: angina pectoris, pulmonary embolism, herpes zoster, myalgia, and oesophagitis immediately cross their minds. In addition, they might consider the presence of a myocardial infarction, pericarditis, aortic aneurysm, pleuritis, neuralgia or non-somatic (psychological or social) problems. Thus, they scan all seven tracts found in this part of the body. Their list of hypotheses will be shorter when they are dealing with complaints that usually relate to no more than one or two tracts, such as dysuria or arthralgia. Proper knowledge of basic medical science, that is, anatomy and pathophysiology, is thus essential during this step.[9] However, further knowledge is needed if a hierarchy is to be imposed on the hypotheses.

Imposing a hierarchy on the diagnostic hypotheses

The process of assessing the individual probabilities of diseases being present involves three steps, in which the so-called contextual factors play a key role.[10] In the first step, the approach is based on known incidences of diseases. Such incidences differ between populations. In general practice, incidences of serious diseases are lower than among hospital populations, while in the hospital, specialists will less frequently see self-limiting, harmless conditions. These incidences are reflected in the predictive values of related signs and symptoms.[8] In general, the lower the incidence of a disease, the lower the probability that the presence of a related complaint predicts the presence of this particular disease. For example, in a general practice setting, pain located in one joint will more often relate to (temporary) overuse of the joint than to the presence of osteoarthritis, and in no more than a few cases does a cough predict the presence of pneumonia. In hospital and outpatient populations, the opposite is usually true.

The second step involves modifying the hierarchy on the basis of age and gender of the patient. Chest pain is more likely to be a sign of angina in a 60-year-old male patient than in a 40-year-old woman, in whom the same complaint might very well signal the presence of oesophagitis. In children up to 14 years of age, fatigue will, in 33 per cent of the cases, relate to diseases of the respiratory tract (mostly recurrent and chronic infections), whereas in the elderly it will often be a side effect of the use of medication. Most doctors are very well aware of these relationships between age, gender, and the likelihood of particular diseases. Medical students, however, will often relate a complaint to what they were taught in a recent lecture. As a result, AIDS or respiratory malignancies may end up high in their diagnostic hierarchies, even in patients not presenting other symptoms of these diseases.

In the third and final step, the hierarchy is adapted to the patient's medical and family history. Up to this stage, knowledge of *diseases* has determined the process of diagnostic reasoning, but now knowledge of the *diseased* is added. Apart from the diseases they sustained, social aspects of the patients' environment (family, job, etc.) and their personalities become important. Chest pain in a 40-year-old female patient who has an elevated cholesterol level and whose father died of a myocardial infarction will lead to a diagnostic hypothesis that differs very much from that in a 25-year-old woman who has three young children and has great trouble in bringing them up.

Establishing a definite diagnosis

After considering all diagnostic hypotheses and adapting their likelihoods to incidence rates, age, gender, medical and family history, and environmental factors, the doctor draws up a final diagnostic hierarchy, and the process of induction ends, while deduction starts. From here on, it becomes important to rule out, one by one, the various hypotheses and end up with the definite diagnosis. Five strategies can be distinguished in this final step of diagnostic reasoning: recognizing diagnostic patterns, using diagnostic algorithms, ruling in or ruling out a particular hypothesis, using a diagnostic dragnet and sequential hypothesis testing. The first three strategies are applicable to those cases in which no more than one or two diagnostic hypotheses have been established. The fourth and fifth strategies are used when a larger number of hypotheses are being considered. In reality, doctors will apply combinations of these five strategies or parts thereof. The more experienced a doctor is, the more sophisticated, efficient and effective these combinations become.

Recognizing diagnostic patterns

As explained above, diagnostic patterns are particularly used by experienced doctors.[11,12] A 70-year-old male patient suffering from fatigue and considerable weight loss, as well as a persistent cough, and having yellow-coloured stains on his fingers, will immediately make the doctor consider the possibility of lung cancer. The clinical picture is so clear that the results of further medical history taking and physical examination can hardly change the doctor's diagnostic hypothesis. Skin diseases in particular often allow doctors to establish a diagnosis at first sight. Furthermore, any experienced doctor immediately recognizes the smell of the breath of a child with tonsillitis, and he or she will quickly recognize the typical cough produced by a child suffering from laryngitis (even its sound over the telephone may be sufficient).

Using diagnostic algorithms

Algorithms, or decision trees, can be constructed around medical problems that lead to a limited number of diagnostic hypotheses and therapeutic possibilities, such as urinary tract infection and lumbosacral radicular syndrome.[13,14] One advantage of algorithms is that they may enable people who are not doctors, including practice nurses and nurse practitioners, to play a role in the management of a particular disease or condition. Highly structured algorithms are currently used in nurse-led telephone advice and diagnosis services in primary care in the United Kingdom and the Netherlands. Diagnostic algorithms are also used in rural settings in the third world and other remote areas.

In particular, algorithms unify the diagnostic and therapeutic reasoning applied by doctors and enable colleagues to follow each other's management, thus minimizing the occurrence of inefficient, ineffective, or even harmful inter-doctor variations in cure and care. However, complicated medical problems can be very difficult to summarize in an algorithm. Moreover, the necessary scientific evidence for developing algorithms is still lacking for many problems. Last but not least, an algorithm will hardly be able to include all infrequent or exceptional problems. Applying the available scientific evidence, summarized in algorithms, in everyday practice, and knowing where and how to depart from the decision tree, will always be the art of medicine.[15,16]

Ruling in or ruling out a particular diagnosis

This approach is followed if the number-one diagnostic hypothesis in the hierarchy has a much greater chance of becoming the definite diagnosis than all other hypotheses, or if one of the other hypotheses, which are less likely to be confirmed, has very important consequences for the patient, such as malignancy. In the first case, a 'ruling in' approach is followed, whereas the second requires 'ruling out' the presence of the disease in question. It is important to distinguish between the two, because certain (laboratory) tests are known to be better at confirming the presence of a disease, while others are known to be better at ruling out a particular disease.[8,17] In statistical terms, the former have a higher positive predictive value, while the latter have a higher negative predictive value. In general, given a fixed sensitivity and specificity, tests tend to have a better negative predictive value if a disease is known to have a low incidence in everyday general practice. As a result, the choice for a particular diagnostic test should preferably be based on its known positive or negative predictive values in general practice. For many tests, however, the discriminating diagnostic abilities remain to be established.

However, using tests to rule in or rule out the presence of a disease involves much more than merely taking blood samples or referring a patient for an X-ray. History taking, in combination with background knowledge held by general practitioners, can be seen as the most important diagnostic test, used for every patient. Furthermore, it is also very accurate and efficient, especially in the hands of skilled doctors. Thus, in the patient mentioned earlier with shoulder pain and vaginal blood loss, who seldomly consults her general practitioner, the simultaneous presence of both symptoms makes the combination of the two signs a very powerful diagnostic test. Time, involving repeated contacts with patients whose diagnoses usually evolve over time, is often used as a second best, but still very efficient, diagnostic tool. A serious infectious or malignant disease will develop more signs and symptoms over time, whereas unexplained signs, symptoms and complaints are normally self-limiting. The examples also illustrate that general practice involves more than efficiently ruling out the presence of serious diseases. It is the (early) detection of harmful conditions using little more than history taking and time that makes the general practitioner an expert in medicine.

Using a diagnostic dragnet

General practitioners, in particular, are frequently consulted for complaints that have a large diagnostic spectrum, such as fatigue, weight loss, or joint pain. In these cases it is often not immediately clear what direction their diagnostic reasoning should take. Screening all body systems one by one may then help to catch the 'diagnostic fish'. This approach, however, is time-consuming and may lead to a series of additional diagnostic tests, which can easily result in abnormal findings unrelated to the complaint presented by the patient. Rather than being reassured, both doctor and patient will then feel increasingly worried and a further series of tests, or hospital referrals may easily follow. The mere fact of doctors being experienced in everyday practice may prevent the development of such unwanted cascades of diagnostic actions, as they know how to communicate with worried patients and have a large number of illness scripts in mind.

Sequential hypothesis testing

This final approach is much more efficient than the trailnet method. It involves all diagnostic hypotheses one by one, following the previously established hierarchy. If none of the hypotheses can be definitely confirmed, the list of diagnostic hypotheses is enlarged and tested again.

Conclusion

Diagnostic reasoning is a complex process in which skills, experience, communication, and doctors' and patients' personalities combine and intertwine to form a network which is difficult to analyze and unravel. It is particularly in general practice, with its enormous variety of presented complaints, that accurate and efficient diagnostic reasoning is crucial for delivering high quality care. Among medical professionals, general practitioners can be seen as high-level performers in this aspect of medicine.

References

1. **Miller, L.** (1985). Sherlock Holmes' method of deductive reasoning applied to medical diagnostics. *The Western Journal of Medicine* **142,** 413–14.
2. **Nurcombe, B. and Fitzhenry-Coor, I.** (1987). Diagnostic reasoning and treatment planning: I. Diagnosis. *The Australian and New Zealand Journal of Psychiatry* **21**, 477–83.
3. **Claessens, H.F. and Boshuizen, H.P.A.** (1985). Recall of medical information by students and doctors. *Medical Education* **19**, 61–7.
4. **Patel, V.L., Groen, G.J., and Frederiksen, C.H.** (1986). Differences between students and physicians in memory of clinical cases. *Medical Education* **20**, 3–9.
5. **Schmidt, H.G., Norman, G.R., and Boshuizen, H.P.** (1990). A cognitive perspective on medical expertise: theory and implication. *Academic Medicine* **65**, 611–21.
6. **Custers, E.J., Boshuizen, H.P., and Schmidt, H.G.** (1996). The influence of medical expertise, case typicality, and illness script component on case processing and disease probability estimates. *Memory & Cognition* **24**, 384–99.
7. **Peyton, J.W.R.** *Teaching and Learning in General Practice.* Herth UK: Manticore Europe Lmt, 1998.
8. **Sackett, D.L., Haynes, B.R., and Tugwell, P.** *Clinical Epidemiology. A Basic Science for Clinical Medicine.* Boston, Toronto: Little Brown and Company, 1985.
9. **Joseph, G.-M. and Patel, V.L.** (1990). Domain knowledge and hypothesis generation in diagnostic reasoning. *Medical Decision Making* **10**, 31–46.
10. **Hobus, P.P.M., Schmidt, H.G., Boshuizen, H.P.A., and Patel, V.L.** (1987). Contextual factors in the activation of first diagnostic hypotheses: expert–novice differences. *Medical Education* **21**, 471–6.
11. **Coughlin, L.D. and Patel, V.L.** (1987). Text comprehension and the effect of expertise in the domain of medicine. *Journal of Medical Education* **62**, 818–28.
12. **Van Leeuwen, Y.D., Mol, S.S.L., Pollemans, M.C., Grol, R., and Van der Vleuten, C.P.M.** (1995). Change in knowledge of general practitioners during their professional career. *Family Practice* **12**, 313–17.
13. **Smeele, I.J.M., Van den Hoogen, J.M.M., Mans, J.M.A., Chavannes, A.W., Fass, A., Koss, S.W., Romeinders, A.C.M., and Van der Laan, J.R.** (1996). NHG Standard 'Lumbosacral radicular syndrome'. *Huisarts en Wetenschap* **39**, 78–89.
14. **Timmermans, A.E., Baselier, P.J.A.M., Winkens, R.A.G., Arets, H., and Wiersma, T.J.** (1999). NHG Standard 'Urinary tract infections'. *Huisarts en Wetenschap* **42**, 613–20.
15. **Knottnerus, J.A. and Dinant, G.J.** (1997). Medicine based evidence, a prerequisite for evidence based medicine. *British Medical Journal* **315**, 1109–10.
16. **Montgomery-Hunter, K.** (1989). A science of individuals: medicine and casuistry. *Journal of Medical Philosophy* **14**, 193–212.
17. **Bordage, G., Grant, J., and Marsden, P.** (1990). Quantitative assessment of diagnostic ability. *Medical Education* **24**, 413–25.

6.3 Clinical judgement

Jane Macnaughton

Introduction

The freedom of clinicians to exercise clinical judgement has come under attack in recent years for a number of reasons. Prominent amongst these has been the rise of the evidence-based medicine movement which has rightly scrutinized the practice of medicine and found it wanting for not implementing good scientific evidence for effective new treatments. Doctors are by nature cautious beings and want to be sure that a new innovation is better than a treatment that they know and have experienced working. To counter this the profession has been inundated over the past 10 years with guidelines and governments have set up agencies to advise doctors on best evidence-based practice. The Australian government was the first to do so in 1998 by establishing its Medical Services Advisory Committee.[1] This was followed in 1999 by the USA's Agency for Healthcare Research and Quality and then by the UK government's National Institute for Clinical Excellence (NICE). The advice handed down to clinicians by these agencies is now, in many cases, beginning to carry more or less statutory authority. In a recent case in the United Kingdom, a GP has had to appear before a tribunal for not following guidelines on the MMR triple vaccine and instead offering separate vaccines to children whose parents have concerns.[2]

What is paradoxical in all this, however, is that at the same time as clinicians are being increasingly told what to think, medical educators are being encouraged to raise a new breed of doctors who are more able to think for themselves.[3] The General Medical Council's 1993 document, *Tomorrow's Doctors*, for example, lists amongst the attitudinal objectives for the new approach to undergraduate education:

> approaches to learning that are based on curiosity and exploration of knowledge rather than on its passive acquisition, and that will be retained throughout professional life.[4]

Similarly, the Australian Medical Council requires students to demonstrate:

> the ability to interpret medical evidence in a critical and scientific manner, and to use libraries and other information resources to pursue independent inquiry relating to medical problems.[5]

How are we to reconcile these two apparently opposing influences on the development of the profession: the one apparently tending to restrict the scope of clinicians to exercise their own judgement in the treatment of their patients, and the other encouraging the development of doctors who regard it as their ethical duty to analyse and assess evidence with which they may be presented? In this chapter I wish to try to answer this question by examining the nature of judgement itself and by comparing the exercise of judgement in various contexts, including in science and the law, with its exercise in medicine. My conclusion will be that judgement is fundamental to all clinical decision-making, and, more fundamental still, to all clinical understanding. I will outline what I think are the skills, knowledge, and attitudes required for good clinical judgements, and I will conclude the chapter by briefly outlining new approaches to medical education which are encouraging doctors of the future to exercise good clinical judgement.

The concept of judgement

'Judgement' is a term in constant use in daily life but it is not an easy concept to describe. I will therefore defer to the view of a thinker from the tradition of Scottish common sense philosophy, Thomas Reid. Reid succeeded Adam Smith as Professor of Moral Philosophy at Glasgow University in 1764 and contributed to the great expansion of intellectual enquiry that was the eighteenth century Scottish Enlightenment. In his *Essay on the Intellectual Powers of Man* (1785) he proposes a definition of judgement as follows:

> it is an act of the mind whereby one thing is affirmed or denied of another;[6]

in other words, to judge is to decide the truth of one proposition over another. He uses the example of a court of law to expand this:

> As a judge, after taking the proper evidence, passes sentence in a cause, and that sentence is called his judgement, so the mind, with regard to whatever is true of false, passes sentence, or determines according to the evidence that appears.
>
> (ref. 6, p. 253)

Reid goes on to make the following observations about judgement:

1. Judgement is to be distinguished from simple apprehension: it involves the mind in an act.
2. Every judgement must be either true or false but
3. one judgement can be contradictory to another and someone can conceive of the two contradictory positions at once but cannot hold the view that each is true.
4. Without some degree of judgement we can form no accurate or distinct notions of things—so one province of judgement is to aid us in forming clear and distinct conceptions of things.[7]

Reid regards judgement as central to the process of reasoning. The mind, says Reid, undergoes a three-fold process to acquire knowledge. Firstly, our senses allow us to apprehend ideas and notions; secondly, by comparing ideas and notions the mind forms its judgements; and thirdly, from forming such judgements the mind comes to conclusions and understands. This process sounds complex but becomes at times almost instantaneous by process of habit. To illustrate this Reid gives the example of looking at an object and being able to describe its colour. Before being able to describe something as yellow we need to have a prior conception of what yellow is in comparison to other colours. We must, in fact, be able to make a judgement that something is yellow rather than red or blue before describing it as such.

Reid, therefore, regards judgement as integral (or intrinsic) to understanding. It differs from simple perception in that it is an active process and the ability to make judgements is what gives us the ability to reason. So far, however, this discussion has dealt with judgement as a theoretical concept; in other words, the implication is that judgement leads only to understanding and does not involve the imperative to action or lead to action. Reid's courtroom analogy suggests that this is not the case: the judgements of the judge require that something happens—that the guilty person gets sent to jail. Judgements can therefore be practical and result in something happening. We are also familiar with the sense that judgements can have a moral force. In the Bible, God is often described as a judge; the understanding here being that judgement will be of a moral kind—between good and evil or good actions and bad.

In summary, therefore, we can distinguish three kinds of judgement. Firstly, there is Reid's simple idea of judgement as deciding between two propositions. This kind of judgement might be regarded as theoretical. Secondly, there is judgement of a legal sort where evidence for or against a proposition is weighed and a decision is made which results in practical action. This kind of judgement is partly theoretical and partly practical. Thirdly, we can describe judgements which have the sense that 'you ought to do such and such' as moral judgements, which are again partly theoretical and partly practical.

We can see from this that judgements do not need to be either theoretical or practical or moral, they can be all three. There are many such examples in clinical practice such as when a doctor discusses giving up smoking with a patient. In this example, the theoretical judgement concludes that the generalizable evidence suggests that smoking is causing the patient's recurrent chest infections. This judgement can be presented to the patient for her to make up her own mind. The doctor may, however, go further and make a moral judgement: 'as your doctor I think you ought to give up smoking'. The doctor may go further still and give practical force to her theoretical and moral judgements by saying: 'these are the facts; you ought to give up and I am now taking away your cigarettes and prescribing a nicotine patch'. This example illustrates the range of judgements open to the clinician but most patients would be deeply dissatisfied with a doctor who did nothing but present the evidence and who never recommended or prescribed treatment. Medicine is a practical profession and its judgements usually have a practical outcome. Let us analyse this further and investigate the unique nature of judgements in the clinical situation.

Judgement and evidence: three models

Dealing with the evidence available in clinical practice is central to the process of making clinical judgements so I wish to compare the handling of evidence in science and in the law in order to draw some conclusions about the unique nature of judgement in the clinical situation.[8]

Scientific model of evidence

Science is characterized by its method which takes the following form:

1. observation;
2. hypothesis formation;
3. experimentation;
4. confirmation or denial of hypothesis;
5. generalization.

How does evidence fit into this scheme? We can say that evidence is the information generated by this scientific method. However, evidence cannot be characterized simply as just 'information'. It is a certain kind of information in that it is related to a specific scientific claim.[(9)] We do not just say 'This is evidence', we say 'This is evidence for something or that something is the case'. Information or data can be about something but they do not suggest that we can assert any claims in their light. If data or findings are to become evidence, then they must firstly be relevant to some scientific claim. This claim can be characterized as a 'hypothesis'.[(10)] A hypothesis unifies relevant information or findings, transforms them into 'evidence' and suggests how further evidence may be found which will count for or against the hypothesis.

In terms of medical science, then, we can now give meaning to 'evidence-based medicine'. It will mean that some anecdotal reports and other observations by clinicians or medical scientists become relevant to hypotheses about the relative success of various treatments which are then tested by trials and other experiments. The conclusions of these can be said to be 'evidence-based' treatments; they are effective for the generality of patients or for some statistically significant percentage of patients.

If this brief account of evidence-based medicine is correct, does it leave any room for judgement? In terms of my analysis of judgement above, it certainly does. If judgement involves deciding the truth of one proposition over another it is central to the process of deciding how far the data derived from the scientific process are directed at the hypothesis and how strongly or weakly they are so directed. In other words, judgement is essential in that someone must carry out the process of weighing or sifting facts, assessing their significance as evidence and drawing generalizable, or at least, statistical significance from them. So even on the science model of evidence there must be a place for human judgement, even if this judgement is theoretical and goes no further than making a judgement about what is or is not the case on the basis of the available evidence. The goal of the process is generalizable scientific truth; the judgements here do not have any normative force nor do they involve any imperative to act.

Detective model of evidence

Scientists are not the only professionals interested in evidence. Detectives are also deeply interested in evidence and its relationship to judgement. In Arthur Conan Doyle's *A Study in Scarlet* Dr Watson upbraids Sherlock Holmes for not paying enough attention to the case they have just set out to investigate:

> 'You don't seem to give much thought to the matter in hand,' I said at last interrupting Holmes's musical disquisition.
>
> 'No data yet,' he answered. 'It is a capital mistake to theorise before you have all the evidence. It biases the judgement.'[(11)]

The role of the detective, as suggested here by Holmes, is to amass all the material relating to a case and then formulate some hypotheses as to its solution. Holmes wrongly suggests, however, that 'data' might be called 'evidence' before the formulation of the hypothesis about the case for in this regard the detective's use of evidence is the same as that of the scientist, as we shall see.

Let us imagine that the Duke is found murdered in the library. The investigating detective takes statements from many people—other family members, maids, gardeners, and the butler. The statements are the data concerning the case. The detective then formulates the hypothesis that it was the Duchess's lover who committed the crime. The information relating to the lover's involvement then turns into evidence because it relates to a particular hypothesis in the case. However, the detective then turns up a convincing piece of counter-evidence, an alibi for the lover. A new hypothesis must be formulated—that the culprit was, in fact, the butler. And so the process goes on.

The 'detective model' of evidence is similar to the scientific model in important respects—the collection of data, the observations, and the chance discoveries, followed by the formulation of hypotheses which transform some of this information into evidence and suggest how other evidence (for or against the hypotheses) might be found. But it is unlike the science model in one important respect: it is not logically possible to generalize. The evidence is relevant to one and only one situation. Both the scientific and the detective models have truth as their goal, but in the one case it is general truth, and in the other it is truth specific to a situation. This is an important difference, but it is not one which removes the need for judgement. Moreover, the nature of the judgement involved seems very like that in the scientific model, for it requires the sifting and evaluation of information and findings and the relating of these to hypotheses. Once again, this sort of judgement is theoretical in nature.

Evidence and judgement in medicine

Let us now look at the application of these models to the medical context. Does the use of evidence and judgement in medicine have more in common with the work of a detective or with that of a scientist? It might seem that medicine uses both models. The work of clinical research involves rigorous application of the scientific model to clinical problems. The aim of research in medicine is to establish truths about clinical diagnosis and treatment which will be true for all common situations. It might also seem that if we look at the work of clinical practice, the work of the individual doctor in the surgery or clinic, this has more in common with the work of the detective. The taking of a clinical history parallels the taking of statements of witnesses to a crime, and the examination process is like the rigorous examination of the crime scene. The doctor is here amassing unstructured data which she will then use to suggest a diagnosis (the hypothesis) and will attempt to establish the truth of that diagnosis by further examination (through X-rays, laboratory testing of blood samples, etc.). These two kinds of activity are quite different but they have this in common: both are concerned with discussing truth, the generalized truth of science or the specific truth of diagnosis, and both involve a similar kind of theoretical judgement.

Clinical practice, however, has two aspects to it: diagnosis and treatment. It is precisely at the point of treatment, of course, that proponents of the supremacy of an evidence-based approach to medicine would say that scientific evidence is relevant; that it is a matter of scientific truth that some treatments are more effective than others. But the clinician is not concerned with treatments in the abstract. The clinician is concerned with treating this specific patient, and the treating of specific patients (as distinct from 'evidence-based' treatments) requires the clinician to be influenced by many factors other than truth, such as the consent of this patient, the meaning of the disease for this patient, how important the side-effects are for this patient, whether the patient has heard of the treatment, the family supports, and perhaps even the cost.[(12)] These factors have nothing to do with truth, whether general or specific. This point about the aim of clinical treatment leads me to propose a third model for evidence as it is used in medicine. This model involves a different sort of judgement which is peculiar to clinical treatment.

A model of evidence in medicine

The third model I will call the 'treatment' model of evidence. Kathryn Hunter described the patient as 'provid[ing] the text that medicine must read and make sense of and explain'.[(13)] She focuses on the importance of the individual patient as the primary source evidence that the doctor needs to assess in the light of the presenting complaint. Her conclusions came from a 2-year study of doctors going about their clinical business—a bit like the conclusions of an anthropologist studying 'doctors in the wild'—and reflects actual practice. The process does not stop at making sense of the 'text' that is the patient, however, as it might in the context of detection or science, as the doctor must then initiate treatment appropriate not only to the specific condition but also to the specific patient. Doctors must, of course, have in their minds a knowledge of evidence-based treatments, but this part of the process also involves an assessment of other sorts of question: will the evidence relating to this patient suggest that they will be able to comply with treatment? Is it clear that the patient understands their condition and trusts the doctor's conclusion sufficiently for the benefits of the placebo effect to come into play?[(14)] Is the treatment appropriate for the social situation of this patient?

This need for individualization of the results of randomized controlled trials is being recognized through the creation of DIPEX, the Database of Individual Patient Experience.[(15)] This database, which has been constructed for use alongside the Cochrane Database for Systematic Reviews, will publish the individual illness experiences of participants in clinical trials. The intention is not to take a snapshot view but to follow the patient's experience throughout the illness from diagnosis through to resolution or progression.

In the context of this model we can now see the paramount importance and peculiar nature of clinical judgement. We have seen how judgement is relevant to assessing data as evidence for or against a hypothesis, but judgement comes into its own when we deal with the range of complex factors in the clinical situation. This is a different sort of judgement and requires different abilities. The judgements of the scientist and the detective are theoretical or technical; that of the clinician is based on what Aristotle calls phronesis or 'practical wisdom'.[(16)] It is certainly true that medicine is in some respects a skill-based activity whose practice requires the exercise of specific skills relating to diagnosis and treatment. It is in this sense that the judgements of medicine are like the theoretical or technical ones of science and detective work and relate to conclusions that are either true or false. But medicine involves more than this; it involves 'a capacity to act with regard to the things that are good or bad for man' (Aristotle). When doctors have to come to a decision about treatments for individual patients—in other words, have to make judgements relating to 'the things that are good or bad for man'—this is not the same as making judgements about what is or is not the case. These judgements have more to do with what is or is not appropriate for this patient with this condition, and at this time.

Summary: clinical judgement

In summary, then, there are several sort of evidence each with its own correlative sort of judgement. In the case of the medical scientist the evidence comes from, say, randomized controlled trials, which suggest the percentage success or failure of treatments. The correlative judgement is theoretical and directed at generalized truth. It is often said that clinical treatment applies this scientific evidence to individual patients.[(17)] This is certainly part of the picture; that part in which diagnosis is like detective work. The correlative judgements of the clinician are in this respect like those of the detective and aim at individualized truth about a given patient. But the other part of the clinical picture concerns treatment. Evidence about what constitutes the best treatment for a given patient involves a wide range of imponderables, but especially a patient's own perspective. The correlative judgement in this case can be only partly theoretical (i.e. based on evidence-based treatments) because it must tap into the belief system of the patient, and, indeed, of the doctor. Hence, the judgements of the good clinician must be more than technical; they must show practical wisdom.

What influences clinical judgement?

I have discussed judgement in the three models above as it relates to the handling of evidence. I have suggested that 'evidence' in medicine must be regarded as coming from a wide variety of sources, including evidence generated by scientific method, such as randomized controlled trials, but also the patient's account of their illness, their beliefs about it, and their social circumstances. This being the case, the doctor's handling of that evidence and her judgements in relation to it will be influenced by many factors. One of the most important of these is the doctor's own beliefs about the efficacy or otherwise of treatments informed by her clinical experience. It has been suggested that one way in which doctors use their clinical experience is by referring to a collection of 'illness scripts' of all the patients they have ever seen who have similar or contrasting clinical stories.[(18)] When the illness script of the patient in front of the doctor at the time deviates from that with which she is familiar, the resulting uncertainty leads to the decision to seek further evidence or the judgement of a colleague whom the doctor believes has greater experience with this problem. It is impossible fully to analyse the process of clinical decision making in an objective way although attempts have been made (ref. 15, p. 251) but experience is an important element in clinical judgement. Experience can also teach the doctor when clinical judgement can be unreliable. For example the clinical diagnosis of anaemia is notoriously inaccurate unless it is supported by haematological results. The important point is that doctors must exercise their judgement when deciding when to rely on inconsistent clinical signs or not. Practical experience of this and the practical wisdom that results from this experience is essential.

The ability of clinicians to make judgements can also be compromised by the quality of the information with which they are presented. Evidence generated by the scientific process has to be adapted for the individual patient's situation, as we have seen. Doctors also have to be able to elicit a reliable history from their patient in order that they can make sensible judgements on this evidence. Patients' accounts of their illness can be riddled with errors of fact or timing which may be crucial to diagnosis.[(19)] The important technical skills to assist the clinician here is that of good history taking; an essential prerequisite for good clinical judgement.

Doctors' decisions, of course, are ultimately worthless without the understanding, agreement, and consent of the patient. Clinicians cannot ignore the patient's judgement concerning their own best interests partly because ultimately the treatment will be ineffective if the patient does not accept it or take it, and partly because obtaining consent is central to the ethical component of clinical judgement.

As we have seen, clinical judgement is a complex concept and is dependent on technical skill, experience, knowledge, and knowing how to deal with that knowledge or evidence about the patient. It is not reducible to algorithms or guidelines, although these may be helpful as contributing to the knowledge available to the clinician. Phronesis—or practical wisdom—is required, with implications for clinical education.

Educating the judgement

As I discussed in the introduction, the General Medical Council and the Australian Medical Council in their recommendations for undergraduate medical education encourage the development of doctors who have an intelligent approach to medical knowledge, rather than a 'memorise all' approach. They encourage the nurturing of good clinical judgement. The exercise of good judgement in medicine requires a range of attributes both technical or scientific and humane (Fig. 1; reproduced from ref. 8, p. 1). On the technical side, clinicians require scientific understanding of how the body works and of how evidence generated by scientific method can contribute to their understanding of treatments. They need to be able to exercise the technical skills of history taking and examination effectively and accurately. To exercise these skills humanely and to be able to deal with the complex human issues which must be taken into account in coming to judgements, doctors need ethical sensitivity and the attributes derived from an effective educational process: adaptability, a broad perspective and personal development. The ability to interpret is also an important attribute for the clinician to acquire, not only for the processes of understanding and sifting scientific evidence but also for understanding the patient's perspective. Insight contributes to understanding in both the scientific and

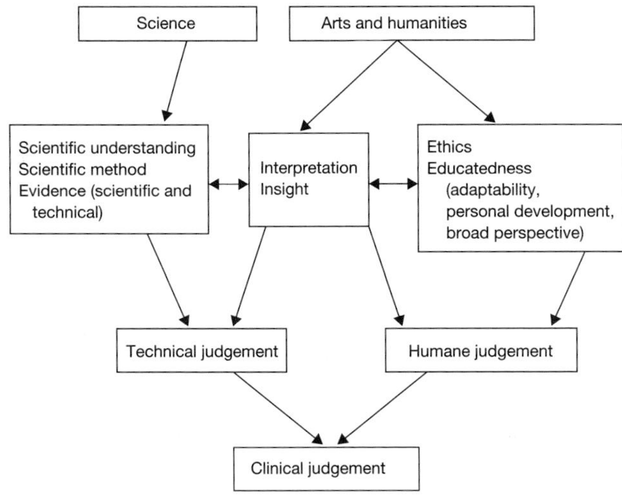

Fig. 1 A range of attributes required for good clinical judgement.

humane sides of medical practice and clinicians need to be open to these flashes of realization which can often help solve clinical dilemmas.

Frank Hulyer's short story, *Sugar*, illustrates the way in which a flash of insight can suddenly make a problem clear.[20] He sees a young child whose presenting complaint is that she 'just isn't acting herself'. Clinical history and examination (in other words, the technical approach) reveals no abnormality, and it is not until Hulyer has his hand on the door of the consulting room and is about to dismiss the child when he has a sudden thought that she might have taken someone else's medication. She has in fact taken one of her grandmother's oral hypoglaecemic tablets and might have lapsed into coma during the night had she gone home. The flash of insight succeeds where the exercise of clinical skills fails!

Undergraduate courses are beginning to address some of the above elements in response to the advice from organizations such as the General Medical Council, Australian Medical Council and the American equivalent, the American Association of Medical Colleges. The challenge for medical education is how these attributes from both the scientific or technical and the humane sides of medicine are to be integrated so they can be engaged seamlessly by the clinician. One developing approach to this is through the emerging discipline of the medical humanities. David Greaves argues against the separation of the attributes required for good clinical judgement into scientific and humane because, he argues, the humanities can contribute to understanding how scientific understanding and humane practice can make up a seamless garment:

> ... the medical humanities perspective raises deeper questions concerning assumptions which are usually taken for granted and are of relevance to the whole of medicine. Promoting medical humanities, then, requires not just an addition to the curriculum but a permeation and change of orientation of the culture of medicine, which will transform not only clinical practice but also the theoretical basis and social structures of medicine and healthcare.[21]

Conclusions

Judgement is a complex concept. It may be described simply as the ability to decide between two propositions (theoretical judgement) but may also have normative and practical force. Judgement in clinical practice can involve all three kinds of judgement and usually requires the clinician to take some practical step (in the treatment model) to help the individual patient she is treating. The exercise of judgement in medicine is complex as it involves decisions to be made not just between two propositions but between many, and to take into account issues involving patients' understanding, fears, and desires as well as those of the clinician and those of society (in the case of rationing). The ability to exercise judgement in this context requires the clinician to be able to integrate a range of knowledge, skills, and attributes derived both from scientific and humane understanding of the human body and of human experience. The new discipline of medical humanities is emerging in undergraduate education as a discipline which might assist students in their ability to draw together the humane and scientific aspects of medical practice into a seamless whole.

References

1. **Medical Services Advisory Committee:** http://www.health.gov.au/msac/index.htm.
2. **Barrat, H.** (2001). MMR vaccine row raises questions of clinical freedom. *British Medical Journal* **323**, 300 (News section).
3. **Maudsley, G. and Scrivens, J.** (2000). 'Science', 'critical thinking' and 'competence' for Tomorrow's Doctors. A review of terms and concepts. *Medical Education* **34**, 53–60.
4. **General Medical Council.** *Tomorrow's Doctors.* London: GMC, 1993, p. 15 (revised guidelines are about to be published).
5. **Australian Medical Council.** *Guidelines for the Assessment and Accreditation of Medical Schools* at http://www.amc.org.au/accredit.asp (also undergoing revision).
6. **Reid, T.** (1975). In *Inquiry and Essays* (ed. K. Lehrer and R. Beanblossom), p. 251. Indianapolis: The Bobbs-Merrill Company, Inc, from Essay Six 'Of Judgement'.
7. **Broadie, A.,** ed. *The Scottish Enlightenment: An Anthology.* Edinburgh: Canongate Classics, 1997, p. 110.
8. **Downie, R.S. and Macnaughton, J.** *Clinical Judgement: Evidence in Practice.* Oxford: Oxford University Press, 2000.
9. **Charlton, B.** (1991). Medical practice and the double-blind randomised controlled trial. *British Journal of General Practice* **41**, 355–6.
10. **Achison, P.,** ed. *The Concept of Evidence.* Oxford: Oxford University Press, 1983, p. 12.
11. **Conan Doyle, A.** *A Study in Scarlet and the Sign of Four.* London: Elder and Co., 1903, p. 39.
12. **Holmberg, L., Baum, M., and Adami, H.O.** (1999). On the scientific inference from clinical trials. *Journal of Evaluation in Clinical Practice* **5**, 157–62.
13. **Hunter, K.M.** *Doctors' Stories: The Narrative Structure of Medical Knowledge.* Princeton NJ: Princeton University Press, 1991, p. 45.
14. **Dixon, M. and Sweeney, K.** *The Human Effect in Medicine.* Oxford: Radcliffe Medical Press, 2000.
15. **Greenhalgh, T. and Hurwitz, B.** *Narrative Based Medicine: Dialogue and Discourse in Clinical Practice.* London: BMJ Books, 1998, p. 212.
16. **Ross, D.,** translator. Aristotle *The Nicomachean Ethics.* Oxford: Oxford University Press, 1980, 1140a and 1140b6.
17. **Sullivan, F.M. and Macnaughton, J.** (1996). Evidence in consultations: interpreted and individualised. *Lancet* **348**, 941–3.
18. **Schmidt, H.G., Norman, G.R., and Boshuizen, H.P.A.** (1990). A cognitive perspective on medical expertise: theory and implications. *Academic Medicine* **65**, 611–21.
19. **Redelmeier, D.A., Schull, M.J., Hux, J.E., Tu, J.V., and Ferris, L.E.** (2001). Problems for clinical judgement: 1. Eliciting an insightful history of present illness. *Canadian Medical Association Journal* **164**, 647–51.
20. **Hulyer, F.** *The Blood of Strangers: True Stories from the Emergency Room.* London: Fourth Estate, 1999, p. 153.
21. **Evans, M. and Finlay, I.,** ed. *Medical Humanities.* London: BMJ Books, 2001, p. 22.

6.4 The therapeutic illusion: self-limiting illness

Pali Hungin

Introduction

The concept of self-limiting illness extends beyond that of the organically defined, short-or medium-term lesion—say, the sore throat, skin abscess, sprained ankle, earache, or viral pneumonia. In such instances, the therapeutic effect is related to the passage of time, the pathological processes, and to the body's own defences and self-healing mechanisms. Here, intervention by the doctor may assist recovery, either by accelerating it with antibiotics or by ameliorating it with analgesics. Rather, the concept of self-limiting illness in this chapter is related chiefly to the category of medical problems that challenge conventional categorization and in which the role of the clinician in influencing an outcome is less clear, although not necessarily any the less involving. Therapeutic interventions are more illusory here;[1] the course of the illness or syndrome is likely to be defined and influenced by factors outside the direct control of the clinician.

A large proportion of the patients presenting to the clinician have no clearly defined organic problem or a specific psychological diagnosis. These patients are often categorized as having either *functional problems* or *unexplained symptoms*. These are sometimes recognized as physiological variations associated with symptoms. In most instances, no abnormality can be demonstrated despite exhaustive tests; the problem can become recurrent and take on the hallmarks of a chronic condition. In between episodes many such patients appear entirely normal, free from the initial complaint, again defying the concept of a chronic disease with its deteriorating effect. Many sufferers report success with the unlikeliest of remedies, a large number of which can be obtained without a prescription.

The extent of the problem

The prevalence of such disorders is underestimated because such patients tend not to fit into clear categories, do not usually require hospitalization, and, when evaluated, tend to be grouped under the nature of the presenting symptoms, such as myalgia. Some are ascribed alleged pathology leading to unnecessary operations such as hysterectomy or appendicectomy.[2] They thus constitute a huge, hidden health problem the cost of which is underestimated.

In most specialities, the workload from these syndromes equals or exceeds that from organically defined lesions;[3] in western general practice the majority of consultations involve non-organic problems and it seems that the incidence of these is rising. The 'symptom and illness iceberg' models which demonstrate explain that only a small proportion of all problems actually present to the physician are based on research indicating widespread unreported physical and psychological morbidity in the community.[4] Self-reported long-standing illness occurs in 40 per cent of the English adult population, rising from a fifth in those aged 16–24 years to two-thirds in those over 75 years. In the United States, up to 50 per cent of those covered by health programmes have unexplained symptoms, 75 per cent of them having sought help from their primary care physician,[5] and nearly one-third of all prevalent symptoms are either psychiatric or unexplained.[6] These figures hide a huge volume of functional and unexplained problems; in hospital practice, for example, up to 25 per cent of all coronary care admissions are due to non-cardiac chest pain.[7]

In general practice, where patients present largely with undifferentiated problems, the symptoms can cut across several systems. These can defy categorization or imply multi-organ involvement for there is no obvious, rational explanation. The differentiation between functional and unexplained problems is usually artificial—the categorization of clusters of symptoms into a recognizable pattern or symptom criteria is often the only difference between *functional* and the *unexplained*. An example of this is the definition of the 'irritable bowel syndrome', a functional bowel disorder, using the Manning or Rome diagnostic criteria. Often the two co-exist, as in the patient with functional bowel disease, who may also have several associated problems, which, in turn, are even more poorly defined and diffuse[8] (Fig. 1). A Nordic review of fibromyalgia confirmed the diagnostic criteria to be subjective and arbitrary with heterogeneity in the patient groups.[9] A characteristic of all these problems is that the most commonly prescribed drugs rarely have an effect greater than that of placebo in well-designed studies.[8]

Furthermore, there is a considerable overlap between functional and organic symptoms in most specialities.[8] A large proportion of patients with one unexplained clinical condition meet the criteria for a second unexplained condition.[10] This is, in part, a consequence of the progressive segregation of the medical disciplines. The need to specialize in different organ systems is linked with the use of specialized technologies and highly specialized personnel, further contributing to the segregation of patients into separate diagnostic–therapeutic areas.[11] This handicaps a cross-disciplinary approach and the general practitioner, therefore, needs to be central in taking a holistic view (Fig. 2).

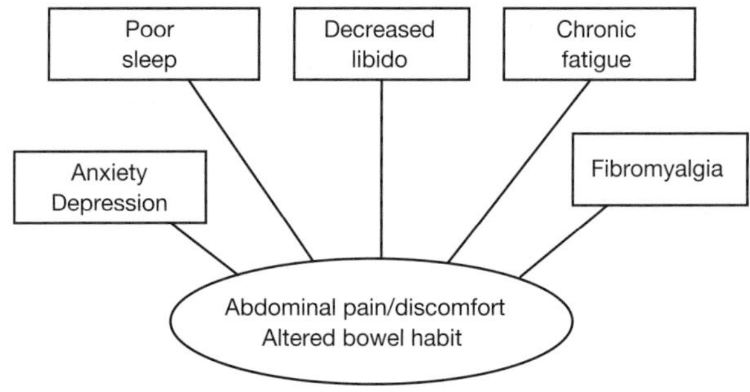

Fig. 1 Common intestinal and extra-intestinal symptoms reported by functional bowel disease patients.[8]

Speciality	Functional syndromes
Gastroenterology	Non-cardiac chest pain Functional gastro-oesophageal reflux Non-ulcer dyspepsia (NUD) Irritable bowel syndrome (IBS)
Gynaecology	Dyspareunia Chronic pelvic pain Premenstrual syndrome
Rheumatology	Fibromyalgia
Urology	Chronic prostatitis Interstitial cystitis
Cardiology	Non-cardiac chest pain
Psychiatry	Somato-visceral symptoms

Fig. 2 Functional syndromes in different specialities.[8]

Origins and mechanisms

Despite their impact on the health care system, the aetiology of functional problems is poorly understood although increasingly thought to be related to autonomic nervous function and mediating mechanisms from the brain.

The social construction of illness and the meaning of health have historically been determined by cultural and philosophical norms. For example, Hippocrates separated health from religion.[12] Current conventional medical training is based on the biomedical model of disease. This implies that health is the absence of a diagnosable disease, that diseases have a specific biomedical process, and that they can be dealt with by finding specific remedies. However, this model is open to challenge if technological advances fail to explain the health problem and to deliver the expected well-being. The competence of the practitioner is then called into question.[13]

The biomedical model recognizes the duality of the body and the mind, accepting cross-influences, but separates them with regard to disease diagnosis and management. Thus, the term 'psychomatic', although universally accepted, is used in a pejorative, negative sense, implying loss of mental control or understanding, a failure of the protective barrier between the mind and the body's physiology, and even a loss of moral fibre. Functional and unexplained problems do not fit comfortably within the biomedical model.

The biopsychosocial model

The duality approach is now augmented by the biopsychosocial model.[14,15] This model explains the brain–body axis in terms of a tangible, biochemical link. It postulates that bodily function is influenced by modulators and mediators released from the brain, which, in turn, are subject to psycho-social factors. In functional bowel disease, psycho-social factors constitute influences from early life experiences and conditioning experiences, including the previous experience of symptoms. Impinging upon these is the individual's own biological disposition (such as genetic and congenital factors), illness reinforcement during childhood, loss and bereavement, and past and current experience of abuse.[15] This is mirrored by social models of disability, which argue that it is their environment that disables people with impairment and that the distinction between able and disabled people is a social construct.

The brain–body link: mechanisms

Evidence for the role of the central nervous system in functional problems comes from knowledge that many patients relate their first onset or the exacerbation of their symptoms to stressful life events; many give a history dating from childhood; therapies aimed at the CNS, such as tricyclic antidepressants, anxiolytics, and psychotherapy, can be effective in symptom relief; and that high placebo responses are common.

Explanations for the basis of the brain–body axis and the experience of symptoms include the discovery of mechanisms that enhance visceral hypersensitivity. This is allied with sensitization of the afferent neurological pathways by acute peripheral tissue irritation. Visceral hypersensitivity has been confirmed in non-cardiac chest pain and irritable bowel syndrome. A large number of naturally occurring chemicals that might fulfill such a role have been identified; prominent amongst these is serotonin (found both in the brain and the body) and other neuropeptides with specific binding sites in the brain. These include bombesin, cholecystokinin, neuropeptide Y, and somatostatin. Some of these have the ability to influence neuromuscular function. This new field of neurobiology may increase our understanding of disorders in this field and holds promise for the development of biochemical interventions.

Placebo and the placebo effect

In their classic piece, 'The Powerful Placebo', Shapiro and Shapiro[16] argue that the effectiveness of procedures and medications through past ages has largely been due to non-specific factors which they liken to the placebo effect. They hold that the history of medical treatment, until recently, has been essentially the history of the placebo effect. Despite the use of ineffective methods, physicians have been respected and honoured because they have been the therapeutic agents for the placebo effect. The placebo has been universal to all cultures throughout history and even in the twenty-first century differentiates cultural attitudes towards health.

What is a placebo?

A placebo as any treatment, including drugs, surgery, psychotherapy, and quack therapy which is used for its ameliorative effect on a symptom or disease but is actually ineffective or is not specifically effective for the condition treated.[16] A placebo therapy may be used with or without the knowledge that it is a placebo and includes therapies given in the belief that they are effective, even though this is not confirmed by objective evaluation. Essentially, a placebo has no specific effect on the condition being treated. Often, the physician is unaware that the drug merely has a placebo effect or that its dosage is inappropriate for the desired specific effect.[16] Such is the belief in some treatments that they are often used in face of clear evidence of their lack of effectiveness.[17,18]

Placebo, placebo effect, and placebo response

A better understanding of this subject requires delineation between the terms *placebo* and *placebo effect*. Historically, placebo has been regarded as a pejorative rather than a scientific term; the term placebo effect having come into medical literature as recently as the mid-twentieth century. The placebo has been described as the agent or procedure and the placebo effect as the response to it.[16] The placebo effect is primarily the non-specific psychological or psychophysiological therapeutic effect but may be a reflection of spontaneous improvement. Where medications or procedures are knowingly used as placebos, the implication is that they are aimed at eliciting a desired effect, known and expected by the prescriber. A distinction has also been proposed between placebo response and placebo effect. The response is considered to be the behavioural change of subjects whilst the effect is only the proportion of change.

The current concept of placebo places it firmly within the domain of the clinical trial, legitimizing it as a research tool. However, the placebo effect is well incorporated into and commonly exploited in clinical practice.[19] Where physicians have no targeted treatment for an illness the door is opened to non-specific management and placebo effects.[16] The tendency for healers (including clinicians) to overvalue the accuracy and veracity of their diagnosis is a major factor contributing to the placebo effect. It can be so powerful that it can cause physicians to reject effective treatment, especially if a new remedy does not fit the dominant medical theory or was created by non-physicians. The delayed use of lemons to prevent scurvy is testament to this.

Yet, people display a remarkable belief in non-specific remedies or in cures that have no demonstrable value. The US Food and Drugs Administration (FDA) estimated in 1993 that 40 million Americans spend US$ 30 billion annually on 'fraudulent treatment', with 10 per cent of users suffering side-effects,[20] remedies ranging from vitamins to unproven anticancer remedies such as Laetrile's apricot pit.

The power of placebo

The powerful effect of placebo was demonstrated as long ago as the 1950s by Beecher,[21,22] who summarized 15 studies of 1082 patients treated with placebo for post-operative wound pain and angina, the common cold, clinically and experimentally induced cough, headache, and various psychological problems. The average relief of symptoms was 35.2 per cent, varying from 21 per cent to 58 per cent. In some of his studies, large doses of morphine relieved pain in 75 per cent of patients, nearly half the effect being attributed to placebo. In other series, those who responded positively to placebo also responded more easily to morphine for pain relief. Kissel and Barrucand,[23] in another classical review, noted a placebo effect of 28.5 per cent in studies on analgesics, 32.3 per cent in migraine, 58 per cent in seasickness, 41 per cent in cough relief, and 49 per cent in rheumatism. In 1993, Roberts et al.,[24] in a retrospective review of data from 6931 patients treated with developing drugs for asthma, duodenal ulcer, and herpes, demonstrated that the placebo or non-specific effects exceeded those reported in publications about the drugs. These clinical studies were uncontrolled, without the use of placebos and used initially promising compounds that later proved to be ineffective. The conditions of these studies mimicked the pragmatic situation of everyday practice—the absence of controls, enthusiastic clinicians and patients, with the prescribing clinicians themselves evaluating the results; it is likely that the effects reported from this study reflect the true magnitude of the placebo effect in routine practice.

This applies not only to drugs used in managing physical ailments but also in psychiatric practice. Psychopharmacology is no less prone to placebo effects in the course of controlled clinical trials—methodological problems are a constant feature of controlled trials in this field. Psychotherapy, regardless of who provides it, is especially subject to placebo effects.[16]

Clinical practice and placebo

The history of medical treatment is characterized by the introduction of new placebos by successive generations of physicians, often accompanied by the derision of those who preferred the previous ones. Studies have demonstrated that physicians attribute the use of placebo to other physicians three times as often as they attribute it to themselves—in a series of questions on what should be included in a definition of placebo, physicians tended to exclude their own therapies: surgeons excluded surgery, internists excluded active medication, and psychoanalysts excluded psychotherapy and psychoanalysis.[25,26]

Healers themselves are often aware of and are subject to the placebo effect of treatment—indeed the physician can start to believe in his placebo. Sir William Osler observed, ‘Faith in the gods or the saints cures one, faith in little pills another, hypnotic suggestion a third, faith in a plain common doctor a fourth ... faith in our drugs and methods, is the great stock in trade of the profession ... the touchstone of success in medicine ... and must be considered in the foundation of therapeutics ... (faith) is a precious commodity without which we would be very badly off’.[16]

Shapiro and Shapiro highlight the continuing importance of the placebo effect in clinical practice:[16] ‘Despite the proliferation of non-placebo drugs and procedures, placebo remedies are likely to fill the gap in knowledge as long as there are illnesses that cannot be treated adequately and the causes of illness are unknown. Moreover, although psychological and emotional factors may be minimized they cannot ever be excluded’. This places the placebo and the placebo effect at the heart of family practice.

The doctor as a therapeutic agent

The ‘drug doctor’, a concept reiterated through Balints's teachings, emanated from Huston's seminal concept in 1938:[27] ‘the physician is a vastly more important institution than the drug store’. George Bernard Shaw in his play, *The Doctor's Dilemma*, describes his doctor as ‘cheering, reassuring, and healing by the mere incompatibility of disease or anxiety with his welcome presence. Even broken bones, it is said, have been known to unite at the sound of his voice’.[19]

Modern clinicians too are well aware of this phenomenon and make use of it even in a world of evidence-based interventions, particularly in situations where the problem is poorly defined or likely to be classed as functional. A positive outcome using this approach is more likely with a patient in whom the meaning attached to his illness is altered in a positive direction. In defining this ‘meaning’, Brody[19] describes three basic components: (a) providing an understandable and satisfying explanation for the illness; (b) demonstrating care and concern; and (c) holding out an enhanced promise of mastery or control over the symptoms.

These concepts, ‘the therapeutic aspects of medical encounters’,[28] are universal to consultations in primary care. They form the basis of vocational training around consultations in general practice, where the exploration of the patient's own fears, concerns, and perceptions is held central. This is an easily recognizable role for the general practitioner faced with a wide variety of undifferentiated problems—sharing or explaining what is happening, or even creating an explanation that fits and is found reassuring, in a manner that expresses concern. It is thus perhaps unsurprising that many doctors whose clinical knowledge might otherwise be judged poor are able to elicit a profound therapeutic effect and that they often have a large and loyal patient following.

The result of these manoeuvres is to make the patient more in control of the symptoms, or else to feel that they need not worry about control because the doctor has taken charge.[19] This ‘meaning’ model is akin to the placebo effect and variations of it can be recognized in all cultures, whether in consultations with a doctor or some other sort of healer. In some circumstances, the healer (and by extrapolation this could be the doctor) is accorded extraordinary influence, such as a form of privileged access to the truth about human function. This can result in the belief that the patient must be healed after an encounter with the healer and any apparent therapeutic failure is the fault of the patient, either due to inattention or due to non-compliance. In some circumstances, the patient will regard themselves as healed, even though, on objective enquiry, the symptoms still remain. These concepts, based on observations of folk healers in Taiwan,[19] resonate with the patient–doctor dynamic in the Western model.

Chronic fatigue syndrome: an evolution from concept to acceptance?

Chronic fatigue syndrome, sometimes known as myalgic encephalopathy (‘ME syndrome’), is commonly recognized from a pattern of symptoms.[29] It typifies within the medical environment the difficulties of coming to terms with a poorly understood problem. In the past, opinions have ranged from this being a form of malingering to an unrecognized physiological disorder or a psychological disorder with somatic manifestations. Some saw it as a disparaging psychiatric disorder: ‘it's all in the mind’. This has been unpalatable to sufferers. Clinicians and patients have been at loggerheads about how to categorize the symptoms.

In an attempt to improve the understanding of the disorder and to recommend management strategies, a British working party, which included clinicians and sufferers, was set up in 1998, reporting in 2001.[30] There was agreement that chronic fatigue syndrome was common and could cause profound, often prolonged, illness and disability, and a significant impact on the individual and the family. It was no longer considered acceptable for clinicians to state that they did not ‘believe’ in the disorder. Graded exercise therapy and cognitive behaviour therapy were considered the best treatments, despite a lack of strong evidence.

Unsurprisingly, there were profound disagreements within the working party. This led to many resignations from the group with some clinicians feeling that there was insufficient evidence for the recommendations and too much reliance on the biopsychosocial model.[31]

The uncertainties surrounding the diagnosis and management of chronic fatigue syndrome and disagreements about its aetiology, or its acceptance as an entity, illustrate the tensions and different understandings of health professionals, lay people and sufferers, set within societal concepts. Traversing the boundaries from recognizing the patterns of a possible disorder, defining it in clinical terms, and formulating responses to it involve interactions between clinicians, the disease entity, and society and can constitute a challenge to established norms of disease and illness. Should only clinicians define a disease?

Medically unexplained symptoms: outcomes

Many clinicians retain a fear that they might have either missed an important diagnosis or have not recognized the early symptoms of a developing problem.

This was enshrined by Slater in 1965 in his 'Diagnosis of Hysteria',[32] which effectively impaired the confidence of doctors to make a definitive non-organic diagnosis, holding that diagnosing hysteria was a 'disguise for ignorance' and a 'fertile source of clinical error'. This doctrine, still pervading much modern medicine, consigned the diagnosis of a non-organic problem in neurology to an inferior and dubious category. However, Crimlisk et al.,[33] in a parallel study, which followed patients for 6 years, concluded that the initial diagnosis was likely to be correct and that the absence of an organic diagnosis was more likely to be associated with a concurrent psychiatric problem. Thus, unexplained organic symptoms, at least in neurological clinics, were not likely to be a prelude to a definitive organic diagnosis. Indeed, the resolution of physical symptoms was often related to the discovery of a co-morbid psychiatric disorder or a change in marital status.

Similar reinforcement comes from primary care research on abdominal complaints. Following up patients a year after presentation, Muris et al.[34] discovered that of those who had unexplained symptoms 68 per cent had experienced complete relief or improvement and that depressive mood was associated with the persistence of symptoms. Another Dutch[35] survey of 229 patients with unexplained symptoms showed that 26 per cent were improved at 3 months and that 15 per cent were receiving psychological help.

Some light on the decision-making of patients and clinicians comes from a qualitative study of gynaecologists and their patients presenting with menstrual problems without confirmed physical pathology.[36] Those who had hysterectomies characterized their subjective symptoms and psychosocial distress as deteriorating in a way that placed responsibility on the gynaecologist. In contrast, interviews with non-hysterectomy patients were characterized by a strategy whereby the gynaecologists established authority by confirming their ability to 'look inside' the uterus and see that it was normal. The patients thus exerted authority by emphasizing their subjective symptoms and the clinicians by their ability to exclude pathology. This suggests that the balance of strategic argument between the patient and the clinician contributes to outcomes.

In the primary care setting, short-term outcomes are likely to be related to the determinants of the consultation, including health-seeking behaviour and expectations based on the individual's fears and perceptions. The level to which an individual is conscious of and monitors their personal health, and the way in which he/she rationalizes the problem plays an important role in deciding whether to seek medical help; not all sufferers consult. Some may seek reassurance, in which case a definitive assessment and, if possible, a positive diagnosis based on specific criteria may be appropriate. In others, investigations are necessary to alleviate fears of more serious disease. Although there is evidence that normal investigative findings are associated with a reduction in subsequent health care resource use in some disorders, there are no data to confirm whether any of these approaches have a sustained effect.

A continuing GP problem?

In the United Kingdom, such patients are perceived to be difficult to manage but most GPs feel that their management should remain in primary care.[37] Providing reassurance, counselling, and acting as a gate keeper to prevent inappropriate investigations is considered an important role. Similar views have been found in the United States; in one study only 14 per cent of physicians expressed satisfaction in dealing with patients with unexplained symptoms. Those who saw themselves as being more effective were more likely to be in single-handed practice and to have practised in the same location for at least 5 years. A common theme is the need to develop newer strategies and the desire to work more closely with psychiatrists.

The therapeutic illusion, though, is perhaps completed by the observation that the patient, not the physician, is in the end the therapeutic agent—the placebo stimulus, whether the physician's behaviour or something else, simply uncorks the internal pharmacopoeia that all humans possess as a biologically programmed tool for self-healing.[19]

References

1. **Thomas, K.B.** (1994). The placebo in general practice. *Lancet* **344**, 1642.
2. **Longstreth, G.F.** (1994). Irritable bowel syndrome and chronic pelvic pain. *Obstetrical and Gynecological Surgery* **94**, 505–7.
3. **Sheehan, J.D.** (1999). The management of medically unexplained symptoms. *Seminars in Gastrointestinal Disease* **10**, 30–6.
4. **Campbell, S. and Roland, M.** (1996). Why do people consult the doctor? *Family Practice* **13**, 75–83.
5. **Hartz, A.J.** et al. (2000). Unexplained symptoms in primary care: perspectives of patients and doctors. *General Hospital Psychiatry* **22**, 144–52.
6. **Kroenke, K. and Price, R.K.** (1993). Symptoms in the community. Prevalence, classification and psychiatric comorbidity. *Archives in Internal Medicine* **153**, 2474–80.
7. **Bennett, J.R. and Atkinson, M.** (1996). The differentiation between oesophageal and cardiac pain. *Lancet* **II**, 1123–7.
8. **Mayer, E.A., Naliboff, B., Munakata, J., and Siverman, D.** (1996). Brain-gut mechanisms of visceral hypersensitivity. In *Neurogastroenterology* (ed. E. Corazziari), pp. 17–31. New York: Walter de Gruyter.
9. **Hilden, J.** (1996). Diagnosis of fibromyalgia: a critical review of the Scandinavian literature. *Nordisk Medicine* **111**, 308–12.
10. **Aaron, L.A. and Buchwald, D.** (2001). A review of the evidence for overlap among unexplained clinical conditions. *Annals of Internal Medicine* **134**, 868–81.
11. **Corazzieri, E.**, ed. *Neurogastroenterology*. New York: Walter de Gruyter, 1996.
12. **Labisch, A.** (1992). The social construction of health. In *The Social Construction of Illness* (ed. J. Lachmund and G. Stollberg), pp. 85–101. Stuggart: Frans steiner verlag.
13. **Bendelow, G.** (2001). Defining disease: determining practice. *Drugs and Therapeutics Bulletin* **39**, 46.
14. **Engel, G.L.** (1977). The need for a new medical model: a challenge for biomedicine. *Science* **196**, 129–36.
15. **Drossman, D.A.** (1999). The biopsychosocial model and chronic gastrointestinal disease. In *Chronic Gastrointestinal Disorders* (ed. E. Corazziari), pp. 33–40. Milan: Messaggi.
16. **Shapiro, A.K. and Shapiro, E.** *The Powerful Placebo. From Ancient Priest to Modern Physician*. Baltimore: John Hopkins University Press, 1997.
17. **Shapiro, A.K. and Shapiro, E.** (1984). Patient–provider relationships and the placebo effect. In *Behavioural Health: A Handbook of Health Enhancement and Disease Prevention* (ed. J.D. Matarrzzo et al.), New York: John Wiley and Sons.
18. **White, L., Tursky, B., and Schwartz, G.E.**, ed. *Placebo: Theory, Research and Mechanisms*. New York: Guildford Press, 1985.
19. **Brody, H.** (1997). The doctor a therapeutic agent: a placebo effect research agenda. In *The Placebo Effect. An Interdisciplinary Exploration* (ed. A. Harrington), Cambridge MA: Harvard University Press.
20. **Henney, J.E.** (1993). Combating medical fraud. *New York State Journal of Medicine* **93**, 86–7.
21. **Beecher, H.K.** (1955). The powerful placebo. *Journal of the American Medical Association* **199**, 1602–6.
22. **Beecher, H.K.** (1959). Experimentation in man. *Journal of the American Medical Association* **169**, 461–78.
23. **Kissel, P. and Barrucand, D.** *Placebo and Placebo Effects in Medicine*. Paris: Masson, 1964.
24. **Roberts, A.H.** et al. (1993). The power of non-specific effects in healing: implications for psychosocial and biological treatment. *Clinical Psychology Review* **13**, 375–91.
25. **Shapiro, A.K. and Struening, E.L.** (1973). The use of placebos: a study of the ethics and physicians' attitudes. *Psychiatric Medicine* **4**, 17–29.
26. **Shapiro, A.K. and Struening, E.L.** (1974). A comparison of the attitudes of a sample of physicians about the effectiveness of their treatment and the treatment of other physicians. *Journal of Psychiatric Research* **10**, 217–29.
27. **Huston, W.R.** (1938). The doctor himself as a therapeutic agent. *Annals of Internal Medicine* **11**, 1416–25.
28. **Novak, D.H.** (1987). Therapeutic aspects of the clinical encounter. *Journal of General Internal Medicine* **2**, 346–55.

29. **Chronic Fatigue Syndrome: Report of a Committee of the Royal Colleges of Physicians, Psychiatrists and General Practitioners.** London: Royal College of Physicians, 1996.
30. **Report of the Working Party on CFS ME to the Chief Medical Officer for England and Wales.** London: Department of Health, 2001.
31. **Clark, C., Buchwald, D., Macintyre, A., Sharpe, M., and Wessely, S.** (2002). Chronic fatigue syndromes: a step towards agreement. *Lancet* **359**, 97–8.
32. **Slater, E.** (1865). Diagnosis of 'hysteria'. *British Medical Journal* **1**, 1395–9.
33. **Crimlisk, H.L., Bhatia, K., Cope, H., David, A., Marsden, C.D., and Ron, M.A.** (1998). Slater revisited: 6 year follow-up study of patients with medically unexplained motor symptoms. *British Medical Journal* **316**, 582–6.
34. **Muris, J.W., Starmans, R., Fijten, G.H., and Knottnerus, J.A.** (1996). One-year prognosis of abdominal complaints in general practice: a prospective study of patients in whom no organic cause is found. *British Journal of General Practice* **46**, 715–19.
35. **Speckens, A.E., van Hemert, A.M., Bolk, J.H., Hawton, K.E., and Rooijmans, H.G.** (1995). The acceptability of psychological treatment in patients with medically unexplained physical symptoms. *Journal of Psychosomatic Research* **39**, 855–63.
36. **Marchant-Haycox, S. and Salmon, P.** (1999). Patients' and doctors' strategies in consultations with unexplained symptoms. Interactions of gynaecologists with women presenting menstrual problems. *Psychosomatics* **38**, 440–50.
37. **Reid, S., Whooley, D., Crayford, T., and Hotopf, M.** (2001). Medically unexplained symptoms—GPs' attitudes towards their cause and management. *Family Practice* **18**, 519–23.

6.5 Diagnostic tests and use of technology

David A. Fitzmaurice

Introduction

Classically the diagnostic process comprises history, examination, and investigation. It has been suggested that within primary care the first two of these processes are most important, yielding around 90 per cent of diagnoses. The specificity of physical signs and symptoms however actually tends to decrease as patients move along the diagnostic pathway from primary to secondary care. This has perhaps led to the devaluing of the physical examination with more reliance on requesting the definitive test to either refute or confirm the suspected diagnosis. This is not always a good idea and all test results must be considered in the light of the history and examination (the so-called pre-test probability). Thus for a patient with suspected deep vein thrombosis, a simple nine point check list can distinguish between a 3 per cent and 75 per cent pre-test probability.[(1)] This will influence the interpretation of a venous ultrasound examination.

This chapter considers investigations as part of the diagnostic process. General issues concerning the use, interpretation, and value of technologies available in primary care are first considered. The main technologies employed in primary care are then considered in turn. Technology covers a broad range of investigations ranging from simple urine dipsticks (or even tasting of urine) to more elaborate investigations such as echocardiography or endoscopy. For the purpose of clarity these have been divided into those tests which are usually available within a primary care setting and those tests which generally require referral to a secondary care centre. Finally, there is a section covering the emerging role of information technology, in particular telemetry, in primary care diagnosis.

The value of diagnostic technologies in primary care

Considerable thought and a limited amount of research has been devoted to considering the value of near patient testing (NPT) in primary care. Although the types of technology considered as NPT most readily encompass the technologies usually available in primary care, the issues apply equally to those usually requiring referral. NPT is more commonly referred to as Point of Care (PoC) tests in the United States. There has been a rapid growth in the area of NPT in recent years, particularly in the United States and Germany, becoming increasingly important in primary care with up to 20 per cent of laboratory tests now performed within primary care settings.

The most clear-cut areas where clinical management would be affected by the availability of an immediate result would be for single test results such as the international normalized ratio (INR) and glycosylated haemoglobin (HBA1C). In these circumstances the usefulness of the result is clear, but important questions remain over the reliability, accuracy, and cost effectiveness of the NPT used.

NPT may be more expensive when tests are performed within primary care (because of the reduced efficiency of low volume activity, training needs, and higher quality control costs). However, this potentially increased direct cost needs to be balanced against the possible reduction in overall costs which may result from delays in receiving results from the laboratory, and the potentially increased number of patient contacts.

The value of a diagnostic test, and NPT in particular, can only be judged by evaluating the test's influence on disease diagnosis, management, or prognosis. For example, with INR measurement, dosing adjustment will be made according to the level of the induced haemostatic deficit, reflected by the INR. The evaluation of INR near patient tests should therefore be closely related to the clinical issues of management and specifically improving the quality of care.

NPT for primary care

The following criteria need to be addressed in clarifying the value of any particular NPT:[(2)]

- Will the result of the test affect management of the patient, by clarifying the diagnosis or by determining therapy or prognosis?
- Is the availability of an immediate result be more useful than waiting for a laboratory result, in terms of value to decision-making?
- Does the near patient test perform sufficiently well, in terms of sensitivity, specificity, predictive values, and reliability, in the appropriate setting?
- Is the near patient test cost-effective compared with the laboratory test?
- Is the near patient test sufficiently reliable in terms of quality control?
- Is the near patient test acceptable to patients?
- Do the users of the test have sufficient clinical knowledge to interpret and use the result effectively in diagnosis, or is support readily available?

As long as the performance characteristics of the test can be adequately determined, it can be seen that an immediate result of, for example a thyroid function test, might enhance clinical management, whilst allaying anxiety for patients who may otherwise have to wait for the result and subsequent advice.

Immediate information will affect the outcomes of medical care

What separates NPT from laboratory-based pathology tests is the (usual) immediate availability of the result and its ability to affect immediate management of the patient. There would be no disagreement over the value of an immediate ECG in the treatment of a patient with a cardio-respiratory arrest or an immediate blood sugar in an unconscious patient. The immediate nature and the value of NPTs in many primary care situations is less clear cut, with other factors being of relevance such as saving time in future consultations or convenience for the patient or practitioner. It may also be postulated that being able to advise patients upon the dose of medication at the time a test is performed may improve patient compliance and allow improved therapeutic control.

Quality assurance

The technical performance of the test, under laboratory conditions and in clinical use, can be grouped under 'quality assurance'. The UK Association of Clinical Biochemists have produced a set of guidelines on the implementation of NPT,[3] concentrating on the issues of quality control, recording of data, training needs of staff using the test, and health and safety issues.

Validity and accuracy

The first question is whether a test actually measures what it aims to. Manufacturers provide performance characteristics for their equipment under ideal conditions in a comparison with an accepted criterion referenced standard (the gold standard) for the test in question. A further question for clinicians is to what extent the measurement of substance 'X' contributes to the diagnosis. For example, different levels of serum glucose during a glucose tolerance test have different predictive values for the diagnosis of diabetes, simplified into the definition of 'impaired glucose tolerance' for the intermediate values.

A problem arises when there is no accepted gold standard for a test, or when a gold standard would be inappropriate in certain settings. For example, if surgical diagnosis were used as a gold standard in a condition which does not invariably require surgery, only the 'worst' cases would receive gold standard validation and the predictive value of the test for less serious cases would remain unknown. The lack of a gold standard is problematic in, for example, INR measurement and *Helicobacter pylori* testing.

Validity and accuracy of can be defined in terms of:

1. Reproducibility of results expressed in terms of coefficients of variance (CVs).
2. Accuracy expressed in terms of CVs.
3. Comparability, expressed in terms of CVs.

Reliability

Reliability includes two quality assurance components: internal reliability, or how consistent are the results of a test on a day to day basis; and external reliability, or how the results compare with an external standard. Some tests need regular calibration using standardized samples, others have their calibration built into the technology or accomplished by the input of a predetermined code for a new set of reagents. The complexity of calibration is a major influence on the degree of staff training and the throughput of tests required to make the near patient test cost-effective.

Precision

Precision describes the statistical variation of a series of results based on the same sample, in the same way that the 95 per cent confidence interval of a statistic describes the distribution of 95 per cent of results of a series of identical experiments. Just as in statistical inference there is no direct relationship with the 'true' test result, this is determined by the accuracy of the test as described above. Precision rather than validity and accuracy is the principle measurement used for comparison of INR measurement technology, due to the absence of a true gold standard.

Local variation of performance

The performance of a diagnostic test may vary considerably in different situations for a number of reasons. The test may be affected by the underlying prevalence of the condition being tested for. Tests with 'poor' likelihood ratios (LRs), that is LR+ less than 10 or LR− more than 0.1 have less ability, in Bayesian terms, to raise a low prior probability to a diagnostically relevant posterior probability. In clinical terms this means that tests with poor LRs will not substantially affect clinical decisions.

Some tests will be sensitive to sampling procedures and therefore potential operator errors, such as the need to collect a quantitative capillary sample, or the timing, preparation or storage of reagents. Other substances, either in the patient (such as drugs) or present as contaminants in swabs, etc. may interfere with the test. These can include lipaemia, haemolysis, icteric samples, raised or lowered haematocrit and serum (as opposed to plasma) samples.

Near patient tests are particularly prone to operator-dependent errors, by virtue of their being performed in a multitude of situations with potential for use in uncontrolled circumstances, by staff with little training, or indeed in the patient's home. Manufacturers need to be particularly aware of the need to make tests simple to use (few operator-dependent steps). The more steps involved, the greater the potential for variability in results between users.

Acceptability to patients

The sampling procedure of a test needs to be acceptable to patients. Acceptability includes the degree of invasiveness of the test: finger-prick samples being less invasive than venous blood sampling (although some patients may prefer venepuncture). However, patients differ in what they deem acceptable.[4]

Cost effectiveness

In all countries, health care expenditure has to compete with other priorities, either personal or national, and budgets are fixed. Diagnostic test expenditure has to be balanced, therefore, against other health needs. Within a fixed budget, if the extra costs of a near patient test cannot be justified by improved quality of care or cost savings elsewhere, the use of that test is not justified. Health economic evaluation of near patient tests needs to be complete, in that costs (both direct and indirect) to the different sectors of health care and to the patient need to be considered.

The measurement of clinical benefit poses special difficulties as all the problems of utility measurement apply. Structural distortions of health care funding can play a key role in determining the local application of particular technologies; such as primary care budget holding organizations in Europe and the United States being able to vire part of their laboratory budget into near patient tests, whilst those with no control over budgets are unable to recover any expenditure the practice makes on such items.

The potential benefits of NPT

Information value of result

The information value of a result in terms of medical diagnosis, is determined by the LR of the test and the balance between the utilities of testing and not testing. Tests have an important value in reducing the uncertainty under which doctors practice. A study of the influence of a rapid transit erythrocyte sedimentation rate on the diagnosis reached by Dutch primary care physicians found that the result confirmed the primary care physicians original diagnosis in 82 per cent of cases and was 'reassuring for both doctor and patient'.[5] Another benefit for the general practitioner is in the increased motivation that some practitioners feel, being able to perform diagnostic tests in-house. INR testing fulfils these criteria, with a clinical decision being directly affected by the result of a test, and allowing a shared management plan to be established between doctor and patient.

Screening

Screening programmes are likely to make more regular use of testing than diagnostic use, thus increasing the economy of scale of NPT. If patients are tested whilst still in the surgery, there are potential savings on administration and ensuring follow up of abnormal results.

Reduction in indirect costs

The main indirect costs to be taken into account within the context of NPT are patient factors such as travelling costs and time off work. Anecdotal evidence suggests that patient travelling and waiting time is reduced by the introduction of NPT, both within the hospital environment and in other situations.

Costs of transport of the specimen to the laboratory, processing the specimen with all the laboratory overheads and the transport of the result to the surgery are avoided. Continuing to provide a laboratory service for hospital and those primary care physicians not using NPT, will reduce the ability to realize cost savings.

Reducing the need for follow-up consultations

If a near patient test is performed while the patient waits, a return visit for further management may be avoided. However, a study of desktop analysers in London revealed that approximately 15 per cent of patients were asked to return to find out their result, even though the analyser was used. A number of primary care physicians used laboratory tests in preference to near patient tests, to provide a delay (using time to resolve a diagnostic problem) whilst still satisfying the need of the patient for symptoms to be taken seriously.

The potential costs of near patient tests in primary care

Direct extra costs of NPT

The cost of capital equipment such as optical readers, centrifuges, or analysers have to be accounted for as well as the recurring costs of reagents and consumables such as capillary tubes. If expensive equipment is infrequently used, the unit costs of an investigation rise sharply.

Opportunity costs

In primary care as in all parts of the health care system, resources are limited. If staff or practitioners are tied up performing near patient tests, they are not available to perform other tasks that might be more appropriate or more effective. This will be particularly true if practitioners choose to test more frequently as a consequence of the technology being available.

Staff, time, and training

The need to train staff appropriately, and the time for the near patient test to be performed, need to be included in the costs of testing. If a test is performed by a family physician, there is obviously a higher unit cost than if the test can be performed by a nurse or a technical assistant. Increasingly, in the United States and Scandinavia, the concept of 'physician's assistant', non-medical personnel, is being utilized to fulfil this kind of role.[6] Centralized laboratories, in contrast, are able to benefit from economies of scale both in equipment costs and also in the delegation of routine tasks to less trained (and less expensive) staff.

Quality control

A primary concern relating to NPT is the quality assurance. Several documents have been produced by pathologists, particularly from clinical chemists, which outline guidelines for decentralized laboratory work.[7–9] Collaboration between pathology laboratories and primary care is essential if NPT is to be safely and effectively utilized.

Primary care practitioners cannot ignore the issues of both internal and external quality control steps in the validation of test results. This will add to the unit costs of testing. Some near patient tests, like pregnancy tests, are single use test strips or cards where the quality control has been built in during manufacture, often taking the form of a visible 'negative test' indicator. Although convenient, these tests would be less cost-effective where many tests are performed daily.

Test availability increases testing

The 'Hawthorne effect' describes a change in the behaviour of subjects when their work is being studied. In a similar fashion, the availability of a test has been shown to increase the usage of that test. It is not known whether such increases in use indicates previously unmet need, are an inappropriate response, or will continue in the long-term. Studies have shown that in practices where desktop analysers have been introduced, the rate of testing increases, but these extra tests do not lead to an alteration in diagnosis or management. However, none of these studies have examined the effect of apparently 'inappropriate' tests on reducing the degree of uncertainty experienced by both doctor and patient.[10]

Specific consideration of tests which are usually available within a primary care setting

Tests usually available within a primary care setting are urine tests, blood tests, electrocardiography (ECG), and others.

Urine tests

The practice of investigating bodily fluids is an ancient one. The ancient Egyptians used the taste of urine as both a measure of physical well-being and also as an augur for future events. The range of tests available for urine today include: glucose as both a screening tool and monitoring aid for diabetes; micro-albuminuria as a method of early detection of renal disease; cytology, for detection of urinary tract cancers; and the most widely used, dip-stick testing for urinary tract infection.

Urinary tract infection

It has been traditional to send urine specimens from all patients suspected of having urinary infections to the microbiology laboratory for examination and culture. It is possible that by using reagent strips and/or low power microscopy, a significant reduction in the number of urine specimens sent to the laboratory can be achieved.

Reagent strips

If reagent strips testing for nitrite, blood, and protein are used, it is possible to predict very accurately which urine needs further analysis. In a clear urine, if all the tests are negative, 98.5 per cent of the samples will not be infected. In a turbid urine, a positive result will detect 80 per cent of infections.[11] Thus, only urines yielding positive results on reagent strip need further examination. Antibiotic treatment should not be started on the evidence of proteinuria alone.

Microscopy

By using low power microscopy to count the number of white cells, it is possible to predict very accurately those urines which are infected and need laboratory analysis. Thus, 95 per cent of urines with white cell counts of less than 18 per low power field (using a Beck microscope with a $6 \times$ eyepiece) will not be infected. It is suggested, therefore, that only urines with white cell counts greater than this are sent to the laboratory.[12]

Laboratory testing

The mainstay of diagnosis remains the mid-stream specimen of urine being examined and cultured in the microbiology laboratory. Bacteriuria is considered 'significant' when a recognized pathogen is isolated with a concentration greater than 10^8 organisms per litre of urine, in a properly collected specimen. More specialized specimens are required for suspected urethritis and prostatitis. Blood cultures are necessary in the investigation of pyelonephritis.

Micro-albuminuria

There is evidence that the use of angiotensin converting enzyme inhibitors (ACEIs) can prevent progression and even reverse renal damage if it is detected early enough, particularly for diabetic patients. Unfortunately, the routine dip-sticks which are used to detect proteinuria need quite a large volume of protein to become positive, indicating significant renal damage which is not reversible with drug treatment. This has led to the development of testing strips for micro-albuminuria. These detect small volume protein molecules which indicates the first stage of renal damage. If micro-albuminuria is detected, this is an indication to start ACEI therapy.

Drug screen

A variety of tests is now available to detect illicit drugs of abuse. Similarly urinary cotinine can be detected which is a marker of tobacco use. These tests tend to be used within specialized clinics which may or may not take place in primary care.

Blood tests

A variety of tests can be performed in the surgery. Some tests can be used for monitoring as well as aiding in the diagnosis of disease. These are generally single test technologies such as INR or blood sugar, but more sophisticated desktop analysers are available which can provide a range of tests which previously could only be performed in hospital laboratories. It is necessary to be aware of why a specific test or group of tests are to be undertaken in the primary care centre rather than a central facility. For example, several commercially available kits measure haemoglobin. Whilst this may be a useful test, the investigation of possible anaemia normally requires a battery of tests. Similarly the haemoglobin level needs to be interpreted as part of a full blood count (FBC). Even if a FBC were available, primary care physicians will often use the ordering of a test such as FBC as part of a 'watchful waiting' management approach. This would not be possible if the result were immediately available. Once again, therefore, we see that the need for an immediately available result is not always clear. Near patient tests are currently available for such things as blood sugar, HBA1C, INR, cholesterol, potassium, creatinine, C-reactive protein, and D-dimer (a marker for thrombosis). These tests can all be seen to be useful within the context of changing patient's management in line with the test results. For example, a negative D-dimer in a patient with a low pretest probability would not need referral for investigation of potential thrombosis. Similarly, a patient with a high blood sugar will benefit from immediate intervention (particularly if ketones are confirmed on urinary dip-stick testing).

Tests which are not currently available but which would theoretically aid clinical practice would include thyroid function tests and serum urate. One exciting development is the role of natriuretic peptide (BNP) as a marker for heart failure due to left ventricular dysfunction. Given the poor sensitivity and specificity of the clinical diagnosis of heart failure the development of a simple near patient BNP test could greatly enhance the diagnostic process.

ECG

The ECG gives a pictorial representation of the electrical conduction through the heart. Interpretation of an ECG is not always straightforward and requires some training although computerized software is now available to assist with this function. Historically, the ECG has been used in order to diagnose acute myocardial infarction. This may not represent the most useful modality for primary care although this may be different in very rural communities. The two main utilities for the ECG in primary care are the diagnosis of arrhythmias and the detection of left ventricular hypertrophy, whilst it is also used for the investigation of chest pain and 'funny turns'. However, the ECG is not always performed within the primary care centre with some centres referring patients to central facilities. The interpretation is even more fraught with many primary care physicians relying on expert (usually cardiologist) interpretation which is fed back in the form of a written report.

Other

The use of further diagnostic technology with a primary care setting will be very much dependent upon the local socio-political position, the economic well-being, and the actual practical make-up of primary care within a given environment. Some tests such as peak flow meters will be readily available in most situations. A peak flow meter gives an objective recording of lung function and can be useful in diagnosing asthma for patients complaining of shortness of breath. The actual peak flow rate (PFR) achieved can be compared to standard charts which give a predicted PFR based on height and gender. An achieved PFR of more than 15 per cent below the predicted is very suggestive of asthma. In order to confirm this diagnosis, however, it is useful to perform spirometry which gives substantially more information than a simple PFR. In a similar manner to the utility of ECG, interpretation of spirometric recordings needs some training and may be regarded as a specialist function in many countries.

Urinary pregnancy tests perhaps represent one of the most widely used near patient test. The role in primary care is unclear, however, with many centres (particularly United Kingdom) not providing routine pregnancy testing as part of their mini-laboratory service. This may be because the demand for this service would swamp request for others. Similarly, with both commercially and secondary care laboratory services available, it may be the urinary pregnancy testing is best managed without the primary care setting.

Specific consideration of tests usually requiring referral to secondary care

1. Echocardiography
2. Upper and lower gastrointestinal endoscopy
3. Radiography and ultrasound
4. Biochemical tests
5. Miscellaneous biopsies
6. Microbiology
7. Other

Primary care is generally perceived as a low-tech environment. If anything more than simple tests are required, this has generally meant referral to a second agency which in most countries predominantly means hospital. This section outlines the kinds of tests available with some indication of how and when they should be employed.

Echocardiography

Echocardiography is a method of inspecting both the structural and functional state of the heart. It uses ultrasonography to visualize the heart and by using a computer-enhanced recording facility can produce films to demonstrate aberrant blood flow through the heart. The role of echocardiography has traditionally been to visualize structural defects of the heart, particularly in paediatrics, but more recently it has become important as the gold standard investigation to diagnose heart failure.

ACEI therapy leads to improvements in both morbidity and mortality for all grades of heart failure due to left ventricular dysfunction (LVSD), and can prevent progression of asymptomatic LVSD to symptomatic heart failure.[13] Clinical diagnosis of heart failure is notoriously unreliable and has led to over-prescription of diuretics with subsequent problems such as electrolyte imbalance. It is important, therefore, that if a diagnosis of heart failure is suspected echocardiography is performed to determine left ventricular function and in this manner determine appropriate treatment. To put this into perspective, the prevalence of heart failure (defined as a left ventricular ejection fraction of $<$40 per cent) is 3.1 per cent (95 per cent CI; 2.6–3.7) in the general population aged 45 and over.[14]

Access to echocardiography is variable and usually requires referral to a specialist, however there are moves, particularly in the United Kingdom and the United States, for open access to echocardiography for primary care physicians.

Upper and lower gastrointestinal endoscopy

Upper gastrointestinal endoscopy

Upper gastrointestinal endoscopy involves inserting a flexible fibre-optic tube into the oesophagus and stomach, whilst more complex procedures can be undertaken by proceeding into the duodenum for visualization of the bile and pancreatic ducts. Endoscopy is valuable in the recognition of anatomical defects, tumours, and for the visualization of gastric and duodenal ulcers. *Helicobacter pylori* (HP) was originally diagnosed from ulcer biopsies. It can also be diagnosed using either blood or breath testing, when combined with the clinical scenario, justifying whether or not endoscopy should be performed. Thus, for patients aged 45 and under, the likelihood of detecting either a malignancy or an ulcer is negligible in the absence of HP. Conversely in a patient older than 45 with symptoms of weight loss, endoscopy should be the investigation of choice (see Vol. II, Chapter 4.1).

HP causes most peptic ulcer disease and non-invasive testing for this organism has emerged as an important alternative to imaging the upper gastrointestinal tract in the management of dyspepsia. The three main non-invasive tests for HP are serology, faecal antigen tests, and the labelled C-urea breath tests.

- Serology measures the antibody response to the organism in patients' serum. It is the cheapest test but also the least accurate with a 80–90 per cent sensitivity and specificity. This technique can be adapted to NPT giving a result within 5 minutes. Local validation of sensitivity and specificity is important before using these kits in primary care.
- The stool antigen test detects HP antigens in stool and is more accurate than serology with a 92–100 per cent sensitivity and 93–95 per cent specificity. The test is more expensive than serology and involves obtaining a stool sample, which is not acceptable to all patients.
- Urea breath tests use the urease activity of HP as the basis for the diagnosis of the infection. Urea labelled with either ^{13}C or ^{14}C is given orally to the patient and if HP infection is present this will be hydrolyzed to isotopically labelled CO_2. Urea breath tests have a sensitivity and specificity of more than 95 per cent. The ^{14}C-urea breath test is simple and cheap, but ^{14}C is radioactive and needs to be administered in a medical physics department, which is not ideal for primary care. ^{13}C is not radioactive so it avoids these problems but it is difficult to detect, requiring expensive mass spectrometry equipment. There have been a number of technological advances in ^{13}C-urea breath tests making analysis cheaper but the test is still expensive compared with other non-invasive alternatives.

Lower gastrointestinal endoscopy

Lower bowel endoscopy ranges from proctoscopy to colonoscopy. Proctoscopy and rigid sigmoidoscopy can be undertaken in the surgery and will exclude around 70 per cent of bowel tumours. The use of total colonoscopy, however, has led to the recognition of ascending colon tumours and also vascular abnormalities responsible for some rectal bleeding. Flexible sigmoidoscopy is increasingly being advocated as a useful procedure as part of a screening programme for colorectal cancer.[15] Whilst colonoscopy remains the gold standard for the diagnosis of both colorectal cancers and adenomas, a combination of flexible sigmoidoscopy and double contrast barium enema may offer a more convenient and equally sensitive approach. The main advantage of this approach, however is the reduction in the number of adverse events, with total colonoscopy having a serious adverse event rate of between 0.4 and 1.2 per cent with an overall mortality of around 0.01 per cent.[16]

Radiography and ultrasound

Radiography remains the mainstay of diagnosis of bony injury, whilst more sophisticated techniques such as spiral CT have become the gold standard diagnostic tools in conditions such as pulmonary embolism. The availability of radiography in some ways dictates its utility. Plain radiographs have limited value in conditions such as chronic airways disease, heart failure, and lower back pain, although if this is the only diagnostic technique available it may still be useful. For example, plain chest X-ray has previously been advised in cases of suspected left ventricular hypertrophy associated with hypertension. If, however, the physician has access to echocardiography then chest X-ray is rendered unnecessary. Even without echocardiography the sensitivity and specificity of plain chest radiography is similar to that of clinical examination (i.e. quite low) such as to make interpretation difficult. There has been an effort to reduce the numbers of X-rays requested from primary care for patients presenting with lower back pain. Around 13 per cent of patients with back pain who consult their primary care physician will receive a lower back X-ray within 3 months. This is a cause for concern as a set of spinal X-rays gives the equivalent of 7 months of natural background radiation (65 times the amount of a chest X-ray). Between 30 and 100 life-time cases of cancer per million may be risked by lumbar spine X-rays (or risk of 1 in 32 000 of a fatal cancer per spine X-ray, or 19 deaths a year in the United Kingdom in 1973). Economic modelling has suggested that management guidelines may provide a 12.5–37.5 per cent reduction in X-rays.

The role of radiography in diagnostic work-up needs to be considered carefully. Requests are often made which will actually have little or no impact on clinical management. The role of patient reassurance cannot be ignored, however patients seem to request X-rays as a kind of panacea and; responsible clinician needs to counsel the patient away from unnecessary investigation. Whilst the case for lower back radiography is quite straightforward there are other occasions where this is not so.

Ultrasound has been used primarily in obstetric care with other applications including Doppler techniques in the diagnosis of deep vein thrombosis and more esoterically for the detection of breast lesions in adolescents. Where primary care takes a lead role in the provision of obstetric care there is evidence that the use of ultrasound within the antenatal period is associated with high quality perinatal outcomes, with primary care reporting a lower incidence of Caesarean section, use of forceps, and low birth weight babies with no difference in the risk profile of the patients.[17]

Biochemical and haematological tests

It is not possible to give an overview of all the possible tests which might assist in diagnosis, but certain principles can be applied in requesting these tests. Numerous tests can be performed in the surgery, but the majority of biochemical tests, whether using blood or urine, require central laboratory analysis. Whereas most near patient tests require individual finger-stick sampling, when more than one test is required it may be preferable from a patient perspective that a venous sample is taken. The range of tests available is immense and well known to most primary care personnel. The most widely requested tests are for serum biochemistry, usually requested as 'urea and electrolytes' (U + Es). This is most often requested alongside a full blood count as a baseline screen. In fact, routine U + E rarely reveals anything of any consequence whereas specific requests for potassium for example, in patients taking diuretics, is much more likely to provide clinically relevant information. This again highlights the issue of pretest probability and the need to critically evaluate the reason for requesting a test. For example, a serum urate level is often requested along with the U + E and liver function test. If the urate level comes back raised in the absence of symptoms, what is its relevance?

A further example is the current role of thrombophilia screening. This may be relevant in young women requesting oral contraception who have a family history of thrombosis. In fact the current situation is less than straightforward. Whilst the prevalence of certain prothrombotic conditions such as Factor V Leiden is well established, its clinical significance is not. Thus, for the primary care physician, the dilemma is whether to request a certain test, such as 'thrombophilia screen', or to refer to a specialist for advice. In this case it is probably wiser to refer for specialist advice unless one is clear about how to respond to a specific situation.

Miscellaneous biopsy

Many lumps and bumps are excised in primary care. Perhaps the commonest of these will be pigmented lesions. Primary care physicians have been criticized in the past for undertaking incomplete excisions which make further surgical intervention necessary but unnecessarily complicated. It is clear therefore that, as in anything else, sufficient training must be undertaken by anyone performing such procedures.

Gynaecological procedures are becoming more commonplace in primary care with cervical cytological sampling being the commonest example. Whilst not formally a biopsy, it is a skilled technique which requires specialized training to ensure adequate sampling. It is also possible to undertake endometrial sampling in primary care which will, in many cases, negate the need for hysteroscopy under anaesthetic.

Microbiology

Microbiological testing is predominantly used in primary care for the diagnosis of urinary tract infections. There is little role for taking swabs for sore throats or wound infections. Tests are available for the detection of streptococcal throat infections and also for C-reactive protein which can aid in distinguishing viral from bacterial causation. The utility of these tests is, however, poor.[(10)] Gynaecological infections (particularly chlamydia) can only be accurately diagnosed by taking swabs for culture.

Other

A number of other diagnostic modalities have not been covered. These include only complex interventions such as MRI scanning or relatively simple interventions such as exercise ECG. These more specialized tests, however, are predominantly organized in the specialist arena and it is rare that a primary care physician will refer for a specific investigation of this nature.

The role of telemetry for primary care diagnosis

The development of information technology and computerization has changed the way in which primary care functions. For example, the prosecution of screening programmes has become much more achievable through being able to identify 'at risk' populations and tracing patients who have not received the appropriate screening test. One more recent development has been the use of telemetry (or telemedicine) which can loosely be defined as 'the delivery of medical care at a distance'.[(18)] One example would be the use of digital images from primary care being streamed to a central facility for the diagnosis of, say, skin rashes. This could use real-time video images or could take the form of transmitted photographic images. Whilst this has become a reality in many countries it is also becoming useful in remote underdeveloped places such as Papua New Guinea.[(18)] This is, however, a relatively new advance in diagnostics and the impact of this technology remains to be formally evaluated.

Acknowledgements

I would like to thank Professors Richard Hobbs and Brendan Delaney for providing invaluable material for this chapter, and also Dr Chris Hyde for his support and help with proof reading.

References

1. **Wells, P.S.** et al. (1997). Value of assessment of pretest probability of deep vein thrombosis in clinical management. *Lancet* **350**, 1795–8.
2. **Dinant, G.J., de Maeseneer, J., and Derese, A.** (1993). How many ROC curves fit into one general practitioner? The paradox between medical decision making and daily general practice. *Huisarts en Wetenschap* **26** (Suppl.), 58–61.
3. **Association of Clinical Biochemists.** *Guidelines for Implementation of Near Patient Testing.* London: Association of Clinical Biochemists, 1993.
4. **Hobbs, F.D.R.** (2000). ABC of colorectal cancer: the role of primary care. *British Medical Journal* **321**, 1068–70.
5. **Dinant, G.J., Knotterus, J.A., and Van Wersch, J.W.J.** (1992). Diagnostic impact of the ESR in general practice: a before–after analysis. *Family Practice* **9**, 28–31.
6. **Asprey, D.P., Zollo, S., and Kienzle, M.** (2000). Implementation and evaluation of a telemedicine course for physician assistants. *Academic Medicine* **76**, 652–5.
7. **Marks, V. and Alberti, K.G.M.M.** *Clinical Biochemistry Nearer the Patient II.* London: Balliere Tindall, 1986.
8. **WHO Regional Office for Europe.** *The Role of Laboratory Medicine in Primary Health Care.* A report from the programme on quality of care and technologies. Copenhagen: WHO, 1989.
9. **Grol, R., Wensing, M., Jacobs, A., and Baker, R.**, ed. Quality assurance in general practice. The state of the art in Europe. Utrecht: Nederlands Huisarten Genootschap, 1993.
10. **Hobbs, F.D.R., Delaney, B.C., Fitzmaurice, D.A., Wilson, S., Hyde, C., Thorpe, G.H., Earl-Slater, A., Jowett, S.M., and Tobias, R.S.** (1997). A systematic review of near patient testing. *Health Technology Assessment* **1** (5), 1–229.
11. **Hiscock, C., Yorall, H., Greig, P., and Lightfoot, N.F.** (1990). Validation of a method for rapid diagnosis of urinary tract infection suitable for use in general practice. *British Journal of General Practice* **40**, 403–5.
12. **Fitzmaurice, D.A.** (1994). Urinary tract infection. In *A Treatment Handbook of Drug Therapy* 51st edn. (ed. F.D.R. Hobbs and L. Beeley). London: Churchill Livingstone.
13. **Garg, R. and Yusuf, S., for the Collaborative Group on ACE inhibitor trials.** (1992). Overview of randomised trial of angiotensin-converting enzyme inhibitors on mortality and morbidity in patients with heart failure. *New England Journal of Medicine* **327**, 685–91.
14. **Davies, M.K., Hobbs, F.D.R., Davis, R.C., Roalfe, A.K., Hare, R., Wosornu, D., and Lancashire, R.J.** (2001). Prevalence of left-ventricular dysfunction and heart failure in the Echocardiographic Heart of England Screening study: a population based study. *Lancet* **358**, 439–44.
15. **Atkin, W.** (1999). Implementing screening for colorectal cancer. *British Medical Journal* **319**, 1212–13.
16. **Waye, J.D., Kahn, O., and Auerbach, M.E.** (1996). Complications of colonoscopy and flexible sigmoidoscopy. *Gastrointestinal Endoscopy Clinics of North America* **6** (2), 343–77(Review).
17. **Deutchman, M.E., Sills, D., and Connor, P.D.** (1995). Perinatal outcomes: a comparison between family physicians and obstetricians. *The Journal of the American Board of Family Practice* **8**, 440–7.
18. **Edworthy, S.M.** (2001). Telemedicine in developing countries. *British Medical Journal* **323**, 524–5.

Further reading

Gives a review of NPT for primary care:

Hobbs, F.D.R., Delaney, B.C., Fitzmaurice, D.A., Wilson, S., Hyde, C., Thorpe, G.H., Earl-Slater, A., Jowett, S.M., and Tobias, R.S. (1997). A systematic review of near patient testing. *Health Technology Assessment* **1** (5), 1–229.

Outlines the difficulties in evaluating the utility of diagnostic tests:

Lijmer, J.G. et al. (1999). Empirical evidence of design related bias in studies of diagnostic tests. *Journal of the American Medical Association* **282**, 1061–6.

Seminal essay putting the context of investigation within the framework of the diagnostic process:

Mcalister, F.A., Strauss, S.E., and Sackett, D.L. (1999). Why we need large, simple studies of the clinical examination: the problem and a proposed solution. *Lancet* **354**, 1721–4.

Useful cost evaluation:

NHS HTA, Grieve, R., Beech, R., Vincent, J., and Mazurkiewicz, J. (1999). Near patient testing in diabetes clinics: appraising the costs and outcomes. *Health Technology Assessment* **3** (15), 1–74.

6.6 Computerized decision support

Jon Emery

> Busy clinicians are caught in an information paradox: overwhelmed with information but unable to find the knowledge they need when they need it.[1]

Introduction

The futuristic vision of computerized diagnosis and management has been discussed for many decades but its realization in clinical practice is only just starting to be seen. Faced by the continuing deluge of information about clinical management and best evidence, how can the busy primary care physician access the right information at the right time? Does the PC on the doctor's desk hold the key through the provision of computer decision support systems? (See Box 1.)

The underlying premise of computer decision support is that human fallibility in the medical decision-making process may, at least partially, be countered by a computer that links information about the patient to its knowledge base and advises the health professional accordingly, thus leading to more cost-effective management. Beneath this premise lie many assumptions that challenge the application of computer decision support in routine practice. This chapter discusses the use of computer decision support systems in primary care, including examples of decision support systems and evidence from systematic reviews of the subject, and ends by discussing some of the challenges facing the application of computer decision support in routine care.

Box 1 Definitions of computer decision support systems

- Active knowledge systems that use two or more items of patient data to generate case-specific advice.[2]
- Software designed to directly aid in clinical decision-making in which characteristics of individual patients are matched to a computerized knowledge base for the purpose of generating patient-specific assessments or recommendations that are presented to clinicians for consideration.[3]

The information gap in the consultation

In a primary care consultation, the traditional approach to decision-making is to rely on past experience and the practitioner's memory of relevant clinical information. The enormous expansion in medical information and the drive to deliver evidence-based clinical practice makes this approach increasingly untenable. By its very nature, primary care practice frequently encounters uncertainty; primary care practitioners report information needs in 20–30 per cent of consultations, most commonly relating to the cause of specific symptoms, drug prescribing, and disease management.[4,5] With the exception of prescribing information, most of these questions go unanswered during the consultation. Computer decision support has the potential to influence and support all stages of the consultation from diagnosis to management and shared decision-making by bridging the information gaps that exist and by presenting information that can be readily shared with the patient.

Potential functions of computer decision support systems

At present, two principal types of computer decision support system are available:

- *Probabilistic systems:* these apply individual patient data to an epidemiological model to inform diagnosis or prognosis or to a pharmacodynamic and pharmacokinetic model to aid prescribing decisions.
- *Rule-based systems:* these depend on the creation of a knowledge base that applies certain clinical features to a series of rules and then offers patient-specific advice. Clearly, they rely on the accuracy and appropriateness of the underlying knowledge base but have the advantage that they can explain the advice given.

Rule-based systems, in particular, have considerable potential to affect clinical behaviour and decision-making through the implementation of clinical guidelines. Concurrent with the evidence-based movement and the drive to reduce variations in clinical practice, the last decade has witnessed the production of a multitude of clinical guidelines aimed at primary care in an attempt to improve the quality of care. Clinical guidelines are meant to embody best medical practice and are expected to change practitioners' decisions towards an ideal level of care.[6] An early systematic review of evaluations of clinical guidelines suggested that guidelines that are developed locally, disseminated using specific educational events, and implemented during the consultation are most likely to succeed.[7] However, a more recent systematic review of the effectiveness of clinical guidelines specifically in primary care found little evidence that they alter patient outcomes.[8] A third review identified a number of barriers to physician adherence to guidelines including lack of awareness of and disagreement with the guideline, difficulties reconciling patient preferences with guideline recommendations, and lack of time to find and apply the guideline.[9] Perhaps the most significant barrier to adopting clinical guidelines is the sheer bulk of information sent to primary care practitioners, principally in paper format. Computer decision support presents a clear opportunity to manage this information overload and implement guidelines during the consultation.

Examples of computer decision support systems

PRODIGY

PRODIGY (Prescribing Rationally with Decision Support in General Practice Study) is a British computer decision support system designed to integrate with general practice electronic patient records and provide patient-specific guidance on drug therapy and non-pharmacological management of a wide range of clinical conditions in primary care.[10] When a diagnosis is entered into the clinical computer system, PRODIGY offers advice on prescribing, investigation, and referral by applying evidence-based recommendations generated by an expert panel. In the future, relevant guidelines from the National Institute for Clinical Excellence will be implemented via PRODIGY.

Risk assessment

Several computer decision support systems exist that calculate risk of specific diseases by entering known risk factors and applying these to a specific risk assessment model.

Cardiovascular disease

A variety of different programmes are available to calculate the risk of cardiovascular disease, most of which apply data from the Framingham populations. These programmes have become increasingly important in supporting primary preventive strategies and treatment decisions based on absolute risks of cardiovascular disease. An example of such a programme is given in Fig. 1 (*Cardiorisk Manager*, BMJ Publishing).[11] Data on standard risk factors such as blood pressure, smoking status, and lipid levels are entered into the programme. Numerical and graphical displays of absolute cardiovascular risk are presented including comparative risks for the general population. The effect of particular risk reduction strategies (e.g. stopping smoking) on the patient's absolute risk can also be demonstrated, which theoretically could help to motivate a patient to reduce their risk.

Genetic risk assessment

The predicted expansion of DNA-based tests, coupled with the minimal training primary care practitioners receive in genetics, has led to proposals that computer decision support could support the delivery of high-quality advice about genetic issues in primary care (see Chapter 9.4). A pedigree-drawing programme that provides patient-specific advice about genetic risk of breast and ovarian cancer has been shown to increase the appropriateness of general practitioners' decisions regarding family history of cancer and the accuracy of pedigrees compared to traditional pen-and-paper methods (Fig. 2).[12]

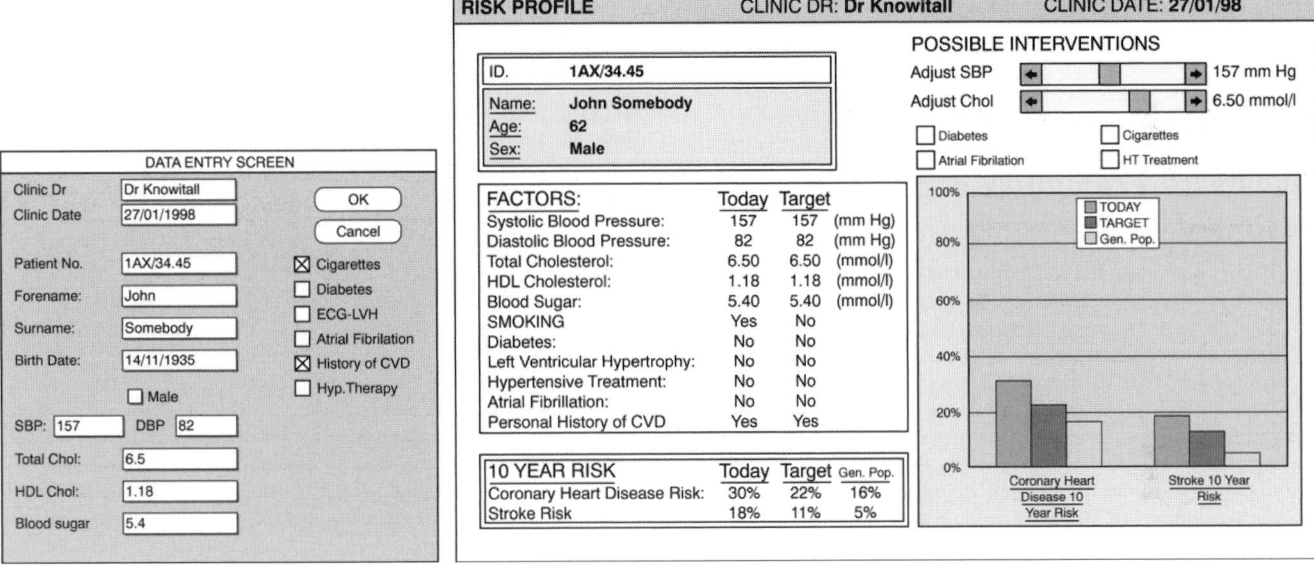

Fig. 1 Example of cardiovascular risk assessment decision support software.[11]

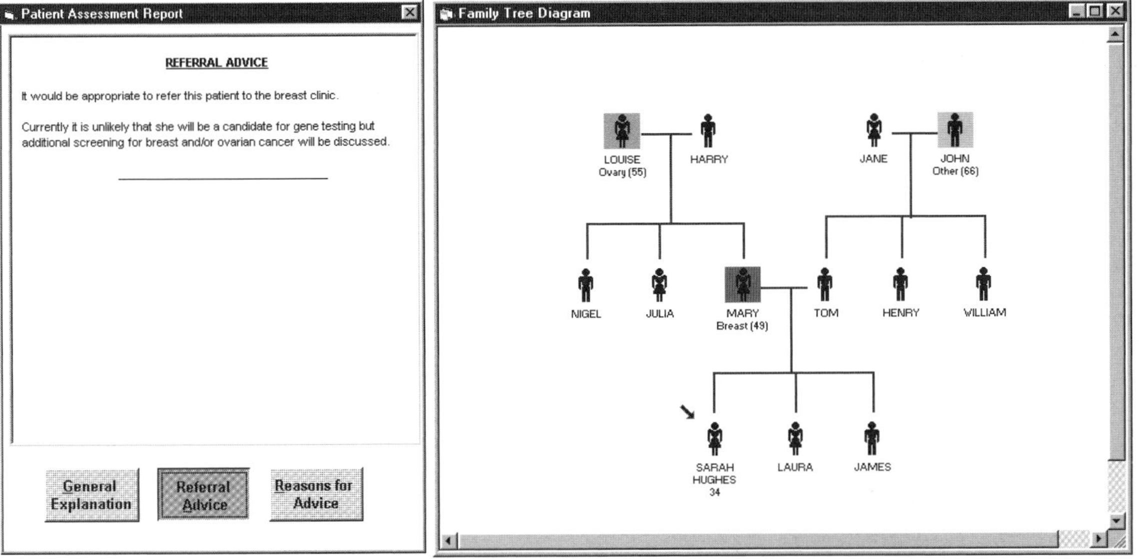

Fig. 2 Example of genetic risk assessment decision support software.[12]

Diagnosis

Computer decision support systems have been developed to assist diagnosis and case-finding for a range of conditions in primary care. PROQSY (PROgrammable Questionnaire SYstem) is a tool to aid recognition of common mental disorders in primary care and consists of a patient-administered computerized assessment.[13] It entails a series of branching questions about symptoms of common mental illnesses and generates a symptom score that prompts primary care practitioners to consider psychological disorders in their diagnosis. In a randomized controlled trial of PROQSY, patients using the system showed modest improvements in clinical outcome at 3 months compared to those receiving standard care.

Chronic disease management

Computer decision support systems have also been developed to support the management of various chronic diseases and conditions in primary care including hypertension, diabetes and anticoagulation. AMSS (Anticoagulation Management Support System) is a computer decision support system to support dosing decisions about warfarin prescribing, by implementing British Society of Haematology Guidelines. In a trial of nurse-led anticoagulation clinics in primary care, patients randomized to management supported by AMSS spent a significantly greater proportion of time within their target INR range than those receiving standard care.[14]

The effect of computer decision support on clinical care

Many different computer decision support systems exist, some of which are commercially available, but how strong is the evidence to support the promise of computer decision support in improving clinical care? There have been several systematic reviews of computer decision support systems that have examined their effect on drug dosage,[15] on clinician performance and patient outcomes.[3,16] and specifically on the effect of computing on clinical care in general practice.[17] Computer decision support systems have been shown in hospital settings to result in higher drug concentrations, reduced time to reach therapeutic control, and fewer unwanted effects.[15] The majority of studies investigating computer decision support on physician performance have demonstrated a beneficial effect, particularly in relation to preventive care, drug dosing, and chronic disease management. However, only a minority of studies have demonstrated positive effects of computer decision support on physician diagnosis or patient outcomes, although this may be due to the limited power of some of these studies.[3]

The Hunt review focused mainly on studies conducted in North American hospitals and health maintenance organizations. A recently updated systematic review of computing predominantly from UK and US primary care also found that computers can improve immunization rates and other preventive tasks (e.g. blood pressure screening and cervical and breast cancer screening), particularly when practitioners were prompted by the computer during the consultation. Use of electronic protocols was associated with the largest improvements in management of chronic diseases such as diabetes and hypertension.

The main use of computers in primary care is currently to support prescribing and the use of computer decision support to aid this process is associated with an increase in generic drug prescribing and a reduction in drug costs. Some of the beneficial effects of using computer decision support were seen especially in general practices serving more deprived populations, suggesting a possible way of reversing the 'inverse care law'. The review found that general practice consultations are lengthened by 48–130 s by the presence of a computer, partly due to increased preventive activities, although this increase in consultation length reduced with time.

Research on the effectiveness of computer decision support systems in primary care has several limitations. There are still relatively few studies that have examined patient outcomes, although those that have showed improvements in diastolic blood pressure, anticoagulation control, and referrals about lipid management. Studies have rarely accounted for cluster randomization or conducted detailed economic evaluations of computer decision support. Randomized controlled trials have often been conducted on poorly developed systems leading to technical failure or software that is unsuitable for primary care practice.

Evidence for a generic benefit of using computer decision support should not be used to imply effectiveness of a specific system. Ideally, each computer decision support system should undergo various stages of evaluation prior to commercial release, and may still require local adaptation once installed. Nonetheless, there is good evidence to support the concept of computer decision support as a method of improving at least the process of clinical care in primary care, while accepting that more rigorous health services research is required to investigate the cost-effectiveness of specific decision support systems in primary care.

The patient perspective

The introduction of the computer and use of decision support potentially adds a 'third person' into the consultation that could alter the consultation dynamics and the doctor–patient relationship. The impact of the computer on the general practice consultation has been described, both in relation to sharing sensitive information on the computer screen and to doctor–patient communication.

In a survey of Dutch patients, 93 per cent felt that their consultation was no less personal when the doctor used a computer but one-third of patients expressed concerns about the security of information held on the computer.[18] Qualitative studies have found that patients do not perceive computers in the consultation as impersonal as long as the doctor maintains eye contact and verbal communication as much as possible,[19] but doctors often become preoccupied with the computer and fall exactly into this trap.[20] Patients feel comfortable viewing only certain types of information about themselves on the general practitioners' computer screen; they find it useful to see information about their own lifestyle (e.g. smoking status) or blood pressure, but do not want to see certain diagnoses on the screen (e.g. mental illness or cancer).[21] Sensitive information about risk of cancer can create difficulties for the practitioner using decision support, especially if new information about disease risk is shared simultaneously with the patient leading to a loss of control of the consultation.[22]

Further work is required to investigate the most effective methods to consult while using a computer. Introducing the computer into the consultation and sharing the screen with the patient may help reduce the 'third-party effect' of the computer, but this depends on careful design of the computer interface so that the practitioner can control the flow of information being shared with the patient, particularly when discussing sensitive issues.[22] Learning how best to share information on the screen with the patient without loss of continuity in the consultation is an art. This art form requires further development to minimize any negative impact on the doctor–patient interaction if use of computer decision support is to become routine.

The future

It is likely that primary care will witness an increase in the number of different types of computer decision support available, many of which will be Internet-based. These will probably remain focused on supporting specific tasks, as has been the general rule for decision support systems. We can also expect to see similar types of programme aimed at the consumer, with patients sharing the results from these programmes with their primary care practitioner.

If computer decision support is truly going to support the provision of high-quality medicine in primary care, a number of important issues must be resolved. Currently, much of the workforce in primary care have relatively few computing skills beyond, for example, the use of a specific clinical computing system to generate prescriptions. The use of a computer mouse and keyboard remains unfamiliar to many primary care practitioners. Most primary medical records in general practice are paper-based and it may take the quantum leap towards electronic health records as the principal repository of the medical record to drive the routine use of computers and acquisition of computing skills in the primary care workforce.

Computer literacy will be less of a problem for the next generation of primary care practitioners. But even with a computer literate workforce, computer decision support systems will need to be carefully designed to facilitate their easy use in a consultation, and provide information that is relevant, accurate, and up to date. Many decision support systems are designed as stand-alone software that do not integrate easily with the clinical computing system. Practitioners resent having to re-enter data that already exist on their computer.

We are moving into a new era of medicine driven by information. If patients and health services are to benefit, primary care practitioners must develop strategies to manage this information. Evidence demonstrates the potential of computer decision support to deliver the right information when it is needed in the consultation. With a well-trained workforce and well-designed software, the promise of high-quality primary care supported by computer decision aids could become a reality.

References

1. **Gray, J.A.** (1998). Where's the chief knowledge officer? To manage the most precious resource of all. *British Medical Journal* **317**, 832.
2. **Wyatt, J. and Spiegelhalter, D.** Field trials of medical decision-aids: potential problems and solutions. *Proceedings of the Annual Symposium on Computer Applications in Medical Care*, 1991, pp. 3–7.
3. **Hunt, D.L., Haynes, R.B., Hanna, S.E., and Smith, K.** (1998). Effects of computer-based clinical decision support systems on physician performance and patient outcomes: a systematic review. *Journal of the American Medical Association* **280**, 1339–46.
4. **Ely, J.W.** et al. (1999). Analysis of questions asked by family doctors regarding patient care. *British Medical Journal* **319**, 358–61.
5. **Barrie, A.R. and Ward, A.M.** (1997). Questioning behaviour in general practice: a pragmatic study. *British Medical Journal* **315**, 1512–15.
6. **Deighan, M. and Hitch, S.** *Clinical Effectiveness from Guidelines to Cost Effective Practice*. Brentwood, Essex: Earlybrave Publications Ltd, 1995.
7. **Grimshaw, J. and Russell, I.** (1993). Effect of clinical guidelines on medical practice: a systematic review of rigorous evaluations. *Lancet* **342**, 1317–22.
8. **Worrall, G., Chaulk, P., and Freake, D.** (1997). The effects of clinical practice guidelines on patient outcomes in primary care: a systematic review. *Canadian Medical Association Journal* **156**, 1705–12.
9. **Cabana, M.** et al. (1999). Why don't physicians follow clinical practice guidelines? *Journal of the American Medical Association* **282**, 1458–65.
10. **PRODIGY.** www.prodigy.nhs.uk (Accessed on 1 May 2001).
11. **Hingorani, A.D. and Vallance, P.** (1999). A simple computer program for guiding management of cardiovascular risk factors and prescribing. *British Medical Journal* **318**, 101–5.
12. **Emery, J.** et al. (2000). Computer support for interpreting family histories of breast and ovarian cancer in primary care: comparative study with simulated cases. *British Medical Journal* **321**, 28–32.
13. **Lewis, G., Sharp, D., Bartholomew, J., and Pelosi, A.J.,** (1996). Computerized assessment of common mental disorders in primary care: effect on clinical outcome. *Family Practice* **13**, 120–6.
14. **Fitzmaurice, D.A., Hobbs, F.D., Murray, E.T., Holder, R.L., Allan, T.F., and Rose, P.E.** (2000). Oral anticoagulation management in primary care with the use of computerized decision support and near-patient testing: a randomized, controlled trial. *Archives of Internal Medicine* **160**, 2343–8.
15. **Walton, R., Dovey, S., Harvey, E., and Freemantle, N.** (1999). Computer support for determining drug dose: systematic review and meta-analysis. *British Medical Journal* **318**, 984–90.
16. **Johnston, M., Langton, K., Haynes, B., and Mathieu, A.** (1994). Effects of computer-based clinical decision support systems on clinician performance and patient outcome. *Annals of Internal Medicine* **120**, 135–42.
17. **Mitchell, E. and Sullivan, F.** (2001). A descriptive feast but an evaluative famine: systematic review of published articles on primary care computing during 1980–97. *British Medical Journal* **322**, 279–82.
18. **Rethans, J.J., Hoppener, P., Wolfs, G., and Diederiks, J.** (1988). Do personal computers make doctors less personal? *British Medical Journal* **296**, 1446–8.
19. **Ridsdale, L. and Hudd, S.** (1994). Computers in the consultation: the patient's view. *British Journal of General Practice* **44**, 367–9.
20. **Greatbatch, D., Heath, C., Campion, P., and Luff, P.** (1995). How do desktop computers affect the doctor-patient interaction? *Family Practice* **12**, 32–6.
21. **Ridsdale, L. and Hudd, S.** (1997). What do patients want and not want to see about themselves on the computer screen: a qualitative study. *Scandinavian Journal of Primary Health Care* **15**, 180–3.
22. **Emery, J., Walton, R., Coulson, A., Glasspool, D., Ziebland, S., and Fox, J.** (1999). A qualitative evaluation of computer support for recording and interpreting family histories of breast and ovarian cancer in primary care (RAGs) using simulated cases. *British Medical Journal* **319**, 32–6.

7

Management of individuals

7 Management of individuals

7.1 Principles of patient management

Wolfgang Himmel, Anja Rogausch, and Michael M. Kochen

Introduction

An ever more popular movement towards strengthening the patient's role (the 'consumer approach') and the increasing economic pressure on primary care doctors has stimulated more rational planning of the management of individuals in general practice.[1] The idea of patient management in primary care, however, is not new and has always been about addressing the patient in his/her biomedical as well as social and psychological context.

The evidence for patient management

Patient management aims to shift the focus from the disease to the sick person,[2] or—as Maimonides, the medieval Jewish physician and thinker, put it 800 years earlier—'the physician should not treat the disease but the patient who is suffering from it'.[3] Such a patient-centred approach is based on a good ('therapeutic') doctor–patient relationship. The quality of the interaction between physician and patient and their expectations may sometimes influence patient outcomes more than specific treatment, for example, with a drug. Moreover, patient-centred practice is associated with increased efficiency of care, involving fewer diagnostic tests and referrals.[4,5]

Engel[6] was one of the first to develop a systematic approach towards the biopsychosocial model.[7] Drawing on systems theory, this model offers a framework of the patient as 'a whole person' with specific emphasis on subjective experience, thoughts, and emotions related to objective data (e.g. medical findings). Consequently, disorders exist at different hierarchical but closely interacting levels (Fig. 1).

Engel's theoretical assumptions are supported by recent evidence from psychoneuroimmunology. The term psychoneuroimmunology expresses the important links between the central nervous and the immune systems. There is a strong bi-directional relationship between the brain and immune systems. Several studies have confirmed the relationship between stressful life events, immunological changes, and adverse health outcomes such as heart disease, cancer, asthma, or infectious disease (Fig. 2).[8]

Supportive relationships are an important mediator and often improve the immunological condition, whereas bereavement, for example, can result in a temporary down-regulation of the immune response.[9] Also, other factors such as chronic stress modulate a variety of immunological activities.

Since immunological processes are embedded within a larger biological, psychological, and social context, it is—as Engel[6] predicted—impossible to practise 'disease management' without taking the patient's concerns and background into consideration.

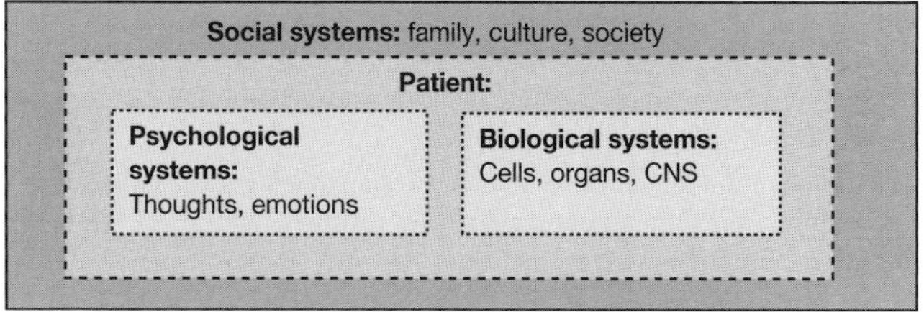

Fig. 1 Levels of the biopsychosocial model.

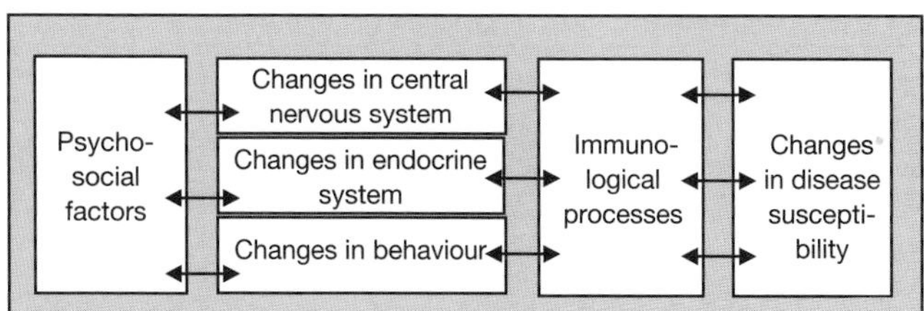

Fig. 2 Psychosocial factors may cause changes in disease susceptibility.[8]

Key principles of patient management

The consultation is at the centre of primary care. Serial consultations establish long-term relationships with patients and knowledge about them, and form the basis for follow-up. It is essential, especially in patients with chronic conditions, not only to structure each consultation but also to develop a structured long-term plan for clinical management.[10–12] Such a plan should include

- collaborative definition of problems,
- action planning (targeting, goal setting),
- information,
- patient education and motivational training,
- scheduled follow-up,
- outcome monitoring,
- adherence monitoring,
- stepped therapy,
- specialty consultation and referral.

Management programmes may improve with active patient participation and shared decision-making. There is evidence that most patients want a patient-centred approach, and are less satisfied, less enabled, and may be more burdened by symptoms if they do not get it.[13,14]

Patient management is also an attempt to overcome clinical inertia: a failure of health care providers to initiate or intensify therapy when indicated.[15] Doctors may thus identify patients and situations in which more intensive management of chronic conditions such as hypertension is appropriate. Moreover, real-world primary care physicians can deliver effective treatment if they are supported by organized systems for patient education, proactive consultation for non-responders, physician education, and patient monitoring, as Katzelnick[16] demonstrated for the management of depression.

Stages and steps of a management plan

A management plan should be based on evidence-based guidelines (if available) for different conditions seen in general practice. The following steps may help to structure a single consultation as well as the long-term doctor–patient relationship (Table 1).

Establishing a relationship

Development of a sustained partnership is an explicit responsibility of GPs and a typical characteristic of primary care (see also Chapter 5.1). Some role allocations should be taken into account: the patients as experts for their life and specific medical conditions, the GP as counsellor and expert in the application of medical knowledge and skills. Both partners maintain responsibility for the process of treatment. Fostering the doctor–patient relationship is a continuing process pervading all stages of a management plan supported by active listening, encouraging narration, providing explanations, and expressing concern.

Eliciting the patient's agenda

In the first consultation with a new patient or at the beginning of a new illness episode, it is a central task to elicit the patient's agenda. Even in well-established patients, their problems should be reassessed from time to time. One of the most prominent reasons for encounter is the patient's need for explanation and not (only) for treatment.[17]

At this stage, the doctor tries to enter the patient's world, get a holistic picture of his or her problems, and obtain the full spectrum of concerns.[18] In addition, information from all levels of the biopsychosocial model (cell–organ, psychological–individual, and family–community) is collected. Information on the patient's symptoms, his or her ideas on the cause of the problem, perception of symptoms, and potential influences on personal and social life are all important. A patient-centred style with open-ended questions as well as the feeling that the doctor listens and understands the problem encourages patients to raise their own concerns and agendas and appears to be most congruent with patient reported quality of primary care.[19]

Table 1 Stages and steps of a management plan

Stages at first or follow-up consultation	Steps ■ binding, □ optional	Consultation style
Establishing a relationship	■ Defining roles, gaining trust, reassurance ■ Formal arrangement; setting	Patient-centred Active listening Refrain from interruptions
Eliciting the patients agenda	■ Screening of complaints and medical condition ■ Hypothesis concerning the patient's reason for encounter	Patient-centred Active listening Structured procedure
Diagnostic procedures History/examinations Context Information	■ Evidence-based examinations, laboratory tests ■ Collecting information about previous diseases (including genetic aspects) ■ Regarding multiple causes and effects of illness ■ The patient's background as well as occupational, social, and personal situation ■ Patient's health beliefs ■ Assessing resources (e.g. social support and the patient's locus of control) ■ Discussing the diagnosis with the patient (name, origin, and consequences of the disease)	Patient-centred Active listening Structured procedure Informing the patient Educational dialogue
Aims of treatment	■ Defining starting point and priorities □ Body/mind area □ Pain (control or reduction) □ Functioning, quality of life □ Understanding, knowledge □ Prevention	Considering patient preferences Educational dialogue Shared decision-making
Planning, choice, and progressive realization of treatment	■ Evidence-based treatment □ Supporting the patient in active and/or emotional coping □ Modification of health behaviour, self-monitoring □ Individualized written action plan (e.g. for use and adjustment of medication)	Motivating Considering patient preferences Concordance/compliance Educational dialogue, instruction
Stepped care	■ Intensification of treatment if needed □ Speciality consultation □ Referral	Considering patient preferences Informing the patient
Evaluation (immediate, intermediate, and long-term outcome)	□ Affective: patient satisfaction □ Behavioural: patient adherence, compliance □ Cognitive: patient recall ■ Health outcome: symptom scores, functional status, pain, quality of life □ Economic: direct and indirect costs (e.g. hospital admission, days off work)	Structured interview Standardized questionnaire Test
End of treatment, follow-up	□ Optimization of outcome □ Preventive activities	To be at the patient's disposal Regular medical review

Diagnostic procedures

In the light of the biopsychosocial model, making a diagnosis is not a mere technical procedure but always a combination of, for example, clinical examinations, laboratory tests, and interpretation of results together with the patient. Diagnostic procedures should be guided by evidence-based information, if available.

Pathology is influenced both by biological and psychological processes and illness itself may affect the patient's psychological and physical well-being (referred to as the multiple-cause–multiple-effect model). For a comprehensive understanding, assessment of situational triggers that promote specific events can be included (e.g. using an asthma diary). Considerations of individual and social resources provide clues for the planning of further treatment.

Especially in general practice, making a diagnosis necessitates communication so that both parties come to a common understanding of the problem, instead of labelling the patient (see Chapter 6). Misunderstanding or dysfunctional health beliefs that make the patient feel helpless (e.g. false conviction of the disease being incurable) can be prevented. Giving the patient comprehensive and understandable information and a perspective on the consequences for daily life is part of a management plan.

Defining and realizing the aims of the treatment

Doctors usually think that their patients expect treatment of their disease according to the state of the art (if it exists). So, why think and talk about the aim of the treatment? First of all, there are different therapeutic options for many conditions. For example, a minor depression may be treated with antidepressants drugs, natural remedies, or psychotherapy, or similar counselling techniques. All of these options may be effective, at least in some patients. Secondly, many treatment options have side-effects and influence the patient's life and well-being in a negative way. For example, antihypertensives may cause dizziness or impotence in some patients. Therefore, the pros and cons of the treatment have to be balanced. Finally, if treatment options require help from others, the doctor must check whether support is really available.

Talking with the patient about the treatment should also include the different dimensions of therapy. A treatment may either address the underlying causes of a disease or simply aim at symptom control, such as pain relief or coping support.

Co-morbidity can be another reason why treatment aims especially in general practice patients are sometimes difficult to determine—or even to realize. For example, 63 per cent of visits made by patients with hypertension are for a range of other reasons and it makes no sense to limit considerations to a single entity in the illness spectrum of these patients.[20] Furthermore, the patient's autonomy often requires doctors to accept his or her choice even when these options are not evidence based or second best.[14]

The management of many conditions seen in general practice requires patient self-management and motivational training to support behavioural change.[21] Following the doctor's advice is only a minor aspect of the patient's cooperation. It seems to be more important to learn to what degree a patient's condition may have been influenced by previous behaviour and how to handle it in the future. Patient self-management should be based on action plans, developed by patients as something they want to do. If necessary, doctors should help patients to make an action plan more realistic in order to avoid failure.[22] Doctors' training and support services include instruction in disease management, help for problem-solving as well as behavioural change (e.g. smoking or dietary interventions), and interventions to cope with emotional demands of chronic disease. It may also include advice on how to document experience with treatment so that a better adjustment of medication is possible. There is substantial evidence that structured self-management and behavioural change programmes improve important outcomes in asthma, diabetes, hypertension, arthritis, coronary heart disease, and other chronic diseases.[21] Doctors can help patients manage their chronic condition by effective communication and information.[23]

Stepped care and support by specialists

One important principle of patient management in general practice is the concept of 'individualized stepped care':[10] simpler, less restrictive, less intensive, or less expensive interventions are tried initially, followed by care based on guidelines for patients who have not responded adequately. Stepped-care principles help to allocate limited professional resources. For example, follow-up visits to report the resolution of a problem may not be necessary for every patient. A management plan, however, should include an agreement on this point.

Clinical responsibilities might also be transferred to specialists in certain patients or conditions.[10] A further important task of the general practitioner is to coordinate and integrate specialist care and prevention of the patient who may otherwise get lost in the technological maze of modern hospitals and clinics.

Outcome evaluation

Immediate outcomes from the consultation include patient satisfaction, recall of the physician's explanations and instructions, and changes in the patient's concern about their symptoms. *Intermediate* outcomes refer to the patient's compliance with the physician's recommendations. Finally, the *long-term* outcome is the change (or not) in the patient's health status. Health outcomes are gaining prominence as validators of the effectiveness of the physician–patient interaction, particularly as brief summary measures of functional status and general well-being have been developed.[24]

The advantage of validated assessment scales, compared to a spontaneous question of how the patient feels, is the multidimensionality and objectivity of such measures. It is important to know whether and to what degree the patient is satisfied with treatment, time spent, practice organization, or communication skills of the doctor. Chapters 14.2–14.6 present and discuss several research tools and outcome measures that are feasible for general practice.

End of treatment; follow-up

In some cases, medical treatment might result in a complete recovery of the patient so that the problem is no longer present. Even in these cases, the doctor should make an agreement with the patient about the evaluation of this aim. In many other cases, follow-up or even life-long consultations will be necessary. On these occasions, the doctor and the patient should talk or check in detail whether the aims have been achieved and what problems still remain. During this time the physician is at the patient's disposal, ready to enter earlier stages of the management plan.

The strength of a management plan

The eight stages in Table 1 represent a logical chain rather than a chronology. The individual stages are strongly interrelated. For example, a good relationship between the doctor and the patient is a prerequisite for eliciting the patient's agenda. At the same time, talking about the patient's problems and health beliefs strengthens this relationship. Talking about how to realize the treatment aims might also support the relationship and may complete the information on the patient's family background and social resources. In some cases, several phases may be compressed or may even be superfluous (e.g. in the management of uncomplicated urinary tract infections or acute respiratory illness).

Future developments

The philosophy of patient management is confronted with, at least, three problems:

1. There appears to be a discrepancy between the strong belief in patient autonomy and the suggestive evidence that many patients do not wish to participate in treatment decisions (even if they may be receptive to greater information exchange).[25] Doctors interested in systematic

methods of patient management will recognize that valid and reliable methods of eliciting patient preferences are still being developed.[26] There is plenty of room for future research (e.g. to find out which patients prefer, or dislike, a more active role in the management of their problem).

2. Patient management has the potential to stimulate doctors to a more active approach, which may, however, conflict with patients' resistance to treatment or to the prescription of evidence-based medicines (especially true in the management of asymptomatic patients). Thus, it seems important to allow individualization of care in patient management plans.[15]
3. Successful patient management may require a redesign of practice. Organizational development includes changes in decision-making process, shape and nature of groups, work procedures, job descriptions (allocation of tasks), and the management of patient contact (appointments, follow-ups, telephone contacts, reminders).[21] Patient management may also create new and important roles for nurse practitioners as case managers.

Patient management offers fascinating opportunities for a more powerful, successful, and satisfying treatment of the patient. History tells us that patient management is fairly straightforward whereas the art of its application is intrinsically challenging: 'The doctor is faced with a particular patient, with a particular bodily constitution, and at a particular point in time' (Maimonides).[3]

References

1. **Rivo, M.L. and Johnson, G.R.** (2002). Managed health care: practicing effectively in the 21st century. In *Textbook of Family Practice* (ed. R.E. Rakel), pp. 1603–14. Philadelphia: Saunders.
2. **Sweeney, K.G., MacAuley, D., and Gray, D.P.** (1998). Personal significance: the third dimension. *Lancet* **351**, 134–6.
3. **Bloch, S.** (2001). Moses Maimonides' contribution to the biopsychosocial approach in clinical medicine. *Lancet* **358**, 829–32.
4. **Stewart, M.** et al. (2000). The impact of patient-centered care on outcomes. *Journal of Family Practice* **49**, 796–804.
5. **Di Blasi, Z., Harkness, E., Ernst, E., Georgiou, A., and Kleijnen, J.** (2001). Influence of context effects on health outcomes: a systematic review. *Lancet* **357**, 757–62.
6. **Engel, G.L.** (1980). The clinical application of the biomedical model. *American Journal of Psychiatry* **137**, 535–44.
7. **Squier, H.A., Brody, H., and Supanich, B.** (1998). Approach to the patient. In *Family Medicine* 5th edn. (ed. R.B. Taylor), pp. 13–18. New York: Springer.
8. **Cohen, S. and Herbert, T.B.** (1996). Health Psychology: psychological factors and physical disease from the perspective of human psychoneuroimmunology. *Annual Reviews Psychology* **47**, 113–42.
9. **Kiecolt-Glaser, J.K. and Glaser, R.** (1995). Psychoneuroimmunology and health consequences: data and shared mechanisms. *Psychosomatic Medicine* **57**, 269–74.
10. **Larsen, J.H., Risor, O., and Putnam, S.** (1997). P-R-A-C-T-I-C-A-L: a step by step model for conducting the consultation in general practice. *Family Practice* **14**, 295–301.
11. **von Korff, M.** (2000). Individualized stepped care of chronic illness. *The Western Journal of Medicine* **172**, 133–7.
12. **Kanfer, F.H. and Grimm, L.G.** (1980). Managing clinical change—a process model of therapy. *Behavior Modification* **4**, 419–44.
13. **Little, P.** et al. (2001). Observational study of effect of patient centeredness and positive approach on outcomes of general practice consultations. *British Medical Journal* **323**, 908–11.
14. **Elwyn, G., Edwards, A., and Kinnersley, P.** (1999). Shared decision-making in primary care: the neglected second half of the consultation. *British Journal of General Practice* **49**, 477–82.
15. **Phillips, L.S.** et al. (2001). Clinical inertia. *Annals of Internal Medicine* **135**, 825–34.
16. **Katzelnick, D.J.** et al. (2000). Randomized trial of a depression management program in high utilizers of medical care. *Archives of Family Medicine* **9**, 345–51.
17. **McCormick, J.S.** (1991). Drugs and placebos in general practice: the view of a sceptic. In *Rational Pharmacotherapy in General Practice* (ed. M.M. Kochen), pp. 227–31. Berlin: Springer.
18. **Larivaara, P., Kiuttu, J., and Taanilia, A.** (2001). The patient-centred interview: the key to biopsychosocial diagnosis and treatment. *Scandinavian Journal of Primary Health Care* **19**, 8–13.
19. **Flocke, S.A., Miller, W.L., and Crabtree, B.F.** (2002). Relationships between physician style, patient satisfaction, and attributes of primary care. *Journal of Family Practice* **51**, 835–40.
20. **Starfield, B.** (2001). New paradigms for quality in primary care. *British Journal of General Practice* **51**, 303–9.
21. **Wagner, E.H., Austin, B.T., and von Korff, M.** (1996). 3. Organizing care for patients with chronic illness. *The Milbank Quarterly* **74**, 511–44.
22. **Bodenheimer, T., Lorig, K., Holman, H., and Grumbach, K.** (2002). Patient self-management of chronic disease in primary care. *Journal of the American Medical Association* **20**, 2469–75.
23. **Heisler, M., Bouknight, R.R., Hayward, R.A., Smith, D.M., and Kerr, E.A.** (2002). The relative importance of physician communication, participatory decision making, and patient understanding in diabetes self-management. *Journal of General Internal Medicine* **17**, 243–52.
24. **McDowell, I. and Newell, C.** *Measuring Health—a Guide to Rating Scales and Questionnaires*. Oxford: Oxford University Press, 1996.
25. **Robinson, A. and Thomson, R.** (2001). Variability in patient preferences for participating in medical decision making: implication for the use of decision support tools. *Quality in Health Care* **10** (Suppl. 1), i34–8.
26. **Bowling, A. and Ebrahim, S.** (2001). Measuring patients' preferences for treatment and perceptions of risk. *Quality in Health Care* **10** (Suppl. 1), i2–8.

7.2 Patient education, advice, and counselling

Leon Piterman

Introduction

It is well known that the term 'doctor' means 'teacher' and comes from the Latin 'docere', 'to teach'. There are many parallels between the role of a doctor in consultation and the doctor–patient relationship, and the role of a teacher in the classroom and the teacher–student relationship. Patients expect their doctors to be knowledgeable and authorative yet kind and empathic. Students have similar expectations of their teachers. Patients expect their doctor to show understanding and respect for their particular viewpoint even if it differs from that of their doctor. Students also expect their teachers to understand and respect them and be tolerant of individual differences. Doctors may conduct consultations in a doctor-centred manner or in a patient-centred manner. Similarly, teachers may adopt a student-centred approach or a teacher-centred approach. In each case compliance with advice or student learning will be influenced positively or negatively.

In adopting a patient-centred approach to a consultation, the doctor will explore the patient's understanding of the problem, their interpretation of the symptoms and signs, their attitudes and beliefs regarding the diagnosis, and their thoughts about management. In doing so the doctor has carried out a form of 'needs analysis' and is able to structure the management phases of the consultation in such a manner that appropriate information is transmitted in a simple, non-judgemental and non-jargonistic fashion, that any misconceptions or misunderstandings are corrected, and that the patient's needs are met. Educators adopting a learner-centred approach to teaching, particularly those using the principles of adult learning[1] will be similarly interested in their students' learning needs and ensure that those needs are met in a non-autocratic and respectful manner.

Insufficient attention has been paid in the past to breaking down the power relationship which exists between health professionals and their patients or clients, and between educators and their students so that one group is perceived as the source of knowledge and the other as the passive recipient of knowledge.

Although the term 'education' may have few connotations with respect to 'power' or power struggles, particularly if the emphasis is on learning-centred processes rather than teacher-centred processes, the same may not be said for the term 'advice' or 'counselling'. These terms, at least on the surface, imply that one party is the repository of useful information and the other party is in search of this information. In commercial terms one is a provider and the other a purchaser. This applies whether advice is being sought from a lawyer, accountant, doctor, or motor mechanic or whether counselling is obtained from a doctor, trained psychotherapist, priest, friend, or relative. Naturally, not all will have commercial implications.

However, the power relationship which I previously referred to need not necessarily apply to advice or counselling. Advisors and counsellors may be just as client-centred in their approach as doctors and teachers.

The terms education, advice, and counselling, will be explored in more detail later in the chapter, however the discussion so far has served to illustrate the potential complexity which exists in these terms and the perceptions which they may conjour in the minds of patients and practitioners.

Although there may be differences in definition, taxonomy, processes, and practices, in any one consultation a mixture of education, advice, and counselling may well take place. This serves to highlight the complex and process rich nature of general practice consultations. Faced, for example, with a patient who wants to give up cigarette smoking, the general practitioner may advise the patient about the dangers of smoking, counsel them about how they might give up and the problems of nicotine withdrawal, and educate them regarding coping strategies with the withdrawal and of patient educational material. This may occur in a space of 5 minutes and the boundaries between education, advise, and counselling may blur and intersect throughout this period of time.

Patient education

Patients derive education about health-related matters from a multitude of sources varying in authenticity, credibility, reliability, and quality. This variability in content and quality poses concerns to health professionals, governments, and consumer groups which have been exacerbated by the explosion of health information on the Internet.[2]

Possible sources of patient education are listed below. No doubt readers may identify additional sources.

- Media
  - television
  - radio
  - print—magazine, newspapers
  - internet
- Family/friends
- Authorative Public Health bodies, for example, National Heart Foundations, Asthma Foundations, Diabetes Foundations
- Consumer support groups (often special interest groups, e.g. Coeliac, Crohn's, Motor Neurone Disease groups)
- Pharmaceutical industry, including manufacturers of supplements
- Health professionals
  - doctors
  - nurses
  - pharmacists
  - dentists
  - other allied health professionals
  - alternate health practitioners

Role of the Internet

The progressive empowerment of patients and consumers in general has seen a shift from dependence on authority figures such as health professionals as the dominant provider of health education, to the media as an important if not the dominant provider. Whilst the traditional print and electronic media continue to have their market share, the most rapid growth has occurred, and no doubt will continue to occur in the Internet and World Wide Web as the major provider of health education. Although the impact of this information on public health and well-being is unknown,[3] concerns are being expressed about quality control of educational material and of promotion of medical remedies and products through the Internet.[4]

Eysenbach et al.[5] in 1999 estimated that more than 100 000 medical websites existed, many of them private companies offering product information or information which is linked to products. They defined 'cybermedicine' as the 'science of applying internet and global networking technologies to medicine and public health, of studying the impact and implications of the internet and of evaluating opportunities and the challenges for health care'. As distinct from telemedicine which focuses on the transfer of confidential information between health professionals or between professionals and patients, cybermedicine has open access and is more concerned with health promotion, public health education, professional medical education, and the evaluation of health information on the Internet. Of major concern to health professionals in general and cybermedicine specialists in particular, is the lack of quality control, lack of standards and lack of social equity in relation to health educational material appearing on the Internet. Increasingly, patient to patient exchanges are occurring, and whilst this may be little different to talking to one's family or friends, the global scale has the potential for wider ramifications. Increasing pressure is also being placed on health professionals, particularly medical practitioners, to comment on information gleaned by patients off the Web. This raises the important issue of the quality and evidence base for information which patients are downloading. Undoubtedly, there is a role for the medical profession and other health professionals to act as 'rating agencies' for the quality of information, including patient educational material, which appears on the Web, (just as Heart Foundations rate food in the supermarket, or magazines rate cars), however, so far there has been a poor response to calls for such activities.[6]

Undoubtedly, this will change over time as Cochrane style reviews of educational material gain wider community acceptance as the Internet provides such universal freedom of access, it would be a pity to have to legislate to block access to materials or use electronic means to do so. In an age when an abundance of patient educational information and information on self-care is available on the Internet, one might well contemplate on the future role of doctors, in particular, general practitioners. Lord Turnberg[7] believes that despite the mass of available material, patients will always need a practitioner to make sense, interpret, and contextualize their symptoms, signs, diagnoses, and management plans in light of an overwhelming plethora of documented therapeutic options.

Research on patient education

Faced with an ever-growing number of patient educational methods, materials, processes, and practitioners it seems reasonable to ask a number of fundamental research questions and search the literature for possible answers. Just as evidence-based medicine should influence clinical practice, so evidence-based education should influence choices in patient education. Research and research findings in relation to patient education are beset with a number of problems.

Definition

As has already been alluded to it is often difficult to unravel patient education from patient advice and simple unnamed counselling techniques.

Confounding bias

Definitional problems lead potentially to confounding bias. This is further complicated by trying to separate the influence of the message (e.g. educational material) from the messenger and the medium. How do we know whether it is the doctor or health practitioner who is providing the educational material or the materials themselves that are providing the benefit? Naturally, when the practitioner is removed from the equation a degree of bias is also removed. This leaves room to examine delivery systems for particular messages.

For example, paper-based delivery such as literature, pamphlets, booklets, and brochures versus electronic forms of delivery. Whilst this might seem reasonable there are the problems of patient selection bias in as much as certain patients will prefer one delivery system to another making true randomization difficult. The problem is further compounded by the fact that people, although accessing educational material electronically, will often resort to printing it out for reading and subsequent reference, making true comparison of media difficult.

An added complication in educational research, and for that matter in most behavioural research, is the difficulty in finding true control groups who are isolated from the intervention altogether. Patients share information and often there are multiple health educational or health promotional programmes operating within communities. One only hopes that control and intervention groups are equally exposed to ambient education.

Validity and reliability

Educational materials and educators themselves are supposed to increase patient knowledge and improve patient health practices. Checking that they do this is a measure of the validity of the intervention and ideally requires comparison with a non intervention or placebo intervention. Although the randomized control trial is the accepted 'gold standard' in biomedical research, it is not as simple to carry out in educational research, resulting in a compartive dirth of rigorously derived findings. This applies to medical education as well as patient education.(8)

Reliability poses even bigger problems. Materials or methods shown to work for one medical condition may not necessarily work for another condition. For example, whilst a patient video may be helpful in educating asthmatics about correct use of inhalers, a video may not be as effective in improving compliance with lipid lowering medical. Equally, materials which have been trialled in a metropolitan area encourage patients with coeliac disease to join patient support groups may not be as effective in rural areas where these groups do not exist.

Reliability may be further compromised by issues of access, equity, and cost. A successful computer based educational program aimed at improving the self management of phobias may be valid and reliable in an educated group of individuals who are computer literate, but may be of limited value in patients from lower socio-economic groups.

Quality of materials and evaluation research

The problems facing quality control of education messages on the Internet has already been discussed. Whilst more care is given to the development of print, video, and audio material, these are often not peer reviewed in the same way as publications in medical journals. This applies less so to materials which have been developed by public health bodies such as heart foundations or anti-cancer councils than it may to materials produced by organizations with commercial interests.

Despite this, it is surprising how little research is devoted to evaluating the quality or impact of these materials. In most cases they are simply produced and disseminated, be it through doctors or hospital waiting rooms, through mail outs or through handouts. The value of the materials is often judged solely by the number of 'repeat orders' rather than by any systematic attempt to examine how they are handed out, how they are used, what consumers thought of their content, and what impact if any they had on changing knowledge, and more importantly behaviour.

Unfortunately, many of the organizations which produce these materials lack the funds and the desire to systematically evaluate them.

Patient input and patient preferences

No patient educational material should be produced without active patient participation. Although input is often provided by consumer representatives from special interest groups, it is important to bear in mind that these representatives may be more educated and have better reading skills than the average consumer. Field testing of materials, usually in focus group situations is essential at the very least, prior to final production and dissemination. Most printed materials are produced at Year 8 (14-year-old) school age readership levels for this reasons. Care must also be taken to ensure that materials translated into other languages are translated accurately with correct use of idiom and tested in the ethnic groups who will use them.

Patients should also be surveyed on their preferred method of learning. Just as in any group of learners there will be preferred styles and preferred media. Some patients prefer video material others prefer to read educational messages.

Providers of written information must ensure that the material produced is simple enough to read by a large segment of the community yet is authorative and supported by a solid evidence base. An instrument known as DISCERN(9) has been produced to enable both patients and information providers to judge quality of written educational tools. Although primarily developed using information on three medical conditions: myocardial infarction, endometriosis, and chronic fatigue syndrome, the instrument has been found to be more generally reliable and valid.

Coulter et al. have stressed the importance of involving patients in the clinical decision management process. In a qualitative study involving review of patient education materials through focus group processes,(10) they found that the patients expressed considerable concern regarding deficiencies in the education material, many of which could have been rectified by early consultation and involvement of patients in the development of materials.

Examples of deficiencies include:

- Inadequate information about causes, consequences, and natural history of conditions.
- Over-optimistic views of outcomes of conditions and interventions, without adequate presentation of possible adverse outcomes or even uncertain outcomes.
- Inadequate information about all treatment options including implementing therapy and self-care.
- Inadequate presentation of the sources of information presented and the evidence base for that information.
- Lack of adequate dating of information so that its currency was certain.
- The use of patronizing language, lack of personally relevant data, and poor layout and presentation of the material.

Table 1 Checklist for patient information materials

The process:
(1) Involve patients throughout the process
(2) Involve a wide range of clinical experts
(3) Be specific about the purpose of the information and the target audience
(4) Consider the information needs of minority groups
(5) Review the clinical research evidence and use systematic reviews wherever possible
(6) Plan how the materials can be used within a wider programme promoting shared decision making
(7) Consider cost and feasibility of distribution and updating when choosing media
(8) Develop a strategy for distribution
(9) Evaluate the materials and their use
(10) Make arrangements for periodic review and up
(11) Publicize the availability of the information materials
The content:
(1) Use patients' questions as the starting point
(2) Ensure that common concerns and misconceptions are addressed
(3) Refer to all the relevant treatment or management options
(4) Include honest information about benefit and risks
(5) Include quantitative information where possible
(6) Include checklists and questions to ask the doctor
(7) Include sources of further information
(8) Use non-alarmist, non-patronizing language in active rather than passive voice
(9) Design should be structured and concise with good illustrations
(10) Be explicit about authorship and sponsorship
(11) Include reference to sources and strengths of evidence
(12) Include the publication date

Source: Coulter, A., Entwistle, V., and Gilbert, D. (1999). *British Medical Journal* **318**, 318–22.

Patient were more concerned about the information in the message rather than its means of presentation with no clear preference for video, audio, computer-based, or printed materials.

Another study[11] has shown that patients are more satisfied with consultations where educational was handed to them by their doctors than by receiving it in the material or through other means in the clinic.

Coulter et al. have developed a useful checklist aimed at facilitating the process of production of materials and improving the quality of materials. This is outlined in Table 1.

Doctors' use of education materials

Doctors purchase or receive free of charge, a myriad of patient education materials which collectively cost millions of dollars each year to produce and distribute. A study examining doctors' use of these materials[12] found that doctors were either 'stockpilers' who called on staff to collect and collate materials or 'personal stashers' who collected a 'smaller pile' that they personally supervised. In all practices, the doctors most commonly handed out the materials but the 'personal stashers' used the materials more often, more efficiently, and in a contextually more relevant manner.

Self-care and self-help materials

Most bookshops are stockpiled with self-care and self-help literature and patient's often receive publicity about such literature in the mail or through the media. Large employers and health insurers, particularly in the United States, have been interested in testing the efficacy and effectiveness of such materials on health outcomes in an effort to reduce costs associated with hospital administrations.[13] Using screening questionnaire, high-risk individuals are identified by these organizations and sent a range of self-help materials related to their area of disability (e.g. arthritis, back pain, hypertension, diabetes, heart disease). Fries and McShane[13] showed an improvement in health risk scores, reduction in physician visits and reduced hospitalization rates as well statistically significant in cost savings in the high-risk group receiving trial and intervention compared with control groups.

Impact of general practitioners' (GPs') education and nurse education on patient education and patient health outcomes

As the gate keeper to the health care system and as the point of both primary treatment and continuing care, GPs are widely perceived to be ideally placed to promote health and well-being in the large number of patients under their care. Professional education and continuing professional development are integral to the professional life of GPs and in many cases are essential for continuing certification or validation of practice.

Whilst GPs engage in a range of educational activities there is dearth of information on the effects of such education in patient education or patient health outcomes.

In a randomized controlled trial of health promotion in general practice for patients at high cardiovascular risk, Cupples and McKnight[14] showed that personal health education carried out every 4 months for 2 years increased exercise, improved dieting patterns, and lessened the frequency of angina thereby removing restrictions in everyday activities. This occurred despite the absence of any significant effect on other cardiovascular risk factors.

In another study involving Australian GPs participating in an educational and clinical audit programme related to health promotion in the elderly, patient education resulting from this programme demonstrated significant changes in their health behaviour.[15] This included an increase in walking by an average of 88 min per fortnight, increased frequency of carrying out pleasurable activities, and improvement in self-rated health compared with the control group.

However, an intervention involving the establishment of an asthma resource centre in which nurse specialists in asthma educated and supported practice nurses to educate patients about asthma failed to improve outcomes of asthmatic patients over a 3-year period.[16]

These studies serve to highlight the variable and unpredictable impact of education by health professional on patients in terms of changing health outcomes. Quite apart from the quality of the message and the quality of the messenger, patient willingness and readiness to accept and comply with educational information is often unpredictable.

Role of the patient and health professional–patient relationship

Patients' responses to educational messages and to health promotion in general are extremely variable. The literature on patient compliance is vast. In a review of the importance of patient education on the compliance process Day[17] highlighted the importance of attitudes, beliefs, and perceptions of patients rather than their demographic features in determining outcomes, and stressed the importance of recognizing the life-long nature of educational processes in influencing change. This requires health professionals to be flexible in their approach, to be patient centred, and to focus on the establishment of a long-term relationship which might produce long-term benefits.[18] This might explain why some of the trials of educational interventions fail to produce desired health outcomes. They are usually of relatively short duration (determined by trial conditions and trial funding) and often involve research staff who only have a transient relationship with the patients whilst the trial is active, but are not involved in ongoing management.

Patient counselling

As indicated earlier in the chapter, the separation of patient education from advice and counselling is at times artificial in the clinical setting. In any one consultation a clinician, particularly a general practitioner, may provide all three and move in an unstructured way from one modality to another. There are, however, highly structured and well-defined forms of patient counselling which have been shown to be effective in management of a number of psychiatric disorders. These are discussed later in the chapter and evidence for their benefit or otherwise is provided. It should, however, be pointed out that the most common form of counselling carried out in practice is supportive therapy which certainly requires good consulting and communication skills but lacks the structure of these listed counselling modalities.

With regard to counselling patients to change health risk behaviours such as smoking, overeating, and lack of exercise, many practitioners use the Prochaska and Di Clemante[19] cycle of change as a framework for conducting the counselling phase of the consultation. The cycle is outlined in Fig. 1. It involves identifying where the patient is with respect to their readiness to change a particular behaviour. The counselling strategy used in the consultation is determined by the phase within the 'stage of change' process and is summarized below. This approach is particularly useful in time-limited consultations characteristic of general practice and acknowledges that there is little point in spending much time counselling patients who are not ready to change or motivated to change (i.e. they are in 'pre-contemplation').

Pre-contemplation:

- Motivate (link with health benefits and costs, e.g. stopping smoking will save the cost of an overseas trip each year)
- Provide patient education handout
- Offer assistance when ready to change
- Spend no more than few minutes

Contemplation:

- Motivate
- Support and provide specific advice

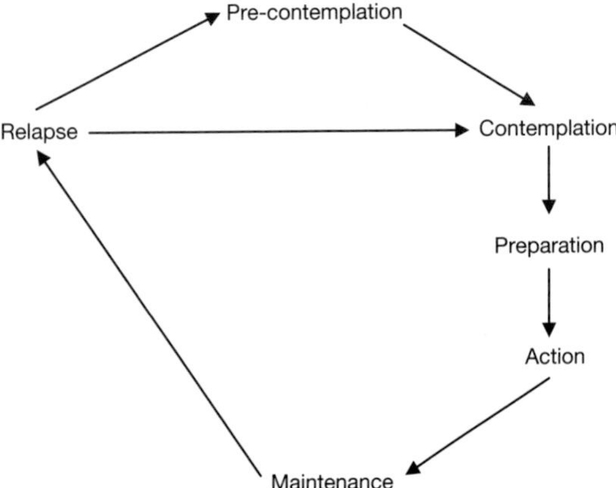

Fig. 1 The Prochaska and Di Clemante cycle of change.[19]

- Provide patient education handout
- Offer assistance and arrange follow up

Preparation:

- Encourage self-monitoring (e.g. diary)
- Identify barriers
- Negotiate short- and long-term goals
- Arrange follow-up

Action:

- Behaviour modification plan
- Patient self-management
- Identify at-risk situations
- Teach practical coping skills (e.g. relaxation techniques)
- Enlist social support
- Review and reward progress

Maintenance:

- Assess and review progress
- Assist patient problem solving
- Reinforce positives and reward progress
- Encourage independence (with further assistance only if needed)

Relapse:

- View as a 'slip-up' on the road to success
- Reframe positively
- Re-establish stage of behaviour change
- Offer assistance

Advice regarding counselling for patients for lifestyle change

The community at large is well aware of the risks associated with a number of lifestyles and possible benefits which might result from changes in these behaviours. There is also general acceptance that health professionals have a role in informing patients and the community of the health consequences of risk-taking behaviour, to counsel high risk taking individuals and to support health promotion programmes directed to a population or a community. In the report of the US Preventive Services Task Force,[20] the range of conditions or behaviours listed below is targeted as suitable for counselling:

- Prevention of tobacco use
- Promotion of physical activity
- Promotion of a healthy diet
- Prevention of motor vehicle injuries
- Prevention of household and recreational injuries
- Prevention of youth violence
- Prevention of back pain
- Prevention of dental and periodental disease
- Prevention of HIA and other extremely terminal diseases
- Prevention of unintended pregnancy
- Prevention of gynaecological cancers

The task force has developed a system of grading each of the recommendations for detection and counselling based on the best available scientific evidence that indictates there is benefit to be derived from an intervention.

On this basis the 'strength of recommendations' are graded from A to E and the 'quality of evidence' to support the recommendation is graded from I to III. This is detailed below:

A. Good evidence supports the recommendation that the condition be specifically considered in a periodic health examination.

B. Fair evidence supports the recommendation that the condition be specifically considered in a periodic health examination.

C. Insufficient evidence to recommend for or against the inclusion in a periodic health examination.

D. Fair evidence supporting evaluation of the condition from previous health examination.

E. Good evidence supporting exclusion from periodic health examination.

Tables 2–4[20] indicate the effects of the appropriateness of this grading system on three principal lifestyles which are closely related to cardiovascular disease, namely smoking, physical activity, and diet.

Naturally these are general recommendations and lack of evidence for the efficacy of an intervention does not mean that it will not be effective in the management of a particular individual. Clinical decision-making, including decisions regarding counselling, should not be solely determined by level of evidence or strength of a recommendation.

In the clinical setting it is most appropriate to apply a model of each of these lifestyle behaviours in deciding who should be counselled and with what degree of intensity depending on their place in cycle of change.

Specific counselling techniques used in primary care psychiatry

Cognitive behavioural therapy (CBT)[21]

This consists of a limited number of structured sessions (normally 15–20 over a 3–4-month period) aimed at changing negative automatic thoughts and dysfunctional beliefs which we are common in depressive disorders.[21] Training is required to carry this out effectively.[22] A systematic of randomized controlled trials has found that CBT is effective and may be more effective than drug treatment in the treatment of people with mild to moderate depression.[23]

Table 2 Counselling to prevent tobacco use

Intervention	Level of evidence	Strength of recommendation
Efficacy of risk reduction		
Avoidance of cessation of tobacco use to reduce the risk of cancer, cardio-vascular and respiratory diseases, adverse pregnancy and neonatal outcomes, and effects of passive smoking	II-2	A
Effectiveness of counselling and other clinical interventions		
Clinical counselling of all patients, including pregnant women, who use tobacco to reduce or stop use	I	A
Nicotine patches or gum as an adjunct to counselling	I	A
Clonidine as an adjunct to counselling	I	C
Clinical counselling of school-aged children and adolescents to avoid tobacco use	III[a]	C

[a] Controlled trials have demonstrated the ability of school-based intervention programmes to delay the initiation of tobacco use in children and adolescents.

Table 3 Counselling to promote physical activity

Intervention	Level of evidence	Strength of recommendation
Efficacy of risk reduction		
Regular physical activity to prevent coronary heart disease, hyper-tension, obesity, and other diseases	II-2	A
Effectiveness of counselling		
Counselling patients to incorporate regular physical activity into their daily routines	I, II-2	C

Table 4 Counselling to promote a healthy diet

Intervention	Level of evidence	Strength of recommendation
Efficacy of risk reduction in the general population		
Limiting intake of dietary fat (especially saturated fat)	I, II-2, II-3	A
Limiting intake of dietary cholesterol	II-2	B
Emphasizing fruits, vegetables, and grain products containing fibre	II-2, II-3	B
Maintaining caloric balance through diet and exercise	II-2	B
Maintaining adequate intake of dietary calcium in women	I, II-1, II-2, II-3	B
Reducing intake of dietary sodium	II-3	C
Increasing intake of dietary iron	II-2, II-3, III	C
Increasing intake of beta-carotene and other anti-oxidants	II-2, II-3	C
Breastfeeding infants	I, II-2	A
Effectiveness of counselling		
Counselling to change dietary habits		
Specially trained educators	I[a]	B
Primary care clinicians	III	C

[a] These trials generally involved specially trained educators such as dieticians delivering intensive interventions (e.g. multiple sessions, tailored materials) to selected patients with known risk factors.

Interpersonal therapy

This is a standardized form of brief psychotherapy normally conducted over 12–16 weekly sessions which are mostly used for the treatment of unipolar depression.

It aims to identify and solve interpersonal difficulties which may underline the depressive episode. These are usually identified in one or more of four categories: role disputes, grief reaction, role transition, and deficits in social skills.

There is weak evidence from randomized controlled trials demonstrating the comparative benefits of interpersonal therapy over drug treatment in the treatment of mild to moderate depression.[24]

References

1. **Knowles, M.** *The Adult Learner* 5th edn. Houston: Gulf Pub, 1998, p. 40.
2. **Yellowlees, P.M.** (2000). Healthcare on the Internet. Buyers beware. *The Medical Journal of Australia* **173**, 629–30.

3. **Coiera, E.** (1998). Information epidemics, economics and immunity on the internet. We still know little about the effect of information on public health. *British Medical Journal* **317**, 1469–70.
4. **Skolnick, A.A.** (1997). WHO considers regulating advertising and sale of medical products on the internet. *Journal of the American Medical Association* **278**, 1723–4.
5. **Eysenbach, G., Sa, E.R., and Diepgan, T.L.** (1999). Shopping around the internet today and tomorrow: towards the millennium of cyber medicine. *British Medical Journal* **319**, 1294.
6. **Bingham, C.M., Higgins, G., Coleman, R., and Van der Weyden, M.B.** (1998). The Medical Journal of Australia internet peer review study. *Lancet* **352**, 441–5.
7. **Lord Turnberg** (2000). Science, society and the perplexed physician. *Journal of the Royal College of Physicians, London* **34**, 569–75.
8. **Davis, D.A., Thomson, M.A., Oxman, A.D., Haynes, A.B., and Brian, R.** (1995). Changing physician performance: a systematic review of the effect of continuing medical education strategies. *Journal of the American Medical Association* **274**, 700–5.
9. **Charnock, D., Shepherd, S., Needham, G., and Gann, R.** (1999). DISCERN: An instrument for judging the quality of written consumer health information on treatment choices. *Journal of Epidemiology and Community Health* **53**, 105–11.
10. **Coulter, A., Entwistle, V., and Gilbert, D.** (1999). Sharing decisions with patients: is the information good enough? *British Medical Journal* **318**, 318–22.
11. **Terry, P.E. and Healey, M.L.** (2000). The physician's role in educating patients. A comparison of mailed versus physician delivered patient education. *Journal of Family Practice* **49**, 327–8.
12. **McVea, K.L., Venugepal, M., Crabtree, B.F., and Aita, V.** (2000). The organization and distribution of patient education materials in family medicine practices. *Journal of Family Practice* **49**, 319–26.
13. **Fries, J.F. and McShane, D.** (1998). Reducing need and demand for medical services in high-risk persons: a health education approach. *The Western Journal of Medicine* **169**, 201–7.
14. **Cupples, M.E. and McKnight, A.** (1994). Randomised controlled trial of health promotion in general practice for patients at high cardiovascular risk. *British Medical Journal* **309**, 993–6.
15. **Kerse, N.M., Flicker, L., Jolley, D., Arroll, B., and Young, D.** (1999). Improving the health behaviours of elderly people: randomized controlled trial of a general practice education programme. *British Medical Journal* **319**, 683–7.
16. **Premaratne, U.N., Sterne, J.A.C., Monks, G.B., Webb, J.R., Azima, H., and Burney, P.G.J.** (1999). Clustered randomized trial of an intervention to improve the management of asthma: Greenwich asthma study. *British Medical Journal* **318**, 1251–5.
17. **Day, J.L.** (1995). Why should patients do what we ask them to do? *Patient Education and Counseling* **26**, 113–18.
18. **Dunn, S.M.** (1995). Barriers and challenges in training health care providers for patient education. *Patient Education and Counseling* **26**, 131–8.
19. **Prochaska, J.D. and Di Clemante, C.C.** (1986). Towards a comprehensive model of change. In *Treating Addictive Behaviours* (ed. W. Miller and N. Heather), pp. 3–27. New York: Plenum Press.
20. **US Preventive Services Task Force.** *Guide to Clinical Preventive Services* 2nd edn. Baltimore: Williams and Wilkins, 1996, pp. 861–78.
21. **Haugh, D.A.F. and Beck, A.T.** (1992). Cognitive therapy. In *Handbook of Affective Disorders* (ed. E.S. Paykel), pp. 511–23. Edinburgh: Churchill Livingstone.
22. **Gloaguen, V.** et al. (1998). A meta-analysis of the effects of cognitive therapy in depressed patients. *Journal of Affective Disorders* **49**, 59–72.
23. **Klerman, G.L. and Weissman, H.** (1992). Interpersonal psychotherapy. In *Handbook of Affective Disorders* (ed. E.S. Paykel), pp. 501–10. Edinburgh: Churchill Livingstone.
24. **Elkins, I.** et al. (1989). National Institute of Mental Health treatment of depression? Research program: general effectiveness of treatments. *Archives of General Psychiatry* **46**, 971–82.

7.3 Communication about risks and benefits of treatment and care options

Adrian Edwards and Glyn Elwyn

Introduction

Risk is the probability that a hazard will give rise to harm.[1] Over recent years the number of publications on risk-related topics has risen exponentially.[2] This reflects the emergence in the late twentieth century of the 'risk society',[3] in which risk is increasingly the focus of attention. This can be seen in news stories, economics, litigation, domestic responsibilities, and environmental influences.

In the field of medicine and health there is a huge volume of literature addressing aspects of risk. Risk information can be used to identify individuals or populations who are at 'high risk' of developing disease. Health care professionals can then intervene to try to reduce these risks by appropriate strategies. It is in using this information that *risk communication* itself is important. This applies, *inter alia*, to communication about risks of disease, treatment, investigation, or familial and genetic risk.

One definition of risk communication is:[4]

> The open two-way exchange of information and *opinion* about risk, leading to better understanding and better risk management decisions.

This definition originates from the field of agriculture, but it is also appropriate for health care.[5] It encapsulates several key characteristics of (good) risk communication—it should be open and honest, a two-way process (between professional and patient), and involves exploring opinions and values ('utilities') about the risks involved, not simply giving information. Finally, there is a focus also on patient understanding and decision-making. The definition also conveys that risk communication is firmly placed in current and progressive developments in health care delivery. These developments include 'patient-centred medicine',[6] 'promoting patient choice',[7] and 'evidence-based patient choice'.[8] As will be described later, risk communication constitutes an important part of shared decision-making.[9]

But what can be said about current practice in primary care? We know that health care professionals spend much of their time discussing risks and benefits of treatments with their patients.[10] This can take the form of describing the broad advantages or disadvantages of options. Alternatively, it may involve using numerical data about the potential outcomes of choosing one treatment or another. But in reality, data are rarely available to professionals when needed.[11] Even when the information is available professionals are unclear about how best to discuss the risks and benefits of treatment most effectively with patients. There are certainly great risks of misleading patients depending on how the information is presented.[12]

The understanding of risk communication

The current concept of risk derives from the 'games of chance' (throwing dice, etc.). After a *subjectivist* interpretation of probability in which the emphasis was on the individual, the *frequentist* interpretation came to view risk as the property of groups of individuals ('the collective').[13] This frequentist paradigm underpins much of modern bio-statistics. The historical evolution of these interpretations of probability included the development of theoretical bases. Attempts could then be made to predict the occurrence of events, such as the typical length of a human life. This has developed into a world-wide industry, in which chance, probability or risk are integral to the understanding of economics, the process of litigation, and the actuarial basis of insurance to name but some.

Theoretical models in the literature

Of more relevance here, however, is risk communication between professionals and their patients. The usual conceptual framework for this is derived from two main strands: cognitive psychology and decision-making theory. In general, the theoretical models seek to provide an understanding of how individuals perceive risk and how this influences behaviour. These models frequently attribute *consequences* in behaviour change to two underlying dimensions: an individual's perception of the *value* of an outcome presented in a health recommendation and perceived *threat* presented by the outcomes in the recommendation.

The Health Belief Model (HBM), Theory of Reasoned Action, Theory of Social Behaviour, and Prospect Theory all emphasize the perceived value of a presented consequence. The Transtheoretical Model ('stages of change') is another model in which interpretation of the likelihood of behaviour change is understood in terms of an individual's *readiness* to change and interventions may be targeted accordingly. Many of these models are indeed the basis for planning several risk communication interventions, as will be seen later.

Research in the field of risk perception is growing particularly rapidly. Important factors affecting an individual's response to a perceived risk include the potential lethality, its controllability through safety measures, the number of people simultaneously exposed, personal familiarity with the consequences of the risks, and the degree of voluntariness of risk exposure.[14] This understanding of risk perception also provides the basis for risk communication interventions in many instances.

The influence of risk information on patients

There is relatively little theoretical work specifically relating to *communication about risks* in the health care setting. However, empirical data are available. The interpretation of risks varies greatly[15] with wide ranges in the meanings or numerical values attributed to verbal descriptions of risks ('rarely', 'sometimes', 'often', and so on). For example, the term 'frequent' was expressed on average as equivalent to nearly 70 per cent in one study looking at information about the probabilities of harm and benefit from treatments, but with a wide range around this figure (from 30 to 90 per cent).[16]

Most people usually prefer numerical presentation of information but approximately one-third of patients prefer verbal descriptions.[17] The type of information preferred and how people understand numerical information is affected by several factors, including the severity of the illness or other outcome concerned, and characteristics such as age, educational level, health status, and recent experience of illness.[18]

Furthermore, people differ not just in their interpretation of the language of risk but also in the meaning or significance they attach to different outcomes.[19] The 'utilities' or values that people will place on different outcomes are likely to affect their use of risk information responding to their own risks. For example, the significance people attach to the term 'breast cancer' may affect motivation to be screened, even if the same information is presented to all such patients. It is important that risk communication interventions address both these aspects of risk communication—the probabilistic information and the significance of the risks to the individual.

The effects of risk communication interventions

A systematic review of the literature[5] sought to identify effective risk communication interventions, and then to identify the characteristics of the most effective interventions—the '*effect modifiers*'. Ninety-seven studies were included in the review. Modest beneficial effects of the interventions were demonstrated across a range of clinical topics (mean effect size 0.3; funnel plot midline of effect sizes was approximately 0.15). This is equivalent, for example, to a study demonstrating that adherence to a screening programme increased from 70 to 83 per cent with the introduction of a risk communication intervention.

The most effective risk communication

Two key 'effect modifiers' were identified. These were '*treatment choice*' clinical topics and the use of *individualized (calculated) risk estimates* in the risk communication process. The 'treatment choices' included topics such as cholesterol lowering therapy, blood pressure therapy, and hormone replacement therapy (HRT). Risk communication interventions were more effective in these situations, where patients were making decisions or expressing treatment preferences, compared with interventions to modify risk behaviour, such as uptake of screening tests or smoking cessation.

The goals of risk communication interventions

In the treatment choices studied, professionals may often be close to 'equipoise'—that is, not having a clear preference about which treatment (or no treatment) the patient chooses.[9] In risk behaviour modification programmes, professionals often have a clear aim: to enhance uptake of tests or reduce risk exposure. This may be at odds with enhancing 'informed choice', but this dilemma needs to be resolved. In keeping with the spirit of partnership with patients and 'evidence-based patient choice' now emerging,[20] perhaps the professional goals of communication should be to enable 'informed choices' by patients, not simply to modify behaviour. This may be despite the fact that conventional public health gains from these newer approaches could be smaller in some situations.[21] For example, more people may decline to take up cervical smear tests if they were fully aware of their actual level of risk (which is low for most women).

Framing

For any method of risk communication, different ways of 'framing' the information have varying effects.[22] Framing itself is defined as presenting 'logically equivalent' information in different ways.[23] For example, the risk of major osteoporotic fractures is 12 per cent in women who take HRT for over 5 years, and 15 per cent in those who do not. This can be framed as a 3 per cent reduction in (absolute) risk, or that fractures are 20 per cent less common in women who take treatment (relative risk reduction). A further derivation from the absolute risk reduction is the 'number-needed-to-treat' (NNT) or its converse the 'number-needed-to-harm'. In the example above, the NNT to prevent a fracture would be 33—that is, 33 people would need to be treated for 5 years to prevent a hip fracture. These presentation formats have both their supporters and detractors, but may be useful in maintaining an accurate perspective on the size of risks or reductions in risks.

Other framing variations include expressing the figures as '3 percent more people remaining free of fractures with HRT' (positive framing) or '3 percent more people suffering fractures if not taking HRT' (negative framing), or converting absolute risk reductions into the 'number needed to screen'.[24] These different expressions have different motivational effects and substantially influence whether individuals choose treatment options or adhere to chosen plans.[25]

The largest effects are evident when relative risk information is presented, as compared with absolute risk data.[22] In addition, 'loss-framing' is more effective in influencing screening uptake behaviours than 'gain-framing'. Studies comparing simpler with more complex information, more data with less, and those comparing numerical with verbal descriptions of risks suggest that providing more information, and which is more understandable to the patient, is associated with improved patient knowledge and a *greater* wariness to take treatments or participate in trials.

Knowing that there are these effects, care is required in deciding whether to use such formats in discussions with patients. People also have different *preferences* for the way they wish information to be presented and discussed with them.[26] For example, some people may not be comfortable with the use of numerical terms and may prefer the same 'facts' to be conveyed descriptively, such as 'fractures are slightly less common in those who take HRT'.

Hux and Naylor concluded that 'multiple complementary formats may be most appropriate'.[27] A *range* of complementary formats could include descriptive, absolute, and relative risk, 'numbers needed to treat' and graphical presentations of information. This is likely to be valued by professionals and patients.[26] Having such information available may facilitate partnerships between professionals and patients in the consultation, in which both are able to make an informed contribution.

It is important that the available data facilitate a sense of perspective. Others propose using 'everyday risks' with which people are familiar (e.g. car driving or others as appropriate) to provide data for people to make informed comparisons of risks.[1,28]

The future

How do these issues help us with risk communication in clinical practice? It appears there may be of most value, at least initially, in concentrating on treatment decision-making.

Ethical principles

Some approaches may enable patients to make informed choices based on the 'whole truth' rather than the 'truth'. This appears close to the 'relationality' ethical principle proposed by Bottorff.[29] Relationality promotes the provision of accurate honest information in the context of the individual situation. It examines the ethics of care in terms of factors such as response, interpretation, accountability, and social solidarity, often counterbalanced against other values such as truth and confidentiality. Using information in this context will enable strides towards 'informed choice' and quality in health care consultations.

Evidence of informed choice and understanding

Such informed choice may not be evident in the conventional cognitive and behavioural outcomes frequently reported in the literature. It is perhaps more likely to be evident in affective outcomes. These include satisfaction with the communication process, understanding of the risks and benefits of the different options, and certainty that the best treatment choice has been made.[30]

We suggest that future strategies to enhance informed choice should be based on methods that portray the decision issues in more depth, but with flexibility to provide the amount of information that the patient desires. The information should be presented (framed) in as fair and balanced a way as reasonably possible. There could be a 'shopping basket' of complementary data formats options, with enough flexibility to address the needs of a great range in requirements of patients.[31]

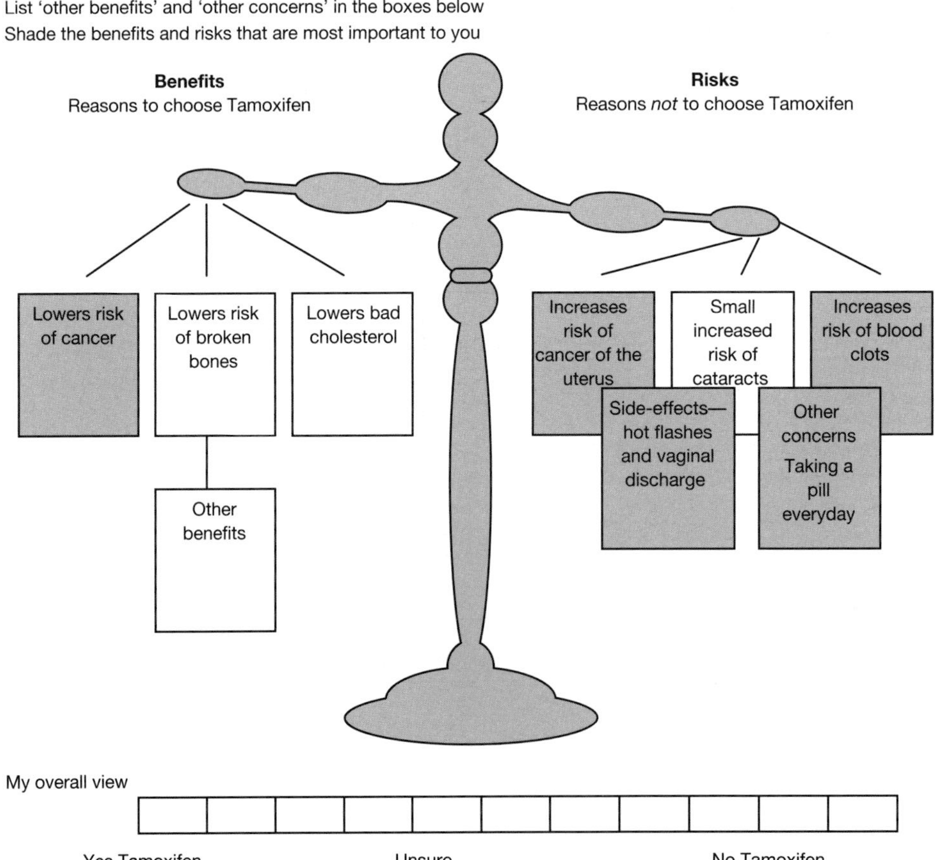

Fig. 1 Example of values clarification exercise using 'weigh scale' depicting the importance a woman at high risk for breast cancer places on tamoxifen outcomes.[34]

Decision aids

This idea is starting to be operationalized in some of the 'decision aids' now available.(32) The common objectives of such aids are to provide information for patients and to facilitate involvement in decisions if patients so desire. Through the use of illustrations (verbal and pictorial), charts, and figures, decision aids portray the relevant treatment options and associated risks and benefits.

Decision aids may use a variety of media including booklets, tapes, videodiscs and interactive computer programmes, paper-based charts, and so on. Some decision aids are provided for patients to work through on their own (outside the consultation or at home), some are specifically intended to provide a platform for discussions in a further consultation. Others form the basis for discussions within consultations, prompting patient questions and so on. Additional components of decision aids include structured counselling approaches for the professional,(33) exploration of the patient's preferred level of involvement in the decision-making itself, and the use of specific approaches to clarify or quantify patient values (e.g. 'weigh scales' or formal utility assessment methods). An example of a weigh scale is shown in Fig. 1.(34)

Figure 2 shows how the weigh scale comprises one of the steps which a patient may or is even encouraged to work through in making a decision about treatment with Tamoxifen for prevention of breast cancer in high-risk individuals.

Information is often presented in a variety of ways, even when considering just graphical formats. Some packages have used simple histograms to show risk and benefit profiles. Two are shown in Figs 3 and 4 from an intervention we are currently evaluating in UK general practice. These charts are made available to professionals (along with numerical and other formats), and may be used if the professional feels it would help the discussion with the individual concerned. Clearly, they are not a substitute for effective communication but support the discussion by providing data in easily assimilated formats.

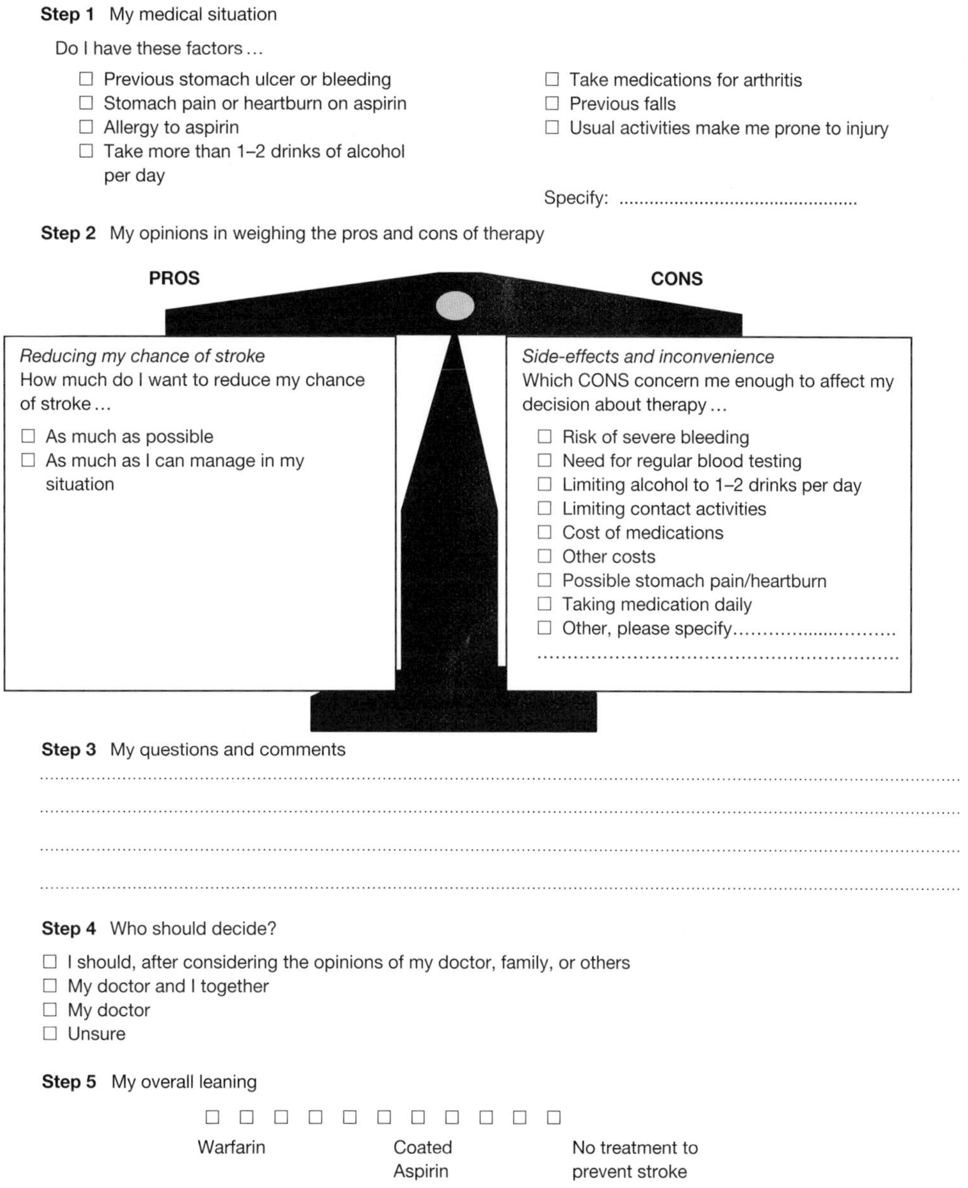

Step 1 My medical situation

Do I have these factors ...

- ☐ Previous stomach ulcer or bleeding
- ☐ Stomach pain or heartburn on aspirin
- ☐ Allergy to aspirin
- ☐ Take more than 1–2 drinks of alcohol per day
- ☐ Take medications for arthritis
- ☐ Previous falls
- ☐ Usual activities make me prone to injury

Specify: ....

Step 2 My opinions in weighing the pros and cons of therapy

PROS

Reducing my chance of stroke
How much do I want to reduce my chance of stroke ...

- ☐ As much as possible
- ☐ As much as I can manage in my situation

CONS

Side-effects and inconvenience
Which CONS concern me enough to affect my decision about therapy ...

- ☐ Risk of severe bleeding
- ☐ Need for regular blood testing
- ☐ Limiting alcohol to 1–2 drinks per day
- ☐ Limiting contact activities
- ☐ Cost of medications
- ☐ Other costs
- ☐ Possible stomach pain/heartburn
- ☐ Taking medication daily
- ☐ Other, please specify..............................

....

Step 3 My questions and comments

....

....

....

....

Step 4 Who should decide?

- ☐ I should, after considering the opinions of my doctor, family, or others
- ☐ My doctor and I together
- ☐ My doctor
- ☐ Unsure

Step 5 My overall leaning

☐ ☐ ☐ ☐ ☐ ☐ ☐ ☐ ☐ ☐ ☐

Warfarin | Coated Aspirin | No treatment to prevent stroke

Fig. 2 Example of personal worksheet guiding people to consider the steps in decision-making.(34)

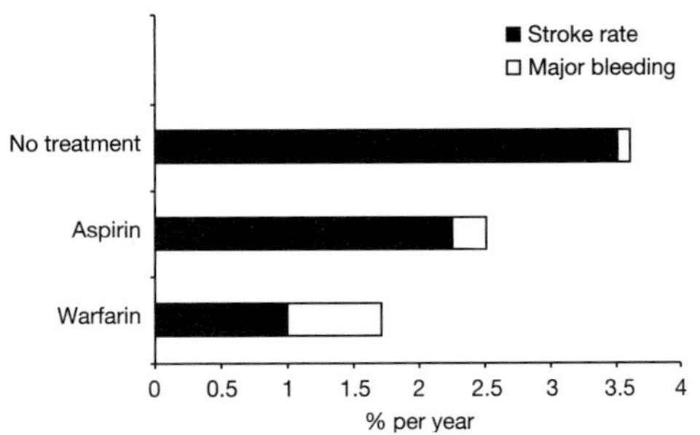

Fig. 3 Histogram depiction of risks and benefits of anticoagulation treatment options for atrial fibrillation.

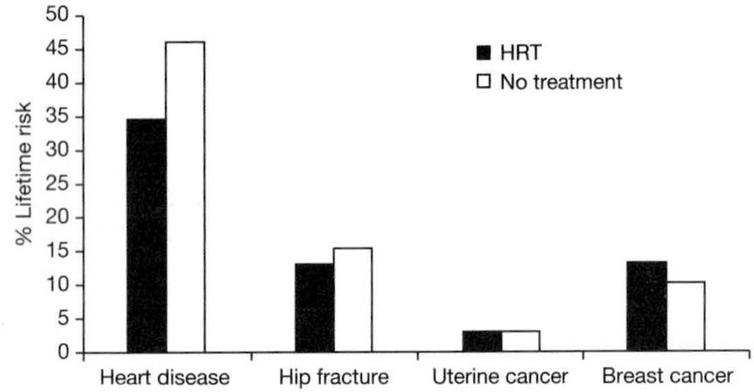

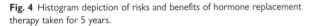

Fig. 4 Histogram depiction of risks and benefits of hormone replacement therapy taken for 5 years.

Other decision aids have used different graphical presentations. 'Population crowd' figures are being increasingly used, perhaps to enhance the reality of the risks and benefits, portraying them as affecting *people* as individuals. Usually, these charts align those affected or unaffected together. Figure 5 shows a potrayal of the baseline risks associated with atrial fibrillation. The harm and benefit profiles of anticoagulation treatments can then be presented and compared in similar diagrams. Figure 6 shows outcome data from a commoner scenario in primary care—whether to have treatment or not with antibiotics for otitis media (middle ear infection) [courtesy of Dr Chris Cates (http://www.cates.cwc.net/ear.htm)].

Other researchers have examined the effects of dispersing the affected individuals more randomly throughout the crowd (see Fig. 7). Whilst this may be true to real life and from statistical perspectives, preliminary work with patients has found that these formats may be more confusing.(35) Further presentation formats include pie charts, thermometer readings, and traffic light colour coding for levels of risk(36) and so on.

Professionals often feel uncertain about *how* to discuss these risks and the language they should use. However, the review cited earlier(5) suggested that beneficial effects of risk communication were evident from a variety of interventions by different professionals and in many clinical settings. Risk communication is not the domain of the specialist. Clinicians should feel confident from this finding and follow their natural inclinations when dealing with individual patients. Particularly when professionals get to know their patients, they are able to understand what would be helpful in the context of an individual consultation and to match the presentation and discussion of information effectively. With risk information available and discussed

Option no.1. Taking no medication to prevent stroke

Chance of HAVING A STROKE in next 2 years

4 out of 100

Chance of NO STROKE in next 2 years

96 out of 100

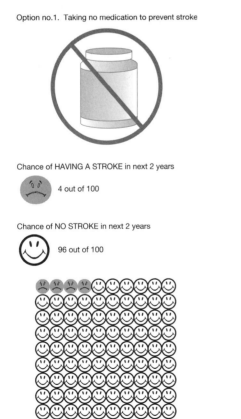

Fig. 5 Example of presenting probabilities of outcomes for patients with atrial fibrilation.(34)

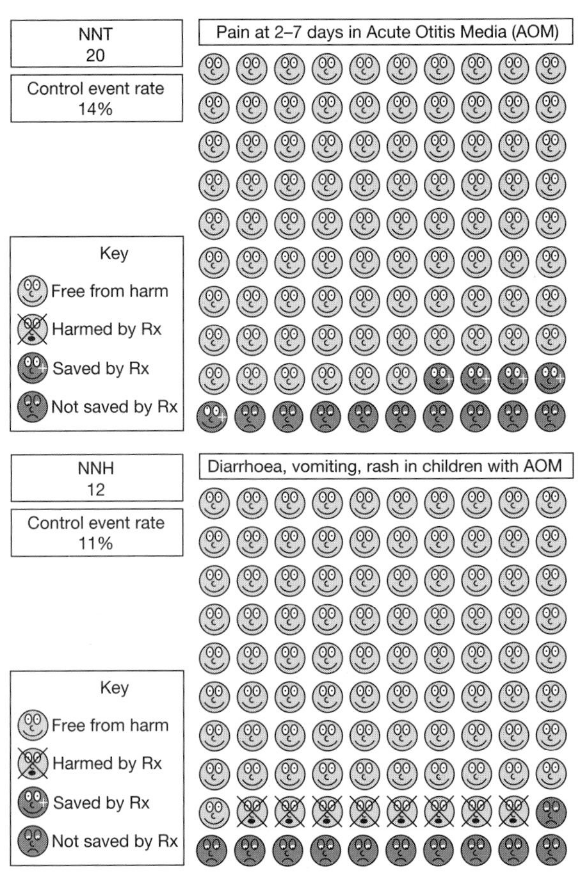

Fig. 6 Outcome data of treatment with antibiotics for patients with otitis media [courtesy of Dr Chris Cates (http://www.cates.cwc.net/ear.htm)].

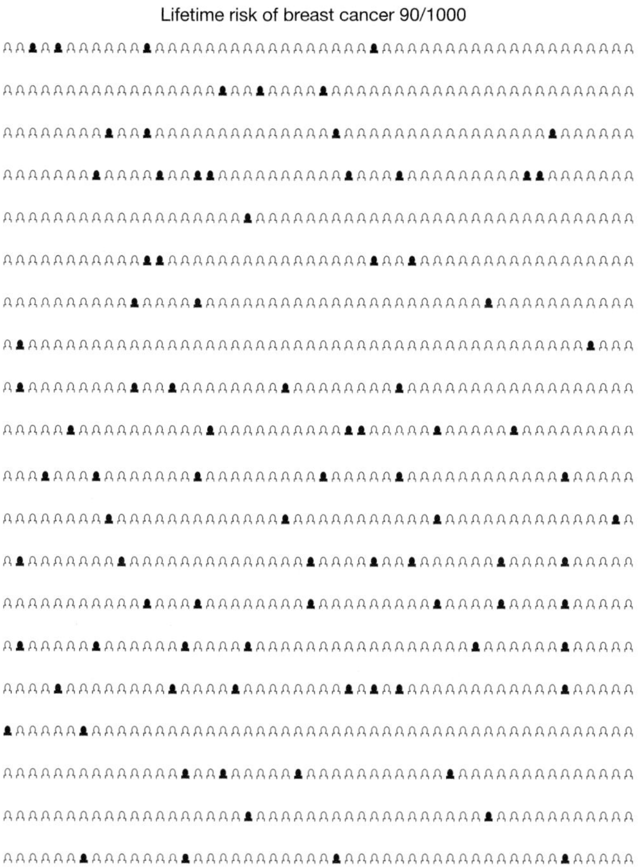

Lifetime risk of breast cancer 90/1000

Fig. 7 Display of risk by population crowd figures, with random placement of affected individuals (courtesy of Dr M.M. Schapira[35]).

(and returning to the definition of risk communication at the start of the chapter), professionals are then also in a better position to explore the meaning and significance of the risks in question to the individual patient. Almost inevitably this will increase the level of patient involvement in the consultation and decision-making.

Implementation

Many professionals are reluctant to use some of the decision aids and other tools now becoming available.[37] Wider implementation is likely to depend on greater promotion of the principles of 'shared decision-making' so that professional attitudinal barriers may be diminished.[37,38] This stimulus may be most effective if it comes from consumers or their representatives rather than professional opinion leaders.[39]

Professionals will also need to be sufficiently familiar with the content of decision aids to use them to maximum benefit. Interactive media may be required to enable individually calculated risks to be used in consultations. This presents practical difficulties of using technological innovations across a range of clinical settings and suggests that interventions must remain simple if they are to be broadly implemented.

For both simple and complex decision aids, professionals will require training, not least to feel confident in their own understanding and ability to use risk information.[11] It is also important for any training to address the ethical issues raised (above), particularly relating to the risk of manipulating patient decisions or behaviour. Raising awareness of these issues should be the first step at least towards reducing the risks of professionals manipulating individual patients with data. In this context there will be a platform from which to discuss risks, to enhance understanding of the risks and potential risk reductions, and to facilitate informed choices by patients.

Summary

Risk communication in practice

- Risk communication is not the domain of the specialist.
- It is found to be helpful in heterogeneous settings and is valued by patients.
- The potential to manipulate patient decisions by framing manipulations is great and should be minimized.
- Clinicians, researchers, and policy makers should note the potential for more informed choices by individual patients to result in lesser or greater use of services; in some situations this may be less likely to maximize health gain in the population.
- Professionals often know their patients well and are often also well placed to understand what would be helpful in the context of an individual consultation.
- Greater flexibility is required in matching information about treatments or care to the needs of individual patients.
- Decision aids are being developed widely, and offer scope to help achieve this.
- They allow balanced information presentation, often with individualized estimates of risk, and can support the current discussions about harms and benefits of treatment options.
- Continuing evaluations are required, assessing their effects on health outcomes, resource use, and whether informed choices and satisfaction with decision-making have been achieved.

References

1. **Mohanna, K. and Chambers, R.**, ed. *Risk Matters in Health Care: Communicating, Explaining and Managing risk* 1st edn. Abingdon, Oxon: Radcliffe Medical Press, 2001. Chapter 1, Risk: what's that all about then? pp. 3–14.
2. **Skolbekken, J.A.** (1995). The risk epidemic in medical journals. *Social Science and Medicine* **40**, 291–305.
3. **Beck, U.** *Risk Society*. London: Sage, 1992.
4. **Ahl, A.S., Acree, J.A., Gipson, P.S., McDowell, R.M., Miller, L., and McElvaine, M.D.** (1993). Standardisation of nomenclature for animal health risk analysis. *Revue Scientifique et Technique (International Office of Epizootics)* **12**, 1045–53.
5. **Edwards, A.G.K.** et al. (2000). The effectiveness of one-to-one risk communication interventions in health care: a systematic review. *Medical Decision Making* **20**, 290–7.
6. **McWhinney, I.** *A Textbook of Family Medicine*. Oxford: Oxford University Press, 1996.
7. **Richards, T.** (1998). Partnership with patients. *British Medical Journal* **316**, 85–6.
8. **Elwyn, G., Edwards, A.G.K., Edwards, A.G.K., and Elwyn, G.**, ed. *Evidence-Based Patient Choice—Inevitable or Impossible?* Oxford: Oxford University Press, 2001. Chapter 1, Evidence-based patient choice? pp. 3–18.
9. **Elwyn, G.J., Edwards, A.G.K., Kinnersley, P., and Grol, R.** (2000). Shared decision-making: defining the 'competences' of involving patients in health care choices. *British Journal of General Practice* **50**, 892–9.

10. **Makoul, G., Arntson, P., and Schofield, T.** (1995). Health promotion in primary care: physician–patient communication and decision making about prescription medications. *Social Science and Medicine* **41**, 1241–54.
11. **Edwards, A.G.K., Matthews, E., Pill, R.M., and Bloor, M.** (1998). Communication about risk: diversity among primary care professionals. *Family Practice* **15**, 296–300.
12. **Skolbekken, J.A.** (1998). Communicating the risk reduction achieved by cholesterol reducing drugs. *British Medical Journal* **316**, 1956–8.
13. **Barnett, V.** *Comparative Statistical Inference* 1st edn. London: John Wiley & Sons, 1972. Chapter 3, Introduction: statistical inference and decision-making, pp. 62–71.
14. **Vlek, C.** (1987). Risk assessment, risk perception and decision making about courses of action involving genetic risk: an overview of concepts and methods. *Birth Defects: Original Article Series* **23**, 171–207.
15. **Mazur, D.J.** (1990). Interpretation of graphic data by patients in a general medical clinic. *Journal of General Internal Medicine* **5**, 402–5.
16. **Woloshin, K.K., Ruffin, M.T.I., and Gorenflo, D.W.** (1994). Patients' interpretation of qualitative probability statements. *Archives of Family Medicine* **3**, 961–6.
17. **Shaw, N.J. and Dear, P.R.F.** (1990). How do parents of babies interpret qualitative expressions of probability. *Archives of Disease in Childhood* **65**, 520–3.
18. **Mazur, D.J. and Merz, J.F.** (1994). Patients interpretations of verbal expressions of probability—implications for securing informed consent to medical interventions. *Behavioral Sciences & The Law* **12**, 417–26.
19. **Edwards, A.G.K., Pill, R.M., and Stott, N.C.H.** (1996). Communicating risk: use of standard terms is unlikely to result in standard communication. *British Medical Journal* **313**, 1483.
20. **Hope, T.** *Evidence-Based Patient Choice.* London: King's Fund, 1996.
21. **Raffle, A.** (2001). Information about screening—is it to achieve high uptake or to ensure informed choice? *Health Expectations* **4**, 92–8.
22. **Edwards, A.G.K., Elwyn, G., Mathews, E., and Pill, R.** (2001). Presenting risk information—a review of the effects of 'framing' and other manipulations on patient outcomes. *Journal of Health Communication* **6**, 61–82.
23. **Wilson, D.K., Purdon, S.E., and Wallston, K.A.** (1988). Compliance to health recommendations: a theoretical overview of message framing. *Health Education Research* **3**, 161–71.
24. **Rembold, C.** (2000). Number needed to screen: development of a statistic for disease screening. *British Medical Journal* **317**, 307–12.
25. **Sarfati, D., Howden-Chapman, P., and Woodward, S.C.** (1998). Does the frame affect the picture? A study into how attitudes to screening for cancer are affected by the way benefits are expressed. *Journal of Medical Screening* **5**, 137–40.
26. **Edwards, A.G.K., Matthews, E.J., Pill, R.M., and Bloor, M.** (1998). Communication about risk: the responses of primary care professionals to standardising the language of risk and communication tools. *Family Practice* **15**, 301–7.
27. **Hux, J.E. and Naylor, C.D.** (1995). Communicating the benefits of chronic preventive therapy: does the format of efficacy data determine patients' acceptance of treatment? *Medical Decision Making* **15**, 152–7.
28. **Paling, J.** *Up to Your Armpits in Alligators: How to Sort Out What Risks Are Worth Worrying About* 1st edn. Gainesville FL: Risk Communication & Environmental Institute, 1997.
29. **Bottorff, J.D.** et al. Uncertainties and challenges. Communicating risk in the context of familial cancer. Report to the National Cancer Institute of Canada, Vancouver; School of Nursing, University of British Columbia, 1996.
30. **Edwards, A.G.K. and Elwyn, G.J.** (1999). How should 'effectiveness' of risk communication to aid patients' decisions be judged? A review of the literature. *Medical Decision Making* **19**, 428–34.
31. **Edwards, A. and Elwyn, G.** (2001). Understanding risk, and lessons for clinical risk communication about treatment preferences. *Quality in Health Care* **10** (Suppl. 1), i9–13.
32. **O'Connor, A.** et al. *Decision aids for people facing health treatment or screening decisions* [*Cochrane Review*]. Oxford: Cochrane Library. Update Software, 2001.
33. **Lerman, C., Biesecker, B., Benkendorf, J.L., Kerner, J., Gomez-Caminero, A., Hughes, C., and Reed, M.M.** (1997). Controlled trial of pretest education approaches to enhance informed decision-making for BRCA1 gene testing. *Journal of the National Cancer Institute* **89**, 148–57.
34. **O'Connor, A.M., Edwards, A.G.K., and Elwyn, G.J.,** ed. *Evidence-based Patient Choice.* Oxford: Oxford University Press, 2001. Chapter 14, The role of decision aids in promoting evidence-based patient choice, pp. 220–42.
35. **Schapira, M.M., Nattinger, A.B., and McHorney, C.A.** (2001). Frequency or probability? A qualitative study of risk communication formats used in health care. *Medical Decision Making* **21**, 459–67.
36. **Lipkus, I.M. and Hollands, J.G.** (1999). The visual communication of risk. *Journal of the National Cancer Institute Monographs* **25**, 149–62.
37. **Elwyn, G.J., Edwards, A.G.K., Gwyn, R., and Grol, R.** (1999). Towards a feasible model for shared decision-making: focus group study with general practice registrars. *British Medical Journal* **319**, 753–6.
38. **Elwyn, G.J., Edwards, A.G.K., and Kinnersley, P.** (1999). Shared decision making in primary care: the neglected second half of the consultation. *British Journal of General Practice* **49**, 477–82.
39. **Edwards, A. and Elwyn, G.** (2001). Developing professional ability to involve patients in their care: pull or push? (editorial). *Quality in Health Care* **10**(3), 129–30.

7.4 Principles of drug prescribing

Les Toop

Introduction

Prescribing is a core activity of primary care physicians. The purpose of this chapter is to explore some of the general principles underlying the prescribing process. The challenge for the prescriber is to recognize the multitude of internal and external influences impacting on prescribing decisions, and to prescribe as effectively and safely as possible. To prescribe well in primary care requires a very broad knowledge base. Well-developed critical and analytical skills are also needed, as is the ability to sift, interpret, and extrapolate from available evidence whilst logically and pragmatically filling in the gaps where there is no evidence. It follows that in many instances there are choices to be made without a definitive or correct answer. The communication skills to engage and involve patients in informed decisions about treatment are equally important to the effective prescriber. Perhaps the greatest challenge through a physician's career is to maintain these critical skills in the face of an ever-increasing technical and evidence base, a global pharmaceutical industry with highly sophisticated and effective marketing strategies, and the changing expectations of an increasingly knowledgeable public.

Why are drugs used?

Drugs are used for many reasons. These include the prevention of illness or undesirable events thereby preventing morbidity or prolonging life, to reduce unpleasant symptoms, to modify the course of an existing illness, to replace a deficiency, or on occasion, to induce an altered state of consciousness.

In all cases, the purpose(s) for taking a particular drug should be clear both to the prescriber and to the patient. In the majority of clinical situations seen in primary medical care, the first step therefore will be to establish a diagnosis and treatment goal. Where this is not possible a clear assessment of the symptom complex to be modified is a necessary minimum. With the increasing popularity of screening a further group of patients will be identified who have one or more risk factors for future disease, for example, high blood pressure or abnormal lipid profile. For these patients the decision to prescribe will be influenced by both the physician's and the patient's interpretation of the risks and benefits of treatment.[1]

The place of drugs in management

Many illnesses seen in primary medical care are self-limiting and the aim of treatment is simply to reduce the duration and severity of symptoms. Often the effects of available medications are modest and other elements of management are of more importance. Lifestyle changes whilst difficult are likely to have a more sustained effect than slimming pills or hypnotics. Diet and exercise may be the most appropriate initial interventions for those found to have mildly raised blood pressure[2] or impaired glucose tolerance.[3] Similarly, the most effective therapeutic intervention for a patient with chronic obstructive airway disease is to stop smoking. In other situations, medication is used together with other non-pharmacological treatments. Muscle strengthening exercises for low back pain, modifying the timing, size, and type of meals in patients with oesophageal reflux or the judicious application of heat in musculoskeletal disorders would be common examples. There is evidence that involving patients actively in their treatment (above and beyond taking a medicine) helps speed recovery.[4] Wherever possible, prescribers should use the therapeutic encounter as an opportunity to give common sense advice on non-pharmaceutical self-management of common ailments. The pharmaceutical market is huge and direct-to-consumer advertising by manufacturers already present in some countries will almost certainly spread to others. Physicians have a responsibility not only to treat where necessary but also to counter the commercially driven medicalization of health when medications are not needed.

Assessment of risk and benefit

Consciously or subconsciously, every prescribing decision involves a consideration of risks and benefits. When the benefits are seen by all to clearly outweigh the possible risks, little time is given to weighing the relative merits, for example the use of antibiotics in the management of bacterial meningitis or the use of aspirin in the secondary prevention of ischaemic heart disease. However, in many if not most prescribing decisions the balance is not so heavily weighted in favour of treatment and consideration should be given to considering the relative risks and benefits of treatment. For instance, the net benefit of taking penicillin for a streptococcal sore throat (assuming it was clear that this was the causative organism at the time of prescribing) relies on an assessment of the benefits and risks of treatment. A decision to treat might be influenced by a desire to reduce the extent and duration of symptoms, to prevent transmission of the organism or to prevent the longer-term complications of rheumatic fever and glomerulonephritis. In a European population both the short- and long-term benefits might be seen as marginal. In contrast, in a Polynesian community with very high rates of rheumatic fever, the potential benefits of aggressively treating sore throats would be seen as much greater. The risks of a course of penicillin might be seen as small to the individual; ranging from gastrointestinal upset or vaginal candidiasis through to rare but life threatening anaphylaxis. Another common example would be weighing up the relative risks and benefits of anticoagulation for someone with chronic atrial fibrillation (AF). The risks of cerebral haemorrhage from over anticoagulation in a young, otherwise fit patient with AF probably outweigh the net benefit of reducing the small risk of cerebral infarction from a mural thrombus. In an elderly patient with AF the risks of embolisation and therefore the potential net benefit of anticoagulation is much greater and may be considered to outweigh the risks of haemorrhage, unless of course the elderly patient is falling in which case the risks of intracerebral haemorrhage increase. The important principle is to ensure wherever possible that a discussion of the net benefits and likely risks takes place with patients and a joint decision is made on treatment. The way in which individual physicians and patients interpret risks and benefits can vary considerably. The way the information is presented can in itself have a major influence on decision-making. It is common practice for those publishing the results of drug trials to maximize the apparent effect by presenting results as relative risk reductions (RRRs), for example, by claiming a 30 per cent reduction in a particular adverse outcome. The effect seems much more modest when it becomes clear that the adverse outcome in the control group was say 1 per cent, giving an absolute risk reduction (ARR) of 0.3 per cent. Taking the reciprocal of the ARR gives the numbers needed to treat (NNT) so that on average one would benefit. In this example NNT would be 330. In one study, three randomly selected groups of patients were presented with the same information on the benefits of a cholesterol-lowering agent in three different ways.[5] More than 80 per cent agreed to take the medication when presented with the large apparent RRR. Far less than half of that number chose to take the medication when presented with the same facts converted to NNT. It should also be remembered that individual physicians and patients vary considerably in their inherent approach to risk taking versus risk aversion and different patient may interpret and make different decisions on the same data. It is important that prescribers understand their own values and do not impose them on their patients. Similarly, physicians vary considerably in their ability to tolerate uncertainty and in their inherent conservatism and willingness to adopt new drugs. Early adopters place their patients at additional risk of suffering rare adverse events that only become apparent after a year or two when large numbers of patients have been exposed to the drug. In recent years, there have been numerous examples of new drugs claiming to be cleaner and safer than existing alternatives that have been withdrawn when a rare but serious side effect subsequently arises. As a general principle, unless a drug truly represents a breakthrough (despite aggressive marketing, few do) and particularly if it is a new chemical group, it is safer to wait a year or two before switching patients who are adequately managed on existing medications.

Choosing drugs

Having made a decision that drug therapy is appropriate and assuming the patient is in agreement, there are a number of steps or questions to answer in the prescribing process (Table 1).

Table 1 Checklist for prescribing decisions

What is the reason for prescribing?
Is drug treatment necessary at this time?
Are there alternative non-pharmaceutical options?
Is the patient prepared to take a drug?
Which drug group(s) would be most suitable?
Which drug is the best choice from this group? (safety, efficacy, compliance, and cost)
Do I need to find out more about this drug?
What formulation, dose frequency, and duration?
How should the drug be monitored and adjusted?
Does the patient understand the potential risks and benefits?

Which drug group should be considered?

In many situations, there are several different drug groups that could be used to achieve the same result. The treatment of blood pressure is perhaps the best example. The prescriber must weigh up the evidence for relative efficacy of the various groups. There may or may not have been direct head to head comparisons between the groups. For long-term preventative outcomes the evidence for newer drugs will not be available and so presumed efficacy will have to be inferred by desirable changes in surrogate endpoints (e.g. reductions in blood pressure or cholesterol level). There also may be patient or disease characteristics that favour one drug group over another: beta blockers are relatively less effective in lowering raised blood pressure in those of African descent and are contraindicated in those with asthma, yet are a good choice in someone with both hypertension and ischaemic heart disease. Thiazide diuretics raise glucose and uric acid and would not be first choice in a patient with gout or diabetes. At other times, the mode of action of different groups makes the choice easier. In an overweight or obese patient with diabetes and relative insulin resistance, the mode of action of metformin makes it a much more logical and effective first choice than a sulfonylurea.

Which drug to choose within a group?

This can be equally problematic and is compounded in many cases by counter-marketing of apparent (often not clinically important) advantages of one drug over another. Those charged with creating preferred medicines lists and preferred formularies usually consider *efficacy, safety, compliance*, and *cost* (often they also consider common usage). Often there is little to choose on any of these criteria. In principle, if this is the case it is better to become familiar with one or two (rather than all) members of a drug group.

Efficacy

When a drug within a group is found to be effective in the treatment of a new condition the question arises: 'Is this property peculiar to that drug alone or is it a class effect?'. In recent years there have been a number of studies showing the beneficial effect of beta blockade in heart failure (a reversal of conventional teaching). The initial large studies used metoprolol. If the beneficial effect is because of beta blockade per se then intuitively it should occur with all beta-blockers. Usually, in time as more and more drugs within a group are shown to have the same beneficial effect the more likely it becomes that indeed it is a class effect. The protective effect of ACE inhibitors on diabetic nephropathy would be a good example of an apparent class effect. The purist approach is clearly only to use those agents for which evidence exists. However, it may be that in some countries these drugs are not available or are very expensive. Similarly, to extend the heart failure example, it may be that a patient is already taking a different beta-blocker at the time of developing heart failure. The decision then is whether to continue with the tolerated drug for which there is not yet evidence (invoking the plausible but not yet proven class effect), or to switch to the drug with proven evidence of efficacy.

Given the enormous range of problems presenting to primary care physicians, there are many times daily when patients present either with conditions that defy a diagnosis or with variations and co-morbidities that would exclude them from any clinical trial. The challenge for the physician in these situations is to extrapolate from what evidence there is to similar conditions and/or to the same conditions in different patient groups or those with other confounding problems. It is useful to remember the maxim 'No evidence of efficacy (trial not done) is NOT the same as evidence of non-efficacy' (trial done with negative effect). Primary care physicians of necessity must prescribe in the former situation daily. It is arguably unethical to continue to prescribe in the latter.

Safety

Different drugs even within the same drug group may have different side-effect profiles and interactions. It is important when considering new drugs for the prescriber to check for possible interactions. The British National Formulary (BNF) provides a readily accessible reference for common side effects. The electronic form can be accessed along with numerous useful links at www.bnf.org.uk . As discussed above, prescribers should be cautious of claims that brand new drugs have few if any side effects or interactions.

Compliance

Most drugs are not taken exactly as prescribed. Remembering to take them is a significant issue and wherever possible drugs that can be taken once daily are best. Other factors such as appearance, size, taste, and immediate gastrointestinal effect can at times dictate the choice of drugs from within a group. A more detailed discussion of compliance and concordance can be found in Chapter 7.5.

Cost

Drug pricing and reimbursement systems vary enormously from country to country. The only constant is that the demand for health care will always be greater than the ability of governments and users to fund it. In those countries where the state pays for the bulk of pharmaceuticals, there is an ethical responsibility for prescribers to use scarce funds wisely. If all else is equal (including the discounting of theoretical but practically and clinically insignificant differences) it is clearly appropriate to choose the cheapest drug within a group.

Choosing and titrating doses

There is no greater source of variation amongst prescribers than in the doses of drugs they use. It is not uncommon within an apparently homogenous group of prescribers caring for apparently similar populations to find a four- or fivefold variation in average doses used. The reasons for this variation are multifactorial.[6] In reviewing utilization data it is clear that some prescribers tend to use much higher doses of drugs across the board than do others. Whilst it is beyond the scope of this chapter to explore clinical pharmacological principles of dosing in depth, it is worth considering the practicalities of initial dose choice and dose titration. Using the example of inhaled steroid therapy in asthma, there are two distinct schools of thought on choice of initial dose. The first and conservative approach is to start with a low dose and titrate the dose upwards until symptoms are controlled. The second approach is to start with a much higher dose with the intention of gaining symptom control quickly and then back titrating the dose. In theory, for similar patients either approach should meet in the middle with the lowest appropriate dose to maintain symptom control. In reality, for most patients the maintenance dose is usually close to the starting dose, so that the patients of the high starting dose prescriber end up on a significantly higher maintenance dose than those served by the prescriber adopting the conservative starting dose approach. Back titration is difficult in practice and happens much less often than upward titration as it involves reducing the dose of an asymptomatic patient back to the point of breakthrough symptoms to determine the lowest effective dose. Mostly this does not happen. Similar variation in starting and maintenance doses is seen in other conditions both acute and chronic.

There is a tension between natural conservatism with a desire to start low and go slow and the evidence based pressure to use similar doses to those reported in studies. Early clinical randomized controlled trials of new drugs are generally designed using the highest tolerated doses deliberately. This is understandable to minimize the possibility of missing an important clinical benefit simply because an inadequate dose was chosen. The original studies demonstrating the increased survival of patients with heart failure given ACE inhibitors used large doses. The prescriber faced with implementing the findings from these trials for an elderly patient in heart failure (who would not have been eligible to enter the study for various reasons) has a problem. Clearly, it is not possible to titrate dose against increased life expectancy in an individual patient. When there is no evidence to support (or refute) the beneficial effect of low dose treatment, it would therefore seem justifiable, with the patient's agreement, to cautiously increase the dose to the maximum tolerated, or the doses used in the relevant trial(s).

In titrating doses against an easily measurable endpoint such as blood pressure or cholesterol level often a single drug will not achieve the target levels. The dose–responses curves of most drugs begin to flatten out well below the maximum recommended doses. The additional benefit of increased doses at the upper end of the range are thus small and adding another agent will often result in greater efficacy than maximal doses of a single agent. In recognising this synergistic effect some drugs (e.g. ACE inhibitors and thiazide diuretics) are marketed as fixed dose combinations. This aids compliance at the expense of limiting the ability to titrate the drugs individually. There are many instances when the standard doses of drugs must be varied. In particular, care is needed when prescribing for children, in the elderly, during pregnancy and lactation, and in those with hepatic or renal impairment. Once again, the BNF is a useful starting reference in these situations.

There are a number of medications where it is necessary to monitor blood levels of the drug. The frequency of testing will depend upon the stability of the results. When monitoring anticoagulants it is the effect of the drug on clotting rather than the drug levels that are measured, but the principle is the same.

Frequency and duration of treatment

The manufacturers' data sheets usually list the recommended frequency of dosing. Compliance improves with less frequent dosing. In recognition of this manufacturers have developed numerous systems of slow or controlled release for drugs with short half-lives. If it is important that drugs are taken at particular times then this should be specified on the prescription. If, for instance, it is important that a thrice-daily drug is evenly spaced then it should be prescribed '8 hourly' rather than 'three times daily' as this usually results in three doses being taken in 12 h followed by a 12-h break. The fluctuation in drug levels that result can lead to sub therapeutic levels in the morning and toxic levels at the end of the day.

Duration of treatment for acute self-limiting conditions, particularly infections, has traditionally been empiric. Community-based randomized controlled trials in many of these conditions are difficult to carry out, witnessed by the attrition rate of studies considered and discarded in most Cochrane systematic reviews. Over time, studies of community-acquired infections have tended to explore shorter courses of higher dose treatment. Analysis of prescriptions however still reflects the empiric digit preference for short courses of 1, 3, 5, 7, 10, and 14 days. Understandably, compliance diminishes with time and many longer courses of treatment are not finished or continued for very long after symptoms abate. In most instances this probably does not matter other than the potential to encourage antibiotic resistance. For more chronic conditions, the decision to stop or withdraw treatment should be made in discussion with the patient and the implications and importance of a relapse (e.g. driving with epilepsy) must be considered. Where the risks of long-term treatment can be significant (e.g. the use of non-steroidal anti-inflammatory medications in the elderly) it is appropriate to periodically review the need for ongoing treatment or consider safer alternatives.

Education of prescribers

Primary care physicians write many prescriptions. In many countries, data from these are collated and fed back to the prescriber, often in comparison with peers.(7) This feedback has been shown to be most useful when explored with one or more peers or a pharmacist acting as a facilitator.(8) The limitation of most of these feedback systems is that they were not designed with education in mind, rather they have been piggybacked onto systems originally designed for pharmacy reimbursement and more recently budget holding. Such information often does not capture the enduring interest of prescribers as there is a common perception of an overemphasis on cost and an accompanying lack of the invaluable additional clinical information that would allow in-depth review, true comparison and reflection. For this reason, written and standardized case studies have become popular and allow more reliable comparison at least to the stated prescribing intentions of peers faced with exactly the same information. For groups of prescribers using fully electronic clinical records much useful information can be extracted directly from practice computers. In many ways this provides more useful educational data as it represents intention to prescribe rather than pooled data from dispensed prescriptions, which do not include those prescriptions, which are never presented to pharmacies. Practice-based prescribing data can be linked to clinical indications and to other referred services, particularly laboratory utilization.

It is clearly not possible for generalists to keep up with all potentially relevant original research publications and therefore it is necessary to seek out respected sources of pre-digested summary information. Traditionally, this has come from didactic lectures and review articles from invited experts, often presented along with advertising of one form or another. Unquestionably these presentations and publications do influence primary care prescribing. As a result, such experts are themselves subject to intense marketing pressure by the manufacturers of pharmaceuticals. Drug information is increasingly available on the Internet and formularies with important prescribing information are also being incorporated into patient management software. Most of the prescribing information on the Internet is available to the public, it is often not peer reviewed and may be funded by the pharmaceutical industry. In those countries which allow direct-to-consumer advertising of prescription only medication, there are further pressures on prescribers to use newer, patented often more expensive drugs.

For the generalist prescriber, the skills to access appropriate independent information quickly are more important than trying to commit an impossibly large and changing knowledge base to memory. Many countries have state-funded centres whose purpose is to produce and disseminate independent comparative reviews and prescribing information.

References

1. **Mohanna, R. and Chambers, R.** *Risk Matters in Healthcare: Communicating, Explaining and Managing Risk.* Oxford: Radcliffe Medical Press, 2000.
2. **Beilin, L.J.** (1994). Non-pharmacological management of hypertension: optimal strategies for reducing cardiovascular risk. *Journal of Hypertension—Supplement* **12** (10), S71–81.
3. **Hamdy, O., Goodyear, L.J., and Horton, E.S.** (2001). Diet and exercise in type 2 diabetes mellitus. *Endocrinology and Metabolism Clinics of North America* **30** (4), 883–907.
4. **Royal Pharmaceutical Society of Great Britain.** *From Compliance to Concordance: Toward Shared Goals in Medicine Taking.* London: Royal Pharmaceutical Society, 1997.
5. **Hux, J.E. and Naylor, C.D.** (1995). Communicating the benefits of chronic preventative therapy: does the format of efficacy data determine patients acceptance of treatment? *Medical Decision Making* **15**, 152–7.
6. **Carthy, P., Harvey, I., Brawn, R., and Watkins, C.** (2000). A study of factors associated with cost and variation in prescribing among GPs. *Family Practice* **17** (1), 36–41.
7. **Thomson O'Brien, M.A., Oxman, A.D., Davis, D.A., Haynes, R.B., Freemantle, N., and Harvey, E.L.** Audit and feedback: effects on professional practice and health care outcomes. [Systematic Review] Cochrane Effective Practice and Organisation of Care Group. *Cochrane Database of Systematic Reviews* Issue 2, 2002.
8. **Thomson O'Brien, M.A., Oxman, A.D., Davis, D.A., Haynes, R.B., Freemantle, N., and Harvey, EL.** Educational outreach visits: effects on professional practice and health care outcomes. [Systematic Review] Cochrane Effective Practice and Organisation of Care Group, *Cochrane Database of Systematic Reviews* Issue 2, 2002.

7.5 Concordance and compliance

Nicky Britten

The problem of non-compliance

The problem of non-compliance (also referred to as non-adherence) is long standing, extensively documented, and largely unsolved. Haynes et al.[1] define adherence as the extent to which patients follow the instructions they are given for prescribed treatments. It continues to generate a large research literature, which confirms the fact that typical adherence rates are about 50 per cent. One review concluded that the search for stable characteristics of non-compliant patients is fruitless since an individual may adhere to some aspects of their treatment but not others.[2] Another review of interventions for helping patients to follow prescriptions, concluded that the full benefits of medications cannot be realised at currently achievable levels of adherence, and that effective ways of helping people follow medical treatments would have far larger effects on health than any treatment itself.[1]

In parallel with the growing literature on non-compliance have been critiques of the assumptions on which the term is based. Stimson[3] criticized the image of the ideal patient in compliance research as a passive, obedient, and unquestioning recipient of medical instructions. Any divergence from this ideal was seen as irrational in the light of medical rationality. The blame for such defaulting could then be seen as lying with the patient rather than the prescriber. Stimson advocated a more active view of patients in which they make their own treatment decisions, have their own ideas and attitudes about medications, and evaluate doctors' actions.

Over 20 years later, Donovan[4] took up the same theme to address much the same problem. She identified a number of assumptions inherent in the ideology of compliance: that doctors know what is best for their patients; that they are able to impart medical information clearly and neutrally; that they prescribe effective treatments rationally; and that they are the principal (or only) contributors to decisions about medications and other treatments. She asserted that patient compliance is a false goal for two reasons. Firstly, patients are not concerned about compliance but make their own decisions based on their own beliefs and the information available to them at the time. Secondly, prescribing is not an exact or neutral science, since prescribers are influenced by commercial and other pressures, and personal experience. Donovan concluded that the traditional concept of compliance is outmoded in modern health care systems in which chronic illness and questioning patients predominate.

Over the years, the literature about medicine taking has evolved. It has moved from a doctor-centred perspective to a more patient-centred perspective; it has shifted its focus from a narrow concern with why patients do not take their medicines properly to broader considerations; and has included qualitative as well as quantitative methods.

Origins of the term concordance

The use of the term 'concordance' in relation to prescribing and medicine taking was introduced in a report published by the Royal Pharmaceutical Society of Great Britain[5] entitled 'From compliance to concordance: towards shared goals in medicine taking' (see Box 1).

While compliance refers to something that patients do or do not do with their medicines, concordance refers to a relationship between two or more parties. A patient can be non-compliant but an individual cannot be non-concordant. Only a consultation, or a discussion, can be non-concordant. Concordance also differs from compliance in acknowledging and valuing the patient's perspective. The two terms are related however, as concordance may well lead to improved prescribing and medicine taking. Indeed the precise relationship between concordance and compliance (or adherence) needs to be carefully researched. What is already clear is that non concordance can lead to non-adherence.[6]

Box 1 Definition of concordance

> Concordance is a new approach to the prescribing and taking of medicines. It is an agreement between a patient and a health care professional that respects the beliefs and wishes of the patient in determining whether, when and how medicines are to be taken. Although reciprocal, this is an alliance in which the health care professionals recognize the primacy of the patient's decisions about taking the recommended medications (www.concordance.org).

The last sentence in the definition of concordance has stimulated debate and misinterpretation. Although it refers to patient autonomy, it also reflects the pragmatic observation that people make their own decisions on a day to day basis about when, where and how to take their medicines. Unless the patient is closely supervised in hospital or undergoing directly observed treatment, health care practitioners cannot force people to take medicines against their will. The point of concordance is to identify any differences in patients' and practitioners' perspectives, whether due to doctors prescribing treatments patients are unwilling to take, or patients wanting treatments doctors are unwilling to prescribe, so that these can be discussed and negotiated. The outcome of a concordant consultation may be an agreement to differ.

Discussions between patients and prescribers, or between patients and pharmacists, have implications for other members of the primary health care team. Any agreement, particularly an agreement to take a medicine in a non-standard way, needs to be communicated to other health care professionals.

Comparison with other models

Concordance is similar to a number of other models of the patient-health professional relationship, but is different from them all, principally in its focus on prescribing and medicine taking. The most obvious of these is shared decision-making (see Chapter 5.5). The shared decision-making model requires both professional and patient to be involved and to share information with one another. However, it is possible to have concordance without shared decision-making, as some patients may not want to share decisions preferring instead that the professional take responsibility. In these situations, engagement with patients' views about medicines is still necessary to avoid misunderstandings which could lead to non-adherence.[6] In the context of long-term treatment of chronic problems, new decisions are not necessarily being made at each consultation. The need for mutual understanding remains, as patients' symptoms or situations may be evolving.

Concordance also shares features with the patient-centred clinical method advocated by Stewart et al.[7] The patient-centred method is concerned with much more than prescribing and medicine taking. Its third element, finding common ground regarding management, comes closest to concordance. However, this does not explicitly include discussion of patients' treatment preferences.

It is the model of clinical negotiation advocated by Katon and Kleinman[8] which comes closest to concordance. This is an eight-stage model of the clinical encounter which begins with the physician eliciting the patient's explanatory model, after which the physician presents his or her explanatory model. Katon and Kleinman explained that the physician needs to elicit the patient's model first, to avoid contaminating or inhibiting the patient by presenting the physician's model first. Following this exchange of views, the model described the steps needed to arrive at a negotiated agreement, acknowledging the possibility that such an agreement might not be possible. However, this model was not about prescribing or medicine taking.

Lastly, concordance should not be confused with the consumer choice model, in which clinicians provide information and consumers make their own treatment choices. Concordance does not mean providing patients with whatever they ask for or want, as this is as one-sided as patients following doctors' orders.

Patients' perspectives on medicines and medicine taking

In contrast to the compliance literature that has tended to ignore or problematize patients' perspectives, a largely qualitative sociological and anthropological literature has explored the meanings of medicines and the ways in which people use them.

The ambivalence felt by many people is reflected in, and influenced by, the polarized media portrayal of drugs as either miracle cures or poisonous chemicals (see Chapter 3.4). Aversion to medicines is a recurring theme, with people saying that they prefer not to take medicines if at all possible. Studies of patients on long-term medication for chronic conditions have revealed the extent to which some people hate taking drugs.[9] In the United Kingdom, Donovan and Blake[10] reported that more than four-fifths of their sample of rheumatology patients spontaneously expressed dislike at having to take drugs at all. There was a general belief that to rely on drugs was a sign of weakness and most respondents only took drugs regularly as a last resort. Many of their fears about drugs sprung not from medical advice but from their own or others' experience of side effects, or from the adverse publicity about withdrawn drugs.

Medicines are perceived by some people as being unnatural and harmful, and are unfavourably compared with self-treatment, no treatment, alternative, or complementary therapies. In a study in Sweden, Fallsberg[11] found that 36 of 90 respondents suffering from long-term pain, asthma, and hypertension spontaneously referred to medicines as poison. Fears of addiction and dependence are also widespread, extending beyond medications known to be pharmacologically addictive.[12]

As well as these negative views, there is much taken for granted acceptance of medicine taking and the efficacy of drug therapy.[12] The balancing of positive and negative views is sometimes explicit. For example, Donovan and Blake[10] found that rheumatology patients carried out theoretical cost–benefit analyses of their medicines and that many put them into practice. Some decided that the risks outweighed the benefits so clearly that they would not even try the medications, and disposed of scripts or drugs. In most cases, drugs were taken 'on trial' for whatever period seemed most appropriate to patients. Drugs such as non-steroidal anti-inflammatories would be tried for a few days, and if clear beneficial effects were not perceived or if side effects were experienced, they would be stopped or the doses reduced. In many cases, patients did not give the drugs sufficient chance to work, but most were unaware of this.

Using a sample of over 500 British patients suffering from a range of chronic illnesses, Horne[2] identified four themes underlying commonly held beliefs about medicines. Core beliefs about prescribed medication are its perceived necessity for maintaining health (specific-necessity) and concerns about the potential for dependence or harmful effects (specific-concerns). General beliefs about medicines fell into two categories: beliefs about intrinsic properties of medicines and the extent to which they are harmful and addictive (general-harm) and beliefs about whether medicines are overused by doctors (general-overuse). Horne showed that age and medication beliefs accounted for over a quarter of the variation in self-reported adherence, with beliefs about prescribed medication contributing 13 per cent to the total variance explained. He found that views about the patient's specific medication regimen were more strongly related to adherence than were general views about medicines.

These studies show that the rationality informing lay views of medicines does not always correspond with medical rationality, for example in the varied meanings of the terms dependence and addiction. The literature also demonstrates the importance of people's social contexts and everyday lives for their decisions about medicine taking. In his influential paper about the meaning of medications for people with epilepsy in the United States, Conrad[9] argued that the context of people's everyday lives was more salient than doctor–patient interaction for understanding why people altered their prescribed medication regimens. He coined the term 'medication practice' to refer to a patient-centred concept of how people manage their medications, and found that people varied their medication practice according to the circumstances of their everyday lives. Self-regulation of medicine taking occurred in nearly half his sample. Sometimes this occurred as a way of testing whether the epilepsy was still there and whether people needed to continue taking their antiepileptic medication. Some people altered their medication as a way of controlling the dependence they experienced, as the medication was symbolic of the dependence created by having epilepsy. Some altered their medication practice as a way of minimizing the stigmatization experienced when taking antiepileptic medication. Others did so in response to practical circumstances such as taking exams or drinking alcohol.

The concept of self-regulation of medicine taking is applicable in a wide range of chronic diseases, from hypertension to schizophrenia to arthritis.[10,13] The most common form of self-regulation appears to be reduction of either dose or frequency, although in some cases patients take more medication than is recommended. The literature also shows that many patients do not discuss their fears about medicines or their medication practices with doctors, and that doctors do not ask.[6] Thus, many doctors remain uninformed about the reasons why patients use medicines in the ways that they do.

Prescribers' perspectives

The original definition of concordance referred to the doctor's professionally informed health beliefs.[5] The exchange of views about prescribing and medicine taking requires the doctor to explain the basis for his or her treatment decisions, and to provide information about any drugs being prescribed. This includes the evidence base for treatment decisions, particularly if doctor and patient disagree about the most appropriate treatment. Other chapters in this book explicate the basis for appropriate prescribing in more detail than is possible here (see Chapter 7.4).

Prescribing decisions are influenced not only by doctors' knowledge and clinical experience but also by their perceptions of patients' expectations. When prescribers are asked about the factors influencing their prescribing decisions, they usually include some reference to patient expectations or patient demand.[14] In particular, studies of antibiotic prescribing have identified the doctor's need to preserve doctor–patient relationships as a factor responsible for the writing of prescriptions that are not clinically indicated.[15] General practitioners' perceptions of patients' expectations for prescriptions have been shown to influence prescribing decisions, so that patients who are perceived as expecting prescriptions are much more likely to receive them than those who are not perceived as expecting prescriptions.[16] In fact, doctors' perceptions are a stronger influence than patients' actual expectations. These perceptions may however be based on guesses and assumptions and are not necessarily accurate.[6] In particular, doctors may be unaware of the relevance of patients' ideas about medicines for appropriate prescribing. This underlines the necessity for doctors to ask about patients' ideas and expectations explicitly, and the need for concordance.

Concordance in the consultation

A comprehensive study of British general practice carried out by Tuckett et al.[17] in the late 1970s showed that most consultations could not be characterized as a meeting between experts. The authors concluded that doctors and patients did not share or exchange ideas to a very great degree, and that the few attempts made to establish the patients' ideas and explanations were brief if not absent. Twenty years later, a study specifically concerned with doctor–patient communication about drugs in British general practice showed that the lack of discussion of patients' ideas about medicines led to misunderstandings and thence to potential or actual non-adherence.[6] A range of misunderstandings were identified, all of which could be characterized by a lack of patient participation in the consultation, and all of which were associated with subsequent problems with medicine taking. Patients' participation in the consultation can take the form of the voicing of expectations and preferences, and the voicing of responses to doctors' actions and decisions. When patients in this study did not express their expectations and preferences, doctors sometimes made assumptions about them based on prior knowledge. While these assumptions were reasonable in themselves, they were not always appropriate for that person at that moment.

In a study of communication about antihypertensive medication in Sweden, doctors and patients were found to talk about medication very differently. Patients talked about the experiences of being on medication while physicians focused on pharmacological effect and dosage. Patients had a very fragmentary understanding of their medication and their questions mainly referred to unwanted effects.[18] In a series of papers based on outpatient settings in the United States and Canada, Sleath et al. investigated patient–physician communication about medication.[19,20] Physicians and patients spent an average of 20 per cent of each medical visit discussing medications. Almost half of the patients did not ask any medication questions at all even though they were currently taking at least one medication. Starting a new medication doubled a patient's likelihood of question asking.[19] A fifth of patients expressed complaints about their medication, and those who did so were twice as likely also to express an adherence problem than patients who did not express a complaint.[20]

Some researchers have analysed consultation transcripts in order to understand the process of communication about medication in more detail. Smith-Dupre and Beck[21] analysed the consultations of a single physician in which patient involvement was facilitated. The physician used self-disclosure as a way of downplaying perceived status differences and facilitating a cooperative approach. This enabled her patients to express their preferences about prescribed medication in the context of non-antagonistic consultations. In another study, Gwyn and Elwyn[22] analysed a single consultation between the parents of a child with tonsillitis for whom antibiotics were not prescribed and a general practitioner who regularly employed shared decision making. In this consultation, the GP's efforts to reach a shared decision were thwarted by a combination of the embedded power imbalance and the conflict between the GP's and the parents' prescription preferences.

Few of the studies of communication about medicines have examined differences in patients' and doctors' perspectives, perhaps because this is rarely addressed in clinical practice.

Impact of concordance

Since the publication of the RPSGB report, the use of the term concordance has become more widespread. For example, in the UK the Department of Health's document on the Expert Patient initiative (www.doh.gov.uk/healthinequalities) refers to concordance in the context of self-management programmes. Unfortunately, it can also be used inappropriately as a politically correct synonym for compliance. Thus Gadsby,[23] in an article which was actually about improving compliance in type 2 diabetes, posed the question 'Why don't patients concord with treatment?'. This misuse of the term concordance is not isolated.[1] In his discussion of patients' failure to carry out prescribers' or dispensers' instructions, Gadsby portrayed them as confused, insufficiently educated, as having problems opening packages or reading labels, or as having busy lifestyles.[23] By characterizing patients in this negative way, Gadsby failed to consider or engage with patients' everyday decision-making processes about diabetes.[24]

A number of criticisms have been made of the concept of concordance. Firstly, many practitioners fear that discussion of patients' views will lead to inordinately long consultations. Some see concordance as a way of giving in to patients' inappropriate 'demands' which is incompatible with evidence-based prescribing. It is claimed by some that concordance shifts responsibility onto patients or alternatively that it privileges patient autonomy. However, the relationship between consultation length and better patient outcomes remains unclear (Chapter 5.6). It is possible that concordance may save time in the longer term through resolution of misunderstandings. The model of concordance emphasizes the importance of prescribers explaining their views as much as the converse, including the reasons why some prescriptions are seen as inappropriate by professionals. Any clinician attempting concordance needs to take account of patients' preferences for shared decision making and the sharing of information.

The point of concordance is not necessarily to change patients' behaviour, as prescribers cannot force patients to take medicines, but to bring these differences into the open for discussion and negotiation.

The way forward

The introduction of the concordance model was intended to move away from the widespread yet unhelpful model of compliance in which patients were merely expected to do as they were told. It is an approach which combines two previous strands in the compliance literature: doctor–patient communication and patients' health beliefs.[9] It represents a model of prescribing and medicine taking which is more in keeping with other developments in health care such as patient participation and shared decision making. The concordance model requires practitioners, educators, and researchers to engage with the now considerable literature on patients' perspectives on prescribing and medicine taking. There are signs that researchers and policy makers have started to do this. However, there remains a considerable research and educational agenda. The evidence suggests that few practitioners are yet conducting concordant consultations,[6] and as a result, the precise link between concordance and subsequent medicine taking remains to be documented.

References

1. **Haynes, R.B., Montague, P., Oliver, T., McKibbon, K.A., Brouwers, M.C., and Kanani, R.** Interventions for helping patients to follow prescriptions for medications (Cochrane Review). In *The Cochrane Library* Issue 1. Update Software, Oxford: Update Software, 2001.
2. **Horne, R.** (1998). Adherence to medication: a review of existing research. In *Adherence to Treatment in Medical Conditions* (ed. L. Myers and K. Midence), pp. 285–310. London: Harwood Academic.
3. **Stimson, G.V.** (1974). Obeying doctor's orders: a view from the other side. *Social Science and Medicine* **8**, 97–104.
4. **Donovan, J.L.** (1995). Patient decision making: the missing ingredient in compliance research. *International Journal of Technology Assessment in Health Care* **11**, 443–55.
5. **Royal Pharmaceutical Society of Great Britain.** *From Compliance to Concordance: Achieving Shared Goals in Medicine Taking.* London: RPSGB, 1997.
6. **Britten, N., Stevenson, F.A., Barry, C.A., Barber, N., and Bradley, C.P.** (2000). Misunderstandings in prescribing decisions in general practice: qualitative study. *British Medical Journal* **320**, 484–8.
7. **Stewart, M., Belle Brown, J., Wayne Weston, W., McWhinney, I.R., McWilliam, C.L., and Freeman, T.R.** (1995). *Patient-Centred Medicine: Transforming the Clinical Method.* Thousand Oaks: Sage Publications.
8. **Katon, W. and Kleinman, A.** (1981). Doctor–patient negotiation and other social science strategies in patient care. In *The Relevance of Social Science for Medicine* (ed. L. Eisenberg and A. Kleinman), pp. 253–79. Dordrecht, Holland: D. Reidel Publishing Company.
9. **Conrad, P.** (1985). The meaning of medications: another look at compliance. *Social Science and Medicine* **20**, 29–37.
10. **Donovan, J.L. and Blake, D.R.** (1992). Patient non-compliance: deviance or reasoned decision making? *Social Science and Medicine* **34**, 507–13.
11. **Fallsberg, M.** Reflections on medicines and medication: a qualitative analysis among people on long-term drug regimens. Linkoping University, Linkoping, Sweden, 1991.
12. **Britten, N.** (1994). Patients' ideas about medicines: a qualitative study in a general practice population. *British Journal of General Practice* **44**, 465–8.

13. **Morgan, M. and Watkins, C.J.** (1988). Managing hypertension: beliefs and responses to medication among cultural groups. *Sociology of Health and Illness* **10**, 561–78.

14. **Weiss, M. and Fitzpatrick, R.** (1997). Challenges to medicine: the case of prescribing. *Sociology of Health and Illness* **19**, 297–327.

15. **Butler, C.C., Rollnick, S., Pill, R., Maggs-Rapport, F., and Stott, N.** (1998). Understanding the culture of prescribing: qualitative study of general practitioners' and patients' perceptions of antibiotics for sore throats. *British Medical Journal* **317**, 637–42.

16. **Britten, N. and Ukoumunne, O.** (1997). The influence of patients' hopes of receiving a prescription on doctors' perceptions and the decision to prescribe: a questionnaire survey. *British Medical Journal* **315**, 1506–10.

17. **Tuckett, D., Boulton, M., Olson, C., and Williams, A.** *Meetings between Experts: An Approach to Sharing Ideas in Medical Consultations.* London: Tavistock Publications.

18. **Kjellgren, K.I., Svensson, S., Ahlner, J., and Saljo, R.** (1998). Antihypertensive medication in clinical encounters. *International Journal of Cardiology* **64**, 161–9.

19. **Sleath, B., Roter, D., Chewning, B., and Svarstad, B.** (1999). Asking questions about medication: analysis of physician–patient interactions and physician perceptions. *Medical Care* **37**, 1169–73.

20. **Sleath, B., Chewning, B., Svarstad, B., and Roter, D.** (2000). Patient expression of complaints and adherence problems with medications during chronic disease medical visits. *Journal of Social and Administrative Pharmacy* **17**, 71–80.

21. **Smith-Dupre, A.A. and Beck, C.S.** (1996). Enabling patients and physicians to pursue multiple goals in health care encounters: a case study. *Health Communication* **8**, 73–90.

22. **Gwyn, R. and Elwyn, G.** (1999). When is a shared decision not (quite) a shared decision? Negotiating preferences in a general practice encounter. *Social Science and Medicine* **49**, 437–47.

23. **Gadsby, R.** (2000). Improving concordance in type 2 diabetes. *Prescriber* (Suppl.), 19 February, 3–6.

24. **Campbell, R., Pound, P., Pope, C., Britten, N., Pill, R., Morgan, M., and Donovan, J.** (2003). Meta-ethnography: a synthesis of qualitative research on lay experiences of diabetes and diabetes care. *Social Science and Medicine* **56**, 671–84.

7.6 Continuity of care

Per Hjortdahl

'Continuity of care' is a phrase often used to describe the extent to which patients see the same practitioner or visit the same facility from one visit to another over a period of time. Continuity has been lauded as a key attribute of primary care for more than 50 years. It is intuitively a significant concept; 'like it is important for a child to have a mother, it is important for a person to have a regular doctor'. At the same time it is a complex issue closely interwoven with other key elements of general practice like accessibility, first-contact care, comprehensiveness, and coordination of care.[1] Continuity of care is thus seldom an isolated or one-dimensional virtue, which can be altered or enhanced without some corresponding or even conflicting effects. Much has been written about the benefits and dangers of continuity of care in the patient–doctor relationship,[2,3] but scant factual evidence is available about its effects. Its essential elements have yet, by and large, to be pinpointed.

The concept of continuity of care is being challenged from several sources.[4] Modern medicine is becoming so complex that it is difficult for individual general practitioners to have a professional grasp of the whole field of medicine, necessitating more referrals and shared care of their patients with other specialists or secondary care. Society at large is changing; the 'patient' patient is becoming a rarity, patients want increasingly to participate actively and exercise choice regarding their own health care. Prompt access to care is sometimes preferred by patients rather than personal continuity of care. The population, including patients and doctors, is becoming more geographically mobile, making continuity over time difficult. General practitioners are increasingly valuing their own free time for their families and for leisure. Professional activities like postgraduate education or teaching commitments increasingly disrupt availability. Many general practitioners seek only to hold part-time positions. In Norway, which has a strong primary health care system, more than 25 per cent of general practitioners now see patients in their offices only 3 days or less a week,[5] necessitating cooperation from colleagues in the practice, or deputizing, open access, walk-in clinics or emergency services. In a study from 1998 covering 30 European countries, it was noted that in 17 of them one quarter or more of the general practitioners held appointments outside their practice.[6] This frequently leads to fragmentation of care; the antithesis of continuity.

Continuity of care is thus an important personal issue to discuss and relate to for each general practitioner and his or her individual doctor–patient relationships. It is equally important to come to terms with on the organizational levels of the practice, locally and nationally. At the same time it is a highly relevant topic for the individual patients and politically for the population at large.

Continuity of care; what is it?

In spite of having been a fundamental principle of general practice for more than half a century, we still lack a common understanding of what 'continuity of care' actually entails, and as part of that, a sensible and agreed upon definition of the term. In the strict sense of the word continuity implies an uninterrupted chain of events. In medicine it has been used as a 'catch all' phrase implying that there is one place, one individual, or one team of associated individuals that serves as the source of care over a period of time, regardless of the presence or absences of particular health-related problems or the type of problem.[1] Continuity may be achieved by a variety of mechanisms; one practitioner who cares individually for the patient, an integrated group of professionals looking after the health needs of the patient, or simply it can be the medical record of the patient reflecting the care given over time.

Hennen broke the overall concept of continuity down into five dimensions:[7]

- interpersonal (relationships between patient and doctor);
- chronological (or longitudinal, temporal);
- geographic (or organizational linked; continuity between sites such as home, office, hospital);
- interdisciplinary (integration and coordination of care between different health care providers); and
- informational (continuity through medical records).

Later, the elements of accessibility of care and stability of the patient's environment were added. Splitting the overall concept into the different dimensions makes it easier to conceptualize the many facets of continuity.

Starfield maintains that 'longitudinality' conveys the spirit of this key characteristic of primary care better than 'continuity', highlighting the importance of the element of long-term personal relationships between practitioners and their patients.[1] In her opinion, continuity is not necessary for this longitudinal relationship to be present; interruptions in the continuity of care for whatever reason need not disrupt the long-term relationship. Fleming states that the concept of continuity commonly is confused with that of being a personal doctor.[4] He takes a different approach to understanding continuity and points out that continuity of care may lead to increased personalization of care in some circumstances, but that continuity of care can and does exist outside personalized care. Hjortdahl focused on continuity as the overall, direct or coordinated responsibility for the different medical needs of the patient.[8] The key words here are responsibility and coordination, in addition to personal care. The doctor cannot be available at all times, or be at several places at the same time, nor can he or she carry out all the different care the patient may need. The doctor is responsible for ensuring continuity of service by a competent deputy and for following through when some aspects of care are delegated to a consultant.

Freeman et al. followed this up with a broad review of continuity of care across all medical disciplines in the year 2000, defining continuity as the experience of a coordinated and smooth progression of care from the patient's point of view.[9] This is achieved when the health service is supplying:

- excellent information transfer following the patient;
- effective communication between professionals and services and with patients;
- flexibility and adjustability to the needs of the individuals over time;
- care from as few professionals as possible, consistent with other needs; and
- one or more named professionals with whom the patient can develop a therapeutic relationship.

Continuity of care, in the strict sense of the word implies the patient seeing the same health care worker or team of health professionals over time. As such it is a tool used by the general practitioner. Together with communication skills and the consultation, continuity of care is probably *the* most important tool of general practice. For a man building a house, a hammer and a saw are important tools, as is the surgeon's knife or the neurologist's reflex hammer. As a tool, continuity is important in itself, but for the concept of general practice it is what this tool is being *used for*, or what it leads *to*, that is crucial. Or to extend the metaphor; it is the kind of house we are building with these tools that matters at the end. In my opinion the final product is establishing and maintaining a curing and caring professional relationship with our patients. In this building process continuity of care may lead to better knowledge about each other, and a sense of responsibility and trust, all of which can be summed up in that rather poetic phrase *Personal doctoring*. There is a close relationship between continuity and personal doctoring, but they should be looked upon as separate entities. The first is a tool, linked to longitudinal continuity or longitudinality, while the second is an outcome, closely linked to relational or personal continuity.

Why continuity of care?

The second component of Hennen's breakdown of continuity is the chronological or longitudinal element, usually understood as the chain of care given by one health care provider over time, related to how often this process is interrupted by non-coordinated care. This is the continuity element most frequently evaluated in health care research, as it is a fairly clear-cut concept that can be objectively measured and evaluated looking at patients' health trajectories. As such it is a useful tool to evaluate and compare the delivery of primary health care locally or nationally, and is often used in health care planning and administration. Several methods have been developed to assess continuity of care in this way: among the better known are usual provider continuity (UPC), continuity of care index (COC), and likelihood of continuity (LICON). Other indexes have been developed to measure continuity and coordination of care. Each of these methods has its strength and weaknesses, described in detail by Starfield.[1] These are purely quantitative measures, however, and tell little about what these contacts over time may lead to in the more qualitative aspects of the individual patient–doctor relationships. It has been postulated that the main outcome of longitudinal care is the development of ongoing relationship that build trust, create a context for healing, and increase the practitioner's and the patient's knowledge of each other.[10]

Sick people have a particular need for trusting others, primarily their family and their doctor. Trust often implies a transfer of power, to a person or a system, to act on one's behalf, in one's best interest.[11] Personal trust grows in ongoing relationships. It evolves between people with names, identities, feelings and faces, and it must be actively gained. Recent studies have shown that higher continuity is associated with a higher level of trust between patient and doctor.[12] A practitioner's sense of responsibility toward his or her patients, in many ways the counterpart of patient trust, increases with the duration of the relationship and with the number of contacts.[8] It has, furthermore, been stated that the developments of personal relationships with patients, within certain limits, are important elements in the job satisfaction of general practitioners.[2]

Two main categories of contextual or personal knowledge are related to an ongoing doctor–patient relationship. The first is linked to the development of a mutual knowledge and understanding of each other. With continuity of care, the patient usually knows what to expect of the doctor before a consultation, and has less fear of the unknown. On the other side, continuous and comprehensive care allows the doctor to build, piece-by-piece, a 'capital' of knowledge about the patient and his or her previous history of illness. In addition to this formal knowledge, most of it usually also documented in the patient's clinical record, the practitioner frequently accumulates a more personal repository of knowledge; a tacit understanding of the patient as a person, family situation, and the social context.[13] Hjortdahl, in a large study from Norway, found a strong link between continuity of personal care and the doctor's accumulated knowledge about the patient.[8] Knowledge accumulated slowly during the first few months of the relationship, increased sharply between 3 and 12 months, then flattened out somewhat, but still increased steadily during the next few years. The frequency of contacts also contributed to the accumulation of knowledge; the major impact being at four to five visits a year. This is not an 'all or none' situation, however. Even though personal knowledge about patients accumulates over time, it is a fallacy to assume that the general practitioner has a comprehensive knowledge of all of his or her patients, even after many years in practice. The doctor's personal knowledge is acquired only as the opportunity arises and when the patient is ready to give it. Only in a minority of patients in a practice does this knowledge amount to a full picture.[14]

The other category of knowledge is of a more general nature and is related to the general practitioner's development of his or her own personal clinical knowledge and skills. You need longitudinal continuity of care to understand illness and disease in a contextual setting. You learn much about health and illness in general practice following your patients over time. This is in my opinion one of the main reasons why 'continuity of information and records' is unlikely to replace personal continuity of care. The record contains mere information, while the doctor possesses integrated knowledge about the patient, the illness and the setting in which it occurs. Much of this knowledge is tacit and gathered from several sources and over time.

Continuity of care; is it worth it?

A crucial question in the debate about continuity and personal doctoring is; does it lead to improved quality of health care, or is it all ideological rhetoric?

There is research evidence for an overall, reasonably strong and consistent association between continuity and patient and doctor satisfaction. One large study involving more than 2000 patients in 89 British general practices found that patients in practices with 'personal' lists were significantly more satisfied with their care than those patients seen in practices with 'group' lists.[15] In a Norwegian study including more than 3000 patients from 133 randomly selected general practices it was demonstrated that the longer the duration of the patient–doctor relationship, the higher the patient satisfaction with the most recent consultation.[16] This was clearly evident even after controlling for such factors as the number of contacts between the patient and doctor during the previous year; the age and sex of the patient; the age, sex, and the reimbursement of the provider (fee-for-service or capitation); location of practice (rural or urban) and type of consultation (scheduled or in-between appointments); reason for encounter (diagnosis); and duration of problem (acute, follow-up or chronic). Satisfaction with a consultation is, however, by itself usually not an adequate measure of the value of continuity, as dissatisfied individuals are more likely to change their practitioners if they are able to do so. Patients with chronic diseases are furthermore over-represented in practice-based surveys; a less biased view is usually obtained when the population at large is approached.

In the same Norwegian study, the doctors evaluated the extent to which prior knowledge of the doctor influenced the diagnostic process and management of the patient in each of the more than 3000 consultations.[17] The general practitioners stated that their prior knowledge contributed more to management than to diagnosis, and more to chronic problems than to short episodes of illness such as minor infections and minor injuries.[18] Prior knowledge reduced the duration of the consultations in 40 per cent of the visits. It was, furthermore, associated with ordering fewer laboratory tests, more use of expectant management, fewer prescriptions written, a more liberal use of sickness certification, and more referrals than when the doctor had no or only scant personal knowledge about a patient before the consultation.[17]

Indications of associations of continuity of care with improved intermediary medical outcomes are also emerging from other countries, such as Australia,[19] the United States,[20] and Great Britain.[21] Patient enablement, participation in the decision-making process in the consultation and compliance with medication and appointments, uptake of preventive care, and use of resources in the consultation, utilization of emergency departments and hospitals, and overall utilization of services and cost of care have been linked positively to continuity. People whose care is longitudinal had fewer emergency hospitalizations and shorter stays while in the hospital, in a study where men over the age of 55 were randomly assigned to two different groups for care, one with continuity of care and the other not.[22] Another American study including patients of all ages and both genders showed that individuals with better continuity during a 1-year period had significantly lower rates of hospitalizations in the subsequent year.[23] Other studies have, among other things, looked for associations between continuity and quality of care for patients with tonsillectomies, pregnancy complications, and utilization and cost of ambulatory care, but failed to demonstrate such links.

In their scoping exercise on continuity of care Freeman et al. identified several studies in the subject areas of cardiovascular disease, diabetes, cancer, care of older people, mental health, maternal care, and primary care, where the intervention involved a strong continuity element.[9] They concluded, however, that because of the lack of specificity few studies have been able to assess the impact of continuity of care in any conclusive manner. They, furthermore, stated that there are few experimental studies where a specific approach to enhancing continuity and assessing the outcome has been subject to rigorous trial in order to make a reasonable deduction of causality.

In summary, there is little evidence linking continuity of care to improved patient mortality or morbidity. There are emerging indications of positive associations between continuity and intermediary medical outcomes such as use of resources and patient behaviour. The strongest links have been demonstrated between patient satisfaction and continuity of care. Continuity is, however a multi-dimensional concept and may conflict with other key attributes of general practice, such as accessibility, coordination of care, and second opinions.

Potential dangers of continuity of care

As in most other important relationships, the greatest dangers of continuity appears when taken to the extreme, becoming 'too much of a good thing'. One example is the general practitioner monopolizing the patients in the name of continuity, not making proper use of referrals or competent colleagues, nor respecting the patient's rights to second opinions. The general practitioner is considered to be at the crossroads of health care, giving him or her a particular responsibility to ensure the integration of care from several sources, being at the same time the coordinator and the main provider of care.[4] In line with this it has been claimed that 'continuity makes blind', or that important diagnoses that develops slowly, like hypothyroidism, are missed by the family doctor seeing the patient frequently, but picked up by the locum looking at the patient with fresh eyes.[2] Patients with chronic conditions, like multiple sclerosis, have voiced the experience that their regular doctor has a tendency to blame all their ailments on the chronic disease, often not taking seriously other complaints or illnesses the patient may develop.

Another potential danger is the doctor–patient relationship becoming too close and intimate. Sharing major life events over time frequently ties strong bonds, making the relationship personal and cordial, which usually is of benefit for both patient and doctor. Sometimes, however the boundary between personal and private involvement is crossed, introducing feelings that disturb the professional relationship, and in the extreme allowing an intimacy that violates the patient's integrity. A lesser degree of the same hazard may take place if the positive attachment in the patient–doctor relationship turns into a dependency on the part of the patient, with the doctor emotionally taking over the responsibility for the patient's health and illness. In the long run, this makes the doctor's professional role difficult, but more important, it negates patients' enablement and responsibility for their own health.

Personalized continuity may in some cases limit patients' choice of health care. A basic assumption has been that continuity of care is an inevitable good for all patients, at all times and to the same degree; 'one size fits all, from cradle to grave'. This is not necessarily so, as is documented by Kearley et al.[24] In their study from England, 64 per cent of the respondents to a mailed questionnaire rated having a personal GP as very or extremely important. Having a personal doctor–patient relationship was highly valued by the patients, particularly for more serious, psychological or family issues where almost 9 out of 10 patients valued a personal relationship more than a convenient appointment. For minor illness it had much less value. Equally interesting is that one-third of the respondents rated the general importance of having a personal practitioner only as moderately, slightly, or not at all. From this it is evident that different groups of patients have different views of the importance of continuity. It is, furthermore, likely that individual patients hold different views on continuity, both over time as they go through different stages of life, or even at the same time for different health care reasons. Patients may wish only an 'on–off' transaction with a virtually anonymous health care worker at key points in their life, such as youth seeking information about contraception or worrying about sexually transmitted diseases. In certain circumstances patients value strangers rather than friends as their health care advisors.

Accessibility to primary care when the patient experiences a need for help is another value that increasingly comes into conflict with the concept of continuity of care. With personal lists the waiting time to see your regular doctor for all your health care needs, acute as well as chronic, minor as well as major, is often experienced as an annoyance for patients. Already in 1967 Cartwright observed that more than one-third of the patients would prefer to see another doctor without waiting, rather than waiting for half an hour for their own doctor.[25] Since then, with the emergence of a global market, increased consumerism and better-informed patients, general practitioners are facing a new brand of impatient patients demanding participation and choice in their own health care. These patients often prefer 'drop-in' clinics where a competent doctor can see them without undue waiting. Furthermore, they increasingly demand direct access to specialist care, eroding the basis of continuity and coordinated care.

Continuity of care; an anachronism in modern health care?

After more than 50 years of faithful service to primary health care service, the concept of continuity is not dead, but in serious need of rehabilitation.

The idea of a single provider available for all primary care needs at all times is outdated, from the point of view of the patient, the doctor and society at large. We need to find ways of combining continuity with personal doctoring, ready access, patient choice, professional competence, and realistic expectations of commitment on the part of the doctor. This is a big challenge for primary care all over the world. Steps are being taken in the right direction.

In many countries, patient rosters or 'lists' are made an integral part of primary care, organized so that there is generally one primary care practitioner for each 1000–3000 persons, depending on the age and illness level of the population and its geographic distribution. Patient lists are the basis for establishing a sense of responsibility for a group of people, and are the means by which practitioners can keep track of their patients' needs and to the extent to which they are met.[1] Such lists are established in the United Kingdom, Italy, the Netherlands, Portugal, and Denmark. The Norwegian government has been implementing, since 2001, a national patient list system modelled after that of the United Kingdom.

Teamwork is another approach being tried out in several countries. Here general practitioners join other primary health care workers in smaller medical teams. Such clinical units share administrative, computing, prescribing, audit, and educational support with each other, while trying to maintain one or more named general practitioners with whom the patient can develop a personal, therapeutic relationship. Teamwork necessitates good communication between the team members, highlighting the importance of a good clinical record as a major source of information. In this record relevant facts, interventions, and treatment are recorded and made available to all members of the health care team. Such a record is a means of ensuring consistency of care within the team, and will increasingly be computer-based and in many cases patient-held.

To date the discussions and research efforts related to continuity have to a large degree been static, doctor-centred, and limited in scope. It is a paradox that most studies to date have been cross sectional when evaluating a process that in its very nature is longitudinal. Longitudinal process-oriented research, where patient trajectories are followed over time, are urgently needed to understand more about barriers to greater personal continuity and what is needed to maintain and improve such continuity.

Continuity of care and personal doctoring are essential parts of good general practice, and they will even gain importance with the population growing older and medicine becoming increasingly complex. But we have to think anew. Continuity of care is costly to deliver in the day to day service and entails expenses in the way of personal commitments from the general practitioner. We should thus focus our research and continuity of care efforts on those who want, need, or deserve it, striking the right balance between continuity and accessibility.

References

1. **Starfield, B.** *Primary Care. Balancing Health Needs, Services and Technology.* New York: Oxford University Press, 1998.
2. **Freeman, G. and Hjortdahl, P.** (1997). What future for continuity of care in general practice? *British Medical Journal* **314**, 1870–3.
3. **Guthrie, B. and Wyke, S.** (2000). Does continuity in general practice really matter? *British Medical Journal* **321**, 734–6.
4. **Fleming, D.M.** (2000). Continuity of care: a concept revisited. *European Journal of General Practice* **6**, 140–5.
5. **Hjortdahl, P.** (1989). General practice and continuity of care, organisational aspects. *Family Practice* **6**, 292–8.
6. **Boerma, W.G.W. and Flemming, D.M.** *The Role of General Practice in Primary Health Care.* Norwich: World Health Organization (Europe), Stationery Office, 1998.
7. **Hennen, B.K.** (1975). Continuity of care in family practice. Part 1: Dimensions of continuity. *Journal of Family Practice* **2**, 371–2.
8. **Hjortdahl, P.** (1992). Continuity of care, general practitioners' knowledge about, and sense of responsibility toward their patients. *Family Practice* **9**, 3–8.
9. **Freeman, G., Shepperd, S., Robinson, I., Ehrich, K., Richards, S.C., and Pitman, P.** *Continuity of Care: Report of a Scoping Exercise,* Summer 2000, for the SDO programme of NHS R&D (Draft). London: NCCSDO, 2001. www.sdo.lshtm.ac.uk.
10. **McWhinney, I.R.** (1998). Core values in a changing world. *British Medical Journal* **316**, 1807–9.
11. **Fugelli, P.** (2001). James Mackenzie Lecture. Trust—in general practice. *British Journal of General Practice* **51**(468), 575–9.
12. **Mainous, A.G., Baker, R., Love, M., Pereira Gray, D., and Gill, J.M.** (2001). Continuity of care and trust in one's physician: evidence from primary care in the United States and the United Kingdom. *Family Medicine* **33**, 22–7.
13. **Gulbrandsen, P., Hjortdahl, P., and Fugelli, P.** (1997). General practitioners' knowledge of their patients' psychosocial problems: multipractice questionnaire survey. *British Medical Journal* **314**, 1014–18.
14. **McWhinney, I.R.** *A Textbook of Family Medicine.* New York: Oxford University Press, 1997.
15. **Baker, R. and Streatfield, J.** (1995). What type of general practice do patients prefer? Exploration of practice characteristics influencing patient satisfaction. *British Journal of General Practice* **45**, 654–9.
16. **Hjortdahl, P. and Laerum, E.** (1992). Continuity of care in general practice: effect on patient satisfaction. *British Medical Journal* **304**, 1287–90.
17. **Hjortdahl, P. and Borchgrevink, C.F.** (1991). Continuity of care, influence of general practitioners' knowledge about their patients on use of resources in consultations. *British Medical Journal* **303**, 1181–4.
18. **Hjortdahl, P.** (1992). The influence of general practitioner's knowledge about their patients on the clinical decision-making process. *Scandinavian Journal of Primary Health Care* **10**, 290–6.
19. **Veale, B.M.** Continuity of care and general practice utilization in Australia. PhD thesis. Australia National University, Canberra, 1996.
20. **Lambrew, J., DeFriese, G., Carey, T., Ricketts, T., and Biddle, A.** (1996). The effects of having a regular doctor or access to primary care. *Medical Care* **34**, 138–51.
21. **Howie, J.G.R., Heaney, D.J., Maxwell, M., Walker, J.J., Freeman, G.K., and Rai, H.** (1999). Quality at general practice consultations: cross sectional survey. *British Medical Journal* **319**, 738–44.
22. **Wasson, J.H., Sauvigne, A.E., Mogielnicki, P., Frey, W., Sox, C., Gaudette, C., and Rockwell, A.** (1984). Continuity of outpatient medical care in elderly men: a randomized trial. *Journal of the American Medical Association* **252**, 2413–17.
23. **Gill, J. and Mainous, A.** (1998). The role of provider continuity in preventing hospitalizations. *Archives of Family Medicine* **7**, 352–7.
24. **Kearley, K.E., Freeman, G.K., and Heath, A.** (2001). An exploration of the value of the personal doctor–patient relationship in general practice. *British Journal of General Practice* **51**(470), 712–18.
25. **Cartwright, A.** *Patients and their Doctors.* London: Routledge & Kegan Paul, 1967.

7.7 Complementary therapies

Andrew Vickers and Catherine E. Zollman

What is complementary medicine?

Complementary medicine (CM) refers to a group of therapeutic and diagnostic disciplines that were developed and have existed largely outside the institutions where conventional health care is taught and provided.

Examples of such therapies include acupuncture, chiropractic, herbal medicine, homeopathy, hypnosis, massage, and yoga. Less common and more unusual techniques may also be described as CM, including therapies such as flower essences, colour healing, iridology, and unconventional dietary practices. In the 1970s and 1980s, these disciplines were often provided as an alternative to conventional health care and hence became known collectively as 'alternative medicine'. The name 'complementary medicine' developed as the two systems began to be used alongside (to 'complement') each other. The term 'integrated medicine'—suggesting incorporation of both conventional and CM into a single treatment plan—has recently become popular.[1] This changing and overlapping terminology explains some of the confusion that surrounds CM.

Though definitions of CM have been attempted, the wide range of disciplines classified as CM makes it difficult to find defining criteria common to all. Many of the assumptions made about CM are simplistic (see Table 1). Nonetheless, some features are shared by most CM disciplines.

Historical development

In most countries of the world, training, research, and practice in conventional health care is supported and regulated by the state. The development of CM has taken place largely in the private sector. Until recently, most complementary practitioners trained in small, privately funded colleges and then worked independently in relative isolation from other clinicians.

Conceptual basis

Many CM therapies invoke concepts that are not recognized in biomedicine. For example, reflexologists believe that areas of the foot correspond to the organs of the body; practitioners of traditional Chinese acupuncture believe that health depends on a body energy called 'Qi'. One consequence is that complementary and conventional clinicians may diagnose the same patient differently, for example, 'deficient liver Qi' (traditional Chinese medicine); 'pulsatilla constitution' (homeopathy), and 'peptic ulcer' (conventional medicine). Confusingly, there is little correlation between the different diagnostic systems: some patients with deficient liver Qi do not have ulcers, and some ulcer patients do not have deficient liver Qi but another traditional Chinese diagnosis.

Training and regulation

CM practitioners are subject to different training and regulation to their counterparts in conventional medicine. Regulation varies from country to country and from therapy to therapy. Standards of training are inadequate in some cases.

Knowledge base

CM practitioners have not generally been concerned with the scientific understanding of their therapy. Their knowledge base is often derived from a tradition of clinical observation and treatment decisions are usually empirical. Some traditional teachings have been handed down in a way that discourages questioning and evolution of practice. Complementary practitioners are often encouraged to base clinical decisions on their own and others' individual anecdotal, clinical, and intuitive experience, although some training institutions are now starting to appreciate and emphasize the role of research and evidence-based practice.

Holistic approach

Many, but not all, complementary practitioners have a multifactorial and multilevel view of human illness. Disease is thought to result from disturbances at a combination of physical, psychological, social, and spiritual levels. The body's capacity for self-repair, given appropriate conditions, is emphasized. According to most complementary practitioners, the purpose of therapeutic intervention is to restore balance and facilitate the body's own healing responses rather than to target individual disease processes or stop troublesome symptoms. They may, therefore, prescribe a package of care, which could include modification of lifestyle, dietary change, and exercise as well as a specific treatment.

Use and users of CM

Surveys in various countries have followed the prevalence of CM use since the early 1990s.[2] Because these studies have used many different methodologies and definitions of CM, precise comparisons over time and between countries are not easy. It appears that in a number of developed countries

Table 1 Unhelpful assumptions about CM

Non-statutory—not provided by the NHS

- Complementary medicine is increasingly available on the NHS
- 40% of general practices provide access to complementary medicine for NHS patients

Unregulated—therapists not regulated by state legislation

- Osteopaths and chiropractors are now state registered and regulated, and other disciplines will probably soon follow
- Substantial amount of complementary medicine is delivered by conventional health professionals

Unconventional—not taught in medical schools

- Disciplines such as physiotherapy and chiropody are also not taught in medical schools
- Some medical schools have a complementary medicine component as part of the curriculum

Natural

- Good conventional medicine also involves rehabilitation with, say, rest, exercise, or diet
- Complementary medicine may involve unnatural practices such as injecting mistletoe or inserting needles into the skin

Holistic—treats the whole person

- Many conventional health care professionals work in a holistic manner
- Complementary therapists can be narrow and reductionist in their approach
- Holism relates more to outlook of practitioner than to the type of medicine practised

Alternative

- Implies use instead of conventional treatment
- Most users of complementary medicine seem not to have abandoned conventional medicine

Unproved

- There is a growing body of evidence that certain complementary therapies are effective in certain clinical conditions
- Many conventional health care practices are not supported by the results of controlled clinical trials

Irrational—no scientific basis

- Scientific research is starting to uncover the mechanisms of some complementary therapies, such as acupuncture, relaxation therapy, and herbal medicine

Harmless

- There are reports of serious adverse effects associated with using complementary medicine

Adapted from Zollman, C. and Vickers, A. (1999). ABC of complementary medicine. What is complementary medicine? *British Medical Journal* **319** (7211), 693–6.

the use of CM has increased significantly over the last decade (e.g. by 47 per cent between 1990 and 1997 in the United States[3]) and now represents a significant proportion of total health expenditure (e.g. 4 per cent or £1.6 billion in the United Kingdom[4]). The popularity of individual therapies differs widely from country to country. This is partly because of cultural and political differences. For example, some disciplines, which are considered complementary in the United Kingdom or North America, are regarded as part of mainstream health care in continental Europe.

In general, demographic comparisons show that CM users are more likely to be female, better educated, and have higher incomes than non-users.[5] However, this may tell us more about these users' ability to access information and pay for treatment rather than indicating a particular preference for CM, as cost and lack of information have been cited as the main reasons for not choosing CM among various patient groups.[6]

A number of studies have looked at patterns of usage and individual patient's reasons for consulting CM practitioners.[7,8] The vast majority (>85 per cent) appear to be using CM alongside conventional medicine to meet health needs. A typical example might be an arthritis patient who consults an acupuncturist while continuing to take analgesics. Many patients appear to be 'shopping for health', discriminating on the grounds of perceived risks and benefits to determine the most appropriate system for managing their individual health problems. Some studies have shown that side-effects and ineffectiveness of conventional medicine lead people to experiment with CM. Others show that a desire to try all available options or a congruence of CM with personal values and beliefs are the factors most strongly associated with CM use. In some patient groups, particularly those with chronic, relapsing conditions, CM use appears higher than in the general population.[8]

How is CM practised?

Much of CM is practised from private clinics in the community. Practitioners generally work from private homes or small clinics in which several different therapies are offered. Such clinics typically provide treatment rooms to independent practitioners and do not often offer a team approach for a particular patient's problem.

CM is also widely and increasingly practised in conventional health settings (see Table 2). In one survey,[9] approximately 40 per cent of GP partnerships in England provided access to some form of complementary therapy for their NHS patients. In about half of these cases, CM was practised by the doctor or by another member of the primary care team. This survey was conducted in the UK in the mid-1990s when fundholding was operational and so CM provision may have changed significantly since then. There do not appear to be comparable studies in secondary care.

An overview of CM therapies

Acupuncture

Acupuncture is the stimulation of special points on the body, usually by the insertion of fine needles. Though originally developing in the context of traditional Chinese medical theories of yin/yang and the flow of Qi energy, many conventionally trained health professionals who practice acupuncture dispense with such traditional concepts. Instead, they view acupuncture points as corresponding to physiological and anatomical features such as trigger points or peripheral nerve junctions, and diagnoses are developed in purely conventional terms.

Table 2 Examples of CM use in conventional health care settings

Setting	Therapy	Provider	Comment
Pain clinics	Acupuncture	Doctors, physiotherapists, CM acupuncturists	Acupuncture thought to be of direct benefit for the treatment of chronic pain
Pain clinics	Hypnosis, relaxation therapies	Clinical psychologists, occupational therapists	Often integrated as part of a package of pain clinic care
Physiotherapy departments, rheumatology	Acupuncture	Physiotherapists, CM acupuncturists	Acupuncture thought to be of direct benefit for the treatment of chronic pain
Physiotherapy departments	Manipulative therapy	Physiotherapists	Physiotherapists learn techniques similar to those of osteopaths and chiropractors
Hospice/palliative care	Massage	CM practitioners, nurses	Massage provides relaxation and improves overall quality of life
Hospital inpatients	Music therapy, massage	CM practitioners	Used to improve mood, decrease feelings of isolation, and alleviate acute anxiety
Psychiatric care	Acupuncture	Doctors, CM practitioners	Widely used for the treatment of substance abuse
Psychiatric care	Massage	CM practitioners	Treat anxiety, improve levels of trust and communication between patients and care providers
Secondary care CM providers	Acupuncture, homeopathy, osteopathy, chiropractic	Doctors, CM practitioners	A number of specialist referrals, including NHS homeopathic hospitals, take referrals from primary care, typically for the treatment of refractory chronic conditions
Primary care	Acupuncture, homeopathy, hypnosis	General practitioners	Many GPs have learnt CM techniques and use these with selected cases
Primary care	Osteopathy, chiropractic	CM practitioners	Typically back and neck pain treated by referral from GP
Primary care	Relaxation, yoga, tai chi	CM practitioners, nurses	Often aimed at patients with mild psychological or chronic physical complaints for which further treatment options are limited
Primary care	Massage	CM practitioners, nurses	Often aimed at patients with mild psychological or chronic physical complaints for which further treatment options are limited

The most well-known indication for acupuncture is pain. There is evidence from randomized trials supporting the value of acupuncture for both acute pain, such as that following dental surgery[10] and chronic pain, such as headache.[11] There is also good evidence that acupuncture is effective for nausea and vomiting.[12,13] Acupuncture is probably not of benefit for smoking cessation,[14] tinnitus,[15] or weight control.[16]

Herbal medicine

Many modern medicines were originally extracted from plant sources: aspirin (from willow bark), quinine (from cinchona bark), and morphine (from the opium poppy) are obvious examples. Herbal medicine differs from conventional pharmaceutical therapy by use of whole plant extracts containing many constituent compounds, reliance on combinations of herbs, and, in some cases, use of unconventional diagnosis such as those based on traditional Chinese principles. Herbal medicine is typically used to treat chronic or recurrent conditions such as eczema, arthritis, fatigue disorders, asthma, migraine, dysmenorrhoea, or mood disorders.

There is good evidence from randomized trials supporting a number of individual herbal treatments including St John's wort for depression,[17] saw palmetto for benign prostatic hyperplasia,[18] ginkgo biloba for intermittent claudication,[19] and a fixed combination of several Chinese herbs for eczema.[20] Far fewer studies have examined herbalism as typically practised where herbs are given in combination and individualized to meet patient needs.

Homeopathy

Homeopaths treat disease using medicines administered according to the principle that 'like should be cured with like'. Practitioners select a drug that would, if given to a healthy volunteer, cause the presenting symptoms of the patient. For example, onions cause irritation to the nose and eyes; a homoeopathic medicine made from onion is, therefore, sometimes prescribed to patients with hay fever. Homeopathy is used to treat similar disorders as herbal medicine (see above). It is also used for some acute conditions such as infantile colic, respiratory infection, adult influenza, teething, and trauma.

Homeopathic medicines are prepared by serial dilution and succussion (shaking). Many are diluted to such a degree that not even a single molecule of the original solute is present. Perhaps surprisingly, there is good evidence from a meta-analysis of randomized controlled trials that homeopathic medicines can have effects different from placebo.[21] This evidence needs to be evaluated in the light of homeopathy's biological implausibility.[22]

Hypnosis

Hypnosis is the induction of a deeply relaxed and focused state, with increased suggestibility and suspension of critical faculties. Once in this state, sometimes called a hypnotic trance, patients are given therapeutic suggestions to encourage changes in behaviour or relief of symptoms. For example, hypnosis for a patient with arthritis might include a suggestion that the pain can be turned down like the volume of a radio.

Hypnosis is typically used to treat anxiety disorders, physical conditions with a strong psychological component (such as asthma and gastrointestinal disturbance), and conditions such as pain that can be modulated by levels of arousal.

Randomized trials support hypnosis for many of its most common indications including anxiety related to medical procedures,[23,24] nausea,[25] asthma,[26,27] irritable bowel syndrome,[28,29] and cancer pain.[23,30]

Relaxation therapies

A variety of different CM techniques are used to bring about relaxation. One commonly used technique is systematic muscle relaxation, in which patients are instructed to tense and relax major muscle groups in sequence. Meditation techniques use a more cognitive approach to relaxation by encouraging a conscious attempt to still the mind. Other relaxation therapies include yoga—postures, breathing exercises, and meditation aimed at improving mental and physical functioning—and tai chi, a series of slow and graceful movements that follow a set pattern. The therapeutic scope of relaxation therapies is broadly comparable to that of hypnosis as is the research base, though there is slightly better evidence for anxiety and perhaps less convincing data on pain.[31–33] Relaxation therapies are often used because they bring about a general feeling of well-being, rather than because they treat a specific symptom.

Osteopathy and chiropractic

Osteopathy and chiropractic are therapies of the musculoskeletal system: practitioners work with bones, muscles, and connective tissue, using their hands to diagnose and treat abnormalities of structure and function. The best known technique is the 'high-velocity thrust', a short, sharp motion usually applied to the spine. This manoeuvre is designed to release structures with a restricted range of movement. Practitioners also use a variety of soft-tissue and functional techniques. Many of the treatment methods used by osteopaths and chiropractors are similar to techniques used by those physiotherapists with additional training in manipulative therapy. From a general practitioner's perspective, there are few important practical differences between the three types of practitioner.

Though both osteopathy and chiropractic were originally regarded as complete systems of medicine, contemporary practitioners concentrate primarily on musculoskeletal disorders. There is considerable evidence from randomized controlled trials of the effectiveness of spinal manipulation for back and neck pain.[34–36] Although this evidence is largely positive, it has been criticized for failing to exclude non-specific effects of treatment.

Massage therapies

Therapeutic massage is the manipulation of the soft tissue of whole body areas to bring about generalized improvements in health, such as relaxation or improved sleep, or specific physical benefits, such as relief of muscular aches and pains. Some practitioners add oils derived from plants to the base massage oil that acts as a lubricant during treatment. This may be described as aromatherapy. Although often used purely for their smell, the oils are claimed, on sparse evidence,[37] to have a wide range of medicinal properties.

There is considerable randomized trial evidence that massage reduces anxiety scores, in the short term at least, in groups as varied as adolescent psychiatric patients,[38] intensive care unit patients,[39] elderly people in care homes,[40] and children suffering post-traumatic stress disorder.[41] In addition to treating anxiety (often described in terms of 'relief from stress'), practitioners also claim to bring about short-term improvements in conditions known to be exacerbated by arousal such as sleep disorders and pain. Feelings of general well-being are commonly reported after massage.

Other CM therapies

A wide variety of other techniques are sometimes described as CM. Some practitioners use unusual diagnostic techniques, such as iris diagnosis ('iridology'), muscle testing ('kinesiology'), and unconventional allergy tests, on the basis of which they prescribe dietary change and herbal medicines. Many of these tests have been shown to be unreliable in systematic research.[42–45] There is a wide spectrum of unconventional nutritional practices. Some of these are specific, well-researched, biochemically understood treatments, such as fish oil for rheumatoid arthritis.[46] Others are unresearched, biochemically implausible interventions popularized by spectacular claims in the lay press and largely used without professional supervision. An example is the Hay diet, the rationale for which is that starch and protein should not be eaten together is that each type of food requires a different pH for optimum digestion. A practice common to many CM nutritional methods is 'elimination dieting'. This is based on the principle that foods particular to each patient may contribute to chronic disease when eaten in normal quantities. Diagnosis consists of eliminating all but a few foods from the diet and then reintroducing foods one by one to see if they provoke symptoms. There is evidence from randomized trials for the effectiveness of this approach in conditions as varied as hyperactivity,[47] rheumatoid arthritis,[48] and migraine.[49]

Some CM therapies have been developed specifically to treat particular conditions, in particular, childhood disability[50] and cancer.[51] Most of these therapies are of highly doubtful efficacy. Serious concerns can be raised about the way in which they are marketed to vulnerable groups of patients.

Ensuring good practice

Which therapy for which condition?

One of the commonest dilemmas for practitioners and patients is the best choice of CM therapy for any particular health problem. In CM there is no one-to-one correspondence between specific diseases and treatments. Many therapies have broad and overlapping indications. For example, evidence shows that acupuncture can be beneficial in conditions as varied as nausea, and chronic pain and that pain can respond to treatments as varied as acupuncture, manipulation, and hypnosis. Data from the growing body of controlled trials and systematic reviews in CM can help make decisions more evidence-based, and a number of recent publications[52,53] and specialist databases (such as the Cochrane Library) help to make this information more accessible. But it is not always easy to apply even the best-quality research findings to individual situations. There is a wide variation in CM treatments given by different practitioners—even within a single discipline—and non-specific factors such as the therapeutic relationship between CM practitioner and patient often have a major influence on the experience, and probably the outcome, of treatment. Determining the right therapy for an individual patient, therefore, usually involves identifying the techniques for which there is the strongest evidence of benefit and selecting the one which has greatest congruence with the patient's health beliefs. Finding the right practitioner—one who is appropriately qualified and insured, and who can communicate well with the patient and the relevant conventional health care workers—is a prime consideration.

Safety of CM

In the minds of the public, CM is generally perceived as natural and therefore safe. The fact that many complementary practitioners are unregulated and many complementary medicines are freely available over the counter, only adds to this impression. In practice, although systematic data collection is extremely limited, most complementary disciplines appear to have a very low risk profile if delivered by experienced, appropriately trained practitioners (see, e.g. Yamashita et al's study of acupuncture[54]). However, it is also true that there have been a number of serious adverse events, including fatalities, related to the use of CM. The precise incidence is difficult to quantify, but many appear to be due to the ways in which CM has been used inappropriately, rather than specific effects of the CM treatment itself (see Table 3). The possibility of interactions between herbal medicines and conventional drugs is a particular concern.[55]

Other negative consequences that can sometimes occur as a result of CM use include: becoming dependent on CM practitioners; feelings of guilt when implicit messages of 'you can heal yourself if you really want to' fail to come true; denial and failure to accept or adjust to a prognosis because of unrealistic hopes from CM; and financial liabilities. Choosing a sensitive and experienced CM practitioner and maintaining a good relationship with other health care professionals, such as a GP or community nurse, reduces the risk of such occurrences.

Regulation of CM

The way that practitioners of CM are trained and regulated varies widely between different countries and between different states in countries like Canada and the United States. The situation ranges from no regulation at all, to statutory regulation where title and practice are protected by legal statute, in the same way as for medical practitioners. In any one country there is also a marked difference in regulation between different complementary disciplines, and sometimes even between different branches of the same, or very similar, complementary therapies (see Table 4). As CM becomes more widespread, regulation of practitioners and medicines is becoming more of an issue for governments across the developed world. In the United Kingdom, there have been official calls for the development of a single lead body which represents all practitioners of a given complementary discipline, even those with conventional health care qualifications such as doctors and nurses. Changes are occurring fastest in those disciplines that have the strongest internal organization (e.g. osteopathy, chiropractic, and acupuncture), or are under greatest threat as having the highest potential for causing harm (e.g. herbal medicine). State regulation of less invasive disciplines such as massage and relaxation is not considered as great a priority.

Table 3 Adverse effects from CM

Type of adverse event	Examples
Adverse events from stopping or avoiding beneficial medication (either patient-initiated or CM practitioner directed)	Seizures after sudden withdrawal of anticonvulsant, or acute asthma attack after sudden withdrawal of bronchodilators; potentially avoidable, serious infection after failure to immunize
Missed or delayed diagnosis	Malignancies or serious infections not treated/treated too late because patient uses CM and does not seeking conventional diagnosis and treatment
Interactions between conventional and complementary treatments	Reduced blood concentration of the HIV-1 protease inhibitor indinavir associated with use of St Johns Wort
Toxic reactions from wrongly labelled CM products	Toxic imported Chinese herbs wrongly identified and mistakenly labelled as therapeutic preparations; herbal or homeopathic preparations contaminated with steroids or other drugs
Disreputable/untrained/malpracticing practitioners	Hepatitis B spread by unregistered acupuncturist re-using unsterilized needles
Direct acute toxicity	Nephrotoxic combination of Chinese herbal products administered via unregistered private slimming clinic
Results of inappropriate long-term or excessive use of CM	Malnutrition in patients on strict nutritional exclusion diet, toxicity from overdose of vitamin or nutritional supplements
Rare but recognized sequelae	Stroke or spinal cord injury after cervical osteopathic or chiropractic manipulation, pneumothorax after acupuncture

Table 4 Different types of regulation of CM

Type of regulation	Examples
CM regulated as part of mainstream medicine	In the UK, homeopathy provided by specifically trained NHS doctors; in Germany, naturopathy provided by specifically trained doctors
CM practice illegal except by state registered health care professional	In the UK, osteopathy and chiropractic can only be practised by practitioners on the register of the General Osteopathic Council and General Chiropractic Council, respectively; in Germany, state registered Heilpraktiker are the only practitioners able to practise CM
Title protected by license	In 30 states of the USA, calling oneself a 'massage therapist' requires state licensure granted on satisfaction of certain fairly stringent qualifying criteria. In the other states, there are less formal requirements or no regulation at all
CM products have a limited license	In the UK, certain herbal products such as *Ephedra sineca* and *Lobelia inflata* are not on the general sales list and need to be dispensed by a doctor, pharmacist or herbalist (SI 2130 of the 1977 revision of the 1968 Medicines act)
Voluntary regulation with main lead body	In the UK, acupuncturists who are members of British Acupuncture Council
No uniform regulation across a discipline	In the UK, hypnotherapy, reflexology, nutritional therapy, massage
CM products regulated only in terms of health claims	In the USA, CM products can be sold as 'dietary health claims supplements' as long as there is no claim to cure specific symptoms or diseases

Communication between CM and conventional medicine

Doctors, particularly in primary care, have an important role in identifying patients who are using CM, minimizing their risk of harm and, as far as possible, in ensuring that their choice of treatment is in their best interests. The key is usually through maintaining good communication with patients, and sometimes with complementary practitioners.

First, a patient needs to feel safe in disclosing their CM use to their doctor. There is evidence that many patients fear a negative response and do not volunteer relevant information unless asked about it specifically and non-judgementally. Second, any discussion needs to be sensitive to the individual underlying reasons for seeking CM. Is the patient concerned about side-effects of conventional medication? Are there difficulties coming to terms with a new diagnosis? Expectations should also be explored—what is the patient hoping CM will provide? Once there is mutual trust and understanding, a primary care physician is in a position to offer helpful, evidence-based advice, suggestions on appropriate referrals, or simply the opportunity for regular review with impartial discussion and monitoring of progress.

Patients with chronic disease or on long-term medication who seek CM should be encouraged to find a complementary practitioner who is happy to liaise and cooperate with their GP. But even with goodwill between conventional and CM clinicians there are a number of barriers to effective communication between practitioners from different backgrounds. They may have different views of illness causation and treatment, and therefore effectively speak different health care 'languages'. They may be looking for different types of health care response, for example, a change in general well-being and emotional state, rather than a disappearance of specific symptoms. Underlying issues of power and control, and private versus NHS settings, may also make communication more difficult. Patients often have less difficulty reconciling these differences than the professionals involved. Written communication, multidisciplinary meetings, or conversations between practitioners involved with the same patient, which focus on the patient perspective, can help ensure a more integrated, and safe, approach to health care.

References

1. **Rees, L. and Weil, A.** (2001). Integrated medicine. *British Medical Journal* **322** (7279), 119–20.
2. **Harris, P. and Rees, R.** (2000). The prevalence of complementary and alternative medicine use among the general population: a systematic review of the literature. *Complementary Therapies in Medicine* **8** (2), 88–96.
3. **Eisenberg, D.M., Davis, R.B., Ettner, S.L., Appel, S., Wilkey, S., Van Rompay, M., and Kessler, R.C.** (1998). Trends in alternative medicine use in the United States, 1990–1997: results of a follow-up national survey. *Journal of the American Medical Association* **280**, 1569–75.
4. **Ernst, E. and White, A.** (2000). The BBC survey of complementary medicine use in the UK. *Complementary Therapies in Medicine* **8** (1), 32–6.
5. **Stevinson, C.** (2001). Why patients use complementary and alternative medicine. In *The Desktop Guide to Complementary and Alternative Medicine* (ed. E. Ernst, M.H. Pittler, C. Stevinson, A.R. White, and D. Eisenberg), pp. 395–403. London: Mosby.
6. **Boon, H., Stewart, M., Kennard, M.A., Gray, R., Sawka, C., Brown, J.B., McWilliam, C., Gavin, A., Baron, R.A., Aaron, D., and Haines Kamka, T.** (2000). Use of complementary/alternative medicine by breast cancer survivors in Ontario: prevalence and perceptions. *Journal of Clinical Oncology* **18** (13), 2515–21.
7. **Furnham, A. and Forey, J.** (1994). The attitudes, behaviors and beliefs of patients of conventional vs. complementary (alternative) medicine. *Journal of Clinical Psychology* **50** (3), 458–69.
8. **Astin, J.A.** (1998). Why patients use alternative medicine: results of a national study. *Journal of the American Medical Association* **279** (19), 1548–53.
9. **Thomas, K.J., Nicholl, J.P., and Fall, M.** (2001). Access to complementary medicine via general practice. *British Journal of General Practice* **51** (462), 25–30.
10. **Ernst, E. and Pittler, M.H.** (1998). The effectiveness of acupuncture in treating acute dental pain: a systematic review. *British Dental Journal* **184** (9), 443–7.
11. **Melchart, D., Linde, K., Fischer, P., White, A., Allais, G., Vickers, A., and Berman, B.** (1999). Acupuncture for recurrent headaches: a systematic review of randomized controlled trials. *Cephalalgia* **19** (9), 779–86.
12. **Lee, A. and Done, M.L.** (1999). The use of nonpharmacologic techniques to prevent postoperative nausea and vomiting: a meta-analysis. *Anesthesia and Analgesia* **88** (6), 1362–9.
13. **Vickers, A.J.** (1996). Can acupuncture have specific effects on health? A systematic review of acupuncture antiemesis trials. *Journal of the Royal Society of Medicine* **89** (6), 303–11.
14. **White, A.R., Rampes, H., and Ernst, E.** Acupuncture for smoking cessation (Cochrane Review). In *The Cochrane Library*. Oxford: Update Software, 2001.
15. **Park, J., White, A.R., and Ernst, E.** (2000). Efficacy of acupuncture as a treatment for tinnitus: a systematic review. *Archives of Otolaryngology—Head and Neck Surgery* **126** (4), 489–92.
16. **Ernst, E.** (1997). Acupuncture/acupressure for weight reduction? A systematic review. *Wiener Klinische Wochenschrift* **109** (2), 60–2.
17. **Linde, K. and Mulrow, C.D.** St John's wort for depression (Cochrane Review). In *The Cochrane Library*. Oxford: Update Software, 2000.

18. **Wilt, T.J., Ishani, A., Stark, G., MacDonald, R., Lau, J., and Mulrow, C.** (1998). Saw palmetto extracts for treatment of benign prostatic hyperplasia: a systematic review. *Journal of the American Medical Association* **280** (18), 1604–9.
19. **Moher, D., Pham, B., Ausejo, M., Saenz, A., Hood, S., and Barber, G.G.** (2000). Pharmacological management of intermittent claudication: a meta-analysis of randomised trials. *Drugs* **59** (5), 1057–70.
20. **Sheehan, M.P., Rustin, M.H., Atherton, D.J., Buckley, C., Harris, D.W., Brostoff, J., Ostlere, L., Dawson, A., and Harris, D.W.** (1992). Efficacy of traditional Chinese herbal therapy in adult atopic dermatitis. *Lancet* **340** (8810), 13–17.
21. **Linde, K., Clausius, N., Ramirez, G., Melchart, D., Eitel, F., Hedges, L.V., and Jonas, W.B.** (1997). Are the clinical effects of homeopathy placebo effects? A meta-analysis of placebo-controlled trials. *Lancet* **350** (9081), 834–43.
22. **Vickers, A.J.** (2000). Clinical trials of homeopathy and placebo: analysis of a scientific debate. *Journal of Alternative and Complementary Medicine* **6** (1), 49–56.
23. **Zeltzer, L. and LeBaron, S.** (1982). Hypnosis and nonhypnotic techniques for reduction of pain and anxiety during painful procedures in children and adolescents with cancer. *Journal of Pediatrics* **101** (6), 1032–5.
24. **Goldmann, L., Ogg, T.W., and Levey, A.B.** (1988). Hypnosis and daycase anaesthesia. A study to reduce pre-operative anxiety and intra-operative anaesthetic requirements. *Anaesthesia* **43** (6), 466–9.
25. **Jacknow, D.S., Tschann, J.M., Link, M.P., and Boyce, W.T.** (1994). Hypnosis in the prevention of chemotherapy-related nausea and vomiting in children: a prospective study. *Journal of Developmental & Behavioral Pediatrics* **15** (4), 258–64.
26. **Ewer, T.C. and Stewart, D.E.** (1986). Improvement in bronchial hyper-responsiveness in patients with moderate asthma after treatment with a hypnotic technique: a randomised controlled trial. *BMJ Clinical Research Edition* **293** (6555), 1129–32.
27. **Anonymous** (1968). Hypnosis for asthma—a controlled trial. A report to the Research Committee of the British Tuberculosis Association. *British Medical Journal* **4** (623), 71–6.
28. **Whorwell, P.J., Prior, A., and Faragher, E.B.** (1984). Controlled trial of hypnotherapy in the treatment of severe refractory irritable-bowel syndrome. *Lancet* **2** (8414), 1232–4.
29. **Harvey, R.F., Hinton, R.A., Gunary, R.M., and Barry, R.E.** (1989). Individual and group hypnotherapy in treatment of refractory irritable bowel syndrome. *Lancet* **1** (8635), 424–5.
30. **Spiegel, D. and Bloom, J.R.** (1983). Group therapy and hypnosis reduce metastatic breast carcinoma pain. *Psychosomatic Medicine* **45** (4), 333–9.
31. **Anonymous** (1996). Integration of behavioral and relaxation approaches into the treatment of chronic pain and insomnia. NIH Technology Assessment Panel on Integration of Behavioral and Relaxation Approaches into the Treatment of Chronic Pain and Insomnia. *Journal of the American Medical Association* **276** (4), 313–18.
32. **Seers, K. and Carroll, D.** (1998). Relaxation techniques for acute pain management: a systematic review. *Journal of Advanced Nursing* **27** (3), 466–75.
33. **Eppley, K.R., Abrams, A.I., and Shear, J.** (1989). Differential effects of relaxation techniques on trait anxiety: a meta-analysis. *Journal of Clinical Psychology* **45** (6), 957–74.
34. **Meade, T.W., Dyer, S., Browne, W., and Frank, A.O.** (1995). Randomised comparison of chiropractic and hospital outpatient management for low back pain: results from extended follow up. *British Medical Journal* **311** (7001), 349–51.
35. **Koes, B.W., Assendelft, W.J., van der Heijen, G.J.M.G., Bouter, L.M., and Knipschild, P.G.** (1991). Spinal manipulation and mobilisation for back and neck pain: a blinded review. *British Medical Journal* **303**, 1298–303.
36. **Shekelle, P.G., Adams, A.H., Chassin, M.R., Hurwitz, E.L., and Brook, R.H.** (1992). Spinal manipulation for low-back pain. *Annals of Internal Medicine* **117** (7), 590–8.
37. **Vickers, A.** *Massage and Aromatherapy: a Guide for Health Professionals.* London: Chapman and Hall, 1996.
38. **Field, T., Morrow, C., Valdeon, C., Larson, S., Kuhn, C., and Schanberg, S.** (1992). Massage reduces anxiety in child and adolescent psychiatric patients. *Journal of the American Academy of Child & Adolescent Psychiatry* **31** (1), 125–31.
39. **Stevensen, C.** (1994). The psychophysiological effects of aromatherapy massage following cardiac surgery. *Complementary Therapies in Medicine* **2** (1), 27–35.
40. **Fraser, J. and Kerr, J.R.** (1996). Psychophysiological effects of back massage on elderly institutionalized patients. *Journal of Advanced Nursing* **18** (2), 238–45.
41. **Field, T., Seligman, S., Scafidi, F., and Schanberg, S.** (1996). Alleviating posttraumatic stress in children following Hurricane Andrew. *Journal of Applied Developmental Psychology* **17** (1), 37–50.
42. **Lewith, G.T., Kenyon, J.N., Broomfield, J., Prescott, P., Goddard, J., and Holgate, S.T.** (2001). Is electrodermal testing as effective as skin prick tests for diagnosing allergies? A double blind, randomised block design study. *British Medical Journal* **322** (7279), 131–4.
43. **Sethi, T.J., Lessof, M.H., Kemeny, D.M., Lambourn, E., Tobin, S., and Bradley, A.** (1987). How reliable are commercial allergy tests? *Lancet* **1** (8524), 92–4.
44. **Kenney, J.J., Clemens, R., and Forsythe, K.D.** (1988). Applied kinesiology unreliable for assessing nutrient status. *Journal of the American Dietetic Association* **88** (6), 698–704.
45. **Knipschild, P.** (1988). Looking for gall bladder disease in the patient's iris. *British Medical Journal* **297** (6663), 1578–81.
46. **Fortin, P.R., Lew, R.A., Liang, M.H., Wright, E.A., Beckett, L.A., Chalmers, T.C., and Sperling, R.I.** (1995). Validation of a meta-analysis: the effects of fish oil in rheumatoid arthritis. *Journal of Clinical Epidemiology* **48** (11), 1379–90.
47. **Schmidt, M.H., Mocks, P., Lay, B., Eisert, H.G., Fojkar, R., Fritz Sigmund, D., Marcus, A., and Musaeus, B.** (1997). Does oligoantigenic diet influence hyperactive/conduct-disordered children—a controlled trial. *European Child & Adolescent Psychiatry* **6**, 88–95.
48. **Darlington, L.G., Ramsey, N.W., and Mansfield, J.R.** (1986). Placebo-controlled, blind study of dietary manipulation therapy in rheumatoid arthritis. *Lancet* **1** (8475), 236–8.
49. **Egger, J., Carter, C.M., Wilson, J., Turner, M.W., and Soothill, J.F.** (1983). Is migraine food allergy? A double-blind controlled trial of oligoantigenic diet treatment. *Lancet* **2** (8355), 865–9.
50. **Vickers, A.** *Health Options: Complementary Therapies for Cerebral Palsy and Related Conditions.* Shaftersbury: Element, 1994.
51. **Vickers, A.J. and Cassileth, B.R.** (2001). A review of unconventional therapies used for treatment of cancer and cancer-related symptoms. *Lancet Oncology* **2**, 226–32.
52. **Ernst, E., Pittler, M.H., Stevinson, C., White, A.R., and Eisenberg, D.** *The Desktop Guide to Complementary and Alternative Medicine.* London: Mosby, 2001.
53. **Zollman, C.E. and Vickers, A.J.** *ABC of Complementary Medicine.* London: BMJ Publishing, 2000.
54. **Yamashita, H., Tsukayama, H., Tanno, Y., and Nishijo, K.** (1999). Adverse events in acupuncture and moxibustion treatment: a six-year survey at a national clinic in Japan. *Journal of Alternative and Complementary Medicine* **5** (3), 229–36.
55. **Miller, L.G.** (1998). Herbal medicinals: selected clinical considerations focusing on known or potential drug–herb interactions. *Archives of Internal Medicine* **158** (20), 2200–11.

7.8 Terminal and palliative care

Irene J. Higginson, Polly Edmonds, Paola Viterbori, Massimo Costantini, and Sarah Cox

Introduction

Throughout the world the nature of illness is changing. Infectious and congenital diseases are more effectively treated, people live to older ages and die later in life following chronic or progressive, rather than acute, illnesses. Thus, palliative and terminal care are of increasing significance. Much can be done for patients whose disease is progressive, to control symptoms, to improve the quality of remaining life, the quality of dying and to support patients and their family. Controlling symptoms and improving the quality of life for patients, even at the end of life, can enhance their existence, and in some instances may extend it.(1) Patients regard this as important in many countries.(2)

When does palliative or terminal care start: rectangles or triangles?

Common definitions are shown in Table 1, and Fig. 1 illustrates two visions of palliative care. In the rectangle, as Fox(3) calls it, palliative care begins only when attempts at cure have been abandoned. But in the triangle, palliative care merges seamlessly with attempts at cure. The World Health Organization definition of palliative care was extended with: 'Many aspects of palliative care are also applicable earlier in the course of the illness, in conjunction with anti-disease curative treatment'. However, in some countries, this approach is difficult. For example, in the United States, entry to hospice care is determined by prognosis and Medicare reimbursement is not available unless patients are predicted to have a prognosis of less than 6 months.

However, not everyone could or should be cared for by a specialist service. Three levels of care are proposed:

- the palliative care approach employed ideally by every doctor and nurse;
- palliative care procedures and techniques (important adjuncts to care that are undertaken by relevant specialists); and
- specialist palliative care—where doctors, nurses and other clinicians are specially trained.

As Fig. 1 indicates, terminal care continues from and is part of good palliative care. The trajectory towards dying can vary: a patient may appear reasonably stable and then deteriorate, but then become stable again (see Chapter 17.1).

Table 1 Definitions of palliative and terminal care

Origins of terms

A *Pallium*, in ancient times, was a rectangular woollen cloak draped over the left shoulder and body. From the word *pallium*, Latin derived *palliare* 'to cover, cloak or protect'

Hospice comes from the same Latin root as words such as 'hotel', 'hostel', and 'hospital', and during medieval times 'hospice' was a place of shelter for travellers

Initially, palliative care services were called hospices. However, in French the term hospice can be used to describe a hospital. For this reason, the term *palliative care* has gained precedence over the term 'hospice'

Definitions today

The World Health Organization definition of palliative care is: the 'active total care of patients whose disease is not responsive to curative treatment'

The terms total and active are important—they indicate a holistic approach, alleviating symptoms, physical, emotional, social, and spiritual concerns, and an active approach, where patients and their families are skilfully assessed, problems are anticipated, and solutions are actively sought using appropriate therapies

Terminal care occurs when the patient's condition suggests that it is extremely likely that death will occur within a matter of days

Specialist services providing palliative care include palliative care teams working in the community (including residential and nursing homes) and in hospitals, and hospices, either inpatient or with home care programmes, such as in the United States

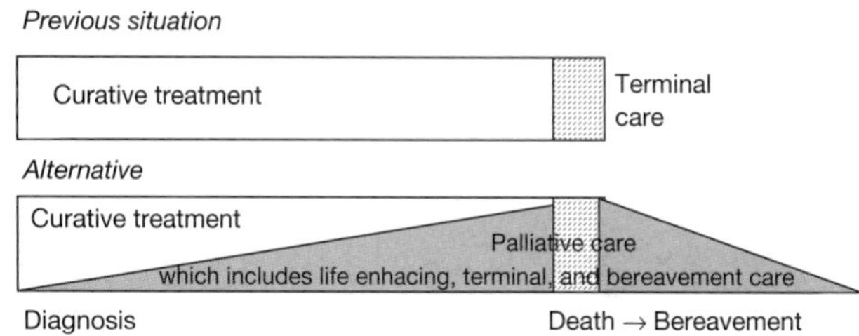

Fig. 1 Models of palliative and terminal care.

Specialist palliative care services

Hospices and specialist palliative care services have increased rapidly in number world-wide. In 2001, there were approximately 3000 hospice or palliative care services in the United States of America, 600 in Canada, over 1500 in 36 countries in Europe, and over 240 in Australasia. In the United Kingdom there were over 210 inpatient hospices, over 400 home care teams and over 260 palliative care teams working in hospitals.(4)

Palliative services and hospices have evolved differently in different countries, influenced by the different health care structures, training and funding mechanisms. In the United Kingdom, palliative care teams usually offer a shared model of care and here 60 per cent of cancer patients who die receive care from some kind of palliative care team or nurse, although non-cancer patients rarely receive this type of care. About 18 per cent of cancer deaths occur in hospices. In the United States, hospices are predominantly home care services, often led by nurses, with either a small number of beds or none. However, once involved, they often provide the whole package of care, including practical nursing in the home. The numbers of patients receiving hospice care varies greatly from state to state, although care among non-cancer patients is slightly more common. Hospital teams are rare and in early states of development.

Despite the difference in models, many of the approaches to care, such as multiprofessional practice, holistic care, pain and symptom control, and support for the patient and family are similar. A Cochrane meta-analysis of the effectiveness of specialist palliative care teams identified randomized controlled trials, comparative and observational studies. Most studies were from the United Kingdom and the United States although there were a few from other countries. The review showed a small significant benefit for patients cared for by a team in terms of improved pain and symptom control and satisfaction with care.(5) There was a trend indicating that patients maintained a higher level of quality of life if they were cared for by teams that had trained multiprofessional specialist staff rather than by 'teams' comprising one or more nurses. Thus, primary care services should ensure that they can access specialist palliative care services for their patients.

Education and research

In almost all countries of the globe, undergraduate medical training in palliative and terminal care is either completely absent or restricted to a brief series of lectures. Most physicians leave medical school unprepared by education or experience to satisfy the palliative or terminal needs of their patients or even how to get them help from other providers of care.[6] This situation is beginning to change, but it progress is slow and patchy. In the United Kingdom, the General Medical Council's recommendations for the training of doctors 'Tomorrow's Doctors' specially included requirements for training in care of the dying, symptom management, and communication. There are also needs for postgraduate education, including updates in practice, and multiprofessional Masters programmes.

Research into many important symptoms is urgently needed, as is work on the best service configurations and methods to support complex emotional and other needs. Too little is known about the nature of symptoms, physical, emotional, social, spiritual, and ethical concerns, how these interact and, most importantly, how problems can be alleviated. Although Palliative Medicine became a specialty within medicine in the United Kingdom in 1987, and this has helped to drive forward the knowledge and skills base, there is a lack of relevant funding and infrastructure for research. Much of the existing work has been on pain, and is based in inpatient rather than community settings. In the United States, projects such as the Project on Death in America and support from the Robert Wood Johnson Foundation, have begun to establish a foundation for research, although much development is still needed. Although these have been an important start, establishing good research in palliative care will be a major quality issue for the future.

Principles of clinical management

The family as the unit of care

Treating the patient and family as the unit of care is an essential element in palliative and terminal care. The term family is meant in its broad sense and encompasses those close to the patient, often a spouse, partner, children or siblings, and close friends who are significant for the patient. The concerns of the family or friends need to be heard and discussed, wherever care is. A systematic review of both descriptive, comparative studies and randomized trials affirmed this.[7]

Skilled assessment and review

Skilled, accurate, and appropriate assessment is essential in palliative and terminal care. However, measurement of pulse, blood pressure, temperature, and functional status are often inappropriate because they do not help to plan care. Appropriate assessment should emphasize pain and symptom control, the quality of life for the patient, fears and anxiety, psychological, social, and spiritual concerns, any future wishes, and the circumstances and needs of the family members or carers. This breadth of assessment requires a multiprofessional approach to care.

It is important to determine the likely cause of the symptom or problem, and to assess its significance to the patient and family to plan treatment. Many patients, particularly older patients, have multiple health problems. So determining which problem is most important and should be dealt with first becomes a priority.

Not all symptoms may be due to the main disease. Symptoms may be caused because of secondary effects of the illness (e.g. weakness or debility), because of side effects of treatment, or because of unrelated, concurrent illness. Good clinical assessment is necessary because in some instances it will affect the treatment used (see Chapter 17.2).

Aids to assessment

Clinical records are often helped by including a body chart on which pain and other symptoms are recorded at each visit. However, these are often charted only when patients are first seen, and re-assessment is missed. This can be improved by continued monitoring of key issues. Several suitable assessment systems are available and several of these have been tested in primary care and or nursing homes as well as in hospices. Examples of assessment systems in common use are: the Support Team Assessment Schedule (STAS), the Cambridge Palliative Assessment Scale (CAMPAS), Edmonton Symptom Assessment System (ESAS), and the Palliative Care Assessment (PACA), and the new Palliative Outcome Scale (Table 2).

Table 2 The Palliative Outcome Scale[8]

Each item is graded 0 (no problem) to 4 (most severe/overwhelming problem); considering the last 3 days	
Open question, patient describes two most important concerns and grades the severity of these	
A checklist then considers:	
Pain	Support
Other symptoms	Depression
Patient anxiety	Self-worth
Family anxiety	Wasted time
Information	Personal affairs

Epidemiology and interactions of symptoms and problems

Determining the prevalence of problems in palliative care, particularly in general practices, is made difficult because most of the studies rely on data collected in selected populations. However, some findings are consistent:

1. Pain, weakness (or asthenia, and associated cachexia), breathlessness, and constipation are all common symptoms, occurring in between 50 and 90 per cent of patients, that require management.
2. Symptoms are usually multiple, and interact with each other. For example depression may lead to anorexia, or exacerbate pain.
3. Symptoms also interact with emotional, social, and spiritual problems, so that pain can be exacerbated by worry, lack of information, fears, anxiety, or any unresolved matters.

The systems of comprehensive assessment, described above, allow analysis of the different and the potential interactions. The prevalence of different symptoms and problems are shown in Chapters 17.1, 17.2, and 17.6.

Management of pain and symptoms

It is beyond the scope of this chapter to give a detailed account of the management of pain and symptoms; Chapters 17.1 (on the dying patient), 17.2 (on pain), and 17.6 (on other symptoms) provide this. In addition, there are many well-researched text books[9–11] and excellent resources on the Internet,[12] which provide guidance on pain and symptom control. The sections below give general guidance for some common symptoms.

Pain

The aim of palliative care is to allow patients to be pain-free or for their pain to be sufficiently controlled that it does not interfere with their ability to function or detract from their quality of life. Pains can be multiple and can result from tumour involvement, anti-cancer treatments, arthritis, cardiovascular pain, musculoskeletal system, or many other causes (Chapter 17.2). Despite the many guidelines for appropriate pain management in cancer, many patients experience considerable pain and approximately half receive inadequate analgesia, in hospitals, the community and nursing homes, even when the symptom has been detected.[13]

Pharmacological treatment based on the regular use of oral opioids for moderate and severe pain results in excellent pain control in the majority of cancer patients (see Chapter 17.2). The World Health Organization analgesic ladder proposes non-opioid analgesics as the first step, followed by a mild opioid (step 2) or strong opioids (step 3) in patients with persistent pain (Chapter 17.2). Non-opioid drugs (including non-steroid anti-inflammatory drugs, or NSAIDs) are effective analgesics for patients with mild cancer pain and can be combined with opioids for moderate to severe pain. Oral morphine remains the opioid of choice, but other opioid agonists, such as hydromorphone and oxycodone, exhibit similar pharmacokinetic and pharmacodynamic properties.

Opioid analgesics may not completely control pain syndromes in some patients, particularly in instances of neuropathic pain. Co-analgesics such as tricyclic antidepressants[14,15] and antiepileptic drugs[16] can be used for neuropathic pain. In patients with bone pain, NSAIDS are often useful (see Chapter 17.2).

Because of the side effect of constipation, stool softeners and laxatives should be prescribed routinely. Sedation and nausea are frequent complications of initial opioid doses, but usually subside spontaneously upon continuation and are rarely a cause for halting analgesic treatment. There is no consistent evidence that one particular opioid agonist has significantly lower prevalence or intensity of sedation, nausea, or constipation compared to other opioid agonists, but individual patients may sometimes benefit from a change in the type of opioid (see Chapter 17.2).

Breathlessness

Breathlessness may become more severe in the last weeks of life, and is often difficult to control. It now may be the most prevalent severe symptom at the end of life.[17,18] It has many potential causes including: lung cancer or metastases, pleural effusion, pulmonary embolism, muscle weakness, anaemia, pneumonia, chronic heart failure, chronic obstructive pulmonary disease, and/or psychological distress.[19] The goal of treatment is to improve the subjective sensation as experienced by the patient, rather than to improve abnormalities in blood gas or pulmonary function. Specific causes—such as pulmonary embolism or pneumonia—should be treated if they are causing symptoms. General measures include ensuring that the patient is comfortable, providing information and discussion, and ensuring that the room is well ventilated. Other therapies can include low dose morphine, oxygen, bronchodilators and methylxanthines, corticosteroids, benzodiazepines, and other anxiolytics and physiotherapy. In some instances a fan is helpful.[20]

Cachexia–anorexia

This syndrome consists of progressive weight loss, lipolysis, loss of visceral and skeletal protein mass, and profound anorexia. Many patients experience this before dying of cancer, HIV/AIDS, and cardiac failure and, it is now believed in some cases, dementia. Recent research has demonstrated that cachexia occurs mostly as a result of major metabolic abnormalities including profound lipolysis and loss of skeletal and visceral proteins due to immune mediators such as tumour necrosis factor and interleukin-6, as well as tumour by-products including lipolytic hormone. In addition to general supportive measures, corticosteroids and progestogens may have beneficial effects on the symptoms of cachexia (omega-3 fatty acids, thalidomide, hydrazine sulphate, and other drugs are currently being tested).

Asthenia, weakness, and fatigue

This syndrome consists of profound tiredness upon usual or minimal efforts, accompanied by an unpleasant anticipatory sensation of generalized weakness. There are many possible causes, including those as for cachexia and anorexia, paraneoplastic syndromes, anaemia, chronic infections, treatment side effects, muscle wasting following prolonged lack of use, neurological disorders, lack of sleep, depression, and psychological problems. Whenever specific causes are identified, their correction will lead to improvement in asthenia. General non-pharmacologic measures such as adapting activities of daily living and occupational therapy will help match clinical function and symptom status with the expectation of patients and families. Consistent with the management of asthenia in chronic fatigue syndrome, in some instances gentle activity rather than rest can be helpful. Pharmacological measures are similar to cachexia.

Constipation

Constipation is common in progressive and terminal illness. Causes include: inactivity, weakness, dehydration, diminished food intake, low-fibre diet, and direct or indirect effects from cancer such as narrowing of the gut, hypercalcaemia or nerve damage. Constipation may also result as a side effect of medication, such as opioids, iron, anticonvulsants, diuretics, vincristine, or antimuscarinics, such as hyoscine. Management of constipation usually requires a combination of a softening agent and a stimulant laxative (except in cases of bowel obstruction).

Emotional responses to progressive and terminal illness

Emotional distress is a normal response to severe illness. It occurs at each transitional point of illness: diagnosis, beginning of treatment, recurrence, treatment failure, and disease progression. Normal responses to the stress of severe illness are characterized by a period of shock and disbelief, followed by confusion and possibly symptoms of anxiety and depression. An impairment of usual daily living, problems in concentrating and carrying out usual activities, and intrusive thoughts of the illness are present. These symptoms usually begin to diminish over several weeks with the support of family and friends or with limited medical care. The adaptive goals of patients with progressive and terminal illness are: managing insecurity and loss of control, mastering existential threats and preserving a meaningful quality of life.

When facing advanced, progressive, and terminal disease, all the range of psychological responses may be present, from little emotional reactions to major psychiatric disturbance. Loss of control is one of the most common and important problems experienced by patients with terminal illness and may lead to a sense of helplessness. Patients may use different strategies to cope with the loss of control such as struggling to maintain control through seeking treatments alternatives or concentrating on areas over which the patient can have control.

The way patients cope with the existential threat of illness depends upon:

- The disease-related determinants such as nature of illness, symptoms, treatments, and side effects.
- Individual variables such as premorbid adjustment, meaning attached to the illness, availability of social support, developmental stage in which cancer occurs, personality characteristics, and ways of coping.
- The social and cultural context.

Denial is often reported in progressive and terminal illness. Denial is a defence mechanism whose goal is to reduce unpleasant affects by disavowing some aspects of reality. Denial can fluctuate in the course of illness and, at some stages, can be an adaptive response which allows the patient to adjust slowly to the situation. Other common emotional responses can include: regression (becoming more child-like), rationalization (providing an alternative everyday explanation for symptoms or feelings), intellectualization (becoming theoretical, is often used by doctors and nurses in painful situations), projection (pushing the problem on to others), displacement (displacing emotional energy into other thoughts and activities), introjection (looking within oneself to find solutions), repression (unconscious suppression of painful memories), and withdrawal and avoidance (withdrawing from and consciously avoiding painful situations).

Recognizing these mechanisms can help staff deal with a patient's and their family's response to illness. The response will often be consistent with the individual's previous ways of coping, and it is often useful to find ways to support the patient within their method of coping and to encourage the more active coping mechanisms. Challenging their mechanism, especially in cases of denial, can be difficult. There is no evidence to suggest whether or not the patient and family would benefit from this.

Maladaptive coping occurs when any of these responses becomes extreme, for example excessive introspection can lead to guilt. Risk factors for maladaptive coping and concomitant psychological problems include: social isolation, low socio-economic status, drug or alcohol abuse, previous psychiatric history, recent losses, rigidity of coping, multiple obligations. Patients with these characteristics may need additional psychological support, for example early referral to a specialist palliative care team (see below) or if particularly at risk, referral to a psychologist or psychiatrist.

On the other hand, some aspects may facilitate adaptation to illness, particularly coping strategies that promote an active response are more effective than passive and helpless responses. Since coping with illness is a dynamic process which changes with the circumstances and the way the patient evaluates the meaning of his/her illness, individuals who are more flexible in responding to changing demands cope more effectively. Social support improves the ability to cope.

Psychiatric disorders

These are more common in patients with a progressive or terminal illness than in the general population. The Psychosocial Collaborative Oncology Group reported that half of the patients (53 per cent) were adjusting adequately to cancer. According to the DSM-III criteria, of the remaining patients, 68 per cent received a diagnosis of adjustment disorders, 13 per cent had a major depression, 8 per cent a organic mental disorder, 7 per cent a personality disorder, and 4 per cent an anxiety disorder. Full information on the management of these disorders are given elsewhere in this textbook; but in designing treatments it is important to choose ones which are likely to work within the remaining life span of the patient. Issues particular to palliative and terminal care are outlined below.

Depression

Different studies have found widely varied prevalence of depression in cancer patients, ranging 1.5–50 per cent. A higher prevalence is found in other advanced diseases, ranging from 23 to 53 per cent. Risk factors for the development of depression include: previous depressive episodes, uncontrolled pain, substance or alcohol abuse, advanced disease, physical impairment, pancreatic cancer, other medical conditions (such as metabolic or endocrinological abnormalities) or some drug treatments (such as steroids or some chemotherapeutic agents).

According to DSM criteria, diagnosis of major depression includes changes in appetite or weight, sleep and psychomotor activity, decreased energy, feelings of worthlessness or guilt, problems in concentrating, recurrent thoughts of death or suicidal ideation. In patients with progressive and terminal illness, somatic symptoms such as anorexia, insomnia, and fatigue may be unreliable signs since they mimic symptoms of the medical condition. Thus, the psychological symptoms of depression, such as hopelessness, guilt, worthlessness, suicidal ideation, helplessness, may be more useful when making a diagnosis. The Endicott Revised Criteria for depression in cancer patients, replaces somatic symptoms with non-somatic alternatives: tearfulness and depressed appearance, social withdrawal and decreased talkativeness, brooding, self-pity, pessimism, lack of reactivity.

Evaluation of the patient is important in determining the potential causes and appropriate management. In addition to assessing the psychological symptoms, as above, it should include:

- Determine whether a medical condition (e.g. hypothyroidism, multiple sclerosis) or medical treatment underlies the depressive syndrome. In this case it may be possible to treat the medical condition directly or change the treatment.
- Evaluate the level of distress and impairment in functioning, that is, how much the depression is affecting the patient and family.
- The transitional point of illness, emotional distress is normal at transitional or crisis points of the illness, and should be distinguished from a continuing depression, as it is likely to respond to increased support and perhaps help in developing appropriate coping strategies.

Anxiety

The prevalence of anxiety in cancer patients ranges from 1 to 44 per cent; as for depression prevalence increases in progressive illness. Risk factors for the development of anxiety include: previous anxiety disorders and pre-morbid adjustment and medical conditions (such as metabolic or endocrinological abnormalities).

Pathological anxiety is characterized by apprehension and worry, and associated anxiety symptoms such as restlessness and feeling keyed up or on edge, difficulty in concentrating, irritability, sleep disturbance, being easily fatigued. Somatic symptoms of autonomic hyperactivity (e.g. shortness of breath, palpitations, dry mouth, diarrhoea) are present. As for depression, the diagnosis of anxiety disorders in medically ill patients is problematic since somatic symptoms of anxiety may be identical to the characteristics signs and symptoms of the medical condition.

Anxiety symptoms may contribute to physical disability and exacerbate cancer symptoms: loss of appetite, fatigue, and pain may worsen with anxiety.

Communication and information

Effective palliative and terminal care are impossible without effective communication, but as Chapter 5.3 discusses in detail, there are many barriers to good communication. Specific general problems in palliative and terminal care include: the general denial of death and dying in contemporary society making this a difficult issue to raise and a lack of experience of death in the family—most adults have not witnessed a previous death. In addition, patients and their families often have fears which they are scared to raise. Professionals have fears about being blamed, about dealing with areas in which they have not been taught, about admitting they do not know, for example, the prognosis, and about expressing emotions. A doctor or nurse may have fears about their own illness or death.

Listening skills, including sitting down, ensuring that patients are comfortable and asking sufficient open questions (see Chapter 5.3), are crucial in palliative care where treatment priorities, the need for information and wishes are highly individual. Specific communication issues in palliative and terminal care are shown in Table 3.

Communicating with the family and with other professionals

In palliative care, the patient and their family or those important to them are regarded as the unit of care. However, this does not mean that carers should be given information before patients; and professionals need to follow the patient's wishes. The fears, anxieties and concerns of the carer can to be explored and their more intimate knowledge of the person drawn out. Asking 'what would worry you particularly about her knowing?' gives an opportunity for this and shows that the listener values the family's opinions. It may also be helpful to discuss with the family the strain that the situation is placing on them and ways in which services and the professionals may help.

Table 3 Specific communication issues in palliative care

Breaking bad news
Therapeutic dialogue
Starting and withdrawing or withholding treatments
Dealing with uncertainty
Planning to live and planning to die
Communicating with the family
Communicating with other health professionals

One of the common concerns of patients in hospitals and in the community is that of receiving mixed messages from different professionals. It is important that all of the team involved in the care of the patient and family are kept fully informed of the important decisions and wishes of the patient and their family or carer. If people are at home and different services are visiting, the carer or patient can sometimes feel that they have a full time job coordinating which services arrive when. It is important in these instances to identify a key worker for that patient and family who helps to take on some of the role of coordination and advocacy—so that the patient and the carer receive the services and benefits to which they are entitled. Similarly, in hospitals patients and carers may ask for information from different nurses—depending on who is with the patient at one time. There may also be different teams involved. This may be particularly likely with palliative care patients—who may be seeing members of the hospital palliative care team as well as their own doctors. When the circumstances and condition of the patient changes rapidly it is especially important that all the team is kept rapidly informed of relevant changes in the treatment plans or in the person's condition or wishes.

Ethical issues in palliative care

Withholding and withdrawing treatments

As treatments become more complex and patients and their families are faced with an increasing array of different options, the process of discussing treatment choices with patients and families is of growing importance. This is made more complex by the fact that many patients are ill and doctors and nurses themselves often feel that it is important that they offer a positive outlook on treatment options—in some instances so that they can maximize the potential benefits of any placebo effect. One first important principle in discussing starting or withdrawing treatments with patients and families is to determine the extent to which patients themselves wish for full information and to make decisions, or where they wish either family members or professionals to make those for them. Individual wishes vary but increasingly in our cultures, patients want a greater role in the process of decision-making. The second role of the doctor, having listened to the patient's wishes, is to try to explain the different treatment options and the potential trade off. It is important to try to avoid jargon and to explain things simply.

Dealing with uncertainty

This is a particular problem among patients with progressive non-cancer conditions, where it is often not clear how long the condition will last, or what the course of progression will be. Common uncertainties include how much treatment there is, its likely benefits, how long before death comes, what will the intervening period be like, and how will death come. Living with uncertainty often creates great anxiety and patients, their carers and professionals may feel the need for concrete statements on some of these issues. In the face of uncertainty, health professionals may think it best to say little, if anything, about the possibility of, for example, the patient dying suddenly or of treatment finishing. This ignores the knowledge patients have of their own bodies and the knowledge they, therefore, acquire about how well they are doing. There is limited evidence about effective strategies, but guidelines suggest that professionals should acknowledge their uncertainties and the difficulties this will cause. They propose a scheme of responses which checks if the enquirer would like to know what signs may herald further deterioration. They also encourage positive use of present time, show of willingness to monitor the situation regularly and a readiness to respond to any emergency. This gives the security of feeling that someone with more experience recognizes the problem and can be called on if there are particular worries or difficulties.

For some the strategy of 'hoping for the best and planning for the worst' is helpful. The approach is sometimes taken in cancer care of thinking with the patient or carer what the situation would be if the best happened and what they would need to consider if the worst happens may be helpful here, although further work is needed to understand its value in non-cancer care.

The family

How we perceive the family and those close to the patient is fundamental to their well-being, but their role has been confused and is ambiguous. The family is often cast in the role as providers of care and information, almost as extensions of the patient. However, the family is in the unique position of both providing and needing support. It is sometimes unclear who is 'the patient'.

Family members may be giving care, not giving care, or may be receiving nursing care themselves. There may be several different family members, with different and sometimes conflicting views and needs. Friends and neighbours are a small but considerable resource, and providers of support services need to ensure that they do not overlook those providing valuable community-based support.

The family is often involved in several complex tasks during the course of illness, although the role of the family varies between cultures and countries. Possible tasks include: provision of emotional support and containment, shared responsibility for decision-making, concrete care-giving, meeting financial and social costs, maintaining stability by filling in for the lost role, managing the demands and losses, meeting the emotional needs of other family members, continuing to perform usual family functions, adapting to changing.

The concerns of family members in palliative care can be different to those in other circumstances. Their concerns include, a time limited illness, progressive loss, the management of disclosure and awareness of disease progression, the medicalization of the home, patchy specialist services, and bereavement support. Additional stress can be experienced by having to observe the disease progress or trying to enhance patient quality of life when prognosis is poor.

There has been a considerable growth of evidence of the needs of family members palliative care settings, demonstrating that these needs are wide-ranging and sometimes acute. Needs are both practical and psychological. These needs remain largely unmet; research has found that family members are overlooked by most health services, and even sometimes by specialist palliative care services.

Families at increased risk of poor psychosocial outcome often exhibit low levels of cohesiveness and high levels of conflict and show poor family relationships. They may be already suffering from poor health, have suffered multiple losses or be in deprived circumstances. Other risk factors in palliative and terminal care include: poor function of the patient and having to provide extensive practical care, younger age, and pre-existing illness in the carer.

Two main types of intervention have been developed to support the family: (i) providing extra practical services and respite care, such as hospice at home, home nursing services, day care, respite admission; and (ii) proving emotional and psychological support to assist coping through one-to-one counselling, support groups, or drop-in centres. Families also have urgent needs for information and guidance if they are to provide care; a need often overlooked. Although there is an abundance of research into the needs of family members, there is a dearth of information on the best mechanisms to support the family. Most reports of interventions are anecdotal or descriptive; and in palliative and terminal care there are no adequate trials of specific interventions to support the family.

Bereavement

Bereavement refers to the loss of a person. Grief describes the feeling resulting from loss at the time of the loss and afterwards. The reaction of grief is characterized by three aspects: the necessity to cry and search for the lost person; the necessity to repress crying or searching; and the necessity to review and modify internal models (see Chapter 17.3).

Key points

- Palliative care is a person-centred approach to care, concentrating on the alleviation of symptoms and emotional, social, and spiritual problems for patients and those close to them.
- Palliative and terminal care are of growing importance world-wide.
- Palliative care should begin early in care, and for many conditions, be a gradually increasing component of care until terminal care and ultimately death.
- Specialist palliative care services, such as inpatient units, hospices, and multiprofessional palliative care teams working in hospitals and at home, can work in collaboration with the primary care team to provide the extra support and expertise needed to care for patients with progressive conditions.
- This model of care is effective in improving care for patients and families.
- Principles of management include:
  - the patient and family being considered as the unit of care;
  - rigorous assessment, review, and anticipatory planning of care;
  - expert symptom management, recognizing the interaction of symptoms, and of symptoms with emotional, social, and spiritual concerns;
  - care of emotional, social, and spiritual needs;
  - excellent listening, communication, and giving of information;
  - attention to ethical considerations;
  - care for the family, including into bereavement.

References

1. **Hanratty, J.** *Palliative Care of the Terminally Ill.* Oxford: Radcliffe Medical Press, 1989.
2. **Higginson, I.J.** (1997). Palliative and terminal care. In *DHA Project: Research Programme. Epidemiologically-based Needs Assessment.* Series 2 (ed. A. Stevens and J. Raftery). Oxford: Radcliffe Medical Press.
3. **Fox, R.** (2001). From rectangles to triangles. *Journal of the Royal Society of Medicine* **94** (9), 427.
4. **Hospice Information Service, International Services** (http://www.hospice-information.co.uk/hospservices/hospservs.asp).
5. **Higginson, I.J., Finlay, I., Goodwin, D.M., Hood, K., Edwards, A.G., Cook, A.M., Douglas, H.-R., and Normand, C.E.** (2003). Is there evidence that palliative care teams alter end-of-life experiences of patients and their caregivers? *Journal of Pain and Symptom Management* **25**, 150–68.
6. **Foley, K. and Gelband, H.** *Improving Palliative Care for Cancer. Summary and Recommendations.* National Academy Press, 2001.
7. **Hearn, J. and Higginson, I.J.** (1998). Do specialist palliative care teams improve outcomes for cancer patients? A systematic literature review of the evidence. *Palliative Medicine* **12**, 317–32.
8. **Hearn, J. and Higginson, I.J.** on behalf of the Palliative Care Audit Project Advisory Group (1999). Development and validation of a core outcome measure for palliative care: the palliative care outcome scale. *Quality in Healthcare* **8**, 219–27.
9. **Doyle, D., Hanks, G.W.C., and MacDonald, N.**, ed. *Oxford Textbook of Palliative Medicine* 2nd edn. Oxford: Oxford University Press, 1998.
10. **Higginson, I.J. and Bruera, E.** (2002). Care of patients who are dying, and their families. In *Oxford Textbook of Oncology* 2nd edn. (ed. Souhami, R., Tannock, I., Hohenberger, P., and Horiot, J.-C.), pp. 1103–20. Oxford: Oxford University Press.
11. **Addington-Hall, J.A. and Higginson, I.J.**, ed. *Palliative Care in Non-malignant Disease.* Oxford: Oxford University Press, 2001.
12. **A particularly useful internet resource, *The Manual of Palliative Care* by Doyle, D. and Woodruff, R.**, available from the International Association of Hospice and Palliative Care, at http://www.hospicecare.com/IAHPC manual.html, 2001.
13. **Bernabei, R.** et al. (1998). Management of pain in elderly patients with cancer. *Journal of the American Medical Association* **279**, 1877–82.
14. **McQuay, H.J., Tramer, M., Nye, B.A., Carroll, D., Wiffen, P.J., and Moore, R.A.** (1996). A systematic review of antidepressants in neuropathic pain. *Pain* **68**, 217–27.
15. **McQuay, H.J. and Moore, R.A.** (1997). Antidepressants and chronic pain. *British Medical Journal* **314**, 763–4.
16. **McQuay, H., Carroll, D., Jadad, A.R., Wiffen, P., and Moore, A.** (1995). Anticonvulsant drugs for management of pain: a systematic review. *British Medical Journal* **311**, 1047–52.
17. **Higginson, I.J. and McCarthy, M.** (1989). Measuring symptoms in terminal cancer: are pain and dyspnoea controlled? *Journal of the Royal Society of Medicine* **82**, 264–7.
18. **Reuben, D.B. and Mor, V.** (1986). Dyspnea in terminally ill cancer patients. *Chest* **89**, 234–6.
19. **Simon, P.M.** et al. (1990). Distinguishable types of dyspnea in patients with shortness of breath. *American Review of Respiratory Disease* **142**, 1009–14.
20. **Schwartzstein, R.M.** et al. (1987). Cold facial stimulation reduces breathlessness induced in normal subjects. *American Review of Respiratory Disease* **136**, 58.

8

Integrated management

8 Integrated management

8.1 Coordination and continuity of care

Wil J.H.M. van den Bosch and George K. Freeman

Introduction

The more complex and specialized medicine becomes, the more important is the role of the general practitioner (GP) as a coordinator. She/he is the health professional with the broadest view of the patient's health care problems in context. This includes family, work, and other social contexts, other primary health care workers, and specialist services in secondary care. Coordination of care is particularly relevant for patients with chronic multisystem problems. It, therefore, tends to be given higher priority by older patients. It appears to be important for patient satisfaction.[1]

Coordination of care can take place for an individual patient but the GP has also the opportunity to coordinate care itself. The potential for GP coordination of health care varies in different parts of the world. There is a difference between countries with a strong GP-structure such as the United Kingdom and the Netherlands and in developing countries where there has to be a great emphasis on basic medical care. In this chapter, we address the state of the art in coordination of care with an emphasis on continuity of care. We will concentrate on the coordination of care within general practice/primary care; the coordination of care between primary and secondary care and details of continuity of care are dealt with in other chapters.

Coordination of care and continuity of care

These concepts are closely related. Coordination of care is often assisted by elements of continuity of care. The ideal is that patients experience their medical care as continuous (sometimes termed 'seamless', without visible interruptions). This means that various elements of care link together well and that there are no problems in transition from one episode to the next or in various providers of care working together.

Continuity of care is a broad concept and has been described as 'not an entity but a relational idea'.[2] Several of its elements are important for coordination of care in general practice:

- The most basic level is availability of relevant information for health care. The medical record itself is an important tool for continuity of *information*. This aids coordination by reducing conflict and duplication of tests and treatments. Usually, a medical record of all the patient's medical problems is held in general practice. But information, though important, is not sufficient in itself. No written record, either paper or electronic, can capture all aspects of care coordination between professionals.
- *Cross-boundary* continuity concerns coordination of a patient's care between specialists and across institutions and involves direct mechanisms and communications to supplement shared records. These communications may be spoken or may be written commentaries or explanations to supplement records. They may be used to modify protocols or guidelines for the best individual care in negotiation with the patient.
- Traditionally, in a small stable community, a patient would receive nearly all their care from the same GP. This *longitudinal continuity*, where all or most contacts are with the same professional has been said to be an essential feature of general practice, but societal and professional change is rapidly reducing it. Patients move more often and feel less dependent on one physician. Professionals, including GPs, work in larger groups with a tendency to specialize and to share workload. It is thus difficult for care to be confined to one GP. Longitudinal continuity in a typical British practice with five GP partners and some doctors in training might be quite low with a mean of less than half of the consultations being with one doctor, a higher proportion in the case of older patients, and a relatively low proportion for young children who often want to see the first available doctor quickly.[3]

Rather than insisting that all contacts should be with one doctor, it is more important that a patient has a constructive therapeutic relationship with at least one doctor (or other professional).[4,5] This is *interpersonal continuity* or continuity of *relationship*. It is not necessary to consult the same professional each time though obviously some contacts are needed to establish and then maintain a trusting therapeutic relationship. This person is likely to have a major role in care coordination because the patient will tend to consult her/him about major medical decisions, including referrals to specialists. Recently, Donaldson has shown how agency theory can be applied to elucidate what is happening in continuity of care. She proposes that a patient needs a trustworthy agent and will gain by building a relationship with that agent to ensure that the agent (here the GP) will indeed work maximally for the patient's own interest.[6]

Coordination of care in general practice/primary care

Patients often have more than one problem and even a single problem can need care from different sources. The GP typically coordinates these elements of medical care including care delivered by medical specialists, primary care colleagues, and non-medical carers including social workers and voluntary workers. He/she may do this in person or by leading or participating in a team which does it. Coordination does not just happen, it requires teamwork and investment of time and resources. Teamwork and coordination are enhanced by *care protocols and critical pathways*, which help members of the team to support each other's care. Regular *team meetings* are essential and these should include both the inner practice team (nurses, doctors, receptionists, and manager) and also the wider primary care team (health visitor, midwife, physiotherapist, social worker, psychiatric nurse, school nurse, dietician, and chiropodist). Continuity and coordination within primary care is enhanced by direct connections between health providers and by a limitation of the number of health providers of a certain discipline involved. Ideally, there is a team of primary care workers, working closely together, knowing each other well, and having easy access to one another. We will discuss the structure of the coordination of care followed by a number of examples of special categories of patients.

Structure

Practice organization

Primary care workers may work within small private practices run by themselves or they can work within bigger structures where others define policies concerning collaboration and coordination. For a GP working in the centre of primary care, the quality of communication is related to the number of primary care workers involved in a certain discipline. In small teams, frequent personal contacts can be a good basis for optimal collaboration. In teams with many different workers there should be a greater emphasis on structured arrangements, protocols, and keeping records of these arrangements. In times where there is a greater chance of discontinuity, continuity of care within the whole team may be more feasible than continuity on a day-to-day basis provided by one doctor. A policy of personal continuity without commitment from all members of the primary care team is not possible. For optimal continuity and coordination of care, the members of the primary care team involved must share the same vision. They have to know each other's competencies, ideas, and potential. There has to be an agreement in the tuning of activities between primary care workers so that all their efforts have the best results. This means respect even more than knowledge.

Reimbursement

A condition for optimal coordination in primary care is a supportive reimbursement system. An adequate system has to stimulate workers to offer high quality care, to discourage activities that are more focused on the worker's income than on the patient's well-being, and must not deter or inhibit the work of other primary care colleagues.

There is some evidence that financial incentives can support coordination of care.[7] These apply both within primary care and to the collaboration between primary and secondary care. Comparable levels of reimbursement are very important in order to avoid envy and bad feeling.[8] Although important, the quality of primary care delivery nevertheless appears to be less dependent on the payment system than on the maintenance of a good patient–physician relationship.[9]

Leadership and the core primary care team

Working in a primary care team in a discrete community, for example, a village or a small area in a town, offers advantages. Where this is not already in place, it may help to set up such small areas for local coordination and cooperation. GPs often initiate these arrangements. The core primary care team consists of general practice, home care, and perhaps social services, depending on national or local policy. The team can also include physiotherapists, speech therapists, midwives, and pharmacists. It is difficult to give an international overview of all the possibilities because there is much variety. In some countries, patients have free access to all members of the primary care team while in others the GP acts as the gate keeper. In most cases, however, leadership will be assigned first and foremost to the GP. This demands specific leadership skills.

Coordination of care is not always the task of the GP alone. Some aspects of coordination can be assigned to practice managers. There is also increasing experience with coordination of care by nurses, especially in the care of the elderly, for patients with chronic diseases, and for patients in need of palliative and terminal care. These nurses can work as the practice nurse in a health centre but can also work in home care or community nursing organizations.[10]

Coordination of prevention and other services

Preventive care and primary care are distinct parts of the health care system in some countries, in others they are strongly related. Primary care, however, has always been a mix of these two ways of thinking. In a well-organized primary care system preventive care can flourish. This demands optimal coordination. High levels of coordination of care are associated with patients being more up to date on screening, immunization, and other preventive activities.[11]

Coordination of care within primary care also can include communication and collaboration with other services and providers outside of the core primary care team, for instance, with schools, social services, municipalities, services related to labour, child protection, police and judiciary organizations, and many others. There is a variable and often ambivalent relationship with people working outside medicine. In most cases, there is relatively little communication and coordination of care between GPs and alternative practitioners.[12]

Communication

Communication between primary care members in some cases is only a result of an initiative of one of the health providers to another. Sometimes, there is more structured contact resulting in regular meetings. A further step is organizing multidisciplinary meetings.

Continuity and coordination of care is also helped by adequate opportunities for communication. Recently, the possibilities for electronic communication have been rapidly increasing. Electronic communication networks for exchanging consultation outcomes significantly increase the completeness of information about the care that patients are receiving.[13]

GPs now have to choose whether they will develop electronic record keeping in their practice only, whether they set up collaborative record keeping across primary care or whether they cross the boundary into secondary care and share these developments with hospitals. As health care becomes more complex, interest in the benefits of coordination of care has increased. Patients who are being treated jointly by more than one physician are especially vulnerable to adverse effects resulting from inadequate coordination and communication. One of the options to improve quality of care is the use of computer-based patient records in a central database.[14]

Good coordination not only includes communication of patient data but also forces health providers to think about mutual goals, about criteria, and about setting quality standards for care between providers. With a primary care based information system there is more scope to share data about chronically ill patients within multidisciplinary care teams, using an electronic data bank.[15] In summary, coordination is a hallmark of primary care. Efforts to improve primary care services should involve assessment of the extent to which coordination is achieved.[16]

Examples of coordination of care in special categories of patients

Children

For children there are often two different systems for the provision of primary health care. The curative one includes an important role for the GP, while the organized preventive one tends to be run separately by child health and/or public health specialists. In some countries, the GP is also involved in this preventive health care. There are regular consultations in well baby clinics or child health centres. Attention is given to nutrition, gaining weight, psychomotor development, parent–child interaction, and all kind of questions of the parents. Vaccinations are given according to national vaccination programmes. Doctors as well as nurses are involved in these activities. Special attention is given to descent of the testes in young boys, signs of deafness, dysplasia of the hips, and heart murmurs. When abnormalities are suspected the child is referred to the GP or to hospital care. Later in childhood one will look to mental development, signs of scoliosis of the spine, refraction problems, and growth problems. It is important that the two systems remain in optimal communication. In special cases, such as suspected sexual abuse, neglecting to communicate, share information, and to keep a consistent policy can lead to serious mistakes.

Women/maternity

Women generally consult with GPs more than men, partly because of maternity care and the medicalized nature of female contraception. Women have a vital parental role and coordinate the care of their children. Women are also more likely to be carers and so consult about those they are looking after. Thus, women have more opportunity to get to know their local practice both as patients and as carers. Just as GPs coordinate medical care, women tend to coordinate family care and so there is a natural alliance. However, while women might be expected to value a personal relationship with a GP more than men, the gender difference in preference for seeing the same doctor is less than expected.[17]

Care of childbirth itself was largely the responsibility of GPs and midwives in the community until very recently, most notably in the Netherlands.[18] Now, maternity care has become increasingly medicalized and institutionalized within hospitals. This has brought problems of incoordination and discontinuity between intrapartum care and ante- and post-natal care. As the GP's role in intrapartum care has reduced, coordination of obstetric issues with other medical aspects has been highlighted as a particular role for GPs. The GP provides a general medical context for the special life event of childbirth.[19,20]

In the last decade of the twentieth century, there was something of a concerted movement by women to reverse the medicalization process. This has been in alliance with midwives. At the same time midwives themselves (like doctors) no longer wish to offer the traditional '24/7' personal availability. This has led to shift working and team working. Sometimes, there has been a separate community team which the mother has to leave if she is admitted to hospital during labour, she then meets a new team of midwives. Even today many labours last more than one 8-h duty shift, so the mother is unable to get exclusive care from one midwife, let alone from the same one that has given preparatory antenatal care. Thus, mothers have had to be offered one of several models of less than total longitudinal continuity. One model is that the same team gives antenatal and intrapartum care and this team crosses the boundary between community and hospital. Even so the mother may meet an unfamiliar midwife for the first time during her labour. Another model keeps the mother to a small community team where she meets all members antenatally. It is difficult for such a small team to straddle the community specialist boundary.

In practice, much depends on other aspects of continuity such as cross-boundary communication. Antenatal care was one of the first specialties to introduce a shared patient-held record for continuity of information. A WHO Bulletin reports the success of such a record across 13 countries in varying stages of health service development, but warns that such a record needs careful introduction through a designated 'champion' who could be in primary care.[21] Considerable academic effort has been directed to showing that enhancing elements of continuity of maternity care improves outcomes.

The needs of older people

As already noted, older people are more likely to have chronic and multiple health care problems and they are known to be more likely to wait and see the same doctor in a group practice.[22] They seem to value relationships more and to feel secure seeing the same professional. This does not mean they are more assertive or more critical. On the contrary, they tend to be more satisfied and may be more willing to tolerate substandard care, perhaps because it meets their expectations. One study of how patients traded off aspects of the care of severe liver disease showed that older people were more likely to trade-off for a better process of care against possibly less good outcomes.[23]

Mental illness

The care of mental illness is a major challenge to GPs, both in the sense of primary mental health problems and in the psychological aspects of all problems. This is exemplified in the 'triple diagnosis' (medical, psychological, and social), which needs to be at least considered for every patient.[24]

Increasingly, depression and anxiety problems are managed entirely in primary care by GPs and their teams, which may include psychologists and counsellors. Counsellors and other mental health workers are increasingly attached to primary health care teams in spite of relatively scant evidence for their cost-effectiveness.[25] Counsellors are popular with patients and with many GPs. Their location within the practice makes communication and coordination of care easy.

Coordination of the care of severe mental illness (SMI) is more challenging. Most SMI, typically schizophrenia, bipolar mood disorder, and psychotic depression, is cared for by specialist mental health teams. Often, communication between secondary and primary care is poor and there is an additional boundary problem with social care. In a study in one of the author's (G.K.F.) own practice, where all known schizophrenic patients were interviewed and their care assessed, there was only a slight correlation between severity of disability and the number of agencies involved. There was wide variation in the frequency of contact between the patient and GPs, psychiatrists, community psychiatric nurses, and social workers. An additional problem was the relatively poor anticipatory physical care of these patients. No one was checking their weight and blood pressure and trying to persuade them to smoke less.[26] Thus, even in a practice where care of SMI is considered a general practice responsibility, the GPs were not co-ordinating care for these patients in an optimal manner. It may be difficult to improve coordination of care of patients with SMI more generally, as long as GPs have considerably differing views about clinical responsibility for these patients. Some GPs feel able to take primary responsibility and refer to specialist teams and social workers as necessary. More often GPs prefer to transfer this responsibility completely to specialists. Their role is then confined to the general medical care of the patients.[27] In spite of differences in attitude to SMI, most GPs are very aware of and comfortable with the complex blend of psychological with general medical problems in their patients. This means that mental health issues are not seen as so separate and 'untouchable' as they are too often in hospital care. The most important coordinating activity might be that which occurs within the consultation where doctor and patient negotiate understanding of the likely mechanisms of often complex problems.

Palliative care

Patients with cancer, AIDS, chronic progressive neurological diseases, and other diseases in need for palliative care often have less than optimal care at the end of their life. One of the most important problems is lack of coordination of care in situations where many different disciplines are involved. Because there is a trend to move care from hospital to primary care settings, a primary care coordinator has to have easy access to the skills of specialists and other providers of hospital care.[28–32]

GPs think their role in palliative care is important. They feel comfortable with their role as coordinator of care but there is dissatisfaction with the collaboration with secondary care providers.[33]

Current and future developments and their implications

Organization of lists—personal lists

GPs have particular opportunities for long-term coordination of care in countries such as the Netherlands and the United Kingdom where virtually all patients are registered with a named GP. This GP holds the patient's lifetime health record. Normally, all other medical care agencies communicate a letter or summary of their medical encounter to the GP for information and this is filed in the patient's record. When the patient moves to a new GP the record follows.

As practices gain more patients, due to population growth and/or professional success, the existing GPs take on new colleagues or partners. This is seldom easy to plan and practices tend to continue slowly with enlarging rather than to reach some planned limit. Organization within such a group practice varies. Most often a patient registered with a particular doctor is able to see any other doctor in the group without the formality of re-registering, this is called a *shared or combined* list system. Shared lists are an important way of offering free and informed choice of professional to patients. Such choice is informed because the patient can sample different doctors without actually committing themselves by formal registration. The result is that a majority of patients identify one or more personal doctors and this is not necessarily the one with whom they are registered.[34,35] The advantage of sharing workload can be added to that of choice. This helps patients by offering a quicker service and the professionals by evening out fluctuations in workload.

But there is one important downside, namely what Pereira Gray has called 'the collusion of anonymity'.[36] If patients are not tied to a particular doctor then it is not clear who is responsible for them. Sometimes the 'buck gets passed' and the need for an important clinical decision is allowed to drift. If the patient has no serious ongoing problems and consults for isolated minor episodes then being seen quickly by any suitably trained GP may suffice. But the patient may be suffering complex, sometimes ill-defined multiple problems where a strange doctor is at a professional disadvantage,[37] although to admit this and insist that the patient sees their usual doctor may cause delay and seem like laziness. Striking the right balance needs a well-formed group whose members trust each other. Unfortunately, such trust is not always optimal.

Some groups of GPs have been sufficiently concerned about the problems of shared lists to insist on a *personal list system* where the patient is only normally allowed to consult with their registered doctor. This can work well and can be popular with patients in spite of often leading to longer mean waiting times for an appointment (2 days rather than 1 day in one study[38]). However, the lack of choice carries paternalistic overtones that are increasingly at odds with evolving societal emphasis on patients' autonomy. Also, there is little evidence that forcing patients to see the same doctor, rather than allowing and encouraging them to do so, leads to better care.[39,40] So, although there is evidence that personal lists may offer something important,[41] it is a greater priority to make it easy for patients to get to know their doctors on a voluntary basis. There is a clear association between patients knowing their doctor well or very well and better enablement after a consultation.[42]

Threats of discontinuity in general practice

While continuity of care in the sense of interpersonal continuity (usually consulting with the personal doctor) is not essential for coordination of care, continuity of care in the sense of an integrated record system and continuity across professional boundaries is indeed essential. There are three main threats to this sort of continuity in general practice.

The first is increasing patient mobility. Every time a patient moves to a new practice there is some delay in transfer of paper records. In some communities some groups of patients stay in one place for a short time, either because of upward social mobility, or, more seriously, because of social instability with problems of social support, housing, employment, and money. This latter group of patients most needs a stable medical reference point and is often least likely to get it. This is another example of Julian Tudor Hart's 'inverse care law'.[43] A patient-held or patient-accessed electronic health record will be particularly helpful here.[44]

The second is poor management within large group practices where it may be difficult to identify who is coordinating a patient's care. This has been discussed under the heading of shared/personal lists (above).

Last comes an unfortunate new development from the United States. The problem *is forced discontinuity* where patients in certain health insurance schemes may be forced to sign on with a new practice each year because the Scheme is seeking the financially most advantageous deal.[45] Hopefully this will be temporary and only last until the adverse consequences are more widely appreciated.

Patients' expectations of coordination in general practice

Patients' expectations are largely governed by their prior experience.[46] However, this may be limited, particularly when the onset of more serious health problems increases the need beyond the patient's previous experience. Most practising GPs will be aware that patients may have very differing views on the overview available to an unfamiliar GP at an initial consultation. Whereas some patients will immediately launch into a detailed update of their medical history, others may either be surprised that the GP does not already have a full copy of their records available or, if these have arrived, that the GP has not already mastered this document in detail!

Expectations can be both individual and shared. Thus, in a stable long-established community there will be good general understanding of the GP's ability to coordinate care both within health boundaries and beyond to social care, housing, and police authorities. On the other hand, in a multiethnic less stable but often very dynamic community, perhaps with many immigrants, understanding of the GP's role in coordinating care may be limited and laced with serious misunderstanding. Longer consultations and good communication from all team members is essential to overcome this disadvantage.

Bypassing the GP: alternative access to primary care

There have always been alternatives to organized general practice. GPs have never held a monopoly even in places where their primary contact and gatekeeper role are institutionalized. Typically, there has always been direct access to hospitals through *accident and emergency departments* (A&E) (often bringing the complaint that such patients are neither 'accidents' nor 'emergencies' from the staff there[47]). In addition, in some large cities there is a long tradition of hospitals providing primary care to the poorer people in their neighbourhood through hospital dispensaries and outpatient departments.[48]

Now, there are an increasing number of alternative types of primary care. One is for A&E departments to 'make a virtue out of necessity' and actively cater for primary care patients, whether attending out of hours care or merely because access to their GP is inconvenient.[49] Here, a common response is to set up a *separate primary care unit within the A&E department* and set up an initial triage, usually staffed by nurses, to direct patients either to the traditional department or to the primary care unit. This logical development has had mixed success in the United Kingdom and communication and coordination with local GPs is not always optimal.[50] Since they do not always save money for the host department, some of the early initiatives have been discontinued.

The development with the most apparent potential to reduce coordination is *Walk-in clinics*. These have been introduced on both sides of the ocean. They are particularly suitable for patients seeking care near their workplace where this is inconveniently far from their home GP, for example, for employees in large cities who commute to work. While this category of users may find a convenient and useful alternative to attending an inner-city A&E department, walk-in centres are potentially useful for a large number of people who find that their own general practice is inaccessible. Such difficulty may be due to seeking care after normal working hours, or because young people, relatively unfamiliar with the process of negotiating access via GP receptionists, may prefer to wait in an anonymous walk-in centre. If they seek an appointment in their practice they risk being told their problem is non-urgent and they must wait several days to see a doctor or even a nurse. Immigrants may also find general practice intimidating.

Many GPs have been hostile to walk-in centres. At the same time, many do find it very difficult to offer quick access via their appointment systems.

Finally, there is *direct telephone access*, either to an out of hours cooperative (common in urban areas world-wide) or perhaps *to a comprehensive telephone advice service* available '24/7'. In the United Kingdom this is called NHS Direct. It is staffed entirely by specially trained nurses working from carefully designed protocols. Again, NHS Direct has had a mixed reception from general practice, being accused of giving inappropriate advice and of needlessly encouraging patients to seek inappropriate appointments. No balanced assessment of NHS Direct is yet available but, without waiting for this, a number of GP out of hours cooperative groups are already arranging that all emergency patient callers are encouraged to contact NHS Direct first as a method of triage.

Coordination with private-sector care

If most health care is delivered through the public sector then private-sector care is reserved for small numbers of patients who are relatively well off. They are usually buying privacy, additional time, and more scope for choosing their practitioner individually. Mechanisms for coordination between the public and private sectors tend to be weak in these countries and indeed the private sector is used as a form of opt-out from health system coordination. The burden of coordination is thus borne entirely by the patient. Often, if they become seriously ill they revert to the public sector.

In the United States, where private medicine is dominant, there are more formal mechanisms for coordination between health care providers but systems for cost re-imbursement between providers may bring perverse incentives for coordination. One example is the case of coordination of care of the mentally ill, where private-sector funding may encourage inpatient institutional care rather than community care coordinated through family doctors.[51]

Influence of payment systems on care delivery

Payments systems have been mentioned several times in this chapter. We have noted that differing payscales may discourage team work and also coordination across the primary/secondary care boundary. Some aspects of 'private medicine' may seem to work against care coordination, as in forced discontinuity and poor access to private inpatient mental health facilities. Another relevant aspect of payment is whether practitioners are directly reimbursed or are salaried. Salaries may be very useful (if generous enough) in encouraging well-qualified staff to work in deprived areas. In the United Kingdom, for example, GPs receive such enhanced payments based on numbers of their patients living in 'underprivileged areas'.[52] Salaries may be less good for encouraging practitioners to take responsibility for their patients' care, perhaps because there is less incentive for the practitioners to ensure that patients return to them personally. In a large sample of Norwegian GPs, Hjortdahl found that those paid by 'fee for service' were more likely to be accessible to their patients and more likely to offer emergency house calls than their salaried colleagues.[53] Thus, there is no perfect system, but all those involved need to be aware of the potential for payment systems to modify coordination of care.

International perspectives

The GP has a potentially important role in the coordination of care in any care system. Just how central this role depends on local history and tradition. At least three patterns can be described.

A GP for all patients who is the gate keeper for specialized care

The United Kingdom and the Netherlands are both in this group. The key feature is that all patients are registered with one (and only one) GP. Access to specialists is then on the recommendation of the GP. The GP is thus in a key position to coordinate all specialized care. Equally, if the patient does access specialized care directly then the specialist can be confident that the patient does indeed have a GP.

Well-funded health service with a highly developed specialist sector

Examples are the United States, where general practice nearly died out before being reborn as family practice, and France. Family practitioners have to share primary health care with internists, paediatricians, and gynaecologists and patients have direct access to any of these as well as to any specialist. The family physician's coordinating role is thus less securely built into the system. While they are very effective as patient advocates and care coordinators in particular in rural areas, they have to earn this role with each patient, and sometimes for each care episode, rather than accept it as a right and a duty. Patients in the United States are not registered unless this is part of an insurance plan such as a Health Maintenance Organization. On the other hand, family physicians often enjoy admitting rights to hospitals and thus have far greater opportunities for care coordination for iller patients than do their British or Dutch colleagues. The position is similar to some extent in other developed economies such as Germany and Sweden, though a registration system has been introduced in Norway and in some Swedish districts.

Countries of the former Soviet Union and its allies

Before 1990 these countries worked in a different tradition using a polyclinic system where the only generalists had very low status without significant clinical responsibility. In the ensuing decade these countries have all to some extent been attempting to introduce an enhanced system of primary care based around GPs. There have been no suitably trained local doctors, which has been a serious challenge because this specialty of all is particularly context dependent. There are now numerous programmes of educational development funded by bodies such as the World Bank. The unifying theme is the training of local GP leaders both at home and in 'donor' countries in the first two categories above. Here, the role of care coordinator is particularly hard to assume because existing teams of specialists have to learn about the GP role as well as the patients having to trust them. But these new general practice systems should be watched. Each one is an experiment in itself and an opportunity to show that there are many contrasting ways of coordinating care in general practice.

Conclusions

Coordination and continuity of care in general practice/primary care are important issues. Both care providers and patients emphasize that both belong to the core activities of general practice. But there are some major threats. Making teams of primary health care providers bigger, shifts from primary to hospital care, splitting daycare and out of hours care, and part-time working of the care providers may all generate discontinuity. Coordination of care transferred from small primary care teams to hospitals, insurance companies, or other bigger organizations also can have negative influences. On the other hand, ICT developments can improve the sharing of information and the communication between different care providers.

In the future, primary care needs to cope with the threats of discontinuity and adopt a shared mission that coordination and continuity of care are core items of general practice care. It is important to look over borders and to learn from experiences in other countries.

References

1. **Flocke, S.A.** (1997). Measuring attributes of primary care: development of a new instrument. *Journal of Family Practice* **45**, 64–74.
2. **Freeman, G., Shepperd, S., Robinson, I., Ehrich, K., and Richards, S.** *Continuity of Care: Report of a Scoping Exercise for the National Coordinating Centre*

for NHS Service Delivery and Organisation R&D (NHSCCSDO). London: NCCSDO, 2001. (http://www.sdo.lshtm.ac.uk/continuity of care.htm)

3. **Freeman, G.K. and Richards, S.C.** (1990). How much personal care in four group practices? *British Medical Journal* **301**, 1028–30.
4. **Kearley, K.E., Freeman, G.K., and Heath, A.** (2001). An exploration of the value of the personal doctor–patient relationship in general practice. *British Journal of General Practice* **51**, 712–18.
5. **Freeman, G. and Hjortdahl, P.** (1997). What future for continuity of care in general practice? *British Medical Journal* **314**, 1870–3.
6. **Donaldson, M.S.** (2001). Continuity of care: a reconceptualisation. *Medical Care Research and Review* **58**, 255–90.
7. **Goldberg, R.J.** (1999). Financial incentives influencing the integration of mental health care and primary care. *Psychiatric Services* **50**, 1071–5.
8. **Boult, C. and Pacala, J.T.** (1999). Integrating healthcare for older populations. *American Journal of Management and Care* **5**, 45–52.
9. **Flocke, S.A., Stange, K.C., and Zyzanski, S.J.** (1997). The impact of insurance type and forced discontinuity on the delivery of primary care. *Journal of Family Practice* **45**, 129–35.
10. **Waszynski, C.M., Murakami, W., and Lewis, M.** (2000). Community care management. Advanced practice nurses as care managers. *Care and Management Journal* **2**, 148–52.
11. **Flocke, S.A., Stange, K.C., and Zyzanski, S.J.** (1998). The association of attributes of primary care with the delivery of clinical preventive services. *Medical Care* **36**, 21–30.
12. **Mainous, A.G., Gill, J.M., Zoller, J.S., and Wolman, M.G.** (2000). Fragmentation of patient care between chiropractors and family physicians. *Archives of Family Medicine* **9**, 446–50.
13. **Branger, P.J.** et al. (1998). Shared care for diabetes: supporting communication between primary and secondary care. *Medinfo* **9**, 1412–16.
14. **Branger, P.J., van't Hooft, A., Duisterhout, J.S., and van den Lei, J.** (1994). A standardized massage for supporting shared care. *Proceedings of the Annual Symposium of Computer Applications in Medical Care* Vol. 33, pp. 473–7.
15. **Moran, W.P.** et al. (1994). A practice based information system for multidisciplinary care of chronically ill patients: what information do we need? *Proceedings of the Annual Symposium of Computer Applications in Medical Care*, pp. 585–9.
16. **Starfield, B.H., Simborg, D.W., Horn, S.D., and Yourtee, S.A.** (1976). Continuity and co-ordination in primary care: their achievement and utility. *Medical Care* **14**, 625–36.
17. **Freeman, G.K. and Richards, S.C.** (1990). How much personal care in four group practices? *British Medical Journal* **301**, 1028–30.
18. **Hingstman, L. and Boon, H.** (1988). Obstetric care in The Netherlands: regional differentiation in home delivery. *Social Science and Medicine* **26**, 71–8.
19. **Brown, S. and Lumley, J.** (1998). Changing childbirth: lessons from an Australian survey of 1336 women. *British Journal of Obstetrics and Gynaecology* **105**, 143–55.
20. **Tucker, J.S., Hall, M.H., Howie, P.W., Reid, M.E., Barbour, R.S., dyFlorey, C.V., and McIlwaine, G.M.** (1996). Should obstetricians see women with normal pregnancies? A multicentre randomised controlled trial of routine antenatal care by general practitioners and midwives compared with shared care led by obstetricians. *British Medical Journal* **312**, 554–9.
21. **Shah, P.M.** et al. (1993). Evaluation of the home-based maternal record: a WHO collaborative study. *Bulletin of the World Health Organization* **71**, 535–48.
22. **Freeman, G.K. and Richards, S.C.** (1990). How much personal care in four group practices? *British Medical Journal* **301**, 1028–30.
23. **Ratcliffe, J. and Buxton, M.** (1999). Patients' preferences regarding the process and outcomes of life-saving technology. An application of conjoint analysis to liver transplantation. *International Journal of Technology Assessment in Health Care* **15**, 340–51.
24. **RCGP Working Party** (1969). Working Party from the Vocational Training subcommittee of the Royal College of General Practitioners. The educational needs of the future general practitioner. *Journal of the Royal College of General Practitioners* **18**, 358–60.
25. **Rowland, N.** (2000). Counselling in primary care: a systematic review of the research evidence. *British Journal of Guidance and Counselling* **28**, 215–31.
26. **Blair, G. and Deaney, C.** (1998). Inner-city GP population of people with schizophrenia. *Psychiatric Bulletin* **22**, 221–5.
27. **Bindman, J., Johnson, S., Wright, S., Szmukler, G., Bebbington, P., Kuipers, E., and Thornicroft, G.** (1997). Integration between primary and secondary services in the care of the severely mentally ill: patients' and general practitioners' views. *British Journal of Psychiatry* **171**, 169–74.
28. **Smith, T.J.** (2000). Future strategies needed for palliative care. *Seminars in Radiation Oncology* **10**, 254–61.
29. **Parker, D., Maddocks, I., and Stern, L.M.** (1999). The role of palliative care in advanced muscular dystrophy and spina muscular atrophy. *Journal of Paediatrics and Child Health* **35**, 245–50.
30. **Smith, T.J.** (1998). Health service studies in the terminally ill cancer patient. *Cancer Treatment Research* **9**, 781–97.
31. **Cherin, D.A., Simmons, W.J., and Hillary, K.** (1998). The transprofessional model: blending intents in terminal care of AIDS. *Home Health Care Services Quarterly* **17**, 31–54.
32. **Sessa, C.** et al. (1996). The last 3 months of life of cancer patients: medical aspects and role of home care services in southern Switzerland. *Supportive Care—Cancer* **4**, 180–5.
33. **Gilbert, R., Willan, A.R., Richardson, S., and Sellick, S.** (1994). Survey of family physicians: what is their role in cancer patient care? *Canadian Journal of Oncology* **4**, 285–90.
34. **Freeman, G.K. and Richards, S.C.** (1990). How much personal care in four group practices? *British Medical Journal* **301**, 1028–30.
35. **Kearley, K.E., Freeman, G.K., and Heath, A.** (2001). An exploration of the value of the personal doctor–patient relationship in general practice. *British Journal of General Practice* **51**, 712–18.
36. **Gray, D.J.P.** (1979). The key to personal care. *Journal of the Royal College of General Practitioners* **29**, 666–78.
37. **Hjortdahl, P.** (1992). Continuity of care: General practitioners' knowledge about and sense of responsibility towards their patients. *Family Practice* **9**, 3–8.
38. **Freeman, G.K. and Richards, S.C.** (1993). Is personal continuity of care compatible with free choice of doctor? Patients' views on seeing the same doctor. *British Journal of General Practice* **43**, 493–7.
39. **Freeman, G.K. and Richards, S.C.** (1994). Personal continuity and the care of patients with epilepsy in general practice. *British Journal of General Practice* **44**, 395–9.
40. **Freeman, G. and Hjortdahl, P.** (1997). What future for continuity of care in general practice? *British Medical Journal* **314**, 1870–3.
41. **Baker, R.** (1997). Will the future GP remain a personal doctor? *British Journal of General Practice* **47**, 831–4.
42. **Howie, J.G.R., Heaney, D.J., Maxwell, M., Walker, J.J., Freeman, G.K., and Rai, H.** (1999). Quality at general practice consultations: cross-sectional survey. *British Medical Journal* **319**, 736–43.
43. **Hart, J.T.** (1971). The inverse care law. *Lancet* **i**, 405–12.
44. **Liaw, T., Lawrence, M., and Rendell, J.** (1996). The effect of a computer-generated patient-held medical record summary and/or a written personal health record on patients' attitudes, knowledge and behaviour concerning health promotion. *Family Practice* **13** (3), 289–93.
45. **Flocke, S.A., Stange, K.C., and Zyzanski, S.J.** (1997). The impact of insurance type and forced discontinuity on the delivery of primary care. *Journal of Family Practice* **45**, 129–35.
46. **Hart, J.T.** (1998). Expectations of health care: promoted, managed or shared? *Health Expectations* **1**, 3–13.
47. **Fry, L.** (1960). Casualties and casuals. *Lancet* **1**, 163–6.
48. **Loudon, I.** (1985). The nature of provincial medical practice in eighteenth-century England. *Medical History* **29**, 1–32.
49. **Robertson-Steel, I.R.S.** (1998). Providing primary care in the accident and emergency department: the end of the inappropriate attender (editorial). *British Medical Journal* **316**, 409–10.
50. **Freeman, G.K., Meakin, R.P., Lawrenson, R.A., Leydon, G.M., and Craig, G.** (1999). Primary care units in A&E departments in North Thames in the 1990's: initial experience and future implications. *British Journal of General Practice* **49**, 107–10.
51. **Bachrach, L.L.** (1983). Planning services for chronically mentally ill patients. *Bulletin of the Menninger Clinic* **47**, 163–88.

52. **Bajekal, M., Alves, B., Jarman, B., and Hurwitz, B.** (2001). Rationale for the new GP deprivation payment scheme in England: effects of moving from electoral ward to enumeration district underprivileged area scores. *British Journal of General Practice* **51**, 451–5.

53. **Hjortdahl, P.** (1989). General practice and continuity of care: organisational aspects. *Family Practice* **6**, 292–8.

8.2 The primary–secondary care interface

Martin Roland

The importance of the gate-keeping role for primary care

The majority of patients who consult a primary care practitioner are dealt with entirely within primary care. In the last major cross national study of referrals, between 2.6 per cent (France) and 8.1 per cent (Norway) of consultations resulted in a specialist referral, with most European countries averaging referrals from between 4 and 6 per cent of consultations.[1] In some countries, such as the United Kingdom, patients require a referral from their general practitioner in order to see a specialist, apart from a small number of specialist services such as accident and emergency and genitourinary medicine departments. In other countries, like the Netherlands, reimbursement has, in the past at least, required referral from a general practitioner. In countries like these, there is a long-standing tradition of generalists controlling patient access to specialists.

In some countries, there has been a dramatic change in the organization of medical care. In Eastern Europe, for example, most countries operated with a system of specialists working in polyclinics whom patients could access directly. Since the early 1990s, most of these countries have changed their systems, trained cadres of primary care practitioners, and controlled access to specialists. Likewise, in the United States, there have been major changes in the role of the primary care physician as gate keeper. While many managed care plans attempted to enforce a strong gate keeper role in the late 1990s, due to negative reactions from patients, many have since abandoned these controls.

In this chapter, some of the features of the gate-keeping role which have made it so attractive to those who organize and fund health care will be described. Also included are descriptions of the different types of relationship which occur at the interface between primary and specialist care, what is known about the factors which affect physician behaviour at this interface, and how quality of care for patients may be maximized when they have a need for referral.

The role of the generalist

Starfield has defined the role of the generalist as being to provide first contact care which is patient focused over time (longitudinality), comprehensive and coordinated.[2] The generalist also provides care for problems which are not limited by age, sex, or condition. Starfield's work has been very influential in demonstrating, through cross-national comparisons, that primary care oriented systems not only appear to be more cost effective than health systems based on specialist care, but they also appear to produce better health outcomes. There is no consensus however, on what balance between primary and specialist provision optimizes the cost effectiveness of a health care system.[3]

While a 'pure' form of generalist occurs in some countries, for example, the United Kingdom, Denmark, and the Netherlands, others have generalists who work in different ways. In Spain, for example, family physicians do not routinely see children or women with gynaecological and obstetric problems. There is therefore a cadre of primary care paediatricians and gynaecologists who work alongside family physicians. In Germany, the general practitioner may initiate the referral, but often does so without direct assessment of the patient or a consultation.[4] In the United States, family practitioners generally see the full range of problems that a patient may present with, but gynaecologists, paediatricians, and internal medicine specialists are also regarded as primary care physicians. Furthermore, some American health plans do not reimburse mental health care from primary care physicians, which effectively takes the care of these problems out of the arena of primary care physicians.

Family physicians also vary greatly between countries in the complexity of tasks which they carry out, and the extent to which they care for patients in hospital (see also Chapter 8.3). In the United States, many primary care physicians have hospital admission rights, whereas this scarcely occurs at all in countries such as the United Kingdom. In rural parts of Australia, general practitioners (GP) may be the only medical staff in a hospital, and will undertake a wide range of surgical and obstetric procedures. In 2001, the UK government announced a major programme to develop specialization within general practice in the United Kingdom. Opinion on such moves is divided between those who see the potential for primary care physicians to provide a greater proportion of overall medical care in a cost-effective manner, and those who believe that increased specialization within primary care undermines and devalues the generalist nature of the discipline. This issue is discussed in more detail in Chapter 8.4.

Advantages and drawbacks of a well-defined primary–secondary care interface

Most health care systems have some sort of distinction between care that is provided by generalists and care provided by specialists. The advantages of such a distinction are clear. Patients know what to expect from different parts of the system, doctors are clear about their responsibilities, and those with responsibility for training are clear about the competencies which need to be developed for any individual discipline. Where systems differ between countries however, this may cause problems, but at least the problems are defined. In the European Union, for example, there is free movement of labour across national boundaries. Trained Spanish family physicians know that they will need extra training in paediatrics, obstetrics, and gynaecology to be general practitioners in the other countries, even though they may have a license to practice the full range of primary care medicine without further experience.

The principal drawback of a rigid boundary between generalists and specialists is that patient care becomes fragmented. This is especially the case in countries where the tasks carried out by general practitioners are more limited. So, for example, a US family physician is likely to manage a chest infection requiring hospital admission in an elderly person, possibly with consultation from a specialist. In the United Kingdom, the care of such a patient would, except in a small number of areas with community hospitals, be transferred to a specialist, with all the attendant problems of lack of continuity, and lack of understanding of the patients home, and social circumstances. There might therefore be an argument for greater involvement of generalists in the care of their patients. The limiting factor is the extent to which adequate skills can be acquired and retained by the generalist, and the availability of sufficient generalists within the health care system. This issue is addressed in different ways in different countries. In Denmark, primary care practitioners are employed as advisors in hospitals, with the specific remit to promote cooperation between generalists and specialists, a role which is being modelled in some accident and emergency departments in the United Kingdom.

There may also be problems in areas where responsibilities are unclear or split. In the United Kingdom, this occurs most frequently over drug prescriptions, especially where patients need very expensive medications that require some degree of specialist supervision. An example of this relates to patients with renal failure who require erythropoetin treatment: there are regular arguments between generalists and specialists about who should prescribe this treatment. These are partly about where appropriate clinical responsibility lies, and partly about attempts to cost shift between primary and secondary sectors.

Where there are clearly defined responsibilities for the tasks to be carried out by generalists and specialists, there will also be opportunities for mutual education across that interface. Specialists involved in schemes such as those described later in this chapter often comment how closer working with general practitioners gives them a better understanding of how to manage their patients. General practitioners for their part look to specialists to contribute to their own education, though there is a tendency for the latter to provide information on new advances in their discipline rather than dealing with issues of more direct relevance to general practitioners.[5]

Improving care at the primary–secondary interface

The approach taken to improving care at the primary–secondary interface will depend on whose perspective the problem is seen through. The payer seeks to reduce costs, the health service manager seeks to reduce waiting times if these are a political priority, the patient seeks coordinated efficient and effective care, the specialist seeks appropriate demands being made of his skills, and the primary care practitioner looks for a secondary care system that is responsive to the many and diverse demands that he might need to make of it. The following sections discuss a number of practical initiatives designed to improve care at the primary–secondary interface.

Variation in referral patterns: maximizing appropriateness of referrals

There is wide variation in the referral rates of individual general practitioners. Attempts to explain these on the basis of the characteristics of the patients have been relatively unsuccessful.[6] Age and sex differences explain little of the differences in rates of referral, though socio-economic factors may be more important, especially when comparing different populations.[7,8] One Dutch study found that casemix explained nearly half the variation in referral rates,[9] though others have found only small differences in casemix of high and low referring doctors.[10] Primary care physicians are widely held to differ in their propensity to refer, but there is little clear relationship between, for example, age or experience and patterns of referral.[6] Some of the variation in referral rates can be explained in terms of measurable psychological characteristics of the doctor such as risk aversion or tolerance of uncertainty,[11] and one Finnish study found that more specialized and more experienced primary care practitioners made fewer referrals to specialists compared to younger doctors and locums.[12] However, rates of referral may also vary markedly between countries.[13] Not surprisingly, models which describe the decision making process which primary care physicians go through when making referrals are complex,[14,15] reflecting the considerable complexity of the actual decisions made. This partly relates to the range of reasons that primary care physicians refer to specialists (Box 1) and the fact that there will often be more than one reason for referral.

Wherever the boundary between primary and specialist care is set in an individual country, care will be most efficient if all those patients who need to be referred are referred, and no patients are referred unless they have a need for specialist care. This, of course is never the case, and some patients will be referred who have nothing to gain from the referral and others will be cared for by their primary care physician where they would benefit from seeing a specialist. These patients represent inefficiency in the health care system, and considerable attention has been paid in some countries to 'inappropriate referrals', especially by those with responsibility for funding specialist services.

Box 1 Reasons for referral from primary care practitioners to specialists

- Referral for diagnosis
- Referral for specific investigation
- Referral for advice on management
- Referral for specific treatment
- Sharing the load of a difficult or demanding patient
- Poor relationship with patient leading to need for second opinion
- Avoidance of malpractice complaint/litigation
- Response to requests from the patient or his/her caregiver
- Reassurance for the doctor or the patient

Variation in referral behaviour is therefore of importance to the extent that it represents inappropriate under- or over-use of specialist resources. Patients inappropriately referred will cost the health care system more, and may be exposed to risk of harm through unnecessary investigation or treatment. Patients who are not referred when they should be might, as a result, be in poorer health. Considerable effort has therefore been expended on trying to improve the situation, and to reduce inappropriate referrals. The results of these efforts have not, however, been entirely satisfactory. First, there has been a failure by governments and payers to understand the extent of random variation that is likely to occur in rates of specialist referral,[16] or to take account of known socio-demographic effects in comparing referral rates from different populations.[7,8] Second, there has been an assumption that a wide range of referral rate means that inappropriate referral is common. In the United Kingdom, this appears not to be the case. Generally, rates of referral defined as inappropriate have been found to be less than 10 per cent.[17–19] A possible exception to this is orthopaedics,[20] but in that specialty there are large differences in the perceptions of patients and specialists as to what constitutes an appropriate referral. In the Netherlands, no difference was found in the appropriateness of referral from high and low referring doctors,[21] and Coulter et al. found that practices with high referral rates were just as likely to have their patients admitted after referral, again casting doubt on the suggesting that high referring practices refer inappropriately.[22] Although examining crude rates of referral tells little about the appropriateness of referral, the wide variation in these rates is one of the stimuli for the development of referral guidelines to try to ensure greatest efficiency at the primary–secondary interface.

Referral guidelines

Referral guidelines have been widely used as a means of improving the appropriateness of referrals. Under- and over-use commonly co-exist in medical care, and referrals are no exception. If guidelines were widely used, it does not therefore follow that referral rates would drop (often the intention of those who write referral guidelines), and indeed, there is some suggestion that they might rise.[16,18] In some instances, referral guidelines have been shown to change behaviour: in Scotland, providing guidelines on infertility investigations increased the number of investigations carried out prior to referral and improved the appropriateness of referral.[23] However, frustratingly, a follow-up trial showed that specialists generally ignored the results of the test previously carried out by the GP, so the referral guidelines produced no overall benefit to patients.[24] Guidelines therefore need to be backed up by methods of measuring and monitoring the quality of care at the interface (i.e. audit), and they should contain specific quality indicators which enable care to be monitored.

Auditing referrals

Specialist referral has been a common subject for audit activity. However, the benefits of this depend on the approach taken. If the impetus comes from managers who wish to reduce rates of referral then the impact is likely to be small. GPs know that information on rates of referral tell little about the quality of clinical care, so when referral rates are fed back on a routine basis, they are likely to be ignored.[25] More promising are approaches which depend on detailed analysis of cases by clinicians in order to identify patients who might have been managed differently. One approach to this would be significant event auditing, choosing cases for discussion in order to identify ways in which care might be improved (see Box 2).

Shared care

One way to maximize the efficiency and effectiveness of care at the primary–secondary interface is for care to be formally shared between the generalist and specialist, that is, both have responsibilities which are (or should be) clearly defined. So, for example, shared care of a patient with diabetes may involve a visit to the medical specialist once a year, with routine care at other times being provided either by the GP or the diabetic specialist nurse. Likewise, in shared obstetric care, in the United Kingdom, the role of the specialist in uncomplicated patients is generally limited to one occasion at the beginning of pregnancy, and one towards the end. It is very hard to make shared care arrangements work effectively unless the roles and responsibilities of each party are well defined and well understood, and the generalist has the skills which enable him or her to undertake the defined roles effectively.

The rationale behind shared care is that the knowledge and expertise of the specialist should be available to patients who are seen principally in primary care, thus extending the benefits of specialist care, especially where specialist resources are limited. The extent to which these work well is crucially dependent on the way in which care is organized. For example, a meta-analysis of diabetes care[26] shows that diabetes care provided principally in primary care can be as good as that provided in specialist settings. However, this only works in the presence of good infrastructure. This is likely to include

- up-to-date registers which are used to recall patients and monitor care;
- clear responsibility for organizing care within the primary care team (often led by a nurse);
- use of computers to prompt reviews and monitor care;
- well defined protocols for care; and
- good routes of communication between generalist and specialist.

Poorly organized primary care produces poor outcomes, especially for chronic diseases, which are potentially the most amenable to a shared care arrangement. The following section describes some special examples of shared care arrangements: in three of them, the aim of the specialist is quite specifically to enhance the role of the GP.

Box 2 Examples of specialist referrals which could form part of significant event audit

Possible unnecessary referral: Referral of a patient to a medical specialist with somatic symptoms that the GP believed to be psycho-somatic. Referral involves increased risk to the patient from unnecessary investigation. Discussion might focus on other approaches the GP could have taken, and how more appropriate options might be discussed with the patient.

Possible late referral: A routine audit of patients with cancer can be used to discuss whether specialist referral took place at the appropriate time, or whether there were delays in primary care, for example, failure to recognize the importance of early symptoms, leading to important conditions remaining undiagnosed or treatment delayed.

Possible failure to refer: A routine audit of patients who have died can be used to discuss whether there were failures in diagnosis which could have led to treatable conditions being referred to a specialist.

Liaison attachment and specialist outreach clinics

A range of approaches have been used to improve communication and effectiveness at the primary care interface by means of direct interaction between specialists and generalists. Especially where specialists and generalists consult jointly with a patient, there are opportunities for joint learning to occur and for the generalist to enhance his or her skills as occurred in a joint clinic for patients with musculo-skeletal problems in the Netherlands.[27] Arrangements designed to promote direct contact between generalist and specialist have most often been used in psychiatry. These vary from those where the psychiatrist comes to the GP's surgery and sees patients, to ones where the psychiatrist comes and carries out a joint consultation with the GP, to ones where the psychiatrist comes to discuss patients with the primary care staff. The aim of these approaches is partly to improve access for patients, and partly to improve communication between primary care practitioners and specialists. The way in which the scheme is organized will determine which of these benefits are likely to occur.

It is clear that improved communication does not occur if the main role of the specialist is to see patients in a community setting. In the United Kingdom in the early 1990s, there was widespread adoption of 'specialist outreach clinics'—in which specialists held regular clinics in GP surgeries, it was suggested that there would be benefits to patients and doctors. Patients would benefit by having easier access to specialists, and the doctors would benefit through opportunities to discuss cases, and to learn from each other. However, the reality was that there was very little communication or learning between GPs and specialists. The specialists travelled to primary care premises, saw the allocated patients, but rarely had any contact with the GP. Although patients found these clinics more convenient, they were not a cost-effective use of health care resources in the way in which they were used,[28,29] and the clinics were not used to increase the management of cases by GPs. Box 3 shows a number of examples of direct liaison between primary care practitioners and specialists, the first three of which increased the skills of the GPs involved, and the last of which had modest benefits for patients alone.

Improving communication between generalists and specialists

Communication is often poor between GPs and specialists. Letters to specialists may not contain information about patients' previous problems or their medication, and communication back is also often poor.[30,31] One crucial aspect of improving care at the interface is for better information sharing, and the completeness of the referral letter has been suggested as a performance indicator for general practice.[32] Specific schemes for sharing information are at present usually limited to specific conditions. For example, shared care arrangements for obstetric care are used in many countries, with the patient retaining all or part of their obstetric record. Similar schemes are used for patients with hypertension and diabetes. If shared electronic records can be established between primary and secondary care, then the opportunities for coordinated care increase greatly. Shared records between community-based primary care clinics and hospitals already exist in some settings (e.g. the Veterans Administration in the United States), and

Box 3 Models of liaison between specialists and GPs

Enhancing the GP's role (1): A psychiatrist in Cambridge offered a liaison service to local GPs. Where a GP had difficulty managing a particular patient, the psychiatrist would arrange to do a joint consultation with himself, the GP, and the patient. Sometimes he would take the lead in such consultations, but sometimes his main role was to sit in on a consultation between the GP and the patient. His aim was to strengthen the GP's own role, and not to take over management of the patient.

Enhancing the GP's role (2): A diabetic specialist came to the diabetic clinic in a South London practice on a regular basis. Initially, he would see the patients with the GPs. Then, increasingly, he sat in the common room doing his own paperwork, just giving advice when needed. Eventually, the GPs were so attuned to his management approaches that he no longer needed to come to the clinic.

Enhancing the GP's role (3): A psychiatrist attended regular primary care team meetings in a Manchester practice, and came with her community psychiatric nurse. They did not see patients when they came, but spent the time discussing patients under the care of both the psychiatrist and the primary care team, or other patients with whom the practice were having difficulty.

Improving patient convenience: An orthopaedic surgeon came to do outreach clinics in a practice in Derbyshire. The practice had a budget for specialist services, so was able to 'buy in' the services of the specialist. Initially, the GPs planned to meet with the specialist when he came. However, they were always too busy, so he simply saw the patients who had been booked. Patients enjoyed the convenience of the service, but the specialist resented the time spent away from his base. When funding ran out, the scheme stopped.

have the potential to be developed in other centrally coordinated care systems (e.g. the British National Health Service).

Advances in information systems that allow better sharing of information across the primary–secondary interface have great potential to improve care in the future. Indeed, Hampson and colleagues[30] argue that sharing information across health sectors (including with pharmacists) is an essential prerequisite for the cultural change that needs to take place if the overall care of patients is to improve.

Improving hospital discharge

This section has so far concentrated on referrals from primary care to specialists. However, they also return, and there may be substantial problems associated with the transfer of care from specialists back to generalists. There are particular problems associated with unplanned discharge of elderly patients from hospital, and poor transfer for information back to the primary care practitioner when he or she resumes responsibility for the patient's care. The recognition that patients may no longer need specialist care at a time when they are still unable fully to care for themselves has led to the development of intermediate care schemes. In these schemes, patients may receive high intensity support, either in their own homes or in a nursing home for a few weeks prior to being able to manage more independently.

The patient's perspective

Much of the research cited in this chapter so far represents professional perspectives on the primary–secondary interface. Patients' views are also of considerable importance, and may not concur with those of their specialist[11] or their primary care practitioner.[33] Patients views are heavily dependent on their expectations and may therefore depend crucially on the health system context. In the United States, for example, the introduction of primary care gate keepers by health plans has been widely resented by patients who have seen this as a method of controlling costs by denying them effective treatments.

Patients also have an important part to play in the primary care practitioner's decision to refer, though the relative importance of this is likely to vary between cultures (prominence of patient versus professional choice), and the extent to which individual practitioners view themselves as advocates for their patients or guardians of scarce specialist resources (in countries where they are scarce).

For those who wish to gain patients' views on referral, Baker et al. have developed a series of questionnaires which can be used to track a patient's progress through the referral system, including information from the GP prior to referral, visits to the specialist, and care after discharge from specialist care. These are combined into a 'patient career diary'.[34]

Referrals outside the health sector

Referrals between primary and secondary care which have been discussed so far in this chapter represent only one type of referral which primary care practitioners make. Their other major interaction is with social care providers, who may be local authority or private providers. Relationships and communication between health and social care sectors are often poor. Where there is specific attachment of a social worker to a primary care practice, relations improve. Joint assessment also helps patients get access to a wider range of services. However, joint ownership of such schemes is necessary for them to operate effectively, and this does not always occur.[35]

In the United Kingdom, one approach to deal with problems of fragmentation between health and social services has been to give patients money to purchase services themselves instead of having to rely on decisions made by professionals. Disabled people do not divide their needs into 'health needs' and 'social care needs' and appear better able to secure integrated services and continuity of care when they are given greater control of the resources for their own care.[36]

Although the success of individual schemes to improve coordination across the health–social care interface show some promise, this remains an area of concern in many countries, and the funding of care for elderly people in particular remains a major problem.

Targets for improvement at the primary–secondary interface

Difficulties at the interface between primary and secondary care are not new. In the early part of the twentieth century in the United Kingdom, there was a very blurred distinction between those who claimed specialist skills (and who might or might not be continuing to see more general and family problems) and those to whom the GP could refer with confidence. 'Poaching' of patients was common, and GPs tried to insist that specialists were only asked to consult (hence their current title of 'consultants') for fear that they would take over actual treatment and deprive GPs of their livelihood.

These and other problems continue into the twenty-first century, and although some are dependent on the operation of an individual health care system, many problems are common across national boundaries.

The European Working Party on Quality in Family Practice (EQuiP) has published a set of ten priorities for improvement at the interface.[37] These are mostly just as relevant for the interface between primary care and social services and non-health sectors and can be summarized as:

- Developing specifically identified clinical leadership with a defined responsibility for the interface: At present, part of the reason for problems at the interface is precisely that it is no-one's problem, with managers, specialists and generalists each looking to their own interests.
- Developing a shared approach for patients seen in both primary and secondary care: local management structures need to encourage rather than impede the process of care at boundaries.

- Creating consensus on explicit task division and job sharing: the individual responsibilities of primary care practitioners and specialists will differ in different countries. Both sides need to know what is expected of them, and have appropriate support to fulfil those roles.
- Developing local guidelines for referral: these need to incorporate national guidelines where they exist, but must be tailored to local circumstances and resources.
- Incorporating the patient's perspective into planning care at the interface: the patient is the one who suffers when poor un-coordinated care occurs at the interface. Patients need to be included in planning and monitoring services.
- Developing better information systems: information systems are currently un-coordinated and fragmented. Where integrated information systems exist (e.g. hand-held cards for patients), they generally relate to one isolated aspect of care (e.g. diabetes). Some examples (e.g. the Veterans Administration in the United States) show how electronic records can become completely shared between primary care practitioners and specialists across many sites.
- Using professional education to improve care at the interface: this involves sharing problems and learning from mistakes. Specialists have just as much to learn as generalists, and learning should have quality improvement as its specific aim.
- Facilitating team working across the interface: for care which inevitably involves a major component at the interface (e.g. palliative care, diabetes, stroke rehabilitation), nothing less than a team approach will produce good care.
- Establishing quality monitoring at the interface: experience shows that, left unattended, care at the interface between primary and secondary care is unlikely to look after itself. Guidelines for care at the interface should therefore be developed to include specific quality indicators that can then be built into the management of the interface.
- Maximizing cost effectiveness: within any individual health system, this means ensuring that patients receive the right care at the right level, at the first try. The other recommendations of the EQuiP group will all work towards ensuring that this happens.

Conclusions

As medicine advances, care will become more complex. The history of the past 30 years is of increasing amounts of care being provided by primary care practitioners. For example, in many countries, it would now be uncommon for the main management of patients with mild hypertension or type 2 diabetes to be carried out by specialists—a situation which has changed radically over the past 30 years. There is likely to be little change in the general trend for care to move from the secondary to the primary sector. The need for good communication between primary care practitioners and specialists will therefore become more important, not less. The problems that arise from the interface being no-one's responsibility need to be addressed. Furthermore, information technology needs to be enhanced to support doctors and patients. We accept without thinking that it is possible to check one's bank account by going to an ATM in almost any country in the world. The health sector needs to catch up in order to provide patients with the care that they need and deserve.

References

1. **Royal College of General Practitioners.** *The European Study of Referrals from Primary to Secondary Care.* Occasional Paper 56. London: RCGP, 1992.
2. **Starfield, B.** (1994). Is primary care essential? *Lancet* **344**, 1129–33.
3. **Coulter, A.** (1996). Why should health services be primary care led? *Journal of Health Services Research and Policy* **1**, 122–4.
4. **Fleming, D.** (1992). The interface between general practice and secondary care in Europe and North America. In *Hospital Referrals* (ed. M.O. Roland and A. Coulter), pp. 30–47. Oxford: Oxford University Press.
5. **Marshall, M.N.** (1998). Qualitative study of educational interaction between general practitioners and specialists. *British Medical Journal* **316**, 442–5.
6. **O'Donnell, C.A.** (2000). Variation in GP referral rates: what can we learn from the literature? *Family Practice* **17**, 462–71.
7. **Hippisley Cox, J., Hardy, C., Pringle, M., Fielding, K., Carlisle, R., and Clivers, C.** (1997). The effect of deprivation on variations in general practitioners' referral rates: a cross sectional study of computerised data on new medical and surgical outpatient referrals in Nottinghamshire. *British Medical Journal* **314**, 1458–61.
8. **Giuffrida, A., Gravelle, H., and Roland, M.** (1999). Measuring quality with routine data: avoiding confusion between performance indicators and health outcomes. *British Medical Journal* **319**, 94–8.
9. **Delnoij, D.M.J. and Spreeuwenberg, P.M.M.** (1997). Variation in GPs' referral rates to specialists in internal medicine. *European Journal of Public Health* **7**, 427–35.
10. **Wilkin, D. and Smith, A.G.** (1987). Variation in general practitioners' referral rates to consultants. *Journal of the Royal College of General Practitioners* **37**, 350–3.
11. **Roland, M., Grimshaw, J., Grol, R., Shanks, D., Johnson, A., Russell, I., and Taylor, R.** (1997). Do general practitioner attitudes and characteristics of their practices explain patterns of specialist referral? *European Journal of General Practice* **3**, 143–7.
12. **Vehvilainen, A.T., Kumpusalo, E.A., Voutilainen, S.O., and Takala, J.K.** (1996). Does the doctor's professional experience reduce referral rates? Evidence from the Finnish referral study. *Scandinavian Journal of Primary Health Care* **14**, 13–20.
13. **Forrest, C.B., Majeed, A., Weiner, J., Carroll, K., and Bindman, A.B.** (2002). Comparison of specialty referral rates in the United Kingdom and United States. *British Medical Journal* **325**, 370–1.
14. **Wilkin, D. and Smith, A.** (1987). Explaining variations in general practitioner referrals to hospital. *Family Practice* **4**, 160–9.
15. **Newton, J., Hayes, V., and Hutchinson, A.** (1991). Factors affecting general practitioners' referral decisions. *Family Practice* **8**, 308–13.
16. **Moore, A.T. and Roland, M.O.** (1989). How much of the variation in general practitioner referral rates is due to chance? *British Medical Journal* **298**, 500–2.
17. **Emmanuel, J. and Walter, N.** (1989). Referrals from general practice to hospital outpatient departments: a strategy for improvement. *British Medical Journal* **299**, 722–4.
18. **Fertig, A., Roland, M.O., King, H., and Moore, A.T.** (1993). Understanding variation in general practitioner referral rates: are inappropriate referrals important, and would guidelines help to reduce rates. *British Medical Journal* **307**, 1467–70.
19. **Jenkins, R.M.** (1993). Quality of general practitioner referrals to outpatients departments: assessment by specialists and a general practitioner. *British Journal of General Practice* **43**, 111–13.
20. **Roland, M.O., Porter, R.W., Matthews, J.G., Redden, J.F., Simonds, G.W., and Bewley, B.** (1991). Improving care: a study of orthopaedic outpatient referrals. *British Medical Journal* **302**, 1124–8.
21. **Knottnerus, J.A., Joosten, J., and Daams, J.** (1990). Comparing the quality of referrals of general practitioners with high and average referral rates: an independent panel review. *British Journal of General Practice* **40**, 187–91.
22. **Coulter, A., Seagroatt, V., and McPherson, K.** (1990). Relation between general practices; outpatient referral rates and rates of elective admission to hospital. *British Medical Journal* **301**, 723–6.
23. **Emslie, C., Grimshaw, J., and Templeton, A.** (1993). Do clinical guidelines improve general practice management and referral of infertile couples? *British Medical Journal* **306**, 1728–31.
24. **Morrison, J., Carroll, L., Twaddle, S., Cameron, I., Grimshaw, J., Leyland, A., Baillie, H., and Watt, G.** (2001). Pragmatic randomised controlled trial to evaluate guidelines for the management of infertility across the primary care–secondary care interface. *British Medical Journal* **322**, 1282–4.
25. **De Marco, P., Dain, C., Lockwood, T., and Roland, M.** (1993). How valuable is feedback of information on hospital referral patterns? Lessons from visits to 92 East Anglian practices. *British Medical Journal* **307**, 1465–6.

26. **Griffin, S.** (1998). Diabetes care in general practice: meta-analysis of randomised controlled trials. *British Medical Journal* **317**, 390–5.
27. **Vierhout, W.P.M., Knottnerus, J.A., van Ooij, Crebolder, H.F.J.M., Pop, P., Wesselingh-Hegens, A.M.K., and Beusmans, G.H.M.I.** (1995). Effectiveness of joint consultation sessions of general practitioners and orthopaedic surgeons for locomotor-system disorders. *Lancet* **346**, 990–4.
28. **Bowling, A. and Bond, M.** (2001). A national evaluation of specialists' clinics in primary care settings. *British Journal of General Practice* **51**, 264–9.
29. **Black, M., Leese, B., Gosden, T., and Meade, N.** (1997). Specialist outreach clinics in general practice: what do they offer? *British Journal of General Practice* **47**, 558–61.
30. **Hampson, J.P., Roberts, R.I., and Morgan, D.A.** (1996). Shared care: a review of the literature. *Family Practice* **13**, 264–79.
31. **Forrest, C.B., Glade, G.B., Baker, A.E., Bocian, A., von Schrader, S., and Starfield, B.** (2000). Co-ordination of specialty referrals and physician satisfaction with referral care. *Archives of Pediatric and Adolescent Medicine* **154**, 499–506.
32. **Elwyn, G.J., Rix, A., Matthews, P., and Stott, N.C.** (1999). Referral for 'prostatism': developing a 'performance indicator' for the threshold between primary and secondary care? *Family Practice* **16**, 140–2.
33. **Grace, J.F. and Armstrong, D.** (1987). Referral to hospital: perceptions of patients, general practitioners and consultants about necessity and suitability of referral. *Family Practice* **4**, 170–5.
34. **Baker, R., Preston, C., Cheater, F., and Hearnshaw, H.** (1999). Measuring patients' attitudes to care across the primary secondary interface: the development of the patient career diary. *Quality in Health Care* **8**, 154–60.
35. **Glendinning, C., Rummery, K., and Clarke, R.** (1998). From collaboration to commissioning: developing relationships between primary care and social services. *British Medical Journal* **317**, 122–5.
36. **Glendinning, C., Rummery, K., Halliwell, S., Jacobs, S., and Tyrer, J.** Buying independence: using direct payments to purchase integrated health and social services. Executive Summary 17. National Primary Research and Development Centre, University of Manchester, 2000. Available at: http://www.npcrdc.man.ac.uk/
37. **Kvamme, O.J., Olesen, F., and Samuelsson, M.** (2001). Improving the interface between primary and secondary care: a statement from the European Working Party on Quality in Family Practice (EQuiP). *Quality in Health Care* **10**, 33–9.

8.3 Generalists in hospitals

Frede Olesen

Introduction

Specialization in hospitals has contributed enormously to the development of modern western medicine over the last 100 years, and it has become necessary due to the ever increasing sum of knowledge and the skills and technology required. One of the consequences of this is that patients need to be in contact with many departments during a care episode. Another side-effect may be a lack of coordination and patient-experienced continuity during each care episode, and a lack of a total assessment of a patient and his disease.(1) The general practitioner (GP) may have a special role as a generalist in this context.(2)

In some countries, for example, the United States and Canada, the GPs enjoy full hospital privileges as partners in decisions about treatment and care. Other countries, for example, the United Kingdom and the Scandinavian countries, maintain a clear separation between primary and secondary care. Although in the United Kingdom substantial numbers of GPs work in hospitals as clinical assistants or hospital practitioners, undertaking outpatient clinics and diagnostic procedures such as gastrointestinal endoscopy. Such health care systems may create a lack of mutual understanding between staff in primary and secondary health care and may cause patients to be left in a limbo between the sectors. It might, therefore, be an idea to employ primary care staff in the secondary sector and vice versa to help bridge the gap between the sectors.

The GP is trained to make a comprehensive assessment of each individual episode of care, and his skills may, therefore, be valuable in two main areas in hospitals even in those countries where there currently is clear separation between primary ambulatory care and secondary hospital care:

- in hospital-based clinical front line functions, for example, in emergency rooms and in ambulatory settings;
- as a partner in a coordinating process designed to ensure seamless episodes of care that cut across traditional primary and secondary care sector boundaries.

This chapter will deal with both areas, but emphasis will be devoted to GPs assuming the role of coordinators of hospital care.

GPs as frontline clinicians in hospitals

All countries experience an increasing demand for accident and emergency (A&E) services in hospitals, and the number of hospital-based open walk-in clinics in the different specialities is growing. The GP may have a special function in these clinics as she/he is trained to make diagnoses in situations with a low disease prevalence and to assess a disease in a broad bio-psychosocial context. She/he is also well informed about the possibilities in primary health care and about what a hospital physician can expect to be done when she/he refers a patient back to general practice and primary health care.

For this reason, several hospitals have used GPs in A&E services for problems resembling those seen in primary care. The advantage is that patients are assessed in this hospital frontline function in the same way as they would normally have been in primary health care. A London health services project demonstrated another advantage of frontline usage of GPs in A&E services: the GPs used fewer resources than young doctors and consultants (Table 1) when caring for a random sample of patients.(3,4) The introduction of GPs did not change patient satisfaction and clinical outcome and may owe its success to the fact that GPs assess the patients' symptoms in a broad perspective with less use of high technology and refer patients back to general practice, hence improving intersectoral cooperation.

The future will undoubtedly see a more widespread introduction of physicians trained to the level of being specialists in general practice in hospital-based frontline care, including special hospital units for primary assessment of acutely referred patients.(4)

GPs might help bridge the gap between the best elements from the generalist function and the best elements from the highly specialized hospital functions. The GP's broad skills in assessing patients' symptoms in a comprehensive light are likely to become even more important in the future as western culture seems to cause a growing number of patients to develop somatizing health care seeking behaviour. An early and broad assessment at the frontline of the hospital function can contribute substantially to reducing hospital workloads.(5)

GPs as coordinators and advisers in hospitals

The fragmentation of hospital care can result in specialized physicians in hospitals being uninformed about the competences and possible management options in primary health care, and GPs may over time lose detailed insight into the complicated process of diagnosis, cure, and care at hospital

Table 1 Costs in relation to types of physicians treating patients attending accident and emergency departments with primary care problems

Cost category	General practitioners (n = 1702)		Senior house officers (n = 2382)		Registrars (n = 557)	
	Cost (£)		Cost (£)		Cost (£)	
	Total	Per case	Total	Per case	Total	Per case
Total, incl. admissions	54 970	32.30	138 745	58.25	24 881	44.68
Total, excl. admissions	19 909	11.70	45 967	19.30	10 004	17.97

Source: Dale, J. et al. (1996). Cost effectiveness of treating primary care patients in accident and emergency: a comparison between general practitioners, senior house officers, and registrars. *British Medical Journal* **312**, 1340–4.

departments. This may reduce the opportunities to create good and well-coordinated care episodes where patients experience a seamless approach to symptoms and diseases and a well-defined task distribution across traditional sectoral barriers of the health care system. Patients often feel left in a limbo between primary and secondary care and this situation will be worsened by an ever shorter turnover time in hospitals and by the involvement of many hospital departments in a care episode. This development calls for a coordinating effort between primary and secondary care and for teaching different stakeholders in the health care system about core values and core functions in other parts of the health care system.

One possible answer to this call for coordination may be to employ GPs as coordinators and advisers in hospitals. The *overall aim* of employing GPs in such positions is to increase cooperation between hospitals and the primary health care physician and other care givers.(6) Furthermore, a GP will be instrumental in strengthening a shared approach to care, raising patient satisfaction with health care and guaranteeing greater cost-effectiveness. The Scandinavian countries, first Denmark and later Sweden and Norway, have decided to use GPs as part-time employed advisers and coordinators in hospital departments. The system, which has developed gradually over the last 15 years, is now seen as a cornerstone in the efforts to create a comprehensive, integrated, seamless health care system within a health care setting where both primary and secondary health care are highly developed, but also quite independent and separate.(6,7) This system with GPs as advisers and coordinators in hospitals will be described in detail as it may inspire those who are involved in comprehensive health care planning under similar administrative conditions.

What are GP coordinators and advisers?

A GP *adviser* is a part-time employed clinically working GP who, for a few hours per week, works as an adviser to the senior staff at a hospital department with regard to the department's cooperation with primary care, especially general practice.

A GP *coordinator* may have the same function in relation to hospital departments, but mainly works within a hospital setting or even a region coordinating hospital or regional functions in relation to primary health care and as a coordinator of the activities performed by the GP advisers at different departments. For some years the Netherlands has had such coordinators attached to hospital laboratories to act as intermediators concerning diagnostic testing and use of diagnostic facilities.

Today, nearly all departments in Denmark that cooperate with general practice have employed a GP adviser. Large hospitals have separate GP coordinators and the same is the case for health care regions (catchment area: some 200 000–600 000 inhabitants). Small hospitals may have the same adviser employed for different departments, and the hospitals may even be so small that they only have one GP coordinator who also acts as adviser to all departments.

A typical GP adviser is employed 6–8 h per month, a coordinator typically 10–60 h per month depending on decisions and experienced needs in the region. Regional coordinators are usually employed for even more hours each month.

A GP adviser is appointed by the head of the involved hospital departments in cooperation with a GP coordinator. The association of general practitioners and the health insurance administrators of the region normally have observers overseeing the employment process, and they have the main responsibility for the appointment of coordinators.

A GP adviser earns a salary that matches what she/he earns as a private GP to make sure that advisory and coordinating functions are not financially unattractive activities.

Tasks of the GP advisers and coordinators

The tasks of the GP advisers and coordinators are many:

- To obtain consensus and explicitly describe the task distribution between hospitals and primary health care with regard to planning of care episodes. This is seen as a tool to promote shared care. This overall task is obtained by:
  - establishing appropriate communication between hospitals and GPs;
  - ensuring high-quality referral and the use of discharge letters as communication tools between general practices and hospitals;
  - discussing and describing care plans with involved stakeholders inside and outside hospitals;
  - finding methods for improved cooperation between primary health care and hospital departments;
  - describing ways of coordination between a hospital department and a GP setting in general and outlining specific care responsibilities for disease groups involving major treatment in a hospital;
  - contributing to disseminating information from general practice to hospitals and information about working conditions inside and outside hospitals;
  - participating in planning of continuous medical education (CME) activities for GPs addressing the needs of the hospital departments and in staff CME activities at hospital departments focusing on functions, needs, and ways of cooperation with general practice.

The GP who is acting as a coordinator also should work towards ensuring coordination between different GP advisers at the hospital and keeping contact and seeking cooperation with the administrative and political hospital chiefs. Most of the coordinators are the final editors of any information material from hospitals to GPs within a district.

A few hospital regions have one or two regional, leading coordinators who serve as advisers to the regional health care officers and the regional politicians and ensure that different hospital coordinators and advisers produce plans in a way that leads to an explicit joint regional approach to the handling of the major diseases in the region.

Specific initiatives from GP advisers

As stated, GP advisers have a wide range of functions, for example:

- Entering into a dialogue between consultants at hospital departments, other members of the medical staff, and GPs in the district. Dialogue has taken place, for example, in joint working groups, joint CME programmes, open department days for GPs, and at arrangements where hospital staff could spend 1 or 2 days in a GP setting.

- Auditing of referral and discharge letters and drawing up of guidelines to secure a good quality of these information initiatives.
- Monitoring of the delay in sending discharge letters from hospitals to GPs and initiatives to reduce unnecessary waiting time.
- Taking steps to negotiate and create consensus with respect to common goals, tasks, and administrative planning between the administrative staff, the consultants, and the GPs in a region.
- Negotiating and setting standards for electronic communication between hospitals and GP settings. (Today more than 85 per cent of all Danish GPs have computers, and most of the communication between hospitals and GPs is in a national standardized electronic format. This process was started by GP coordinators.)
- Translating national guidelines into regional action plans based on consensus between administrative staff, hospital staff, and GPs in a region and based on explicit task distribution.
- Creating local guidelines on the basis of equal cooperation between local stakeholders where national guidelines do not exist.
- Creating, implementing, and monitoring quality-improvement activities, for example, within the field of prescribing and the use of laboratory tests and diagnostic imaging.
- Describing recommended pre-hospital investigation plans for patients who later should be referred to hospital.
- Describing the logistics of hospital investigations and other hospital procedures upon patient referral.
- Describing expected follow-up from GPs when patients with special diseases, for example, rheumatic diseases, are referred back to general practice.
- Participating in joint regional information exchange on web-pages. One region (Aarhus County, Denmark) has produced a comprehensive web-page for all GPs in the region. The regional GP coordinators and advisers have the main responsibility for the correct input to this web-page from all hospital and health departments in the region.

Teaching and training

As stated, hospital GPs only work part-time at the hospital and spend the rest of their time in their own clinical setting. These conditions carry the risk that they are weak partners in the cooperation with the hospital staff. It is, therefore, essential that GP advisers and coordinators create mutually stimulating networks. This is done in a regional setting through regular meetings two to four times a year headed by the coordinator. At these meetings, which are supported by the national college of GPs, plans, achievements, working methods, and problems can be discussed and experiences can be exchanged.

Political support

The system of GP advisers and coordinators needs major early support from those chief physicians at hospitals who see their own goals and tasks as taking leadership in creating a comprehensive regional approach to the major health care problems within their region. Some department heads may be sceptical of the system with GP advisers because it has entailed a measure of shared decision-making with primary health care. In this situation, it is crucial that the GP advisers are well trained as described above, but it is also crucial that the system enjoys strong support from the administrative hospital chiefs, the regional administrative chiefs, and the regional and national politicians. In Denmark, these important stakeholders have seen the system with GP advisers as a tool for making care more effective, seamless, and coordinated; a tool instrumental in ensuring good patient evaluation of care, cost-effective care, and further commitment of health care staff to good coordination in different parts of the health care system.

It is also important that the system receives political support from the GPs' association and its regional boards.

Weaknesses of the system

The system of GPs as advisers can contribute substantially to creating a comprehensive health care system with mutual respect between different physicians. The weak points of the system are, however, that GPs are only spending a short time in the hospital settings, and if GP advisers are not well trained they may be taken hostage to departmental policy. Health care planners should always be aware that GPs acting as advisers work together with hospital chiefs on equal terms. Another weakness of the system is that integration with other CME and quality improvement activities in the region has occasionally been lacking and contact with the research basis for general practice activities has also to some extent been lacking.

Coordination with other quality assurance and research activities may be weak unless initiatives are taken to ensure good coordination between primary health care research, teaching, and quality improvement activities. These activities should include joint CME activities between hospital staff and primary health care staff.

Conclusion

The system was developed in Denmark, but it has now spread to Sweden and Norway, two countries with quite similar health care systems, and the principles described seem suitable for health care settings where there is a wish to bridge the gap between primary health care and hospital care.

Other countries where GPs have been less involved in co-ordinating hospital care, for example, the United Kingdom, are also establishing initiatives to increase cooperation between primary and secondary care. They have taken the approach of health planning through Primary Care Trusts. These initiatives are based on an equal negotiation between primary and secondary care while the system described here with GPs as advisers is a more consensus-seeking procedure. The ultimate aim is, however, the same—to create a comprehensive health care system where patients feel that they are well taken care of irrespective of whether they are in contact with primary or secondary care.

References

1. **Kvamme, O.J., Olesen, F., and Samuelsson, M.** (2001). Improving the interface between primary and secondary care: a statement from the European Working Party on Quality in Family Practice (EQuiP). *Quality in Health Care* **10**, 33–9.
2. **Olesen, F., Dickinson, J., and Hjortdahl, P.** (2000). General practice—time for a new definition (editorial). *British Medical Journal* **320**, 354–7.
3. **Dale, J.** et al. (1996). Cost effectiveness of treating primary care patients in accident and emergency: a comparison between general practitioners, senior house officers, and registrars. *British Medical Journal* **312**, 1340–4.
4. **Bindman, A.B.** (1995). Triage in accident and emergency departments (editorial; comment). *British Medical Journal* **311**, 404.
5. **Fink, P.** et al. (1999). Somatization in primary care. Prevalence, utilization of health care and GP recognition. *Psychosomatics* **40**, 330–8.
6. **Forsom, L., Grinsted, P., and Ralov, H.**, ed. *Praksiskonsulentordningen i Danmark. Statusrapport 2000 (General Practitioners as Advisers in Hospitals. Status report 2000).* Copenhagen: Praksiskonsulentordningen, 2001.
7. **Olesen, F.** et al. (1998). General practitioners as advisers and coordinators in hospitals. *Quality in Health Care* **7**, 42–7.

8.4 Clinical specialization

Yvonne D. van Leeuwen, Jo Baggen, and Roger Jones

Introduction

Specialization in primary health care may, on first sight, appear a contradiction in terms. One of the unique features of primary medical care and general practice is generalism itself, with an orientation to whole person illness, rather than to specific diseases. It might, for example, be argued that the link between care and cure conflicts in many ways with compartmentalization of patients and their problems. However, specialization of various kinds in primary care is a reality, and an interesting development that warrants analysis.

Concepts of specialization in primary care are likely to vary between different health care systems, in which there are differing relationships between primary and secondary care. For example, in Scandinavia, the Netherlands, and the United Kingdom the interface between primary and secondary care is fairly sharply defined. General practice and primary medical care are themselves specialisms, with highly structured postgraduate training and continuing professional development requirements for qualification and accreditation, and in some of these countries the way in which health services are funded further differentiates specialists and generalists. In other health care systems, such as those in other parts of Europe and the United States, the distinction between generalists and specialists is more blurred and patients often have direct access to specialists without the need for referral from primary care physicians, particularly in non-capitated systems. Under these circumstances specialists may, by virtue of acting as the first point of medical contact, themselves function as primary care physicians—the primary care gastroenterologist or cardiologist.

Another setting in which generalism and specialism become less distinct is that of the rural primary care physician, who, because of geographical isolation and other factors, may need to be expert in a wide range of diagnostic skills and interventional techniques which might, in an urban setting, be regarded as the province of the specialist.

It is also important to recognize that specialism in primary care is not an attribute solely of doctors, but of other health care workers as well, including nurses, health visitors, public health nurses and others.[(1–3)] It is now commonplace for nurses to develop particular clinical skills in topics such as diabetes, asthma, and cardiovascular disease and to lead chronic disease management clinics in these areas. The diagnostic role of the nurse—nurse triage and the development of nurse practitioners—is now being reported in a number of health care settings, and the physician's assistant concept is important in the provision of primary medical care in a number of countries. Health visitors and public health nurses may develop particular expertise and focus on the care of families, infants or the elderly, and nurses working in the community may develop particular skills and expertise in other topics including, for example, palliative care, the management of varicose ulceration and the support of carers of patients with physical and psychological illness.

In this chapter we consider different aspects and models of specialization in primary care and the ways in which they might contribute to the provision of health care in the future.[(4–6)]

Characteristics of specialization in primary care

It is difficult to provide a generally accepted definition of specialization in general practice, because the concept will be dependent to a large extent on the health care system in question. Specialization does, however, suggest an above-average expertise in a certain domain of activity. General practitioners with special clinical interests (GPSCIs) is, perhaps, the most useful term that can be applied to primary care physicians who dedicate part of their time working on a specialized area. They are not, however, the same as specialists working in the community. Specialists and GPSCIs differ in their training and because of the different kinds of patients and problems encountered in primary and secondary care settings and the diagnostic and therapeutic tasks involved.[(7–9)] A general practitioner with a special clinical interest in asthma will treat an entirely different patient population from a hospital doctor specializing in respiratory illness; the general practitioner may be particularly focused on acquiring expertise in the diagnosis and management of early and mild to moderate asthma, in order to optimize detection and to ensure a good quality of life. The respiratory specialist is likely to focus on the pharmacology and management of more severe cases in order to avoid disability and death.

The roots of specialization in primary care are complex. Many GPSCIs are likely to have acquired an expertise during hospital training and specialist posts and have recognized that this knowledge can also usefully be applied in the primary care setting.[(10)] A GP may realize that certain patient problems encountered in primary care are not adequately managed there, and recognize the need to develop particular interests to deal with these problems. Under these circumstances, the pattern of primary care provision will emerge with features determined by the needs and characteristics of patient populations, rather than by the physicians' professional backgrounds, as in the first model.

It is interesting to consider the knowledge base which distinguishes specialists from GPSCIs. Although both share the knowledge gleaned in undergraduate medical education (although most undergraduate medical education remains hospital-based), their postgraduate development is likely to be quite different. Whilst much of secondary care medicine rests on a fairly firm base of evidence, the evidence base for many primary care interventions is still lacking. Although both specialists and GPSCIs will undergo continuing professional development, the respective experiences on which this development is based will be quite different, further differentiating them.[(11,12)]

General practitioners with special clinical interests

Few data are available about the extent to which GPs pursue particular clinical interests in different health care settings, but a survey from the United Kingdom provides information which may well prove generalizable, at least in principle, to other health care services, particularly those in which a patient registration system has been established. In a cross-sectional survey of a random sample of GPs working in the United Kingdom and members of a number of primary care specialists societies, as discussed below, it appeared that the majority of GPs are able to identify at least one special clinical interest and that around 16 per cent of them are involved in delivering clinical services related to this interest. Some of these GPs provide in-practice clinical expertise, in areas such as diabetes, family planning, asthma, and minor surgery, whilst others work in acute hospital and community settings, where as well as providing expert opinions and a primary care referral service, they also perform specialized techniques such as gastrointestinal endoscopy and cardiac ultrasonography. The clinical interests and clinical sessions provided by the GPs surveyed in this study[(13)] are shown in Table 1. A further substantial number of GPs provide services in general practitioner and community hospitals; similar models of working are found in the community hospitals in Finland and in rural hospitals in North America, where GPs often have admitting privileges.

Task differentiation

Specialization in general practice will often lead to task differentiation within the professional unit, so that the specialized GP may begin to fulfil the role of

Table 1 Top 10 special clinical interests and special clinical sessions of respondents ($n = 390$)

Clinical interests ($n = 282$)	*n*	%	Clinical sessions ($n = 152$)	*n*	%
Diabetes	57	20	Diabetes	26	17
Dermatology	41	15	Dermatology	16	11
Family planning	34	12	Minor surgery	13	9
Paediatrics	25	9	Family planning	12	8
Gynaecology	25	9	Occupational health	11	7
Minor surgery	23	8	Gynaecology	8	5
Cardiology	20	7	Cardiology	7	5
Psychiatry	18	6	Endoscopy	6	4
Acupuncture	18	6	Acupuncture	6	4
Drug addiction	17	6	Geriatrics, orthopaedics, paediatrics, palliative care sports medicine	5	3

a consultant for his or her colleagues, although the 'mixed portfolio' described above, where GPs spend the majority of their time delivering primary care services and only perhaps 1–3 half-days a week working in their specialist clinical area, enables them to sustain both roles. In a number of countries, many specialized GPs work in group practices or medical centres, facilitating access and interpersonal communication.

The scope of GP specialism

The ways in which GPSCIs will be integrated into health policy development in the future are still developing, and will vary from country to country. In the UK joint work between the Royal Colleges of General Practitioners and Physicians has delineated three types of task which GPSCIs might fulfil, as follows:

1. The provision of a local referral service, in which an opinion is provided to primary care colleagues about a patient referred either within the practice or within the locality. These GPs could be situated either within medical centres or acute hospitals.
2. The provision of a clinical skill or technique. This could include, in the primary care setting, minor surgery, joint injection and possibly ultrasonographic techniques and, in the hospital setting, gastrointestinal endoscopy, cardiac ultrasonography, outpatient hysteroscopy, and other procedures.
3. Coordination of care in a particular clinical area. In this situation the GPSCI would be responsible for working across the primary–secondary care interface to provide an appropriate mix of services for the local population. Examples of this role in the United Kingdom include the 'cancer leads' established to coordinate the care of patients with malignant disease in primary care.

Training and accreditation

Training and accreditation represent significant challenges for GPSCIs, and, again, the solution to these problems will vary from country to country.[14–17] The generic issues are, however, the need to provide a level of training which is acceptable to both primary and secondary care colleagues, to establish an accreditation system based on this training and to assure continuing professional development and, if necessary, re-accreditation. The incorporation of advanced clinical training in existing masters courses and the establishment of new courses, with primary and secondary care contributions, is one approach to this. The more difficult question, however, is the identification and training of 'new' GPSCIs, who may not have spent a prolonged period of time in hospital posts, but who are interested in developing a primary care specialist service. All of these issues demand close working between professional bodies in generalist and specialist medicine.[18–20]

Philosophical concerns

At least three philosophical and theoretical concerns stem from the phenomenon of specialization and task differentiation in primary care. First is the danger to the 'core business' of generalism in general practice, and to the orientation to patients with diseases rather than diseases themselves. There is concern that expertise gained in a specialist field may lead to preoccupation (by fascination) with the disease, reinforced by task differentiation, which may result in consultations where the doctor hardly knows the patient. Continuity of care may be at risk and diagnostic bias may be introduced, strikingly described by the expression 'if your only tool is a hammer, then everything looks like a nail'.

The remedy to both of these concerns probably consists in ensuring that GPs developing special interests continue to maintain a mixed portfolio of work, in which traditional generalist patient care is combined with specialist work. The disruption of continuity of care may be a more difficult problem, and in non-capitated systems may be exacerbated by patients shopping between one doctor and another, depending on the symptoms concerned. This clearly needs to be avoided, and mechanisms need to be put in place to avoid duplication of care and failure of continuity.

A third concern, perhaps more prevalent in European countries than in Australasia and North America, is that of the increasing use of technology in primary care, which some fear may compromise the doctor–patient relationship. Both UK and Dutch general practice have been, almost self-consciously 'low tech', with technology being considered to interfere with the romantic idea that a GP should diagnose without tools, know without study, and treat without appropriate equipment. This is clearly at odds with a more sophisticated concept of the diagnostic and therapeutic role of the GP, essential in rural practice and some of the other settings mentioned earlier. It may be argued, equally, that a closer engagement with patients, through the use of invasive diagnostic and therapeutic technologies, might strengthen, rather than weaken, the doctor–patient relationship.

Professional policy development

Is it possible to develop a generalized policy within primary care on the topic of GP specialism? Should there be incentives for specialization or, on the contrary, some form of discouragement? It is important to realize that specialization in primary care is, as discussed earlier, predominantly a bottom-up development, based on a desire amongst GPs to change, to discover and to sustain skills learnt in other settings.[21] It may also, of course, be a potent remedy for burn-out. Variety and change are likely to be important in ensuring professional refreshment, and there is some evidence that the provision of 'mixed portfolio' job descriptions does indeed enhance recruitment and retention of GPs in health care settings where these have traditionally been problems. Given that patients' access to care and the use of resources may both be improved by the provision of GPSCIs working at an intermediate level in health care systems, it would be inappropriate to discourage specialism within general practice, but it is important to establish a system in which GP specialism is used optimally and produces minimal side-effects.

Optimal use may include the creation of new masters courses, described above, which could lead to a 'critical mass' of GPSCIs which could contribute to raising the standard of care for general practice as a whole. It would be possible to incorporate such courses either during or following on from vocational training, which may itself enhance the attractiveness and innovative appeal of training courses, in which traditional hospital-based components could, perhaps, be replaced by community-based specialist clinical teaching.

Primary care specialist societies have developed quite extensively in the United Kingdom and internationally over the last decade. They involve specialities such as gastroenterology, cardiology, asthma, diabetes, and rheumatology, and are another approach to concentrate and enhance expertise and facilitate professional exchange. At present, over 5000 GPs in the United Kingdom (about 16 per cent) are members of these societies which are able to provide support for postgraduate teaching and continuing professional development and to advise on practice-based diagnostic and therapeutic facilities. Perhaps most importantly they have had a significant effect on the way in which primary care problems are viewed by specialist colleagues, through facilitating interchange and discussion between generalists and specialists.

The most worrying potential side-effects of GP specialization are, perhaps, the development of diagnostic bias and the loss of the generalist frame of reference of patient care.[22] Although there is no easy antidote to this, the 'mixed portfolio' approach described above is likely to be important, and it will also be necessary to attempt to minimize referral of patients to colleagues and to maximize pre-referral consultation between generalists.

Conclusions

In summary, much may be gained by specialization in primary care, with little risk as long as the generalist and long-term dimensions of primary care are retained. Changes in skill mix and the roles of doctors, nurses and other primary care workers are inevitable, and it will be important in the future to maximize the enthusiasms, skills, and expertise of all members of the team. Recruitment and retention of general practice is frequently a problem, and providing new approaches to training and new methods of working is likely to enhance the attractiveness of primary care as a professional option.

Further research, however, is likely to be the key. It is important to find out from patients what they think about seeing another GP or a nurse practitioner, rather than their regular doctor, and to look carefully at the clinical outcomes and health economic consequences of setting up intrapractice, interpractice and other forms of referral systems between generalists and GPSCIs. Each country is likely to have much to learn from others in which different forms of specialization have been developed, and there seems little doubt to us that specialization in primary care deserves further attention in the development of twenty-first century health care policy.

References

1. **Richards, A., Carley, J., Jenkins-Clarke, S., and Richards, D.A.** (2000). Skill mix between nurses and doctors working in primary care-delegation or allocation: a review of the literature. *International Journal of Nursing Studies* **37**, 185–97.
2. **Jenkins-Clarcke, S., Carr-Hill, R., and Dixon, P.** (1998). Teams and seams: skill mix in primary care. *Journal of Advanced Nursing* **28**, 1120–6.
3. **Cornwell, C. and Chiverton, P.** (1997). The Psychiatric Advanced Practice Nurse with prescriptive authority: role development, practice issues and outcome measurement. *Archives of Psychiatric Nursing* **11**, 57–65.
4. **Donaldson, M.S., Yordy, K.D., Lohr, K.N., and Vanselow, N.A.** *Primary Care: America's Health in a New Era.* Washington DC: IOM, National Academy Press, 1996.
5. **IOM 25th Anniversary Symposium:** 2020 Vision. *Health in the 21st Century.* Washington DC: IOM, National Academy Press, 1996.
6. **Phelps, G.** (1994). Adaptability or extinction: trends in generalist and subspecialty medicine. *American Family Physician* **49**, 1055–8.
7. **Donohoe, M.T.** (1998). Comparing generalist and specialist care. Discrepancies, deficiencies and excesses. *Archives of Internal Medicine* **158**, 1596–608.
8. **Lowe, J., Candlish, P., Henry, D., Wlodarccyk, J., and Fletcher, P.** (2000). Specialist or generalist care? A study of the impact of a selective admitting policy for patients with cardiac failure. *International Journal for Quality in Health Care* **12**, 339–45.
9. **Grumbach, K., Selby, J.V., Schittdiel, J.A., and Quesenberry, C.P.** (1999). Quality of primary care practice in a large HMO according to physician specialty. *Health Services Research* **34**, 485–502.
10. **Kearley, K.** (1990). An evaluation of the hospital component of general practice vocational training. *British Journal of General Practice* **40**, 409–14.
11. **Ericsson, K.A., Krampe, R.Th., and Tesch-Römer, C.** (1993). The role of deliberate practice in the acquisition of expert performance. *Psychological Review* **100**, 363–406.
12. **Fox, R.D., Mazmanian, P.E., and Wayne Putman, R.**, ed. *Changing and Learning in the Lives of Physicians.* London: Praeger, 1989.
13. **Jones, R. and Bartholomew, J.** (2002). General practitioners with special clinical interests: a cross-sectional survey. *British Journal of General Practice* **52**, 833–4.
14. **Koppel, J.I. and Pietroni, R.G.** *Higher Professional Education Courses in the United Kingdom* (occasional paper). London: Royal College of General Practitioners, 1991.
15. **Dinant, G.J., Filion-Laporte, L., Op't Root, J., and Crebolder, H.** (1995). The Dutch advanced training programme for general practitioners; an international initiative. *European Journal of General Practice* **1**, 121–3.
16. **Van Zwanenberg, T., Pringle, M.** et al. (2001). The case for strengthening education and training for general practice. *British Journal of General Practice* **51**, 349–50 (editorial).
17. **Crebolder, H. and Op't Root, J.**, ed. The Dutch (experimental) SGO core training for general practitioners. Final reports of the participants. Report, Maastricht University, 1996.
18. **Smith, L.F.G.P.** (1994). Higher professional training in general practice: provision of master's degree courses in the United Kingdom in 1993. *British Medical Journal* **308**, 1679–82.
19. **Peyton, J.W.R.** *Appraisal and Assessment in Medical Practice.* Silver Birches, Heronsgate, Rickmansworth, Herts: Manticore Europe Ltd, 2000.
20. **Peck, C., McCall, M., McLaren, B., and Rotem, T.** (2000). Continuing medical education and continuing professional development: international comparisons. *British Medical Journal* **320**, 432–5.
21. **Thew, R.J.** (1982). Leicestershire: encouraging specialization in a general practice. *British Medical Journal* **284**, 949–51.
22. **Moore, G.** (1992). The case of the disappearing generalist. Does it need to be solved? *The Milbank Quarterly* **70**, 361–79.

8.5 Interprofessional communication

Ron Winkens and Paul Wallace

Working together means acknowledging that all participants bring equally valid knowledge and expertise from their professional and personal experience. Affirmations, acknowledgement and recognition are important, but it is the questions and challenges that arise from the differences that are vital. A diverse group can arrive at a place no individual and no like-minded group would have reached.[1]

Introduction

As long as clinicians treat patients, they need to communicate. They communicate with patients, with colleagues, and with other health care professionals.

Communication is needed to collect information, to provide information, and to learn. Not all problems that primary care professionals encounter can be managed and solved without assistance, and sometimes transitions in care are needed, with the involvement of other health care professionals.

As primary care professionals, we need to communicate with other members of our own profession, with other professionals in primary care such as practice nurses, pharmacists, physiotherapists, home nurses, nurse practitioners, and with specialist colleagues in secondary health care.

Sometimes, primary care professionals communicate via the telephone or through direct personal contact. Such communication can be facilitated by the organization of meetings, in the general practice or elsewhere. For example, physicians may make contact while taking part in continuing medical education meetings. The benefits of becoming familiar with colleagues is likely to be substantial, but unfortunately the evidence is difficult to obtain. Face to face meetings are often not possible or convenient, and in the majority of cases, the transfer of patient information to other professionals is done in writing, as in the case of referral, admission, and discharge letters. The use of facsimile is becoming increasingly widespread, and may be especially helpful in situations where patients need to be triaged or after discharge from hospital, when the primary care professional needs to be informed rapidly of the status of the patient.

To date, however, more sophisticated information communication technologies such as voice mail, e-mail, video-conferencing (telemedicine), and 'store and forward technologies' are available. So far, they have played a relatively minor role in communication between health care professionals, and there is little information in the literature about the impact of such rapid information transfer systems.[(2)] We envisage, however that such technologies will become increasingly important as use of electronic medical record systems becomes more widespread in both primary and secondary care. This chapter is about interprofessional communication of all kinds, discusses different models of communication and the problems related to it in daily practice. It reviews potential solutions and ethical and legal issues related to information sharing. It specifically addresses communication between primary and secondary care, largely in relation to communication between general practitioners (GPs) and specialists.

Problems with interprofessional communication

In daily practice, most primary care professionals will have experienced the negative impact of poor communication, and some may themselves have contributed to these problems. GPs and specialists often do not communicate adequately, and sometimes do not communicate at all. Deficiencies in interprofessional communication may impair the quality of care provided. These may result in the overuse of health care resources, such as the unnecessary ordering of tests or duplication of treatment, with the potential risk of iatrogenic damage. It may also lead to lack of information, an underuse of tests, and to delays in treatment, and it is self-evident that patients may suffer as a result. For example, failure to transfer information effectively between doctors at stages of transition in care may result in patients undergoing unnecessary repeated examinations or diagnostic tests.

Despite the importance of this topic, there is a dearth of reliable data about the influence of the quality of communication between GPs and other primary care professionals. In a Cochrane systematic review by Zwarenstein and Bryant, no studies in primary care were found.[(3)] A number of observational studies on written correspondence found that communication of relevant patient data was frequently inadequate, if not absent. Westerman, for example, found that referral letters by GPs were prompt, but more than half contained insufficient information.[(4)] Discharge information by specialists, though usually comprehensive and complete, often arrived too late or not at all.[(5)] In one Spanish study, GPs received a discharge letter in only one-fourth of cases.[(6)] In another, specific questions raised in referral letters to orthopaedic surgeons were answered only in 44 per cent of cases.[(7)] In his study, Jenkins found a clear relation between the quality of the information provided and the appropriateness of the referral, with the percentage of inappropriate referrals being highest in referral letters with the least information.[(8)] Improved communication has been demonstrated in a hospital setting to have a clear effect on several process outcomes, such as the length of stay after hospital admission. Although these data came from hospital care, the findings may be relevant to primary care as an example of what can be achieved when the level and quality of communication is improved.

As for communication between GPs and non-medical health care professionals, such as nurse practitioners, physiotherapists, and social workers, the need for appropriate communication is even greater, because of the differences in setting, background, patient-related tasks, knowledge, and expertise. This may require the exchange of information on aspects beyond strictly medical issues. Here, the problems of communication are similar to those between physicians, yet strengthened by separate cultures of professional decision-making.[(9)] With the growing importance of shared care in disease management, the different professionals involved will have to communicate more effectively.

Innovative ways of improving standard methods of communicating

There have been many attempts to improve communication. Some of these interventions have been designed to improve the quality and comprehensiveness of the information provided with transitions in care. Others are meant to provide innovative alternatives to the current standard forms of consultation. Some make use of the technological imperative, and rely on the potential of information and communication technologies. Others still aim at changing doctors' attitudes towards communication, in an attempt to find alternatives to traditional methods. A few are presented below.

Standardized referral letters

There have been various attempts to improve the quality of paper-based communication by organizing and structuring the content of letters. In several countries, structured referral letters were developed, including recommendations about what a good referral letter should contain. One example is the standard referral letter developed by the Dutch College of General Practitioners.[(10)] The addition of a note of what the patient understands about the referral should be considered.

It is likely that communication will benefit from referrals containing such data. However, despite the general consensus about the contents of a good referral letter, evidence about the effects on the quality of communication is absent. As lack of time is likely to be the principal reason preventing doctors from providing information at the appropriate level of detail to a colleague, more effective implementation strategies are needed to stimulate the use of standard referral letters.

A prototype referral letter should contain as a minimum:

- personal information about the patient;
- doctor identification;
- signs and symptoms of the patient;
- the reason for referral.

In case of referral to a non-surgical specialty, information should be added:

- data such as test results;
- drug use;
- family history.

Source: Dutch College of General Practitioners[(10)]

Domiciliary visits

A number of methods not involving written communication have evolved to overcome difficulties in communication between GPs and specialists. The domiciliary visit, where the hospital specialist visits the patient at home, sometimes in the presence of the GP, is probably the longest established mode of specialist consultation. In the past, this was commonly used for consultations with specialists in care of the elderly, but because this is time consuming for both the specialist and the GP, it is now rarely used, except when the patient is unable or unwilling to leave home. More recently, specialists have been brought into primary care through the outreach clinic, which in the United Kingdom came into favour during the period of general practice fundholding. Here, practices contracted with specialists through their provider hospital trusts to see patients referred to them within the general practice premises of the referring GP. There was initially much expectation that this would lead to better communication between GPs and specialists, with potential educational as well as clinical benefits, but most studies have indicated that this was rarely achieved because of the lack of GP involvement.[11]

Patient-held records

Where the exchange of information between one health care professional and another is problematic, it is conceivable that more efficient data exchange can be achieved when the data accompany the patient. A good example is the patient-held medical record. The patient-held record has been tried out extensively for many years and several benefits are described in literature, varying from indirect positive effects on the health of patients (e.g. through better adherence to preventive care) to time-savings.[12,13] It seems especially valuable in cases where multiple institutions or health care workers are needed, such as in antenatal care, oncology, and palliative care.[14,15] Clear-cut effects of the patient-held record on the quality of communication have so far not been found, due, at least in part, to the absence of sufficient randomized trials focusing on this subject.[16]

Joint consultations

A promising instrument to improve communication and cooperation between GPs and specialists is the joint consultation, an interesting alternative to the usual referral of patients with problems that GPs cannot handle without the help of a specialist. In this consultation procedure, the GP is present when the patient is seen by a specialist, and responsibility for the care of the patient remains with the GP. Though potentially time consuming, such joint consultations can be especially helpful in the many cases where the GP needs advice from the specialist, rather than to transfer the patient for hospital care. In the Maastricht studies series, the joint consultations were organized as monthly meeting between a group of GPs (four to five) with one specialist in the practice of one of the GPs. During the monthly $1\frac{1}{2}$-h sessions each GP could bring in one or two patients. These patients were re-assessed in the practice, together with the other GPs and the consulting specialist. Such consultations were organized with orthopaedic surgeons, cardiologists, and dermatologists. Overall, the acceptance of the joint consultations was high, and they appeared to have a direct effect on the management of the patient and communication.[17] There was a reduction in the number of patients subsequently referred to specialist care and another effect was that in a large number of cases GPs were capable of managing the patient problem on their own after the joint consultation. A clear spin-off of the joint consultations was an improvement in diagnostic and therapeutic skills of the GPs, and the data also indicated that they helped to overcome difficulties in communication between GPs and specialists.

Solutions from information and communications technologies

Since primary care is characterized by the dispersed nature of the different professionals involved, the major challenge is to achieve the seamless delivery of care to patients across geographical and professional boundaries; information and communication technologies appear to offer some very attractive potential solutions.

Telephones

The use of telephones has been adopted to a very variable degree in different countries, probably in relation to cultural and socio-economic factors.[18] In several countries, national and regional telephone services have been established, manned by nurses who respond to patient calls using clinical protocols.[19] Additional use has been made of the telephone to deal with the follow-up of outpatients and to review patients after their discharge from hospital, and further studies have demonstrated the effectiveness of telephone calls as a means of increasing patient compliance with prescribed medication.

Voice mail

In many countries, the use of voice mail for exchanging information is widespread in daily health care. Voice mail has a potential role in the exchange of patient information in cases of referral and discharge. It allows a rapid exchange of information; if the speed of exchange is combined with prompt feedback, it may be very helpful in triaging patients, in order to reduce waiting lists and to save time of health professionals. In the literature, many descriptive papers, notes, and comments can be found, but surprisingly, trials on the effects of voice mail communication are hard to find. By and large, the published studies on voice mail communication concern those where patients can provide information, for example, to monitor adverse drug effects or to promote self-management for diabetes care.[20]

Electronic mail and store and forward transmission of images

Electronic mail and other electronic messaging systems provide opportunities for different professionals to exchange communications promptly, with the potential for simultaneous transmission to several professionals. This provides substantial potential to improve both the level of communication between professionals and its timeliness. Practical examples are the electronic exchange of laboratory data (test results from laboratory to practice) or the immediate distribution of patient data with little effort in cases of centralized out-of-office-hours primary care centres that now exist in Denmark and the Netherlands.

The transmission of images through electronic networks can be achieved either as real-time transmission of moving pictures, or through 'store and forward' transmission of fixed images. These may be X-rays and other radiological investigations, or actual digital photographs, preferably of high resolution. In primary care, the predominant clinical application is in dermatology, though it has also been used for retinal imaging. Although the transfer of images is technically feasible, first research findings give the impression that the impact of 'remote' specialist consultations through digital images may be limited. The desired effect, fewer patient referrals to outpatient clinics after a triage system via these images plus a quicker referral of those cases where doctors delay has serious consequences, is only partially achieved. For example, in cases of potentially dangerous skin lesions, the dermatologist does not seem to rely sufficiently on the digital image to conclude it is safe enough to wait. In the majority of cases, the specialist still recommends that the patient is referred. This form of telemedicine may be considered at present as promising and feasible from a technical viewpoint, but it is too early to make definitive conclusions about the likely effects on communication and the health status of patients, as was shown in a recent Cochrane review.[21]

Video-conferencing technologies

Video-conferencing technologies make it possible to achieve 'virtual outreach', in which a virtual meeting takes place between patients and different health care professionals, without the necessity for all to travel to the same place. This has potentially great advantages in facilitating communication. The major disadvantage in relation to the store and forward technologies described above is that all the parties need to be present simultaneously, something which for busy health professionals may be very difficult to achieve. A number of rather small-scale studies have been carried out, exploring the potential of teleconferenced medical consultations in a range of clinical areas, including dermatology, orthopaedics, cardiology, and psychiatry.[22] The main finding from these studies was high levels of patient satisfaction, though the validity of these findings has been questioned.[23] Teledermatology has been widely used, though doubt remains about its cost-effectiveness, except over large distances.[24] In Australia and the United States, there is increasing implementation of teleconferencing networks to aid communication between professionals across large distances.[25] In England and Wales, a large multicentre trial has been carried out to assess the effectiveness and economic implications of undertaking virtual outreach for a range of specialty referrals.[26] The trial showed that while this kind of technology may be useful as an alternative to the routine outpatient consultation, its main impact is likely to be restricted to selected types of referral, especially those where advice about management and long-term care is needed, and where there is a limited requirement for the specialist to examine the patient.[27] These consultations may also be very useful for 'triage'.

The electronic health care record

The electronic health care record constitutes a powerful tool to enable pooling of relevant data from different sources relating to a particular patient. Providing that appropriate standards are developed and implemented, such records could in theory be made universally accessible at all points of health care provision, with the potential to extend this further to social care providers. Such systems have the potential to provide all the professionals involved with the ability to access and act on pre-existing information about the patient. They can be generated for use within dedicated clinical care systems (such as the many computer systems now being used across Europe and the United States), but frequently there is inability for the different systems to 'speak to' each other.[28] In addition, there has been a great deal of interest in electronic patient records, employing microchip technologies similar to those of a standard credit card. Although the amount of data that can be stored is limited, these have the advantage of travelling with the patient, and thus being available to all professionals with whom the patient has contact. However, the success of such systems is dependent on adherence to standards, and the availability of electronic reading systems that could deal with different types of cards at all the relevant health care provision points. Finally, there appears to be a real potential to develop web-based health care records. Here, information is posted on a site, either on a dedicated intranet, or on the World Wide Web. Such systems are engineered to ensure that only those with the appropriate permission and rights are able to gain access, but there are complex technical issues in defining and implementing these arrangements, and ensuring confidentiality and security of these records. All of these systems provide major potential advantages, but depend crucially on adequate provision for safeguarding confidentiality, and the willingness and ability of patient and health and social care providers to share information (see below).[29]

Medico-legal and ethical considerations

Given the developments described above, it is inevitable that in the future more and more patient information will be exchanged and stored in different databases. From a medico-legal and ethical viewpoint it may be questioned whether the benefits of the increased exchange of patient data outweigh the negative side-effects that may arise. Sharing of data has a clear and overt function in the primary process of care for the individual patient, as well as in the potential to improve interprofessional joint working in transitions in care. On the other hand, with the growing exchange of information between different health care professionals, there are significant risks involved. First of all there is the question of privacy. There should be guarantees and technical provisions to ensure that exchanged data are available only to those professionals directly involved in the primary process of care for the patient. Passwords and secure exchange protocols are a first prerequisite to ensure this. On the other hand, increased possibilities for data exchange make it likely that more data may be exchanged than strictly necessary. Furthermore, these data can (and often will) be stored in several databases, with the risk of the so-called 'orphan' data.

Uniform guidelines to identify relevant, potentially relevant, and irrelevant data should be assembled first by the professionals involved. Also, patient, organizations should be involved in this development process to ensure that the protocols meet the needs of the doctor and the patient. In the case of patient-held data, the situation is easier. Here, data are kept by the patient, who thus becomes the legitimate custodian. Keeping data with the patients makes it easier for them to exercise control about whether information should be kept or destroyed once it is no longer needed. Gilhooly studied the ethical aspects of the patient-held record and found no drawbacks.[30]

In summary, it may be concluded that, as long as defined criteria are met, there is no medico-legal reason to refrain from increasing the exchange of patient data, especially when the ultimate goal is to improve the quality of care.

Conclusions and recommendations for the future

In this chapter, we have described potentially powerful innovations to improve communication and collaboration. By and large such innovations are still 'under construction' and their use is far from widespread. However, we envisage that, with the inevitable increase in the deployment of electronic information systems in health care, systems will integrate more and more, and it will be easier to exchange data between different health care providers. Written communications, such as referrals, hospital admission requests, test ordering, discharge letters, and prescriptions, will increasingly be undertaken electronically. However, given the importance of personal contact, other ways of communicating such as phones and face-to-face exchanges will continue to be essential. Indeed, personal contact may well become more important and grow, if the barriers between primary care and hospital care gradually fade, and specialists act increasingly as consultants to provide support in disease management for primary care.

References

1. **Davies, C.** (2000). Getting health professionals to work together. *British Medical Journal* **320**, 1021–2.
2. **van der Kam, W.J., Moorman, P.W., and Koppejan-Mulder, M.J.** (2000). Effects of electronic communication in general practice. *International Journal of Medical Information* **60**, 59–70.
3. **Zwarenstein, M. and Bryant, W.** (2001). Interventions to promote collaboration between nurses and doctors (Cochrane Review). In *The Cochrane Library* Issue 2. Oxford: Update Software.
4. **Westerman, R.F., Hull, F.M., Bezemer, P.D., and Gort, G.** (1990). A study of communication between general practitioners and specialists. *British Journal of General Practice* **40**, 445–9.
5. **Branger, P.J., van der Wouden, J.C., Duisterhout, J.S., and van der Lei, J.** (1995). Problems in communication between general practitioners and internal medicine consultants. *Medical Information* **20**, 45–51.
6. **Irazabal Olabarrieta, L. and Gutierrez Ruiz, B.** (1996). Does the communication between primary and secondary levels function? *Atention Primaria* **17**, 376–81.
7. **Jacobs, L.G.H. and Pringle, M.A.** (1990). Referral letters and replies from orthopaedic departments: opportunities missed. *British Medical Journal* **301**, 470–3.

8. **Jenkins, R.M.** (1993). Quality of general practitioner referrals to outpatient departments: assessment by specialists and a general practitioner. *British Journal of General Practice* **43**, 111–13.
9. **Walby, S., Greenwell, J., Mackay, L., and Soothill, K.** *Medicine and Nursing: Professions in a Changing Health Service.* London: Sage, 1994.
10. **Sips, A.J.B.I., Smeele, I., and van der Voort, J.P.M.** (1989). NHG-Standaard de verwijsbrief naar de tweede lijn. *Huisarts Wet* **32**, 102–5.
11. **Bowling, A. and Bond, M.** (2001). A national evaluation of specialists' clinics in primary care settings. *British Journal of General Practice* **51**, 264–70.
12. **Stevens, M.M.** (1992). 'Shuttle sheet': a patient-held medical record for pediatric oncology families. *Medical and Pediatric Oncology* **20**, 330–5.
13. **Dickey, L.L.** (1993). Promoting preventive care with patient-held minirecords: a review. *Patient Education and Counselling* **20**, 37–47.
14. **Liaw, S.T., Radford, A.J., and Maddocks, I.** (1998). The impact of a computer generated patient held health record. *Australian Family Physician* **27** (Suppl. 1S), 39–43.
15. **Finlay, I.G. and Wyatt, P.** (1999). Randomised cross-over study of patient-held records in oncology and palliative care. *Lancet* **353**, 558–9.
16. **Henderson, C. and Laugharne, R.** (2001). Patient held clinical information for people with psychotic illnesses (Cochrane Review). In *The Cochrane Library* Issue 2. Oxford: Update Software.
17. **Vierhout, W.P.M., Knottnerus, J.A., van Ooij, A.** et al. (1995). Effectiveness of joint consultation sessions of general practitioners and orthopaedic surgeons for locomotor-system disorders. *Lancet* **346**, 990–4.
18. **Foster, J.** et al. (1999). Concerns and confidence of general practitioners in providing telephone consultations. *British Medical Journal* **49**, 111–13.
19. **Florin, D. and Rosen, R.** (1999). Evaluating NHS Direct. *British Medical Journal* **319**, 5–6.
20. **Piette, J.D.** (1997). Moving diabetes management from clinic to community: development of a prototype based on automated voice messaging. *Diabetes Education* **23**, 672–80.
21. **Currell, R., Urquhart, C., Wainwright, P., and Lewis, R.** (2001). Telemedicine versus face to face patient care: effects on professional practice and health care outcomes (Cochrane Review). In *The Cochrane Library* Issue 2. Oxford: Update Software.
22. **Perednia, D.M. and Allan, A.M.** (1995). Telemedicine technology and clinical applications. *Journal of the American Medical Association* **273**, 483–8.
23. **Mair, F. and Whitten, P.** (2000). Systematic review of studies of patient satisfaction with telemedicine. *British Medical Journal* **320**, 1517–20.
24. **Wootton, R.** et al. (2000). Multicentre randomised control trial comparing real time teledermatology with conventional outpatient dermatological care: societal cost benefit analysis. *British Medical Journal* **320**, 1252–6.
25. **Yellowlees, P.M.** (2000). Intelligent health systems and third millenium medicine in Australia. *Telemedicine Journal* **6** (2), 197–200.
26. **Wallace, P.G.** et al. (2002). Putting telemedicine to the test; design and performance of a multi-centre randomised controlled trial and economic evaluation of joint tele-consultations. *BMC Family Practice* **3**, 1.
27. **Wallace, P., Haines, A., Harrison, R., Barber, J., Thompson, S.** et al. (2002). Joint teleconsultations (virtual ontreach) versus standard outpatients appointments for patients referred by their general practitioner for a specialist opinion: a randomised trial. *Lancet* **359**, 1961–8.
28. **Branger, P.J.** et al. (1992). Electronic communication between providers of primary and secondary care. *British Medical Journal* **305**, 1068–70.
29. **Luke, S.G., Gallagher, A., and Lloyd, B.W.** (1999). Staff and family attitudes to keeping joint medical and nursing notes at the foot of the bed; questionnaire survey. *British Medical Journal* **319**, 735.
30. **Gilhooly, M.L. and McGhee, S.M.** (1991). Medical records: practicalities and principles of patient possession. *Journal of Medical Ethics* **17**, 138–43.

8.6 Getting beyond disease-specific management

John H. Wasson and Leif I. Solberg

Introduction

What is disease management?

Traditional disease management programmes have been aimed at patients with a single chronic disease condition in an individual practice, a care delivery system, or a managed care plan membership. These programmes typically have contained structured components of care for patients with that disease, often combining four elements:

- practice guidelines (consensus about the best ways to care for a clinical problem);
- care management protocols for nurses and other non-physician care providers to follow those guidelines for treatment, monitoring, and patient self-management;
- supervision of those providers by specialist physicians; and
- health education services for patients.[1]

Disease management programmes were developed because chronic conditions are very costly and the existing quality of care for them is far from ideal. In the United States, for example, non-institutionalized people with chronic illnesses account for 75 per cent of all direct health care expenses.[2] Many studies have documented the continuing failure of usual care settings to match either best practices as identified in clinical guidelines or desirable outcomes. Since disease management programmes have been shown to improve the quality of care and reduce costs, they have been very popular in the United States.[3–5] Some have been established within an existing care delivery system but many have been promoted by entrepreneurial sub-specialty physicians or by proprietary companies.

Why traditional disease management is not enough

Despite its initial promise, disease management is now criticized for three reasons. First, it is focused on a single disease. In diabetes, for example, we have learned that cardiovascular disease is a much more important reason for health care costs, morbidity, and mortality, than is glycaemic control or screening for the usual microvascular complications of diabetes (eye, kidney, and extremity problems).[6] Endocrinologists who lead disease management programmes are not necessarily effective at managing such cardiovascular risk factors or diseases, nor are they particularly appropriate care providers for general preventive services or other medical problems. Furthermore, a disease management programme typically cares for only a subset of patients with the particular chronic condition in a population because disease management is often referral rather than population-based.

Second, disease management is disease- and not patient-centred. For example, most patients with diabetes will have pain, important psychosocial problems, and non-medical needs. Self-management support for the many problems that afflict patients with a disease is often inadequate.

The third criticism is the inherent inefficiency of single disease management programmes. Disease management programmes are additions to the usual care of a primary care clinician. These programmes are not built into everyday primary care practice. As a result, communication breakdowns and conflicts are common. For example, there may be different case managers for each programme, practices and patients may be involved with several programmes, and the programmes may use different expert recommendations and materials.

Despite these limitations, the concepts behind disease management programmes deserve understanding and support by primary care clinicians. After all, within their narrow area of focus, they do work. However, for the reasons listed above, disease management is not enough. In the remaining sections of this chapter, we describe how a busy primary care practice can get beyond the limitations of disease management programmes.

The Planned (Chronic) Care Model

Those who have studied various strategies to improve the quality of medical care over the past 25 years have largely focused on trying to change the behaviour of individual clinicians. There have been so many controlled trials of these strategies that there are nearly 50 systematic reviews of the literature on these trials and at least three overviews of these reviews.[7–10] The general conclusion from all of this work is that passive dissemination of information is generally ineffective, that reminder systems in the course of patient care are the most effective, and that multifaceted interventions seem to be more effective than any single strategy. There is a growing realization that most of these studies may have missed the point, and that is to think systematically about what is needed to foster an informed activated patient, and to make a prepared, proactive practice team efficient and effective.

What might such a systematic approach look like?

The Planned (Chronic) Care Model is based on a comprehensive review of approaches that have been demonstrated in clinical trials to improve clinical outcomes and patient function (see Fig. 1). When a care delivery organization systematically combines key, patient-oriented components of the model to improve the interaction, better patient outcomes are much more likely to follow. Table 1 lists critical components of the Planned Care Model.

An increasing number of medical practices in many countries are implementing various components of the model, although few, if any, have put them all in place as yet. Various health care organizations, governmental bodies, and professional groups are also making efforts to help primary care practices build and implement these components.

Several references[4,5,11,12] describe the Planned Care/Chronic Care Model in greater detail (www.improvingchroniccare.org).

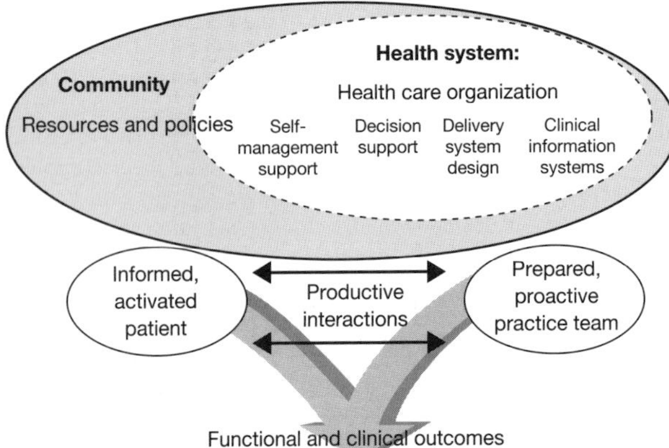

Fig. 1 The Planned (Chronic) Care Model. The critical components of the model support a productive interaction between an informed, activated patient, and a practice team. The effect of a productive interaction is improved patient outcomes; refer to Table 1 for more details of the components. (*From:* Wagner, E.H. (1998). Chronic disease management: what will it take to improve care for chronic illness? *Effective Clinical Practice* **1**, 2–4, with permission.)

Putting planned care into practice

Primary care clinicians are in an ideal position to combine the best components of the Planned Care Model to serve all of their patients' needs. Although some clinicians may assume that the Planned Care Model is too formidable to implement in their practice without many more resources, there is no basis to substantiate such assumptions. In fact, small practices achieve fundamental change easier than large multisite medical groups with their inertia and bureaucratic organizational structures. Whether a practice unit is large or small, three elements of the model are central to transforming the actual care process and are most clearly under the control of the local care system: delivery system design, self-management support, and clinical information systems.

Table 1 Critical components of the Planned Care Model

Health care organization
Include measurable goals for chronic illnesses as part of the organization's business plan
Design benefits to promote good chronic illness care by patients
Create incentives for providers to improve chronic illness care
Use effective improvement strategies that drive comprehensive system change
Senior leaders visibly support improvement in chronic care as an organizational priority
Community resources and policies
Identify effective community patient support programmes and encourage participation
Form partnerships with community organizations and integrate their services into your planned care
Encourage health plans to coordinate their chronic illness guidelines, quality measures, and care resources
Self-management support
Perform standardized assessments of the self-management knowledge, skill, confidence, supports and barriers of your patients with chronic conditions
Emphasize the patient's active and central role in managing their illness
Assure regular collaborative care-planning and assistance with personalized problem-solving
Decision support
Embed evidence-based guidelines into daily practice
Integrate specialist expertise into primary care
Inform patients of guidelines pertinent to their care
Delivery system design
Define roles and delegate tasks so that care becomes a team process
Emphasize and integrate the role of RNs as educators and self-management supporters of patients
Use reminder systems to assure that tests and follow-up occur at desired frequencies
Use the registry or chart labels to take advantage of acute visits for updating chronic illness and prevention needs
Do pre-visit planning, even for same day visits
Be proactive, reaching out to patients who do not visit or who need specific services
Share relevant clinical information (including the care plan) with other team members and the patient
Consider group visits and non-visit care (phone, mail, and e-mail)
Clinical information systems
Establish a continually updated registry that provides both proactive population-based care reminders and summaries for use during encounters for other reasons
Build in care reminders and feedback to both providers and patients
Enable the identification and proactive care of relevant patient sub-groups within the registry
Facilitate individual patient care planning

Delivery system design

As noted in Table 1, there are a number of ways in which the current approach to delivering care can be altered to provide better management of individual patient's diseases. Most involve information management and can be implemented relatively easily if there is an effective reconfiguration of staff roles.

First, registered nurses can take on new tasks such as monitoring patient understanding and self-care, educating, coordinating various resources, and making follow-up phone calls. The results of controlled clinical trials document registered nurse impact for better diabetic control,[13] improved secondary prevention measures in coronary heart patients,[14] reduced smoking rates,[15] and higher rates of recovery from depression and chronic pain.[16–20]

Second, it is important to identify nursing functions that can be done very well by relatively less educated nurses such as Licensed Practical Nurses (LPNs) or non-nurses such as Certified Medical Assistants (CMAs). In current practice, LPNs and CMAs typically prepare patients for the office visit, assist with procedures, provide immunizations, and distribute educational materials as ordered by the clinician. But they can also perform pre-visit review of the chart, questionnaire completion while rooming, and providing or arranging delegated services.

The real challenge is to create an environment in such a way that both the more- and less-trained nurses function with a physician in a well-integrated team that does not fragment care. Fullard et al. in the United Kingdom have successfully been working on this for a long time.[21] There is an extensive literature on the issues surrounding such teams, summarized by Taplin along with a description of how his practice uses this model.[22] Additional information about the organization of optimum teams can be found at www.clinicalmicrosystem.org.

Self-management support

In the early 1990s, only about 50 per cent of the patients with chronic diseases recalled having received any instruction in self-care from their physician.[23] For many important limitations, physician awareness is poor and self-management support remains inadequate. For example, less than 50 per cent of those who are limited by emotional problems report that their clinician is aware and only 60 per cent of those who report an aware clinician report a good explanation about it. Studies that involve direct observation of physicians confirm that when asking patients to make important decisions, they directly ask if the patient has understood the subject of discussion less than 10 per cent of the time.[24]

Patients need knowledge, confidence, and skills to adequately manage their illness. Table 1 lists the behavioural objectives of self-management support. The job of the practice is to optimize co-management of problems with their patients. How might a practice best achieve those objectives?

Some practices still believe that providing self-management support is distributing brochures. However, the mere addition of information is not likely to result in better management and outcomes.

Better is the assignment of a staff member to be 'in charge' of diabetic teaching, nutrition, counselling, etc. But for optimum impact, the information must have a direct and obvious link to effective action. One efficient way to support this linkage is through the expanded role of nurses described above as part of Delivery System Design.

Another proven approach is to take advantage of group visits and thereby empower patients and their peers as the agents for change and sources of useful information. The group may be condition- or population-specific. An optimum group size ranges from 9 to 15 patients and the time frame for sessions is 1.5–2 h. Group visits can be organized for a cohort of patients who spend many sessions together, or they can be held as single sessions. Clinicians, expanded-role nurses, or specially trained peers can supervise group visits.[25,26] For more information about group visits, see www.improvingchroniccare.org.

Clinical information systems

Clinical information systems provide the glue for Planned Care. Large health systems with clinical information systems are often able to generate a registry list of patients' diagnoses, test results, and medications. Clinicians can use such registries to gather data on patient populations, automate reminders, plan care, and track care for individuals and populations. But current clinical information systems are seldom patient-centred.

Web-based 'interaction technology' enables practices to make Planned Care patient-centred. Interaction technology supports:

- Patient preparation for an office visit. The technology directs age- and gender-specific inquiries about symptomatic, functional, and condition-specific needs. Single page chronic condition management forms are tailor-made for the use of individual patients.
- Practice team preparation for an office visit. The technology generates an action-oriented summary of the patient's issues and a summary of the past health care received for these issues.
- Quality improvement. The technology provides immediate, on line cumulative feedback of all patients' response for the clinical staff. For example, a typical practice can generate on line a list of 125 variables for patients aged 19–69. These variables are cross-tabulated by six gender/age groups, income, and six common chronic conditions. The technology also offers options for the clinical staff to customize questions for their patients and invite patients to participate in condition management programmes.[27,28]

Clinical trials have shown that the use of this technology improves the process of care and patient outcomes, particularly when reinforced by clinicians.[20,29] The approach is also applicable for use in schools and cities.[27,30] An example of multilingual (English, Spanish, and several other languages) Web-based support to which practices can refer their patients is www.howsyourhealth.org.

E-mail is another patient-centred technology. However, the practice needs to be very clear about how it will and will not be able to respond to e-mail from its patients (http://www.hippocrates.com/archive/november2000/llfeatures/llfeat_email.html).

A checklist of useful concepts for practice change

Underlying the six groupings of strategies in the Planned Care Model (Fig. 1) and the components listed in Table 1 are several concepts that are as applicable for effective management of disease as they are for clinical preventive services.[31] These concepts constitute a useful checklist for the primary care team that plans on putting Planned Care into practice:

1. take a patient/population viewpoint;
2. integrate care components or processes into one system;
3. take advantage of missed opportunities and reduce waste;
4. use delegation and teamwork;
5. reduce unwanted variation by standardizing; and
6. routinely check progress.

Population viewpoint

A patient-centred viewpoint is fundamental for Planned Care. About 20 per cent of patients in adult practices have moderate or severe pain and 15 per cent have bothersome emotional problems. How does the practice now identify these issues, assist the patient with self-management, offer treatments, and ensure follow-up? How might the practice make care of these types of problems more predictable in the future?

Integrated systems

In the same way that single disease management programmes result in fragmenting the care of patients with chronic diseases, applying unrelated solutions or programmes is at least inefficient and usually less effective than when they are integrated.

An example of how a primary care practice can become accomplished in systems thinking is provided by a Web-based 'Microsystem Action Guide' (www.clinicalmicrosystems.org). It disseminates the principles, processes, and methods used by exemplary health care teams (clinical microsystems) to provide superior care in a cost-effective manner. This workbook enables the primary care practice to redefine team roles, eliminate waste, and improve practice efficiency.

Missed opportunities and waste

As a practice begins to think of itself as a system, it will uncover many forms of waste. For example, many patients with chronic conditions do not have regular visits to monitor and improve their management of their conditions. However, those same patients usually appear more frequently and make other phone contacts for care of acute problems. We have found that healthPartners members with diabetes are seen in their clinic an average of eight times a year, but only two of the visits are for diabetes care follow-up. If clinicians (or more importantly other staff) knew at these other visits that the patient had diabetes too, they could schedule a diabetes visit or arrange for screening tests as needed.

Delegation and teamwork

Since physicians are typically the rate-limiting factor in medical care, and most are primarily oriented toward diagnostic and therapeutic decision-making, the monitoring and education needed by patients with chronic diseases often gets short-shrift. Therefore, using guideline-based standing orders for other staff and interactions with nurses to accomplish desired care goals would be more successful.

Figure 2 illustrates an easy method to blend the traditional roles of certified medical assistants (CMA) and licensed practical nurses (LPN) with interaction technology and planned care. Instead of just checking the patient's weight, blood pressure, or pulse before sending the patient to the physician, the LPN or CMA checks for other important preventive and patient-relevant issues. For patients aged 19–69, the nurse would usually inquire about the presence of three to five common chronic conditions, pain, health habits, feelings, and medication problems. (Examples of Planned Care Vital Sign Forms for common age groups and in several languages can be obtained on www.howsyourhealth.org.)

When an issue is identified during this 'Planned Care Vital Sign' process, the nurse informs the patient about valuable resources for self-management and brings the issue to the attention of the clinician. The clinician is in a powerful position to further reinforce and direct patient self-management. After the clinic visit the Planned Care Vital Sign form is given to the patient as a reminder to use the practice's interaction technology before the next office visit. Figure 2 contrasts usual care to the multiple opportunities this method offers for support of patient self-management.

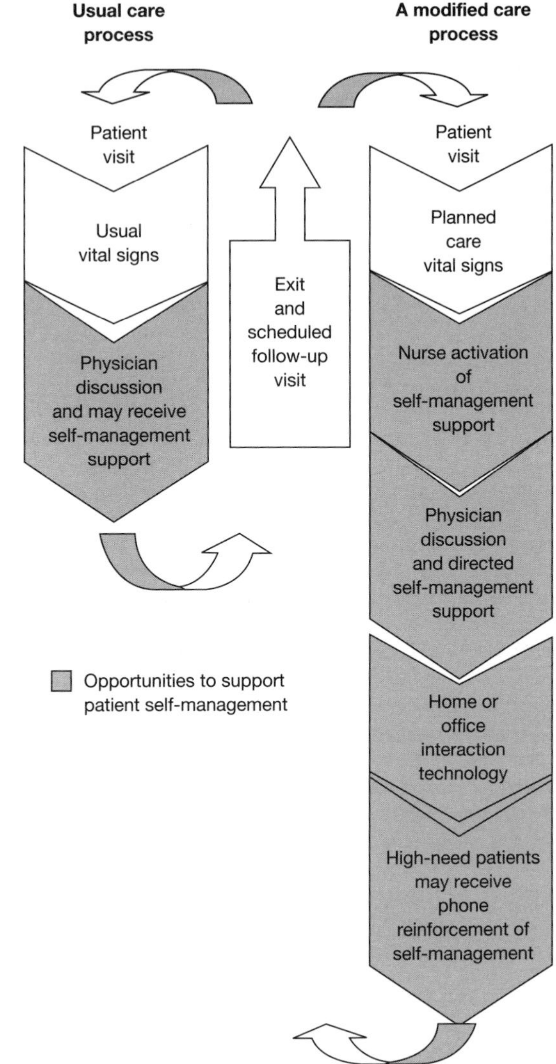

Fig. 2 One easy method to increase opportunities for patient self-management support. This method extends the traditional roles of CMA and LPN and blends this new role with interaction technology and planned care; refer to text for more details about this method.

Standardization

In order to accomplish the conversion to an integrated system of care that takes advantage of every opportunity, uses delegation and teamwork, and adds a proactive population approach to medical care, practices must adopt a degree of standardization of their work.

Guidelines can provide us with an evidence-based basis for intelligent standardization, but moving in this direction will require a broader understanding of the problems of undesirable variation explicitly described by Berwick.[32]

Technology will increasingly enable a standard of care customized to the needs of individual patient. The 'Planned Care Vital Sign' process illustrates how currently available interaction technology can minimize unwanted variation and maximize patient-centred care.

Measurement for process improvement

Planned care requires ongoing evaluation and process improvement.

An easy way to measure progress is to routinely ask a small sample of patients if the new approaches are meeting their needs. Open-ended patient inquiries are particularly helpful because the patients often suggest ways to reduce waste, increase communication, and improve the relevancy of self-management efforts. Formal surveys or interaction technology can also be used to see how the practice is doing. For standard measures of process improvement, readers are urged to visit www.clinicalmicrosystem.org.

Summary

Disease-specific and patient-centred outcomes will improve if the Planned Care Model is built in to everyday primary care practice. To be successful in bringing planned care to their patients, practices must, at a minimum, test different delivery systems designs, routinely support patient self-management, and adopt appropriate information technologies. We also suggest that primary care practices make sure they are:

- taking a patient/population viewpoint;
- integrating care components or processes into one system;
- taking advantage of missed opportunities and reduce waste;
- using delegation and teamwork;
- reducing unwanted variation by standardizing; and
- routinely check progress.

References

1. **Bodenheimer, T.** (1999). Disease management—promises and pitfalls. *New England Journal of Medicine* **340**, 1202–5.
2. **Hoffman, C., Rice, D., and Sung, H.** (1996). Persons with chronic conditions: their prevalence and costs. *Journal of the American Medical Association* **276**, 1473–9.
3. **Rich, M.W., Beckham, V., Wittenberg, C., Leven, C.L., Freedland, K.E., and Carney, R.M.** (1995). A multidisciplinary intervention to prevent the readmission of elderly patients with congestive heart failure. *New England Journal of Medicine* **33**, 1190–5.
4. **Wagner, E.H.** (1998). Chronic disease management: what will it take to improve care for chronic illness? *Effective Clinical Practice* **1**, 2–4.
5. **Wagner, E.H., Davis, C., Schaefer, J., Von Korff, M., and Austin, B.** (1999). A survey of leading chronic disease management programs: are they consistent with the literature? *Managed Care Quarterly* **7**, 56–66.
6. **Gilmer, T.P., O'Connor, P.J., Manning, W.G., and Rush, W.A.** (1997). The cost to health plans of poor glycemic control. *Diabetes Care* **20** (12), 1–7.
7. **Solberg, L.I.** (2000). Guideline implementation: what the literature doesn't tell us. *The Joint Commission Journal on Quality Improvement* **26** (9), 525–37.
8. **Bero, L.A., Grilli, R., Grimshaw, J.M., Harvey, E., Oxman, A.D., and Thomson, M.A.** (1998). Closing the gap between research and practice: an overview of systematic reviews of interventions to promote the implementation of research findings, *British Medical Journal* **317**, 465–8.
9. **NHS Centre for Reviews and Dissemination** (1999). Getting evidence into practice. *Effective Health Care* **5** (1), 1–16.
10. **Grol, R.** (2001). Improving the quality of medical care. *Journal of the American Medical Association* **284**, 2578–85.
11. **Wagner, E.H., Austin, B.T., and Von Korff, M.** (1996). Organizing care for patients with chronic illness. *The Milbank Quarterly* **74**, 511–44.
12. **Von Korff, M., Gruman, J., Schaefer, J., Curry, S.J., and Wagner, E.H.** (1997). Collaborative management of chronic illness. *Annals of Internal Medicine* **127**, 1097–102.
13. **Aubert, R.E.** et al. (1998). Nurse case management to improve glycemic control in diabetic patients in a health maintenance organization. *Annals of Internal Medicine* **129**, 605–12.
14. **Campbell, N.C.** et al. (1998). Secondary prevention in coronary heart disease: a randomised trial of nurse led clinics in primary care. *Heart* **80**, 447–52.
15. **Hollis, J.F., Vogt, T.M., Steven, V., Biglan, A., Severson, H., and Lichtenstein, E.** (1994). The Tobacco Reduction and Cancer Control (TRACC) Program: team approaches to counseling in medical and dental settings. In *Tobacco and the Clinician: Interventions for Medical and Dental Practice* (ed. D.R. Shopland and D.M. Burns), pp. 143–67. Washington DC: National Institutes of Health.
16. **Hunkeler, E.M.** et al. (2000). Efficacy of nurse telehealth care and peer support in augmenting treatment of depression in primary care. *Archives of Family Medicine* **9** (8), 700–8.
17. **Wells, K.B.** et al. (2000). Impact of disseminating quality improvement programs for depression in managed primary care: a randomized controlled trial. *Journal of the American Medical Association* **283**, 212–20.
18. **Rubenstein, L.V.** et al. (1999). Evidence-based care for depression in managed primary care practices. *Health Affairs* **18** (5), 89–105.
19. **Dietrich, A.J.** (2000). The telephone as a new weapon in the battle against depression. *Effective Clinical Practice* **3**, 191–3.
20. **Ahles, T.A.** (2001). Panel-based pain management in primary care. *Journal of Pain and Symptom Management* **22** (1), 584–90.
21. **Fullard, E., Fowler, G., and Gray, M.** (1987). Promoting prevention in primary care: controlled trial of low technology, low cost approach. *British Medical Journal* **294**, 1080–2.
22. **Taplin, S.H., Galvin, M.S., Payne, T., Coole, D., and Wagner, E.** (1998). Putting population-based care into practice: real option or rhetoric. *Journal of the American Board of Family Practice* **11** (2), 116–26.
23. **Kravitz, R.L.** et al. (1993). Recall of recommendations and adherence to advice among patients with chronic medical conditions. *Archives of Internal Medicine* **153**, 1869–78.
24. **Braddock, C.H., Edwards, K.A., Hasenberg, N.M., Laidley, T.L., and Lewinson, W.** (1999). Informed decision-making in outpatient practice: time to get back to basics. *Journal of the American Medical Association* **282**, 2313–20.
25. **Lorig, K.R.** et al. (1999). Evidence suggesting that a chronic disease self-management program can improve health status while reducing hospitalization: a randomized trial. *Medical Care* **37**, 5–14.
26. **Coleman, E.A., Eilertsen, T.B., Kramer, A.M., Magid, D.J., Beck, A., and Conner, D.** (2001). Reducing emergency visits in older adults with chronic illness. *Effective Clinical Practice* **4**, 49–57.
27. **Wasson, J.H. and James, C.** (2001). Implementation of a Web-based interaction technology to improve the quality of a city's health care. *Journal of Alternative and Complementary Medicine* **24**, 1–12.
28. **Wasson, J.H., Jette, A.J., Johnson, D.J., Mohr, J.J., and Nelson, E.C.** (1997). A replicable and customizable approach to improve ambulatory care and research. *Journal of Ambulatory Care Management* **20** (1), 17–27.
29. **Wasson, J.H., Stukel, T.A., Weiss, J.E., Hays, R.D., Jette, A.M., and Nelson, E.C.** (1999). A randomized trial of using patient self-assessment data to improve community practices. *Effective Clinical Practice* **2**, 1–10.
30. **Bracken, A.C., Hersh, A.L., and Johnson, D.J.** (1998). A computerized school-based health assessment with rapid feedback to improve adolescent health. *Clinical Pediatrics* **37**, 677–83.
31. **Solberg, L.I., Kottke, T.E., Brekke, M.L., Conn, S.A., Calomeni, C.A., and Conboy, K.** (1997). Delivering clinical preventive services is a systems problem. *Annals of Behavioral Medicine* **19** (3), 271–8.
32. **Berwick, D.M.** (1991). Controlling variation in health care: a consultation from Walter Shewhart. *Medical Care* **29**, 1212–25.

8.7 Collaboration between professional and lay care

Myrra Vernooij-Dassen and Maaike Dautzenberg

Introduction

Most chronic patients with severe illnesses such as stroke or cancer live in the community, in their own homes. It has been reported that over 80 per cent of the care received by the frail elderly is provided by informal carers: spouses, relatives, friends, and neighbours.[1] Besides informal carers, other voluntary lay carers and a variety of professional carers might be involved in care. Optimizing the collaboration between professional and lay carers offers substantial opportunities for the improvement of the quality of care and, hence, the quality of life of chronically ill patients.

The responsibility for taking care of a frail or sick relative does not fall equally on all informal carers. Usually one informal carer, the primary carer, is mostly involved and takes the overall responsibility for the care. Primary carers prefer to share care responsibilities rather than hand over the care task completely to professional carers. Schneider[2] found that in Europe primary carers of dementia patients received on average 6 h of assistance per week from other lay carers and 4 h of help from professional carers. The professional carers most involved are general practitioners (GPs), community nurses, and home helps. Primary carers not only prefer to share responsibilities, but often opt for a division of tasks between the various types of carers. In particular, care tasks that require higher levels of physical intimacy, such as washing and dressing a patient, are preferably handed over to professional carers.[3]

From a humanitarian point of view, an optimal collaboration between professional and lay care offers substantial opportunities for the improvement of the quality of life of both chronic patients and their primary carers. For both providers and receivers, such a collaboration will enhance feelings of being valued and esteemed and belonging to a network with mutual obligations. From a cost-effectiveness point of view, well-organized cooperation between various carers may shield lay carers from burnout, hence reducing patients' rate of institutionalization.

This chapter focuses on the characteristics of collaboration between professional and lay care, models for collaboration, impediments to collaboration, and opportunities for improving effective collaboration.

Characteristics of the cooperation between professional and lay care

Professional carers cooperate with several types of lay carers: informal carers, volunteers, and patient organizations. Each of these types of collaboration has its own characteristics and problems.

Cooperation with informal carers

The role of GPs includes providing care not only to the patient, but also to the informal carer. Systems theory draws attention to the impact of a patient's disease in the family. Rather than focusing on patients as individuals, it focuses on patients as being part of a system, that is, of their family.[4] Families are considered as a system of interacting personalities and as a system of interacting roles and expectations.[5] Persons depend on each other to a large extent.[6] According to this theory, changes in the life of a family member, for example, becoming a chronically ill patient, have consequences for other family members, especially for the persons acquiring the role of primary carer.

In line with this perspective, the GP has a moral obligation to protect the quality of life of both the individual patient and the lay carers who are part of the patient's system. This causes a duality in the collaboration between GPs and primary carers: collaboration with the primary carer to support the patient, and protection of the primary carer against caregiving stress. This duality might be experienced as conflicting. On the one hand, it is in a GP's interest to encourage maximum input from a lay carer. Family carers are required to assess, monitor, and deliver complex therapeutic interventions such as pain and symptom control, and the administration of complex medical regimens.[7] On the other hand, the GP should ensure that lay carers are not overwhelmed by care tasks. Carers feeling over-burdened and unable to care for the patient are at risk of burnout and depression.[8]

Most GPs indeed may perceive it as their task to manage the problems of primary carers: only 6 per cent of GPs saw *no* role for professionals in helping informal carers without specific medical problems.[9] However, in practice, only 25 per cent were proactive in paying attention to informal carers without medical complaints.[9] The quality of care for chronically ill patients can be improved by a collaboration in which the professional carer is proactive and acknowledges the delicacy of the balance between caring together *with* the primary carer and caring *for* the primary carer.

Cooperation with patient organizations and volunteers

Other groups of potential collaborators in care to be taken into account by professional carers are patient organizations and volunteers. Patient organizations operate from the patient's perspective.[10] Such organizations represent specific patient groups and often their carers too. They are usually organized around one specific type of disease or disability, such as diabetes or COPD. Activities include providing an opportunity for members to contact others in similar situations, advocating on behalf of individual members, campaigning on behalf of members as a group, and providing information to patients, professionals, and citizens.[10,11] Patient organizations organize face-to-face peer groups, but also use information technology to promote contacts. IT services include online support groups, chat groups, news groups, discussion groups, narrative sites, bulletin boards, and mailbases.[11] The new technologies have the potential to enable, liberate, and broaden the social network of patients and carers whose social horizons are very limited, being confined to their homes because of their disease; patients should be advised to make use of them. However, it must also be borne in mind that new technologies have the potential to isolate people. The new technologies have not yet been used widely in new approaches in supporting patients; the value of IT in this respect is yet to be fully tested.[11]

Patient organizations also try to influence national health policy and the laws and regulations that affect the patient groups they represent.[10] In the Netherlands, for example, 220 patient organizations operated and collaborated under the umbrella of a national patient and consumers federation in 2001.[10] They have a strong political influence. Patient organizations have the limitation that they are often not fully representative of their members. White, middle-class perspectives dominate and only a minority of members are active. Another limitation is that although patients may be well aware of patient organizations, their actual involvement in the various activities is often low.[11]

The importance of volunteers has been recognized internationally. The United Nations declared 2001 as the Year of the Volunteer, aiming at the recognition, support, exchange, and promotion of voluntary work. Volunteers do not necessarily lack professional knowledge or skills; they might be retired professionals, or have become experts through experience. Yet, volunteers without adequate training might become overinvolved in care or respond to family situations based on their own experience, which might not be appropriate. GPs might, on the one hand, have a role in protecting patients from volunteers who act inappropriately. On the other hand, it is crucial that professional carers reward volunteers by showing appreciation and respect for their work. Voluntary do not receive any remuneration for their work and rely completely on their intrinsic motivation.

Collaboration of professionals with volunteers in primary care might resemble cooperation with colleagues, for example, collaborating with home care services. However, often there is no real cooperation, it is just bringing patients into contact with voluntary services. Yet, it is important for GPs to be fully aware of the support that local volunteer services can offer to patients and primary carers. The opportunities that are provided by their support in improving the quality of care should be fully utilized.

Models for collaboration between professional and informal care

The models available for promoting collaboration of GPs with informal carers range from a general and comprehensive model that describes all important aspects of collaboration to a specific model that focuses only on the assessment of problems of carers. The general comprehensive model describes a variety of actions to improve the collaboration with carers: (a) conducting periodic assessments of the carer as well as of the patient; (b) using a home-based approach to care and services; (c) providing training to carers, particularly in managing difficult behaviour; (d) validating the role of the carer; and (e) acting as a case manager.[12] This model includes the main elements of caring with and for carers by GPs. However, it might also be perceived as being too time consuming.

Recently, Cohen proposed a more limited approach that seems more feasible. This model comprises three components: education, support for the carer, and assistance in mobilizing support networks.[13] *Education* refers to the provision of information on prognosis and treatment, on financial and living arrangements, and on approaches to common problems that usually occur when caring for a chronically ill patient.[8] Education offers an opportunity for the carer to get more insight into the changes that have occurred because of the patient's deteriorated condition and indicates how the carer might adapt to this new situation. *Support for the carer* usually aims at giving emotional and practical support to carers. A variety of programmes may support carers. The majority is directed at supporting carers of dementia patients. Most effective were those which tailored professional care to the needs of informal carers. It has been reported that they relieved the burden of care and reduced nursing home placements.[14,15] Most programmes are meant to be used by local health services and are not feasible to be used by GPs. Therefore, it is an important task of GPs to provide assistance in *mobilizing support networks*. This is in accordance with their role as gate keepers in health care. GPs should know which services may help carers, including voluntary services, and inform carers accordingly. It is neither necessary nor feasible for GPs to solve all problems of carers themselves.

GPs might be willing to collaborate with carers and consider actions to support them, but it has been reported that it is not the routine of GPs to focus proactively at the needs of carers.[9] Furthermore, GPs often find it difficult to unravel the need for support of carers.[16] Some models offer the opportunity for a systematic investigation of the problems that carers have. Among those models is the Short Sense of Competence Questionnaire (SSCQ), offering the opportunity to identify key caregiving problems and to provide strategies to deal with these problems (Box 1).[17] The SSCQ may help the GP to identify to what extent the carer feels that he/she is able to care for the patient. The SSCQ (seven items) is a shortened version of a larger questionnaire (27 items). In the shorter version, the original structure with three domains of problems of carers has been maintained. The first domain refers to the satisfaction of the carer with the patient as a recipient of care. The second domain refers to the satisfaction of the carer with his/her own performance as a carer. The third domain focuses on the negative consequences that the care task has for the social and personal life of the carer.[5] The SSCQ enables GPs to select the proper strategy for the carer to manage each domain of problems. As shown in Box 1, when a carer indicates that he/she feels manipulated by the patient, the carer needs, in particular, information on the illness-related behaviour and on how to deal with this behaviour. The GP can provide this information or refer to a medical specialist who can give detailed information.

In another model, the carers diagnose their own problems and their needs for support. Carers indicate in a checklist what problems and needs for care they have. This checklist is known as the Problems and Needs in Palliative Care checklist (PNPC),[18] and starts from the viewpoint of the carer rather than that of the professional. An example of problems that may be addressed in the checklist is presented in Box 2. The model applies the following procedure: the carer fills in a checklist at home; the problems and needs for care that are indicated in the checklist are discussed in a next consultation with the GP and actions to meet the needs are discussed. The PNPC proved to be suitable for identifying and prioritizing person-focused problems. Furthermore, it eases communication and screens for hidden problems.[19]

The presented models promote the collaboration between GPs and carers by describing the actions that can be undertaken and by offering tools that can be used easily in the daily routine of GPs.

Box 1 Short Sense of Competence Questionnaire

Short Sense of Competence Questionnaire (SSCQ)	Domain
1. I feel that my . . . behaves the way s/he does to have her/his own way	1
2. I feel that my . . . behaves the way s/he does to annoy me	1
3. I feel that my . . . tries to manipulate me	1
4. I feel strained in my interaction with my . . .	2
5. I wish that my . . . and I had a better relationship	2
6. I feel stressed between my responsibilities for my . . . as well as for my other family members, my job, etc.	3
7. I feel that the present situation with my . . . does not allow me as much privacy as I'd like	3

Strategies for management

Items referring to

- *Domain 1* Lack of satisfaction with the demented person as a recipient of care: clarify how the patient's behaviour is related to the dementia syndrome.
- *Domain 2* Lack of satisfaction with one's own performance as a carer: open a dialogue on expectation of carers, the resources they have access to, and the conflicts they experience.
- *Domain 3* Consequences of involvement in care for the personal life of the carer: define an acceptable level of involvement. Organize additional professional support.

When the problems of a carer are related to the domain 'satisfaction with the patient as a recipient of care', the carer might need more information. The GP can provide this information or refer to a medical specialist who can give detailed information.

Problems related to the carer's own performance, such as feeling strained in the interaction with the patient, can be relieved by the GP providing the carer the opportunity to express what the carer thinks he or she should do. This often includes expressing feelings of guilt and not being able to perform according to their own demands. It also includes helping the carer to reflect on the (im)possibility to act upon their own expectations and resources.

For problems of the carer related to the consequences of the care task for their personal life, the GP may assist in defining acceptable levels of involvement. Furthermore, the GP may organize additional support of professionals, volunteers, and patient organizations.

Impediments to collaboration

Impediments to collaboration between GPs and primary carers can be found both on a micro- and a macro-level. At the micro-level, an obstacle is that informal carers often ignore their own complaints and are reluctant to ask for help until a crisis occurs. Furthermore, GPs are usually not proactive in paying attention to carers.[9] At the macro-level, a special barrier is that most doctors are not trained to pay attention to carers; only 10 per cent of the GPs had received training about issues important for informal carers.[9] These impediments in collaboration between GPs and primary carers are unfortunate, since in many countries GPs are the formal or informal gate keepers of other professional health services. Another problem is that the use of volunteer services in health care and of special programmes to support informal carers depends on the local availability of these services, and these may be absent.

Box 2 An example of problems addressed in the PNPC checklist

Answer categories:
Is this a problem?
Do you want attention for this problem?

- How to bathe and dress the patient and attend to any other of her/his physical needs
- How to deal with the patient's pain
- How to handle the patient's diet
- To know which symptoms of the patient demand my attention
- How to find someone who can take over the care for the patient every now and then
- How to support the patient to fill in and structure daily activities

More specific impediments to the use of collaborative programmes such as shared decision-making and methods for tailoring interventions to the needs of *patients* have also been studied. These barriers may also apply to the use of collaborative programmes with *lay carers*. The barriers to the use of shared decision-making include time constraints, threat to the 'power' relationship between doctor and patient, lack of training of physicians, lack of skill in 'sharing' and 'involving' patients in decision-making, lack of tools to convey information about risks and benefits, and patients disliking 'doctor uncertainty'.[20] The constraints to the use of methods for tailoring interventions to the specific needs of patients are a lack of knowledge of collaborative models and GPs having difficulties in discovering problems and needs for care.[16,20]

Conclusions: opportunities for improving collaboration between professional and lay care

We will conclude this chapter by using elements discussed earlier to build a checklist for successful collaboration between GPs and lay carers (Box 3). The checklist includes the following aspects: focus of care, methods to analyse the problem, and quality improvement methods.

A GP may focus not only on the patient, but also on the carer with regard to the illness experience, their need for support, and preferred treatment. Most GPs would agree to focus on these aspects, but it is not their common practice to focus also on carers' perceived problems or needs for care.

Obviously, the main tool to identify problems for professional carers and, in particular, for GPs, is to listen. For more specific problem analyses the previously mentioned models can be helpful.[17,18] We acknowledge that more tools suitable for other illnesses are needed.

The improvement of quality of care by using methods to respond to problems and needs for care is hampered by pessimism. When cure is no longer possible, physicians often feel they have nothing more to offer.[21] However, a key task of physicians is to offer relief.[22] One effective way of doing this is to start from the point of view that, particularly when major problems occur in chronically ill patients, goals should be limited in scope, concrete, and feasible. GPs may encourage patients and carers to get enough sleep, to meet loved ones, to relieve pain, and so forth.[5] It should be emphasized that mobilizing networks, including volunteers and patient organizations, may improve the quality of care and simultaneously decrease GPs' workload. Even when limited goals are reached, an unbearable situation may change into one where there is still some enjoyment of life.

Last but not least, the responsibility for successful cooperation between professional and lay carers should not rest only on the shoulders of professional carers. Lay carers can also contribute to the collaboration by providing honest and sufficient information and by sharing responsibility for agreements jointly made. The final outcome of successful cooperation might not only be an improvement in the quality of care and the quality of life for patients and lay carers, but also more job satisfaction and enhanced feelings of competence for the professional carers.

Box 3 Checklist for collaboration between professional and lay carers

Professional carer focuses on:

- Collaboration with the carer in order to support the patient and to protect the carer from becoming overburdened
- The objective facts about the condition of the patient *and* the subjective meaning carers attribute to the situation
- Patients' and carers' needs for care and preferences for treatment

Problem analysis by professional carer:

- Listening to patients and primary carers
- Use of tools to detect individual problems and needs for care

Quality improvement methods:

- Education, tailored to the needs of patients and carers (e.g. information on how to deal with patient's behavioural problems)
- Support for carers (e.g in helping to define acceptable goals of involvement)
- Assistance in mobilizing support networks, including volunteers and patient organizations and support from home help services

References

1. **Dautzenberg, M.G.H.** *Daughters Caring for Elderly Parents.* University of Maastricht, 2000.
2. **Schneider, J.** et al. (1999). Eurocare: a cross-national study of co-resident spouse carers for people with Alzheimer's disease: I—factors associated with carer burden. *International Journal of Geriatric Psychiatry* **14**, 651–61.
3. **Stommel, M.** et al. (1995). The impact of the frequency of care activities on the division of labor between primary caregivers and other care providers. *Research on Aging* **17**, 412–33.
4. **Parsons, T.A.** (1958). The kinship system of the contemporary United States. In *Essays in Sociological Theory* (ed. T.A. Parsons), pp. 177–96. Glencoe IL: The Free Press.
5. **Bengtson, V.L. and Kuypers, J.** (1985). The family support cycle: psychosocial issues in the aging family. In *Life-span and Change in a Gerontological Perspective* (ed. J.M.A. Munnichs, E. Dibrich, P. Mussen, and P.G. Coleman), pp. 257–73. New York: Academic Press.
6. **Elias, N.** *Wat is sociologie? (What is Sociology?).* Utrecht/Antwerpen: Het Spectrum, 1972.
7. **Aranda, S.K. and Hayman-White, K.** (2001). Home caregivers of the person with advanced cancer. *Cancer Nursing* **24**, 300–7.
8. **Burns, A. and Rabins, P.** (2000). Carer burden in dementia. *International Journal of Geriatric Psychiatry* **15**, 9–13.
9. **Simon, C. and Kendrich, T.** (2001). Informal carers and the role of general practitioners and district nurses. *British Journal of General Practice* **52**, 655–7.
10. **Nederlandse Patiënten Consumentenfederatie (Dutch Patiënt Federation).** *Gids patiënteninformatie (Guide for Patient Information).* Utrecht, 2001.
11. **Small, N. and Rhodes, P.** *Too Ill to Talk? User Involvement and Palliative Care.* London: Routledge, 2000.
12. **Council on Scientific Affairs A.M.A.** (1993). Physicians and family caregivers. A model for partnership. *Journal of the American Medical Assocation* **269**, 1282–4.
13. **Cohen, C.A., Pringle, D., and LeDuc, L.** (2001). Dementia caregiving: the role of the primary care physician. *Canadian Journal of Neurological Sciences* **28**, 72–6.
14. **Hepburn, K.W.** et al. (2001). Dementia family caregiver training: affecting beliefs about caregiving and caregiver outcomes. *Journal of the American Geriatrics Society* **49**, 450–7.
15. **Vernooij-Dassen, M.J.F.J.** et al. (2000). Prognostic factors of effectiveness of a support program for caregivers of dementia patients. *International Journal of Aging and Human Development* **51**, 259–74.
16. **Vernooij-Dassen, M.J.F.J.** et al. (2000). Quality assessment in general practice trainers. *Medical Education* **34**, 1001–2.
17. **Vernooij-Dassen, M.J.F.J.** (1999). Assessment of caregivers competence in dealing with the burden of caregiving for a dementia patient: a short sense of competence questionnaire (SSCQ) suitable for clinical practice. *Journal of the American Geriatrics Society* **47**, 256–62.
18. **Osse, B.H., Vernooij-Dassen, M.J., Schadé, E., and Grol, R.P.** (2003). Towards a new clinical tool for needs assessment in palliative care of cancer patients; the PNPC instrument. Submitted.

19. **Vernooij-Dassen, M.J.F.J., Osse, B.H.P., Schadé, E., and Grol, R.P.T.M.** (1999). Implementatie van een communicatie instrument in de palliatieve zorg: een pilotstudie in de huisartspraktijk (Implementation of a communication tool in palliative care: a pilot study in general practice). University of Nijmegan.
20. **Elwyn, G., Edwards, A., and Kinnersley, P.** (1999). Shared decision-making in primary care: the neglected second half of the consultation. *British Journal of General Practice* **49**, 477–82.
21. **Van Hout, H.P.J.** et al. (2000). General practitioners on dementia: tasks, practices and obstacles. *Patient Education and Counseling* **39**, 219–25.
22. **Crul, B.J.P. and van Weel, C.** (2001). 'Verlichten: vaak'; aandacht voor palliatieve zorg in Nederland (Providing regular relief; drawing attention to palliative care in the Netherlands). *Nederlands Tijdschrift voor Geneeskunde* **145**, 2011–14.

9

Family medicine

9 Family medicine

9.1 Working with families in primary care

Thomas L. Campbell and Pekka Larivaara

Working with families is one of the defining characteristics of family practice. Despite rapid societal changes in the structure and function of families, the family remains the most important relational unit and provides individuals with their most basic need for physical and emotional safety, health, and well-being. Families are the primary context within which most health problems and illnesses occur. Family members, not health professionals, provide most of the health care for patients. The ability to work effectively with families and use them as a resource in patient care is an essential skill for all primary care physicians.

Family theory and primary health care have developed from two different traditions. The roots of family science are primarily in social sciences and systems theory whereas primary health care has roots mainly in Cartesian biomedicine. The Peckham Experiment in Southeast London was the first concerted effort to provide family-centred care to a community.[1] It was developed in the early 1920s and led to an articulation of family-centred principles, but received little attention in medicine. In Europe, general practitioners' work began to change towards a holistic direction in 1950s when Michael Balint started his revolutionary work with general practitioners.[2] Balint emphasized the importance of the doctor–patient relationship and encouraged GPs to carefully listen to the patient's story and gradually reveal the real reasons for the visit to the doctor. However, the Balint tradition has remained individually oriented and not until 1990s were family issues and systemic perspectives addressed in general practice.[3,4] Some European family therapy pioneers have used a family systems approach in their work with GPs in the 1970s and 1980s.[5]

In the 1930s, the Macy Foundation funded the first study of families and health in the United States. Researchers at Cornell Medical School intensively studied 15 families and their health problems for 2 years. In his book, *Patients have Families*, Richardson describes the research findings and his conclusion:

> The idea of disease as an entity which is limited to one person and can be transmitted to another fades into the background and disease becomes an integral part of the continuous process of living. The family is the unit of illness because it is the unit of living. (ref. 6, p. 76)

In the United States and Canada there has been an increasing interest in the role of the family since the development of the specialty of Family Practice in the late 1960s.[7–9] Family practice has been influenced by family therapy theories and practices.[10,11] Both family practice and family therapy were developed primarily as clinical disciplines in response to the fragmentation and subspecialization in biomedicine and the dominance of psychoanalytic theory in psychiatry.

This chapter will provide an overview of the opportunities and challenges of working with families in primary care. The research on the impact of families on health will be briefly reviewed. The principles and some of the concepts of a family-oriented approach will be addressed. We will conclude with some suggestions for how to work with families in primary care. This chapter also serves as an introduction for this section of the textbook. We have referred the reader to other chapters in the section which cover some of these topics in more detail. We recognize that in some countries and in some settings, economic pressures have shortened the length of visit, making it more difficult to integrate family issues into primary care.

Research on families and health

What is the evidence to support working with families in primary care? A substantial body of research now demonstrates that the family and other intimate social relationships have a powerful influence on all aspects of health, including health promotion, adherence to medical recommendations, management of chronic disease, and overall morbidity and mortality.[12] A growing number of studies have also shown the effectiveness of family interventions for physical disorders.[13]

Family health promotion and risk reduction

The World Health Organization has characterized the family as the 'primary social agent in the promotion of health and well being'. A healthy lifestyle is usually developed, maintained, or changed within the family setting. Behavioural health risk factors cluster within families, as family members tend to share similar diets, physical activities, and use of substances (e.g. tobacco, alcohol, and illicit drugs).[14] Parents' health-related behaviours strongly influence whether a child or adolescent will adopt a healthy behaviour, and family support is an important determinant of an individual's ability to change an unhealthy lifestyle.

Like other health behaviours, the initiation, maintenance, and cessation of smoking is strongly influenced by the family. A teenager who has a parent and older sibling who smokes is five times more likely to smoke than a teenager from a non-smoking family. Smokers are much more likely to marry other smokers, to smoke the same number of cigarettes as their spouses, and to quit at the same time. Smokers who are married to non-smokers or ex-smokers are more likely to quit and to remain abstinent, than smokers who are married to smokers. Supportive behaviours involving cooperative participation, such as talking the smoker out of smoking a cigarette, and reinforcement, such as expressing pleasure at the smoker's efforts to quit, predict successful quitting. Negative behaviours such as nagging the smoker and complaining about the smoking predict relapse.[15]

Nutrition is an obvious family activity. Family members usually share the same diet and ingest similar amounts of salt, calories, cholesterol, and saturated fats. Eating behaviours and obesity can play important homeostatic functions within families, and the family plays an important role in the development and treatment of the major eating disorders, anorexia nervosa, and bulimia. Parents often use food as a reward or punishment for their children. Dietary interventions directed at an individual in the family, often influence the nutrition of other family members. School-based child nutrition programmes have resulted in improvements in the parent's diet, and the wives of men in cardiac risk reduction programmes tend to improve their nutrition as well. Several family-focused cardiac risk factor trials have resulted in healthier lifestyles across the entire family.[16]

This research demonstrates that families influence most health-related behaviours and should encourage primary care physicians to move beyond thinking just about healthy individuals, to promoting healthy families, and directing our prevention efforts at families as well as individuals.

Family stress and support

There is ample research demonstrating that psycho-social factors can affect an individual's susceptibility to disease, whether it is the common cold or cancer. Studies of stress and social support provides convincing evidence that the family is often the most important source of stress or support and has a potent influence on health.

Most of the stressful life events that have been associated with poor health outcomes occur within the family, and 10 of the 15 most stressful events are family events.[17] Children in chronically stressed families have been shown to have higher rates of streptococcal pharyngitis, more frequent respiratory illnesses, visits to the physician, and hospital admissions for a wide range of conditions.

The death of a spouse and divorce are both associated with poor health outcomes. Bereavement is associated with an increased mortality in the surviving spouse, especially for men within the first 6 months. Divorced and widowed individuals have higher death rates than married persons from all diseases. Research in psychoimmunology has demonstrated a decrease in cellular immunity (T-lymphocyte stimulation) during bereavement and poorer immune functioning for divorced or separated individuals.[18] Poor marital quality is associated with both depression and decreased immunity.

An extensive body of research has shown that family and social supports can directly improve health, as well as buffer the adverse effects of stress. In an article in *Science*, sociologist James House reviewed the research on social support and health and concluded:

> The evidence regarding social relationships and health increasingly approximates the evidence in the 1964 Surgeon General's report that established cigarette smoking as a cause or risk factor for mortality and morbidity from a range of diseases. The age-adjusted relative risk ratios are stronger than the relative risks for all cause mortality reported for cigarette smoking.[19]

The relative importance of different aspects of family support may change over the life span. Elderly persons with impaired social supports have two to three times the death rate of those with good supports. The presence and number of living children are the most powerful predictors of survival in the elderly. This finding suggests that adult children become the most important source of social support in older populations.

Family support and family stress, especially bereavement, can have a powerful influence on health and mortality. An understanding of the family and potential sources of stress and support can provide health care professionals with ways to reduce family stress, bolster family supports and improve health.

Families and chronic illness

During the past few decades, there has been an increasing number of studies on the influence of the family on chronic illnesses, including asthma, chronic renal failure, neurological diseases, diabetes, cancer, and others. In most of these studies, family dysfunction is associated with poor coping of patients and family members, lower adherence with medical treatments and adverse health outcomes. More recently, researchers have designed and tested family interventions for chronic illnesses, especially for childhood diseases and family caregivers.[20] Family psycho-education appears to be the most effective type of family intervention for chronic illness. It involves providing information and support to families: information about the chronic illness and how to cope with it; and instrumental and emotional support through family counselling, family support groups, and self-help organizations. This type of intervention has been shown to improve the physical and emotional health of children and their families with diabetes, asthma, sickle cell disease, and cystic fibrosis.

A family intervention with dramatic impact has been used with the family caregivers of patients with Alzheimer's disease. Mittelman developed a programme that included family psycho-educational sessions with individual families and groups of families, on-going family support groups, and crisis counselling for family caregivers.[21] The family caregivers in the group that received this multifaceted intervention had improved physical and mental health, and the patients were placed in a nursing home almost 1 year later than those in the control group, resulting in enormous financial savings. This intervention serves as a model for other family programmes for chronic illness and should be part of the routine care of all dementia patients.

Principles of a family-oriented approach

There are three basic principles for working with families. They are derived from family systems theory, are supported by research, and help guide a family-oriented approach.

A family-oriented approach is based on a biopsychosocial model of health care in which there is an inter-relationship between biological, psychological, and social processes

This approach places the patient and the illness in a larger framework involving multiple systems. The family-oriented physician must recognize and address the psycho-social factors as well as the biomedical factors in understanding a patient and his or her illness. A systems approach emphasizes the interaction among the different levels of the larger systems and the importance of continuous and reciprocal feedback.

The family has an influence on physical and psychological health and well-being

This principle is well supported by research and has important implications for clinical practice. Clinicians must understand how the family can positively and negatively influence health and use the information to improve health care. There are several corollaries to this basic premise:

1. The family is a primary source of many health beliefs and behaviours.
2. The family is an important source of stress and social support.
3. Physical symptoms may have an adaptive function within a family and be maintained by family patterns.

The family is the primary social context in which health care issues are addressed

Although the patient is the primary focus of medical care, the family is often the most important social context that must be understood and considered when delivering health care. It is not useful to think of the family as 'the unit of care'. Family physicians treat individuals within families, not families themselves. They must consider the family context and address family relationships when they influence health problems. This is important whether a physician cares for only one or every member of a family.

Family systems concepts

All families are unique. However, when working with families certain concepts are useful for understanding family structure, functioning, and development. From the systemic point of view, the family is more than the sum of its parts. A change in one family member affects other family members and the family as a whole. The primary care physician often has to address who has the power and authority in the family, often called the *family hierarchy*. When a child holds too much responsibility or power in a family, he or she can be considered *parentified* and at risk for physical and mental health problems. The child might also function as a *scapegoat* in a family where his or her symptoms reflect problems for the family as a whole.

Boundaries, alliances, and coalitions describe the structure of the family and are helpful concepts for working with families. *Boundaries* define a family into functional sub-groups: the marital sub-group, the sub-groups of children and grandparents. If the boundaries are obscure or unclear in the family system, the doctor may expect functional problems and symptoms in family members. An *alliance* occurs when two or more family members are working constructively together and not against someone else, such as a well-functioning parental alliance. On the other hand, a *coalition* results when two or more individuals join together against a third person, such as the coalition of one parent and a child against another parent. A coalition can cross the generational boundaries with a grandparent taking sides with the children against one or both parents.

Family therapists often use the concepts of enmeshment, disengagement, and triangulation. *Enmeshment* and *disengagement* refer to the extremes of family closeness or cohesion. Individuals in enmeshed families have little or no separateness or autonomy and overreact to the thoughts and emotions of other family members. In these families, adolescents and young adults have a difficult time becoming independent and leaving home. Members of enmeshed families are at increased risk for developing psychosomatic symptoms. In disengaged families, individuals are emotionally distant and unresponsive from each other. The fears and concerns are not shared and there is little family support or caregiving for chronically ill family members. *Triangulation* occurs when a family member or health care professional is drawn into a conflict between two other persons. Family members will often attempt to get their family physician to take sides in any family conflict.

Application of a family-oriented approach

Based upon the principles of a family-oriented approach and the research on families and health, one can derive several ways to implement a family systems approach in daily clinical practice. These applications can be used to 'bring the family into family practice'.

Consider the family context of routine visits by using the genogram

The family tree or genogram is the simplest and most efficient method for understanding the family context of a patient encounter.[22] It should be part of the database for every patient. It provides a 'biopsychosocial snapshot' of the patient and family. It also provides crucial information about the family history of serious illnesses and genetic risks. With the development of the 'genetic revolution', the genogram with genetic information will be an essential part of the database for every patient (see Chapter 9.4 for further discussion on the use of the family tree in genetics). Ideally, the genogram should include both genetic and psycho-social information.

The genogram can be started at an initial visit and added to during subsequent encounters. It may be quite simple and only include current household and family history of serious diseases or provide more detailed information about family events and relationships. There are self-administered genograms and computerized genogram programmes that can be part of an electronic medical record.

Use a family-oriented approach when seeing individual patient

Even for the most family-oriented physician, most office visits will be with individual patients and not include family members. The family-oriented individual interview builds and expands upon most individual interviewing approaches, including patient-centred interviewing, by asking questions about context and interpersonal interaction about health and illness behaviours.

Since family physicians meet with individual patients more often than with family members, having a family-oriented interviewing approach to all patients is an important skill. This approach complements a patient-centred approach in which the physician explores the patient's experience of illness, an experience that occurs in a family or relational context. The patient's presenting complaint can be thought of as an entrance or window into understanding the patient in the context of the family. By exploring the patient's symptoms and illness, the physician can learn more about the patient's family, its relationship to the presenting complaint and how the family can be used as resource in treatment.

In addition to using genograms, using family-oriented questions can metaphorically bring the family into the exam room. A key is choosing appropriate questions to learn about the psychosocial and family related issues without the patient feeling that the physician is intruding or suggesting that the problem is 'all in your head'. Some of the more useful questions are:[23]

1. Has anyone else in your family had this problem?
2. What do your family members believe caused the problem or could treat the problem?
3. Who in your family is most concerned about the problem?
4. Along with your illness (or symptoms), have there been any other recent changes in your family?
5. How can your family be helpful to you in dealing with this problem?

These questions can be integrated into a routine 15-min office visit and provide valuable family information relevant to the presenting problem.

Involve family members in routine office visits, when appropriate

Most of physicians' encounters with family members occur when a family member accompanies the patient to a routine office visit. Family members are present during approximately one-third of all office visits. They might also accompany the patient to the physician's office, but remain in the waiting room. Children, adolescents, and the elderly are commonly accompanied by family members to an office visit.

There are many times when a family physician may want to invite another family member to the next office visit. Partners and spouses are routinely invited to prenatal visits. Fathers should be invited to well child visits, especially when the child has a health or behaviour problem. Whenever there is a diagnosis of a serious medical illness or concerns about adherence to medical treatments, it is helpful to invite the patient's spouse or other important family members to come for the next visit. Elderly couples are usually highly dependent on each other. It can be particularly effective and efficient to see them together for their routine visits. Each can provide information on how the other one is doing and help with implementation of treatment recommendations.

The physician must have basic family interviewing skills to effectively deal with family members who accompany the patient to a routine visit. Table 1 includes some guidelines for interviewing family members.

For more serious health or family problems, consider convening a family meeting or conference

Chapter 9.3 addresses some of the indications for a family conference and how to convene and conduct one.

Table 1 Dos and don'ts of family interviewing

Dos
Greet and shake hands with each family member
Affirm the importance of each person's contribution
Recognize and acknowledge any emotions expressed
Encourage family members to be specific
Maintain an empathic and non-critical stance with each person
Emphasize individual and family strengths
Block persistent interruptions
Don'ts
Let any one person monopolize the conversation
Allow family members to speak for each other
Offer advice or interpretations early in a family interview
Breach patient confidentiality
Take sides in a family conflict, unless someone's safety is involved

Adapted with permission from McDaniel et al. *Family Oriented Primary Care* 2nd edn. New York: Springer-Verlag, 2003.

Table 2 When to treat and when to refer

Primary care counselling	Referral to mental health
Coping with new diagnosis	Suicidal or homicidal ideation or behaviour
Adjustment disorders	Psychosis
Crises of limited duration/severity	Physical or sexual abuse
Child behaviour problems	Substance abuse
Mild to moderate depression	Moderate to severe depression
Mild marital or sexual problems	Moderate to severe marital problems
Uncomplicated grief reactions	Multiproblem families
	Problems that do not respond to primary care counselling

Adapted with permission from McDaniel et al. *Family Oriented Primary Care* 2nd edn. New York: Springer-Verlag, 2003.

Develop a collaborative relationship with a family therapist or other mental health professional

About 4.5–10 per cent of patients frequently visit doctors' offices or surgeries.[(24)] These 'heavy users' of medical care constitute about 21–43 per cent of all visits to doctors and these patients' visits are unrelated to the severity of their illnesses. Over-half of these high utilizers have mental health as well as physical health problems and need the holistic, biopsychosocial model based treatment. Heavy users of medical care and other patients with psychiatric and psycho-social problems are difficult for any primary care physician to treat alone and without assistance. Collaboration between primary care physicians and mental health professionals has generated much interest and enthusiasm in recent years.[(25)]

When working alone with a challenging family, it can be difficult to remain neutral and not take sides. A mental health or family therapy co-worker can be a valuable resource for the primary care physician in three ways. The physician may consult with the mental health co-worker about a difficult, confusing or complex patient or family. He/she might want to refer more difficult cases to the therapist or, on occasion see the patient or family together in co-therapy. Co-therapy can be particularly helpful with somatizing patients who may be reluctant to be referred to a therapist.

Family physicians need to know when and how to refer families for family therapy and be skilled at working collaboratively with behavioural health clinicians. The decision to refer a patient or family to a mental health professional will depend upon the severity and chronicity of the problem, the physician's skills and the patient and family's desires. Family physicians with the time, interest and skills in primary care counselling may chose to manage some patients with family and behavioural problems. Table 2 lists the common types of problems that can be managed solely by a family physician and those that should be referred.

Family physicians should develop collaborative relationships with a wide range of behavioural health clinicians in their community, including family therapists. It is harder to get to know behavioural health clinicians who usually do not work in hospital settings where physicians usually develop working relationships with other specialists. The most effective collaboration occurs when the physician and the therapist work as a team at the same site. Whether on- or off-site, regular communication in person, by phone or letter is essential for good integrated care.

Training professionals for collaboration

Traditionally family physicians and therapists have trained separately and have not developed the skills to work effectively together. During the last few decades, there has been growing interest in collaborative models of care in which mental health professionals practice in primary care. In the United States, this movement evolved into an organization, the Collaborative Family Healthcare Association, whose mission is the promotion of family-oriented, collaborative health care. New models of collaboration and training have been developed,[(25)] and traditional health and mental health training programmes are expanding their curricula and clinical training opportunities in this area.

Towards the end of the 1980s in Europe and especially in Finland, many medical educators and GPs believed that instruction in medical schools was too biomedical and ignored the family and psycho-social context of patients' illnesses. Medical school graduates were not adequately trained to deal with their patients' complicated problems.[(24)] In Finland, a 2-year systemic family medicine training programme for experienced GPs was developed in cooperation with several American colleagues. The principles of systemic family medicine and the biopsychosocial model were adopted as the theoretical framework for these training programmes. The primary goal of this training was to enhance GPs' skills in working with families. From 1989 up until now, courses have been taught in several Finnish cities. Evaluation of these programmes demonstrated that the graduates integrated a system-oriented biopsychosocial model into their clinical practices. However, it was difficult for these physicians to change the routines of their health care organization. Therefore the training programme was adapted and implemented at entire health centres. In the autumn of 2000, a 2-year family- and community-oriented training programme for multi-disciplinary teams in health centres was started in the Province of Oulu, Finland.[(26)]

The future of working with families

Advances in medical technology and changes in health care delivery have major implications for families in primary care. Family caregiving, end of life decision-making, and advances in genetics represent new opportunities and challenges for involving families in primary care.

The ageing of the population and changes in our health care delivery system have resulted in a dramatic increase in family caregiving. Unfortunately, adequate services have not been provided to families to manage these increased demands, making it more challenging for families to cope with chronic illness. Caring for a chronically ill family member can be very stressful and burdensome and result in poor physical and mental health for many caregivers. Primary care physicians need to assess how family caregivers are coping and assess their health. Interventions and programmes to assist family caregivers, such as those developed for Alzheimer's disease, need to be developed for other chronic diseases.

As medical advances allow United States to prolong life, more attention has been paid to end of life decision-making. Only recently has the role of the fam-ily in these decisions been addressed. The development of health care proxy laws has allowed patients to identify an individual, usually a close family member, to make medical decisions if the patient is unable to. Very little is known about how patients make these choices, what they discuss with family members, whether family members follow the wishes of the patient and what the impact of end of life decision making has on family relationships. When addressing end of life decisions, primary care physicians must meet with families to elicit their opinions and garner their support.

As discussed in Chapter 9.4, the genetic revolution will have profound effects on the practice of primary care. Physicians will soon have the ability to screen for hundreds of genetic disorders. The impact of genetic technology on families is just beginning to be examined. For example, consider a woman found to carry one of the BRAC genes that puts her at higher risk of breast and ovarian cancer. Should she tell her sisters? What is the impact of testing on the other family members? Should they have been consulted about whether genetic testing should be done, since the results will have major implications for other family members? Genetic counselling not only needs to address the genetic risks of the individual, but the implications for other family members. Primary care physicians will play a critical role in counselling patients and their families about genetic disorders and testing.

One of the unique and distinguishing characteristics of family medicine is its emphasis on the family. No other medical specialty has a family focus or uses a family-oriented approach. Under changing health care systems, there is increasing recognition of the importance and cost-effectiveness of involving the family in all aspects of medical care. New models of care are being developed that emphasize teamwork, prevention and collaboration with patients and their families. A family approach provides a conceptual paradigm, clinical skills, and support from research for an approach to medicine that is consonant with our health care needs in the twenty-first century.

References

1. **Pearse, I.H. and Crocker, L.** *The Peckham Experiment: A Study in the Living Structure of Society.* London: Allen & Unwin, 1943.
2. **Balint, M.** *The Doctor, his Patient, and the Illness.* London: Tavistock Publications, 1957.
3. **Larivaara, P., Vaeisaenen, E., Vaeisaenen, L., and Kiuttu, J.** (1995). Training general practitioners in family systems medicine. *Nordic Journal of Psychiatry* **49** (3), 197.
4. **Launer, J. and Lindsey, C.** (1997). Training for systemic general practice: a new approach from the Tavistock Clinic. *British Journal of General Practice* **47** (420), 453–6.
5. **Andersen, T.** (1987). The general practitioner and consulting psychiatrist as a team with 'stuck' families. *Family Systems Medicine* **5** (4), 481.
6. **Richardson, H.** *Patients have Families.* New York: Commonwealth Fund, 1948.
7. **Medalie, J.** *Family Medicine: Principles and Applications.* Baltimore MD: Williams and Wilkins, Co., 1978.
8. **Doherty, W.J. and Baird, M.A.** *Family Therapy and Family Medicine: Toward the Primary Care of Families.* New York: Guilford Press, 1983.
9. **Christie-Seely, J.** *Working with the Family in Primary Care: A Systems Approach to Health and Illness.* New York: Praeger Press, 1984.
10. **Doherty, W.A. and Campbell, T.L.** *Families and Health.* Beverly Hills CA: Sage Press, 1988.
11. **McDaniel, S.H., Campbell, T.L., and Seaburn, D.B.** *Family-Oriented Primary Care: A Manual for Medical Providers.* New York: Springer-Verlag, 1990.
12. **Campbell, T.L.** (1986). The family's impact on health: A critical review and annotated bibliography. *Family Systems Medicine* **4** (2/3), 135–328.
13. **Campbell, T.L. and Patterson, J.M.** (1995). The effectiveness of family interventions in the treatment of physical illness. *Journal of Marital and Family Therapy* **21** (4), 545–83.
14. **Doherty, W.J. and Campbell, T.L.** *Families and Health.* Thousand Oaks CA: Sage Publications, 1988, p. 159.
15. **Cohen, S. and Lichtenstein, E.** (1990). Partner behaviours that support quitting smoking. *Journal of Consulting & Clinical Psychology* **58** (3), Jun 309.
16. **Knutsen, S.F. and Knutsen, R.** (1991). The Tromso Survey: the Family Intervention study—the effect of intervention on some coronary risk factors and dietary habits, a 6-year follow-up. *Preventive Medicine* **20** (2), 197–212.
17. **Holmes, T.H. and Rahe, R.H.** (1967). The Social Readjustment Rating Scale. *Journal of Psychosomatic Research* **11** (2), 213–18.
18. **Kiecolt-Glaser, J.K., Fisher, L.D., Ogrocki, P., Stout, J.C., Speicher, C.E., and Glaser, R.** (1987). Marital quality, marital disruption, and immune function. *Psychosomatic Medicine* **49** (1), 13–34.
19. **House, J.S., Landis, K.R., and Umberson, D.** (1988). Social relationships and health. *Science* **241** (4865), 540–5.
20. **Weihs, K., Fisher, L., and Baird, M.A.** Families, health and behavior. *Families, Systems & Health* (in press).
21. **Mittelman, M.S., Ferris, S.H., Shulman, E., Steinberg, G., and Levin, B.** (1996). A family intervention to delay nursing home placement of patients with Alzheimer disease. A randomized controlled trial (see comments). *Journal of the American Medical Association* **276** (21), 1725–31.
22. **McGoldrick, M., Gerson, R., and Shellenberger, S.** *Genograms: Assessment and intervention* 2nd edn. New York: W.W. Norton & Co, Inc, 1999.
23. **Cole-Kelly, K. and Seaburn, D.** (1999). Five areas of questioning to promote a family-oriented approach in primary care. *Families, Systems & Health* **17** (3), 348.
24. **Larivaara, P.** Frequent attenders at doctors' surgeries in a Finnish health care center. Acta Universitatis Ouluensis, Oulu, Finland, 1987.
25. **Seaburn, D.B., Lorenz, A., Campbell, T.L., and Winfield, M.A.** (1996). A mother's death: family stories of illness, loss, and healing. *Family Systems Medicine* **14** (2), 207–21.
26. **Taanila, A., Larivaara, P., Korpio, A., and Kalliokoski, R.** (2002). Evaluation of a family-oriented continuing medical education course for general practitioners. *Medical Education* **36**, 248–57.

9.2 Families, health, and cultural diversity

Eliana C. Korin and Patricia Lebensohn

Health professionals all over the world are challenged to provide appropriate care for an increasingly culturally diverse population. Social and demographic changes and political/ethnic upheavals in many nations have caused unexpected waves of migration and dislocation among people and intensified cultural exchange among countries and ethnic groups. Consequently, cross-cultural encounters are becoming increasingly common, if not the norm, in many health care settings all over the world. In this context, a socio-cultural perspective becomes necessary to the practice of medicine, so that physicians can respond appropriately to the needs of a culturally diverse population.

Beliefs and attitudes about health and illness differ greatly among ethnic and socio-cultural groups thus affecting therapeutic relationships, diagnosis, and treatment outcomes. Clinical impasses, such as poor response to treat ment, non-adherence to treatment and doctor–patient–family conflicts, are likely to occur when cultural orientations between patients and their families, physicians and/or the medical system clash. In addition, many legal and administrative medical dilemmas faced by physicians and institutions these days seem to be related to cultural misunderstandings involving patients/families, physicians' values and beliefs, and western health practices. Physicians can minimize such conflicts by increasing their awareness and understanding of the ethnic and socio-cultural groups they serve and by becoming more culturally knowledgeable and skilful.

Learning about culture involves a lifelong and interactive process that includes both discovering other cultures and re-discovering one's own. This process should be complemented by self-awareness, as well as reflection about one's own values, biases, and subjectivities. This chapter will offer a schema or roadmap to guide physicians along a process of cultural examination of the clinical encounter in order to facilitate positive interactions with physician/patient/family and maximize health outcomes. After reviewing the concept of culture and its implications for medical practice, we will focus on discussing how particular challenges or barriers caused by cross-cultural differences are likely to affect the physician–patient–family relationship and the broader management of health problems.

Culture and medicine

Culture can be described as a set of socially learned behaviours, values, and customs that influence the way people think, feel, and act regarding many areas of their lives, including their behaviours and beliefs about health and illness. In addition to cultural heritage, social determinants, such as age, gender, class, race, language, religion, nationality, and sexual orientation among others, are important dimensions of culture. Depending on a particular context, one of these dimensions, or cultural identities, might be more or less significant in determining an action or behaviour. For instance, from a cultural perspective a patient's refusal of a referral for a mammogram could be mostly related to her religious beliefs (religious culture), or to a preference for alternative approaches to care (ethnicity), or to concerns about her health insurance coverage (socio-economic factors), and so on.

Culture also varies among subgroups, among individuals within groups, and over time. A Turkish middle-class immigrant living in England might be more similar to a middle-class Latin American immigrant regarding her health beliefs and practices than another immigrant woman also born in Turkey but coming from a poor background. *Intracultural* differences are as important as are *intercultural* similarities.

Culture is neither seamless nor static. Apparently conflicting beliefs can co-exist in the lives of the same patient or family. For instance, a study on health beliefs and folk models of diabetes in British Bangladeshis showed that while the patients held to strong religious (Muslim) views and explained events in terms of 'God's will', such views did not exclude acceptance of individual responsibility for the illness.(1) A patient from an Indian background may maintain a vegetarian diet at home while allowing a non-vegetarian diet when eating out.

Health professionals need to learn about the predominant values or practices of a particular cultural group or community they serve. However, knowledge about cultural values or practices of a particular ethnic group is useful only as long as it works as a map or framework to generate questions or hypotheses about the patient, and does not become a schema to interpret a specific patient's behaviour or attitude. Descriptions of cultural practices usually describe basic norms for a group but do not explain an individual's behaviour. Cultural assumptions about an ethnic group or patient need to be examined at every encounter as a particular physician interacts with a particular patient to avoid stereotyping.

Culture, family, and illness: case vignette

The following case highlights how family, culture, and health are intertwined realities. More specifically, it illustrates how cross-cultural differences related to values, to communication styles, and also, to notions about families affecting the therapeutic relationship and treatment decisions:

> An European-American physician in the United States approached a 65-year-old woman, an immigrant from Trinidad of African descent, hospitalized with terminal cancer, to tell the patient her diagnosis. However the patient was unwilling to talk about her illness, and deferred treatment decisions to her family. The physician, concerned that the patient was unaware, or in denial of her condition, tried to elicit her daughters' support. To his surprise, they insisted that he not tell their mother the diagnosis.

The family as the unit of care

The doctor in this case was guided by a belief predominant in many Western cultures—and clearly emphasized in United States medicine—where preservation of autonomy is a highly valued principle. Illness is understood mostly as an individual issue: one that should be dealt with mainly by doctors and their individual patients. Because the patient avoided discussing her illness and deferred it to the family, the physician therefore misinterpreted it as denial, ignoring the possibility of other meanings for her reaction. In ethnic or socio-cultural groups, in which values of interdependence and mutuality are predominant, health and illness are most likely considered family matters, not individual issues. The family is an active participant in the treatment process, and often takes charge of treatment decisions for the ill relative. In the face of serious illness, close relatives are expected to protect the patient, who is often shielded from 'bad news'. As we will show below, the patient apparently knew the 'bad news' but delegated to her family the ultimate decisions for her treatment and avoided talking directly about it. An understanding of the patient's and family's cultural beliefs and values regarding illness and health is crucial in order to avoid clinical impasses and to promote appropriate medical care. When the family is involved in the decision-making and treatment plan, there is greater likelihood of avoiding conflicts and promoting the patient's positive responses to treatment.

> Disagreeing with the physician's opinion of the futility of treatment, the patient's daughters insisted that she be given chemotherapy. Later, the physician found out that an older daughter, informally adopted by the patient when a child, was emotionally closer to the patient, and, therefore, more informed about the patient's wishes and more understanding of her illness. Contrary to the physician's impressions, the patient understood her condition to be terminal despite her avoidance of the word 'cancer'. She had expressed her wishes to receive only enough treatment to enable her to return to her country of birth, where she wanted to die. The conflict around the treatment plan was diffused when the physician brought the family together for a conference, explored the reasons behind the younger daughters' requests for more treatment, and invited the adopted daughter to clarify the patients' wishes.

The request for chemotherapy by the daughters was based on their concern that such treatment had been 'denied' because of their mother's socio-economic and insurance status. Disagreements with doctors by patients and families over treatment decisions often reflect mistrust related to possible socio-economic and/or racial discrimination. As patients and families become more socially conscious of patterns of discrimination and exclusion in the helping systems, they might become more guarded in their contacts with professionals. In this case, the physician's openness and interest in understanding their position allowed the family to share previous negative experiences with the health care system and become more trusting of his recommendations.

Defining family

When convening a family meeting, it is important that the physician understands that the definitions of family vary greatly across cultures. In many groups family involves more than blood relatives and encompasses an extended network of relatives and community. In the case above, the physician was initially misled by his culturally limited definition of family, which for him included only the patient's biological daughters. Among patients of African descent, 'fictive kin', those informally adopted by the family for sustained periods, are often considered family, as this case demonstrates. For most Chinese and Vietnamese patients, the family also includes their ancestors, whose legacies are respected and honoured in special family occasions.(2)

Ethnic and socio-cultural groups also vary regarding the organization/prioritization of family relations. This must be considered by the physician when he/she is defining the unit of care or deciding who to call for a meeting. For instance, when dealing with pre-natal care or child care issues, physicians tend to give primacy to the marital dyad. However, in collectivistic cultures, characterized by close family and communal bonds, the marital dyad is not necessarily the centre of family power. In deciding on health or other life matters, a patient might rely more on a parent or on a sibling than on the husband or wife, as the main source of support or decision-making. The influence of the family of origin often takes precedence over the marital dyad or nuclear family. A grandmother's opinion might be more influential than the father's in determining a family's adherence to a sick child's treatment.

Overcoming cross-cultural barriers in the medical encounter

Clinical problems are likely to occur when the physician's and the patient's cultural models clash and when the physician is therefore not able to recognize and negotiate differences. For instance, cases involving a patient's 'poor compliance' with treatment are frequently related to a mismatch with the physician's expectations and values. To avoid misunderstandings, physicians need to examine their own values and beliefs in relation to those of the patient and the family, before attributing a particular meaning to their behaviour. To build trust and confidence in the relationship with a patient/family culturally different from themselves, physicians need to reflect and explore potential areas of differences related to cultural norms, health beliefs, and practices and show sensitivity and flexibility in how to integrate the patient's and their own perspectives. However, trust and confidence can only be built in cross-cultural relationships when physicians acknowledge the patient's culture or include it as part of the clinical dialogue by engaging in a conversation about potential areas of differences.

But how can physicians promote and focus on such dialogue? Self-awareness and reflection about their cultural values, beliefs, and social location is a first requisite, plus a posture of genuine curiosity and 'cultural humility'[3] vis-a-vis the patient's/family's culture.

The following descriptions of the typical areas of physician/patient/family differences that often lead to misunderstandings will assist physicians in how to focus this *self-reflective process* and *cultural dialogue.* When cross-cultural misunderstandings occur, they are usually related to five areas: (a) differences in belief systems; (b) differences in worldviews or normative values; (c) differences of communication styles; (d) differences related to the concept of family; and (e) issues of trust/distrust.

Differences of belief systems in dealing with health and illness

The different ways in which patients and physicians often explain illness are described by Kleinman as *explanatory models for health and illness.*[4]

These models can differ in the following:[5]

1. their beliefs about the cause of their symptoms and illness;
2. what they label as a symptom;
3. how they express discomfort and represent illness;
4. their attitudes and preferences towards seeking help; and
5. the treatment they desire or expect.

There are important differences between the predominant medical model in industrialized societies and the values and beliefs of many patients they served by this model. Western physicians become accultured to the dominant biomedical belief system as they go through their training. They understand the *disease* processes as having a pathophysiological basis, and learn how to diagnose and treat them based on the latest technology or on evidence-based medicine. On the other hand, patients experience *illness,* which represents the personal, interpersonal, and cultural reaction to *disease.* How people perceive, experience, and cope with disease is based on their explanation of sickness, which is shaped both by the social position they occupy and by the systems of meaning available in their culture. When the physician is able to understand and accept the patient's explanatory models of illness, he/she is better equipped to negotiate differences and address the clinical problem.

The differences in the meaning of suffering and disability in many ethnic and socio-cultural groups often conflict with the traditional model in which physicians operate. Most doctors think that treatment should include intervention and that biological anomalies should be corrected. However, some ethnic and socio-cultural groups view disability as a spiritual rather than a physical phenomenon, and might believe that disability itself is a blessing or reward for ancestral tribulations. Suffering is also seen in some groups as redemptive.[6] Among some Christians, for instance, it is considered an experience to be endured rather than avoided.[7] But cultural beliefs are not necessarily rigid; as the patient and family integrate into new social environments, these meanings tend to evolve—or be 'contextualized'—to incorporate new perspectives. For instance, if an immigrant parent is skeptical about treating a child's correctable disability, the physician should explore if some family/parent member in their community might think differently, or if treatment might be accepted under some circumstances. Negotiation between belief systems can occur over time *between* doctors/patients and families, as well as *within* patients, families, and communities.

Table 1 Helpful questions

What do you/your family think caused these symptoms?
What do your friends, family, and other people you know say about your condition?
Do you know anyone else who has the same problem?
Did you learn about the problem from a newspaper, radio, or TV?
What concerns you/your family the most about your problem?

Adapted from Like, R.C. and Steiner, R.P. (1986). Medical anthropology and the family physician. *Family Medicine* **18**, 87–92; and Kleinman, A. *Patients and Healers in the Context of the Culture: An Exploration of the Borderland between Anthropology, Medicine and Psychiatry.* Berkeley: University of California Press, 1980.

Both how an illness is presented, and how people react to it, are largely socio-culturally determined. For instance, recent research suggests that somatization is a very common expression of distress worldwide but that its prevalence and specific features vary considerably among cultures.[8] In contrast to the Western view of a mind/body dichotomy, the distinction between psychological and somatic symptoms is not obvious in many cultures. In many so-called culture-bound syndromes, somatic idioms of distress commonly incorporate somatic, emotional, and also social meanings and are, therefore, truly a biopsychosocial phenomenon that challenges Western medicine's dichotomous conceptualizations. 'Heart distress' among Iranians can be characterized as a culturally determined manifestation of a host of personal and social concerns primarily related to loss and grief.[9] Indeed, the body is an impressive metaphor through which to communicate emotions. The heart, in particular, is a powerful symbol that conveys an array of basic emotions throughout cultures. Somatic symptoms can serve to reconfigure family relationships and other social roles. For instance, a Latina woman's 'ataque de nervios' might be the only means for her to ascertain her authority vis-a-vis her adolescent children.

Socio-cultural differences also influence the 'help-seeking process'. When a patient seeks medical help, and what they expect from the physician, is largely determined by socio-cultural factors. The use of culturally oriented questions (Table 1) to elicit the patient's explanatory model of illness can be most helpful to physicians in eliciting the socio-cultural context of the visit. With regard to treatment, physicians are often unaware of patients' use of herbal remedies, special foods, or traditional healers. Physicians can benefit from learning about alternative forms of healing used by their patients and accepting their use as an adjunct part of treatment. A helpful tool to guide the physician in this process of identification and negotiation of treatment is ETHNIC[10] (Table 2). Many times, the involvement of a religious counsellor or healer can facilitate the medical treatment.

Differences of worldviews or normative values

Most physicians around the world are socialized within a Western medical tradition that is based on a set of assumptions and values informed by ideals of *individualism, autonomy, and self-reliance* (Table 3). In contrast, many

Table 2 ETHNIC: a framework for culturally competent clinical practice

E: Explanation	What do you think may be the reason you have these symptoms? What do friends, family, others say about these symptoms? Do you know anyone else who has had or who has this kind of problem? Have you heard about/read/seen it on TV/radio/newspaper? (If patient cannot offer explanation, ask what most concerns them about their problems)
T: Treatment	What kinds of medicines, home remedies, or other treatments have you tried for this illness? Is there anything you eat, drink, or do (or avoid) on a regular basis to stay healthy? Tell me about it? What kind of treatment are you seeking from me?
H: Healers	Have you sought any advice from alternative/folk healers, friends, or other people (non-doctors) for help with your problems? Tell me about it?
N: Negotiate	Negotiate options that will be *mutually acceptable* to you and your patient and that do not contradict, but rather incorporate your patient's beliefs Ask what are the most important results your patient hopes to achieve from this intervention
I: Intervention	Determine an intervention with your patient. May include incorporation of alternative treatments, spirituality, and healers as well as other cultural practices (e.g. foods eaten or avoided in general, and when sick)
C: Collaboration	Collaborate with the patient, family members, other health care team members, healers, and community resources

From: Levin, S.J., Like, R.C., and Gottlieb, J.E. (2000). ETHNIC: a framework for culturally competent clinical practice. In Appendix: useful clinical interviewing mnemonics. *Patient Care* **34**, 188–9.

Table 3 Common cultural conflicts

Emphasis on the individual	Emphasis on the family
Individualism/autonomy	Communal style
Self-reliance	Interdependence
Direct communication	Indirect communication
Linear relation with professionals	Hierarchical relationships
Valued 'what you do'	Valued 'who you are'

Adapted from Friedman, H.L. (1999). Guest editorial: Culture and adolescent development. *Journal of Adolescent Health* **25**, 1–6.

patients they serve come from collectivistic societies that espouse values of *interdependence and mutuality*. These contrasting views challenge predominant medical notions about confidentiality, decision-making, caregiving, and definitions of the self.

As discussed earlier, in many ethnic and socio-cultural groups illness is both a family and an individual issue as well as a social and personal event. When a family member, such as a spouse or a parent, comes to see a doctor who has been consulted by another family member, he/she might expect the physician to comment on the health condition or agreed-upon treatment plan. The assumption is that the patient's best interests are the same as those of the family or the kinship group, and appropriate treatment is defined in terms of the patient as *a member of* a family or community. The family expects to be recognized as a caregiver and to be given pertinent information.

But how can a physician be sensitive to these cultural values and also be respectful of the principles of autonomy and self-determination advocated in Western medicine? Acknowledging and exploring the family member's concerns but not sharing sensitive information without the patient's authorization might solve this dilemma. As the physician becomes more culturally competent, he/she often anticipates these situations and addresses beforehand the individual patient's preferences regarding family participation in the treatment. This questioning about the patient's views becomes relevant not simply to respect confidentiality but also to assess where a particular patient, or family, is on the *continuum of cultural change*. In other words, the question is: how is this patient/family integrating two sets of differing cultural values as they move in or adjust to a new cultural context?

One of the areas of potential conflict in terms of autonomy/interdependence is medical decision-making. Some patients from a Latino or Asian background may not share the value of patient autonomy in decisions about resuscitation and truth-telling regarding end-of-life issues. In a study by Morrison et al.,[11] 67 per cent of elderly Latino patients believed that health care proxies were not needed (versus 12 per cent whites and 19 per cent of African Americans). Another study found that Korean American (57 per cent) and Mexican American (45 per cent) elderly individuals were more than twice as likely as elderly European Americans (20 per cent) and African Americans (24 per cent) to believe that the family should be the primary decision-maker.[12]

In collectivistic societies, ideals of responsibility for others—especially vulnerable others—and for a group, or community, supersede the ideals of self-interest and autonomy. In many African, Asian, and Latin American cultures, family members are expected to provide assistance and support to their old, frail, and younger members. Findings suggest that African American caregivers, for instance, perceive the provision of care to impaired elders in the families to be less of a burden than do Anglo American caregivers.[13] The institutionalization of disabled or ill relatives is usually avoided within many ethnic and socio-cultural groups and hospice is usually not accepted because accepting care from outsiders may dishonour the dying parents by sending the message to the community that the family is unable to provide adequate care.[7] Interestingly, there is no exact translation for the words *privacy*, *caregiver*, and *assertiveness* in Latin languages.

Anglo and Northern European cultures promote notions of self-fulfilment, self-development, and self-actualization that are based on a concept of the Self as an autonomous entity-seeking. These concepts, which permeate professional theories about human nature, are rendered meaningless in cultures that define the Self as a *relational self:* the Self is only understood in terms of social roles and in the context of social interactions. An individual sense of fulfilment or actualization occurs as a result of positive interactions with others. One is most valued, therefore, by '*what one is*', and not by '*what one does*'. Qualities that stress responsibility for others and affectional ties are valued in cultures that promote interdependence and mutuality among family members. Regarding child-rearing practices, for instance, a parent in an Anglo Saxon culture might discipline a child by reinforcing their performance in a task ('*You did a good job*'); a Latin American parent might prefer to highlight the impact of their behaviour vis-a-vis others ('*People do not like you when you do this*'). Avoiding shame and preserving honour are important related concepts guiding behaviour in many collectivistic cultures. However, when dealing with a particular family, physicians should be careful to examine how that family incorporates its cultural norms along a *value continuum* (see Table 3), in this case, the continuum individual versus communal orientation. It is important to be aware that, depending on their orientation and preferences, an Anglo Saxon family might place greater value on relational responsibility than on individual achievement. Conversely, a Latino family might also stress individual achievement to their children as an important value.

Differences of communication styles

Language barriers and cultural differences in communication styles often lead to multiple misunderstandings among patient, family, and physician. Clinical impasses are sometimes attributed to cultural beliefs when the real problem might be one of poor communication.

In Western cultures, direct, 'honest' communication is often the norm. Yet in collectivistic cultures, the preferred mode of communication tends to be indirect, implicit, or non-verbal. Social harmony and conflict avoidance are important ideals. Many Latinos, for instance, publicly agree—or at least do not disagree—in order 'to get along' and not make others uncomfortable.[14] Conversely, assertiveness, open differences of opinion, and direct demands for clarification are frequently seen as rude or insensitive to others' feelings. For example, many Asians typically understand direct questions as intrusive and are reserved about sharing personal information.[15] Eye contact, taught in most medical interviewing courses as a sign of appropriate communication, is avoided in traditionally oriented cultures—such as many Asian, Latin American, and Native American groups—especially when interacting with authority figures. Direct eye contact might be seen as a sign of hostility or disrespect as opposed to the expression of honesty and trustworthiness. But in the same cultural group or family, two sets of communication styles might co-exist, as individuals acculturate and adopt new ways to communicate. For instance, a younger second-generation immigrant might surprise her physician with her active role in the medical interview when compared to older women in her family.

Expression of emotion is usually regarded positively in certain cultural groups, such as Southern European, Latinos, and Middle Easterners, while Northern Europeans and Asians tend to value stoicism and self-control. In Western cultures, denial is often seen as a deterrent to patients' progression through the grief process. In contrast, denial and repression of emotions are an integral part of other cultures, such as Japanese and other Asian cultures.[16] Western psychological theories that promote the verbalization of feelings in the face of psycho-social stressors conflict with the ways many patients coming from other areas in the world express themselves.

Clearly, it is not possible for physicians to learn about all cultural modes of communication, but increased self-awareness about their own styles and greater attention to their patients' reactions will help them to identify and explore potential areas for misunderstandings.

Attempts with non-Western patients to promote the patient's autonomy might be undermined by some of these patients' views of the doctor's role as the knowledgeable authority. When asked for their own opinions, such patients might be surprised and interpret this gesture as a sign of physician's weakness or insecurity about the proper treatment rather than an expression of consideration and inclusion. A more hierarchical approach in the initial interview might be more effective with some patients. According to their cultural norms, many patients are often unwilling to disagree openly or say no to people in positions of authority. Physicians should, of course, be aware of their position of privilege and power when dealing with any patient. However, this awareness is especially relevant when working with patients from hierarchically oriented cultures or from marginalized groups. A 'yes' from such a patient does not necessarily mean, 'I agree'. To facilitate positive responses to treatment, physicians should not assume a patient's clear understanding of his or her treatment and illness.

In the United States and other Western countries, direct communication and open disclosure of diagnosis and prognosis to patients are advocated as the ethical way to practice. As discussed in the case presented earlier, this approach often conflicts with the patient's and family's beliefs. By avoiding a discussion about her illness, the patient in the case was not necessarily denying the illness; rather, she was dealing with the illness in a less direct way. The custom of avoiding the name of a 'bad' or stigmatizing illness is not uncommon in some groups as a way to promote hope and positive thinking about the patient's condition.[17] Although 'truth-telling' or open disclosure of diagnosis and prognosis is increasingly the norm in Western medicine, in many countries, such as Italy and Japan, physicians and patients are reluctant to tell the patient the diagnosis of a terminal disease, seeing this as a way to protect the ill patient from an additional burden.[18] Many non-Westerners find the Western practice of informed consent to be a burden on the patient, who they believe should, as a consequence of being ill, be relieved of such decision-making responsibilities.[15]

When physicians and patients speak different languages the possibility of miscommunication is significant. Seldom is a professional interpreter available. Instead, the physician often depends on the assistance of an untrained interpreter or family member to translate. The patient often withholds sensitive information when the interpreter is someone they know, and frequently, the interpreter, in attempting to be helpful, merges his/her own views with the patient's verbalizations. Children often become the interpreter for their parents and therefore have access to otherwise privileged information and the private feelings of their parents. This can create disruption of family relations: parental authority is undermined and children become overburdened with responsibilities usually delegated to the elders. The use of professional interpreters—or, if not possible, of telephone translating services—is the best approach when working with a patient who speaks a different language.

Differences related to the concept of family

Illness, disability, and death are universal experiences confronted by families. However, families respond differently to these challenges according to their organization and resources, as well as the circumstances of the particular stressing event. Preferences regarding family arrangements and access to or the availability of resources vary according to socio-cultural factors. Often, when evaluating family reactions to illness, physicians might inadvertently pathologize some behaviours by not taking into account the relational and socio-cultural context in which they occur. Behaviours are evaluated according to the standards of the host culture even if there is conflict between the two sets of standards. Practices that were normative in the culture of origin might be scrutinized if they differ from the dominant culture.[19] For instance, reports of child abuse are sometimes made to authorities without a proper evaluation of the interpersonal and social context in which the parent physically punished the child. A referral to authorities might be inevitable for ethical/legal reasons. However, an understanding of the incident from a family and socio-cultural perspective, and the continuing involvement of the physician with the family, might facilitate a positive outcome.

Family relations in different cultures vary according to preferred levels of connectedness and separateness, gender and generational hierarchies, styles of communication, and problem-solving among family members and outsiders. Strong intergenerational bonds characterize many extended family arrangements in which connectedness is valued over individuation, interdependence over autonomy, and compliance over authority rather than assertion of individual rights and needs. Frail and sick older immigrant family members are often disappointed by the decreased involvement of their adult children in their affairs. They (as well as, sometimes, physicians) misinterpret their children's diminished availability as abandonment rather than adaptive responses to the pressures of daily living and social mobility in a new social context. Elderly depression can be successfully addressed in many cases by facilitating a family dialogue to bring about mutual support and better understanding about these issues.

Family roles, rules, and power dynamics change as families reorganize in the process of cultural transition: a depressed man with uncontrolled hypertension might be having trouble with adjusting to his new role as the main caretaker for his children after his wife has become the primary provider. Supportive ties might become less available because of geographic distance and the multiple demands that must be faced in the process of succeeding in a new environment.

Culture influences the individual and family life-cycle at every stage. The definition of the timing of life-cycle stages and the tasks appropriate at each stage, and the traditions, rituals, and ceremonies that mark life-cycle transitions are determined and shaped by culture.[20] 'Leaving home' or 'empty nest' are not familiar concepts in cultures where children, as they become adults, create new lives differentiated from their parents without necessarily separating themselves emotionally or physically from their family of origin. In many cultures, respect for parents and parent–child involvement are expected throughout life. A physician concerned with a patient with uncontrolled high blood pressure and diabetes might be more successful in motivating self-care behaviours by telling the patient that 'your children need you to be well' than by suggesting that she 'focus on her needs and be less concerned with her (adult) children'.

Families and individuals are especially vulnerable at times of life transitions, which often trigger family conflicts and symptoms. But problems are amplified when cultural transitions overlap with life-cycle transitions.[21] For instance, in families whose cultures of origin are distinct from the dominant culture, cultural clashes tend to exacerbate intergenerational conflicts when parents and adolescents become polarized between the two sets of values. These conflicts are often expressed through adolescent acting-out behaviours, such as suicidal attempts and risky sexual activity, in addition to depression and somatization. The intergenerational conflict needs to be understood in the context of cultural transition and reframed or interpreted as it relates to cultural differences between the host and culture of origin. With this approach, mutual blame and hostility can be diffused.

The experience of migration affects and can alter a family's developmental progression by changing its structure and dynamics as it forces separations from loved ones, postpones reunions, and creates other family disruptions. Many somatic and psycho-social symptoms presented in medical clinics are responses to feelings of loss, grief, and anxiety, as well as to experiences of trauma caused by the migration process. The reasons and circumstances of migration need to be explored by the physician, as they affect family relations and be related to psychological and physical symptoms. Families migrate for many reasons: political, economic, personal, etc., and not all family members necessarily chose to immigrate. In any case, the meaning that people give to their migration and the experiences they have in the host country will largely determine how they deal with migration stressors.

Among immigrant families, intergenerational and gender-based family conflicts often emerge as the family struggles to negotiate values while adapting to the new culture. Physicians often find themselves caught in these conflicts as they mediate between acting-out adolescents and parents, or between unhappy spouses. Some typical clinical presentations are: parents bringing their daughter to the doctor to check if she is still a virgin; a patient complaining of her husband's increased alcohol use after she took a job; or a husband blaming the wife for supporting the children's new social pursuits. Reframing the family problem as a cultural conflict, and examining together with the family the differing cultural norms of the cultures in question, helps to diffuse blame and bring about understanding.

The use of the *genogram*,[22] with a focus on developmental and cultural transitions and multigenerational legacies, can be a useful tool when working with immigrant families. It can serve to reinforce the therapeutic alliance as the patient and family feel their culture and migration experiences validated—and depathologized—by the physician. Moreover, it can encourage individual patients and families to gain a new perspective into their problems as they are examined within a historical and developmental context.

Issues of trust and distrust

There is an implicit assumption in each clinical encounter that the patient will be essentially receptive to the physician's views and recommendations. However, when socio-cultural differences are present in the clinical relationship, this is not necessarily the case. Because of past and on-going experiences of discrimination in their dealings with some professionals and health care systems, some socio-cultural groups might not be ready to establish an initial trusting relationship with their physicians. For example, an ethnographic study examining attitudes of older people from diverse ethnic backgrounds documented that African Americans expressed 'distrust toward the health care system and a fear that health care was based on one's ability to pay' (ref. 23, p. 1779). Misunderstandings regarding treatment recommendations, poor responses to treatment, refusal to participate in research trials, and other behaviours might represent self-protective responses against the possibility of discrimination.

In recent years, disparities in health and access to health care have become increasingly recognized among racial and ethnic minorities, women, homosexuals, and the elderly.[24] For instance, African Americans, when compared with white Americans have less access to coronary angiography, thrombolysis, and coronary angioplasty.[25] Similarly, other studies on treatment for lung cancer, pain management, access to medications, and some treatment modalities have also shown patterns of discrimination.[25] Health care for ethnic and racial minorities, the poor, and the elderly is different and, in some cases, less than optimal than care available to more socially and economically privileged groups. Mortality and morbidity are more prevalent among disadvantaged groups due to social and environmental disparities.[26]

In conclusion, it is important to consider structural factors *other than* cultural ones in the effort to understand patients'/families' *and* physicians' behaviours and attitudes, in order to avoid clinical impasses and improve health outcomes. Cultural competence, then, involves the consideration of many socio-cultural dimensions involving patients, physicians, institutions, and society in general. The challenge for the physician is to determine which socio-cultural dimensions might be more or less relevant to a particular clinical context.

Finally, it is important to be reminded that the best learning always comes from the best teachers: our patients.

Acknowledgements

We thank Robert Like, MD, MS, and Victoria Gorski, MD, for their valuable comments on an earlier version of this manuscript.

References

1. **Greenhalgh, T., Helman, C.G., and Chowdhury, A.M.** (1998). Health beliefs and folk models in British Bangladeshis: a qualitative study. *British Medical Journal* **316**, 878–83.
2. **McGoldrick, M. and Giordano, J.** (1996). Overview: ethnicity and family therapy. In *Ethnicity and Family Therapy* 2nd edn. (ed. M. McGoldrick, J. Giordano, and J.K. Pearce), pp. 1–27. New York: Guilford Press.
3. **Tervalon, M. and Murray Garcia, J.** (1998). Cultural humility versus cultural competence: a critical distinction in defining physician training outcomes in multicultural education. *Journal for Health Care of the Poor and Underserved* **9**, 117–24.
4. **Kleinman, A.** *Patients and Healers in the Context of Culture: An Exploration of the Borderland between Anthropology, Medicine, and Psychiatry*. Berkeley: University of California Press, 1980.
5. **Helman, C.G.** *Culture, Health and Illness* 4th edn. Oxford: Oxford University Press, 2000.
6. **Crawley, L.** et al. (2000). Palliative and end-of-life care in the African-American community. *Journal of the American Medical Association* **284**, 2518–21.
7. **Kagawa-Singer, M. and Blackhall, L.** (2001). Negotiating cross-cultural issues at the end-of-life. *Journal of the American Medical Association* **286**, 2993–3001.
8. **Kirmayer, L. and Younge, A.** (1998). Culture and somatization: clinical, epidemiological, and ethnographic perspectives. *Psychosomatic Medicine* **60**, 420–30.
9. **Good, B.J.** (1977). The heart of what's the matter: the semantics of illness in Iran. *Cultural Medicine and Psychiatry* **1**, 25–58.
10. **Levin, S.J., Like, R.C., and Gottlieb, J.E.** (2000). ETHNIC: a framework for culturally competent clinical practice. In Appendix: useful interviewing mnemonics. *Patient Care* **34**, 188–9.
11. **Morrison, S.R.** et al. (1998). Barriers to completion of health care proxies: an examination of ethnic differences. *Archives of Internal Medicine* **158**, 2493–7.
12. **Blackhall, L.J.** et al. (1995). Ethnicity and attitudes towards patient autonomy. *Journal of the American Medical Association* **274**, 820–5.
13. **Haley, W.E.** et al. (1996). Appraisal, coping, and social support as mediators of well-being in Black and White family caregivers of patients of Alzheimer's disease. *Journal of Counseling and Clinical Psychology* **64**, 121–9.
14. **Falicov, C.J.** *Latino Families in Therapy: A Guide for Multicultural Practice*. New York: The Guilford Press, 1998.
15. **Heitman, E.** (1993). Cultural diversity and the clinical encounter: intercultural dialogue in multi-ethnic patient care. In *Theological Analyses of the Clinical Encounter* (ed. G.P. McKenny and J.R. Sande), pp. 203–23. Dordrecht: Kluwer Academic Publishers.

16. **Pickett, M.** (1993). Cultural awareness in the context of terminal illness. *Cancer Nursing* **16**, 102–6.
17. **Beyene, Y.** (1992). Medical disclosure and refugees: telling the bad news to Ethiopian patients. *Western Journal of Medicine* **157**, 328–32.
18. **Holland, J.C.** (1987). An international survey of physician attitude and practice in regarding to revealing the diagnosis of cancer. *Cancer Investigation* **5**, 151–4.
19. **Patcher, L.M. and Harwood, R.L.** (1996). Culture and child behavior and psychosocial development. *Developmental and Behavioral Pediatrics* **17**, 191–8.
20. **Carter, B. and McGoldrick, M.**, ed. *The Expanded Family Life Cycle: Individual, Family, and Social Perspectives* 3rd edn. New York: Allyn and Bacon, 1999.
21. **Korin, E.C., McGoldrick, M., and Watson, W.** (2002). The individual and family life cycle. In *Fundamentals of Clinical Practice* 2nd edn. (ed. M. Mengel, W. Holleman, and S. Fields), pp. 19–45. New York: Kluwer/Plenum Press.
22. **McGoldrick, M., Gerson, R., and Shellenberger, S.** *Genograms: Assessment and Intervention* 2nd edn. New York: W.W. Norton & Company, 1998.
23. **Blackhall, L.J.** et al. (1999). Ethnicity and attitudes towards life sustaining technology. *Social Science and Medicine* **48**, 1779–89.
24. **Kerridge, I.H.** et al. (2001). Discrimination in medicine: the uncertain role of values. *Internal Medicine Journal* **31**, 541–3.
25. **Crawley, L.** (2001). Palliative care in African American communities. *Innovations in End-of-Life Care* (http://www.edc.org/lastfacts). Accessibility verified, 3 January, 2002.
26. **Krieger, N.** (1993). Analysing socioeconomic and racial/ethnic patterns in health care. *American Journal of Public Health* **83**, 1086–7.

9.3 Family interviewing and assessment

Macaran A. Baird and Alon P.A. Margalit

Why involve families?

Prior chapters have reviewed many reasons why primary care physicians usefully involve family members directly in the care of individual patients. The usual medical interview involving only the physician and patient is similar to an optical illusion since the individual patient is really part of a family system always present in one way or another. This is 'the illusion of the dyad in medical practice'. The family's influence is powerful and similar to a 'ghost in the room'. Doherty and Baird have labelled this the 'therapeutic triangle' in medicine (Fig. 1).[1]

Families are almost always involved in some way when any family member is ill and/or is seeking health care services as explained in earlier chapters. Although families are not always involved directly in the physician–patient discussion except immediately following surgical procedures, there are many opportunities in ambulatory and hospital care when families are available in the waiting room and could be invited to join the medical interview in a productive manner. If physicians are skilled and confident about formal and informal family interviews, they may take advantage of this family resource to improve the care of the patient. In many instances, the family member might simply accompany an ageing parent, a spouse, or an adolescent on a routine visit. For example, parents are present for almost all child visits. Therefore, families are present in up to 30 per cent of routine primary care visits. This chapter will explore some practical issues involved when families are part of the medical interview.

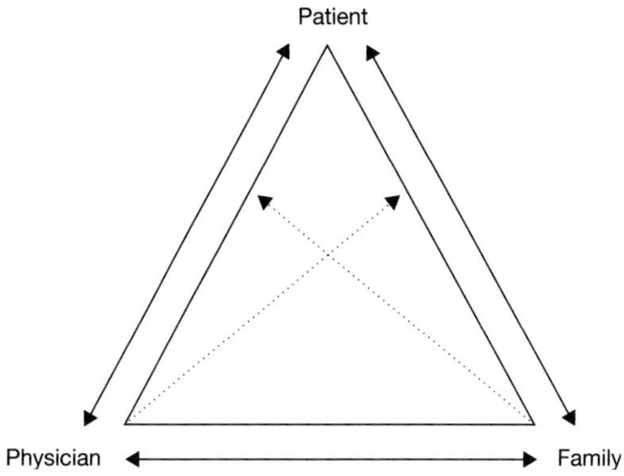

Fig. 1 The therapeutic triangle in medicine.[1]

Individual interviewing methods that elicit family themes

On many occasions, the physician is faced with a need to understand the family influences and context of the individual patient but does not have the opportunity for a family interview. The most common way to introduce family themes into the individual interview is to create a genogram. This 'family tree' or 'family map' can be done briefly to gather medical information in a family context or can be used in detail to explore family dynamics.[2] Using a genogram routinely with patients improves the primary care physician's understanding of family themes important to the individual patient (see Chapter 9.4).

Another interviewing technique designed to elicit family themes is to ask the individual patient to answer in place of others. This introduces the idea of family involvement in a non-threatening manner. These are often called 'circular questions' in that they have no correct answer.[3,4] Such questions invite the patient to hypothesize about the perspectives of others in the family regarding the patient's condition. The accuracy of these hypothesized views is not important. Such questions and the resulting answers help the physician to construct a therapeutic suggestion that will fit the patient as well as the family.

For example: *If your wife were here what would she say about this problem?* Some family members' opinions are more influential than others. Doherty and Baird[1] used the term 'informal family health advisor' to describe that person within the family or close social network who has high credibility regarding matters of health. This influential person has the ability to support or undermine the physician's recommendations.

When to ask for a family interview?

Primary care physicians seek ways to involve family members in the care of individual patients when that option contributes to improved care. This is done to understand more completely individual patients and how best to diagnose and manage the patient's complaint. For example, the physician may want to gain a more accurate diagnosis of a behavioural problem, or want to improve the patient's ability to adhere to the medical or surgical treatment. Sometimes, the primary care physician needs to enlist the patient's family or very close friends to facilitate coping with a chronic or serious acute illness. A family interview can help enormously when the physician needs to ensure that the diagnosis or treatment is fully understood by everyone involved in the patient's life, or when the psycho-social dimension of a medical problem is an influential part of the treatment or

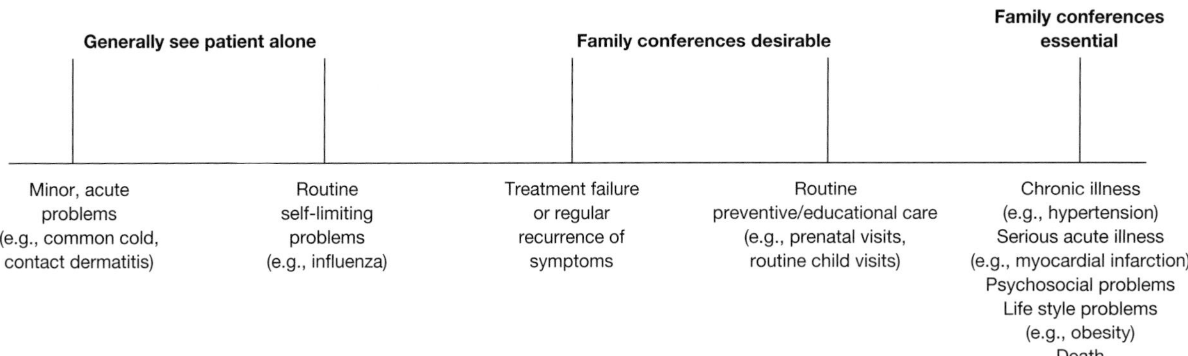

Fig. 2 When to assemble the family.[1]

diagnostic plan.[5] There is a spectrum of indications for direct family involvement as noted in Fig. 2.

How and whom to invite

The physician must have permission from the individual patient to invite anyone else into the next interview. Most patients would agree to include one or more family members to join the medical interview if this expansion of the interaction was perceived as sensible. A straightforward approach works best when the inviting physician addresses logical questions related to gaining permission to involve families such as: Which member to invite? How to invite them? Should the whole family be invited? Should children be included?

Sometimes, there is no need for a formal invitation. As noted above, patients are often accompanied by a family member. The presence of another family member in the waiting room is an important clue for the physician. The physician may refer to this clue by simply asking for the patient's permission to invite the family member to join the patient in the examination room, or by discussing with the patient the significance of this family member in this clinic visit. Adult children who are accompanying an ill and ageing parent might suggest the possibility of an exhausted young parent who does not have enough support at home to care for the older parent (grandparent) as well as balance caring for young children or active adolescents. This 'middle' generation or 'squeezed' generation faces many strains in today's busy world. Sometimes, generational boundaries are blurred due to illness, divorce, or economic challenges. When a spouse accompanies the patient it may imply support or can raise the possibility of family anxiety regarding the patient's health. A parent still supervising the visit of a young adult may suggest parental difficulty with 'letting go' of the young adult or persistent dependence of the young adult on parental reassurance. In some instances both themes would be mutually reinforcing. The physician alert to these possibilities would want to clarify the significance of the parental presence rather than assume any meaning. A skilled family interview would be one way to gain an understanding of the family dynamics for any of these situations.

Many studies [1,2,6–10] point out that inviting the relevant family members shortens the road to satisfactory treatment. Involving families empowers the family and improves cooperation between physician and patient. It helps the primary care physician to be a better physician for the patient. Sometimes, there is a need for an invitation for a family meeting. The invitation can be direct and simple.

For example: The physician was discussing weight loss with a female patient. While constructing her genogram, it became clear that the woman's husband shared the same problem of being overweight and so the physician suggested the husband be included in the following meeting:

> What do you think about inviting your husband to our next meeting and together looking for ways to overcome similar issues?

The key is to feel comfortable inviting those family members relevant to the patient and to the patient's problem. For marital conflict and sexual dysfunction usually the children would not be invited. However, to understand a child's or parent's new cancer diagnosis it would be appropriate to invite all family members to the interview.

How to invite and why?

The physician can anticipate common variations in how patients might interpret the initial invitation to expand the medical interview. Research suggests that most patients view a family interview very positively. (It is seen as an appropriate and logical extension of the one-on-one interaction of a caring physician and patient.) Such interviews can be very brief and informal as when a family member accompanies the patient for a routine or non-threatening office visit. Alternatively, the family interview could be a planned 'family conference' regarding a life-threatening condition, substance abuse, or transfer to a care centre for the elderly. The depth and complexity of involvement with the family is addressed later in this chapter (five levels of involvement with families). Formally inviting a family member to join the patient for a future medical visit sometimes invokes unintended reactions. In other words, even invitations of the family may have side-effects. But they can be managed successfully.[4,6,7] For example, the patient might misinterpret the physician's intentions:

- The doctor is hiding some grave information that he wishes to tell the family;
- The doctor thinks I am not reliable and therefore wants to invite my family;
- The doctor believes that my pains are connected to relationships in the family and not to some defect in my own body.

Even the invited family might misinterpret the invitation:

- The doctor wants to tell us about some severe illness;
- The doctor is blaming us for the sickness or for not treating the patient well enough;
- The doctor does not trust the patient to inform us correctly.

Consequently, the way the invitation is delivered is of high importance. Mostly it is advisable to issue the invitation in a biomedical context in order to decrease both threat and anxiety.

The following examples illustrate how one justifies an invitation to the family:

> *For taking responsibility:*
> The decision to undergo a surgical procedure is difficult and complicated. I would suggest that we all meet to discuss the pros and cons.
>
> *For an explanation:*
> My guess is that your husband would also like to know how smoking affects the children's health and what effective ways there are to stop smoking.

For integration of treatments:
In view of the fact that several cases of asthma exist in your family, I would suggest that we have a family meeting in order to discuss ways of preventing any worsening of the disease.

For decreasing anxiety:
I understand from what you tell me that your family is worried about you and, therefore, I believe that by meeting with them I will be able to assist them to overcome this worry.

For cooperation with treatment:
I have learned from my experience that participation of other family members in the weight loss and fitness building program heightens the probability of success.

In order to avoid later inconveniences, the clinician can practice the way the invitation is to be delivered with the patient.[3,6,11] One may, for instance, ask the patient to repeat what she/he is planning to tell the family in the coming meeting and let the patient predict their expected reactions. Other options are to send a letter of explanation to the family, to call them at home in the patient's presence, or to arrange for a house call at a time when most of the family is there—in their natural surroundings. Of course, these formalities are rarely needed if the family members are simply already present in the office with the patient arriving for a straightforward problem. Under those common conditions the family interview can be an informal, non-threatening interaction in which everyone gets to know one another in a new 'family' context.

Conducting a family interview

How does one conduct a family interview? The physician's principal role in the family meeting is to *listen* to the opinions of the family members, to *reflect* their feelings, to *empathize* with their reactions, and to *discuss* their suggestions. This way the physician assists the family in organizing towards a functional adjustment without the physician having to intervene substantively in the family relationships. The physician's questions serve as an 'invitation to the family to step in'.[12]

Before the interview make sure there is enough room for everyone to sit comfortably. Conference rooms in clinics and hospitals empty waiting rooms, or large offices with extra chairs can be satisfactory. Develop goals for the conference using the guidelines noted below.

Structure helps get things started and adjustments can be made as one gains confidence in the process of the family interview. The following interview structure is derived from a variety of sources:[1,3,11,13–19]

1. Join with all family members: Greet every person by name. Begin with the most senior family member. Socialize for 1 or 2 min to make everyone comfortable.
2. Establish behavioural rules for the conference: Each person has the right to speak without interruption. Everyone's voice and opinion is important. All participants will remain respectful. The session will end on time. A session might be planned to last 20–60 min.
3. Clarify what information will be included in the medical record: This relieves the worry that intimate family details will be discoverable in the medical record. Generally, only agreed upon information would be included in the medical chart. Examples of commonly included items would be the diagnosis, the names of family members present, how long the interview lasted, major worries that were discussed, and what next steps are planned.
4. Define the nature of the problem: With the patient's approval give clear medical information about the medical problem. Primary care physicians should use everyday language to explain the medical aspects of the patient's problem and invite questions to ensure that everyone understands. Several rounds of questioning are often needed to address everyone's most important concerns. At other times, the most penetrating questions come quickly. It is appropriate to answer honestly, of course, when the primary care physician has no answer or must ask other experts about some aspects of the patient's care.
5. Invite everyone to express something regarding the topic under discussion: Not only spouses but children and grandparents often have interesting and challenging perspectives on the patient's issues. The adept primary care physician seeks everyone's input, thereby showing respect for the entire family.
6. Identify resources within the family or the community: Such resources help the family cope with the illness or challenge at hand. At first family members may need encouragement in identifying a family resource.[20] For example, some families may not recognize surviving a past trauma as evidence of having a family resource now titled 'survivorship' or 'courage'. With help such a family could develop pride in themselves as having this newly labelled characteristic. By maintaining a positive and encouraging stance the primary care physician helps a family identify previously unrecognized strengths and other resources. Identifying these family resources involves active listening and testing metaphors and analogies with the family for accuracy and validity.
7. Establish a plan or next steps for the family and patient: This plan is a negotiation process that addresses patient's and family's expectations, needs, and resources. What does the patient/family expect next? What is the family to do to cope with this issue? How can this goal be accomplished? Are other medical tests, treatments, or consultations needed? Where can they find information to read about this illness? Is there a trusted World Wide Web site? Will the family meet again with the primary care physician? Are there support groups or educational programmes to be recommended?

Sometimes, the patient does not agree with other family members or there are multiple different perspectives to balance. The most common professional stance is that the physician's primary role is to support the identified patient. If that is in conflict with the physician's best judgement, then the family meeting moves to a higher level of complexity addressed more completely in the next section.

If the family conflict runs deep, is chronic, and reaches well beyond the medical question at hand, it becomes a matter of helping a family deal with those more long-standing issues first. Then, they might be able to deal more positively with the pressing medical question. Managing that higher level of family conflict may take more than one family conference. Resolving the conflict may evolve into the realization that the next step will demand more complete sharing of information, to sharing feelings among family members, or the physician may want to support a brief 'intervention' intended to move the patient toward specific treatment for an addiction. In some cases, the physician may want to move the family toward family therapy to help them resolve fundamental conflicts that reach well beyond the medical question originally bringing the group together. Those next steps would be addressed in the mutually created plan for the patient.

8. Close the family meeting: family members should feel that the family meeting made a difference in the way they relate to the patient or the illness. It is recommended, therefore, that the primary care physician will sum-up what was learned from the meeting, and ask the family whether and how this meeting was of any help to them. Family members should be empowered and encouraged to take farther steps in coping with the illness as a team. Sometimes, a follow-up meeting is scheduled and assignments allocated to be done before the next meeting.[4]

After the family interview

Once the family interview has been completed, the primary care physician should complete the process with several action steps:[2,14]

1. Record relevant information about the family interview according to the agreement made early in the interview: For example, who was present, how long was the family interview, the diagnosis, and discrete information about the family understanding of the problem discussed. Note the treatment plan and next steps. Record family and community resources.

2. Record or revise the genogram: Electronic charts and paper charts offer different challenges and opportunities in documenting genograms. However, primary care physicians can record this type of information in a variety of ways.
3. Debrief with a colleague about what happened and what was learned, especially when the physician wants to reflect more fully upon what she did in the meeting or when he feels emotionally charged or upset from this encounter: This can be done with a physician, nurse, or nearby therapist. This would rarely be needed following brief or informal family interviews. An upsetting family interview would be an occasion to debrief. Occasionally, a family interview will trigger new or uncomfortable feelings within the primary care physician. It is important to discuss such feelings with a trusted professional to ensure the continued growth and development of a primary care physician who touches the heart of families facing serious health and other challenges. Interviews that focus upon substance abuse, family violence, serious medical errors, or unexpected death would commonly warrant post-interview discussion.
4. Stay within appropriate professional limits of his/her time, training, and skills. Set limits on the number of planned interviews with a specific family and then contemplate the degree of involvement that might be needed for a given family early in the process. Then review those estimates periodically: Especially when the family interview is a very positive experience it is important to set clear limits on the subsequent number of primary care family interviews. A maximum of five or six sessions is reasonable and more than that may not be appropriate for most primary care physicians. By that time the family changes that are likely to occur within a primary care setting will have been stimulated. Prolonged engagement with a specific family not yielding the intended results runs the risk of adding stability to a family system needing change. The savvy physician is wise to avoid drifting or being led unintentionally towards family therapy that requires advanced training and longer-term challenges for both the family and the therapist. But how can a physician decide how much to become involved with a specific family? The next section outlines one model for understanding various degrees or 'Levels' of involvement with families.

How involved with the family?

This section recommends ways to conduct a family interview in a medical setting. This is not family therapy but a family conference to improve everyone's understanding of and ability to cope with the patient's medical problem. How does the primary care physician decide 'how far to go' during a family interview? Even with the outline above a family interview could become quite complicated. Doherty and Baird have suggested that there are five possible 'Levels of Involvement' with families.[21,22] The organizing principle is that physicians may have qualitatively different degrees or *levels of involvement* with families *based upon the family's needs* and the *physician's knowledge, personal development, and skills.* In a parallel manner, primary care physicians demonstrate different levels of participation in medical and surgical care with few doing a full range of care in all categories. The different levels of involvement with families are manifest most clearly during family interviews but are demonstrable during individual interviews as well.[16]

Table 1 outlines the model with a specific knowledge base, personal development, and skills appropriate for each level. Level I suggests that the physician meet with families for only medico-legal reasons and to explain medical information in a one-dimensional manner. This is often seen at post-surgical family explanations of care while all participants are standing in a hospital hallway or waiting room. The model goes through all five levels to clarify the utility and dimensions of the mid-range of family involvement. At Level V, the physician is actually doing family therapy to challenge deeply imbedded dysfunctional family patterns. This would be unrealistic for all but a few physicians with extensive training in family therapy. The appropriate level for a specific patient/family is determined by the needs of the patient/family, the knowledge, personal development, and skills of the physician and the other circumstances relevant to the case.

Level I family interview

Level I is the most common level of involvement with families in medical settings.[23] It is time efficient in the short run and achieves the purpose of demonstrating to families and patients that the physician will take some time to explain the patient's problem, however briefly. All primary care physicians use this type of interaction when circumstances restrict other options. For example, at Level I a physician would briefly explain a medical problem to the patient and rarely seek planned interactions with the patient's family. If family members were present, the physician in this role would talk almost exclusively to the patient, avoid prolonged discussions with family members, not seek family member input, and would try systematically to understand the perspective of other family members regarding the identified patient's health. This level is useful when physicians have no discretionary time and are not able to reach beyond the minimum in understanding or managing the social context of the individual patient. Making early morning hospital visits is one way to avoid family contact and stay within this minimal level of involvement with families. This level of involvement with families is reinforced by office consultation rooms that do not have seating for anyone beyond the patient and physician. It does have the disadvantage of not making the family available as a resource to the physician or patient.

Level II family interview

Planned family interviews really begin at Level II. This represents a more interactive option in which all participants would be seated for a planned time together. The physician would use this option whenever the need arose in daily practice, especially if a patient had been hospitalized. The physician would have a *collaborative stance* and would be comfortable asking participants about their opinions and understanding of the medical problem. At this level of involvement the physician must comprehend that she is functioning as part of the family system. This triangular relationship between the patient–family–physician can be a 'therapeutic triangle' (Fig. 1).

The care of chronic or serious medical conditions can almost always be improved with this collaborative, family-centered approach. A family interview at Level II can be brief (10–20 min) and can often improve the patient and family's confidence as well as cooperation with the medical plan.[24,25]

Level III family interview

At Level III, the primary care physician would conduct a planned family interview intended to share the medical and family information collaboratively *and explore patient and family members' feelings* about the medical situation. A key to this level of family interview is for the physician to avoid premature reassurance of the family in order to allay the physician's own discomfort. Feelings may spill out quickly once family members are asked. At that moment the physician interviewer may be tempted to make 'the pain in the room go away' by resorting to premature reassurance. Remaining respectfully silent is a wise and therapeutic behaviour after a patient or family member expresses sorrow or pain. Example:

'Don't worry, it will all be OK.'

Physicians can usually avoid this mistake by having a reliable way to process her/his own feelings about this patient or situation. This can be achieved by anticipating what might occur and talking about the possible patient and family feelings of discomfort before the meeting with a collaborative therapist, nurse, or other similarly oriented provider. In an ideal practice setting, a family therapist or other psychotherapist who is trained in interviewing families and understands family systems would be available for this discussion before or after the family interview. Having this therapist as a partner and geographically located within the ambulatory practice is

Table 1 Levels of physician involvement with families

Level I: minimal emphasis on family	Level II: ongoing medical information and advice	Level III: feelings and support	Level IV: systematic assessment and planned intervention	Level V: family therapy
This baseline level of involvement consists of dealing with families only as necessary for practical and medico-legal reasons, but not viewing communicating with families as integral to the physician's role or as involving skills for the physician to develop. This level presumably characterizes most medical school training in which biomedical issues are the sole conscious focus of the patient	*Knowledge base:* Primarily medical, plus awareness of the triangular dimension of the physician–patient–family relationship *Personal development:* Openness to engage patients and families in a collaborative way *Skills:* 1. Regularly and clearly communicating medical findings and treatment options to family members 2. Asking family members questions that elicit relevant diagnostic and treatment information 3. Attentively listening to family members' questions and concerns 4. Advising families about how to handle the medical and rehabilitation needs of the patient 5. For large or demanding families, knowing how to channel communication through one or two key members 6. Identifying gross family dysfunction that interferes with medical treatment, and referring the family to a therapist	*Knowledge base:* Normal family development and reactions to stress *Personal development:* Awareness of one's own feelings in relationship to the patient and family *Skills:* 1. Asking questions that elicit family members' expressions of concerns and feelings related to the patient's condition and its effect on the family 2. Empathetically listening to family members' concerns and feelings, and normalizing them where appropriate 3. Forming a preliminary assessment of the family's level of functioning as it relates to the patient's problem 4. Encouraging family members in their efforts to cope as a family with their situation 5. Tailoring medical advice to the unique needs, concerns, and feelings of the family 6. Identifying family dysfunction and fitting a referral recommendation to the unique situation of the family	*Knowledge base:* Family systems *Personal development:* Awareness of one's own participation in systems including the therapeutic triangle, the medical system, one's own family system, and larger community systems *Skills:* 1. Engaging family members, including reluctant ones, in a planned family conference or a series of conferences 2. Structuring a conference with even a poorly communicating family in such a way that all members have a chance to express themselves 3. Systematically assessing the family's level of functioning 4. Supporting individual members while avoiding coalitions 5. Reframing the family's definition of their problem in a way that makes problem solving more achievable 6. Helping the family members view their difficulty as one that requires new forms of collaborative efforts 7. Helping family members generate alternative, mutually acceptable ways to cope with their difficulty 8. Helping the family balance their coping efforts by calibrating their various roles in a way that allows support without sacrificing anyone's autonomy Identifying family dysfunction that lies beyond primary care treatment and orchestrating a referral by educating the family and the therapist about what to expect from one another	*Knowledge base:* Family systems and patterns whereby dysfunctional families interact with professionals and other health care systems *Personal development:* Ability to handle intense emotions in families and self and to maintain neutrality in the face of strong pressure from family members or other professionals *Skills:* The following is not an exhaustive list of family therapy skills but rather a list of several key skills that distinguish Level V involvement from primary care involvement with families: 1. Interviewing families or family members who are quite difficult to engage 2. Efficiently generating and testing hypotheses about the family's difficulties and interaction patterns 3. Escalating conflict in the family in order to break a family impasse 4. Temporarily siding with one family member against another 5. Constructively dealing with a family's strong resistance to change Negotiating collaborative relationships with other professionals and other systems who are working with the family, even when these groups are at odds with one another

the highest level of collaboration. However, a similar therapist available in the community and available by phone is a more common alternative.[26]

At Level III, the physician *would understand normal family development and predictable reactions to stress.* Many primary care physicians would be in contact with a family over months and years. The primary care physician may assume a quasi-family role as advisor, confidante, and, of course, medical care provider. During the family interview, this acquired leadership role can be a therapeutic resource for a distressed family. However, managing this trust to the benefit of the patient and family works best if the physician is aware of her own feelings and reactions to this situation and remains in an objective and professional stance. Then, exploring the patient's and family's emotional response to an illness can be addressed from a balanced perspective. Reflecting the family's comments back to them and asking functional questions help the physician move into the meaning of the patient's complaint or illness and move past technical details.[3,4,27]

Examples of functional questions might be:

Is this condition temporary or a long term problem?
How are you feeling about all of this?
How has this affected each of you?
How are you each coping with this?
What will happen if there is no effective treatment right now?
Do you believe the planned treatment will improve the functional impairment?

Level IV family interview

A Level IV family conference would be an option for primary care physicians with a *solid understanding of family systems and trained to work with moderately challenging family issues* that may have been blocking a patient and family from coping with a serious illness or behavioural problem. With one or a few family conferences the physician at this level would *be able to structure a family interview with a family not eager to openly discuss the relevant issue.* Illustrating this level of involvement is the complex example of a patient with a pain-related disorder who is not responding to conventional treatment. Another example would be drug or alcohol abuse.[28]

The Level IV family interview would be *a systematic assessment of the patient and family.* In these situations, a planned intervention might be needed to help the patient and family change their approach to a stubborn patient problem. The outcome would be a common understanding of the problem and new options for treatment. Previously unspoken fears, concerns, and feelings would be explored respectfully and openly. Sometimes, parallel problems for other family members could be clarified. The family and the physician would have shared an intimate and change-oriented experience.[11,29] The family systems-trained physician would demonstrate respect for shared and divergent stories and suggestions for further evaluation or treatment.[30–32]

Level V family interview—family therapy

Level V involvement with families is rarely needed and not often a realistic option for primary care physicians. Among the tasks within family therapy are: management of intense emotions, generating and testing hypotheses about the family's difficulties, and constructively dealing with the family's strong resistance to change.[7,33,34] Fellowship training or master's degree training in family therapy is required for this level of involvement.

Clinicians can use the 'Five Levels of Involvement with Families' in two ways:

1. To plan for a family interview by establishing goals for that interview: For example: 'Today I want to understand how other family members are feeling as they cope with one person's illness' (Level III) or 'We don't have much time today so I will be careful to share information but not ask questions about how you are all feeling about this problem until I have more time' (Level II).
2. For self-assessment for understanding the limits of one's overall knowledge base, personal development, and skills related to family interviewing which might be apparent before (planning) or after (debriefing) a family conference: This assessment of the physician's knowledge, skills, and attitudes can be used to understand why a specific family interview seemed successful in reaching positive goals versus a dissatisfying or less than positive interview that did not reach goals thought to be appropriate before the interview.

For example, a physician might plan a family conference with an understanding that it would be more than routine and might demand the physician or other interviewer to create a brief but influential intervention:

'This family is struggling with alcohol addiction that is apparently a problem for several family members. My goal for today will be to help them all consider this a problem worthy of future discussion with an alcoholism counselor.' This would be a way to plan a conference at Level IV. The goal of the interview would be to help the family to accept consultation with a trained addiction counsellor to begin the long journey towards recovery from alcohol addiction or abuse.

Alternatively, the 'Levels' can help with a debriefing after a family conference:

'This family interview became uncomfortable for me and possibly everyone when alcohol addiction surfaced as a problem for several people. I couldn't keep track of what happened after that, and the interview just seemed to end abruptly.' In this example, the physician was debriefing after a family conference and processing what had transpired. In this case the family interview demanded a Level IV intervention (alcoholism intervention), which was beyond the physician's Level III skills and knowledge. However, up to the point of the discussion of alcohol addiction the interview may have gone well.

By clarifying several different degrees of depth and complexity, the Levels of Involvement concept helps clinicians *plan* and *process* the rich but fluid experience of interviewing families. This model provides some structure to explain why processing feelings is different than collaboratively sharing medical information. It outlines the knowledge base, personal development, and skills appropriate for each level. A primary care physician might use this model to understand the high clinical value of collaboratively sharing information (Level II), and guiding an open discussion of feelings or emotional responses to illness (Level III). It also illuminates the difference between short-term intervention (Level IV) and long-term family therapy (Level V).

Training options for learning more

Interviewing families to explore feelings and understanding normal family development and reactions to stress is within the scope of many primary care training programmes and continuing education workshops (Levels II and III). However, brief interventions intended to create significant change in how families cope with more serious illnesses and successfully challenging embedded patterns of behaviour (Level IV) as well as formal family therapy (Level V) requires more advanced and more lengthy training. Such training normally would include direct supervision of family interviews, exploration of the related professional literature, and developing self-awareness beyond what routine primary care training can offer.

Many family physicians have learned a variety of skills related to family interviewing through years of rich practice experience. Some have expanded their knowledge base and attitudes through reading available books and journals and by participating in conferences and workshops. Fellowships in family systems and medical family therapy are available and offer structured opportunities for advanced training.[7,8,11] Very few current primary care postgraduate training programmes offer training in formal family therapy with the required level of education and skill development. However, many family practice residencies provide supervision and training in family interviewing up to Level IV. More advanced postresidency training is increasingly available in addition to workshops and distance supervision provided by some academic medical centres. There are numerous master's degree and doctoral degree programmes in family therapy but few primary care clinicians would be inclined to seek that level of training. The websites noted in the box are sources of current information on advanced training options.

A primary care physician who just wants to see what family therapy is like might join with a therapist for one or two sessions with a family referred for therapy. Participating in early therapy sessions helps transfer the family's trust and speeds the process of the therapist joining with the family. Thereafter, by remaining outside the therapy role the primary care physician can reinforce the therapy process by supporting the family's continued involvement with a therapist.[22,35]

Primary care physicians with an interest in understanding and working with families are important resources for families. The following websites have more information about training programmes and networks of primary care physicians and therapists with interests and knowledge regarding this topic:

Websites for advanced training in family interviewing:

- www.cfha.net—Collaborative Family Healthcare Association
- www.stfm.org—Society of Teachers of Family Medicine
- www.FSH.org—The journal, *Families, Systems and Health*
- www.cpct.co.uk—The Counseling in Primary Care Trust Website

Summary

Family interviews enrich the role of primary care physicians by engaging families directly in the care of a loved one. The goals of such group interviews can be modest. At a minimum the physician and family will learn collaboratively. Families may share their feelings about the patient and about the illness. Sometimes, the interview leads to changes in the care plan. It may improve the family's ability to cope with illness or loss. Occasionally, the entire thrust of the medical intervention may change based upon new insights gained. Family interviews help patients and medical care providers become more competent in coping with illness, life, recovery, adaptation, and death. Interviewing families can be an unusually rewarding aspect to a balanced primary care practice.[36,37]

References

1. **Doherty, W.J. and Baird, M.A.** *Family Therapy and Family Medicine: Toward the Primary Care of Families.* New York: Guilford Press, 1983.
2. **Christie-Seely, J.** *Working with the Family in Primary Care: A Systems Approach to Health and Illness.* New York: Praeger, 1984.
3. **Eshet, I., Margalit, A., and Almagor, G.** (1993). 'SFAT-AM'—treatment approach in 10–15 minute encounters. *Family Practice* **10** (2), 178–87.
4. **Margalit, A. and Eshet, I.** *'SFAT-AM'—A Biopsychosocial Handbook for Primary Care Providers.* Tel-Aviv: Heiliger, 1997 (in Hebrew).
5. **Kushner, K.** et. al. (1986). The family conference: what do patients want? *Journal of Family Practice* **23**, 463–7.
6. **McDaniel, S.** et al. *Family Oriented Primary Care: A Manual for Medical Providers.* New York: Springer-Verlag, 1990.
7. **McDaniels, S.H.** et al. *Medical Family Therapy.* New York: Basic Books, 1992.
8. **Asen, K.E. and Tomson, P.** *Family Solutions in Family Practice.* Lancaster: Quay Publishing, 1993.
9. **Van Doorn, H.** (1990). Integrating family counseling into general practice. *Australian Family Physician* **19**, 467–71.
10. **Holloway, R.L.**, ed. (2001). Clinics in family practice. *Behavioral Medicine in Family Practice* **3**(1).
11. **Bloom, M.V. and Smith, D.A.** *Brief Mental Health Interventions for the Family Physician.* New York: Springer-Verlag, 2001.
12. **Neighbour, R.** (1982). Family therapy by family doctors. *Journal of the Royal College of General Practitioners* **32**, 737–42.
13. **Campbell, T.L. and McDaniel, S.H.** *Conducting a Family Interview. The Medical Interview: Clinical Care, Education, and Research.* New York: Springer-Verlag, 1995, pp. 178–86.
14. **Campbell, T.L. and McDaniel, S.H.** (2001). Family systems in family medicine. *Clinics in Family Practice* **3** (1), 13–33.
15. **Marchand, L.** et al. (1997). Getting to the heart of the family conference: the residents' perspective. *Family, Systems, and Health* **15**, 305–19.
16. **Marvel, M.K., Doherty, W.J., and Baird, M.A.** (1993). Levels of physician involvement with psychosocial concerns of individual patients: a developmental model. *Family Medicine* **25**, 337–42.
17. **Meyer, D.L.** et al. (1989). Family conferences: reasons, levels of involvement and perceived usefulness. *Journal of Family Practice* **29**, 401–5.
18. **Craigie, F.C.** et al. (1990). Perceived social support and family meeting attendance preferences among family medicine outpatients. *Journal of Family Practice* **31**, 65–8.
19. **Erstling, S.S.** et al. (1989). The single session family interview. *Journal of Family Practice* **28**, 556–60.
20. **Baird, M.A. and Doherty, W.J.** (1986). Family resources in coping with serious illness. In *Family Resources* (ed. M. Karpel), pp. 359–83. New York: Guilford Press.
21. **Doherty, W.J.** et al. (1986). Developmental levels in family-centered medical care. *Family Medicine* **18**, 153–6.
22. **Doherty, W.J. and Baird, M.A.**, ed. *Family-Centered Medical Care: A Clinical Casebook.* New York: Guilford Press, 1987.
23. **Marvel, K.** et. al (1994). Levels of physician involvement with patients and their families: a model for teaching and research. *Journal of Family Practice* **39**, 535–44.
24. **Cole-Kelly, K.** et al. (1998). Integrating the family into routine patient care. *Journal of Family Practice* **47**, 440–5.
25. **Crouch, M.A. and Roberts, L.** *The Family in Medical Practice.* New York: Springer-Verlag, 1987.
26. **Doherty, W.H., McDaniel, S.H., and Baird, M.A.** (1996). Five levels of primary care/behavioral healthcare collaboration. *Behavioral Healthcare Tomorrow,* October, 25–7.
27. **Rolland, J.** *Families, Illness, and Disability: An Integrative Treatment Model.* New York: Basic Books, 1994.
28. **Baird, M.A.** (1992). Addictive disorders: a practical guide to treatment. In *Care of Family Members and Other Affected Persons* (ed. M. Fleming and K. Barry), pp. 195–210. Mosby Year Book. St. Louis MO: Mosby.
29. **Watzlawick, P.** et al. *Change: Principles of Problem Formation and Problem Resolution.* New York: Norton, 1974.
30. **Doherty, W.J. and Burge, S.K.** (1987). Attending to the context of family treatment: pitfalls and prospects. *Journal of Marriage and Family Therapy* **13**, 37–47.
31. **Weakland, J.H. and Fisch, R.** (1984). Cases that 'don't make sense': brief strategic treatment in medicine practice. *Family Systems Medicine* **2**, 125–36.
32. **Jacobs, B.** *Partnering with Patients' Loved Ones.* Hippocrates, 2000, pp. 39–42.
33. **McDaniel, S.H., Hepworth, J., and Doherty, W.J.** *The Shared Experience of Illness.* New York: Basic Books, 1997.
34. **Wood, B.L.** (1993). Beyond the 'psychosomatic family': a biobehavioral family model of pediatric illness. *Family Process* **32**, 261–78.
35. **Baird, M.A.** (1992). Family medicine: a time for clarity. In *Family Health Care* (ed. J.S. Russell), pp. 167–85. Newbury Park: Sage Publications.
36. **Baird, M.A. and Doherty, W.J.** (1990). Risks and benefits of a family systems approach to medical care. *Family Medicine,* September–October **22**(5) 396–403.
37. **Baird, M.A.** (2001). Introduction to family-oriented care in the new millennium. *Holloway, Family Practice Clinics of North America* **3** (1), 59–61.

9.4 Assessment and management of genetic risk

Peter Rose and Jon Emery

Introduction

The announcement of the complete sequencing of the human genome in 2001 was the culmination of 30 years of rapid expansion in our knowledge of genes and the development of techniques to identify the function of normal and abnormal genes. Although much of this work is still in the hands of laboratory scientists, some of the applications of this new knowledge are beginning to trickle down to primary care.(1) The excitement of these genetic discoveries is tempered by the lack of training in genetics for many primary care practitioners and uncertainties about how best to apply this new knowledge in primary care.

Genetics has begun to make an impact on primary care in two main areas. Firstly, in relation to patients' concerns about the possible impact of their family history on their own health. Secondly, in ante-natal care and the increasing number of tests available to pregnant women to identify genetic disorders in the foetus. In the future we are likely to see an expansion in the number of genetic tests that predict risk of common disease such as cardiovascular disease and diabetes, and pharmacogenetic tests that will help tailor drug dosage and selection.

This section includes information on the main skills and knowledge required by a primary care practitioner to undertake consultations in genetic medicine:

- The construction and assessment of a family history, the main assessment tool.
- An outline of the primary care practitioner's role in two common presentations to primary care-cancer genetics and pre-natal diagnosis.
- The services available in secondary care to guide appropriate referrals.

Genetic mechanisms

It is beyond the scope of this chapter to discuss genetic mechanisms in detail, but it is essential to have some knowledge of the way that different abnormalities in genes and chromosomes result in disease. Fuller discussion of this subject can be found in a genetic textbook, for example, Rose and Lucassen.(2)

Genetic disorders can be classified as follows:

- chromosomal disorders;
- single gene disorders;
  - autosomal dominant,
  - autosomal recessive,
  - X-linked,
  - non-classical inheritance including mitochondrial inheritance and imprinting,
- multifactorial disorders.

There are 23 pairs of chromosomes in the human somatic cell. Twenty-two of these are matched pairs and two are sex chromosomes (matched in females –XX– and unmatched in males –XY). Thus, with the exception of genes on the Y chromosome, there are two copies of each gene in a somatic cell.

Chromosomal disorders are caused when a cell has either too many chromosomes (Down syndrome), too few (Turner's syndrome), or parts of a chromosome are missing, duplicated or in the wrong place (translocation). Translocations are sometimes carried by an individual without clinical effects. However, if the translocation is passed to this person's offspring, it might then result in a clinical problem. For example, 3 per cent of cases of Down syndrome are inherited due to a translocation in one of the parents.

Autosomal dominant disorders are caused by a mutation in one copy of a gene (e.g. Huntington's disease). An individual will pass this mutation onto 50 per cent of their offspring.

Autosomal recessive disorders are caused when there is a mutation in both copies of a gene (e.g. cystic fibrosis). A person who has only one copy of the abnormal gene is healthy and is called a carrier. If two carriers produce children there is a one in four chance that a child will inherit both mutations and develop the condition.

X-linked disorders result from a mutation in a gene on the X chromosome (e.g. classical haemophilia). A male with a mutation on his single X chromosome will develop disease. A female with the mutation does not develop the disease (because she has one healthy X chromosome) but can pass the mutation on to 50 per cent of her sons, who will all be affected and 50 per cent of her daughters, who will be carriers.

Multifactorial disorders result from interactions between a gene or genes and environmental factors to cause the disease. Heart disease is an example where we know that some people have an inherited element to their disease. However, this susceptibility interacts with environmental factors (diet, smoking, etc.) to result in disease.

There is one other genetic phenomenon which affects genetic assessment, that of penetrance. This is usually expressed as the percentage lifetime risk that someone carrying a mutation will develop the associated disease. For example, the penetrance of mutations causing hereditary non-polyposis colon cancer (HNPCC) is 80–85 per cent.

The family history

The main tool for the assessment of genetic risk in primary care is the family history. It is important to differentiate its use as a genetic assessment tool from its other uses:

- A genetic assessment tool—'the pedigree'. This could be used in response to an enquiry from a patient about their risk of disease.
- A screening tool, for example when a patient registers with a new practice. The information gathered might be useful when meeting new patients for a variety of reasons, but as discussed later, the family history does not fulfil all the criteria of a screening test, with the exception of a few rare diseases (see below).
- A risk factor in the diagnostic process. The presence of a family history of breast cancer is one of several risk factors to take into account when assessing a woman with a breast lump.
- A socio-cultural tool. Historically, this is how most primary care practitioners would use the family history. Knowledge of diseases that have occurred in a patient's family, whether they have originated by chance, through sharing a common environment or due to genetic factors helps to understand the patterns of presentation of diseases. People present with a concern that they might be developing the same disease as a relative, for example, a headache might be associated with a brain tumour if another member of the family had such a presentation (see Chapter 9.1 for further discussion of the genogram).

Taking and interpreting the family history

A detailed family history (pedigree) is normally required to assess whether a presenting problem is likely to have a genetic component. Concerns are often expressed about time constraints, but it should be possible to take a family history over three generations in about 10 minutes providing the family is not large or the history too complex. The alternative is to re-schedule this task when more time is available, as might happen with assessment of a complex psychological problem.

Currently, the commonest reasons for constructing a pedigree would be at the ante-natal booking appointment or in response to a patient with concerns about their family history of cancer. A family physician with 2000 patients will have 40–50 patients with at least one first-degree relative affected by breast, ovarian, colorectal, or endometrial cancer.[3] In a US survey, 42 per cent of primary care physicians had discussed genetic testing for cancer with their patients[4] and in the United Kingdom and Holland one to two patients per month per family practitioner discuss their concerns about a family history of cancer.[5,6] How this might change as public awareness of genetic testing increases is unclear, for example, through media influences including the Internet.

The skill of taking a family history requires some practice. There are a number of important steps to consider when recording a pedigree:

- The family history should be dated to allow future amendments as the history develops.
- The presenting patient (known as the proband) is identified with an arrow.
- Ethnic origin should be recorded since it is important for many conditions (e.g. haemoglobinopathies, breast cancer).
- Move across a generation (i.e. from the patient to his/her siblings) and then move up or down to next generation (children and parents and their siblings).
- For those alive, record sex, age/date of birth, medical history. If you are interested in assessing one illness, concentrate on this and related illnesses only. For example, if the patient is concerned about a family history of breast cancer, the main diseases of concern will be breast and ovarian cancer and other related cancers. You might wish to record members of the family who had heart disease but this will not affect your overall assessment.
- For those who are dead, record sex, age at death, and cause of death.
- For significant illnesses record age at diagnosis (in both live and dead relatives), this is more important than whether the disease was fatal.
- Aim for first- and second-degree relatives over 3 generations. This might need to be extended if a suspicious pattern develops.
- Consanguinity (marriage between second cousins or closer) is important in autosomal recessive diseases.
- Specific questions might be necessary about children who have died, physically/mentally handicapped relatives, adoptions, miscarriages, still births, and half-siblings because these details might not be offered spontaneously.

The standard symbols that are used in a pedigree are found in Fig. 1.

Patients' recollections of diseases in relatives are sometimes vague, particularly concerning the primary site of internal tumours or the exact name of rare syndromes. It might be necessary to ask patients to do some homework on their pedigree by speaking to other family members or consulting death certificates. Primary care practitioners can approach hospitals or cancer registries for confirmation of histology but this would usually be done routinely by clinical genetics departments.

The family history can reveal patterns of inheritance suggestive of a single gene disorder or a multifactorial disease occurring more frequently than would be expected by chance. The brief description of single gene disorders above gives a guide to their pattern of inheritance. For example, for an autosomal dominant condition you would expect about 50 per cent of each generation to be affected with an equal distribution between men and women. If the gene has less than 100 per cent penetrance the figure will be lower than 50 per cent.

Primary care computer systems are not yet programmed to record family history data of sufficient complexity. Computerized pedigree drawing programs are available, however, and computer decision support has been shown to improve the accuracy of risk assessment for family history of cancer and the quality of family history recording compared to traditional pen-and-paper methods[7] (see Chapter 6.6).

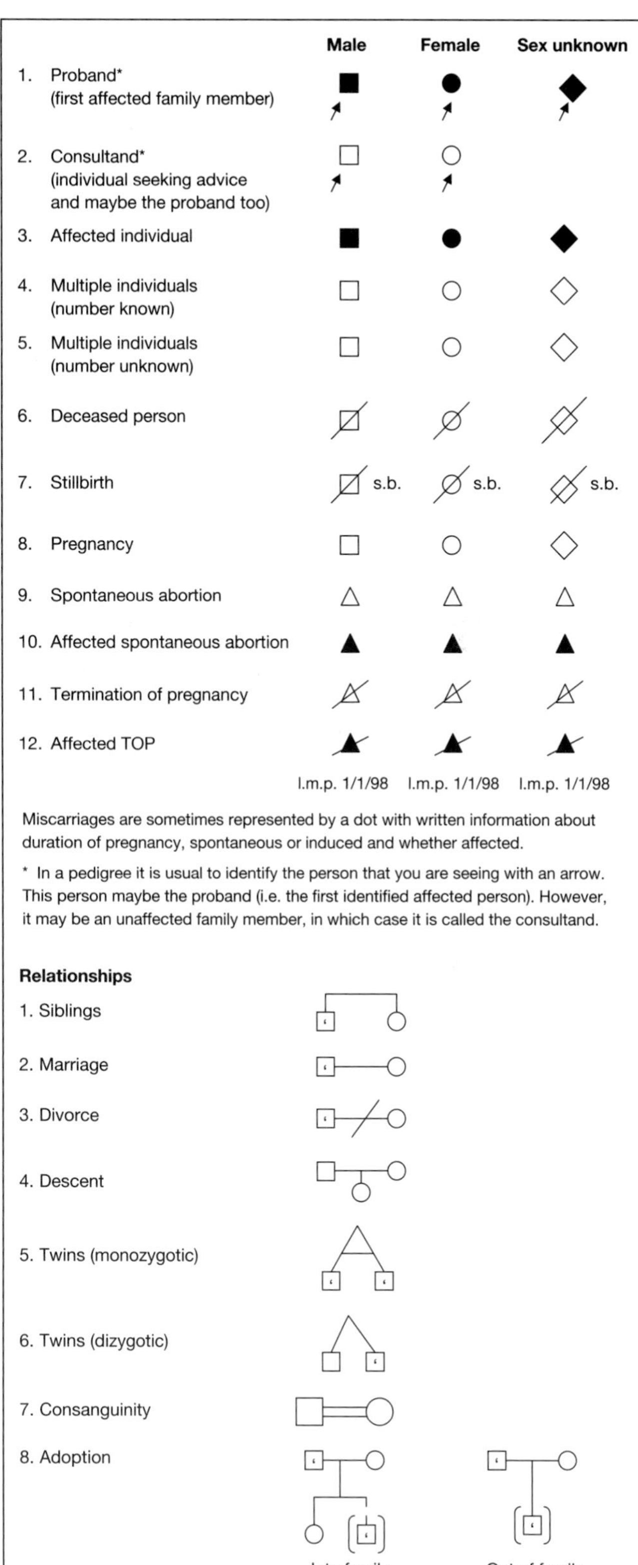

Fig. 1 Symbols used in a pedigree.

Genetic counselling

Definition

Genetic counselling is the process by which patients or relatives at risk of a disorder that can be inherited are advised of the consequences of the disorder, the probability of developing or transmitting it, and of the ways this can be prevented, avoided or ameliorated.[8]

There are many instances in current practice where primary care practitioners undertake genetic counselling without recognizing it as such. It is routine practice to elicit a family history of cardiovascular disease and use this knowledge, together with other factors, to discuss cardiovascular risk with a patient. Discussing the Guthrie test for phenylketonuria or pre- and post-test counselling for the Down syndrome screening are other examples.

Why is genetic counselling perceived as different?

There are a number of reasons why genetic counselling can be perceived as different from other counselling situations:

- Many primary care physicians have not had basic training in genetics and so do not possess important background knowledge and skills.
- Knowledge is advancing rapidly in this field and therefore it is more difficult for a generalist to keep up to date.
- It is perceived as time consuming and therefore does not fit easily into a 10-minute consultation.
- Primary care practitioners do not feel confident to assess risk on which the counselling is based.
- Initial assessments often result in a risk score rather than a definitive result. A patient might need to make a decision based on this risk, for example, whether to proceed to amniocentesis if the triple test risk is high. Patients' perceptions of risk vary, making the counselling process more difficult.
- Once genetic information about an individual is known, this is immutable. Therefore, the consequences of a wrong decision about whether to be tested are lifelong and so might have more lasting effects on the doctor–patient relationship.
- Genetic information affects families not individuals, some of whom will not be registered with the same primary care practitioner.
- There are difficult ethical issues around genetics, some of which remain unresolved (see below).

Despite these difficulties, primary care professionals are increasingly becoming involved in this work, knowingly or unknowingly. Suchard et al. showed that although only 15 per cent of English general practitioners felt sufficiently prepared to counsel patients about genetic test results, 50 per cent had actually done so in the previous year.[9] With the probable rise in number of different genetic tests and increased patient demand for information about their family history and disease risk, genetic counselling will become an increasingly important task in primary care.

Primary care role in genetic counselling

Roles will include:

- Reassuring those at background risk of potentially inherited disease.
- Discussing and organizing referral for those at increased risk including an explanation of the process involved and what a clinical geneticist might be able to offer.
- Supporting patients who have been referred and clarifying information that the patient has been given by specialist geneticists.
- Explanation of genetic mechanisms to patients and families to support informed decision-making.
- Pre- and post-test counselling for genetic tests. The number of tests undertaken by primary care physicians will vary according to each practitioner's knowledge and confidence. For example, screening for cystic fibrosis and haemoglobinopathy carriers has been undertaken satisfactorily in primary care.[10,11]

Familial cancers

The inherited cancers (see Box 1), and in particular breast, ovarian, and colorectal cancer provide a clear example of the potential clinical applications of research arising from the Human Genome Project. In the last decade, several genes have been identified that, when mutated, place an individual at very high lifetime risk of developing specific cancers (see Table 1). These mutations are rare in the general population and account for only a small proportion of such cancers even in patients with a family history of cancer.

The key issue facing primary care practitioners at present is to identify patients with a family history of cancer who are at increased risk of carrying a mutation, for example in BRCA1 or BRCA2, and reassuring the majority of patients for whom genetic testing, early or more frequent cancer screening or prophylactic treatments offer no benefit.[12] A range of referral criteria exist nationally and locally to help primary care practitioners assess inherited risk of breast, ovarian, and colorectal cancer (see Table 2). The important factors to consider are:

- Does the family history of cancer fit an autosomal dominant pattern?
- Family history of cancer is more likely to be due to a mutation in a cancer predisposing gene in the following circumstances:
  - multiple cases with early onset disease (e.g. below the age of 50 years);
  - certain ethnic groups (e.g. Ashkenazi Jews, BRCA1, and BRCA2);
  - certain cancer clusters (e.g. colorectal, endometrial cancer, and HNPCC mutations).

An important point when discussing inherited cancer with patients is the therapeutic gap that currently exists for mutation carriers. There is reasonable evidence to support total colectomy for people with familial adenomatous polyposis, and for regular colonoscopy and removal of polyps in HNPCC.

Box 1 Examples

Case 1

A 23-year-old woman came to her family physician for a routine contraceptive pill check. She told the doctor that she was planning to stop the pill in the near future with a view to becoming pregnant. However, her older sister had just given birth to a baby with Down syndrome and she was concerned about the possibility that this could affect her pregnancy too. There were no other cases of Down syndrome in the woman's family and no other relevant history. Her sister had a blood test to confirm that her own chromosomes were normal. In consequence the doctor was able to reassure the woman that she was not at increased risk of having a child with Down syndrome. The doctor took the opportunity to discuss ante-natal screening for Down syndrome, other screening tests in the ante-natal period and the benefits of folic acid.

Case 2

A 46-year-old woman presented to her family physician with a concern about her risk of breast cancer. Her eldest sister aged 58 had recently been diagnosed with breast cancer. She had read in a magazine that breast cancer is hereditary. Her second sister aged 55 and her mother who was 80 were both well. No other immediate family members had suffered from cancer. The doctor consulted the guidelines for referral circulated by the local clinical genetics department and was able to reassure the woman that she was not at significantly increased risk. He discussed the population risk of breast cancer (approximately 1 in 12 lifetime risk) and advised her that she should have regular mammograms in the national screening programme.

Table 1 Summary of the more common inherited cancers

Genes (chromosomal location)	Associated features	Interventions
BRCA1 (17q)	Breast, ovarian, colorectal, and prostate cancer	Prophylactic mastectomy Chemoprevention
BRCA2 (13q)	Breast (including male breast cancer), prostate, ovarian, pancreas cancer (risk of ovarian cancer less than BRCA1)	?Tamoxifen ?raloxifene ?Mammography ?MRI breast screening ?CA125 and transvaginal ultrasound for ovarian cancer screening ?Prophylactic oophorectomy ?COCP for ovarian cancer
APC (familial adenomatous polyposis) (5q)	Multiple colonic and gastroduodenal polyps with malignant potential Epidermoid cysts, retinal pigmentation, desmoid tumours	Colonoscopy Prophylactic colectomy ?Upper gastrointestinal surveillance ?COX-2 inhibitors
MLH1 (3p), MSH2 (2p) PMS1 (7q), PMS2 (2q), MSH6 (2p) (hereditary non-polyposis colorectalcancer HNPCC)	Colorectal cancer (especially proximal or multiple tumours) Endometrial, ovarian, ureteric, and gastric cancers	Colonoscopy ?Chemoprevention ?Endometrial screening ?Prophylactic colectomy

Table 2 An example of referral guidelines for patients with a family history of breast cancer

UK Cancer Family Study Group guidelines for referral and screening mammography[a](13)

- One relative[b] with breast cancer diagnosed <40 years
- Two relatives with breast cancer average age of diagnosis 40–49 years
- Three relatives with breast cancer average age of diagnosis 50–60 years
- One relative with breast cancer diagnosed <50 years and one or more relatives with ovarian cancer diagnosed at any age or one relative with both breast and ovarian cancer

[a] See original paper for breakdown of moderate and high risk groups.

[b] Relative includes first-degree relative and their first-degree relatives (parent, sibling, child).

Considerable doubt exists however about the effectiveness of mammography, prophylactic tamoxifen, prophylactic surgery, and ovarian cancer screening in young women with a mutation in BRCA1 or BRCA2.

Routine family history screening of asymptomatic patients is currently performed by many primary care practitioners for any type of cancer. But this approach does not meet accepted criteria for deployment of a screening test given the limited evidence for interventions to manage the increased risk of most cancers. In the future, screening in primary care for a family history of specific cancers will be appropriate once stronger evidence exists for at least one intervention for that specific cancer, be it chemoprevention, screening, or prophylactic surgery. We may never have evidence from randomized controlled trials for all such interventions, so primary care practitioners will need to discuss the uncertainties about other management options with patients whom they identify through family history screening.

Pre-natal diagnosis

There are two situations in primary care where it is appropriate to discuss genetic issues relating to unborn children: pre-conception and in the early ante-natal period. The issues in both these situations are similar:

- identify those people who are at increased risk of passing on a genetic condition who might need assessment and investigation in secondary care;
- identify those people at population risk who might wish to pursue ante-natal screening tests; and
- discuss with the couple the pros and cons of being tested.

Pre-conception assessment and management

Pre-conception advice is usually given as part of contraceptive services. Very few primary care practices run separate pre-conception clinics but it is feasible to invite women for pre-conception assessment, using the family history as a genetic assessment tool.(14) This method was shown to be acceptable to patients and did not raise anxieties. It was also an opportunity to reassure patients who had concerns about their family history.

If the family history reveals the possibility of a chromosomal or single gene disorder, the patient should be referred for further assessment. If the couple is proven to have an increased risk of a child with a genetic disorder there are several possible management options:

- Testing one or both partners, for example, where there is a close relative with cystic fibrosis.
- Pre-implantation diagnosis: the foetus is conceived by *in vitro* fertilization and a single cell is removed and tested at the 8-cell stage to see if the embryo has inherited the condition. An unaffected embryo can then be implanted.
- Ante-natal testing: chromosome or genetic mutation testing of foetal material obtained by chorionic villous sampling (CVS) or amniocentesis (see below).
- Testing to identify a condition that can be treated *in utero* or when delivery in a unit with special expertise for that condition is indicated.
- Discussion about adoption or *in vitro* fertilization as an alternative to natural conception.

Ante-natal assessment and management

The family history is the usual assessment tool to identify patients at increased risk although this of course is a less sensitive test for risk of recessive conditions. Patients can be considered in four categories. Referral is appropriate for the first three categories for assessment, counselling, and testing if indicated:

1. Those with a high risk of a chromosomal disorder or single gene mutation, for example, a previous child with or family history of muscular dystrophy.
2. Those with an increased risk that is less likely to be due to an inherited chromosomal or single gene disorder, for example, a previous child with spina bifida, Down syndrome, heart defect, or cleft lip.
3. Those at high risk due to another risk factor, for example, maternal age or abnormal maternal serum screening test for Down syndrome (see Table 3).
4. Those at normal risk who are considering screening tests such as nuchal translucency ultrasound scan, serum screening for spina bifida, and Down syndrome, and the anomaly ultrasound scan. Carrier testing for common autosomal recessive conditions will soon become part of this gamut of ante-natal tests to discuss, for example, for haemoglobinopathies in specific ethnic groups and for cystic fibrosis. The feasibility of offering such a carrier testing service in primary care is well documented(10,11) but to provide first trimester diagnosis routinely requires carefully organized ante-natal services to enable discussion of these issues early in pregnancy.

The role of the primary care team for people in this final category involves both pre- and post-test counselling.

Table 3 Risk of conceiving child with Down syndrome according to maternal age

Maternal age (years)	Risk of having Down syndrome baby
25	1 in 1400
30	1 in 900
35	1 in 400
40	1 in 100
45	1 in 30

Pre-test counselling includes explaining:

- what condition the test is trying to detect;
- the implications of having a child with this condition and explore the parents' feeling about this;
- that the test only helps to identify people at lower and higher risk of the condition and that further testing will be necessary to confirm the diagnosis;
- that the test will give false positive and false negative results;
- that definitive tests (CVS or amniocentesis) can cause miscarriage;
- that most conditions detected will not have specific treatment, so parents might need to consider a termination of pregnancy;
- when the result is expected and how it will be communicated.

Post-test counselling

Some test results are not conclusive. For example, the triple test gives a risk for carrying a baby with Down syndrome and carrier screening for cystic fibrosis will not detect all known mutations. Many patients are not familiar with the interpretation of a risk figure, and it may require a range of techniques to help patients understand the meaning of their result.

Primary–secondary interface

Traditionally, clinical genetics has been concerned with the identification and management of rare single gene disorders. Referrals for these disorders tended to be from other hospital specialities. Referrals from primary care to clinical genetics departments have risen considerably in the last few years, mainly due to referrals in cancer genetics or for ante-natal testing.

The scope of genetic services in secondary care

The services provided include:

- Diagnosis of inherited syndromes.
- Assessment of genetic risk, including confirmation of diagnoses in other family members through hospital or cancer registry networks.
- Genetic testing where appropriate to confirm disease risk, including pre-test counselling and post-test follow up (e.g. testing for cancer predisposition and Huntington's disease mutations).
- Testing for mutation status in relatives of patients with a known problem. This might involve liaison with other clinical genetics departments.
- Counselling and support of patients with inherited diseases.
- Laboratory facilities for detecting both single gene mutations and chromosomal abnormality.
- Keeping registers of patients with genetic diseases to ensure appropriate follow-up for them and their family members and to enable future contact if significant treatment advances are made.
- Storage of samples (blood or tissue) in families suspected of an inherited disease if genetic testing became available.

Referrals from primary care

As with all referrals, the need to refer will depend on a combination of three factors: the presenting problem, the patient's views about referral (including anxiety about the problem), and the primary care practitioner's knowledge and skills. The third factor is currently very significant when considering referrals for genetic problems. Patients' expectations might be raised inappropriately if patients at low risk are referred. To avoid this many departments have produced guidelines to assist in the referral process. In a recent UK study, the appropriateness of referrals to a cancer genetics clinic improved in the 8 months after sending guidelines to local general practices.[15]

When referring for genetic testing, it is important to understand the difference between a diagnostic test to confirm a suspected genetic disease and a predictive test to identify the presence of a mutation that might lead to a disease in the future. In the context of inherited cancers, diagnostic testing is initially performed on individuals who have already developed cancer and are at high risk of carrying a mutation. If a mutation is identified in the affected subject, then predictive testing, in which only that specific mutation is sought, can be offered to their unaffected relatives.

Ethical issues

The basic principles of ethics apply equally to genetics as they do to any other medical situation. However, there are additional considerations in genetics:

- The results of any intervention, for example assessing a family history or performing a genetic test, have implications beyond the person being tested. This can create conflict between the right to this knowledge for one family member and the choice of a relative not to know.
- The result of a genetic test can enable a patient to make better informed choices about a situation, for example, to undergo prophylactic mastectomy or to avoid pregnancy. However, unless gene therapy were to become possible, the mutation itself is present for life and so is the knowledge of their test result. This is why pre-test counselling for conditions like Huntington's disease, where no treatment is available, is so rigorous.
- Results of genetic testing can lead to discrimination or stigmatization, as happened in the 1970s when sickle cell testing was mandatory for black Americans. There are also concerns about the use of genetic test results by employers and insurance companies. In many US states, the use of genetic information by employers has been banned. The debate will continue however about the right balance between the needs of the insurers, the protection of the individual and the threat of creating a genetic underclass.
- Genetic testing of a foetus or child presents particular difficulties. The parents' decision to test can be more easily justified if knowledge of the result might prevent illness or death before the child is able to give informed consent. However, the conflict between the rights of the child and the desires of the parents is much greater in conditions which do not present until later in life. A parent might wish to know (and even terminate a pregnancy) to prevent a child inheriting Huntington's disease or a cancer predisposing gene but this must be balanced against uncertain disease penetrance and the possibility that treatment might become available before the child is affected.

The future of genetics in primary care

There are reasonable doubts as to how quickly the new genetics will deliver clinically useful tests and knowledge to primary care, and whether it will initially raise more questions than provide answers.[16] Concerns about potential harm from inappropriate use of genetic testing in primary care have been expressed[17] as has reluctance by primary care practitioners to adopt these new responsibilities. For the next few years, genetics in primary care will centre around ante-natal counselling, including carrier screening for haemoglobinopathies and cystic fibrosis, and risk assessment for certain cancers. Beyond that there will be increasing use of pharmacogenetic information to tailor drug selection and dosage and to predict risk of common conditions such as diabetes and cardiovascular disease. Changes in undergraduate and postgraduate training, implementation of management guidelines and computerized genetic risk assessment will be needed to prepare the current and future primary care workforce for this new knowledge in clinical practice.

References

1. **Emery, J. and Hayflick, S.** (2001). The challenge of integrating genetic medicine into primary care. *British Medical Journal* **322**, 1027–30.
2. **Rose, P. and Lucassen, A.** *Practical Genetics for Primary Care*. Oxford: Oxford University Press, 1999.
3. **Johnson, N., Lancaster, T., Fuller, A., and Hodgson, S.V.** (1995). The prevalence of a family history of cancer in general practice. *Family Practice* **12**, 287–9.
4. **Friedman, L.C., Plon, S.E., Cooper, H.P., and Weinberg, A.D.** (1997). Cancer genetics—survey of primary care physicians' attitudes and practices. *Journal of Cancer Education* **12**, 199–203.
5. **Hyland, F.** et al. (2001). Raising concerns about family history of breast cancer in primary care consultations: prospective, population based study. Women's Concerns Study Group. *British Medical Journal* **322**, 27–8.
6. **Emery, J., Watson, E., Rose, P., and Andermann, A.** (1999). A systematic review of the literature exploring the role of primary care in genetic services. *Family Practice* **16**, 426–45.
7. **Emery, J.** et al. (2000). Computer support for interpreting family histories of breast and ovarian cancer in primary care: comparative study with simulated cases. *British Medical Journal* **321**, 28–32.
8. **Harper, P.** *Practical Genetic Counseling*. Oxford: Butterworth Heinemann, 1998.
9. **Suchard, M., Yudkin, P., Sinsheimer, J., and Fowler, G.** (1999). General practitioners' views on genetic screening for common diseases. *British Journal of General Practice* **49**, 45–6.
10. **Harris, H., Scotcher, D., Hartley, N., Wallace, A., Craufurd, D., and Harris, R.** (1993). Cystic fibrosis carrier testing in early pregnancy by general practitioners. *British Medical Journal* **306**, 1580–3.
11. **Rowley, P.T., Loader, S., Sutera, C.J., and Kozyra, A.** (1995). Prenatal genetic counseling for hemoglobinopathy carriers: a comparison of primary providers of prenatal care and professional genetic counselors. *American Journal of Human Genetics* **56**, 769–76.
12. **Emery, J., Lucassen, A., and Murphy, M.** (2001). The common hereditary cancers and the implications for primary care. *Lancet* **358**, 56–63.
13. **Eccles, D., Evans, D., and Mackay, J.** (2000). Guidelines for managing women with a family history of breast cancer. *Journal of Medical Genetics* **37**, 203–9.
14. **Rose, P., Humm, E., Hey, K., Jones, L., and Huson, S.** (1998). Family history taking and genetic counseling in primary care. *Family Practice* **16**, 78–83.
15. **Lucassen, A., Watson, E., Harcourt, J., Rose, P., and O'Grady, J.** (2000). Guidelines for referral to a regional genetics service: GPs respond by referring more appropriate cases. *Family Practice* **18**, 135–40.
16. **Holtzman, N.A. and Marteau, T.M.** (2000). Will genetics revolutionize medicine? *New England Journal of Medicine* **343**, 141–4.
17. **Giardiello, F.M.** et al. (1997). The use and interpretation of commercial APC gene testing for familial adenomatous polyposis. *New England Journal of Medicine* **336**, 823–7.

9.5 Working with families with chronic medical disorders

Jack H. Medalie, Thomas M. Mettee, Kathleen Cole-Kelly, Jeffrey M. Borkan, and Mary P. Hogan

Background

The family has universally been the basic unit of society throughout history,[1] able to adapt and adjust its functioning to meet the demands of changing environments. Many, however, believe that currently, in some places, the family is not fulfilling many of its key functions, thus laying the foundation for destructive forces like family violence, drug abuse, etc. However, whether it is a haven or a destructive place, the family is still the principal caring place for people with severe or chronic health problems.

Up to the late 1970s and early 1980s, the belief was that due to the advances in medicine and public health, major infectious diseases were on the road to elimination. Unfortunately, the recent epidemic of the new infectious diseases, AIDS, and the resurgence of tuberculosis have torpedoed those ideas. At the same time, despite the advances in medicine, there has been a remarkable parallel increase in chronic conditions, such as ischaemic heart disease, cerebrovascular events, cancer of varying types, Alzheimer's dementia, neurological conditions, depression, and other mental conditions. In many parts of the world, these chronic conditions have replaced infectious diseases as the leading causes of morbidity and mortality.[2]

In this chapter, our objective is threefold. First, we shall discuss factors related to the increase in chronic diseases and the importance of the family's role in chronic illness. Second, we propose a model for collaborative care for the patient and his/her family by a group of primary and secondary caregivers. Finally, we describe a home care programme that is part of a primary care practice, as an illustration of the practical application of the themes and principles discussed in this and the preceding chapters.

Definitions

The definitions of chronic disease, family, caregiver, and home are given elsewhere in this book, but we must emphasize that chronic disorders consist of at least two elements, the disease and the illness. Illness is the experience of symptoms and signs by the patient with or without any objective findings; the everyday reality of symptoms and suffering. Disease, on the other hand, relates to the conceptualization of symptoms, signs, laboratory, and other technological results into a classification of disease categories, related to abnormalities in the structure and functioning of body organs, as defined by physicians. In addition to this important clinical differentiation, both illnesses and diseases have a psycho-social element that affects the emotional life and functioning of the patient, other individuals, and systems interacted with at home, at work, and in the wider community.

Factors related to increased prevalence of chronic diseases

The increase in chronic disease can be ascribed to a complex interacting set of demographic, medical, economic, and cultural factors. Some of these factors include the increase in total population with a marked increase in the proportion of elderly; the decrease in infant and total mortality (except in countries where AIDS is rampant), leading to an increase in total population; increased length of life, wherever AIDS has not decimated the young; decreased hospitalizations and decreased length of stay for most conditions, driven by economic forces as well as advances in medicine; the ability (due to medical advances) to keep alive people who some years ago would have died; and early discharge of psychiatric patients from the hospital into the community.

The increase has not been uniform. Great differences exist between countries, as well as within countries, where ethnic and cultural minorities and lower socio-economic groups bear the brunt of chronic diseases. In some countries, all this has led to an increased availability of home care and ambulatory programmes for patients with chronic diseases who are disabled or housebound.

This increase of people with chronic illnesses and/or diseases, together with decreased hospitalizations, has led to an upsurge of patients with chronic diseases. It is estimated that in 2000, there were about 105 million people in the United States who had chronic conditions, out of a total population of 280 million.[3] The vast majority of these live in the community. This has increased the responsibility of the family in providing medical, nursing, rehabilitative, and support care for their sick members. While many groups all over the world accept this as their cultural responsibility, many, if not most families, whether they accept this responsibility or not, are unprepared for these roles. The attempt to fulfil these roles often leads to stress, resulting in dysfunction and conflict within the whole family system.

Types and stages of chronic diseases

All chronic disorders have some common elements, but they differ substantially depending on the *type* and *stage* of the disease. For example, chronic conditions with mental/brain dysfunction, such as Alzheimer's or multi-infarct dementia, mental retardation, and schizophrenia, pose very different problems and stresses than those patients with normal cognitive ability. Then, there are the groups of congenital and early childhood chronic diseases, which have problems relating to developmental issues, in addition to others. These diseases, as well as those that do not fall into one of these two groups, have many psycho-social problems relating to the patient, the caregiver, the family, and friends. The most disabling conditions are purportedly related to mental retardation, paralysis of extremities, blindness, respiratory conditions (cancer and chronic obstructive pulmonary disease), and multiple sclerosis.[3]

In addition to the type of illness described above, another important facet is the *illness cycle* or *course* and the *stage* of the cycle at any given time.[4] Some chronic diseases, such as amyotrophic lateral sclerosis and end-stage renal disease, are *slowly progressive* to marked disability and death. Others are of the *relapsing* type, in which stable periods alternate with relapses and crises, for example, multiple sclerosis, diabetes, and bipolar psychiatric conditions. Still others are *mixed*, for example, a progressive condition with periods of crisis. These different types and stages of the disease, together with the *family and community resources available*, will direct the type of care and service required. In many countries, numerous types of chronic care services are available (not always well coordinated), including inpatient and outpatient medical and nursing care, home health care, homemaker services, nursing home care, adult day care, rehabilitative services, but the main burden usually rests with the family.

The family's ability to care for an individual member with a chronic condition is dependent on a number of interrelated factors discussed below.

The family

The context of care for a patient coping with chronic disorders is the family within their own social, cultural, and economic milieu. Whether or not the family are members of the same medical practice, it is important to learn the patient's context.[5] If assessment is confined solely to the individual patient and the status of his/her chronic disease, it restricts the physician's understanding and access to the most important collaborators in the patient's care.

Understanding the family's relationship to the patient and the significant family caregivers is critical for the health care provider. As mentioned earlier, different chronic diseases have different courses, and families are challenged to adjust to the idiosyncratic changes in the course of the illness. The caregiver is usually part of the biological family (spouse or daughter), but other significant family members, friends, neighbours, or hired help may assume care taking roles in response to the situation. This caregiving group has been called the 'functional family'.[6]

To understand the background of the family and who the participants in the 'functional family' are, an assessment of the family is very helpful. This assessment includes an assessment of their health status, development (life-cycle) stage, strengths and support, functioning, and health beliefs.

Understanding the stage of the family's life-cycle is important since the life-cycle stage often determines family experiences. If the family is at the stage of the life-cycle of bearing children, a parent's chronic illness, especially if it is disabling, can be disruptive to the nurturing and development of the children. If the chronic illness affects one of the younger children and the family is mainly coping with adolescent children, different behavioural and health problems can become more pronounced in the family system. If the chronic illness affects parents at a later stage of the family life-cycle, strains and tensions can arise in the adult children trying to balance their own family and work demands, leading to economic, emotional, and physical distress.

Assessment of family function should accompany any physical evaluation of the patient and of other family members involved with the chronically ill member. Primary care physicians who have a longstanding relationship with their patients can assess their patients and families accurately. Today, however, with the emphasis placed on cost-effectiveness and productivity, there is less time for this relationship to develop, so physicians might want to use questionnaires or other professionals, such as social workers or nurses, to aid their assessment and gain a better understanding of the family. Some of the instruments are referred to in the 'Further reading' section.

The caregiver is the key to the care of a chronically ill patient, and if the caregiver does not receive adequate support, she/he is at risk of becoming a 'hidden patient'[7] and developing overt or covert disease by neglecting her/his own health needs. Besides the caregiver, the hidden patient could be another member of the family, for example, a child who is ignored while the sick member receives all of the family and professional attention. If the hidden patient is not identified, acknowledged, and attended to, multiple problems can arise. These possible situations underscore the importance of the physician focusing not only on the patient, but on the caregiver and the whole family system. The family is called a system because, like all systems, if one individual (or part) is disabled or diseased, it affects all the family members and the family (or system) as a whole.

Most health care providers are more adept at noticing pathology than noticing strengths. The benefits of identifying *family strengths* are twofold: the health care provider can comment and reinforce the strengths that exist; and also can remind the family, when it is struggling, of strengths that it may have overlooked. Being able to comment on a family's history of resiliency, of their ability to carry on with important family rituals in the midst of challenging chronic illness, or their being able to remobilize former resources, can be instrumental in the family's coping with a new or existing chronic illness. Olsen identified family characteristics that were markers of the family's functioning and their way of structuring relationships by emphasizing family cohesion and family adaptability.[8]

Family cohesion (closeness) defines how close family members are to each other. Understanding the degree of closeness can help when a physician is working with a family with a chronically ill member. Usually, families come closer together during crises, but have difficulties over the long haul.[9] Learning about the degree of involvement of different family members can be useful. Less involved members might be encouraged to be more involved with the patients, in hopes of minimizing burnout of a more burdened family member in the main caretaker role.

Some families tend to exclude the patient (even when cognitively able) from information and decision-making. Discouraging this usually suffices to improve or even 'cure' this marginalization. Sometimes, if this process occurs with a family member other than the patient, attention needs to be focused on integrating that member into family activities, including the family health care team. Sometimes, this can be done just by learning about the relationship dynamics and commenting on them. Otherwise, if this is having serious deleterious effects on the family's relationships and organization is very rigid and difficult to change, it may be important to consider delving deeper into the family dynamics or getting a family therapist involved.

An important factor for health care providers to consider is the *family's ability to adapt to change*. Some families are very good in some stages and not in others. For example, a family might do well in a crisis, but be less adaptable when the chronic disease continues over a long period of time. Learning how families cope with change is important when matching that with the idiosyncratic demands of the chronic illness being treated. For the family that is unable to make constant shifts and adaptations to changes, dealing with a steadily declining member with Alzheimer's dementia could be much harder than if the chronically ill member had a permanent but relatively unchanging disability with no cognitive impairment.

Stages of acceptance

Families' reactions to the losses and severe changes involved with a chronically ill member can vary. The stages of grief—shock, denial, anger, bargaining, and acceptance—are commonly experienced by all family members, but in varying order or intensity, depending on other individual and family issues.[10] Not all family members go through the grief stages in the same order or at the same time, which can cause confusion and even conflict.

The *family's belief* about the cause of the illness—their explanatory model[11]—is based on their culture, ethnicity, education, and individual beliefs. Fadiman describes a striking example in California of a Hmong family's belief that spirits caused their daughter's epilepsy.[12] All medical interventions, despite their good intentions and based on well-documented scientific evidence, were traumatic for this family wed to their Hmong culture and traditions. These beliefs may also cover treatment and prognostic expectations, so it is incumbent on a physician to learn the source of the family's beliefs about the illness. Without that understanding, the physician and family can be working at cross-purposes. Without eliciting each family member's belief, important feelings between family members might not be exposed.

An important aspect of family functioning, in addition to those mentioned above, is the *communication pattern* in the family. This pattern is important for the content (facts, opinions, feelings), as well as the clues it presents about relationships between the communicators and the governance of the family. All verbal and non-verbal behaviours, including silence, convey interpersonal messages. Silence and what is not talked about reveals some beliefs and subjects that the family find difficult to discuss. However, the patient or others might be able to discuss certain subjects like anticipated loss with some family members, but not with others. In general, a couple's relationship and the communication pattern between them dictates the communication pattern of the rest of the family.[9] Finally, it must be stressed that there are many different communication patterns in families that are compatible with good family functioning in respect to the member with a chronic disease.

Characteristics of 'chronic disease families'

Steinglass and others working with American families with a member with a chronic disease identified four common characteristics of these families:[13] the disease tends to dominate family life, while other needs are neglected; new coalitions between members are developed, or old ones intensified; the family's coping response becomes rigid and any suggested change is regarded with suspicion; and finally, families tend to isolate themselves.

This tendency towards *isolation* is often overlooked. Learning about the community context of care for the family is crucial in helping families not feel they are battling the chronic illness alone. Learning about nursing and home care services, about community support groups (e.g. CAN COPE cancer support group), or groups targeted specifically for the chronic illness, the family member has can help buffer the families' isolation and support their coping strategies. In this community context, a continuing readily available contact with a family physician is of extreme importance.

Another outcome of the potential sense of isolation and coping challenges can be the development of *depression*, a common co-morbidity with chronic illness. Too often, much attention is being focused on the patient's disease process and too little on the psychological and emotional impact on the patient or other family members. Health care providers need to be adept at diagnosing depression in either the chronically ill patient or the family member burdened by the demands of caretaking, or another family member feeling neglected in the midst of the attention on the chronically ill patient. Often, depression with chronic illness as seen in primary care differs from the diagnostic classification of DSM IV and is thus overlooked.[14] It must be emphasized that even well-functioning families have difficulties at various times and need and often welcome support and help.

We must stress that the diagnosis and assessment of the patient and family is, in essence, the beginning of and an important part of the care process.

Model of collaborative care

In pluralistic multicultural societies, there is a broad range of diverse family forms and styles of organization and functioning. This includes nuclear, extended, single parent, grandparent, foster, reconstituted, and same sex family types, all of which may function in a paternalistic or maternalistic autocratic manner, or in a more democratic way, or have a laissez-faire process, where generational boundaries are all but eliminated. It is important to realize that all or any of these styles of organization and functioning may be compatible with healthy family development and adjustment to a member with a chronic disease or illness. On the other hand, some forms, like an autocratic governed family may cope well with certain stages of chronic disease, such as a crisis, but have difficulty with other stages where more flexibility and role modifications are needed.

Similarly, the patient's and physician's roles change during the course of the disease. During a crisis resulting in hospitalization, the patient and family are largely dependent on the physician's judgement, knowledge, and skills. During other, more stable phases, the patient is more independent and autonomous, while the physician and health care team are more in a 'partnership' mode. With appropriate discussions and consultations between the physician, the health care team, the patient, the caregiver, and the family, important decisions can be made.

In many areas of the world, a person with a chronic disease can only depend on his/her family, perhaps assisted by a physician, nurse, or a traditional healer, since no other resources are available. However, in other parts of the globe, the multiplicity of needs has led to the development of multiple resources in the home, workplace, educational facilities, as well as in the community. These resources aid people with chronic diseases, particularly with disabilities. How a community and society deal with their disabled members is usually a good indication of their social beliefs, modified somewhat by their economic resources. 'Sickness' may be defined as the social construction of the disease/illness; that is, how society addresses patients with disease or moulds the experience for the individual; access for the handicapped, work, and educational opportunities, etc.

In identifying a model of care for the patient with chronic disease, there are some principles that define our orientation and the reasons for our family oriented, primary and secondary model.

The primary and secondary group model

Our approach is not disease-centred or patient-centred, but deals with the patient in the context of the family or with the family as the unit of care. In other words, our orientation is family-centred.[4,10,13]

The core model includes a primary group of care providers or participants. The group is primary in the sense that it is a universal model occurring in most cultures, and consists of the patient, the illness/disease, the patient's family including the main caregiver, and a physician with the health care team (Fig. 1). This model is a modification of Rolland's Therapeutic Quadrangle.[15] The members of the health care team will vary depending on need and available resources, but almost always includes a nurse or nurse's aide.

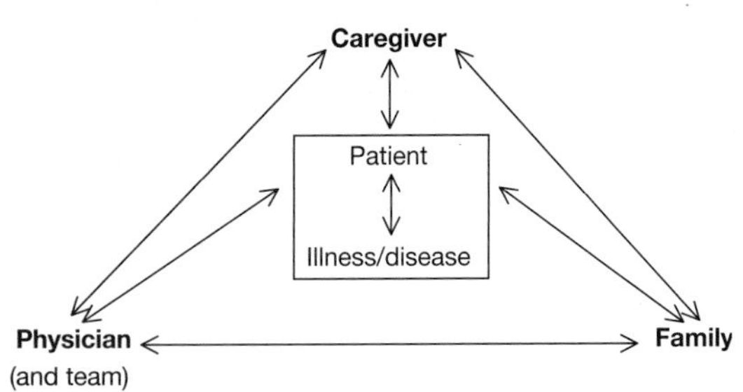

Fig. 1 Primary group of chronic care participants.

Table 1 The secondary group of chronic disease participants—actual or potential, with direct or indirect influence

Nurses—of varying types and training (some may be part of the primary team)
Medical specialists—oncologists, surgeons, etc.
Mental health—social workers, psychiatrists, etc.
Anciliary personnel—physical and occupational therapists, dietitians
Alternative healers—folk and traditional
Social support network—friends, neighbours, religious congregations, specific disease support groups
Volunteer groups—Meals on Wheels, self-help groups, etc.
Medical insurance companies
Public institutions—national, state, and local
Private institutions—hospice, home care agencies
Environmental influences—physical: air, water, and soil pollution; social: attitudes and behaviour towards people with chronic diseases and disabilities at work, school, recreation, and public institutions
Health care system—universal coverage, patchwork, or non-existent; medical and technological resources available

Note: in the United Kingdom there are health visitors, who seem to fulfil some roles of both nurses and social workers.

Supporting the primary group are a number of other providers who vary depending on availability of local resources and the stage of the disease. We call this group the secondary group of care providers/participants (Table 1). Sometimes, one of the secondary group occupies such an important role in the care process that he/she becomes part of the primary group.

Let us now consider these two groups in more detail, from the perspective of the tasks required for the primary care physician, who concentrates on the family in which at least one member has a chronic disease, while coping with his/her own multiple roles over a prolonged time.

The primary group (Fig. 1)

The patient

Assess current health status, including co-morbid conditions; obtain family's medical history, relevant to the patient; assess patient's personality—optimistic/pessimistic, rigid/flexible to new ideas or pleasant/unpleasant to work with; identify stage of life-cycle and future transitions; explore patient's understanding of and reaction to the disease, and beliefs about causation, prognosis, and treatment; understand relationship to caregiver, family, friends, as well as to physician and other health care personnel; encourage independence in functioning and medication use; and encourage participation in family, work, and social activities.

The disease/illness

Assess type of disease (life-threatening, relapsing, progressive, constant or relatively stable, and does it affect cognitive ability and/or development of patient); identify stage of disease (onset, terminal, etc.); and estimate the amount of disability, incapacitation, and financial difficulties the illness or disease is causing or will cause.

The caregiver

It has been estimated that caregivers provide about 80 per cent of home health care, especially to the frail elderly. This group is progressively increasing in numbers with the ageing of the population, while fewer workers seem to be available for the task of care. Caregiver burdens have been well documented. Despite doing all they can in providing for their loved one, the outcome is often nursing home placement or death. Caregivers are prone to anxiety and depression and other symptoms relating to the stress of their work.[7] It has been documented that their immune functions may deplete, making them more susceptible to health problems and even mortality.[16] Particularly troublesome patient problems include incontinence of bladder or bowel and dementia (often with aggressive behaviour), which challenge the level of tolerance and self-perceived competence of the caregiver. Special interventions for caregiver relief, in addition to the support of the caregiver team, include support groups, individual counselling, educational programmes, stress reduction techniques, and respite care. No single one of these interventions has proven completely successful in preventing caregiver burnout.[17,18]

Therefore, the factors that the primary care physician needs to attend to regarding the caregiver include: identify relationship to patient, family physician, and nurses; diagnose current health status and long-term prognosis; assess knowledge of and reaction to disease, ability to detect changes in patient's condition, and inclination to ask for and accept help when needed; learn about ability to withstand demands of situation and whether she/he is receiving adequate support from family and patient; make sure the caregiver feels an integral part of health care team, feels her/his work is appreciated, and is free to express her/his feelings to the physician and also that in emergencies, she/he has immediate access to the nurse or physician; and encourage her/him to take 'respite intervals' and continue own social participation.

The family

Assess the understanding of and reaction to the patient and the disease, and the ability to adjust to different stages of the disease, which includes the relationship to and ability to cope with the patient while allowing for his/her continuing development and participation in social activities; assess the level of support for the main caregiver and the functioning of family regarding the patient and functioning of the rest of the family according to the stage of their life-cycle; explore whether the family can balance needs of the patient with those of the rest of the family; assess the family's relationship to the physician and nurses and their ability to voice opinions and feelings and explore their knowledge of and readiness to use community resources and accept help from outside people, like home aides; confirm that the family is up to date with information about the patient and is involved in discussions and decisions about the patient; and determine family members' explanatory models and beliefs regarding cause and treatment of the disease.

The physician (or physician–nurse team)

Needs to keep up to date about the disease in order to treat the patient and help the patient, caregiver, and family with relevant information; feels at ease about referring the patient for consultation to various specialists when the need arises; shifts focus from 'cure' to improvement of function and alleviation of pain and suffering and includes the patient, caregiver, and family in a 'partnership' mode as part of the comprehensive health care team; needs to make plans to cover all contingencies, that is, care plans during all stages of the disease, including end-of-life stage and plans to maintain health and functioning of the caregiver; needs to organize a system where the doctor or nurse is readily available for urgent and emergency situations, as well as a system of monitoring the progress of the patient, the disease, and the rest of the primary team; needs to provide educational information and support to the patient, caregiver, and family while maintaining relationships and dealing with attempts at 'triangulation' and 'taking sides'; maintains or improves knowledge of and ability to work with relevant community resources; needs to encourage periodic 'respite intervals and care' for caregiver and family; encourages, if culture allows, periodic family discussions and conferences; and maintains adequate boundaries between his/her personal and professional life; accepts and deals with 'loss', and if necessary, obtains counselling if there is a feeling of 'burnout'.

The secondary group (Table 1)

Without detailing the activities of each of the secondary participants, a few general points are given below.

The secondary group participants often play important roles in the support and occasionally in the obstruction of the primary group. This support can be directed to the patient or to one of the other members of the primary group. A nurse or oncologist gives direct aid to the patient, while a social worker might give direct aid to many in the group. Nurses often take leading roles in the care of chronically disabled patients and their families (see the Section on Home care), thereby becoming an important integral part of the primary group. Sometimes, direct aid to the patient occurs with or without the knowledge of and/or the cooperation of the other primary group members. This might occur with the use of alternative remedies or healers.

For economic and other reasons, public and private institutions, like the health care system and health insurance companies, have their own agendas, priorities, and rules. These influence many aspects of hospitalizations, nursing home and hospice admissions, as well as types of operation, examination, medication, or remuneration allowed. Unfortunately, these rules are not always to the benefit of the patient.

Environmental factors have direct and indirect influence. Air pollution directly affects the breathing of elderly patients with COPD, while a newly diagnosed diabetic bus driver might lose his job due to the company's policy of not employing diabetic or alcoholic drivers. Disabled people are sometimes limited in their activities when no facilities exist for wheelchairs.

Family home care

In recent years, there have been numerous pilot projects to improve the care of chronically ill elderly patients, through improvements in their hospital care, their transitional care from hospital to home, day hospital, home hospitals, and home care programmes.[19,20]

Complementary to these improvements, the physician and health care team tending to family care in chronic disease will, at some stage, have to concentrate their efforts in the home of the patient. This can be part of everyday primary care practice (the custom in many countries) or by special arrangements. The studies of outcome measures of home care programmes have shown conflicting results, but studies of integrated home care programmes have consistently shown marked improvements in patient and family satisfaction, decreased use of emergency rooms and hospitals, improved functional abilities, and reduction of total costs.[21,22] The improvement for the patients and the reduction of costs should and will make home visiting and care more important in the overall health systems. Thus, very appropriately, McWhinney issued a call to action for family and other primary care physicians to expand their care into the home.[23] To quote from his article, 'The home is where a family's values are expressed. It is in the home that people can be themselves. The history of the family—its story, its joys and sorrows, its memories and aspirations are there on the walls'. Much earlier, too, Florence Nightingale emphasized the importance of the physician's home visit and the inclusion of the patient in the physician's discussions.[24] Home visiting to see the patient and family in their 'natural' environment is the best place to assess their functioning, beliefs, desires, resources, and needs. In addition, the understanding of the caregiver and her/his needs is much easier when knowing the home environment in which the patient functions.[25,26]

To illustrate the practical application of the principles discussed earlier, we shall review some of the workings of an integrated home care programme that is an integral part of a family doctor's practice.

The home visiting programme has dealt with nearly 200 homebound patients since its inception in 1989. The physician and the practice nurse responsible for the coordination of the programme (an important member of the primary care team) visit their patients regularly for the equivalent of one and a half days per month, besides some follow-up visits in between their rounds. Home agency nurses and others involved, for example, physical therapists and social workers, participate in these visits as do medical students during their clerkship rotations. In between the organized visits, there is always open communication (telephone, beepers) between the patient/caregiver and the office-based nurse, the home care agency, and the physician. This communication and ready availability of the health care team is a source of satisfaction and empowerment for the patient, the caregiver, and family and also keeps the team current with any health changes.

The major conditions that create the homebound status are arthritis, cancer, dementia, heart disease (CHF and IHD), COPD, neurological conditions, para- and quadriplegias, and fractures in the frail elderly. Spinal conditions (disc and joint diseases) aggravate the conditions and lead to increased immobility. Those living alone complicate many of the other conditions and are a challenge to the health care team.

The patient and family assessment of patients previously known to the physician is not a problem, but for new patients the assessment starts with the initial visit and continues through follow-up encounters. The initial home visit is usually an extended one and includes the patient's history and physical examination by the physician in the presence of the primary caregiver and sometimes other family members, in addition to the nurses. This facilitates common understanding by everyone present and allows for questions and discussion. At this and subsequent visits, attention is also paid to the home environment, especially the bedroom, bathroom, kitchen, and lighting at night, to allow for easier access and prevention of accidents.

At subsequent visits, the team reviews the activities of daily living (ADL—bathing, dressing, eating, toilet, mobility), instrumental activities of daily living (IADL—paying bills, preparing meals, light housework, use of telephone), and specific functional activities like walking and stair climbing.

Throughout the activities of the home care programme, primary attention is on the patient in the context of her/his family and home environment, with particular attention to the primary caregiver. The caregiver's inclusion as an integral part of the health care team with easily accessed communication and availability of the coordinating nurse and physician goes a long way to making her/his job and the whole process less stressful and more manageable and satisfying.

Based on a biopsychosocial approach,[6,10,27] the focus is often on emotional, social, and family problems directly or indirectly related to the patient's condition, in addition to the biological concerns of pain, bladder and bowel function, nutrition, and a review of all medications. These visits, too, include many educational aspects of the disease for family members. At the end of each visit, all members of the team, including the patient (if cognitively able) and the caregiver, discuss findings, plans for diagnostic tests, medication changes, emotional status, and other relevant parameters, such as community resources like Meals on Wheels, that might be involved.

When important decisions have to be made, other family members will usually be involved in the family–health care team conference. This proactive approach by the physician–nurse–caregiver team reduces family crises to a rare event. They do occasionally occur, however, and one example of a crisis requiring patient–family decision-making is bowel incontinence. Failure to manage this problem is a common reason for caregiver burnout and transfer of the patient to another setting. Innovative solutions to keep the patient at home, such as elective colostomy, can only happen with the consent of the patient and family, and the support of the health care team. Another occasion when crises occur is when the primary caregiver is taking a well-earned rest and is replaced by someone who is not used to dealing with the emergencies of the patient.

In summary, changes in demographic, economic, and medical processes have led to an increase in people with chronic diseases, most of whom live at home and not in institutions. This has led to more responsibility, role changes, and stress on the families in which there is a chronically ill member. The physician, therefore, has to pay attention not only to the patient, but also to the caregiver and the rest of the family. The important points of care for the chronically ill are: the importance of the family and caregiver for the patient's total care, and the physician's understanding of the family's functioning and beliefs, including the changes that occur as disease progresses; the collaborative primary partnership team of the patient, caregiver, family, and physician–nurse care team; the ready availability of the physician or nurse in times of crisis and emergency; and collaboration with and use of community resources.

References

1. **Adams, B.N.** *The Family: A Sociological Interpretation* 4th edn. San Diego CA: Harcourt Brace Jovanovich, 1986.
2. **Brownson, R.C., Remington, P.L., and Davis, J.R.**, ed. *Chronic Disease Epidemiology and Control* 2nd edn. Washington DC: American Public Health Association, 1998.
3. **Hoffman, C. and Rice, D.P.** *Chronic Care in America: A 21st Century* Challenge. Princeton NJ: Robert Wood Johnson Foundation, 1996.
4. **Medalie, J.H.** (1997). The patient and family adjustment to chronic disease in the home. *Disability and Rehabilitation* **19**, 163–70.
5. **Cole-Kelly, K., Yanoshik, K., Campbell, J., and Flynn, S.** (1998). Integrating a family oriented approach with the individual patient. *Journal of Family Practice* **47**, 440–5.
6. **Medalie, J.H. and Cole-Kelly, K.** (2002). The clinical importance of defining family. *American Family Physician* **65** (7), 1277–9.
7. **Medalie, J.H.** (1994). The caregiver as the hidden patient: challenges for medical practice. In *Family Caregiving Across the Lifespan* (ed. E. Kahana, D.E. Biegel, and M.L. Wykle), pp. 312–30. Thousand Oaks CA: Sage Publications.
8. **Olson, D.H.** (1993). Circumplex model of marital and family systems: assessing family functioning. In *Normal Family Processes* 2nd edn. (ed. F. Walsh), New York: Norton.
9. **Rolland, J.S.** *Families, Illness and Disability.* New York: Basic Books—Harper Collins, 1994.
10. **McDaniel, S., Campbell, T.L., and Seaburn, D.B.** *Family Oriented Primary Care.* New York: Springer-Verlag, 1990.
11. **Kleinman, A.** *Patients and Healers in the Context of Culture.* Berkeley: University of California Press, 1980.
12. **Fadiman, A.** *The Spirit Catches You and You Fall Down.* New York: Noonday Press, 1997.
13. **Gonzales, S., Steinglass, P., and Reiss, D.** (1990). Family-centered interventions for people with chronic physical disabilities. In *Family Oriented Primary Care* (ed. S. McDaniel, T.L. Campbell, and D.B. Seaburn), p. 998. New York: Springer-Verlag.
14. **deGruy, F.V. III.** (1997). Mental health care in the primary care setting: a paradigm problem. *Families, Systems and Health* **15**, 3–26.
15. **Rolland, J.S.** (1987). Family systems and chronic illness. *Journal of Psychotherapy and Family* **3**, 164–8.
16. **Schulz, R. and Beach, S.R.** (1999). Caregiving as a risk factor for mortality. *Journal of the American Medical Association* **282**, 2215–19.
17. **Council on Scientific Affairs—American Medical Association** (1993). Physicians and family caregivers: a model for partnership. *Journal of the American Medical Association* **269**, 1280–4.
18. **Parks, S.M. and Novielli, K.D.** (2000). A practical guide to caring for caregivers. *American Family Physician* **62**, 2613–19.
19. **Boult, C., Kane, R.P., Pacala, J.T., and Wagner, E.H.** (1999). Innovative healthcare for chronically ill older persons: results of a national survey. *American Journal of Managed Care* **5**, 1162–72.
20. **Calkins, E., Boult, C., Wagner, E.H., and Pacala, J.T.** *New Ways to Care for Older People: Building Systems Based on Evidence.* New York: Springer, 1998.
21. **Cummings, J.E.** et al. (1990). Cost-effectiveness of veterans administration hospital-based home care: a randomized controlled trial. *Archives of Internal Medicine* **150**, 1274–80.
22. **Melin, A., Hakansson, S., and Bygren, L.** (1993). The cost-effectiveness of rehabilitation in the home; a study of Swedish elderly. *American Journal of Public Health* **83**, 356–62.
23. **McWhinney, I.R.** (1997). The doctor, the patient and the home: returning to our roots. *Journal of the American Board of Family Practice* **10**, 430–5.
24. **Nightingale, F.** *Notes on Nursing.* London: Doves Publications, 1969.
25. **Urwin, B.K. and Jerant, A.F.** (1999). The home visit. *American Family Physician* **60**, 1481–8.
26. **McWhinney, I.R.** (2001). Home care. In *Textbook of Rural Medicine* (ed. J.P. Geyman, T.E. Morris, and G. Hart), pp. 167–79. New York: McGraw-Hill.
27. **Doescher, M.P., Franks, P., and Saver, B.G.** (1999). Is family care associated with reduced health care expenditures? *Journal of Family Practice* **48**, 608–14.

Further reading

For those readers who are interested in measurements of family factors and variables, we recommend these reference books:

Grotevant, H.D. and Carlson, C.I. *Family Assessment: A Guide to Methods and Measures.* New York: Guilford Press, 1989.

McCubbin, H.I. and Thompson, A.I., ed. *Family Assessment Inventories for Research and Practice.* Madison WI: University of Wisconsin Press, 1987.

Touliatos, J., Perlmutter, B.F., and Straus, M.A., ed. *Handbook of Family Measurement Techniques.* Newbury Park CA: Sage Publications, 1990.

9.6 Family violence

Sandra K. Burge, Colleen Fogarty, and Charles Mouton

The problem

Family violence is widespread and causes serious physical harm. Child abuse affects 40 million children aged 0–14 years worldwide.[1] In some countries, child abuse causes as many as 10–20 deaths per 100 000 children under age 5. Intimate partner violence affects 1.3–52 per cent of women around the world each year (median 17 per cent).[2] In the United States, this act kills 1.5 women per 100 000 annually. Among those who survive, 27 per cent require medical care and 15 per cent require hospitalization.[3] Elder mistreatment harms approximately 3–6 per cent of all adults over age 65 in the United States, Canada, and Great Britain.[4] Abused elders have a poorer chance of survival than self-neglected and non-affected elders.[5] Violent acts are not isolated nor independent, but are interwoven across generations. In families with child abuse, one can often detect wife abuse, and vice versa. Perpetrators of all types family violence are more likely than nonperpetrators to have been victims of abuse as children.

The causes

Several theories address the causes of family violence. Sociological theories observe that societies with high rates of violence contain attitudes and structures that support those violent behaviours. Societies which devalue particular groups of people, such as female children, wives, ethnic minorities, elders, and disabled persons, have higher rates of violence against those people, even within families. While most societies prohibit violence against family members, the abuse is often effectively condoned by the passivity of legal authorities and helping institutions. Physical aggression toward children is one such example. In many countries, this is widely accepted as a method of shaping children's behaviour. Arrests for hitting children are rare except in the most egregious circumstances. After Kempe published the landmark article on the 'Battered Child Syndrome' in 1962,[6] the United States drew the line against the most severe types of harm toward children. Sweden banned corporal punishment of children altogether, and eight other European countries have followed suit.

Psychological theories have posit that the cause lies within the individual abuser, who must have psychological or emotional problems. Research indicates that parents who batter children have poor anger management and ineffective childrearing techniques. Men who batter women have higher rates of alcoholism and drug dependence, anti-social personality disorder, depression, and borderline personality disorder. 'Stress' is a proposed cause; abusers tend to have lower educational attainment, higher unemployment, lower socio-economic status, or more caregiver strain.

Social psychological theories note the influence of social interactions on individual behaviour. Social Exchange Theory posits that violence occurs because 'it works'. It stops an argument or controls the other person's behaviour, and inherently reinforces continued use of aggression. Social Learning Theory states that children model behaviours seen in adult family members, and test them in their relationships with others. The 'intergenerational transmission of violence' supports this theory. Individuals who witness parental violence during childhood or who are physically abused are more likely to become perpetrators of violence against spouses, children, and elders.

Child abuse

Definitions

Child abuse is a broad term encompassing many types of maltreatment: physical, emotional, and sexual aggression, and neglect. 'Neglect' is often defined as an act of omission, while 'abuse' is an act of commission. The World Health Organization does not make that distinction, but defines all types of child abuse as acts of omission and commission. *Physical abuse* of a child is an interaction which results in actual or potential physical harm. There may be single or repeated incidents. *Emotional abuse* includes the failure to provide a developmentally appropriate, supportive environment, but also includes acts that have a high probability of causing harm to the child's health or development. Acts include restriction of movement, belittling, scapegoating, threatening, or other non-physical forms of hostile or rejecting treatment. *Child sexual abuse* is the involvement of a child in sexual activity which he or she does not fully comprehend and cannot consent. The perpetrator can be an adult or another child who is in a relationship of responsibility, trust or power; the goal of the activity is to gratify the needs of the perpetrator. *Neglect* is the failure to provide for the development of the child in all spheres: health, education, emotional development, nutrition, shelter, and safe living conditions.

The victim

The definition of a child is an individual who has not yet attained the age of majority, typically age 18 in most Western nations. Most victims of severe forms of physical abuse are children under the age of 2 years. Worldwide, certain types of children are more likely to be abused: those in poor health, females, unwanted children, children with devalued traits, or children born under conditions of rapid socio-economic change.[7]

The perpetrator

The majority of adults who commit child abuse are family members of the child; 87 per cent are parents. Most abuse occurs within the child's home. Day care settings account for only 0.9 per cent of child abuse.[8] More women than men are perpetrators of neglect and physical abuse, while more men than women are perpetrators of sexual abuse.[1] Risk factors for perpetrating physical abuse can be identified at several levels of the biopsychosocial model (Table 1). They include: male child, life stressors, maternal psychiatric impairment, low maternal educational attainment, lack of pre-natal classes, substance abuse, and low religious attendance. Parental sociopathic behaviour and substance abuse are risk indicators for neglect; young maternal age and parental death are risk indicators for sexual abuse.[9]

Table 1 Biopsychosocial risk factors for child abuse

Victim risk factors
Sex
Prematurity
Unwanted child
Disability
Perpetrator risk factors
Young age
Single parent
Unwanted pregnancy
Poor parenting skills
Early exposure to violence
Substance abuse
Inadequate pre-natal care
Physical or mental illness
Relationship difficulties
Family risk factors
Large family size (high family density)
Poverty
Social isolation
High stress
Family violence history
Community and society risk factors
Inadequate child protection laws (unenforced or non-existent)
Decreased value of children (gender, minority, and disability status),
Social inequities
Organized violence
High social acceptance of violence and corporal punishment
Media violence
Cultural norms

The consequences

Long-term consequences of child abuse are protean, and include depression, anxiety disorders, and post-traumatic stress disorder.[10] In addition, childhood abuse is strongly correlated with increased incidence of risky behaviours (substance abuse, sexual risks, physical inactivity, and obesity), diagnosed medical conditions (including ischaemic heart disease, cancer, chronic lung disease, skeletal, and liver disease) and criminal arrests in adolescence and adulthood.[11] Child sexual abuse may be a risk factor for early pregnancy.[12] Some hypothesize that these associations have a biological basis in an overactive hypothalamic–pituitary axis as a result of repetitive exposure to traumatic events.[13]

Diagnosis

Neglect is the most prevalent form of child abuse and can be difficult to diagnose. Child neglect can be broadly viewed as a failure to meet a child's basic needs, which can involve social entities other than the parents. Possible signs of neglect are listed in Table 2.

Physical abuse can result in severe injuries affecting several different organ systems including: neurological, musculoskeletal, and skin (Table 3).

Table 2 Features of neglect

Features of neglect
Health care
Non-adherence
Delay or failure to access health care
Food and nutrition
Hunger
Failure to thrive
Exposures
Drugs (in utero or in home environment)
Poisonings
Education
Nurturance
Emotional deprivation/abuse
Apathy
Abandonment
Home and protection
Homelessness
Inadequate shelter
Inadequate protection and supervision
Clothing and hygiene
Inadequate clothing for climate
Excessively soiled or torn clothing
Poor hygiene
Physical
Failure to thrive/poor growth
Recurrent or persistent minor infections
Severe diaper rash
Development
Developmental delay
Language delay
Limited attention span
Socio-emotional immaturity
Behavioural
Attachment disorder
Anxious, avoidant
Lack of social responsiveness
Indiscriminate friendliness
Impulsivity
Aggressivity

Table 3 Signs of physical abuse

Signs of physical abuse
Skin
Bruises on unusual body surfaces
Blunt instrument marks
Burns: immersion, circumferential, cigarette
Human hand marks
Human bite marks
Musculo-skeletal
Metaphyseal 'Bucket-handle' fracture
Posterior rib fracture
Scapula fracture
Spinous process fracture
Sternal fracture
Neurological
Closed head trauma
Retinal haemorrhage
General
Poor care
Failure to thrive
Multiple injuries in various stages of healing

'Shaken baby syndrome' refers to the severe intracranial injury resulting from violent shaking of an infant. This is characterized by lethargy, weak cry, vomiting, irritability, and seizures, and may be accompanied by intracranial haemorrhage and retinal haemorrhage. A United Kingdom case series of infants with subdural haemorrhage showed that 82 per cent were likely caused by abuse.[14]

The fractures listed in Table 3 have high specificity for child abuse. Fractures of different ages, bilateral, epiphyseal separations, digital fractures, and skull fractures are moderately specific for child abuse.

In evaluating a child for suspected child abuse, the primary care clinician must take a detailed biopsychosocial history and attempt to corroborate the history reported by the caregiver. In addition, careful medical record documentation, including photographs, is important for criminal legal proceedings. A skeletal survey should be done in all children under the age of 2 years in whom child abuse is suspected and, when clinically appropriate, in children under age 5 years. A 'bodygram' or 'babygram' is not sufficiently accurate to identify subtle injury in the context of suspected abuse.

Clinical interventions

In the United States, all health care providers are mandated to report any suspected child abuse to the local child protective agency. The physician is not obligated to prove or substantiate any suspicions, but should be prepared to provide medical records for review by the local child protective authority. Family physicians must act as an advocate for the child in cases of suspected abuse and continue to maintain an alliance with the whole family during the process of investigating potential child abuse. Many programmes of child protection have an evaluation component that can help with determining the likelihood of abuse. In cases of severe physical injury the child should be hospitalized with an interdisciplinary team working to assess the child's physical health (through diagnostic testing discussed above), mental health, family situation and social situation, with an emphasis on ensuring a safe discharge plan for the child. In cases of neglect, when the neglect appears to be at a systems level (e.g. poverty and unemployment resulting in inadequate money to purchase appropriate food and clothing) the child and family may be referred to local social service agencies to assist with provision of basic needs.

Intimate partner violence

Definitions

Intimate partner violence refers to the infliction of harm by an individual toward the spouse or intimate partner, with the intention of causing pain or controlling the other's behaviour. Some call this act domestic violence, wife abuse, or woman battering. *Moderate* physical violence refers to grabbing, slapping, pushing, or slapping someone, or throwing things with the intention of hitting the other. *Severe* violence refers to punching, kicking, choking, forced sex, threatening use of weapons, or actual use of weapons.[15] 'Psychological abuse' or 'emotional abuse' usually accompany physical aggression and can include threats, intimidation, destruction of property, degradation, constant criticism, extreme possessiveness, social isolation, and lying.

The victim

Violence can be perpetrated by males or females, in both heterosexual and homosexual couples; however, findings from emergency rooms, battered women's shelters, and law enforcement authorities indicate that intimate partner violence is primarily men's violence directed against women.[3,16] Risk factors for victimization include young age, unmarried cohabitation, and witnessing parental violence during childhood.[17] Many have proposed that pregnant women are at particularly high risk; however, studies indicate that it is *not* pregnancy that puts women at risk for abuse, but their young age.[15] However, for those who are already in battering relationships, violence may escalate during pregnancy.

The perpetrator

Compared to non-violent men, men who batter are more likely to have 'high stress': lower income, lower education, and fewer socio-economic resources. They have more difficulties with intimacy, impulsivity, problem-solving skills, anxiety, depression, substance abuse, and personality disorders. Many witnessed parental violence during their childhoods, and many hurt children as well as women.[17]

The consequences

Victimization by an intimate partner has psychological and medical consequences for women and their children (Table 4). The psychological effects of victimization are significant. Symptom severity is related to: severity and the recency of the violence; life threats within the relationship; low personal resources related to education, employment, and social support.[18] Medical consequences are both acute and long term, and signify increased visits to both emergency departments and primary care providers. In violent families, children are at greater risk for abuse. Even when physically unharmed, they are affected by the dangerousness in their families and exhibit psychological and social dysfunction.[19]

Table 4 Consequences of intimate partner violence

Psychological consequences
Depression
Anxiety
Anger and aggression
Low self-esteem
Impaired ability to trust
Elevated MMPI scores on depression, confusion, fearfulness, paranoia, social introversion
Substance abuse
Post traumatic stress disorder
Suicide attempts
Acute medical consequences
Death
Traumatic injury
Injuries to face, breasts, abdomen
Visits to Emergency Department
Multiple injuries
Injuries in various stages of healing
Long-term medical consequences
High health care utilization and costs
Somatic complaints such as insomnia, fatigue, gastrointestinal symptoms, premenstrual symptoms, chronic pain, headaches
Anaemia
Miscarriages, stillbirths, low birthweight newborns
Eating disorders
Substance abuse
Sexually transmitted diseases
HIV
Effects on children
Victimization by adults
Among infants:
poorer health and sleeping habits, excessive screaming
Among pre-schoolers:
signs of terror exhibited as yelling, irritable behaviour, hiding, shaking, stuttering
Among school-age children:
somatic complaints, regression to earlier stages
Among adolescents:
use of aggression to solve problems, projecting blame onto others, anxiety
Among adult offspring:
violent relationships

Screening and diagnosis

Talking about violence in relationships requires a sensitive and confidential approach. Physicians should not wait for the patient to raise the topic, but routinely screen for family violence. One can gently initiate discussions by setting a context for questions ('In my practice I am concerned about safety …'), by asking general questions ('How would you describe your relationship?'), or by including an item on a health screening survey ('During the past 4 weeks, how often have problems in your household led to: Insulting or swearing? Yelling? Threatening? Hitting or Pushing?'). Focused questions should include concrete behavioural terms ('hit' or 'hurt'), not abstract words ('abuse' or 'assault'). Physicians should also be alert to social and somatic clues related to victimization, such as a history of childhood abuse, depression, anxiety, chronic headaches, or chronic pelvic or abdominal pain.

Recent research suggests that two types of violent relationships exist: one far more dangerous than the other.[20] *Common couple violence* is characterized by occasional outbursts for the purpose of winning an argument. In this type of relationship, women are just as likely to hit as men, and violent behaviours tend to be of low severity and low frequency. This aggression is generally not controlling and does not escalate over time. Individuals are not afraid of their partners. In contrast, *patriarchal terrorism* is unidirectional, man-to-woman aggression that escalates in severity and frequency over time. *Patriarchal terrorism is characterized by a man who is extremely dangerous and controlling.* In addition to physical assaults, these men use a pattern of strategies to control their partner's behaviours and to keep them in the relationship: intimidation; coercion and threats; emotional abuse; economic abuse; social isolation; minimizing, denying, and blaming others; using children; and invoking male privilege. When women try to leave these relationships, their partners often escalate the controlling behaviours, making leaving particularly dangerous.

To distinguish between patriarchal terrorism and common couple violence, physicians can begin with the patient's level of fear ('Are you afraid of your husband/partner?'). Other signs of patriarchal terrorism include severe physical violence (beating, choking, kicking, using fists, threatening with weapons); escalating severity over time; and extremely controlling behaviours. Victims in these dangerous relationships are at high risk for lethality during life transitions such as pregnancy, separation or divorce, or when the partner abuses drugs or alcohol, owns a weapon, or has a history of suicide attempts. Patriarchal terrorism requires urgent and comprehensive interventions.

The research on common couple violence is scarce. Only its prevalence is known, about 11–12 per cent among all couples, compared to 1–3 per cent for patriarchal terrorism.[15] The etiology, risk factors, and health consequences of common couple violence have not yet been studied. Is it an early stage of patriarchal terrorism, or a separate phenomena? Until more is known, physicians should closely follow women who are in hitting relationships and routinely assess the dangerousness in their households.

Clinical interventions

The process of change

The 'transtheoretical model' of health behaviour change can explain abused women's movement toward or away from help-seeking behaviours. Stages of change include: pre-contemplation, contemplation, preparation, action, maintenance, and relapse.[21] 'Pre-contemplators' may believe the violence in their relationship is normal, especially if the frequency and severity is low, or if she also hits, as in common couple violence. 'Contemplators' are ambivalent. They recognize victimization as a problem, but find the costs of leaving too high. They feel incapable of action due to low self-esteem, depression, lack of support, or terror. 'Preparers' are saving money, seeking employment, or planning a very careful escape. In the 'Action' stage, individuals discover the costs of change: loneliness, uncertainty, poor finances, and the entire burden of childrearing. In addition, partners may 'turn on the charm' to lure the individual back into the relationship. This phase is the most dangerous for women; extremely controlling men will exaggerate measures of coercion when challenged by separation. Thus 'Relapse,' a return to the relationship, is normal but discouraging to those who are trying to keep victims safe. When violence re-emerges, most victims will try to leave again.

Piling advice on a patient who feels helpless or ambivalent can promote resistance to change. Instead, physicians should encourage patients to do the talking—to think out loud about their own reasons and strategies for change. In the pre-contemplation stage, elicit the patient's thoughts: 'Tell me about your relationship'. Then, 'How does the hitting fit in?' In the contemplation stage, address ambivalence: 'What are the good things about your relationship? What are the not-so-good things?' One should assess the patient's own attempts at problem-solving, and offer other resources if the patient is interested. After drawing her out, summarize the patient's comments and ask 'What do you think of all this?' Allow her to draw her own conclusions, without advice or judgement. Then continue the conversation at follow-up visits.

Develop a 'safe-plan'

One concrete task a physician can do to improve the patient's safety, even when the patient chooses to stay with a violent partner, is to develop an emergency escape plan—a 'safe-plan'. This plan can protect the patient while allowing her time to evaluate her situation and marshal resources. The safe-plan should: identify early stages of violent episodes; plan escape routes, transportation, and destination; and determine who and what to take away (children, clothes, money, important papers). The physician can help patients ascertain personal resources, such as friends and family to provide shelter and support, and direct them to local agencies who can provide services and shelter.

Offer referrals

Another important service physicians can provide is referral to community resources that address partner violence. For *all women* in hitting relationships, physicians should recommend individual psychotherapy. Marital therapy may be helpful for some couples with common couple violence; ask the psychotherapist to determine if marital or separate individual therapy is most appropriate. However, *couples therapy is NOT recommended for relationships with patriarchal terrorism.* Abused women are not free to speak their minds when the abuser is present, and may be physically punished for things they say to the therapist. Other useful community agencies can provide basic resources such as food, shelter, jobs, legal assistance, and support groups. Many communities have treatment programmes for men who batter.

Documentation

Well-documented medical records are important for follow-up of any health problem, but in the case of intimate partner violence, they may also represent legal evidence about the violence. In the note, use the patient's words to describe the violent event and causes of the injuries. One can state an opinion about the adequacy of the patient's explanations, but avoid interpretations (e.g. 'The patient was abused'). Describe injuries in detail, using a body-map if possible. Photographs can be useful if they show clear evidence of injury. Use colour film with a colour standard, and photograph from different angles, full body and close-up. Include the patient's face in at least one picture. Mark the photos precisely, including the patient's name, date, and location of the injury. Finally, report medical treatment, referrals to community resources, and follow-up plans.

When both partners are in the practice, family physicians may question how to proceed. An expert consensus panel from Canada developed guidelines for handling this situation:[22]

> . . . it is not a conflict of interest to deal actively with the issue [of abuse] with one or both of the partners. For example, discussing a safety plan or providing information about domestic violence is not championing one patient more than the other; these options ensure quality of care . . .'. (p. 851)

The guidelines recommend dealing with each patient separately and independently; information from one should not be shared with the other without prior permission. Likewise, information from one patient should not be entered into the other's medical record.

Elder mistreatment

Definitions

The National Center on Elder Abuse defines five types of elder mistreatment: (i) *physical abuse*, referring to the infliction of physical pain, injury, or physical coercion, and involving at least one act of violence including beating, slapping, hitting, burning, cutting, physical restraint use, or intentional over-medication; (ii) *psychological abuse*, including the infliction of mental anguish through yelling, screaming, threatening, humiliating, infantilizing, or provoking intentional fear; (iii) *sexual abuse*, defined as molestation or forced sexual actions; (iv) *financial/material exploitation* defined as the illegal exploitation of monetary or material assets; and (v) *neglect*, including the failure of a caregiver to meet an elder's health care needs.

The victim

Studies show that advanced age (greater than 75 years old), functional dependency, shared living arrangements, social isolation, personality disorder or excessive use of drugs or alcohol places an older adult at risk for elder mistreatment. In Manitoba, Canada, victims were more likely to be women, older than 75 years, physically dependent, and cognitively impaired.[23] In the United States, reports of elder mistreatment were associated with non-White race, ADL impairments, and cognitive impairment.[24] Another study found social isolation, confusion, and depression in the victim to be associated with abuse or neglect.[25] Depression can contribute to elder mistreatment in the form of self-neglect. Of the total cases of confirmed abuse, most carry a diagnosis of self-neglect; these individuals are three times more likely to have a diagnosis of depression and four times more likely to have dementia.[26]

The perpetrator

Certain perpetrator characteristics lead to elder mistreatment. In the United States, perpetrators are more likely to be White and caregivers of the victims. Thirty-nine per cent are adult children of the victim, and 14 per cent are married to the victim.[27] Substance abuse and financial dependence are the most common 'barriers to self-sufficiency' seen in the perpetrators. In Britain, perpetrators are more likely to consume alcohol and have more depressive symptomatology.[28]

Abuse complaints against professional caregivers are associated with having a patient ombudsman at the facility.[29] Nurses aides make up 61 per cent of professionals who perpetrate abuse with male employees almost twice as likely as females to be perpetrators (63 per cent versus 37 per cent).

The consequences

Elder mistreatment is associated with premature mortality in older adults. Victims have poorer survival than non-victims (9 versus 40 per cent), with a risk of death that is three times higher.[30] Victims of elder mistreatment also have higher levels of psychological distress (2.4 point difference on the Global Health Questionnaire) and poorer social support.[31] Examining United States Justice Department Statistics for adult victims of violence over 65 years old, 22.1 per cent were injured and 10.9 per cent required medical treatment. Of all older victims of violence, 2.9 per cent were treated at site of injury, 2.1 per cent were treated at a doctor's office, 5.6 per cent were hospitalized, and 0.9 per cent were hospitalized overnight.

Data on health care utilization and costs related to elder mistreatment are sparse. In one study, 114 victims of elder mistreatment accounted for 628 emergency department visits over 5 years; 30.6 per cent of these visits resulted in a hospital admission.[32] One study of intimate partner violence showed an average annual difference of $1775 in health expenditures when comparing victims of violence with non-victims.[33]

Screening and diagnosis

Researchers and clinicians have developed several different methods to screen for elder mistreatment. The Indicators of Abuse (IOA) discriminates abuse cases from non-abuse cases 84.4 per cent of the time.[34] The Hwalek–Sengstock elder abuse screening test is a 15-item instrument designed to detect abuse exposure, with a sensitivity of 64 per cent and specificity of 91 per cent.[35] The Domestic Violence Screening Questionnaire (DVSQ)[36] measures exposure to mistreatment in functionally independent older adults. Test–retest reliability demonstrated kappa statistics ranging from 0.65 to 0.91.

In the clinic, in a private area away from the perpetrator, the physician can ask a suspected victim of elder mistreatment about daily routines, problems at home, and feelings of safety around their caregiver. These questions can lead into more direct questions about physical, psychological, financial, and sexual abuse. Questions about unmet needs can reveal instances of neglect. The American Medical Association recommends the following screening questions for detecting elder mistreatment.

1. Have you ever been hit, punched, kicked, slapped or otherwise physically abused?
2. Have you been yelled at, screamed at, threatened, scolded, or otherwise verbally abused?
3. Has anyone neglected to take care of you when you needed help?
4. Does anyone use your money or property against your wishes?

Besides screening for the occurrence of elder mistreatment, clinicians should also screen the caregivers of older adults for undue stress in their caregiving activities. The Caregiver Strain Index and the Zarit Burden Interview are measures of caregiver stress that may be useful.[37,38]

In addition to verbal or written screening for elder mistreatment, clinicians should perform a thorough physical examination including a complete skin assessment and pelvic exam for cases of suspected sexual abuse. A complete geriatric assessment should also be performed and should include evaluation of physical function (ADL, IADL, Bartel Index), gait, cognition (Mini-Mental State Exam, Clock Drawing Test), assessment for affective disorders (Geriatric Depression Scale, Hamilton D).

Clinical interventions

In addition to screening, several experts recommend protocols for assessment and intervention for elder mistreatment. Interventions can be indirect or direct. Indirect intervention on the part of the clinician includes documentation of the abuse and referral to Adult Protective Services. In the United States, all 50 states require health professionals to report suspected cases of elder mistreatment.

Documentation of abuse is as important as the assessment process. Exact statements from the victim should be recorded along with detailed descriptions and diagrams of any injuries detected. All descriptions of injuries should include the size, colour, shape, and location of injury. If necessary, a colour picture of injuries should be considered to include date and time of photograph.

The clinician should provide a therapeutic message, referrals to social support services, as well as caregiver support and respite. A therapeutic message uses the detection of elder mistreatment as an opportunity to let the older victim know that abuse is not normal or acceptable. This allows the older victim to recognize mistreatment as a problem. Adult Protective Services and social support services referrals allow the victim to access systems which assure continuity of care. Caregiver support and respite provide a break for the caregiver and allow the rest time that may be necessary to keep a stressful caregiving situation from deteriorating into violence.

Direct clinical intervention uses a diagnostic plan (home visit, short hospital stay) and therapeutic plan (repeated home visits or follow-up office appointments) to manage elder mistreatment. Continuity of home visits and/or frequent follow-up office visits may be used to manage older victims of elder mistreatment, particularly self-neglect.

Primary prevention in primary care settings

The intergenerational nature of family violence indicates that primary prevention should begin in childhood to prevent 'downstream' aggression toward future children, partners, and elder parents. Many community-based interventions have focused on parent support and education as a method to prevent child abuse. Likewise, primary care physicians can support parents and provide information related to non-violent childrearing. Young adolescents should receive targeted guidance related to non-violence. Research in New Zealand found that intimate partner violence in adulthood was predicted by problems documented at age 15: substance abuse, poor parent–child attachment, conduct problems, and school problems.[39] Finally, physicians should attend to stressors in patients' lives—such as caregiver exhaustion, serious marital conflict, school difficulties, and financial hardships—and guide families to community resources that can provide assistance and relief.

Cross-cultural issues

Nearly every culture on our planet has reported the existence of family violence. Across the world, across their life spans, women especially are at risk of victimization: sex-selective abortion or infanticide; forced marriage, prostitution, or bonded labor; incest and physical abuse; female genital mutilation; wife abuse, rape, or murder; dowry-related violence, *sati* (burning the widow on her husbands' funeral pyre), and honour killings. The United Nations declared domestic violence as a violation as early as 1948, under the Universal Declaration of Human Rights. Since that time, they have reinforced protections for women and children under the Convention on the Elimination of All Forms of Discrimination Against Women (1979) and the Convention on the Rights of the Child (1989). By the year 2000, 44 countries had adopted specific legislation on domestic violence, 12 from Latin America.

While the term 'family violence' has no universal definition across cultures, the laws and norms in most societies reflect a broad understanding that extremely violent behaviors, such as those in patriarchal terrorism, are *not* acceptable. In Ghana, physical 'discipline' of a wife by a husband is considered an acceptable behaviour within marriage; however, 'excessive beating' of a woman is not.[40] The definition of excessive violence is nearly always linked to fears about physical harm. Only those in fear for their lives can overcome deep shame about victimization to tell others.

Physicians who work across cultures should make it their business to learn about societal beliefs and traditions that can impact patients' health, and interventions that can maintain patients' ties to the community. In the case of family violence, what is tolerated, and what is considered excessive? What structures provide support for victims and what controls are in place for the perpetrators? Many countries have developed formal systems to protect women and children. In Brazil, Argentina, Colombia, Costa Rica, Peru, Uruguay, Venezuela, Malaysia, Spain, Pakistan, and India, special women's police stations make legal resources more accessible to women. In communities where formal support structures are lacking, informal networks may intervene on behalf of victims. Women, children, and frail elders are the most vulnerable when they are isolated, when abuses are invisible to extended kin and the rest of the community. Rallying natural support systems can provide comfort and protection for the victim as well as correction for the perpetrator.

In the face of cultural norms that oppress women, children or elders, physicians may feel helpless to intervene with family violence. Under these circumstances, clinical treatments are inadequate and community interventions are required. Physicians can utilize community-oriented primary care (COPC) methods to join with concerned community members, examine the impact of violence as a team, and jointly develop interventions that fit the local customs and values. In many areas around the globe, grassroots efforts like these have created effective resources for victims of violence.

Conclusion

Primary care physicians are in an ideal position to contribute to violence prevention. In the context of sustained doctor–patient relationships, where all aspects of health are addressed—biomedical, psychological, and social—primary care physicians can identify patterns across the life cycle that indicate risk of victimization. Families are well served by providers who routinely ask about violence and victimization, treat health consequences of abuse, provide information and encouragement, guide both victims and perpetrators to effective community resources, and offer emotional support through the long journey to end violence.

References

1. **National Clearinghouse on Child Abuse and Neglect Information.** Highlights from Child Maltreatment 1999: Reports from the States to the National Child Abuse and Neglect Data System. US Dept of Health and Human Services. 4-12-2001. US Government Printing Office. 6-11-2001.
2. **Anonymous.** Prevalence of violence against women by an intimate male partner. World Health Organization, 7 February 2001.
3. **United States Department of Justice.** Violence between Intimates. 149259.94. Washington DC: Bureau of Justice Statistics, 1994.
4. **Podnieks, E.** (1993). Elder abuse and neglect: a concern for the dental profession. *Journal of the Canadian Dental Association* **59**, 915–20.
5. **Lachs, M.S., Williams, C.S., O'Brien, S., Pillemer, K.A., and Charlson, M.E.** (1998). The mortality of elder mistreatment. *Journal of the American Medical Association* **280**, 428–32.
6. **Kempe, C.H., Silverman, F.N., Steele, B.F., Droegemueller, W., and Silver, H.K.** (1984). Landmark article July 7, 1962: The battered-child syndrome. *Journal of the American Medical Association* **251**, 3288–94.
7. **Finkelhor, D. and Korbin, J.** (1988). Child abuse as an international issue. *Child Abuse & Neglect* **12**, 3–23.
8. **DiScala, C., Sege, R., Li, G., and Reece, R.M.** (2000). Child abuse and unintentional injuries: a 10-year retrospective. *Archives of Pediatrics & Adolescent Medicine* **154**, 16–22.
9. **MacMillan, H.L.** (2000). Canadian Task Force on Preventive Health C. Preventive health care, 2000 update: prevention of child maltreatment. *Canadian Medical Association Journal* **163**, 1451–8.
10. **Ackerman, P.T., Newton, J.E., McPherson, W.B., Jones, J.G., and Dykman, R.A.** (1998). Prevalence of post traumatic stress disorder and other psychiatric diagnoses in three groups of abused children (sexual, physical, and both). *Child Abuse & Neglect* **22**, 759–74.
11. **Felitti, V.J.** et al. (1998). Relationship of childhood abuse and household dysfunction to many of the leading causes of death in The Adverse Childhood Experiences (ACE) Study (see comments). *American Journal of Preventive Medicine* **14**, 245–58.
12. **Fiscella, K., Kitzman, H.J., Cole, R.E., Sidora, K.J., and Olds, D.** (1998). Does child abuse predict adolescent pregnancy? *Pediatrics* **101**, 620–4.
13. **Heim, C.** et al. (2000). Pituitary–adrenal and autonomic responses to stress in women after and physical abuse in childhood. *Journal of the American Medical Association* **284**, 592–7.
14. **Jayawant, S.** et al. (1998). Subdural haemorrhages in infants: population based study. *British Medical Journal* **317**, 1558–61.
15. **Straus, M.A. and Gelles, R.J.** *Physical Violence in American Families: Risk Factors and Adaptations to Violence in 8,145 Families.* New Brunswick NJ: Transaction Publishers, 1995.
16. **Roberts, G.L., O'Toole, B.I., Raphael, B., Lawrence, J.M., and Ashby, R.** (1996). Prevalence study of domestic violence victims in an emergency department. *Annals of Emergency Medicine* **27**, 741–53.
17. **Hotaling, G.R. and Sugarman, D.B.** (1986). Analysis of risk markers in husband-to-wife: the current state of knowledge. *Violence and victims* **1**, 101–24.
18. **Astin, M.C., Lawrence, K.J., and Foy, D.W.** (1993). Posttraumatic stress disorder among battered women: risk and resiliency factors. *Violence and Victims* **8**, 17–28.
19. **Jaffe, P.G., Wolfe, D.A., and Wilson, S.K.** *Children of Battered Women.* Newbury Park CA: Sage Publications, 1990.
20. **Johnson, M.P.** (1995). Patriarchal terrorism and common couple violence: two forms of violence against women. *Journal of Marriage and the Family* **57**, 283–94.
21. **Prochaska, J.O.** et al. (1994). Stages of change and decisional balance for 12 problem behaviors. *Health Psychology* **13**, 39–46.
22. **Ferris, L.E., Norton, P.G., Dunn, E.V., Gort, E.H., and Degani, N.** (1997). Guidelines for managing domestic abuse when male and female partners are patients of the same physician. The Delphi Panel and the Consulting Group. *Journal of the American Medical Association* **278**, 851–7.
23. **Shell, D.** *Elder Abuse: Summary of Result—Manitoba in Abuse of the Elderly: Issues and Bibliography.* Toronto, Ontario: University of Toronto Press, 1988.
24. **Lachs, M.S., Williams, C., O'Brien, S., Hurst, L., and Horwitz, R.** (1997). Risk factors for reported elder abuse and neglect: a nine-year observational cohort study. *Gerontologist* **37**, 469–74.
25. **National Center on Elder Abuse.** National Elder Abuse Incidence Study: Final Report 1998. Washington DC: American Public Human Services Association, 2001.
26. **Dyer, C.B., Pavlik, V.N., Murphy, K.P., and Hyman, D.J.** (2000). The high prevalence of depression and dementia in elder abuse or neglect. *Journal of the American Geriatrics Society* **48**, 205–8.
27. **Hwalek, M.A., Neale, A.V., Goodrich, C.S., and Quinn, K.** (1996). The association of elder abuse and substance abuse in the Illinois Elder Abuse System. *Gerontologist* **36**, 694–700.
28. **Homer, A.C. and Gilleard, C.** (1990). Abuse of elderly people by their carers. *British Medical Journal* **301**, 1359–62.
29. **Nelson, H.W., Huber, R., and Walter, K.L.** (1995). The relationship between volunteer long-term care ombudsmen and regulatory nursing home actions. *Gerontologist* **35**, 509–14.
30. **Lachs, M.S., Williams, C.S., O'Brien, S., Pillemer K.A., and Charlson, M.E.** (1998). The mortality of elder mistreatment. *Journal of the American Medical Association* **280**, 428–32.
31. **Comijs, H.C., Pot, A.M., Smit, J.H., Bouter, L.M., and Jonker, C.** (1998). Elder abuse in the community: prevalence and consequences. *Journal of the American Geriatrics Society* **46**, 885–8.
32. **Lachs, M.S.** et al. (1997). ED use by older victims of family violence. *Annals of Emergency Medicine* **30**, 448–54.
33. **Wisner, C.L., Gilmer, T.P., Saltzman, L.E., and Zink, T.M.** (1999). Intimate partner violence against women: do victims cost health plans more? *Journal of Family Practice* **48**, 439–43.
34. **Reis, M. and Nahmiash, D.** (1998). Validation of the indicators of abuse (IOA) screen. *Gerontologist* **38**, 471–80.
35. **Neale, A.V., Hwalek, M.A., Scott, R.O., Sengstock, M.C., and Stahl, C.** (1991). Validation of the Hwalek–Sengstock Elder Abuse Screening Test. *Journal of Applied Gerontology* **10**, 406–18.
36. **Mouton, C.P., Rovi, S., Furniss, K., and Lasser, N.L.** (1999). The associations between health and domestic violence in older women: results of a pilot study. *Journal of Women's Health & Gender-based Medicine* **8**, 1173–9.
37. **Robinson, B.C.** (1983). Validation of a Caregiver Strain Index. *Journal of Gerontology* **38**, 344–8.
38. **Zarit, S.W., Reever, K.E., and Bach-Peterson, J.** (1980). Relatives of impaired elderly: correlates of feelings of burden. *Gerontologist* **10**, 649–55.
39. **Magdol, L., Moffitt, T.E., Caspi, A., and Silva, P.A.** (1998). Developmental antecedents of partner abuse: a prospective-longitudinal study. *Journal of Abnormal Psychology* **107**, 375–89.
40. **Fischbach, R.L. and Herbert, B.A.** (1997). Domestic violence and mental health: correlates and conundrums within and across cultures. *Social Science and Medicine* **45**, 1161–76.

10

Managing the practice population

10 Managing the practice population

10.1 The individual and the population

Philip Hannaford

Introduction

Primary care is about providing continuous, comprehensive personal health care at the first point of contact. In the United Kingdom, everyone is entitled to register with a named general practitioner who contracts with the local health authority/board to provide front-line general medical services or, when necessary, ensure that another health care professional provides the required care. These obligations may mean making sure that another member of the primary health care team provides the required front-line care, or ensuring that primary care is supplemented by more specialized, secondary or tertiary care. Although the number, and locale, of professionals providing community-based health care has expanded dramatically in recent years, general practitioners remain the principal gate keepers to specialist care. Countries with similar 'gate-keeping' systems tend to have lower health expenditure per capita than those with non-gate-keeping systems, and appear to be better able to contain the growing cost of outpatient hospital care.[1] Many managed-care organizations in the United States of America also put their primary care physicians in a gate-keeping role.

The defined practice list offers a framework for the primary health care team to provide appropriate diagnostic, therapeutic, and preventive services to individuals and families in the consulting room, and to the rest of the registered population.

Managing the individual

Making a diagnosis

Individuals seeking help from the primary health care team present with a diverse range of symptoms, of varying severity, duration, urgency, and impact. A complex mix of physical, psychological, and social factors contribute to symptom occurrence, as well as the individual's response to the symptom(s) (and their family and practitioner's response). Many of the problems presented are mild, ill defined, poorly expressed, and of short duration. Indeed, it has been suggested that 60 per cent of problems presented to general practice or primary care cannot be labelled as disease.[2]

A key task of the practitioner during the consultation is to determine whether the problem presented is the real reason for the encounter. Another is to identify problems that would benefit from early investigation or referral to another health care professional. Neither task is easy, particularly since symptoms seen in primary care have a wide variety of causes, few of which have serious, long-term implications. Furthermore, much of our understanding of the epidemiology of disease is derived from specialist-based studies which can distort perceptions about the relative value of different symptoms, signs, and investigations in primary care.

The positive predictive value of a symptom, sign or test is the proportion of individuals with the symptom, sign or positive test result who actually have the disease. Predictive values are useful because they reflect the underlying prevalence of disease in the population being studied. The general practitioner's gate-keeping role filters, shapes, and controls demands on specialist care, altering the pattern of disease seen at different points of the health care system. This, in turn, affects the positive predictive value of symptoms, signs and tests in the different settings. When disease prevalence is low (the usual case in primary care, at least for serious disease), the positive predictive value of associated symptoms, signs or tests is also low; meaning that a large number of individuals have to be assessed in order to detect one case. In a literature review of studies of overt rectal bleeding and colorectal cancer, the estimated positive predictive value of this symptom was less than 1 per 1000 in the general population, 2 per 100 among those presenting the symptom to their family doctor and 36 per 100 among patients referred to hospital for investigation of the symptom.[3]

By themselves, most symptoms seen in primary care have low predictive values, especially symptoms that are ill defined or which are associated with a large number of causes. The likelihood of serious disease increases when particular clusters of symptoms occur, especially when these include symptoms such as bleeding, weight loss, anorexia, or general malaise. Time may also help when making a diagnosis; the probability of serious illness increases when symptoms persist, progress, recur, or develop in an unusual fashion. The ability to observe how symptoms or clusters of symptoms change over time is frequently used by primary care practitioners when making decisions about whom to investigate, treat further, or refer. Given the non-specific nature of many problems presented to primary care practitioners it is perhaps not surprising that they often manage these problems symptomatically without attributing a formal diagnosis, especially when treatments are the same irrespective of any diagnostic labels used. Some clinical features may be sought because they provide information about prognosis or aid treatment decisions rather than because they assist in reaching a diagnosis. For example, restricted flexion is a prognostic sign rather than a diagnostic pointer in back pain, and signs and symptoms of compression of the cauda equina are important indicators that surgery might be useful. The low predictive value of most symptoms and signs, however, means that in primary care there is usually little added value from undertaking an extensive history or examination.

Using risk markers

As well as assessing presented symptoms and signs, clinicians use other 'risk markers' of susceptibility to identify individuals with a higher probability of having disease. These markers (also called risk factors) are genetic, environmental, and behavioural determinants of disease found in epidemiological studies. Similar markers can be used opportunistically to screen asymptomatic individuals in the consulting room for previously unknown

Table 1 Rate of first ever venous thrombosis among women aged 15–49 (rate per 10 000 woman-years)[5]

	Number	% of cases	Rate	Relative risk
Factor V Leiden negative				
Not using COC[a]	36	23	0.8	1.0[b]
Using COC	84	54	3.0	3.8
Factor V Leiden positive				
Not using COC	10	6	5.7	7.2
Using COC	25	16	28.5	35.6

[a] COC: combined oral contraception.

[b] Reference group for the relative risks.

disease or for clinical features (such as raised blood pressure or abnormal lipid levels) which predict a higher risk of disease in the future. Before undertaking such activities, there must be worthwhile interventions available to modify any problems detected, and evidence that early treatment of asymptomatic disease makes a clinical difference. Simply labelling someone as being 'at risk' without being able to do anything about it is unethical.

Although risk markers identify individuals with higher susceptibility to disease, they have two important limitations. First, most disease occurs in individuals apparently at low risk of the event. For example, less than 20 per cent of women who develop breast cancer have a known risk marker for this carcinoma apart from age and most cases of myocardial infarction occur in individuals at the lower end of the cholesterol distribution. Our understanding of disease aetiology remains poor, often restricted to broad statements such as 'multifactorial in origin'. Although a risk marker may be strongly associated with a particular disease, it may still only contribute to a small proportion of cases. For instance, the two breast cancer genes, *BRCA1* and *BRCA2*, are present in a substantial number of women with a very strong family history (i.e. those with four or more close relatives affected by breast or ovarian cancer), yet only 5–10 per cent of all cases of breast cancer are of the inherited type. Second, most people with a risk marker remain free of the associated disease; risk markers are poor at pinpointing exactly those who will develop the condition, and when. This leads to the 'prevention paradox' whereby a large number of individuals need to be treated in order to prevent an event in a few.[4]

A study of combined oral contraceptive use, carriage of the haemostatic abnormality, factor V Leiden mutation, and venous thrombosis[5] illustrates these points. In this study, women without the abnormality who used the pill and women with the defect who did not use the pill had a higher risk of venous thrombosis than women without the defect not using oral contraception (relative risk 3.8 and 7.1, respectively; Table 1). Women with both risk markers had a much higher risk of venous thrombosis (relative risk 35.6). These results should be interpreted as suggesting that every woman wishing to use combined oral contraception should be tested for the factor V Leiden mutation beforehand. Such arguments, however, ignore the fact that approximately three-quarters of all events in the study occurred in women without the clotting abnormality; women with a negative test result could be falsely reassured that they will not experience a venous thrombosis. On the other hand, only 16 per cent of cases occurred in women with the defect who used the pill, a tiny fraction of women with the mutation. Since we cannot pinpoint which women with the mutation will develop a thrombosis while using the pill, and given that there are currently no treatments for this genetic abnormality, the only way to minimize the risk would be to deny the contraceptive pill to all women with this clotting defect; perhaps 6 per cent of the general population in Europe[6] (a striking example of the 'prevention paradox').

Average versus specific effects

Epidemiological studies investigate average effects within specified populations. Thus, observational studies examine the average effects (e.g. risk of disease) associated with particular factors, and randomized trials investigate the average effects (usually benefits) of interventions. Clinicians, however, are not interested in average effects; they need information about specific risks and benefits faced by individual patients consulting them. In an ideal world, clinicians would base their management decisions upon robust information from epidemiological studies conducted in populations similar to their own practice population. In reality, the available evidence is derived from populations that rarely match the practice population. Randomized clinical trials may be particularly prone to problems of applicability.[7] Women, the elderly, those of low socio-economic status, and minority ethnic groups are often poorly represented in clinical trials.

These observations mean that some extrapolation of evidence is required in the consulting room. When making inferences from other populations, it is important not to assume an equal distribution of risk across the entire population. For example, a number of studies have found that myocardial infarction and stroke occur predominantly in combined oral contraceptive users with other risk factors for cardiovascular disease, notably smokers and those with raised blood pressure.[8] As a consequence, overall estimates of arterial disease risk among all users of combined oral contraception grossly exaggerate the risk among healthy non-smoking users.

Absolute versus relative risk

Clinicians also need information about the clinical significance of effects found in epidemiological studies. Although relative risks and odds ratios from epidemiological studies provide information about the strength of any associations, they provide no information about the clinical importance of the findings. This is because relative risks are uninformative about the background risk of the outcome of interest in the study population. In cohort studies and randomized trials, the clinical importance of an effect can be assessed directly by determining the difference in risk between exposed and non-exposed groups (also known as the absolute risk). In our earlier example, for instance, the absolute risk of venous thrombosis among pill users without factor V Leiden mutation was 2.2 per 10 000 person-years (i.e. 3.0 minus 0.8 per 10 000; Table 1). The reciprocal of the absolute risk gives the number needed to treat; the average number of individuals who need to be treated before someone benefits. When studying adverse effects, the reciprocal of the absolute risk gives the number needed to harm; the average number of people who need to be treated before someone is harmed. Using data from Table 1, the number needed to harm for women using the pill without factor V Leiden mutation was 4545 [$(1/2.2) \times 10\,000$]. In other words, 4545 women would need to use another method of contraception in order to avoid one case of venous thrombosis (assuming, of course, that the new method is not itself associated with an increased thrombotic risk).

Although relative risks might be similar among different subgroups of a population, the absolute risk in each group may be dramatically different. For example, comparisons of the relationship between death and blood pressure among men of different ages show that in each age group the relative risk of death increases as blood pressure rises, with slightly steeper gradients in younger men.[4] On the other hand, the absolute risk of death associated with high blood pressure is very much greater among older men. This is because older men have a higher risk of death than younger men, regardless of whether their blood pressure is raised. Strong associations with an uncommon event result in few new cases, whereas weaker associations with a common event result in many new cases. The same principle means that less effective interventions applied to a high-risk group can often produce greater clinical benefits than the application of more effective interventions to a low-risk group. Increasingly, clinical guidelines are being developed based on absolute rather than relative risk.[9] These guidelines also emphasize the need to consider all relevant risk markers when categorizing individuals, not just one or two single markers.

Perceptions about the risks and benefits from observational studies and clinical trials are heavily influenced by the way in which they are presented. Both clinicians and patients appear to be more willing to act when relative risks are presented rather than when absolute risks or numbers needed to treat are used.[10,11]

Making management decisions

In spite of their limitations, epidemiological data have a valuable role in guiding clinical practice. Indeed, a key purpose of epidemiology is to inform decisions about the control of health problems. Important considerations when making clinical management decisions include: the strength of available evidence; current knowledge about absolute risks; the hopes, concerns, and expressed wishes of patients and their families; and the type and costs of possible actions resulting from the decision.

In general, actions that result from the removal of an undesirable factor to restore 'normality' tend to be regarded as safe and reasonable.[4] Actions which require the introduction of another factor in order to offer protection or benefit are viewed more cautiously; harm may be introduced as well as benefit. In fact, there is an inherent bias against clinicians providing such services. Individuals protected from an event cannot thank their health care providers since those who would have got the condition cannot be specified in the first place. Conversely, individuals experiencing real, or perceived, harm from an intervention often seem only too ready to disclose this event to their family, clinician, the media, and the legal profession! Even screening programmes with solid evidence of overall benefit are associated with important adverse effects in a significant proportion of participants.[12]

Consistent, albeit imprecise, evidence from epidemiological studies[8] supports the recommendation that women wishing to use the contraceptive pill should avoid smoking in order to minimize their arterial risk.[13] It is difficult to think of major harm coming from such advice. Similar, consistent but imprecise evidence of a link between blood pressure and arterial risk in oral contraceptive users,[8] together with the ready availability of screening equipment, the relative ease and acceptability of the testing procedure, and strong evidence of benefits from the treatment of raised blood pressure,[14] support the recommendation that women should have their blood pressure checked before using combined oral contraception.[13] Other epidemiological data that venous thrombosis rarely occurs in young women,[5] and estimates showing that the positive predictive value of currently available tests is extremely low (varying between 1 in 1000 and 1 in 19 000),[15] informs clinicians that it is inappropriate to routinely screen all women for haemostatic abnormalities prior to their use of the contraceptive pill.[13]

Managing the population

Identifying individuals for preventive services

The defined practice list provides a valuable opportunity to systematically offer primary and secondary preventive services to the practice population. The primary care team is well placed to identify individuals who should be invited to participate in particular programmes. The eligibility criteria for some programmes may be based on simple demographic features such as age and gender (e.g. immunization programmes for children; cervical and breast cancer screening initiatives for selected women). Other programmes might be aimed at individuals with specific clinical features (e.g. hepatitis B vaccination for haemophiliacs or intravenous drug misusers; secondary prevention clinics for individuals with ischaemic heart disease). Some initiatives may be triggered by the absence of information in a patient's medical record (e.g. the checking of blood pressure in middle aged adults who do not seem to have had this done in the past 5 years). Others may be triggered by the presence of disease or risk markers in another member of the family.

The ability of the primary care team to access comprehensive clinical data complied over an individual's lifetime increases the appropriateness of invitation; optimizing uptake rates and minimizing distress from insensitive invites. Increased computerization within primary care has reduced the workload associated with identifying and inviting individuals to participate in preventive programmes. Even without extensive computerization, however, high quality comprehensive services can be provided, especially if practices maintain good manual records and separate disease registers.

Several studies have demonstrated the importance of managing chronic conditions systematically with structured follow-up.[16–19] Without a systematic approach, many patients have an incomplete assessment of risk and sub-optimal treatment of disease. By itself, the compilation of a register of patients eligible for recall appears to be an important step towards increased follow-up and improved assessment of patients.[19,20] Recall of patients to a health care professional for assessment brings additional benefits, at least with respect to assessment of risk markers, if not clinical outcomes.[19] Review by nurses is as good, if not better, than review by a general practitioner, emphasizing the need to adopt a team approach when providing systematic care for chronic conditions.

Methods for compiling disease registers include the identification of patients through repeat prescribing data, opportunistic contact, hospital correspondence, and the hand searching of practice records.[20] Each approach has its advantages and disadvantages, but higher levels of registration are achieved if several methods are used. Identifying patients with disease who are not in regular contact with the practice is important, partly because these individuals remain at risk.

Optimizing uptake of preventive services

Of course, it would be wrong to suggest that the defined practice list is a prerequisite for a successful preventive programme. Clear evidence against such a notion is the successful implementation of preventive services in health care systems without a strong primary care component. Nonetheless, the defined practice list provides an important framework in which non-responders can be readily identified and approached to maximize uptake. Different members of the primary care team (including doctors, nurses, and administrative staff) can target individuals at particular risk. In addition, non-participation in a preventive programme can be discussed opportunistically when non-responders are seen in the practice. Given the large proportion of the practice population that consults each year, there is ample opportunity for such discussions. These discussions build upon the trust that usually develops when individuals know each other for many years, and are enhanced by the health care professional's detailed knowledge of an individual's medical, family, and social circumstances. Decisions by patients to agree or decline to participate in preventative services may be more informed when made in primary care rather than in another health care setting. The consultation also provides the opportunity to introduce targeted preventive advice to patients presenting with a related illness, thereby increasing the chances of uptake. For example, the provision of smoking cessation advice when a patient attends because of an exacerbation of chronic obstructive pulmonary disease.

Moving into the community

We have known for many years that only a fraction of symptoms and illness occurring in the community is presented to health care services.[21] The phenomenon is not confined to mild, self-limiting health problems; accumulating evidence shows that it also occurs with serious disease.[22,23] Awareness of this problem sometimes leads practices to using their practice list as a sampling frame for special initiatives such as health surveys or population-based needs assessments. In effect, practices embarking upon such activities are conducting population screening. The intention is to identify disease that is current unknown to the practice (sometimes referred to as 'unmet need') on the assumption that unknown disease is clinically important. In other words, it is assumed that the clinical impact (e.g. prognostic significance, effect on quality of life, etc.) of unknown illness is similar to, or worse than, that of known illness. In many instances, evidence to support such assumptions is lacking. All screening activities have their costs, both to those screened and to the health care services. Screening also raises important ethical issues, such as whether there are adequate resources to treat those with newly detected disease. Practices need to consider these points carefully before embarking upon such activities.

Monitoring performance

Clinical audit is now an essential tool for practices wishing to provide high-quality care. It is important that audits are based upon the complete ascertainment of those with the disease of interest; audits based on partial registration of patients tend to overestimate the quality of care being provided. Practice performance in successfully identifying those with particular conditions can be assessed by comparing practice prevalence rates with figures from other practices or from epidemiological surveys. When making such comparisons it is important to remember that discrepancies can arise from differences in the populations compared, the level of ascertainment and the diagnostic criteria used. Care provided to identified patients should be regularly audited to see whether pre-determined standards are being met. Area-wide audits are powerful tools for comparing practice performance with peers, and for planning future service developments.

Conclusions

Primary care practitioners have responsibilities to individuals in the consulting room and the rest of the practice population. Individuals seeking help want their problem(s) dealt with in a timely and efficient fashion, by the most appropriate health care professional. They also often want to know if they will develop disease in the future, frequently on the assumption that action taken early can prevent disease onset or minimize its impact. The strategy of identifying risk markers, however, is not without its problems, especially when subsequent actions are based on relative rather than absolute risk. Clear understanding by health care professionals of the limitations of the approach is essential if patients are not to be misinformed about our ability to predict future events, or about the personal and societal costs of adopting this approach. An understanding of the epidemiological issues is also helpful when trying to balance the competing needs and demands of individuals against those of the entire practice population. Restrictions on resources available to primary care require the careful targeting of services to those most likely to benefit.

The defined practice list provides a valuable opportunity to systematically offer primary and secondary preventive services to appropriate sections of the practice population. Thus, the primary care team can construct registers of individuals eligible for recall, facilitating the provision of structured assessment, follow-up, and treatment; assess the completeness of ascertainment of everyone with the condition of interest; and monitor performance in the provision of care.

References

1. **Delnoij, D.** et al. (2000). Does general practitioner gatekeeping curb health care expenditure? *Journal of Health Sciences Research & Policy* **5**, 22–6.
2. **White, K.L.** (1997). The ecology of medical care: origins and implications for population-based healthcare research. *Health Services Research* **32**, 11–21.
3. **Fijten, G.H., Blijham, G.H., and Knottnerus, J.A.** (1994). Occurrence and clinical significance of overt blood loss per rectum in the general population and in medical practice. *British Journal of General Practice* **44**, 320–5.
4. **Rose, G.** (1981). Strategy of prevention: lessons from cardiovascular disease. *British Medical Journal* **282**, 1847–51.
5. **Vandenbroucke, J.P.** et al. (1994). Increased risk of venous thrombosis in oral-contraceptive users who are carriers of factor V Leiden mutation. *Lancet* **344**, 1453–7.
6. **Rees, D.C., Cox, M., and Clegg, J.B.** (1995). World distribution of factor V Leiden. *Lancet* **346**, 1133–4.
7. **Sniderman, A.D.** (1999). Clinical trials, consensus conferences, and clinical practice. *Lancet* **354**, 327–30.
8. **WHO Scientific Group on Cardiovascular Disease and Steroid Hormone Contraception.** *Cardiovascular Disease and Steroid Hormone Contraception: Report of a WHO Scientific Group.* WHO technical report series: 877. WHO: Geneva, Switzerland, 1998.
9. **Jackson, R.** (2000). Guidelines on preventing cardiovascular disease in clinical practice. *British Medical Journal* **320**, 659–61.
10. **Bobbio, M., Demichellis, B., and Giustello, G.** (1994). Completeness of reporting trial results: effect on physicians' willingness to prescribe. *Lancet* **343**, 1209–11.
11. **Misselbrook, D. and Armstrong, D.** (2001). Patients' responses to risk information about the benefits of treating hypertension. *British Journal of General Practice* **51**, 276–9.
12. **Brett, J. and Austoker, J.** (2001). Women who are recalled for further investigation for breast screening: psychological consequences 3 years after recall and factors affecting re-attendance. *Journal of Public Health Medicine* **23**, 292–300.
13. **Hannaford, P.C. and Webb, A.M.C.** (1996). Evidence-guided prescribing of combined oral contraceptives: consensus statement. *Contraception* **54**, 125–9.
14. **Collins, R.** et al. (1990). Blood pressure, stroke, and coronary heart disease. Part 2. Short-term reductions in blood pressure: overview of randomised drug trials in their epidemiological context. *Lancet* **335**, 827–38.
15. **Winkler, U.H.** (1996). Role of screening for vascular disease in pill users: the haemostatic system. In *Evidence-Guided Prescribing of the Pill* (ed. P.C. Hannaford and A.M.C. Webb), pp. 109–20. Carnforth UK: Parthenon Publishing Group.
16. **Pierce, M.** et al. (1989). Prospective randomised controlled trial of methods of call and recall for cervical cytology screening. *British Medical Journal* **299**, 160–2.
17. **Feder, G.** et al. (1995). Do clinical guidelines introduced with practice based education improve care of asthmatic and diabetic patients? A randomised controlled trial in general practices in east London. *British Medical Journal* **311**, 1473–8.
18. **Campbell, N.** et al. (1998). Secondary prevention clinics for coronary heart disease: randomised trial of effect on health. *British Medical Journal* **316**, 1434–7.
19. **Moher, M.** et al. (2001). Cluster randomised controlled trial to compare three methods of promoting secondary prevention of coronary heart disease in primary care. *British Medical Journal* **322**, 1–7.
20. **Moher, M.** et al. (2000). An assessment of morbidity registers for coronary heart disease in primary care. *British Journal of General Practice* **50**, 706–9.
21. **Last, J.** (1963). The iceberg: 'completing the clinical picture' in general practice. *Lancet* **i**, 120–5.
22. **Richards, H.** et al. (2000). Social and gender variation in the prevalence, presentation and general practitioner provisional diagnosis of chest pain. *Journal of Epidemiology and Community Health* **54**, 714–18.
23. **Lawrence, J.M.** et al. (2001). Screening for diabetes in general practice: cross sectional population study. *British Medical Journal* **323**, 548–51.

10.2 Defining the population: registration and record linkage

John Newton

Registration—a special relationship

In this age of competitive markets, it is increasingly unusual to be the sole provider of a professional service to a defined group of clients. In countries such as the United Kingdom, New Zealand, Denmark, and the Netherlands primary care professionals are in just that position. Patients register with a specific practice from which it is expected they will receive comprehensive primary medical care. Registration goes hand in hand with a capitation system of allocation where practices receive payments based mainly on numbers and type of registered patients rather than measures of activity.

Other countries, such as Canada and Australia, which also have universal state-funded health care, allow patients to choose their primary care provider and practices are paid on a fee for service basis (see Chapter 10.8). However, registration systems have been considered in these countries too, often combined with other structural reforms to health services.[1]

The perceived advantages of registration, or rostering or listing, are based on achieving greater continuity of care[1] as well as cost containment through capitation payment. In a comparative 'trans-Atlantic' survey, only 8 per cent of US adults had had their regular primary care physician for 6 years or more compared with 70 per cent of UK patients.[2]

An established relationship based on registration with a single provider can improve access to care. In a fee-for-service system providers are often selective in what they offer.[3] They may, for example, choose not to offer a full out-of-hours service. In the United Kingdom, practices in receipt of capitation payment are obliged to offer a comprehensive service to their patients.

Registration may also increase appropriateness of care. There is evidence that patients with a long-term relationship with a primary care physician make fewer visits to neighbouring hospital Accident and Emergency departments.[4]

Registration imposes constraints on patients as well as providers. Where patients may choose between a range of primary care providers they tend to exercise that choice. In Canada, only 38 per cent of patients in urban areas, and 60 per cent in rural areas, chose to use the same practice for more than 75 per cent of their primary care visits.[3] Nevertheless, when asked, 97 per cent of Canadians reported having an identified family physician.[3] In Australia, 69 per cent of patients in Western Australia had only attended one practice in a 6-month period but again there was a good deal of variation between practices.[5]

In the ideal world, the relationship defined by registration is one of trust rather than dependency or faith.[6] Not dependency, because the individual could choose to be registered elsewhere. Not faith, because that choice is based on some form of objective evidence that care will be acceptable. Continuity of care is likely to increase levels of trust.[2]

For individuals, registration with a primary care practice represents *inclusion* in the prevailing system of health care. Implicitly, it signifies a willingness to accept the conditions under which that care is provided. It is important, therefore, that those conditions are communicated effectively at the outset—for example, in regard to policy on the sharing of personal data with third parties. In return for the promise of care and other assurances, the registered individual undertakes to use the system appropriately. Both parties know that removal from the 'list' remains a powerful sanction against the patient who abuses the system.

The obverse of the above is that those who are not registered, either by choice or circumstance, risk being *excluded*. They may be seen to have rejected the offer of health care, refused to accept the responsibilities of a registered patient and, to some extent, to have forfeited their rights to equal care.

In countries such as the United Kingdom, where levels of registration approach 100 per cent, it is important that these few unregistered individuals or families are not marginalized. This population will include many homeless or travelling people and others with more than their share of substance abuse, mental illness, and social deprivation. For a variety of reasons, therefore, this hard to reach group will be in particular need of careful and sympathetic health care.[7]

Provision of additional primary care facilities, available to all on a drop-in basis, may improve access for marginal groups.[7] However, this policy risks undermining the model of primary care as sole advocate for a registered population and as gate keeper to secondary care. Considerations of access might be deemed an overriding consideration for important public health priorities such as contraception, substance abuse, sexual health, child health, and infectious diseases. For chronic health problems, parallel systems for access to secondary care services may be confusing, produce inequity of access and encourage inappropriate consulting behaviour.

For practices, the registered population defines their responsibilities and determines their remuneration whether by a capitation allowance or through fees paid for specific services (e.g. contraceptive advice). The number of patients registered per doctor has been falling gradually in the United Kingdom since about 1970 (see Fig. 1). This is partly an artefact due to list

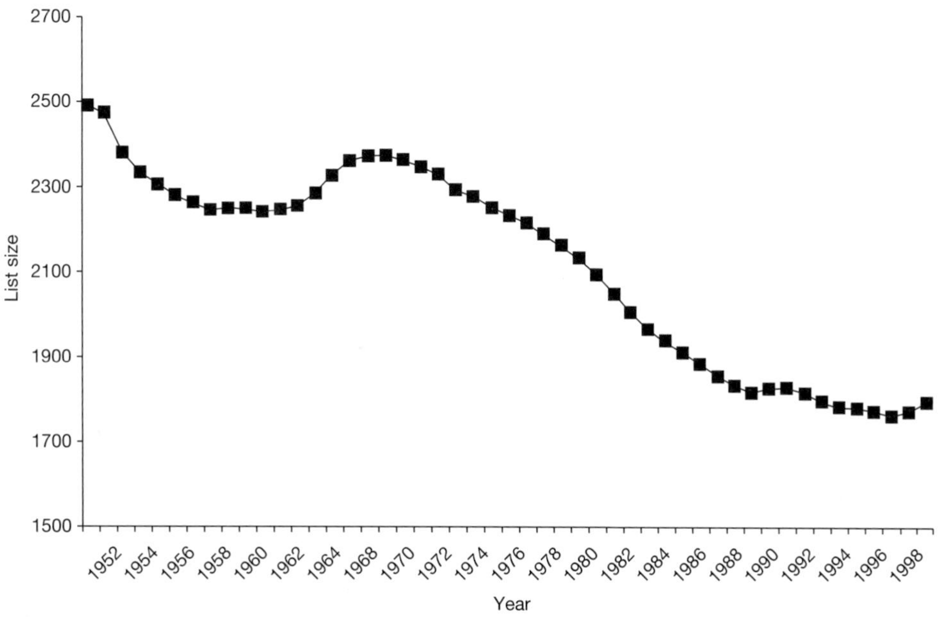

Fig. 1 Resident population per unrestricted principal, United Kingdom 1951–1999. (*Sources:* Department of Health, Scottish Health Statistics, Health Statistics Wales, Northern Ireland Common Services Authority, Office for National Statistics.)

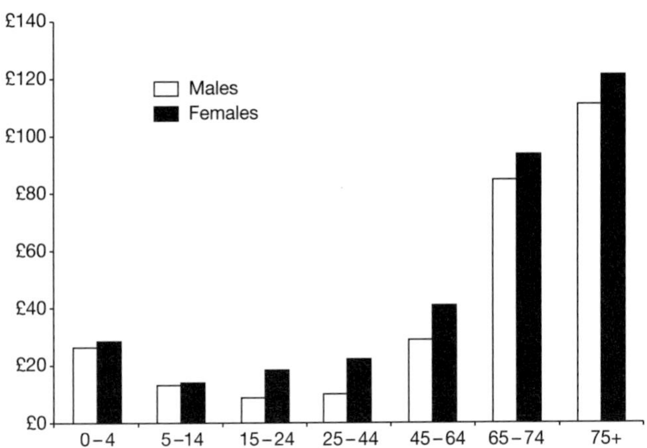

Fig. 2 Mean prescribing costs in 1992 for a sample of practices in Surrey, England: costs in £ sterling per patient per year by age-group and sex. (*Source:* Sleator, D.J. (1993). *British Journal of General Practice* **43**, 102–6).

validation but also reflects the increasing volume and intensity of care expected from practices.

The cost of providing care to a given population is heavily influenced not only by its size but also by its age structure.[(8)] Figure 2 shows the average cost of prescriptions per patient per year broken down by age and sex group.

Collectively, the registered population may also determine the practice's status and influence in the wider local health 'economy'. In England, as a matter of government policy, the registered primary care population is to be used as the vehicle for resource allocation for secondary care services as well as for primary care. This is despite evident problems in defining robust practice populations and in relating them to patterns of need for secondary care.[(9)] By 2004, the British Government will allocate 70 per cent of the National Health Service budget to primary care organizations according to the size and nature of their registered populations. They will use this money to secure the most appropriate services for their patients. The Government is convinced that primary care based organizations will understand the needs of their patients better than more remote agencies.

Practice populations are also the building blocks of much larger health care information systems.[(10)] Many statistical or research processes require more information about the individuals in the denominator than can be obtained from administrative sources such as population censuses. Practice populations can often provide this information. They have the added advantage of being continuously updated and validated. This is particularly important for any work that requires long-term follow-up information. In fact, no other health care information system can reliably relate the group that uses health care to the population from which they are drawn.

Range of information to be recorded

Early attempts to analyse practice populations were hampered by the limitations of 80-column punch cards.[(11)] In those days, it took 3 man-months to punch the records for a single practice (6725 patients) before any analysis could be undertaken. The massive expansion in primary care computing has made highly complex information systems feasible in routine primary care settings. There are clear advantages for practices in this development although evidence that the new systems have improved patient care remains surprisingly sparse.[(12)]

Current computerized practice systems mostly operate as relational databases, one component of which is the registration file (other files would normally hold clinical data, prescribing data and free text, linked via the patient's practice ID). Each system, and there are many, has its idiosyncrasies but information in any registration file would be similar to that shown in Fig. 3.

Field	Description
Practice patient number	A number unique to that patient used only within the practice
Registration category	Full/temporary/other
Registration status	Registered/suspended
Surname	May change over time and in context
Birth surname	Does not normally change
Forenames	
Calling name	Name by which they are known/nickname
Date of birth	Day/month/year
Title	Mr/Mrs/Dr etc.
House name or number	
Street	
Village	
Town	
Post code	
Telephone number	
NHS number	A number unique to that patient used throughout the NHS
Hospital number	An ID number used by a specific hospital before the NHS number was introduced
Surgery normally attends	Usually where paper records are kept
Registered doctor	Doctor with whom the patient is formally registered
Usual doctor	Doctor that normally sees the patient
Rural miles	Distance from surgery (may increase practice payment)

Fig. 3 Content of a typical practice registration file.

Special fields may be added to identify sub-groups of patients, for example, those for which the practice can also dispense medication because there is no pharmacy near where they live. Students or the families of armed forces personnel may be registered for limited purposes such as vaccination. Also, patients included in some research studies or disease registers might be flagged by adding a field to the register file.

It is almost always helpful to collect additional socio-economic data in order to interpret patterns of consultation or morbidity. However, in routine systems these fields are rarely completed satisfactorily.

One of the most important variables derived from the registration data is the number of *person years at risk* for each patient. This is calculated from the number of days that each patient was registered with the practice during the study period and represents the proportionate contribution that each patient makes to the denominator when it comes to calculating rates of occurrence. It can be derived from a series of status records held in the registration file. Each time status changes, a new status record is generated which records the date and the nature of the change. Most systems never delete the information held on old patients even after death.

Category of registration is also important. Many patients register temporarily with a practice while maintaining their full registration elsewhere. This is partly for the convenience of the patients who do not then have to give their details each time they attend but also so that practices can be rewarded for the additional workload. Table 1 shows the age distribution of full and temporary patients in a group of practices in Oxfordshire, England. Young adults and the elderly can be seen to be substantially over represented among temporary residents. Many of the young adults in this population are likely to be students. Elderly temporary residents may be staying with relatives away from home or may be residents of institutions. The phenomenon of seasonally mobile elderly populations is well described in other populations[(13)] and represents a potential challenge for capitation-based health systems.

The 'denominator problem' in primary care

Accurate denominators are crucial to any epidemiological or health utilization studies performed in primary care. Although registration systems are

Table 1 Proportion (%) of registered population by age group according to registration category (patients registered in nine Oxfordshire practices in June 1995)

Age group	Fully registered	Temporary residents	Difference
0–4	5.8	3.7	−2.1
5–14	11.3	8.0	−3.3
15–24	14.7	27.1	+12.4
25–34	17.7	23.9	+6.2
35–44	13.5	9.1	−4.4
45–54	13.4	6.2	−7.2
55–64	9.7	5.4	−4.3
65–74	7.5	3.8	−3.7
75–84	4.6	6.5	+1.9
85+	1.8	6.3	+4.5

Fully registered, N = 65 082 (100%); temporary residents, N = 1094 (100%).

Table 2 Rates of respiratory illnesses reported by the Royal College of General Practitioners Research Unit weekly monitoring service

	Rate per 100 000 per week	First and new episodes
Acute otitis media	71.5	379
Common cold	203.1	1076
Flu/flu-like illness	42.3	224
Acute tonsillitis	103.4	548
Acute sinusitis	44.4	235
Laryngitis/acute tracheitis	17.6	93
Pneumonia/pneumonitis	3.0	16
Acute bronchitis	153.4	813
Pleurisy	2.6	14
Asthma	29.1	154
Allergic rhinitis	4.5	24

Population at risk = 529 822; number of practices = 64; period = 28/01/02 to 03/02/02.

the envy of those who do not have them,[14] they are by no means the perfect solution to the so-called 'denominator problem' in primary care.[15]

Estimates of practice populations may be inaccurate due to both list inflation and deflation.[16] Lists are inflated when patients move away without informing the practice or when they die and the practice is not made aware of the fact. Deflation occurs when patients who move in to an area wait until they are ill before registering or when children are born.[16] Deflation and inflation due to mobility should in theory cancel themselves out.[16] However, this is clearly not the case in practice. Inflation has at times reached levels of 20–30 per cent in inner city areas in the United Kingdom due largely to patient mobility.[17] Delays and imperfect information systems meant that many sets of records did not catch up with the relevant patients. In a purely capitation-funded system there is little incentive for the practices to strive to eliminate these 'ghost' patients.

In other areas of the United Kingdom, list inflation was much less of a problem than it was in London.[16] Rates of inflation were generally found to be less than 10 per cent and could be as low as 2 per cent in some practices.[18]

The situation in the United Kingdom is now thought to be much improved.[10,14] Some years ago, practice payments became partly determined by rates of coverage of preventive care. Ghost patients tend not to attend for breast screening no matter how persuasive the letter of invitation, nor do they bring their children for vaccination or attend health checks!

However, it would be unfair to conclude that financial incentive was the only reason for recent improvements in the accuracy of registration statistics. The introduction of electronic links to administrative population registers has also helped a lot. Electronic transfer of data can now make practices automatically aware of a patient's death within days of the event.

Apart from any remaining inaccuracy, registered populations make excellent denominators when the numerator data are also from primary care; for example, when used to calculate rates of presentation of respiratory illnesses in the community (see Table 2). They may be less good for assessing the need for care in the population. In the United Kingdom demographic data based on practice populations will include an unknown but variable proportion of patients who also have private health insurance. This group will have a reduced need for state-funded care. In the Netherlands, the problem is compounded because only people below a certain level of income are required to register with a GP.[14]

Registered populations overlap almost all geographical and administrative boundaries (except perhaps the coastline). Also, they can fluctuate rapidly in size (e.g. seasonally or when practices reconfigure). Finally, numerator data may not contain practice information which sometimes makes it difficult to relate a numerator to the appropriate denominator. For example, the catchment population of a secondary care provider will not map on to practice populations with any precision. Routine death data do not normally give the name of the usual primary care physician.

Uses of registration information

Generating meaningful morbidity information

In the United Kingdom, a number of sources of morbidity information rely on primary care registration data for their denominators. The most comprehensive are the decennial morbidity surveys of which four have been reported since 1956.[19] In the last survey, information was collected from 60 practices across England and Wales. Denominator information was taken from practice registration files but where duplicates were found the records were amalgamated.

Information was enhanced by ensuring that practices supplied complete data on socio-economic variables.[20] In addition to normal registration data, practices were asked to record the data items shown in the left-hand column of Fig. 4. These data items and others were used to derive the information given in the right-hand column, for example, by using standard tables to allocate social class codes to occupations.

Continuous morbidity information is also provided from sentinel practice systems on a more immediate basis. The Royal College of General Practitioners Research Unit in Birmingham, England, currently receives data electronically each week from approximately 78 general practices in England and Wales. Practices report episodes for a wide range of diseases using the current registered practice population as a denominator (see Chapter 10.3). Results are posted on the World Wide Web (www.rcgpbru.demon.co.uk).

The British Public Health Laboratory Service also runs a comparable system aimed at infectious disease episodes. Similar networks of sentinel practices have been successfully established in other countries with registered GP populations.[21]

Morbidity data from more 'standard' primary care systems can be useful but a good deal of effort is required to obtain data of sufficient quality.[22,23] In a study of 41 practices in Scotland, most could only identify about half of their patients with angina, depression, or stroke from the routine computerized record.[24] The information that was recorded was nearly always reliable.

It is probably unrealistic to expect high levels of completeness for clinical data to be achieved routinely and continuously. If sensitivity is an important consideration, algorithms can be constructed based on

Data collected	Derived variables
♦ Marital status	♦ Social class of men
♦ Cohabiting status	♦ Partner's social class for women
♦ Housing tenure	♦ Own social class for women
♦ Ethnic group	♦ Parent's/guardian's social class (for children)
♦ Sole adult in household	♦ Urban/rural indicator
♦ Children (no.) in household	
♦ Smoking status	
♦ Economic position	
♦ Occupation	
♦ Employment status	
♦ Children living with sole adult	

Fig. 4 Socio-economic and lifestyle variables collected in the Fourth National Morbidity Survey and derived socio-economic variables.

a combination of prescribing data and diagnostic data in order to identify an acceptable proportion of cases. This is a useful strategy but will only work for conditions that are closely linked to specific medications, such as epilepsy, acne, or glaucoma.

Disease-specific registers

Many practices find it helpful to maintain registers of patients with particular conditions. These registers have a number of functions in patient care, public health, technology assessment, and research.[25]

The most obvious use of such a register is in the management of patients who have a continuing need for health care. Regular review may be necessary because they receive long-term therapy (e.g. patients with epilepsy, leprosy, diabetes, hydrocephalus, or acne), because they need to be screened for treatable complications of their disease (e.g. patients with diabetes, renal failure, inflammatory bowel disease, lichen sclerosus, polyposis coli, or melanoma) or to encourage and educate patients to adopt a health-promoting lifestyle (e.g. patients at risk of heart disease or who have a mental health problem).

In general, a register of some sort is probably a prerequisite to the provision of structured and comprehensive care to a defined population. It is definitely required to know whether that aim has been achieved. The most common example of registers being used in this way is in the care of patients with diabetes. Similar registers are currently being set up in the United Kingdom for coronary heart disease although there are problems in deciding which patients to include. These registers will be used, for example, to ensure that all patients discharged from hospital after a myocardial infarction receive appropriate secondary prevention advice and treatment.

Registers can also help the practice monitor patients who are at high risk of complications due to some specific exposure (e.g. patients who have had thyroid treatment, have been treated with human growth hormone, or patients who have received radiotherapy).

Registers may act as a focus for a community-wide collaborative approach to the management of particular groups of patients. The existence of a register leads to the sharing of information about practice, and the standardization of practice around explicit clinical guidelines or a consensus standard. The register also encourages audit and research. An example of this approach is the early use of a diabetic register in Poole, England to encourage shared care between hospital and primary care.[26]

Registers used only for patient care within the practice can be relatively undemanding in terms of case definitions and other information needs. When shared by a group of practices it is important to specify standard definitions and practices in order to maintain comparability. However, the potential to use shared databases for comparative audit may well justify the extra work involved.

Internal migration statistics

One surprising use of primary care registration data is for official estimates of internal migration in England and Wales. Measuring migration is not straightforward, as there is no compulsory system within the United Kingdom to record the movement of the population. Based on registration returns from practices, the National Health Service records net movements of patients between former Family Health Service Authority Areas. More recently, internal migration estimates by age and gender are being made available for all local and health authority areas.

Research uses

There is a long tradition in the United Kingdom and elsewhere of observational epidemiology based on primary care data. Much of this would be impossible without registration.

One of the particular strengths of registration data is in obtaining complete follow-up for individuals included in cohort studies. For example, in 1978 the British Regional Heart Study recruited 7735 men from general practice age–sex registers.[27] Over the next 20 years practices were paid to review the notes of study participants every 2 years and report all cardiovascular events. When a patient moved practices, the study centre was able to trace the subject to the new practice. Information was obtained in this way on 99.5 per cent of the surviving men.[27]

Another very important role of practice registers is as a sampling frame for controls in case-control studies. Almost whatever method has been used for ascertaining cases, it is usually possible to identify a number of potential controls from the age–sex registers of the cases' primary care practice. Information available on the register allows controls to be matched to cases according to potential confounding variables such as age, sex, locality of residence, and medical history.

In addition to the above, researchers have access to a number of databases that combine anonymous records from a large number of practices. The most extensively used system in the United Kingdom is the General Practice Research Database based on the VAMP Medical system.[10] Currently, over 400 practices in the United Kingdom contribute data to this database provided they satisfy the required quality criteria.

Prescribing data in these databases is particularly good being approximately 95 per cent complete. This makes them ideal for pharmacoepidemiology, particularly rapid case-control studies where the exposure of interest is a drug.[10] They are also one of the best sources of information on absolute incidence rates of unusual side-effects of drugs because they provide accurate denominator information.

Potential for record linkage

In general, there is remarkably little overlap between information systems in primary and secondary care. The common element in these systems is, however, the patient. Information systems that relate data collected in different settings to defined groups of individuals might allow the evaluation of services in a way that is both more complete in scope and more meaningful.

Studies based on manual reviews of paper records have shown the value of comparing GP and hospital activity.[28] However, very little work has been done using person-based data derived from general practice linked to hospital computer systems. Nevertheless, in New Zealand, GP data have been successfully linked to information from hospital systems and vital records.[29]

The potential benefits of record linkage outside the practice are:

- *Avoidance of double-counting:* for example if many practices are linked together.
- *Monitoring outcomes:* the impact of care can be established using a more complete set of outcomes.
- *Validation:* comparison of data from more than one source improves accuracy and completeness.

Information on practice systems is already person-based because records are linked together for each patient using a common identifying number. Standard methods for record linkage could be used to link the practice data to hospital activity data, vital statistics, or cancer registrations.[30]

There are two main methods for record linkage. The *exact* method can be used when a unique identifier is available for each record and the quality of the identifying data is high. This might be the case, for example, in Scandinavian countries where personal identification numbers are widely used. Otherwise a *probabilistic* method must be used. This method compares records from the input files and works out whether they should be linked, not linked or possibly linked according to a set of probability-based criteria.[30] The accuracy of the linkage will ultimately depend on the completeness and quality of the identifying information on the relevant input files.

Confidentiality

One of the main obstacles to record linkage using primary care data is the need to release sensitive personal data outside the practice.

Public concern over the appropriate use of confidential data has increased significantly in most countries. As a result, the regulatory environment in which personal data are used has become much more restrictive. Fortunately, legislators and the judiciary recognize that the individual's right to privacy is not absolute and is balanced by a certain duty to society.

Circumstances may arise when it is in the public interest to use personal data without the explicit consent of the individual. For this to be justifiable, the objective must be legitimate and useful and there must be no practicable alternative method of achieving the same objective.

In relation to practice registration data there are two general situations in which personal data might be released. Firstly, in connection with the care of the individual patient, when their consent should almost always be obtained. Secondly, for some other purpose unrelated to their own care such as surveillance by a cancer registry or service evaluation. In this second case, patients should be made aware in general terms that their data may be released for this purpose and they should be given the opportunity to object. However, most authorities recognize that it is impractical to ask for explicit consent from every patient for every release of personal data.

Whenever identifiable personal data are released, there is an obligation on all parties to respect the interests of the data subject. This requires that only individuals with an established duty of confidence to the subjects should have access to the identifiable data and that appropriate data security policies should be applied consistently.

References

1. **Ostbye, T. and Hunskaar, S.** (1997). A new primary care rostering and capitation system in Norway: lessons for Canada? *Canadian Medical Association Journal* **157**, 45–50.
2. **Mainous, A.G., III, Baker, R., Love, M.M., Gray, D.P., and Gill, J.M.** (2001). Continuity of care and trust in one's physician: evidence from primary care in the United States and the United Kingdom. *Family Medicine* **33**, 22–7.
3. **Menec, V., Black, C., Roos, N., and Bogdanovic, B.** (2001). What is the potential for formal patient registration in Canadian primary care? The scale of 'informal registration' in Manitoba. *Journal of Health Services Research Policy* **6**, 202–6.
4. **Gill, J.M., Mainous, A.G., III, and Nsereko, M.** (2000). The effect of continuity of care on emergency department use. *Archives of Family Medicine* **9**, 333–8.
5. **Ward, A.M., Underwood, P.J., Fatovich, B.S., Wood, A., and Bourke, T.J.** (1995). Attendance patterns in general practice. *Medical Journal of Australia* **162**, 37, 40–1.
6. **Davies, H.T. and Rundall, T.G.** (2000). Managing patient trust in managed care. *The Milbank Quarterly* **78**, 609–24, iv–v.
7. **O'Toole, T.P., Gibbon, J.L., Hanusa, B.H., and Fine, M.J.** (1999). Preferences for sites of care among urban homeless and housed poor adults. *Journal of General Internal Medicine* **14**, 599–605.
8. **Sleator, D.J.** (1993). Towards accurate prescribing analysis in general practice: accounting for the effects of practice demography. *British Journal of General Practice* **43**, 102–6.
9. **Gilley, J.** (1999). Meeting the information and budgetary requirements of primary care groups. *British Medical Journal* **318**, 168–9; discussion 169–70.
10. **Lawrenson, R., Williams, T., and Farmer, R.** (1999). Clinical information for research; the use of general practice databases. *Journal of Public Health Medicine* **21**, 299–304.
11. **Acheson, E.D. and Forbes, J.A.** (1968). Experiment in the retrieval of information in general practice: a preliminary report. *British Journal of Preventive and Social Medicine* **22**, 105–9.
12. **Mitchell, E. and Sullivan, F.** (2001). A descriptive feast but an evaluative famine: systematic review of published articles on primary care computing during 1980–97. *British Medical Journal* **322**, 279–82.
13. **Marshall, V.W., Longino, C.F., Jr, Tucker, R., and Mullins, L.** (1989). Health care utilization of Canadian snowbirds: an example of strategic planning. *Journal of Aging and Health* **1**, 150–68.
14. **Schlaud, M., Brenner, M.H., Hoopmann, M., and Schwartz, F.W.** (1998). Approaches to the denominator in practice-based epidemiology: a critical overview. *Journal of Epidemiology and Community Health* **52** (Suppl. 1), 13S–19S.
15. **Cherkin, D.C., Berg, A.O., and Phillips, W.R.** (1982). In search of a solution to the primary care denominator problem. *Journal of Family Practice* **14**, 301–9.
16. **Fraser, R.C.** (1978). The reliability and validity of the age–sex register as a population denominator in general practice. *Journal of the Royal College of General Practitioners* **28**, 283–6.
17. **Robson, J. and Falshaw, M.** (1995). Audit of preventive activities in 16 inner London practices using a validated measure of patient population, the 'active patient' denominator. Healthy Eastenders Project. *British Journal of General Practice* **45**, 463–6.
18. **Sheldon, M.G., Rector, A.L., and Barnes, P.A.** (1984). The accuracy of age–sex registers in general practice. *Journal of the Royal College of General Practitioners* **34**, 269–71.
19. **Fleming, D.M.** (1993). Morbidity registration and the fourth general practice morbidity survey in England and Wales. *Scandinavian Journal of Primary Health Care Supplement* **2**, 37–41.
20. **Fleming, D.M., McCormick, A., and Charlton, J.** (1996). The capture of socioeconomic data in general practice. *British Journal of General Practice* **46** (405), 217–20.
21. **Middelkoop, B.J., Bohnen, A.M., Duisterhout, J.S., Hoes, A.W., Pleumeekers, H.J., and Prins, A.** (1995) Rotterdam general practitioners report (ROHAPRO): a computerised network of general practices in Rotterdam, The Netherlands. Rotterdam's HuisArtsen Project. *Journal of Epidemiology and Community Health* **49** (3), 231–3.
22. **Pearson, N., O'Brien, J., Thomas, H., Ewings, P., Gallier, L., and Bussey, A.** (1996). Collecting morbidity data in general practice: the Somerset morbidity project. *British Medical Journal* **312**, 1517–20.
23. **Scobie, S., Basnett, I., and McCartney, P.** (1995). Can general practice data be used for needs assessment and health care planning in an inner-London district? *Journal of Public Health Medicine* **17**, 475–83.
24. **Whitelaw, F.G., Nevin, S.L., Milne, R.M., Taylor, R.J., Taylor, M.W., and Watt, A.H.** (1996). Completeness and accuracy of morbidity and repeat prescribing records held on general practice computers in Scotland. *British Journal of General Practice* **46**, 181–6.
25. **Newton, J. and Garner, S.** *Disease Registers in England.* Oxford: Institute of Health Sciences, 2002.
26. **Hill, R.D.** (1976). Community care service for diabetics in the Poole area. *British Medical Journal* **1**, 1137–9.
27. **Walker, M., Shaper, A.G., Lennon, L., and Whincup, P.H.** (2000). Twenty year follow-up of a cohort based in general practices in 24 British towns. *Journal of Public Health Medicine* **22**, 479–85.
28. **Coulter, A., Bradlow, J., Martin Bates, C., Agass, M., and Tulloch, A.** (1991). Outcome of general practitioner referrals to specialist outpatient clinics for back pain. *British Journal of General Practice* **41** (352), 450–3, 960–1643.

29. **Tilyard, M.W., Phillips, D.E., Dovey, S.M., Skelly, L., and Whitney, R.K.** (1991). The health services utilisation of a general practice population. *New Zealand Medical Journal* **104** (923), 463–5.

30. **Gill, L.** Methods for automatic record matching and linkage and their use in national statistics. *National Statistics Methodological Series No. 25*. London: HMSO, 2001.

10.3 Health surveillance

Douglas M. Fleming and Andrew Ross

> I must begin with a good body of facts and not from a principle (in which I always suspect some fallacy) and then as much deduction as you please
>
> (Charles Darwin, 1874)

Introduction

At its simplest, surveillance is the action of monitoring particular events or activities. In the context of *health*, the events are usually concerned with the incidence of disease or factors bearing on such incidence. In the context of *infectious diseases*, surveillance has been defined as 'the continued watchfulness over the distribution and trends of incidence through the systematic collection, consolidation and evaluation of morbidity and mortality reports, and other relevant data'.[1] In its broadest sense, surveillance in *primary care* means collecting information on health-related events as they interface with this environment. The direct purpose of surveillance is to prompt or plan action in order that adverse consequences can be mitigated. Surveillance is not hypothesis-driven research, though surveillance data can be used for research. Data can be used to estimate the burden of illness attributable to a particular disease.

If surveillance is primarily to prompt action, then it follows that surveillance data must be available in time for action. For some matters, timing is not as critical as others. The International Classification of Diseases was generated out of a desire to compare the causes of death in differing countries with a view to planning interventions where there were unusual patterns of mortality.[2] This sort of planning involved long-term strategic decisions. Even now in some countries annual mortality data by cause are often not available until well after the year-end. On the other hand, surveillance of communicable diseases with implications for local spread must produce timely information if action is to be taken. It does not always follow that any action is possible, but at least health care providers should be prepared for the consequences. For particular diseases (especially those for which statutory notification is required) outbreak control procedures are in place, but for a wide range of less severe diseases such as influenza, head lice, chicken pox, scabies, or fifth disease (parvovirus), they do not exist in quite the same way. However, for a condition such as influenza, there are considerable public health consequences and commensurate needs for reliable surveillance information.

Surveillance can be considered in many different ways. Raska listed three basic characteristics:[3] systematic collection of data; consolidation and analysis of the collected data; dissemination of information by means of narrative epidemiological reports. In some instances, all general practitioners participate in surveillance, but in others, networks of general practitioners generate proxy information for the whole population.[4–10] Usually, surveillance is a continuous process but occasionally it is intermittent, particularly where the need to provide information is driven by current issues. Often, general practitioners are closely involved in the collection of data but sometimes only peripherally, as for example in the surveillance of deaths by cause or the surveillance of prescribing data. Surveillance of health related issues does not automatically involve general practitioners working in primary care. For some purposes, it is more appropriate to survey population or household samples from the community, for example, General Household Surveys,[11] labour force surveys,[12] etc.

Conducting surveillance in primary care

Ideally, surveillance is best conducted using well-defined diagnostic criteria and for most serious physical illnesses, criteria for diagnosis are commonly agreed. Such an approach is essential for the conduct of clinical trials but is too limited in surveillance, particularly in primary care, where the inclusion of all relevant consultations is desirable. In the routine provision of medical care, it is also often the case that the doctor or practice undertaking the surveillance is reporting on cases diagnosed elsewhere by another doctor. Some diseases may also be active for a number of years and then disappear (e.g. asthma); others never disappear completely but may have very long asymptomatic periods (e.g. multiple sclerosis). Diagnostic criteria appropriate to a particular condition vary with the duration of symptoms at the point of consultation, by age and according to the virulence of the organism. Objective criteria may not exist and the observer is dependent on the historical details reported by the patient. The recording doctor therefore has to make the most of the information available to him at the time of that consultation.

Using routine data

Examples of surveillance included in this chapter are taken chiefly from the Royal College of General Practitioners Weekly Returns Service (WRS). Data are collected on the doctor's working diagnosis from a network of practices (presently 74) covering a population of approximately 660 000 persons and recording all consultations in primary care. Information is received from practices using five different computer systems. Most practitioners input data directly onto the computer themselves, but in some practices clerks input data. The validity of this approach has been demonstrated in several ways: by comparison with virological data;[13] by comparison with hospital episode data;[14] from associations with mortality data;[15] and by internal consistency by region.[16]

One of the strengths of long-term surveillance based on working diagnoses is the relative stability of this evaluation. In particular, the notion that observational time series databases such as the WRS are less useful for research than 'gold-standard' randomized double-blind controlled trials (RCTs) has recently been challenged.[17,18] However, in relation to infectious disease, the quality of diagnostic tests for the identification of causative organisms has improved dramatically over recent years. Advances in investigation techniques using molecular based methods are likely to lead to increased numbers of cases attributable to specific pathogens and ultimately to the identification and greater understanding of the role of hitherto unrecognized pathogens.[19]

Presenting and analysing data

Effective surveillance commonly involves the collection of data from more than one source. Recent work with influenza and respiratory syncytial virus undertaken within the WRS and Public Health Laboratory Service is a good example.[20] Information particularly on influenza is based both on community dwelling persons presenting with flu-like illnesses and on the examination of virological specimens submitted from a subset of the same community. This pattern of surveillance is now established in many European countries.

The science of epidemiology has defined the incidence and prevalence of disease in ways that are not easily applicable to routine operational research. We here suggest suitable measurements for the presentation of data obtained from routine operational research in general practice.

The *disease episode incidence* is the number of new cases of disease identified within a given time period. It is this statistic that is reported by the WRS. This measure recognizes that disease status may become quiescent, but there is of course the potential to count the same person twice. Disease episode incidence is most useful as a measure of acute diseases, which are usually short-lived. The number of pneumonia, otitis media, or acute myocardial infarction episodes experienced in a community is probably a more relevant statistic than the number of persons affected. The converse is true for chronic diseases where numbers of persons are more useful than disease episodes. A particular problem arises for conditions where incidence is low, but prevalence relatively high, for example, cerebrovascular disease and diabetes mellitus. If patients are inappropriately assigned the status of having a new episode of disease, rather than an ongoing one; incidence rates for chronic diseases may rapidly become inflated. Care has to be used with computer data entry systems to avoid this, particularly where analysis involves the extraction of tabular summaries and does not retain individual person identity.

The *annual period prevalence* is the strictest definition of prevalence and is concerned with the number of people with recognizable disease at any one time. Some of the excessively high prevalence statistics quoted for asthma arise because of the use of cumulative prevalence and are based on the principle 'once an asthmatic always an asthmatic'. Currently (July 2001), in our practice of 10 400 registered patients 1514 patients who are still registered have been seen with a diagnosis of asthma in the preceding 12 years, but just 382 of these patients have consulted with asthma in the last 12 months. This comparison highlights the importance of time in defining prevalence data.

The concept of prevalence as seen from a general practitioner with the task of treating patients over many years is that of the annual period prevalence. It is a measure of persons with disease, which is active by manifesting itself in the need for consultation or treatment in a 1-year period. Whilst this statistic underestimates the number of patients in the community with the condition in question, it allows comparison of data between practices and year by year.

Morbidity coding systems

The collection and analysis of consultation-related data involves the coding and classification of primary data. However, where computerized systems are used as the basis for the medical record, data storage is an even more important consideration. For routine medical purposes, it is necessary to store data at a precise level of detail and only subsequently group it for analysis. Historically, classification systems in medicine have been mainly concerned with issues relating to grouping for analysis. This remains important but the emphasis has switched to efficient data storage and from that, classification can be automated. In this regard the introduction of the READ Coding System[21] into British general practice has proved a major advance. It has facilitated automated disease coding through menu-driven software offering recording doctors a thesaurus of medical terminology rather than a list of classification codes.

For health monitoring purposes, the classification system of disease is often completely irrelevant. There needs to be a clear understanding of what information is required. If the use of classification systems makes it easier to capture and analyse the data, the most appropriate classification system for the purpose should be employed. However, an underlying need for the comparability of data between health care sectors within a country and with primary care in other countries must be recognized.

When considering the choice of a classification system, the primary purpose of surveillance is paramount; surveillance of a disease process(es) means that the primary focus of recording must be on the disease; surveillance for adverse events may be focused on presenting symptoms; surveillance of accidents may be focused on the circumstance of the injury; surveillance for health care utilization may be focused on the doctor and his interpretation of health problems or on the patient and his interpretation. The surveillance exercise must recognize that the recording discipline must be observed continuously and consistently. Theoretically, a recording system could be so comprehensive that all purposes might be achieved in a single recording system. In reality, practice-based information systems operate at a minimum level where the recording requirement is kept at a manageable level especially in relation to the time available for consultation.

Surveillance networks

Whilst surveillance of a particular local health problem may be organized within a practice, routine surveillance of disease is usually based on a network of practices. Sentinel networks must aim to achieve representativeness of the population and practices under surveillance. Networks should be encouraged towards the comprehensive monitoring of all morbidity. If they cannot achieve this, then data should be collected with enough information to allow standardization. Where for practical purposes a network collects data on selected diseases, the number of conditions should be sufficient to ensure regular input of data. Infrequent reporting leads to frequent forgetting. The word sentinel has several meanings but the warning function is uppermost.

Not all practice networks are designed for or geared to the surveillance function.[22] There is a danger associated with the belief that a practice-based network can be adapted to serve purposes beyond the primary objective. A sentinel network is not a research network though practices included in a sentinel network may also contribute to research and data gathered in a sentinel network used for research. Collaboration is not confined to practice networks; it is often important for efforts to be combined with other agencies, particularly hospital and public health laboratories and 'on call' agencies.

Telephone contact surveillance

The UK government recently introduced a national telephone advice service—'NHS Direct'.[23] There has been interest in using information derived from NHS Direct to monitor the extent of respiratory problems during the winter. Whilst NHS Direct has the potential advantage of producing daily data on a timely basis, there are a number of drawbacks: the volume of calls received per unit population is only a small fraction of contacts with general practice (about one-fortieth); denominators for calculation of rates are difficult to define and the diagnostic assessment of a doctor or nurse is not available. The highest rates of activity for respiratory infections reported by NHS Direct in 2000–2001 occurred when there were very few influenza viruses circulating in the community, 7 weeks before the peak of the influenza outbreak as reported by the WRS (clinical data) and the Public Health Laboratory Service (virological data) (Fig. 1). The lack of age standardization is particularly important; the numbers of episodes of differing respiratory syndromes which make up total respiratory infections reported by the WRS show striking variation by age group (Fig. 2). In children, upper respiratory tract infections (URTI) dominate within the perspective of total respiratory infections, whereas in the elderly, acute bronchitis is the commonest diagnosis.

Why undertake surveillance

Surveillance is needed to define the burden of illness presenting to health services, to provide an alert for contingency planning and to identify new problems or changing patterns in recognized problems. In a wider sense it is needed to monitor the equitable distribution of health care.[24,25] 'Postcode prescribing' has become a slogan for anyone wanting to demonstrate inequity, but prescribing is not the main issue: the concern is primarily with disease incidence. Prescribing data without underlying morbidity data have very limited value.

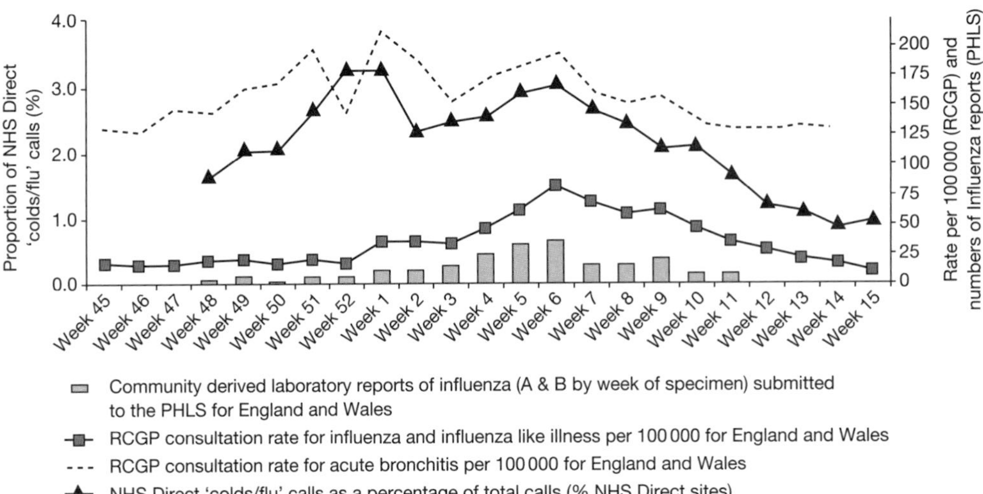

Fig. 1 Comparison of NHS Direct, Royal College of General Practitioner, and Public Health Laboratory Service data 2000–2001. (*Source:* NHS Direct, RCGP Weekly Returns Service, and RCGP/ERVL and PHLS.)

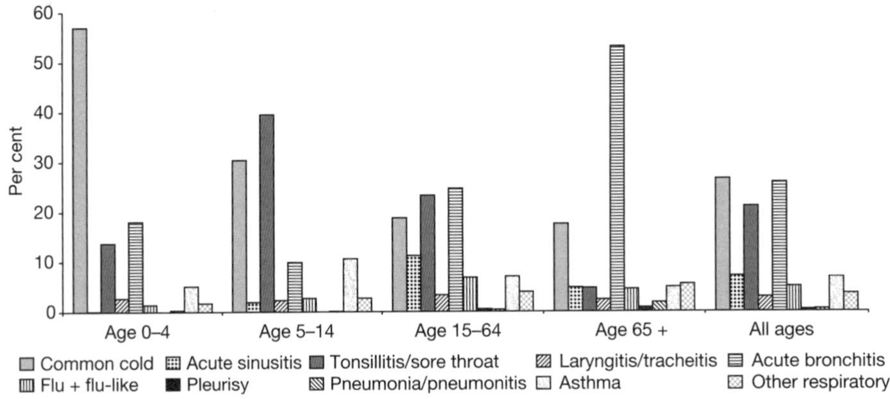

Fig. 2 Episodes of acute respiratory conditions presenting in sentinel practices: percentage distribution by diagnosis. (*Source:* Weekly Returns Service, Annual Report 2000.)

To assist in health care planning

Surveillance data have to be interpreted in a meaningful way and it is here that British general practice has the great advantage of a clearly defined population. Many other health care systems face the difficulty of defining a population denominator. The interpretation of surveillance data for common diseases requires reliable age-specific denominators. However, denominator information is not essential for outbreak control and for rare and serious diseases where proxy based estimates of the denominator may be sufficient.

By way of example, in the last two winters, the National Health Service (NHS) has been particularly concerned with 'winter pressures',[26] generally taken to mean the pressures of illness on health care provision particularly on hospital beds. Surveillance of relevant events needs to contribute to quantifying the pressure (by region, age group, etc.) and to provide an insight into its cause. The pressures on hospital beds at the turn of the year are particularly relevant; whilst influenza is undoubtedly a major contributor, it is certainly not the only cause. Any plan to minimize the pressures calls for action not only on influenza, but also on all related respiratory illnesses. The incidence of episodes of respiratory infection around the turn of the year illustrates this problem. In Fig. 3, we present the average weekly incidence of all respiratory infections combined for persons aged 65 years and over (details of method in ref. 27). This shows the high level of respiratory infections at the turn of the year whether influenza viruses are circulating or not with a peak in the early New Year. The peak in the elderly is synchronous with the peak of deaths in most winters though the pathogen involved is less certain.[28]

A primary purpose of national morbidity surveys stems from concern about *inequalities in health*, be they socio-economic, regional, racial, age, or gender based. Morbidity surveys actually describe health care utilization patterns rather than need, though by suitable interpretation can be used to address issues of need. In the fourth national morbidity survey[6] illnesses were categorized serious, intermediate, and minor (trivial in the third survey[5]). By using this classification, more marked socio-economic gradients in the prevalence of serious disease than of minor disease were demonstrated. By this means the observed inequalities reflected the assessment of true need as made by the doctor when recording diagnoses rather than simply the demand which may be apparent in minor illness. Carr-Hill et al.[29] analysed data from the fourth national morbidity survey, finding demographic and social factors could act as powerful predictors of consultation patterns, and that characteristics of individual patients were much more powerful predictors of consulting patterns than the characteristics of the areas in which the patients lived.

To describe trends over time

The WRS as at present organized is chiefly concerned with the incidence of disease by week but its long history has also provided an opportunity

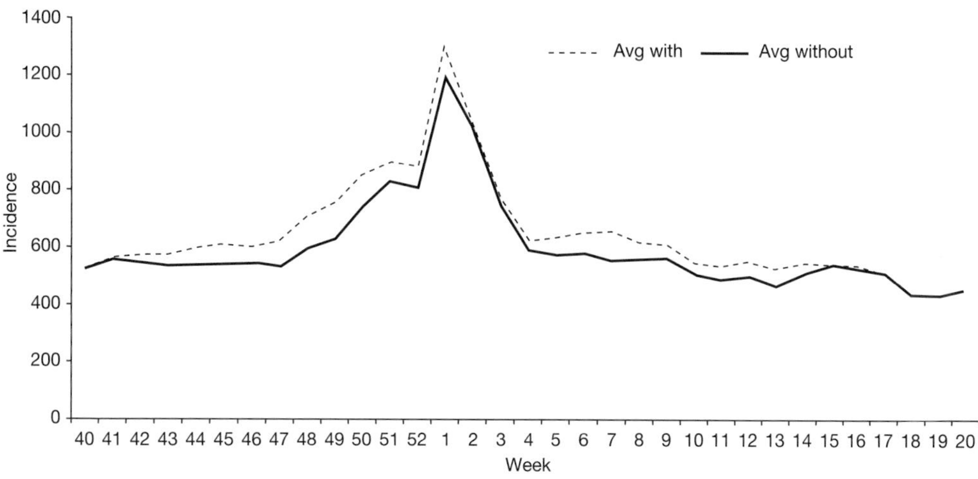

Fig. 3 Average weekly incidence of all respiratory infections in persons 65 years and over calculated with and without the incidence of influenza like illness.

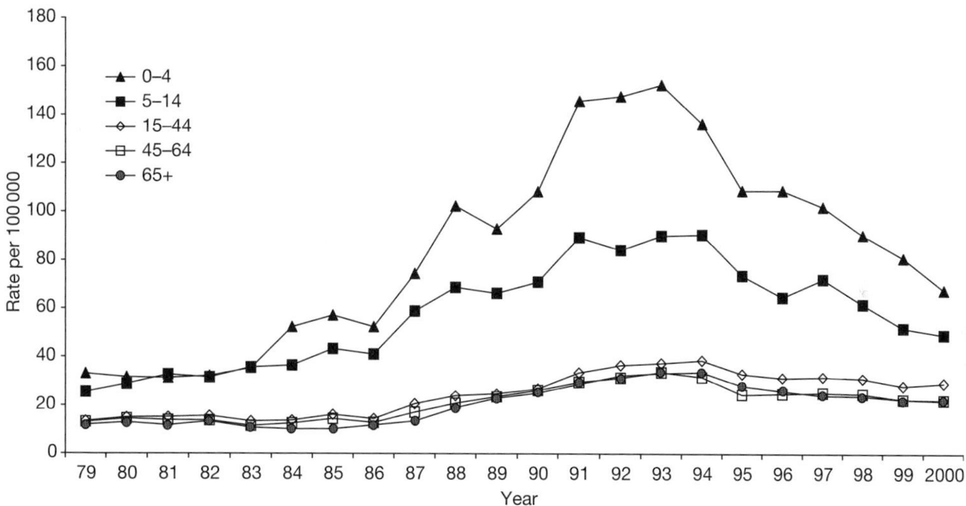

Fig. 4 Episodes of asthma presenting in sentinel practices. Mean weekly incidence by age group, 1979–2000.

to examine trends over time. Secular[30,31] and seasonal[14] trends in *the incidence of asthma* have recently been described using WRS data demonstrating the importance of long-term surveillance to the identification of trends. The declining incidence of asthma since 1993 is found in all age groups (Fig. 4). The incidence of acute bronchitis has also declined, suggesting that the decline in asthma is not due to diagnostic shift. The similarity of the seasonal patterns of asthma attacks in general practice and hospital admissions with asthma is quite striking (data shown only for age group 0–4, Fig. 5). On the vertical axis, unity represents the average weekly incidence/hospital admission rate in each year (1990–1997). In children, asthma attacks presenting to GPs and hospital admissions peak during school terms, troughs occur during school holidays, especially the summer. In the elderly (data not presented), asthma attacks are commoner in winter and the summer peak is absent. An intermediate pattern is found in adults aged 5–44 and 45–64 years.

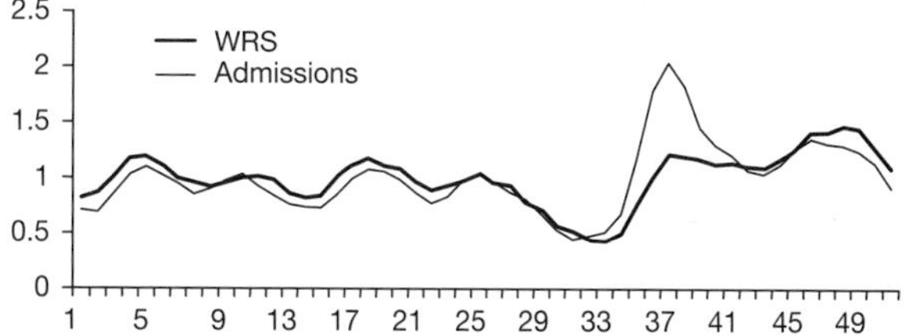

Fig. 5 Weekly seasonal indices of episodes of asthma presenting in sentinel practices and of hospital admissions (national data) for age group 0–4 years (1990–1997). Data points indicate ratio of weekly incidence and hospital admissions to respective yearly averages.

Recent changes in the *incidence of chickenpox* have been reported from the WRS.[32] The age distribution of cases was relatively consistent by year until 1986, but thereafter incidence in children aged 0–4 years increased, and incidence in children aged 5–14 years decreased. By 1999, rates in the younger age group were double those in the older one, having been equal in 1986 (Fig. 6). It is likely this shift was due to the increasing number of pre-school aged children attending nurseries.

The *surveillance of accidents* in primary care is a neglected area. In England and Wales, accidents are the commonest cause of death in persons aged under 35 years and account for 7 per cent of NHS expenditure.[33]

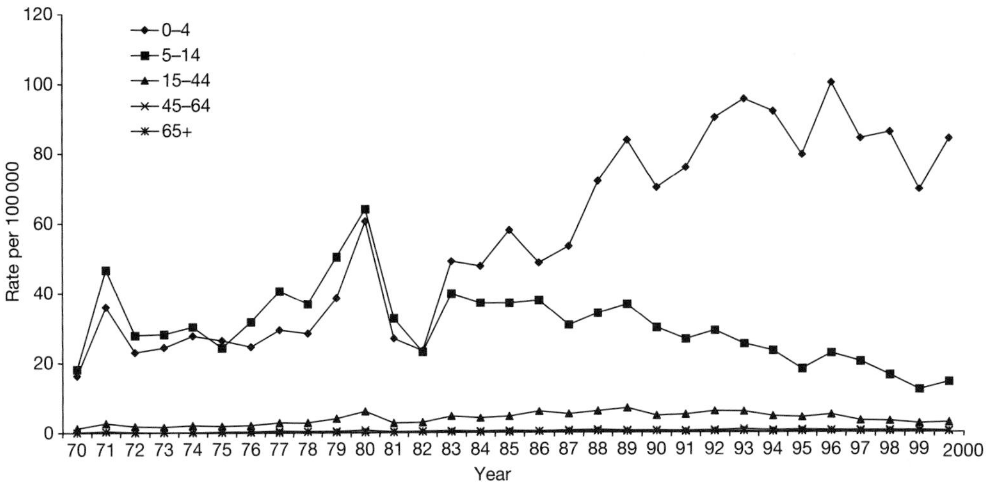

Fig. 6 Episodes of chickenpox presenting in sentinel practices. Mean weekly incidence by age group 1970–2000.

Each year approximately one-fifth of the population receive medical treatment for accidents.(11) The Department of Trade and Industry collects information on home and leisure accidents presenting to 18 hospital A&E departments in the United Kingdom,(34) but no comparable system exists in general practice, despite the publication in 1998 of a Green Paper entitled 'Our Healthier Nation'(35) in which a target was given 'to reduce accidents (defined here as one which involves a hospital visit or *consultation with a family doctor*) by at least a fifth by the year 2010'. The area of accident surveillance in primary care is neglected partly because surveillance requires the capture of information not normally collected by GPs. Data collection is further hampered by limitations of READ codes and the ICD, which focus on the effects rather than the mechanism of an accident.

We carried out a pilot study in 1997–1998 where six large practices captured additional information on accidents.(36) The following conclusions were drawn:

1. Approximately nine-tenths of injuries presenting to primary care were trivial or minor, many patients with more serious injuries were referred on to accident and emergency (A&E) departments.
2. There were similarities between GP and A&E patients concerning the mechanism or location of injury, but GPs see proportionately more elderly, more females and more persons with bites and stings. Proportionately more patients with fractures are seen in A&E.
3. Approximately six times as many persons with home or leisure accident episodes present to A&E compared with general practice.
4. The collection of information on accidents presenting to primary care was feasible, but strategies were required to ensure high-quality recording.

When considering events causing injury there are four dimensions of interest, the event itself, the offending article, the nature of the injury(ies) sustained and the management of the condition. Prevention is concerned chiefly with the first two dimensions and health care with the latter two. The challenge for accident surveillance is that a good surveillance system must provide information on all four dimensions, though health care providers do not normally interrogate patients in a structured way for the preventive aspects.

To allow international comparison

Influenza is a truly international disease. The modern day propensity for travel means that an individual country is not isolated from what is going on in the rest of the world. The stepwise march of influenza across Europe in the winter of 1993–1994 as documented by the European Influenza Sentinel Surveillance project(37) including the WRS is shown in Fig. 7. It has been speculated that the severity of an influenza outbreak in the United Kingdom is influenced by weather conditions. However, these are probably only a relatively minor factor; a virulent strain of influenza establishing itself in one part of the world is likely to spread to others irrespective of climatic conditions.

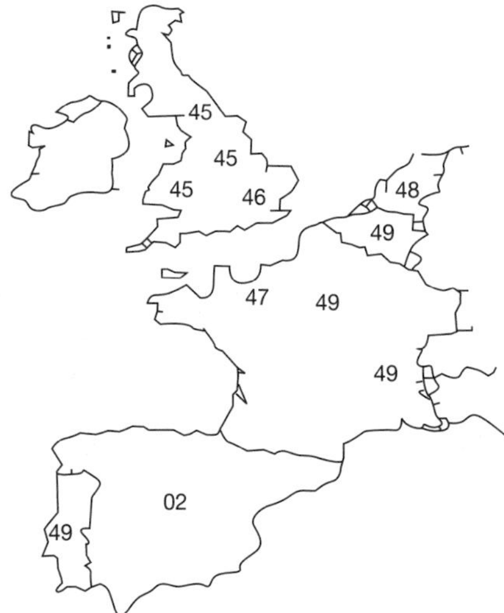

Fig. 7 Map showing the peak week of incidence of influenza like illness in European sentinel practice networks during the influenza epidemic of 1993/94.

In a recent comparison of consultation patterns between Slovenia and England and Wales (E&W)(38) disclosed as part of routine morbidity surveillance, a striking similarity was found for most conditions. However, differences were found in areas; eye diseases, (more in Slovenia) mental illness (more in England and Wales). Differences will sometimes be explained by minor differences in health care structure but equally sometimes occur because of underlying differences in illness predisposition or illness management routines. For example, we believe there is an increased likelihood of cataracts in combination with higher ultraviolet light exposure and that the threshold for recognizing mental illness and methods of management may differ in Slovenia from those in E&W.(39)

To generate and examine hypotheses

Surveillance data may be used as an investigative tool for examining associations between events and diseases. Care must be taken in proposing causal associations, but often surveillance data validate other data sources. The decline in incidence of mumps following the introduction of MMR vaccine in 1988 is a good example (Fig. 8). Data on measles were in accord with statutory notifications. Mumps, however, was not a notifiable condition and there was only limited notification of rubella at the time the MMR vaccine was introduced in 1988, highlighting the value of primary care based surveillance.

Surveillance data may help substantiate hypotheses regarding common, everyday problems in primary care. For example, one might hypothesize that otitis media and conjunctivitis are often secondary to viral upper respiratory tract infections (common cold). Presumably, nasal catarrh caused by a cold results in blockage of the Eustachian tube or naso-lacrimal duct giving rise to otitis media or conjunctivitis, respectively. The seasonality of these conditions is remarkably similar (Fig. 9) supporting the original hypothesis. The timing of assessments and operations for the insertion of ventilation tubes for childhood middle ear disease might be beneficially influenced by consideration of these seasonal effects.

Conclusions

For many diseases where surveillance is considered important, there is no option other than to collect information from primary care. It is important that there is a good discipline for data capture with established recording protocols, even if rigid diagnostic criteria cannot be applied. Surveillance in the setting of routine healthcare delivery requires appropriate descriptive presentation. Organized surveillance should have representative populations. If this is not the case, then data should be collected with enough information to allow standardization. Surveillance over many years, as illustrated by the RCGP Weekly Returns Service in the United Kingdom, provides useful descriptions of trends over time, which are increasingly recognized as scientifically valid.

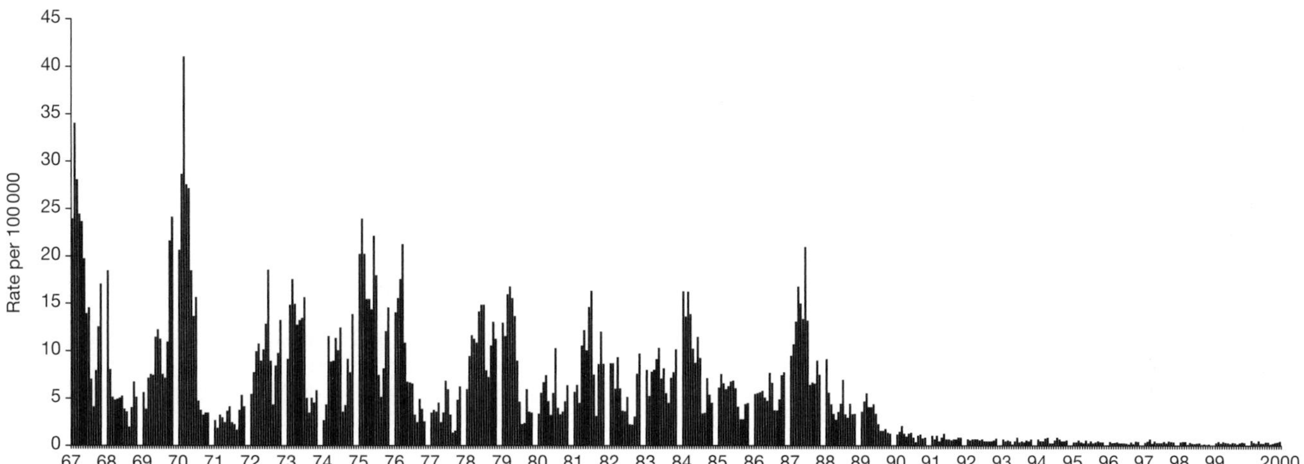

Fig. 8 Episodes of mumps presenting in sentinel practices: mean weekly incidence per 100 000 persons in each 4 week period, 1967–2000 (year end indicated by gap in histogram).

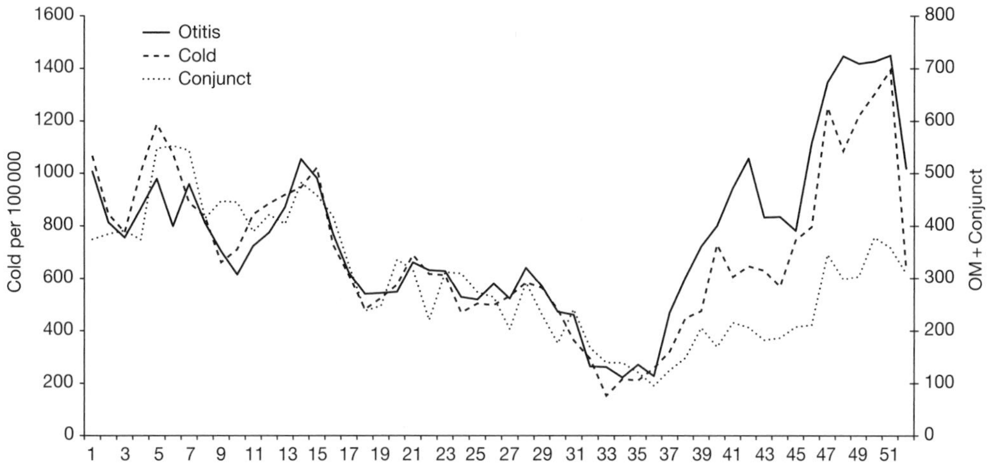

Fig. 9 Episodes of otitis media, common cold, and acute conjunctivitis presenting in sentinel practices in age group 0–4 years. Weekly incidence in year 2000.

References

1. **Langmuir, A.D.** (1963). The surveillance of communicable diseases of national importance. *New England Journal of Medicine* **268**, 182–92.
2. **International Classification of Disease** (1965). London: HMSO, 1967.
3. **Raska, K.** (1969). The concept of epidemiological surveillance. In *Communicable Diseases: Methods of Surveillance*, p. 2. Report on a seminar convened by the Regional Office for Europe of the World Health Organisation. Copenhagen: WHO.
4. **Fleming, D.M.** (1999). Weekly Returns Service of the Royal College of General Practitioners. *Communicable Disease and Public Health* **2**, 96–100.
5. **Royal College of General Practitioners, Office of Population Censuses and Surveys, Department of Health and Social Security.** *Morbidity Statistics from General Practice.* Third national study, 1981–82. Series MB5, no. 1. London: HMSO, 1986.
6. **RCGP, OPCS, and DOH.** *Morbidity Statistics from General Practice.* Fourth national study, 1991–92. Series MB5, no. 3. London: HMSO, 1995.
7. **Pearson, N., Obrien, J., Thomas, H., Ewings, P., Gallier, L., and Bussey, A.** (1996). Collecting morbidity data in general practice: the Somerset morbidity project. *British Medical Journal* **312**, 1517–20.
8. **Jick, H., Jick, S.S., and Derby, L.E.** (1991). Validation of information recorded on general practitioner based computerised data resource in the United Kingdom. *British Medical Journal* **302**, 766–8.
9. **Milne, R.M., Taylor, M.W., and Duncan, R.** (1991). An assessment of computing activity by GPASS users in Scottish general practice. *Health Bulletin (Edinburgh)* **49**, 151–60.
10. **Evans, J.M.** et al. (1995). Topical non-steroidal anti-inflammatory drugs and hospitalisation for upper gastrointestinal bleeding and perforation. *British Medical Journal* **311**, 22–6.
11. **Health Survey for England.** Social and Community Planning Research (SCPR). Department of Epidemiology and Public Health, University College London. London: The Stationery Office, 1996.
12. **OPCS.** *Labour Force Survey 1990 and 1991.* London: HMSO, 1992.
13. **Fleming, D.M., Zambon, M., Bartelds, A.I.M., and de Jong, J.C.** (1999). The duration and magnitude of influenza epidemics: a study of surveillance data from sentinel general practices in England, Wales and the Netherlands. *European Journal of Epidemiology* **15**, 467–73.
14. **Fleming, D.M., Cross, K.W., Sunderland, R., and Ross, A.M.** (2000). Comparison of the seasonal patterns of asthma identified in general practitioner episodes, hospital admissions, and deaths. *Thorax* **55** (8), 662–5.
15. **Fleming, D.M., Cross, K.W., Crombie, D.L., and Lancashire, R.J.** (1993). Respiratory illness and mortality in England and Wales. *European Journal of Epidemiology* **9**, 571–6.
16. **Ross, A.M. and Fleming, D.M.** (1994). Incidence of allergic rhinitis in general practice 1982–92. *British Medical Journal* **308**, 897–900.
17. **Benson, K. and Hartz, A.J.** (2000). A comparison of observational studies and randomized controlled trials. *New England Journal of Medicine* **342**, 1876–86.
18. **Ioannidis, J., Haidich, A., and Lau, J.** (2001). Any casualties in the clash of randomised and observational evidence? *British Medical Journal* **322**, 879–80.
19. **Van Den Hoogen, B.G., de Jong, J.C., Groen, J., Kuiken, T., de Groot, R., Fouchier, A.M., and Osterhaus, A.D.M.E.** (2001). A newly discovered human pneumovirus isolated from young children with respiratory tract disease. *Nature Medicine* **7** (6), 719–24.
20. **Zambon, M.C., Stockton, J.S., Clewley, J., and Fleming, D.M.** Influenza or RSV? Community cases of influenza like illness: an observational study. *Lancet* **358**, 1410–16.
21. **Read, J.D. and Benson, T.J.R.** (1986). Comprehensive coding. *British Journal of Health Care Computing* **3**, 22–5.
22. **Fleming, D.M.** (1998). The role of research networks in primary care. *European Journal of General Practice* **4**, 96–9.
23. **Munro, J., Nicholl, J., O'Caithain, A., and Knowles, E.** (2000). Impact of NHS Direct on demand for immediate care: observational study. *British Medical Journal* **321**, 150–3.
24. **Health 21: The Health for All Policy Framework for the WHO Region.** *European Health for All Series*, no. 6.
25. **Heath, I. and Smeeth, L.** (1999). Tackling health inequalities in primary care. *British Medical Journal* **318**, 1020–1 (editorial).
26. **Hanratty, B. and Robinson, M.** (1999). Coping with the winter bed crisis. *British Medical Journal* **319**, 1511–12.
27. **Fleming, D.M.** (2000). The contribution of influenza to combined acute respiratory infections, hospital admissions, and deaths in winter. *Communicable Disease and Public Health* **3**, 32–8.
28. **Fleming, D.M. and Cross, K.W.** (1993). Respiratory syncytial virus or influenza? *Lancet* **342**, 1507–10.
29. **Carr-Hill, R.A., Rice, N., and Roland, M.** (1996). Socio-economic determinants of rates of consultation in general practice based on fourth national morbidity survey of general practices. *British Medical Journal* **312**, 1008–12.
30. **Fleming, D.M., Sunderland, R., Cross, K.W., and Ross, A.M.** (2000). Declining incidence of episodes of asthma: a study of trends in new episodes presenting to general practitioners in the period 1989–98. *Thorax* **55** (8), 657–61.
31. **LAIA (Lung and Asthma Information Agency).** Factsheet 2000/1, August 2000.
32. **Ross, A.M. and Fleming, D.M.** (2000). Chickenpox increasingly affects pre-school children. *Communicable Disease and Public Health* **3**, 213–15.
33. **Department of Health.** *The Health of the Nation*, Key Area Handbook, Accidents. Department of Health. London: HMSO, 1993.
34. **Home Accident and Surveillance System.** 20th Annual Report 1998. Department of Trade and Industry, 1998.
35. **Department of Health.** *Our Healthier Nation: A Contract for Health.* London: HMSO, 1998.
36. **Ross, A.M. and Fleming, D.M.** The surveillance of accidents presenting in general practice: a feasibility study. *British Journal of General Practice* (accepted for publication).
37. **Fleming, D.M. and Cohen, J.M.** (1996). Experience of European collaboration in influenza surveillance in the winter of 1993–1994. *Journal of Public Health Medicine* **18** (2), 133–42.
38. **Fleming, D.M and Rotar Pavlic, D.** (2002). Information from primary care: its importance and value. A comparison of information from Slovenia and England and Wales, viewed from the 'Health 21' perspective. *European Journal of Public Health* **12**, 249–53.
39. **Car, J., Kersnik, J., Švab, I., and Rotar Pavlic, D.** Management of depression in the elderly by general practitioners: use of antidepressants. In *WONCA 2000: Final Programme and Abstracts* (Vienna: Austrian Society of General Practice and Family Medicine, p.126).

10.4 Community interventions—physical health

Julian Tudor Hart

This chapter is based on experience of continuing proactive care for the whole population of Glyncorrwg, a small industrial village in South Wales, UK, through 26 years, using a systems approach and an augmented team.[1] This included mental health problems. Though these are excluded from this chapter, the same systems approach was useful.

Our programme preceded larger but usually less comprehensive programmes in the past 10 years, which provide most of the evidence now used for developing national guidelines for proactive care. Developed mainly by epidemiologists and hospital-based specialists, these have often failed to connect with local realities.

As our work preceded local computer-held records, we had to depend on simple but rigorous procedures for recording and retrieving data, and for maintaining contact with our population of less than 2000. This is primitive evidence from which to develop local strategies 40 years later, but even recently developed national strategies are themselves primitive, at least in the United Kingdom and the United States, because they fail to take account of co-morbidity, social complexity, and resource constraints, particularly staff time. In Finland and Cuba, local primary care units have clearly defined responsibility for implementing nationwide plans, and are resourced accordingly. In other developed economies, there is as yet little evidence that centrally devised measures for health promotion and proactive primary care have been implemented long enough or widely enough to have an important impact on public health. With these exceptions, experience of pioneering units is all we have.

Though our study population was small and in many ways exceptional, it has two almost unique advantages: virtually complete records and follow-up over more than 25 years, and controlled evidence that it probably reduced mortality. The lessons we learned were simple and universal. We depended on high detection rates in the ordinary course of continuing care, but with proactive case-finding, follow-up, and audit, sustained over more than 25 years, and an exceptionally rigorous record system. This planned proactive care was apparently more effective than care prompted only by patient demand. In the last decade of those 25 years, health outcomes were substantially better in our target population in Glyncorrwg, than in a socially similar control population in Blaengwynfi receiving only good reactive care. Age-standardized death rates under 65 were 28 per cent lower in Glyncorrwg, with reductions mainly in infant mortality and cardiorespiratory causes of death. This is the expected pattern where care is more effective.[2]

Care in the neighbouring control practice was of higher quality than was then generally available in mining areas of South Wales. This also was associated with lower than expected mortality, though less so than systematic proactive care. In 1981–1999, ranking all 55 electoral wards in the County of West Glamorgan, both villages lay in the five most deprived wards (measured by Townsend Index). Ranking the same 55 wards for age-standardized mortality under 65, Glyncorrwg reached the third place (among the most affluent areas of Swansea), Blaengwynfi 32nd. Good reactive care evidently made a difference, but was more effective when supplemented by systematic proactive care, with active search, active recall, and forward planning of clinical policies applied to the whole population.

This evidence is limited by small numbers, and its 'natural experiment' design. Perfect matching of test and control populations was not possible. Two other studies compared outcomes of planned proactive with reactive care using large randomly sampled populations, randomly allocated to proactive or usual care. The New York Welfare Medical Care Study lasted only 2 years.[3] It had no significant effect on infant or adult mortality, but there were substantial gains in patient satisfaction and detection rates. The Hypertension Detection and Follow-up Program (HDFP) had large and unexpected impacts on all-causes mortality as well as cardiovascular mortality. Cardiovascular mortality was most reduced in the least hypertensive group,[4] and in black more than white patients,[5] all suggesting substantial effects outside antihypertensive treatment. Though seldom regarded as such, the HDFP was a remarkable study of two modes of care delivery, reaching far beyond management of hypertension as a single risk. The nurse-practitioners of the HDFP, like all experienced primary care workers, helped their patients with whatever problems they wished to discuss, going beyond the constraints of the study protocol. Had they not done so, they would not have won and retained the loyalty of their participants.

The period of study is crucial. If an improved care system yields only a 1 per cent added reduction in mortality annually, a normal medical lifetime may achieve a 30 per cent reduction. Conventional short-term studies cannot detect such small differences, which take years to reach statistical significance.

Taking action

Effective delivery of continuing care for common health problems in whole populations makes huge added demands on medical, nursing, and office staff, still insufficiently resourced. This remains the key issue for anyone concerned to reduce the huge gap between what existing knowledge makes possible, and the care most people actually receive.[6]

Box 1 Six-point plan

1. Provide reactive care visibly better than people expect from local experience.
2. Edit and amend medical records for the whole target population to include all basic data in retrievable form.
3. Prioritize main local health problems.
4. Mobilize labour from all possible sources, including research funding.
5. Design and implement a project for 5 years.
6. Repeat this expanding cycle.

Proactive care for whole populations begins from local planning, using locally researched data derived from medical records, census returns, and name and address lists of electors, from the telephone directory, and any other source you can find, updated weekly from local gossip. Plans must include informed estimates of what is possible over a period of (say) 5 years ahead, what is most important (as seen by professionals, as seen by individual patients, and as seen by the local community), and a clear view of where successive plans are intended to lead. In the first few years, you choose simple, readily understood targets, likely to yield early evidence of success.

It is also important to understand that complete detection of needs is a trivial task, compared with the cumulative workload generated by follow-up of what you have found. Staff know this. Unless this consequent workload is understood and resourced by service authorities, few will look for more work than they already have.

Starting from a practice operating from a small wooden shed, with virtually no useful records other than hospital letters in random date order, my wife and I adopted the six-point plan outlined in Box 1, more or less in overlapping sequence.

Without at least some advance beyond what people have had in the past, in terms they already understand, all plans for proactive care will fail. For example, unless traditionally conducted consultations reach an average 10 min or more, it is extremely difficult to introduce proactive care, or for patients to participate in decisions.[7,8] Nor is it possible to steal time from home visiting. Doctors may persuade themselves that their time is too valuable to be used anywhere except on their office thrones, but they do not persuade their patients. To escape from ineffective drudgery, family doctors must somehow find ways to do even more than they already do, before they see light at the end of the tunnel. Part of the answer must be to make longer consulting times a serious professional demand (more time is more important than more money),[9] and this is now beginning to happen. But most of the answer lies in mobilizing more people to share work and expand its scope—partly nurses and other practice staff, but mainly patients themselves. Patients must move beyond their old status as passive consumers, to become critical (and self-critical) co-producers of their own health.[10] They learn that continuity matters, and that health care is more than a disconnected series of 'curative' interventions.

Keeping good records

Basic data include name, date of birth, address, telephone number, principal skills, and current occupation; a cumulative summary of major life events and illness; current treatment; inward and outward referral correspondence in date order; and an entry of some kind, however brief, at every contact with team staff, including every clinical decision, even outside such contacts. For planned care, records must act as proxies for patients themselves, so that accurate decisions can be taken outside consultations, based on groups and on small random samples.

Such records take at least a year to achieve and much staff time to maintain. The most challenging part—summarizing major events—cannot be fully delegated. The knowledge required to construct summaries safely and effectively requires a broad knowledge of health, illness, and social realities possessed by few staff other than doctors or fully trained and experienced nurse practitioners. Though patients or their families can supply much of the basic information, few can do this without help from experienced practice administrative staff, and these need special training. On the other hand, when staff have completed this task, they have greatly expanded and deepened their knowledge of the population they serve, and thus improved their efficiency.

A summary of major events provides each patient with a personal story. To be effective, both reactive and proactive clinical interventions need to be understood not as isolated events, but as decision-points within continuing stories. Without this context, staff cannot be sure that their decisions are relevant to patients' problems, and patients cannot participate intelligently in their own care. To professionals, decisions taken in ignorance of at least the outlines of a personal story encourage hasty and inaccurate firing of magic bullets, as likely to hit their patients as to hit disease.

Once such summaries have been constructed for the whole population, and verified and supplemented by patients, keeping them up to date is relatively easy, depending on defined staff responsibilities. Annual distribution of copies of these summaries to patients can help to verify data. This is the simplest and most effective step towards systematic participation of patients in their own care, in reality rather than rhetoric.

Computer-held records, making it much easier to structure information, and magically easy to access or copy it for other purposes (including copies for patients) have speeded and simplified all these tasks. Working before desktop personal computers existed, virtually all our work had to be done by hand, using simple systems such as colour coding or marginal perforated (needle-sorted) cards to identify groups with specific risks or risk-combinations. For primary health workers in systems which cannot yet afford computers, these simple manual methods can be effective. They are laborious, but through their use staff gain a rich personal knowledge of their target population, of immense value for continuing care and low drop-out. Manual methods also provide an excellent educational background for staff when they finally obtain computer-held records. Computers perform the same tasks much faster, but still depend on the same disciplined adherence to agreed criteria for definitions, obsessionally accurate measurements, and meticulous recording of data. All these habits can be acquired through manual methods, at least as a first stage.

Prioritizing local problems

When family doctors serving poorest and sickest populations are asked to name their biggest problem, most choose high consultation rates for trivial problems. Studying over 1000 people registered at a Sheffield health centre in the early 1970s, Hannay and Maddox found 23 per cent had at least one severe or apparently serious medical symptom during the previous 2 weeks for which they had not consulted their doctor. In the same 2 weeks, 9 per cent had consulted their doctor for a medical symptom causing insignificant pain or disability, not apparently serious.[11] Consultations for trivial reasons existed, but so did more than twice as many people with important reasons for consulting, but who failed to do so. In a proactive practice, 'trivial' consultations are opportunities for unpressured assessment of future risks, and shared discussion of personal problems. We saw about 85 per cent of our patients each year, and about 95 per cent over 5 years. Hundred per cent contact over 5 years required some additional effort, but not much.

In the early 1960s, coronary heart disease was thought to affect the rich more than the poor, and sedentary workers more than heavy manual workers. Among our miners, steelworkers, and railwaymen, fatal coronary disease was common in men even in their 40s. This was unexpected. Analysis of local mortality statistics confirmed that men under 65 in the Glamorgan valleys were at much higher risk for both coronary deaths and stroke, than the average for England and Wales.[12] Three powerful contributory causes of coronary disease were then known. Two (high arterial pressure and tobacco) already seemed treatable. In the 1960s, high blood cholesterol was hard to treat, and measurements were often inaccurate. We had an apparently exceptional local problem, and relatively simple means available to tackle it: systematic advice on smoking, and systematic case-finding followed by continued treatment for high blood pressure.

This programme was a readily understood priority for everyone, staff and patients, but there were others. Between 1961 and 1965, three women in our village died from invasive cancer of the cervix. By 1966, our District General Hospital laboratory was able to accept cervical smears for risk assessment, several years before NHS fees were introduced for a national programme. Early diagnosis of pre-cancerous change in the cervix was readily accepted as another priority target by our local community. Policies were discussed individually within consultations, informally with our practice staff (all locally recruited), at several public meetings, and after 1974, by a patients' committee elected annually at a public meeting.

Easy and effective contraception also began to be available in the United Kingdom in the early 1960s, at a pace largely determined by the personal beliefs of doctors. Of all possible means to prevent unnecessary misery, planned parenthood seemed the most obvious and most likely to be effective. If every child were a wanted child, there should be huge social benefits and health gains. We adopted an energetic proactive policy, raising the question with teenagers as they appeared to become sexually active, during every pregnancy, and again after childbirth. The effectiveness of this campaign was monitored by a student who interviewed a random sample of women in 1973,[13] from which we learned a lot about how women actually used the pill, as opposed to what they told doctors or nurses. We also learned the limitations as well as the advantages of public and group work, as distinct from personal discussion within consultations.

As we extended proactive search and follow-up to more health problems, detection rates rose. Once detected, all the problems we looked for required lifelong control—mainly by patients, but requiring periodic monitoring and audit until death, so this workload was cumulative. By 1985, in adults aged over 20, prevalence of diabetes was 2 per cent, alcohol problems 7 per cent (12 per cent in men), moderate/severe hypertension (mean pre-treatment diastolic pressure $\geq$105 mmHg) 10 per cent, body mass index greater than or equal to 30, 16 per cent, peak expiratory flow rate less than 300 l/min and/or augmented greater than or equal to 20 per cent by alpha-agonist 22 per cent, regular smokers (positive urine cotinine or expired CO) 28 per cent. These very high caseloads were mostly followed-up in ordinary clinical sessions, with records of non-attenders reviewed afterwards with team staff. Selective decisions had to be taken about active pursuit of these non-attenders, based on extremely personal knowledge.

This was a paternalist strategy: all initiatives came from staff, and mostly from doctors. In the circumstances of the time, this seemed better than no strategy at all, no leadership from anyone aware of the possibilities and limitations of medical knowledge. We began from above down, but ended more or less sideways, aiming at an ideal of fraternal care. We made at least some progress along that path. Through our elected Patients' Committee we did our best to create an elected local institution from which collective participation in development of health strategies could emerge. This was less effective than we had all hoped. Such committees can easily become self-perpetuating, hoarding their knowledge and power rather than sharing it.

More effective might be specific user groups such as the mothers of asthmatic children, obese men, epileptics, and so on, with more fluid membership and more realistic motives. There is now a wealth of information available for special interest groups of all kinds, notably Herxheimer and McPherson's Database of Patient Experiences of Ilness (DIPEx) based at Oxford University.[14] Participative democracy needs time and resources to grow. The most important thing is to make a material start, and get beyond rhetoric.

Case finding

Planned continuing anticipatory care of whole populations depends on initial proactive case finding, followed by negotiated treatment or observation, active recall, and periodic monitoring. Obviously suitable problems include hyperlipidaemias, hypertension, type 2 diabetes, central obesity, smoking, airways obstruction, and alcohol and/or other drug dependence. In the 1960s, hypertension provided the most obvious model, and this was our main thrust for the first 5 years (1968–1973). Over the next 13 years, we developed similar programmes for all these problem sets and combinations, with proactive case finding, our own increasingly nurse-run problem-specific clinics, and active recall. There is no room here to give a detailed account of these programmes. They would in any case be different starting in 2001 rather than they were in 1968. A full account of our hypertension control programme is available, and was intended as a model for management of all continuously distributed health impairments, including the multiple impairments usually present.[15]

Our rule was to start from where we were with the people and customs we already had, so our programme began from expanded day-to-day doctor–patient or nurse–patient contacts. We flagged the records of patients who had not yet had a measurement. When the flag was removed, this meant the measurement had been done. To reach 100 per cent of a target population, every 5 years or so this systematic case finding was supplemented by active pursuit of patients who had not consulted. This turned up some remarkable cases of health, and also of neglected physical and social pathology. Four or five patients objected to this intrusive approach, but their views were respected and their names dropped from the proactive list. Eventually, all but one joined their neighbours in the programme.

Raised systolic pressure in the elderly (with or without diastolic hypertension) is more immediately dangerous, and more rewardingly treatable, than in any other age group. One of the best randomized trials comparing treatment with watchful waiting in the age-range 70–84 showed a 43 per cent reduction in all-causes mortality in the actively managed group.[16] Initiation of treatment over 85 is seldom effective,[17] but in a well-managed population will rarely be needed.

We included everyone over 20 (100 per cent of the men and 98 per cent of the women), aiming to repeat this every 5 years.[18] Over the 21 years 1968–1989, in a population averaging 1945, we found 25 men and 16 women aged less than 40 with sustained systolic pressures greater than or equal to 160 mmHg or diastolic pressures greater than or equal to 100 mmHg.[19] All 41 of these hypertensives were at over 30 per cent risk of cardiovascular mortality in the 10 years following detection, using Sheffield tables for combined coronary risks.[20] Though we lowered group mean male pressures from 164/110 to 148/89 mmHg, and group mean female pressures from 172/107 to 145/86 mmHg, five of the men and one woman died, and 14 suffered non-fatal cardiovascular events. In our population, serious hypertension under 40 seemed to be common and dangerous.

This situation may now be rare. A recent study of a statistical model population of 100 000, using data from the 1994 English Health Survey, concluded that 'Almost nobody under the age of 45 years has raised blood pressure and a 10-year cardiovascular risk of greater than 30 per cent', and there was therefore no point in screening for undetected hypertension (or other risk indicators for cardiovascular disease) under 45 years of age in a typical practice.[21] There is some evidence of a secular fall in pressures over the last few decades, at least in Scottish university students,[22] and both stroke and heart attack rates are falling in all developed economies except Eastern Europe and the former USSR. The fall everywhere has been in event rates rather than event-mortality, suggesting shifts in causes and perhaps earlier detection and treatment of risk factors, rather than more effective crisis interventions.[23] All three stages of the rule of halves (half are undetected, half those detected are untreated, half those treated are uncontrolled) still applied to hypertension through the 1980s, but by the late 1990s detection and inception of treatment were much improved even at population level. In the early 1990s, poor control still accounted for about one-fifth of all strokes under 80[24] and an accelerated deterioration in about one-third of patients in renal failure.[25]

National guidelines necessarily assume that all practices are typical, but we know they are not. Areas of post-industrial dereliction continue to exist, concentrating high morbidity, high drop-out rates from treatment, and often low detection rates. Their health is improving in absolute terms, but the health gap between affluent and poor areas is widening. For example, between 1979–1983 and 1989–1993, all-causes mortality in Glasgow fell by 14.5 per cent for men and 10.5 per cent for women, but in Edinburgh it fell by 24.5 and 20.4 per cent, respectively. Reasons for this widening gap seem to include quality of medical care, particularly for cardiovascular disease.[26] Without exceptional resources, exceptional needs will neither be recognized nor addressed. One size never fits all.

It is also important to recognize that for optimally efficient production of health gain, particularly in areas of social deprivation, health care needs to be seen as a community enterprise, not a consumer industry. Active, intelligent participation of patients, far beyond the passive role of consumers, is essential for efficient production of health gain, even for these apparently simple processes.[27] To develop and retain motivation, professional staff need continually to expand their roles to embrace wider responsibilities, deeper judgements, and more imaginative perception of their own work within a collective context. The products of health care are for personal use and community gain, not for exchange; they are personal and social use-values, not market commodities. Care should indeed be organized rationally, but through cooperation, mutual respect, and trust.

Dealing with co-morbidity

To many, arterial pressure control seems one of the simplest processes within the continuing care model. In our population, 100 per cent screened within a continuing 5-year cycle, we searched the records of 154 consecutive men and women with sustained pressures above thresholds for mandatory treatment, for evidence of 12 potential complicating factors: total plasma cholesterol greater than 6.6 mmol, ischaemic event within the year preceding treatment, chronic joint pain, airways obstruction, body mass index 30+, recurrent depression or psychosis, alcohol problem, impaired renal function, peptic ulcer, diabetes, gout, and erectile failure. Only 3 per cent of men and 7 per cent of women had hypertension uncomplicated by any of these problems. We had not searched for unhappy marriages, work insecurity, unemployment, or any of the other features that should modify effective decisions.

This paradox, the more obvious complexity of problems seen by generalists compared with those seen by specialists, lies at the heart of the different skills needed by each.[28] Depending on variable criteria for diagnosis, and even more variably incomplete searches, the proportion of all consultations involving two or more different diagnoses varies from less than 1 to over 60 per cent.[29,30] All these definitions are arbitrary, mainly determined by staff needs to make decisions within resources available, rather than the needs of patients to improve their lives. Obviously, in populations where for example, 15 per cent of adults meet criteria for mandatory treatment of hypertension, 25 per cent are overweight, 25 per cent of women live or have lived with domestic violence,[31] and 34 per cent of women (11 per cent of men) have at some time experienced sexual abuse,[32] truly uncomplicated presentations of virtually any problem must be exceptional. If this conflicts with the literature on reported co-morbidity, this tells us more about the limitations of reactive workload studies than about the real world. Overworked GPs do not want to see that reality is even more complex and demanding than the already too complicated and demanding problems for which they already accept responsibility.

Divisions of labour between hospital-based specialists, and pharmaceutical marketing strategies based on associating diagnostic labels with prescribing, and on vertically integrated care for specific diseases,[33] all reinforce the historical tendency of community generalists to accept definitions of ill health derived from hospital rather than community experience. This fragmentation of diagnosis ignores mounting evidence that some preventable causes of death might more usefully be grouped within wider categories, which do not correspond with the boundaries of traditional specialties or subspecialties.

For example, since the 1980s[34] we have known that insulin resistance is a common causal feature of central obesity,[35] type 2 diabetes, hypertension, hypertriglyceridaemia, low HDL cholesterolaemia, raised fibrinogen, and raised apoliprotein B.[36] Recent research has added a variety of chronic inflammatory processes.[37] All these quantifiable health impairments share a common management, educational, and monitoring agenda. Their cardiovascular consequences are all accelerated by tobacco, thus linking them with impaired respiratory function as measured by FEV1, an independent predictor of early all-causes mortality as powerful as any of the recognized cardiovascular risk factors.[38] Disease labels refer not to biologically defined independent species, but to groups of people with shared clinical needs. The label 'hypertension' has no more eternal validity in the twenty-first century than 'fever' had in the nineteenth century.

We must think about what we do, with both socially and biologically informed imagination. Long before it was 'discovered' by epidemiologists, thoughtful and experienced family doctors knew that eventually most type 2 diabetics became hypertensive, most centrally obese hypertensives became diabetic, and both were at exceptional risk from coronary disease. The unified problem and management bundles were obvious, but we seemed generally incapable of applying them. We were, and mostly still are, held back by three factors. Firstly, epidemiologists who plan strategies on our behalf, particularly in the United Kingdom, are still influenced by the null hypothesis of McKeown,[39] who reassured us that as nothing we did could improve public health significantly, so clinical innovation was unimportant. Though scepticism can be healthy, it may support lethal complacency. Secondly, primary generalists still fail to understand that primary care deals with early health impairments with an extremely wide range of future possibilities, in which premature containment within customary disease labels is inappropriate and often counterproductive. Thirdly, the pharmaceutical industry makes a lot of its money by selling sledgehammers developed in the world of advanced disease to crack peanuts in the world of health impairments—we must, therefore, contend with a powerful, advanced disease oriented, dyseducational force.

Once incorporated into official guidelines and information technologies, all these irrational tendencies may accelerate. It may become even more difficult to develop proactive population care in terms that make sense to those who actually live and work in communities, either as health professionals or as patients. Experienced workers in primary care must, therefore, accept more responsibility for developing more widely informed and more socially sensitive local guidelines. Every member of the primary care team should be engaged in a shared enterprise that everyone understands, instead of splitting their functions into dumbed-down mass production of component parts.

Starting from where we are, with the people we have

All of us must start within the systems we find, including those of us compelled to be businessmen and employers, but for proactive care we must somehow put these roles behind us. If we do not, we can forget about real teamwork, and without teams this work is impossible.

In real teams, work is divided by consensus agreement, with a task-mix sufficiently diverse to maintain imagination. Objectives of work are agreed by consensus. All members are accepted as equal professionals, allowed to reach objectives in their own way, working at their own speed. Opinions are valued according to evidence advanced in their support. All members of the team contribute information to the practice record system, and all can extract information about how the unit performs. Such teams meet regularly, take collective decisions, and verify that decisions have either been implemented or will be revised.

Such teams need development and leadership. If staff with particular responsibilities are given time to visit other units tackling the same problems, and have authority to develop their own ideas, the team keeps moving and generates its own leaders. In the end, most of these will be doctors or well-qualified nurses, because of their wider knowledge.

These criteria are rarely met in full, but unless we at least move toward their full implementation, we cannot be serious about full application of new knowledge to whole populations. None of us lives in an ideal society, so we can start only from where we are. But it helps to know where we intend to go.

References

1. **Hart, J.T., Thomas, C., Gibbons, B., Edwards, C., Hart, M., Jones, J., Jones, M., and Walton, P.** (1991). Twenty five years of audited screening in a socially deprived community. *British Medical Journal* **302**, 1509–13.
2. **Kaul, S.** (1991). Twenty five years of case finding and audit. *British Medical Journal* **303**, 524–5.
3. **Goodrich, C.H., Olendski, M.C., and Reader, G.G.** *Welfare Medical Care: An Experiment.* Massachussets: Harvard University Press, 1970.
4. **Hypertension Detection & Follow-up Program Co-operative Group** (1979). Five-year findings of the HDFP. I. Reduction in mortality of persons with high blood pressure, including mild hypertension. *Journal of the American Medical Association* **242**, 2562–71.
5. **Hypertension Detection & Follow-up Program Co-operative Group** (1979). Five-year findings of the HDFP. II. Mortality by race, sex and age. *Journal of the American Medical Association* **242**, 2572–7.
6. **Hart, J.T.** (2001). Commentary: Can health outputs of routine practice approach those of clinical trials? *International Journal of Epidemiology* **30**, 1263–7.
7. **Savage, R. and Armstrong, D.** (1990). Effect of a general practitioner's consulting style on patients' satisfaction: a controlled study. *British Medical Journal* **301**, 968–70.
8. **Howie, J.G., Heaney, D.J., and Maxwell, M.** *Measuring Quality in General Practice.* Occasional Paper no. 75. London: Royal College of General Practitioners, 1997.
9. **Hart, J.T.** (1995). Innovative consultation time as a common European currency. *European Journal of General Practice* **1**, 34–7.
10. **Hart, J.T.** (1992). Two paths for medical practice. *Lancet* **340**, 772–5.
11. **Hannay, D.R. and Maddox, E.J.** (1975). Incongruous referrals. *Lancet* **ii**, 1195–7.
12. **Hart, J.T.** (1970). The distribution of mortality from coronary heart disease in South Wales. *Journal of the Royal College of General Practitioners* **19**, 258–68.
13. **Matthews, R.** (1974). A study of fertility in a Welsh mining village: Glyncorrwg in the Afan Valley. Thesis for Degree BEd.
14. www.dipex.org and dipex@dphpc.ox.ac.uk
15. **Hart, J.T.** *Hypertension: Community Control of High Blood Pressure* 3rd edn. Oxford: Radcliffe Medical Press, 1993.
16. **Dahlof, B., Lindholm, L.H., Hansson, L., Schersten, B., Ekbom, T., and Wester, P.-O.** (1991). Morbidity and mortality in the Swedish Trial in Old Patients with Hypertension (STOP-Hypertension). *Lancet* **338**, 1281–4.
17. **Gueyflier, F.** et al. (1999). Antihypertensive drugs in very old people: a subgroup meta-analysis of randomised controlled trials. *Lancet* **353**, 796.
18. **Hart, J.T.** (1974). The marriage of primary care and epidemiology: continuous anticipatory care of whole populations in a state medical service (Milroy lecture). *Journal of the Royal College of Physicians of London* **8**, 299–314.
19. **Hart, J.T., Edwards, C., Haines, A.P., Hart, M., Jones, J., Jones, M., and Watt, G.C.M.** (1993). Screen detected high blood pressure under 40: a general practice population followed up for 21 years. *British Medical Journal* **306**, 437–40.
20. **Haq, I.U., Jackson, P.R., Yeo, W.W., and Ramsay, L.E.** (1995). Sheffield risk and treatment table for cholesterol lowering for primary prevention of coronary heart disease. *Lancet* **346**, 1467–71.

21. **Marshall, T. and Rouse, A.** (2001). Meeting the National Service Framework for coronary heart disease: which patients have untreated high blood pressure? *British Journal of General Practice* **51**, 571–4.
22. **McCarron, P., Okasha, M., McEwen, J., and Smith, G.D.** (2001). Changes in blood pressure among students attending Glasgow University between 1948 and 1968: analyses of cross sectional surveys. *British Medical Journal* **322**, 885–9.
23. **Tunstall-Pedoe, H.** et al. (1999). Contribution of trends in survival and coronary-event rates to changes in coronary heart disease mortality: 10-year results from 37 WHO MONICA Project populations. *Lancet* **353**, 1547–57.
24. **Xianglin, D.** et al. (1997). Case–control study of stroke and the quality of hypertension control in north west England. *British Medical Journal* **314**, 272–6.
25. **Dasgupta, I., Madeley, R.J., Pringle, M.A.L., Savill, J., and Burden, R.P.** (1999). Management of hypertension in patients developing end-stage renal failure. *Quarterly Journal of Medicine* **92**, 519–25.
26. **Watt, G.C.M. and Ecob, R.** (2000). Analysis of falling mortality rates in Edinburgh and Glasgow. *Journal of Public Health Medicine* **22**, 330–6.
27. **Kaplan, S.H., Greenfield, S., Gandek, B., Rogers, W.H., and Ware, J.E.** (1996). Characteristics of physicians with participatory decision-making styles. *Annals of Internal Medicine* **124**, 497–504.
28. **Horder, J.P.** (1997). Physicians and family doctors: a new relationship. *Journal of the Royal College of General Practitioners* **27**, 391–7. Published simultaneously in *Journal of the Royal College of Physicians of London.*
29. **van den Acker, M., Buntinx, F., and Knottnerus, J.A.** (1996). Comorbidity or multimorbidity: what's in a name? A review of literature. *European Journal of General Practice* **2**, 65–70.
30. **van den Bos, G.A.M.** (1995). The burden of chronic diseases in terms of disability, use of health care and healthy life expectancies. *European Journal of Public Health* **5**, 29–34.
31. **Richardson, J. and Feder, G.** (1996). Domestic violence: a hidden problem for general practice. *British Journal of General Practice* **46**, 239–42.
32. **Halpérin, D.S.** et al. (1996). Prevalence of child sexual abuse among adolescents in Geneva: results of a cross sectional survey. *British Medical Journal* **312**, 1326–9.
33. **Richards, T.** (1998). Disease management in Europe. *British Medical Journal* **317**, 426–7.
34. **Reaven, G.M.** (1998). Role of insulin resistance in human disease. Banting Lecture 1988. *Diabetes* **37**, 1595–607.
35. **Després, J.-P., Lemieux, I., and Prud'homme, D.** (2001). Treatment of obesity: need to focus on high risk abdominally obese patients. *British Medical Journal* **322**, 716–20.
36. **Lamarche, B.** et al. (1998). Fasting insulin and apolipoprotein B levels and LDL particle size as risk factors for ischaemic heart disease. *Journal of the American Medical Association* **279**, 1955–61.
37. **Schmidt, M.I.** et al (1999). Markers of inflammation and prediction of diabetes mellitus in adults (Atherosclerosis in Communities Study): a cohort study. *Lancet* **353**, 1649–52.
38. **Hole, D.J.** et al. (1996). Impaired lung function and mortality risk in men and women: findings from the Renfrew and Paisley prospective population study. *British Medical Journal* **313**, 711–16.
39. **McKeown, T.** *The Role of Medicine.* Oxford: Blackwell, 1979.

10.5 Community interventions—mental health

Jeremy Anderson

Introduction

Until recently, primary care practitioners needed to know considerably less about mental health issues than they do today. Three factors created this change:

- Internationally, patterns of mental health service delivery now emphasize care in the community instead of in large psychiatric institutions.[1]
- There is increased recognition of the importance of mental disorders in primary care. A large, international, WHO study found that 25 per cent of primary care patients had symptoms indicative of a psychiatric diagnosis,[2] and primary care provides 90 per cent of all mental health care.[3] Concurrently, there is recognition that primary care psychiatry is not the same as specialized psychiatry in general practice.[4]
- Primary care practitioners and their patients now have access to a variety of treatment approaches for mental health problems, including new models of care and new pharmacological, social, psychological, and complementary therapies.

These changes challenge primary care practitioners about their mental health knowledge, their recognition of disorder, and their provision of appropriate treatment.[5] To supplement their individual knowledge and skills with appropriate community interventions, each primary care practitioner faces three questions:

- Do effective community interventions exist for this patient?
- Is an appropriate, effective, intervention available for this patient locally?
- How do I access it?

While this chapter deals exclusively with the first question, this theoretical knowledge will make no difference to patients without application of the practical, local, knowledge implied in the last two. No textbook can provide this local knowledge—it is the responsibility of individual practitioners.

For primary care practitioners, the most effective management of many patients with mental health problems will involve liaison with appropriate community resources.[6] In some cases these will be mental health services that operate in the community according to specific models of care delivery, in other cases particular types of interventions delivered in the community that are not necessarily provided by mental health services. This distinction between service models and interventions is artificial to some extent but it reflects historical factors that are still relevant in primary care.

This chapter will examine what is known about the effectiveness of both these types of care. For clarity, it does not examine interventions that are not community-centred, for example, pharmacological treatments or day-hospital programmes.

Any overview of this kind must deal with the major international differences that exist in mental health service policy, funding, and delivery. This chapter draws mainly on research from the United Kingdom, the United States, and Australasia, but similar conclusions have arisen from other countries.

Community interventions in mental health have so far reflected mental health service priorities more than primary care ones. The majority of research in the field has studied 'severe mental disorder',[7] in practice almost entirely people with schizophrenia or bipolar affective disorder. While up to 30 per cent of people with chronic psychotic disorders are managed solely in primary care,[8] they remain a small minority of primary care patients with mental health problems.[9]

Models of mental health care delivery

Introduction

The international wave of psychiatric hospital closures over the last 30 years has produced service models that tend to reflect political developments rather more than clinical ones.[1] Their most common feature is the establishment of 'sectorized services' that offer mental health services to a defined catchment population, usually aimed at people with 'severe mental illness'. Even services that share the same name, however, may differ significantly in practical implementation.

Sectorized services

Two of the models of community-based mental health services described here derive from the pioneering work of Stein and Test,[10] which sought to provide alternatives to psychiatric hospitalization. Each is relevant to an extreme of mental disorder chronicity, namely community treatment of psychiatric crises (crisis management teams) and long-term management of chronic, severe, mental disorder (assertive community treatment).

Crisis management teams

Experimental studies offering intensive home treatment by multidisciplinary teams to acutely unwell patients have followed similar research designs: random allocation of patients who presented seeking an acute psychiatric inpatient admission to either a standard inpatient admission or treatment at home by intensive support from a specialized 'crisis management team'. The team provided a mobile, 24-h, service that had both acute care and rehabilitation elements. Almost all of the patients received psychiatric medication.

A Cochrane systematic review summarizes the results of five trials.[11] Despite the intention of the programmes, 45 per cent of the crisis intervention patients were admitted, although they were less likely to be readmitted. Crisis intervention reduces losses to follow-up, reduces family burden, and is a more satisfactory form of care for both patients and families. There were no differences in deaths or mental state outcomes. All the individual studies found crisis intervention to be less costly than standard care but no formal comparison was possible due to differences in methodology and service context.

Assertive community treatment

Assertive community treatment is the most exhaustively researched of any model of community mental health service delivery.[12,13] The patients invariably suffer from 'severe mental illness'. The service is assertive, since staff actively seek out the patients, and team-based, such that the team shares responsibility for patient care. High staff/patient ratios enable frequent contact with patients in their own environments. The programme aims are to manage the patients' illnesses, encourage treatment adherence, enhance a supportive environment for patients, and assist them with tasks of community living.

Assertive community treatment has demonstrated consistently positive outcomes in different countries and with the most seriously disabled patient groups.[12] Compared to standard community management, a systematic review[14] found that patients receiving assertive community treatment had fewer hospital admissions, spent less time in hospital, and were more likely to remain in follow-up. Assertive community treatment had positive effects on social outcomes with no negative effects on mental state or social functioning. It reduced the cost of hospital care, but did not have a clear advantage over standard care when other costs were taken into account.

Like crisis management teams, assertive community treatment services are now well established internationally, especially in the United States. Recent policy developments suggest an increasing role for them in the United Kingdom.

Case management

Case management is the community mental health intervention with the least satisfactory definition, yet it is also the most widespread. In general usage, it is a term used to describe the work of multidisciplinary community mental health teams, the most common form of sectorized mental health service, in particular, their assessment, care coordination, and treatment activities. The lack of a precise definition makes evaluating the effectiveness of case management difficult.

Two meta-analyses show varied results. Marshall and Lockwood[14] suggest that case management increases hospital admissions and contact with services, but acknowledge that the heterogeneity of treatment interventions may confound these results. Tyrer et al.[15] describe more positive results from their general review of community mental health teams but acknowledge the effects are small.

Thornicroft et al.[16] undertook a controlled, prospective, observational comparison of patient outcomes between 'real world' community teams and local hospital-oriented interventions. They conclude that the health and social gains reported from community-based services in experimental studies are replicable in ordinary clinical settings, although these benefits are diluted.

Taken together, the research evidence provides tentative support for case management in general community-based mental health services, which are likely to be the most widespread form of care delivery in the future. Regrettably, it offers little advice for primary care practitioners aiming to tailor service provision to patient need.

'Shared care' between primary care practitioners and mental health services

While 'shared care' between primary care practitioners and secondary care is widespread in many health systems in some circumstances (e.g. obstetrics), various approaches to integrating primary care and mental health services have not achieved widespread acceptance despite promising individual studies and increasing pressure from policy makers.[17]

A careful systematic review of 38 controlled trials[18] indicates that 'replacement' models, where mental health workers (e.g. case managers) replace primary practitioners as providers of mental health care, do not cause identifiable changes in behaviour of primary care practitioners. 'Consultation–liaison' strategies, aimed at collaborative care between mental health workers and primary practitioners, can change practitioner behaviour but only in the short term. The impact of either of these models on patient outcomes is unclear.

Other care delivery models

Supported employment

People with severe mental illness express a preference for ordinary employment, yet their unemployment rates are high (61–73 per cent in the United Kingdom). Reviews of traditional vocational rehabilitation, based on sheltered workshop or pre-vocational skills training, suggest patient outcomes are comparable to no intervention at all.[19]

In contrast, recent 'supported employment' programmes have greater success. They involve close integration between the vocational team and mental health services, undertake rapid job searches for 'real world' jobs, and provide continuing support after job placement. A recent systematic review of 18 randomized controlled trials demonstrates strongly positive outcomes, with employment rates at 18 months of 34 per cent in supported employment compared with 12 per cent in pre-vocational training.[19] Unfortunately, all the research evidence for supported employment programmes comes from the United States, raising questions of both generalizability and access.

Integrated treatment of substance abuse and mental disorders

There is increased international recognition of the high prevalence of substance abuse amongst people with severe mental illness (current or recent use around 20–40 per cent in the United States), and the negative implications of this co-morbidity for clinical and social outcomes.[20]

Recently, interest has moved from separate specialized teams, operating on either mental health or substance abuse problems, to integrated services where staff operate specific substance abuse interventions within standard models of community mental health care. Narrative reviews reported positive outcomes from integrated treatment approaches, which led some authors to promote them as 'evidence-based' interventions in schizophrenia.[21]

A Cochrane systematic review[22] questions this conclusion, pointing out the methodological shortcomings and inconclusive pooled results from the six randomized controlled trials it identified. Recently, a small but well-designed randomized controlled trial from the United Kingdom has reported positive results in a comparison of clearly defined, integrated, psycho-social interventions with standard care.[20]

This is an evolving field. It is likely that the perceived success of integrated programmes in the United States will provide continued support for their use, which may precede conclusive evidence of their effectiveness.

Particular interventions delivered in the community

Research about particular mental health interventions is more variable, harder to define, and more difficult to summarize than research about models of mental health care delivery.

Less rigorous research exists about particular mental health interventions than research about care delivery models, and it involves a different range of participants and diagnoses. Large-scale epidemiological surveys demonstrate not only a broader range of diagnoses in community samples than in specialized care but also different patterns of service use according to diagnosis, particularly between those categorized as 'severe' and 'non-severe' mental illnesses.[23] Patients also present differently—in primary care depression and anxiety often have a mixed clinical picture and more frequently present with somatic symptoms than is the case in specialized care.[4]

Socially based interventions

Social skills training

Social skills training is formal training in aspects of social functioning such as maintaining personal relationships, role functioning, and self-care skills. Accordingly, it is most commonly used for people with severe mental illness, where profound social deficits are common.[24]

A systematic review by Dilk and Bond[25] demonstrates that social skills training improves interpersonal skills and reduce symptoms amongst severely mentally ill inpatients, although its effect on relapse is less clear.

Although elements of social skills training form a component of some generic rehabilitation programmes for severe mental illness, specialized social skills programmes are uncommon outside the United States.

Family intervention, psycho-education

Research concerning the various forms of family intervention and psycho-education in community settings provides evidence of their effectiveness in a range of mental disorders.

Several models of family intervention exist: individual consultation and psycho-education provided by a mental health professional; forms of traditional family therapy; short-term family education programmes; and support groups run by non-clinical mental health interest groups. Each of these approaches receives some support from experimental research.[26]

The strongest research evidence comes from studies of single- and multi-family group interventions in schizophrenia, which demonstrate reductions in relapse and rehospitalization rates and other social outcomes.[27] When subjected to rigorous meta-analysis, the effect on relapse rates remains although the strength of the findings diminishes, tending toward the null over time.[28] Another systematic review found that any kind of psycho-education also reduced relapse and readmission rates.[29] Taking an overall view, the World Schizophrenia Fellowship has enthusiastically sponsored family intervention and, in collaboration with international clinical leaders in the field, has formulated a strategy to encourage its more widespread use.[30]

Controlled studies also support the value of family intervention and psycho-education for other mental disorders including bipolar disorder, obsessive–compulsive disorder, anorexia nervosa, and borderline personality disorder.[26]

Despite evidence of efficacy, family interventions are not widely available outside research programmes. Several barriers exist to hinder its more widespread use including relatively small effect sizes, clinician preconceptions, logistic problems, and opportunity costs.[26]

Self-help and support groups

Self-help programmes and support groups involve a variety of approaches that often overlap.

Self-help programmes have a more specifically therapeutic focus and may occur on either an individual or a group basis. The interventions vary widely, from computerized, individual, anxiety management programmes[31] to well-known, '12-step', group programmes such as Alcoholics Anonymous.

The heterogeneity of the various interventions studied makes evaluating them difficult, but some relevant systematic reviews are available. Most descriptions of self-help programmes concern their use in alcohol and substance abuse disorders but their effectiveness is questionable. A meta-analysis of the available controlled research showed that attending Alcoholics Anonymous produced worse outcomes than alternative interventions, including no treatment, but did support some treatment components including peer-led self-help therapy groups. Methodological problems limited interpretation of these conclusions.[32]

The evidence is more robust for self-help programmes provided for anxiety and depression[33] and bulimia[34] where systematic reviews demonstrate moderate but positive effects.

The essential feature of support groups is the collaborative involvement of people who have mental health problems with their peers for a common purpose. Psycho-education (see above) is a common focus. Support groups operate according to a number of models that vary most significantly by their level of interaction with mental health professionals,[35] from 'partnership' models to 'separatist' groups that exist as an alternative to formal mental health care systems.

Little research evaluation of support groups exists. In part, this reflects an ambiguity about appropriate outcome measures. In the United States, the National Alliance for the Mentally Ill operates the Family-to-Family Education Program to support carers of people with mental health problems.[36] Preliminary studies report encouraging results for carers, but outcomes for patients are unclear.[26]

Internationally, major non-governmental mental health interest groups such as MIND in the United Kingdom, the National Alliance for the Mentally Ill (NAMI) in the United States, and SANE in Australia, all undertake extensive support programmes that are widely accessible. They provide a significant community resource for primary care practitioners who treat people with mental health problems.

Psychologically based interventions

Counselling

Counselling involves a range of interpersonal interventions, provided by a range of health professionals, usually on a one-to-one basis for a relatively brief duration (6–12 sessions). It is defined as 'a systematic process which gives individuals an opportunity to explore, discover and clarify ways of living more resourcefully, with a greater sense of well-being'.[37] Counselling in primary care is a particular issue in the United Kingdom, where approximately half of all general practices employ a counsellor.[38] In most countries, access to counselling and other forms of interpersonal therapy requires referral outside the primary care setting.

Primary care physicians refer patients with stress and anxiety, depression, and relationship, self-esteem, or bereavement problems to counsellors. Severity of illness and disability may be significant in this group. A large-scale survey in the United Kingdom found that 76 per cent of patients referred to primary care counsellors had problems severe enough to place them in a 'clinical' population.[39]

In the United Kingdom, the Department of Health has issued evidence-based clinical guidelines for psychological therapies.[37] They recommend counselling in primary care for mild stress-related problems, and adjustment to life events, illnesses, and losses. They recommend referral to specialized services (community mental health teams, psycho-therapy services) for patients with a history of severe trauma, complex social problems, severe depression, anxiety or co-morbidity, and previous failed primary care treatment.

The focus on primary care counselling in the United Kingdom has generated considerable evaluative research, recently summarized in authoritative reviews.[37,39] Patients' level of satisfaction with counselling is high. Counselling can be useful in the treatment of mild to moderate mental health problems in the short-term (up to 6 months), but in the longer term there are no outcome differences between counselling and other primary care (including antidepressants and cognitive interventions). The limited available information about cost-effectiveness suggests that costs are comparable between counselling and alternative interventions.

Cognitive therapy

Cognitive therapy is a brief structured treatment aimed at changing the dysfunctional beliefs and styles of information processing that characterize mental health disorders. It requires high levels of therapist training and is commonly practiced by clinical psychologists.[40]

Alone or in combination with behaviour therapy, research evidence supports the effectiveness of cognitive interventions in a variety of mental health problems relevant to primary care. These include depression, anxiety disorders including obsessive–compulsive disorder and post-traumatic stress disorder, and bulimia.[37]

Cognitive therapy is also useful in the treatment of severe mental illness. Five controlled studies of cognitive therapy for persistent psychotic symptoms, such as delusions and hallucinations, have demonstrated positive effects on symptom severity,[24] although a systematic review provided only limited evidence of an effect on relapse rates.[41]

Furthermore, cognitive approaches are effective for some disorders that present with somatic symptoms in primary care. Systematic reviews support cognitive interventions in chronic fatigue syndrome and chronic pain, and some controlled evidence supports their use in irritable bowel syndrome and pre-menstrual syndrome.[37]

The high training requirements for cognitive therapists restrict access to this treatment. However, the structured nature of cognitive therapy lends itself to multimedia training and delivery systems. For example, the Royal College of Psychiatrists maintains a website of Internet resources for cognitive–behaviour therapy.[42] Such initiatives promise to increase access to cognitive treatments considerably.

References

1. **Thornicroft, G. and Bebbington, P.** (1989). Deinstitutionalisation—from hospital closure to service development. *British Journal of Psychiatry* **155**, 739–53.
2. **Usten, T.B. and Sartorius, N.** *Mental Illness in General Health Care: An International Study*. Chichester: John Wiley and Sons, 1995.
3. **Goldberg, D. and Huxley, P.** *Common Mental Disorders: A Biosocial Model.* London: Routledge, 1992.
4. **Hickie, I.** (1999). Primay care psychiatry is not specialist psychiatry in general practice. *Medical Journal of Australia* **170**, 170–3.
5. **Naismith, S.L.** et al. (2001). Effects of mental health training and clinical audit on general practitioners' management of common mental disorders. *Medical Journal of Australia* **175**, S42–7.
6. **Department of Health.** Workforce Planning, Education and Training Underpinning Programme: Adult Mental Health Services. Special Report from the Primary Care Key Area Group. In *Mental Health National Service Framework*, 26 October 2001 (http://www.doh.gov.uk/mentalhealth/watspecialreport.pdf).
7. **Reggeri, M.** et al. (2000). Definition and prevalence of severe and persistent mental illness. *British Journal of Psychiatry* **177**, 149–55.
8. **Melzer, D., Hale, A.S., and Malik, S.J.** (1991). Community care for patients with schizophrenia one year after hospital discharge. *British Medical Journal* **302**, 1023–5.
9. **Tansella, M. and Thornicroft, G.**, ed. *Common Mental Disorders in Primary Care*. London: Routledge, 1999.
10. **Stein, L.I. and Test, M.A.** (1980). Alternatives to mental hospital treatment. I. Conceptual model, treatment program, and clinical evaluation. *Archives of General Psychiatry* **37** (4), 392–7.
11. **Joy, C.B., Adams, C.E., and Rice, K.** (2001). Crisis intervention for people with severe mental illness (Cochrane Review). In *The Cochrane Library* Vol. 3. Oxford: Update Software.
12. **Mueser, K.T.** et al. (1998). Models of community care for severe mental illness: a review of research on case management (Review). *Schizophrenia Bulletin* **24** (1), 37–74.
13. **Olfson, M.** (1990). Assertive community treatment: an evaluation of the experimental evidence. *Hospital and Community Psychiatry* **41**, 634–41.
14. **Marshall, M. and Lockwood, A.** (2001). Assertive community treatment for people with severe mental disorders (Cochrane Review). In *The Cochrane Library* Vol. 3. Oxford: Update Software.
15. **Tyrer, P.** et al. (2001). Community mental health teams (CMHTs) for people with severe mental illnesses and disordered personality (Cochrane Review). In *The Cochrane Library* Vol. 4. Oxford: Update Software.
16. **Thornicroft, G.** et al. (1998). From efficacy to effectiveness in community mental health services. PRiSM Psychosis Study. 10. *British Journal of Psychiatry* **173**, 423–7.
17. **Gask, L., Sibbald, B., and Creed, F.** (1997). Evaluating models of working at the interface between mental health services and primary care. *British Journal of Psychiatry* **170**, 6–11.
18. **Bower, P. and Sibbald, B.** (2001). On-site mental health workers in primary care: effects on professional practice (Cochrane Review). In *The Cochrane Library* Vol. 4. Oxford: Update Software.
19. **Crowther, R.** et al. (2001). Vocational rehabilitation for people with severe mental illness (Cochrane Review). In *The Cochrane Library* Vol. 4. Oxford: Update Software.
20. **Barrowclough, C.** et al. (2001). Randomized controlled trial of motivational interviewing, cognitive behavior therapy, and family intervention for patients with comorbid schizophrenia and substance use disorders. *American Journal of Psychiatry* **158**, 1706–13.
21. **Drake, R.E.** et al. (2000). Evidence-based treatment of schizophrenia. *Current Psychiatry Reports* **2**, 393–7.
22. **Ley, A.** et al. (2001). Treatment programmes for people with both severe mental illness and substance misuse (Cochrane Review). In *The Cochrane Library* Vol. 4. Oxford: Update Software.
23. **Narrow, W.E.** et al. (2000). Mental health service use by Americans with severe mental illness. *Social Psychiatry & Psychiatric Epidemiology* **35**, 147–55.
24. **Mueser, K.T., Bond, G.R., and Drake, R.E.** Community-based treatment of schizophrenia and other severe mental disorders: treatment outcomes? In *Medscape Mental Health*, 26 October 2001 (http://www.medscape.com/Medscape/psychiatry/journal/2001/v06.n01/mh3418.mues.html).
25. **Dilk, M.N. and Bond, G.R.** (1996). Meta-analytic evaluation of social skills research for individuals with severe mental illness. *Journal of Consulting and Clinical Psychology* **64**, 1337–46.
26. **Dixon, L.** et al. (2001). Evidence-based practice for services to families of people with psychiatric disabilities. *Psychiatric Services* **52**, 903–10.
27. **Penn, L.D. and Mueser, K.T.** (1996). Research update on the psychosocial treatment of schizophrenia. *American Journal of Psychiatry* **153**, 607–17.
28. **Pharoah, F.M., Mari, J.J., and Streiner, D.** (2001). Family intervention for schizophrenia (Cochrane Review). In *The Cochrane Library* Vol. 4. Oxford: Update Software.
29. **Pekkala, E. and Merinder, L.** (2001). Psychoeducation for schizophrenia (Cochrane Review). In *The Cochrane Library* Vol. 3. Oxford: Update Software.
30. **World Schizophrenia Fellowship.** *Families as Partners in Care: A Document Designed to Launch a Strategy for the Implementation of Programs of Family Education, Training and Support.* Toronto: World Schizophrenia Fellowship, 1998.

31. **Kenwright, M., Liness, S., and Marks, I.** (2001). Reducing demands on clinicians by offering computer-aided self-help for phobia/panic: feasibility study. *British Journal of Psychiatry* **179**, 456–9.
32. **Kownacki, R.J. and Shadish, W.R.** (1999). Does Alcoholics Anonymous work? The results from a meta-analysis of controlled experiments. *Substance Use and Misuse* **34**, 1897–916.
33. **Bower, P., Richards, D., and Lovell, K.** (2001). The clinical and cost-effectiveness of self-help treatments for anxiety and depressive disorders. *British Journal of General Practice* **51**, 838–45.
34. **Hay, P.J. and Bacaltchuk, J.** (2001). Psychotherapy for bulimia nervosa and bingeing (Cochrane Review). In *The Cochrane Library* Vol. 4. Oxford: Update Software.
35. **Emerick, R.E.** (1990). Self-help groups for former patients: relations with mental health professionals. *Hospital and Community Psychiatry* **41**, 401–7.
36. **Burland, J.F.** (1998). Family-to-family: a trauma and recovery model of family education. *New Directions for Mental Health Services* **77**, 33–44.
37. **Department of Health.** *Treatment Choice in Psychological Therapies and Counselling*. London: Department of Health, 2001.
38. **Mellor-Clark, J., Sims-Ellis, R., and Burton, M.** *National Survey of Counsellors in Primary Care: Evidence for Growing Professionalisation*. London: Royal College of General Practitioners, 2001.
39. **NHS Centre for Reviews and Dissemination.** Counselling in primary care. In *Effectiveness Matters* Vol. 5. York: University of York, 2001 (www.york.ac.uk/inst/ird/em52.htm).
40. **Haaga, D.A.F. and Beck, A.T.** (1992). Cognitive therapy. In *Handbook of the Affective Disorders* (ed. E.S. Paykel), pp. 511–23. Edinburgh: Churchill Livingstone.
41. **Jones, C. et al.** (2001). Cognitive behavioural therapy for schizophrenia. In *The Cochrane Library* Vol. 4. Oxford: Update Software.
42. **Royal College of Psychiatrists.** Webguide: Internet resources for cognitive behaviour therapy. In *Royal College of Psychiatrists*, 26 October 2001 (http://www.rcpsych.ac.uk/info/webguide/cogthe.htm).

10.6 Social care and its place in primary care

Sally Baldwin

The ambitious agenda currently set for primary care views 'social' care as an integral part of its remit. But what exactly *is* social care? Why is it needed? Who, within primary care, should be responsible for delivering it? Are there obstacles to doing that well? What do we know about overcoming them? These are the questions I address in this chapter from the perspective of a social scientist working in social policy, and as the Director of a research unit whose work is concerned with the experience and impact of chronic illness, disability and ageing.

Stella—a case history

I begin with a case history (see Box 1) to illustrate the kinds of need arising from conditions which, while complex, are not unusual at a population level. It is drawn from my own research experience and will, I hope, provide a meaningful context for the ensuing discussion. This family were not well supported, either by their GP practice or by local social workers. They said they would benefit from clearer discussion of Stella's condition and the possibility of behaviour modification; practical support; breaks from coping with Stella; financial support; better housing; discussion of the future; a space to discuss their feelings, and much more. They felt very isolated, and that none of the professionals with whom they came into contact fully understood their situation, communicated with each other about the support the family needed, or was willing to take overall responsibility for their needs. Stella's parents described their attempts to obtain the support they, and Stella, needed as 'a constant battle'.

Box 1 Case history

Stella is a 14-year-old girl with epilepsy and associated learning difficulties and extremely challenging behaviour. She also suffers from asthma. Stella lives with her mother and father, 12-year-old brother, and 10-year-old sister in a small house on an estate in an industrial town. Stella's epilepsy is not well controlled at present. She experiences frequent fits, and sometimes has to be taken to hospital for emergency treatment. Her behaviour is aggressive and destructive. She seems quite incapable of feeling, or showing, affection. Stella needs constant supervision to prevent her destroying her own, and her siblings', clothes and possessions, furnishings, decoration, and so on. She eats constantly and throws her food around. Stella attends a special school, but her attendance is intermittent and her mother is regularly called to school to take her home. Her family are extremely fond of Stella, and their lives revolve around her. Nevertheless, they are adversely affected in many ways by the demands of caring for her. Both parents' employment prospects and earnings have suffered: her father's because he has withdrawn from seeking promotion and regularly loses money from having to take time off to take Stella to appointments, go home in a crisis or give her mother a break; her mother's because she has had to abandon ambitions to train as a nurse, and makes do with casual, low paid, work. From their reduced income, the family has to meet many extra costs created by Stella's condition: for transport, replacing items she destroys, extra food, adaptations to their home to create a safe place for Stella to play and a protected space for her siblings, and much more. Her parents worry constantly: about Stella's medical condition and her future; their own ability to go on coping; the effect of her behaviour, and their own lack of time, on her siblings; and about their financial problems. Stella's mother experiences bouts of anxiety and feels very depressed from time to time. She and her husband never have time to spend together; life is very difficult and they see no prospect of improvement.

As those working in primary care will recognize, this example could be replicated many times over—in respect of frail older people, those with enduring mental health problems, and so on. Such people clearly need not only clinical interventions, but a response to their situations as a whole. They also need interventions to prevent some needs arising in the first place, or in such acute forms—higher incomes, better housing, better employment conditions, investment to increase the capacity of local communities to support people with chronic health conditions. Most countries now recognize the importance of bringing together strands in policy and service provision which have, until now, been separate: national, structural, responses to poverty and ill health, and local strategies for improving social capital; public health and social inclusion strategies. The need for services that integrate health and social care is also widely recognized. This is partly because it is what patients want, is more efficient and delivers better outcomes. It is also because services that respond in an integrated way to health and social needs seem likely to deliver better outcomes in both domains. Qureshi[1] observes that finding an adult with mental health problems a stable place to live may be a necessary precondition for ensuring that medication is taken regularly. Likewise, financial assistance may be needed for a poor family whose child has diabetes to get to regular practice and hospital check-ups. In both cases well integrated clinical and social care will maximize the patient's and family, ability to manage the illness positively. However, progress towards such integration is exceedingly slow. Why is this?

Clinical and social traditions

A good starting point for tackling this question is a recognition that, while the concept of primary care as a multidisciplinary activity is relatively new, it builds on two long-standing traditions—the clinical and the social. Each, in its different way, represents society's collective response to the difficulties of human existence, and to the diswelfares that occur, and are unequally distributed, as countries develop and industrialize. Illness is a dominant human problem and its investigation and treatment the domain of medicine and the professions allied to medicine. As the example above shows, poor health carries both clinical and social consequences. The task of helping people to manage the personal and social consequence of illness is the domain of the social care professions. It is often necessary for both clinical and social perspectives to be brought to bear on a patient's situation. However, relations between the professionals who occupy the territories of health and social care have long been difficult. Given these tensions we need to probe further what is implied by the term social care, and to clarify who, within primary care, should do what in providing it.

What is social care?

Taken for granted understandings of social care tend to invoke notions of the support people need when ill health threatens their ability to function independently. We think of it as the practical and psychological support people need, alongside health care, to modify the effects of illness or disability on their lives. More concretely, we probably think of it in terms of advice, information, counselling, practical help with things like housework, help to avoid isolation, and so on. We might, beyond that, conceive of it as a set of services, provided by agencies outside the health service, for which social workers act as gate keepers and arrangers. These are useful, and relatively accurate, conceptions. However, they do not tell the whole story. There is value in thinking further about a concept which is often used in ways that are vague and ambiguous. Care is itself an ambiguous concept; academics have written at length about its complexity and the mix of positive and negative connotations it carries. Care can be benevolent. It can also be oppressive and controlling. It can be provided voluntarily, but also from duty and as the discharge of professional obligations. It carries connotations of love, but requires hard physical labour. *Social* care shares this complexity.

Aldgate,[2] for example, distinguishes four different perspectives on social care:

- as a universal concept within everyday relations;
- as a policy concept;
- as a set of roles relations—professional and informal; and
- as a set of services offered in different settings.

For our purposes, the last three are particularly salient. However, the universality of the concept of care within everyday relations is a large part of what makes social care as a policy or professional activity so difficult to pin down.

Given our acceptance of collective responsibility for responding to social need, governments clearly have obligations to create policies to do so. In policy terms, 'social care' covers our response to a much wider set of needs than those created by ill health. At the broadest level, it describes all the interventions we collectively make to respond to the needs of individuals who, for whatever reason, are unable independently to manage their lives to the levels judged acceptable in particular societies at particular times.[3]

On this view, social care covers policies relating to a wide range of circumstances. Our particular focus is on needs created by frailty and ill health. Even so, this broader perspective signals important dimensions of social care which are highly relevant to primary care. One of these is the range, and diversity, of the activities it potentially includes. Essentially, social care includes whatever is necessary for maintaining a life which is as meaningful and as fully integrated as possible in the community—all the things mentioned above but also sufficient income, employment, housing, leisure, meaningful occupation, and rewarding human relationships. Another is the range of actors and agencies potentially involved in providing it. As Daly and Lewis[3] point out, social care is provided by, and at the intersection of state, family, market, and voluntary sectors—not by statutory agencies alone. A key role is played by the so-called 'informal' sector of welfare—relatives in particular, but also friends and neighbours. As a large body of research evidence demonstrates, only a small proportion of the care of even the most dependent individuals is provided by professionals, the great majority by kin. Policy increasingly recognizes the importance of strategies both for incorporating informal carers as partners and for responding to their needs, though success in doing so at the level of practice is patchy.

Roles and responsibilities

Looking at social care in terms of the roles and responsibilities of the different professionals involved highlights the need for clarity about appropriate divisions of labour. Clinicians working in primary care quite accurately see themselves as in one way or another providing social care. Doctors, for example, are influenced by ideas of good practice which require them to interpret symptoms in the context of the patient's life as a whole and pay attention, in their response, to the interplay of clinical and social factors. Nursing and the therapies have a long-standing commitment to holistic practice. Moreover, the values which underpin clinical practice in all these professions mean that practitioners are well placed to respond to patients' social, as well as clinical, needs. For social work, on the other hand, social care forms the core of its work. It therefore claims a particular, specialist, role within primary care. How are we to distinguish between these understandings and agree a sensible division of labour?

It is useful to distinguish between social care as one element of clinical practice and as a systematic response to the human consequences of illness. Following from that we can distinguish between the professions whose skills lie primarily in investigating and treating illness and those whose skills lie primarily in responding to its personal and social consequences. On this basis medicine, nursing, and the therapies lie in the first category, social work in the second. Clearly, clinicians have scope to respond to a patient's social, as well as clinical, needs. However, a skilled, and coherent, response is more possible for social workers. In practical terms this is because they are free from competing clinical responsibilities. More importantly, it is because social work's distinctive orientation, knowledge, and value base equips it to do so. Where the clinical professions' primary orientation is to the investigation and reduction of symptoms, social work's is to the person as a whole and to the maintenance of a meaningful life. Its knowledge base is 'woven together from management, psychology, social policy, philosophy, counselling, and the law.[4] It is eclectic, but highly appropriate for delivering social care defined as a coherent response to the multiplicity of ways in which illness and impairment affect people's lives. Social work's distinctive value base is similarly appropriate, characterized by a strong commitment to empowering the client to understand and manage their situation and to support with all aspects of that situation.

The important point here is not that social work per se is recognized as the profession which should take the lead with regard to social care. Rather, it is to establish that, like health care, social care is a complex, specialist, field. Providing it to an acceptable standard requires the acquisition of a body of knowledge, specialist skills, and a value base rooted in commitment to social inclusion and the importance of empowering clients to manage their own lives. As the professions working within primary care develop and change, it may well become less obvious that social work should take the lead.

Boundary disputes

In considering social care as a set of services, a different set of issues comes into play. Here, disputes are more likely to involve agencies denying responsibility for social care services than claiming ownership. Key struggles revolve around which agency is responsible for meeting particular needs; who decides this; who can assess, or refer, a client for a service; who pays; who organizes; where does accountability lie? We are all familiar with sterile debates about whether an individual's need for a bath is a 'health' or 'social' need; which agency is to pay the bill for rehabilitation for a younger person who has a stroke; who is to pay for domiciliary support for an older person occupying an acute bed but capable of living at home.

As a depressingly large body of research has demonstrated, failing to resolve such disputes has had miserable consequences for patients and their relatives and perverse consequences for the service system as a whole. There is abundant evidence of important needs going unmet at the boundary between health and social care, but also of duplication of effort and the delivery of a patchwork of services by a multiplicity of providers—not designed around the patient's needs, not integrated with each other and not fitting into the patient's life or that of relatives involved in providing support.

Dominant themes that emerge from the literature on health and social care concern the importance of understanding its nature and scope, clarity about who is responsible for which aspects of it, and the value of respect, collaboration and good communication between the agencies and professions involved. Until recently it would have been true to say that the need for all of these was acknowledged in principle, but rarely acted on in practice. There is now a much stronger policy commitment to an integrated response to ill health and its consequences, delivered via partnership and collaboration between the agencies and professionals involved, and with primary care playing a central role. In the United Kingdom, further impetus is provided by a set of new mechanisms—pooled budgets, new and flexible ways of jointly providing services—which should make this easier to deliver. Resources will now depend on progress towards this new way of working, and sanctions be applied to those who cannot demonstrate this. It would be naïve, however, to believe that long established patterns can be transformed merely by policy diktat and budgetary flexibility. Real progress requires a clear understanding of what lies behind our failure thus far to deliver the kind of holistic, well integrated, primary care that most practitioners want to be involved in providing.

There is no shortage of reasons. A large number of commentators point to the difficulty of making significant changes in working practices, amidst the turbulence and sheer volume of work that has characterized recent years. They also point to organizations' different purposes, and need to respond to sometimes conflicting demands from government. The requirement to collaborate has to be reconciled with each agency's separate managerial agenda and performance indicators. In health, for example, demands to meet targets on throughput, waiting times, numbers of immunizations and so on sit uneasily alongside demands to develop new ways of working with social care agencies, professionals, and patients. Self-interest, and survival, can conflict with developing common strategies and joint working. Different patterns of employment and accountability complicate matters further, as does the difference between the health sector's more universal approach to service provision and the openly selective ethos of social care. The lack of a strong tradition of user involvement in health can act as a barrier to joint working with social care, as does the difficulty of bringing together a mainly free service and one based on means testing and charging. The absence of a population perspective in primary care causes difficulties in enabling it to work strategically with other local agencies. It is not surprising, then, to find arguments against integrated services, based on assertions that health and social care agencies, and those who work in them, do not understand or respect each other, have incompatible objectives and ways of working, and are locked into current arrangements because of inflexible rules about how money can be spent and the shunting of responsibilities from one agency to another.[5]

All of this is recognizably true. Moreover providing holistic, flexible, well-coordinated care to large numbers of people with very individual needs is an extraordinarily difficult logistical exercise—as Baldock[6] argues with respect to older people. However, the danger of thinking mainly in terms of such immediate, practical difficulties is that we neglect their root causes. Here, the sophisticated analysis carried out by Twigg[7] as part of her study of how bathing for older people in the community is managed and experience, is illuminating.

Twigg identifies three underlying features of the boundary between health and social care which explain why it is so problematic.

- It is not one division, but four: institutional, financial, professional, and ideological. These build on, and reinforce each other.
- It is not fixed but 'has moved historically and across welfare systems' (ref. 7, p. 107). The same service is defined as 'health' at one time and 'social care' at another. This movement, often dictated by finance, creates 'a grey area for provision and responsibility' where the care of people with chronic conditions is typically located.
- The relationship between the medical and the social in this grey area is asymmetric, and the dominance of the medical creates problems.

Twigg unravels how differences in financing and governance have created two very different institutions: health—generally universal, free and governed by national policy; social care—rationed, means-tested, and locally governed. These differences cause practical difficulties for joint working. They also reflect, and sustain, inequalities in the status of clinical activities and those which constitute social care.

Professional and ideological differences are, Twigg argues, a deep-rooted source of difficulty—not only in terms of predictable struggles for territory and power, but also of conflicts between two very different epistemologies and cultures. Clinical practice, resting on the biomedical model, is focused on the body, and oriented to cure and the use of sophisticated technological interventions. Social care, by contrast, rests on belief in work with the whole person, the interaction of mind and body, the therapeutic deployment of interpersonal skills and the use of low tech, practical, interventions. Clinical practice has a prestige which derives from its association with science; social care is perceived as unscientific and carries lower status by virtue of its closeness to ordinary life. The potential for a clash of cultures between the two is particularly strong in primary care. Here the scope for 'cure' and for high tech medicine is limited for patients with chronic conditions, the potential impact of social care large. Yet the status of medicine, and clinical interventions generally, and their power to attract resources, remains higher, even when the limitations of practice based on the biomedical model are widely acknowledged.

Coordinating care

There are clearly long-standing difficulties of many kinds to overcome, then, in delivering the promise of the 'new' primary care—delivering measurable gains in both the health status and quality of life of patients and family carers. However, it is as important to avoid excessive pessimism as naïve optimism. Three grounds for (cautious) optimism are worthy of note. One is the growing convergence of ideas on what primary care is about, and the outcomes it should aim to achieve. Longino (ref. 8, p. 39), for example, argues that we are witnessing 'the emergence of a new paradigm (of medical practice) which combines scientific knowledge with a humanistic approach'. Having dealt successfully with infectious disease medicine now has to respond to a growing volume of chronic disease and disability. This demands a move beyond the biomedical model towards approaches 'which focus more broadly, on health rather than only on medical interventions, (and) understand health to be both holistic and environmental' (ref. 8, p. 43). Most doctors working in primary care are receptive to this way of thinking, as are nursing and the therapies. Moreover, some areas of practice are already based on this approach. Good practice in mental health, for example, is widely accepted as requiring a concerted response to the patient's social as well as health needs, delivered via a truly integrated, multidisciplinary team.

A second cause for hope lies in recent changes in how health and related problems are perceived, and tackled, by local communities. These are complex developments.[9] In simplistic terms, recent years have seen the emergence of a consensus that new approaches are needed to deal with the kinds of difficult, inter-related, problems many communities face—for example, poverty, crime, environmental issues, and numerous forms of inequality (notably in health). Elected authorities are increasingly developing joint approaches to strategic thinking, planning, and problem-solving which involve all the relevant agencies in the area—including the private sector. The strategies that emerge are based on reducing social exclusion and social inequalities, creating healthy communities and promoting public health. They involve a mix of approaches: structural change; initiatives to build social capital; community led initiatives with devolved budgets and so on. Crucially health, in all its manifestations, is now seen as central to such local strategies for economic and social well-being. The very different ethos that now pervades local discussions of 'health' and 'social' care could thus be an important force in unblocking long-standing barriers to integrated services.

A third cause for hope lies in the sheer volume of joint working happening on the ground, and the growth of knowledge as to what makes different ways of delivering holistic, 'seamless' care more possible, and more and less effective. In the United Kingdom, for example, we can find a huge range of local initiatives based on joint working between agencies and professionals. In one county, Wiltshire, 27 such projects were identified 5 years ago, and the number will have grown since.[5] Evaluation and analysis is forcing a clearer, more systematic, understanding of the ideas on which such projects are based—potentially fuzzy concepts such as 'partnership' and 'collaboration'. One recent typology, for example, distinguishes four different types of partnership (competition, cooperation, coordination, and co-evolution), and stresses the need for clarity about which is being used and the value of 'whole systems' thinking to optimize the benefits of each.[10] A recent review of the literature on interprofessional collaboration[11] discerns four models (competition, cooperation, coordination, and co-evolution) and draws out current knowledge of the factors promoting, and inhibiting, collaboration and joint working. Both stress the importance of factors such as identified purpose, consensus, reciprocity and trust, and the time, hard work and skills that are needed for effective partnership working. Hudson[11] concludes that while the evidence base for the effectiveness of team working in general is strong 'primary health care team work, and team working across the primary health care, social care boundary is typically inadequate' at this stage. There is much to learn, then, about the effectiveness of different organizational structures and processes in delivering good outcomes for patients. Fortunately, in view of the current rush to implement joint working, an evidence base is beginning to accumulate.

Conclusion

On balance I am optimistic that the inadequacies and gaps in the health and social care available to the family in the example earlier in this chapter will be very different from our response in ten years time. This is not to say that it will be a perfect, seamless, whole—simply that some of the barbarisms and fault lines that have characterized it thus far will widely be perceived as unacceptable. The concepts and principles which underpin that response have already changed fundamentally. Practice will follow in due course, albeit slowly.

References

1. **Qureshi, H.** Outcomes for social care. Unpublished conference paper, personal communication, 1998.
2. **Aldgate, J.** What is care? Unpublished work in draft, personal communication, 2001.
3. **Daly, M. and Lewis, J.** (2000). The concept of social care and the analysis of contemporary welfare states. *British Journal of Sociology* **51** (2), 281–98.
4. **Barton, R.** *The Territory of Social Care.* K202 Care Welfare and Community. Open University Press, 2001.
5. **Warner, M. and Macallister-Smith, E.** (1996). Integrating health and social care. In *A Primary Care Led NHS: Putting it into Practice* (ed. G. Meads), pp. 103–15. New York: Churchill Livingstone.
6. **Baldock, J.** (1997). Social care in old age: more than a funding problem. *Social Policy and Administration* **31** (1), 171–89.
7. **Twigg, J.** *Bathing, the Body and Community Care.* London: Routledge, 2000.
8. **Longino, C.F.** (2000). Beyond the body: an emerging medical paradigm. In *Care Services for Later Life: Transformations and Critiques* (ed. L. Warren and M. Nolan), pp. 39–53. London: Jessica Kingsley.
9. **Stewart, J.** (2000). New approaches to local governance. In *The Changing Role of Social Care. Research Highlights 37* (ed. B. Hudson), pp. 17–29. London: Jessica Kingsley.
10. **Pratt, J., Gordon, P., and Plampling, D.** *Working Whole Systems.* London: Kings Fund Publishing, 1999.
11. **Hudson, B.**, ed. *The Changing Role of Social Care. Research Highlights in Social Work 37'.* London: Jessica Kingsley, 2000.

Further reading

Davies, C., Hudson, B., and Hardy, B. *Working Towards Partnership.* K202 Care Welfare and Community. Open University Press, 2001.

Hudson, B. (1999). Primary health care and social care: working across professional boundaries. Part one: the changing context of inter-professional relationships. *Managing Community Care* **7** (1), 15–22.

Hudson, B. (1999). Primary health care and social care: working across professional boundaries. Part two: models of inter-professional collaboration. *Managing Community Care* **7** (2), 15–20.

Hudson, B. et al. (1999). In pursuit of inter-agency collaboration in the public sector: what is the contribution of theory and research. *Public Management* **1**, 235–60.

Meads, G., ed. *A Primary Care Led NHS: Putting it into Practice.* New York: Churchill Livingstone, 1996.

Rummery, K. and Glendinning, C. *Primary Care and Social Services: Developing New Partnerships for Older People.* Oxford: Radcliffe Medical Press, 2000.

10.7 Allocating and managing resources

Macaran A. Baird

Introduction

What is the appropriate role for primary care physicians in the overall effort to manage scarce and expensive resources wisely and allocate priority expenditures for managing the health of defined populations? What are the principles that a primary care physician can use to manage resources wisely? This chapter will explore Seven Principles of Managing Health Care Resources that can assist the primary care physician with this dilemma.

The actual cost of all health care services is largely determined by the age of a specific population, the disease burden of that population, the local availability of health care resources such as ambulatory clinics, health care personnel, hospitals, and academic medical centres, and the relative cost of each resource.[1] In the United States, the costs and mortality are heavily influenced by the burden of chronic illness, many of which are secondary to an unhealthy lifestyle.[2] It is now understood that health care resources are used more often if they are more available whether or not they are 'needed'. Therefore, health services costs do not follow the usual 'law of supply and demand' wherein more expensive resources are used more sparingly. In fact, the United States most clearly demonstrates that abundant health and health technology resources create increased demand for use of these expensive resources out of proportion to what would be predicted by the age and other relevant characteristics of the population.[3] Increasingly, patients' expectation that sophisticated diagnostic testing and/or treatment is indicated does not match the scientific opinion of the clinician. Agreeing to the patient requests can contribute to escalating health care costs.

This chapter will discuss allocation and managing resources with the assumption that excess expensive resources are available for the clinician and population being served. Therefore, there is a need to use such resources wisely and in a manner that would tend to maximize health benefits at the lowest cost. In this manner, the task of primary care clinicians and health care systems has expanded beyond the care of individual patients towards management of the health of defined populations.[4] Even in areas where most health resources are scarce, many of these principles would apply. This chapter will focus upon choices reasonably within the influence of primary care physicians. There are macro-level strategies that shape broad health care policies and reach beyond individual providers and groups of physicians. Those societal and political choices have a profound influence upon overall health and health care expenditures.[5] For example, in several European countries and in Britain, universal health insurance and public system strategies dominate the health care systems and shape efforts to simultaneously conserve resources or improve quality.[6] In contrast, the US system is influenced heavily by a combination of privately funded health insurance systems for most working families, government insurance systems, and large populations of uninsured persons who have poor access to an otherwise overly abundant array of health services. In less-developed nations, even basic health care resources are scarce and overwhelmed by the demands of providing fundamental care services. Other nations in Africa are devastated by the wide spread impact of HIV and AIDS. A thorough discussion of macro-level, political, and economic forces upon health care resource utilization is beyond the scope of this chapter.

In this chapter, the author is assuming a relative abundance of options for health care services, which creates the dilemma of how to use those resources most wisely. There are seven principles that primary care physicians and teams of primary care providers can follow to have a significant positive impact on the wise use of health care resources.

The seven principles of Primary Care Resource Management are:

1. Prescribe medications based upon science not advertising.
2. Expand non-office-based care.
3. Provide access to health information and care options day and night, 7 days per week, 365 days per year.
4. Integrate hospital-based physicians into primary care practices.
5. Integrate behavioural health/mental health services into primary care practices.
6. Build prevention into primary care.
7. Create and maintain a database of patient diagnoses, utilization, and cost patterns and share it with providers.

Prescribe medications based upon science not advertisments

No matter how a practice is organized, whether in large multi-specialty groups or in a solo practice, the primary care physician must use pharmaceutical products in a prudent manner. Among all short-term cost factors, this one is most directly under the physician's control. There are several strategies for using pharmaceutical products that apply to primary care physicians in any kind of practice.

1. *Avoid over-use of antibiotics:*[7] Not only is it expensive to overprescribe antibiotics, but a pattern of overuse has created widespread resistance to common antibiotics. The most common prescribing error is use of broad-spectrum antibiotics for treatment of viral respiratory infections. Sinus congestion, cough, nasal congestion, and bronchitis are most often viral infections. The duration of these self-limited illnesses is 7–10 days and is not shortened by use of antibiotics.[8]
2. *Ensure that patients understand why they are using medications for chronic conditions such as asthma, hypertension and diabetes:* The wise physician ensures that patients have access to education regarding medication use via direct discussion in the office, nurse visits, nurse phone calls to follow-up office appointments, and Internet resources when available. For example, there are Internet World Wide Web sites on which patients can find reliable information about almost all chronic illnesses. Patients can read why specific medications may be needed for prolonged improvement in health.[9] WebMD.com and MayoClinic.com are two of many reliable web sites that have full information that is updated regularly.
3. *Use evidence-based medical care to select medications:* In each drug category there are many choices. Primary care physicians can find reliable information on cost-effective treatment strategies on several evidence-based websites. For example, the Cochrane Consortium is an international cooperative dedicated to sharing the latest scientific evaluation of medical care. The Cochrane Library lists the most recent review of the medical literature and clarifies the strength of the evidence to support a specific treatment. The *British Medical Journal* has created a website documenting evidence for effective healthcare (www.clinicalevidence.org). The Institute for Clinical Systems Improvement (ICSI) is a collaborative effort based in Minnesota (USA) that has established evidence-based protocols for the management of many common medical conditions. In 2001, all health plans and large insurance carriers in the state of Minnesota agreed to support ICSI in

Internet Resources:

http://hiru.mcmaster.ca/COCHRANE/—Cochrane Collaboration
www.webmd.com—commercial health information site
www.mayoclinic.com—Mayo Clinic public site for health information
www.clinicalevidence.org—British Medical Journal Publishing Group site for evidence-based medicine reviews
www.icsi.org—Institute for Clinical Systems Improvement
www.nofreelunch.org—free website for information regarding the influence of the pharmaceutical industry
www.cpct.co.uk—Counselling in Primary Care Trust website
www.cdc.gov/wonder/prevguid.org—Center for Disease Control website for prevention guidelines
www.ctfphc.org—Canadian Task Force on Preventive Health Care
www.ashp.org—American Society of Health-System Pharmacists
www.medletter.com—The Medical Letter on Drugs and Therapeutics
www.fda.gov—US Department of Health and Human Services Food and Drug Administration

order to create a state-wide standard for care for common medical problems ranging from low back pain to myocardial infarction.[10] In many cases, a less expensive medication or less use of any medication is the best care according to these research-based guidelines.

One of the goals of evidence-based medical care is to use research-based evidence to shape the care of acute and chronic illness management decisions.[11] Careful selection of pharmaceutical products has an especially large impact on overall costs in the management of chronic illnesses.[12]

4. *Reduce the influence of the advertising and economic incentives from the powerful pharmaceutical industry:* Many newer medications are simply more expensive variations of existing products. These 'me too' drugs can be used sparingly if they offer fewer side-effects. However, there are also exciting breakthroughs in the development of new medications. The complex interplay of innovation and profit are difficult for a clinician to interpret.[13] However, advertising leads physicians and patients to overestimate the indications and benefits of the newer, and usually more expensive, medications. Evaluating industry claims versus scientific evidence is a complex task. Physicians and patients may benefit from the ongoing efforts of local pharmacy and therapeutics committees whose task it is to evaluate the costs and benefits of pharmaceutical products. It is clear that the drug industry spends billions of dollars in advertising, special gifts for physicians, and meals to influence physicians' prescribing behaviour. For an irreverent review of this problem physician's can review an interesting website that challenges the influence of the pharmaceutical industry (www.nofreelunch.com).

Expand non-office-based care

At least in industrialized nations PCPs can reduce costs by decreasing the percentage of care provided to patients solely by direct visits to the office.[14] In chronic illnesses, a primary goal is to help patients 'take charge' of their illness and shift toward more 'self-directed' care.[15] By choosing more carefully how often to see patients with chronic conditions, the primary care physician can facilitate increased patient-centredness and improve access for other patients. Use of outreach calls by both physicians and nurses in place of office visits are realistic options now for pre-paid practices and HMO staff model clinics.[16] Under pre-paid arrangements clinicians are paid per patient per month whether or not the patient is seen. Therefore, the patient does not have to 'cross the threshold' of the physician's office in order to generate the payment for care delivered. A pre-paid arrangement allows the providing team to be more creative in how to reach the patient and 'manage health'. One cost-efficient tool is to call patients or set up scheduled 'phone-based visits'. These outreach calls save time for everyone and reduce the more costly office visits. Patients avoid waiting in the office, travelling to the office, missing time from work, etc. Disease management companies have used this phone-based care to create an entire industry in the United States. By following physician-approved protocols, the nurses and physicians involved in disease management reach patients at home (or at work) to enhance patient adherence with medical treatment, educate patients about a medical condition, and identify treatment failures earlier.[17]

If primary care physicians can arrange for payment for managing patients by phone or by pre-paid contracts, patient care in the office can be improved by phone-based follow-up. The Internet also permits similar care-at-a-distance options if the physician and patient understand the problem of limited security protection of the Internet.[18]

Non-office-based care can be delivered via telephone or e-mail to help reduce office visits and improve patient adherence to chronic care. These same options are useful for managing less serious acute care needs as well. In the United States, pre-paid practices and some large practices have formalized phone-based care strategies for low back pain, simple urinary tract infections, and sinusitis.[19] Under these protocols, the diagnosis is made by phone and treatment prescribed by phone according to physician-created protocols.[20] This is especially useful for conditions for which the diagnosis is documented to rely primarily upon the history rather than physical examination.

Provide access to information and care options day and night, 7 days per week, 365 days per year

Throughout the United States and in some other industrialized nations, practices have learned to reduce unneeded visits to the emergency room and urgent care centres by providing nurse triage services to these practice populations after usual office hours have ended.[17] Of course, this simply recognizes that patients may need care at any time of the day or night. Efficiently meeting this unyielding universal demand for access to care has only recently been a priority in many practices. This type of service demand can most reasonably be met via 24-h access to well-trained registered nurses who work from carefully constructed protocols to assist patients in deciding what to do with their health concerns after the doctor's office closes. The cost of such services is covered by the pre-paid practice or by the employer in 'self-insured' medical insurance. The cost savings are created by working with the patient on the phone to choose the most appropriate option for the immediate care of a problem. Self-limited problems are identified by working through a protocol of severity assessment on the phone that would lead to self-management or safely waiting until the next day to see the doctor. Problems that need more immediate professional evaluation or management are identified via the same protocol. For some problems, the patient is directed to an urgent care centre or emergency room depending upon the severity of the problem and the actual access to urgent care during nighttime or weekend hours.[16] Some large practices with computerized medical records have the phone nurse review the patient's electronic medical record, verify medication allergies, reinforce chronic medical care plans, and treat minor problems immediately by phone-based protocol.

Integrate hospital-based physicians into primary care practices

The British model for primary care has long ago identified the need for hospital-based physicians. In the United States, this pattern of physician role separation by location of care is more recent. However, the use of 'hospitalists' is spreading rapidly in the United States for a variety of reasons.[21] Principally, the complexity of hospital care now demands seeing the patient more than once per day. Efficiency and cost-reduction demands that patients are in the hospital as briefly as possible and receive aggressive and highly technical care while there. If the patient needs primarily intravenous medications or wound care, much of that can now be provided at home. Therefore, hospitalized patients require more technical care or monitoring. The complexity of providing sophisticated hospital care with the greatest efficiency puts unprecedented demands upon the physicians providing this care. Hospital protocols and standards of care change frequently. Fewer and fewer primary care physicians in the United States can keep up with these rapidly changing circumstances.

The pattern of visiting patients before and after office hours is still possible for those primary care physicians with ambulatory offices located adjacent to the hospital. These primary care physicians can also quickly visit the unstable hospitalized patient at other times during the day. However, the majority of the primary care physicians in the United States find it too great a challenge to interrupt office practice to visit hospitalized patients more than once per day. Rotating to the hospital for 1 or 2 weeks every 2 months is still an option for some in the United States. However, this interrupts ambulatory access and continuity. In all of these scenarios it is increasingly difficult for primary care physicians to provide continuity of care in both ambulatory and hospitalized settings.[22] The combination of these factors has created a gradual shift towards the use of full-time hospital-based physicians with a demonstrable improvement in the use of expensive hospital resources.

Integrate behavioural/mental health services into primary care practices

Many primary care practices do not have ready access to behavioural/mental health services. Commonly, this behavioural health care has been provided by a variety of 'off-site' professionals including social workers, family counsellors, psychologists, substance abuse counsellors, psychiatrists, and health psychologists. These behavioural health professionals have specific skills and training to assist patients with a variety of common problems that primary care patients experience regularly.(23) Artificially separating access to such services away from routine primary medical services is inefficient and impairs wise use of professional resources. Such separation of medical and mental health professionals also leads to overuse of medical resources as primary care clinicians struggle to manage patients who present with biopsychosocial dilemmas. Cummings(24) was among the first to demonstrate the cost savings of integrating mental health and primary medical services. The Counseling in Primary Care Trust (www.cpct.co.uk) in Britain has recently demonstrated the cost savings of placing specially trained primary mental health counsellors into GP practices.(25) Large-scale pre-paid practices in the United States are moving gradually to ensure that well-organized primary care practices have a balance of on-site mental health clinicians to share the responsibility of care for defined populations. There is a growing scientific literature that documents the benefits of addressing the psycho-social issues patients have in order to more effectively and efficiently manage their overall health needs.(26)

There are numerous ways to integrate behavioural health and mental health care. At a basic level, all primary care practices need ready access to behavioural clinicians via phone or referral and consultation on specific patients. A more easily accessible model places behavioural health clinicians directly into the local primary care practice with a shared chart, shared appointment system, and adjacent offices. This arrangement offers frequent informal interactions as well as easily achieved joint consultations and shared visits. The level of integration is determined by local organizational, economic, and political issues.(27)

Build prevention into primary care

Ultimately, controlling the costs of health care for specific groups of people involves reducing their burden of disease.(28) For many years, the World Health Organization, national governments, and HMOs have understood that disease prevention via immunization and health education are cost-effective methods to reduce the burden of illness. Prevention programmes range from routine childhood and adult immunization to education regarding the benefits of a healthy diet and regular exercise. The obvious benefits of prevention efforts are reduced acute infectious illnesses, decreases in risk-taking behaviour such as driving automobiles without seatbelts, reduced injuries from drunken drivers, and improved diet and exercise. Some of these efforts happen outside primary care practices. For example, public policy that raises taxes on cigarettes is known to reduce cigarette use by youths and adults. Public health promotion messages on radio and television reinforcing the hazards of tobacco use are major civic steps on the road to reducing illness and injuries.(5)

Primary care practices also play an important role in the journey toward improved public health. However, reaching established goals for ensuring that all patients benefit from practice-related prevention opportunities is a complex challenge. The guidelines for prevention are now published by a variety of governmental (www.wonder.cdc.gov) and non-government health care organizations (www.icsi.org, www.clinicalevidence.org). However, consistently applying these guidelines in a manner that reliably reaches all appropriate patients remains a difficult challenge for most primary care practices. The Quality Improvement model has been a commonly used tool for meeting this challenge.(29) Borrowing from other industries the methods for systematic improvement in work-related outcomes, health systems have gone past blaming individuals for failing to reach specific clinical targets. Now the theme is building fail-safe systems of care that reinforce human potential and recognize human limitations. For example, practices cannot succeed in improving immunization rates if they rely upon physicians to remember to immunize children and adults.(30) Instead, protocols must be established to routinely immunize all patients at every opportunity. Also, alternative options for immunization must be created to simplify the process for young parents and older adults to become immunized. Some practices sponsor specific days in the office when less waiting is required, or immunizations are taken to schools, elderly high apartments, or grocery stores to improve the access to such health services.

Just as airlines have learned to create automated methods to ensure airplane maintenance, practices need to build standing protocols for immunization and health education. Such practice improvements require administrative teamwork to create routine physician orders that nurses and other staff can follow even when the physician is not 'remembering' to ask for the immunization or health education discussion, pamphlet, or video.(31)

Create and maintain a database of patient diagnoses, utilization, and cost patterns and share it with providers

As this twenty-first century progresses, it will be necessary for primary care physicians to know more and more about the population being served. Standard information can be created and managed within the practice via an integrated electronic medical record or via information gathered from insurance companies. The cost of either system will be part of the cost of caring for those patients. Maintaining and constantly updating such information has created a whole new profession, the medical data analyst. Small practices may choose to rely upon the data being managed by those who pay for the care, such as insurance companies or government agencies. Larger group practices and health maintenance organizations create their own data management infrastructure. Common elements of population-based data include much more than age and gender distribution.(32) Each primary care physician is usually assigned responsibility for managing a 'panel' of patients. British GPs manage a 'patch' or geographically determined group of patients. In the United States, most primary care physicians manage a panel of approximately 1500–2500 patients. The size of the panel is larger or smaller depending upon age, severity of illness, and the nature of the team of nurses, nurse-practitioners, or physician assistants working with the primary care physician.(33) Feedback about the patterns of care delivered by each physician or team does influence future performance in a positive manner.(34)

Although the information shared with the primary care physician can be customized, data useful for providers managing a panel of patients includes the following summary data:(35)

Age
Sex
Top 20 medical diagnoses
Top 20 most costly patients
Top categories of common chronic illnesses and conditions including:
- Diabetes
- Cardiovascular disease/hypertension
- Depression
- Migraine headaches
- Hyperlipidaemia
- Asthma
- Mechanical low back pain

Cost data	*Utilization data*
Total costs pmpm	Office visits per 1000 patients
Pharmacy costs pmpm	Hospital admissions per 1000 patients
Consultant costs pmpm	ER visits per 1000 patients
Lab and diagnostic services pmpm	Prescriptions per patient

Ultimately, allocating and managing health care resources is a collaborative process and a shared responsibility for teams of primary care providers and their patients. This challenge has always been important but the complexity of the choices is greater now than for past generations. It is our newly understood responsibility to manage health care resources wisely or risk that others will do so without the best interests of our patients as a top priority.[36–39] Medical education systems must ensure the next generation of primary care physicians is well prepared for this challenging and growing aspect of primary care.[40] Primary care physicians can manage health care resources wisely if dedicated to the principles outlined in this chapter.

References

1. Ray, G.T. et al. (2000). The cost of health conditions in a health maintenance organization. *Medical Care Research and Review* **57** (1), 92–109.
2. **McGinnis, J.M. and Foege, W.H.** (1993). Actual causes of death in the United States. *Journal of the American Medical Association* **270** (18), 2207–12.
3. **Wennberg, J.E.** *The Dartmouth Atlas of Health Care in the United States.* Hanover NH: Trustees of Dartmouth College, 1998.
4. **Kindig, D.A.** (1997). Managing population health. *The Physician Executive,* September/October, **23** (7).
5. **Health and Behavioral Report.** *The Interplay of Biological, Behavioral, and Societal Influences.* Washington DC: Institute of Medicine, 2001.
6. **The Joint Commission Journal of Quality Improvement** (1999). International Improvement (entire issue), **25** (11), November.
7. **McCaig, L.F. and Hughes, J.M.** (1995). Trends in antimicrobial drug prescribing among office-based physicians in the United States. *Journal of the American Medical Association* **273**, 214–19.
8. **Gonzales, R., Steiner, J.F., and Sande, M.A.** (1997). Antibiotic prescribing for adults with colds, upper respiratory tract infections, and bronchitis by ambulatory care physicians. *Journal of the American Medical Association* **278**, 901–4.
9. **Maly, R.C., Bourque, L.B., and Engelhardt, R.F.** (1999). A randomized controlled trial of facilitating information giving to patients with chronic medical conditions. *Journal of Family Practice* **48** (5), 356–63.
10. **Lerner, M. and Howatt, G.** Minnesota Health Plans agree to fund quality initiative. *Star Tribune*, Minneapolis, MN, 13 March 2001.
11. **Sackett, D.L.** et al. *Evidence-Based Medicine: How to Practice & Teach EBM* 2nd edn. London: Churchill Livingstone, 2000.
12. **Fishman, P., Von Korff, M., Lozano, P., and Hecht, J.** (1997). Chronic care costs in managed care. The first single-plan comparison of chronic care costs shows why cost-effective clinical approaches are critical to managed care success. *Health Affairs* **16** (3), 239–47.
13. **Vogel, R.J.** International price controls and the protection of intellectual property rights for the pharmaceutical industry. Center for Health Outcomes & PharmacoEconomic Research, Summer, 2001.
14. **Walczak, S.** (2000). Redesigning the medical office for improved efficiency: an object-oriented event-driven messaging system. *Journal of Medical Systems* **24** (1), 29–37.
15. **Braddock, C.H., III** et al. (1999). Informed decision making in outpatient practice: time to get back to basics. *Journal of the American Medical Association* **282** (24), 2313–20.
16. **Mardsen, J.** (2000). An evaluation of the safety and effectiveness of telephone triage as a method of patient prioritization in an ophthalmic accident and emergency service. *Journal of Advanced Nursing* **31** (2), 401–9.
17. **Nauright, L.P., Moneyham, L., and Williamson, J.** (2000). Telephone triage and consultation: an emerging role for nurses. *Nursing Outlook* **47** (5), 219–26.
18. **McKay, H.G.** et al. (1998). Feasibility and use of an internet support service for diabetes self-management. *The Diabetes Educator* **24** (2), 174–9.
19. **O'Connor, P.J.** et al. (1996). Mechanism of action and impact of a cystitis clinical practice guideline on outcomes and costs of care in an HMO. *Joint Commission Journal Quality Improvement* **22** (10), 673–82.
20. **Von Korff, M. and Moore, J.C.** (2001). Stepped care for back pain: activating approaches for primary care. *Annals of Internal Medicine* **134** (9), 911–17.
21. **Hoff, T.** et al. (2001). Characteristics and work experiences of hospitalists in the United States. *Archives of Internal Medicine* **161** (6), 851–8.
22. **Guyn, T.** (1999). The family physician as a hospitalist. *American Family Physician* **60** (2), 402, 404.
23. **DeGruy, F.V. III.** (1997). Mental healthcare in the primary care setting: a paradigm problem. *Families, Systems & Health* **15**, 3–26.
24. **Cummings, N.A., Cummings, J.L., and Johnson, J.N.** *Behavioral Health in Primary Care: A Guide for Clinical Integration.* Madison CT: Psychosocial Press, 1997.
25. **Brown, G.** et al. (1998). Economic evaluation of community based care; lessons from twelve studies in Ontario. *Journal of Evaluation in Clinical Practice* **6** (3), 1–19.
26. **Sobel, D.** (1995). Rethinking medicine: improving health outcomes with cost-effective psychosocial interventions. *Psychosomatic Medicine* **57**, 234–44.
27. **Doherty, W.J., McDaniel, S.H., and Baird, M.A.** (1996). Five levels of primary care/behavioral healthcare collaboration. *Behavioral Healthcare Tomorrow*, p. 25.
28. **Gold, M.R., Siegel, J.E., Russell, L.B., and Weinstein, M.C.**, ed. *Cost-Effectiveness in Health & Medicine.* New York: Oxford University Press, 1996.
29. **Mosser, G.** (1996). Clinical process improvement: engage first, measure later. *Quality Management in Health Care* **4** (4), 11–20.
30. **Crabtree, B.** et al. (1998). Primary care practice organization and preventive services delivery; a qualitative analysis. *Journal of Family Practice* **46** (5), 404–9.
31. **Weed, L.J.** *Knowledge Coupling: New Premises and New Tools for Medical Care and Education.* New York NY: Springer-Verlag, 1991.
32. **Corrigan, J.M. and Nielsen, D.M.** (1993). Toward the development of uniform reporting standards for managed care organizations: the health plan employer data and information set. *Joint Commission Journal of Quality Improvement* **19**, 566–75.
33. **Wagner, E.H.** (2000). The role of patient care teams in chronic disease management. *British Medical Journal* **320**, 569–72.
34. **Buntinx, F.** et al. (1993). Influencing diagnostic and preventative performance in ambulatory care by feedback and reminders: a review. *Family Practice* **10** (2), 219–28.
35. **Harris, J.R., Caldwell, B., and Cahill, K.** (1998). Measuring the public's health in an era of accountability: lessons from HEDIS. *American Journal of Preventive Medicine* **14** (Suppl. 3), 9–13.
36. **O'Connor, P.J., Solberg, L.I., and Baird, M.** (1998). The future of primary care. The enhanced primary care model. *Journal of Family Practice* **47**, 62–7.
37. **Weed, L.J.** (1999). Clinical judgement revisited. *Methods of Information in Medicine* **38**, 279–86.
38. **Ellrodt, G.** et al. (1997). Evidence-based disease management. *Journal of the American Medical Association* **278** (20), 1687–892.
39. **Kravitz, R.L.** (2001). Measuring patients' expectations and requests. *Annals of Internal Medicine* **134**, 881–8.
40. **Council on Graduate Medical Education Thirteenth Report.** *Physician Education for a Changing Health Care Environment.* US Department of Health and Human Services, 1999.

11

Prevention and health promotion

11 Prevention and health promotion

11.1 Principles of prevention

David Mant

The health gap between rich and poor nations, and between rich and poor people within nations, is shameful. Life expectancy in much of sub-Saharan Africa is now half that in Northern Europe. In the United Kingdom, life expectancy is still 9 years longer for men in social class I than in social class V. It is naive to think that medicine can prevent this situation. The fundamental step in achieving good health remains the elimination of poverty, with consequent access to food, sanitation, education, and shelter. But the power of medicine lies in the scientific understanding it provides of the disease process. Preventive medicine uses this understanding both to try to reduce the risk of disease and to detect and appropriately treat emergent disease before it does damage.

What is the scope for prevention? Figure 1 shows the number of women expected to die at different ages if 10 000 were subject to the age-specific death rates in England and Wales of today compared to the 1870s (the pattern is similar for men). The dramatic fall in deaths during childhood and early adulthood has meant that the modal age of death is now over 80 years. However, what medicine cannot offer is immortality. The proportion of women surviving to age 65 who live on to age 100 is still very low, about 0.5 per cent. So there seems to be a reasonable expectation that effective preventive medicine might make death before age 70 or 80 years uncommon—but the objective is delay of death, and hopefully better quality of life before death, rather than absolute prevention of death.[1]

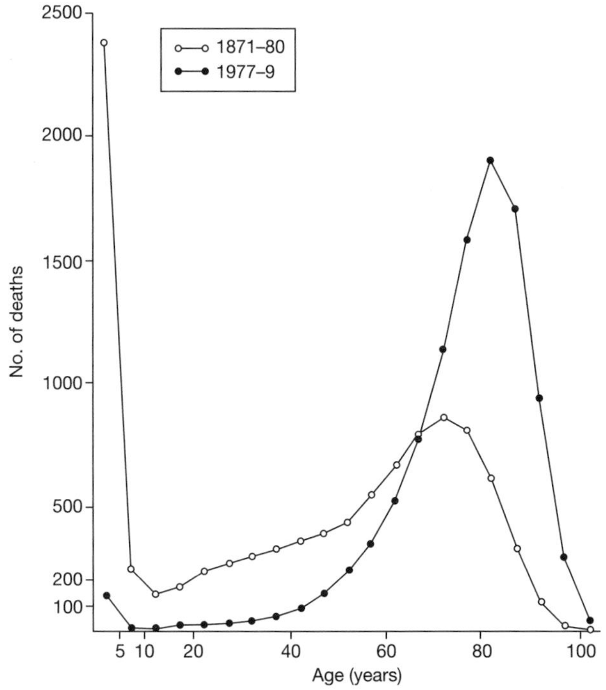

Fig. 1 Numbers of women dying at different ages if 10 000 were subject from birth to the mortality rates current in 1871–1880 and in 2000. (*Source:* Doll, R. (1983). *British Medical Journal* **286**, 445–53.)

Preventive strategies

The prevention paradox

The main difference between preventive and curative medicine is the focus on risk. Preventive medicine aims to reduce the risk of disease and the risk of further morbidity and mortality in those who develop disease. It offers hope for the future rather than immediate benefit. The benefit from preventive medicine is the absence of future disease. This is a difficult benefit to champion, particularly to the individual. As Geoffrey Rose pointed out many years ago, not only is the benefit intangible but many people must take precautions in order to prevent illness in only a few. Even in a country where diphtheria is common, several hundred children must be immunized to prevent one death. Rose called this the prevention paradox—a preventive measure which brings large benefits to the community may offer little to each participating individual.[2]

The risk paradox

The best way to minimize the prevention paradox is to target preventive activity at people at high risk of disease, but this strategy is in itself paradoxical. For example, one of the risk factors for cardiovascular disease is a high blood cholesterol level. Figure 2 shows the prevalence of high cholesterol in the UK population, the death rate associated with each cholesterol level (shown by broken line), and the proportion of all cholesterol attributable deaths occurring at each level (% given above each column). The risk paradox is that although those with a blood cholesterol greater than or equal to 7.5 mmol/l are at highest individual risk of disease, the population at highest risk is that associated with a cholesterol level of 5.5–6.0 mmol/l. This is simply because of the number of people at risk—there are far fewer people in the high than in the moderate risk group. Targeting just the high-risk group will have relatively little impact on the total number of deaths.

Defining and identifying the at-risk population

As preventive medicine seeks to reduce future disease, its patients are usually identified by characteristics that predict risk of developing the disease. Some public health interventions can be applied without identifying the at-risk population—you can pass seat belt legislation and increase the tax on tobacco without identifying either drivers or smokers. However, most interventions in

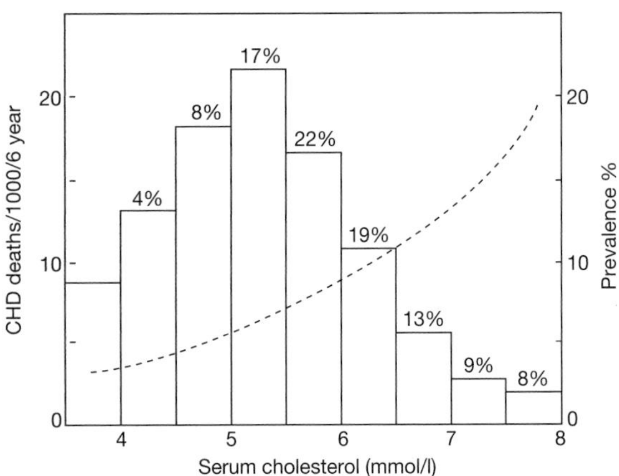

Fig. 2 Proportion of coronary heart disease deaths attributable to raised serum cholesterol occurring at each level (figures above columns). Columns show the prevalence of different levels of cholesterol in the population. The broken line shows coronary heart disease mortality at each level. (Reproduced from Rose, G. *The Strategy of Preventive Medicine*. Oxford: Oxford University Press, 1992, p. 23.)

Box 1 Finding those who need preventive care

- *Registration*—Most socialized health systems keep registers. These may be simply demographic (e.g. age, sex, and address) or contain phenotypic or genetic details of individuals. Effective preventive medicine is much easier where registration exists and its accuracy is systematically maintained.
- *Screening*—The objective of screening is to identify early disease or high risk of disease (e.g. neoplastic dysplasia) before significant morbidity occurs. It can do harm as well as good—it may generate 'false alarms' and detect disease that would not otherwise present during the patient's lifetime. Its benefit needs to be carefully assessed, normally in a randomized trial. Population screening is most efficient when based on an accurate population register.
- *Case-finding*—This involves identifying at-risk individuals during routine clinical work (normally in clinical consultations, but sometimes through contact or family tracing). It is less efficient than systematic population screening, but sometimes provides better access to socially disadvantaged groups who may respond poorly to screening invitations or have no registered address. It also allows some interventions to be given at a particularly appropriate moment (e.g. smoking cessation advice at a consultation for cough or contraceptive advice after termination of pregnancy).

clinical preventive medicine in primary care are delivered to individuals. It is, therefore, necessary not only to define the at-risk population but also to identify the individuals within it. You do not just need to know that smokers are at risk, you need to know who smokes. This is usually done in one of three ways—registration, screening, and case-finding (see Box 1).

Interventions to modify risk

The marked improvements in health that have been achieved in economically developed countries over the past 200 years are not attributable to medicine. Primary care professionals should not pretend to themselves that preventive care for the individual is an alternative to effective public health action. Nevertheless, preventive medicine is an important and integral part of good curative medicine. All doctors have a responsibility to think about why someone is ill. Whatever cause is identified (physiological, social, or psychological) the question of whether the cause can be prevented and the risk of future disease reduced should be addressed. Doctors who work in a primary care role, particularly those with a registered population, have the added responsibility to ask themselves whether the risk should be addressed at a population rather than just an individual patient level. A classic description of how a primary care practitioner can adopt a population approach is given in Tudor Hart's book, *A New Kind of Doctor.*[3]

Box 2 Primary and secondary prevention

- *Primary prevention*—interventions to reduce the risk of disease in healthy people (e.g. use of seat belts to prevent injury in car accidents; tobacco control to prevent the occurrence of smoking related disease; immunization against infectious disease).
- *Secondary prevention*—interventions to prevent avoidable morbidity in people with disease (e.g. treatment of vascular disease with aspirin; screening for early cancer).

Primary and secondary prevention

Preventive interventions have traditionally been categorized as primary, secondary, and tertiary depending on their objectives. However, the term secondary prevention is now often used to cover both secondary and tertiary categories (see Box 2). It is immediately obvious that the distinction between primary and secondary is sometimes difficult. Some interventions can fall into more than one category (e.g. stopping smoking reduces the progression as well as the onset of many smoking-related diseases) and the definition of disease is not absolute (e.g. many apparently healthy people will have undetected disease). Nevertheless, the pragmatic categorization of preventive interventions into primary and secondary is often useful in practice.

Immunization

One preventive intervention that spans primary and secondary prevention is immunization (see Chapter 11.2). It can be a very effective preventive strategy. It is arguably the most important medical contribution to disease prevention, and an important task for primary care in all countries. Vaccination against smallpox has led to global eradication of the disease; eradication of polio seems a feasible global objective in the next decade. Vaccination against many other diseases, particularly diseases of childhood, such as measles, diphtheria and polio, has led to rapid and dramatic falls in disease incidence. A number of new and important vaccines are on the horizon—for example, a malaria vaccine. However, the key point to remember is that the existence of an effective vaccine does not guarantee the success of an immunization programme. This depends on the effective delivery of the vaccine to the at-risk population.

Prophylactic treatment

Although most people think of medicines as cures for current illness, many medicines are prescribed with a view to preventing future illness. Inhaled steroids are given to prevent asthma, uricosuric agents to prevent gout, anticoagulants to prevent stroke, and lipid lowering agents and beta-blockers to prevent heart attacks. Many, perhaps most, drugs have the potential to be used for prevention as well as cure. In some cases (e.g. treatment of diabetes), the distinction between prevention and cure is unhelpful—treatment aims to prevent morbidity in both the short and long-term. However, prophylactic treatment with drugs is less helpful when a high-risk population cannot be easily defined. It is almost always inappropriate to use prophylactic treatment to reduce population risk for three reasons—the strategy is seldom cost-effective, increasing the reliance of the population on medicine is an adverse social outcome, and uncommon adverse effects can easily outweigh any clinical benefit. The use of aspirin to prevent heart disease provides an interesting case study in which costs are low but cardiovascular benefit needs to be balanced against the risk of haemorrhage.(4)

Changing behaviour

Environmental factors contribute substantially to differences in premature morbidity and mortality. Many of these environmental factors reflect individual behaviour. Eating more healthily, taking more exercise, and avoiding riding on a motorcycle are all effective ways of preventing disease. People do listen to doctors, and a number of clinical trials have shown advice on behaviour modification to be cost-effective, even though the effect size may be small (e.g. in most studies only about one in 20–30 smokers given brief advice to stop smoking actually quit). Brief advice is most effective if practical in nature (giving guidance on how change can be achieved) and if backed up by written advice to take home. A review of the evidence for the effectiveness of primary care based interventions to influence individual behaviour is given in Chapters 11.4–11.6 and in the sources cited below.

Environmental change

Many environmental causes of disease are best modified on a public health rather than an individual basis. Such factors include the safety of the workplace, environmental pollution, transport safety, food hygiene, and provision of clean water. However, a number of diseases have environmental causes that can be recognized and avoided by the individual patient. On a global scale, avoidance of insect and other disease vectors (e.g. by netting) and attention to nutritional hygiene (e.g. by filtering water) are probably the most important. In economically developed countries, the most common diseases amenable to individual environmental intervention are those associated with atopy—such as asthma and eczema. Not all patients have an identifiable allergenic cause for their symptoms and, even if one is identified, avoidance (e.g. of house dust mite in asthma) may not be easy. But dramatic improvement can occur and treating contact dermatitis without giving advice on contact avoidance, or treating louse bites without giving advice on how to rid clothes of lice, is bad clinical practice.

What is achievable?

What interventions work?

This chapter is about the principles of prevention—much of the evidence about the effectiveness of primary care interventions is summarized in other chapters, both in this section of Volume 1 and in relation to specific diseases in Volume 2. Nevertheless, it is worth drawing attention to the three best sources of evidence on prevention in primary care. The first is the Task Force Reports from Canada[5] and the United States,[6] which focus on issues of importance in economically developed countries. The Canadian Task Force on Preventive Health Care is probably the most accessible—it is easy to read, regularly updated, and available free on the Internet. It categorizes preventive interventions by their target group (i.e. mother and baby, children, adolescents, adults, and the elderly) and summarizes the evidence for clinical effectiveness.

The second good source of evidence on effectiveness is the International Cochrane Library, which contains a number of very good cumulative meta-analysis on issues of importance to prevention in primary care, ranging from vaccine efficacy to control of smoking through retail tobacco sales. Specific reference to reviews contained on this database are given in other chapters, but there is one general review on the effect of different strategies to implement prevention in primary care.[7]

The newest source of evidence is the *British Medical Journal* sponsored publication *Clinical Evidence*, which is published and updated quarterly in both paper and electronic formats. This tries to provide summarized and evidence-based answers to questions that clinicians face in everyday practice. A good example of the format in which answers are provided is provided by the article on behavioural interventions to reduce the risk of vascular disease cited below.[8]

Programme effectiveness

These three sources of evidence on effectiveness all report the results of clinical trials. However, clinical trials are often done in settings far removed from everyday life in primary care—participants are compliant, those delivering the intervention are highly trained, the technology is of high specification, and quality control is rigorous. These conditions may not hold on a wet Tuesday morning in a poorly resourced practice in a deprived area. When preventive interventions fail, the most common reason is lack of effective implementation of the programme, rather than lack of effectiveness of the intervention itself.

The importance of considering programme effectiveness is seen most vividly in relation to immunization and screening programmes. The three most important issues that determine programme effectiveness are shown in Box 3. The effect on programme effectiveness of failure in just one of these areas is well documented in the United Kingdom in relation both to immunization (e.g. the resurgence of pertussis after media publicity about potential adverse effects of the vaccine led to a fall in uptake) and to cervical screening (e.g. lack of quality control in cervical sampling and cytological assessment led to false negative results and avoidable mortality).

Cultural constraints

Many preventive interventions aim to change behaviour. Most behaviour has a strong socio-cultural component and reflects prevalent attitudes and norms in society. Preventive interventions are severely constrained by this social context—convincing individuals to stop smoking, eat less salt, drink less beer, or drive more slowly is difficult if everyone else is doing the opposite. For example, the mean blood cholesterol level in Finland is almost twice that in Japan (Fig. 3). Migrant studies suggest that this difference is dietary rather than genetic in origin and so medical advice to reduce fat consumption should have the potential to reduce substantially blood cholesterol level. However, even in the context of a clinical trial, dietary advice from health professionals in a community setting seldom achieves a reduction in blood cholesterol of more than 3–5 per cent. Trials of salt restriction (to lower blood pressure) show a similar result—a substantial reduction of 188 mmol/day (6.7 g) is on average necessary to achieve a fall of 4 mmHg in systolic blood pressure,[8] and many find this degree of salt restriction unpalatable. Counter-cultural change is difficult to achieve.

Time effects

Things change over time. The North Karelia project was a large-scale long-term programme to reduce mortality from cardiovascular disease in Northern Finland started in 1972 which involved both public health and individual intervention.[9] Figure 4 compares mortality from cardiovascular disease in North Karelia with that in 10 other provinces in Finland before and during the intervention by plotting two regression lines. The difference in slope of these two lines shows that the intervention was to some extent

Box 3 Key issues determining preventive programme effectiveness

- *Coverage*—what proportion of the population at risk receive the intervention?
- *Delivery*—are factors that effect the delivery of the intervention (like the maintenance of equipment, the training of staff, and the storage of biological materials) up to scratch?
- *Quality control*—are standards set and monitored for key indicators of the intervention process (e.g. immune response or predictive value of screening).

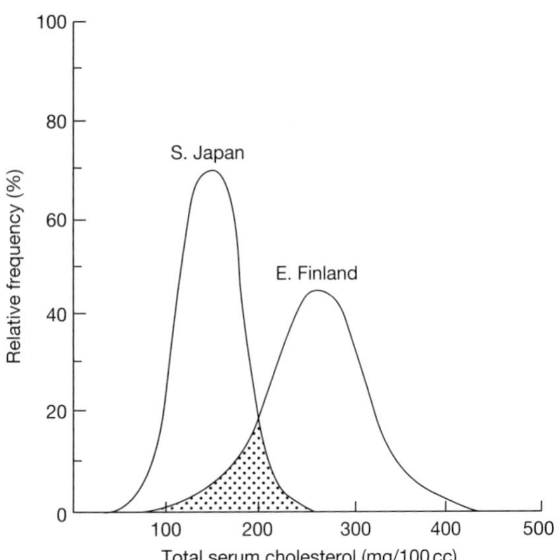

Fig. 3 Distribution of serum cholesterol in southern Japan and eastern Finland. (Reproduced from Rose, G. *Strategy of Prevention*. Oxford: Oxford University Press, 1992, p. 57.)

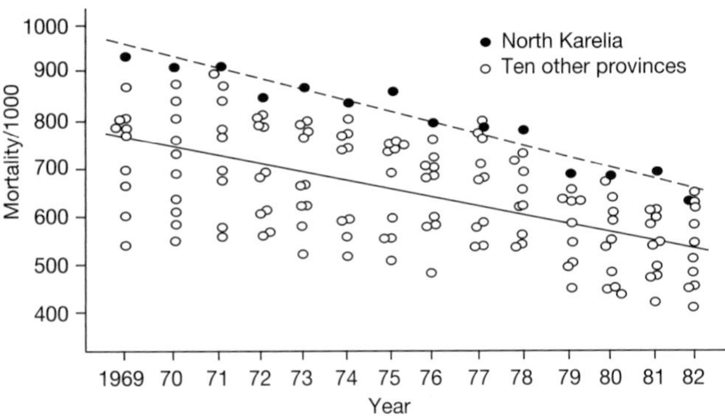

Fig. 4 The North Karelia Project. Age standardized annual mortality from cardiovascular disease in men aged 35–64 in Finland, 1969–1982. (Redrawn from original data published by Tuomilehto, J. et al. (1986). *British Medical Journal* **293**, 1068–71.)

effective. However, far more impressive in magnitude is the absolute fall in mortality over time in both North Karelia and the other provinces. The lessons for preventive medicine are twofold. The effect of medical intervention may be small in relation to the effect of other economic and social influences. And the change in baseline risk and social context over time may be so rapid that it will substantially influence the absolute benefit of any preventive intervention.

Learning from mistakes

Primary care must learn from its mistakes—in relation to prevention, they are numerous.(10) The main lessons are shown in Box 4. The first and most important lesson is that identification of risk is not enough—modifying the risk is the hard bit that requires a commitment of time and energy, which is sometimes beyond the resources of primary care. Identifying risk without being able to do anything effective to ameliorate it is unethical, and we still do it all the time. The second lesson is that effective prevention needs to be systematic and organized, with register-based call and recall. The charge made by the *Lancet* against the UK cervical screening programme of 'Death by Incompetence' was not undeserved at the time and needs to be remembered.(11) The third lesson is that it is important both to set and audit achievement targets, and to ensure that they are achievable. Preventive care is littered with unfulfilled enthusiasms and unrealistic dreams. Lastly, most effective interventions in primary care have involved non-medical staff, in both support and front-line roles. Medical staff often have the benefit of authority, but non-medical staff often have the benefit of being more systematic in their approach, having received specific training in prevention, and having more time. Prevention is an area for teamwork.

Box 4 Four lessons for delivering effective preventive care

- Do not just identify risk
- Be systematic
- Set achievable targets
- Involve non-medical staff

Conclusion

Preventive medicine is an integral part of clinical practice for all primary care doctors. It is our responsibility as clinicians not only to cure the presenting illness but also to take action where possible to prevent future morbidity. We must seek the potential for prevention in each clinical consultation. However, we must also recognize that medicine is not the main determinant of health. Our ability to prevent disease through individual health care is constrained by the cultural and economic environment in which we practice. Therefore, we also have a unique and powerful responsibility to act as advocates for our patients in seeking to ensure that the environmental and social causes of ill-health are addressed. Good clinical practice entails preventive medicine, but good preventive medicine is more than just good clinical practice.

References

1. **Doll, R.** (1983). Prospects for prevention. *British Medical Journal* **286**, 445–52.
2. **Rose, G.** *The Strategy of Preventive Medicine.* Oxford: Oxford University Press, 1992.
3. **Hart, J.T.** *A New Kind of Doctor.* London: Merlin Press, 1988.
4. **Sudlow, C.** (2000). What is the role of antithrombotic treatment in asymptomatic people? *Clinical Evidence* **4**, 70–1 (electronic version at www.clinicalevidence.org).
5. **The Canadian Guide to Preventive Health Care.** Ottawa: Canadian Government Publishing, 1994 (reprinted 1998; electronic version at www.fedpubs.com/subject/health/clinpre.htm).
6. **Guide to Clinical Preventive Services,** 2nd edn. Report of the US Preventive Services Task Force. Washington: US Department of Health and Human Services, 1995 (updated electronic version at www.odphp.osophs.dhhs.gov/pubs/guidecps).
7. **Hulscher, M., Wensing M., van der Weijden, T., and Grol, R.** (2001). Interventions to implement prevention in primary care (Cochrane Review). In *The Cochrane Library* Issue 2. Oxford: Update Software.
8. **Mulrow, C. and Jackson, R.** (2000). What are the effects of lifestyle changes in asymptomatic people with primary hypertension. *Clinical Evidence* **4**, 61–5 (electronic version at www.clinicalevidence.org).
9. **Tuomilehto, J.** et al. (1986). Decline in cardiovascular mortality in North Karelia and other parts of Finland. *British Medical Journal* **293**, 1068–71.
10. **Mant, D.** (1994). Prevention. *Lancet* **344**, 1343–6.
11. **Editorial** (1985). Death by incompetence. *Lancet* **ii**, 363–4.

11.2 Immunization and vaccination

Claire Parker

Introduction

The goal

Immunization against infectious disease is one of the most important preventive health interventions known, second only to a clean water supply. Its goal is the reduction of human suffering and economic loss. In particular, the prevention of common, serious, childhood infections associated with high morbidity and mortality makes an enormous impact on the health of a population and its subsequent economic productivity. Immunization prevents the development of invasive infection or toxicity, rather than treating its complications. It is therefore a method of primary prevention.

Advances in understanding the molecular basis of protective immune responses, the pathogenesis of infections, and the population dynamics of their spread, have all led to improvements in the design of vaccines and programmes for their delivery. The repertoire of vaccine-preventable infections has steadily increased throughout the twentieth and into the twenty-first century (Table 1). The success of many immunization programmes has made the development of vaccines a goal for the prevention of virulent infections, new and old, for which effective immuno-prophylaxis does not yet exist.

The basis

Active immunization, or vaccination, works by harnessing the mechanisms of adaptive (antigen-specific) immunity which when successful, link the activation of innate processes which eliminate infection to pathogen-specific stimulation. The rationale is that individual immune protection is provided artificially in advance of natural exposure, at very minimal risk compared with the risks associated with naturally occurring infection, and at affordable cost.

In addition, vaccines which reduce transmission or carriage of communicable diseases contribute to population immunity. At high levels of vaccine uptake, this is very important in curtailing endemic circulation and epidemic spread. Ultimately, sustained population immunity can lead to the extinction of communicable pathogens if there are no other reservoirs of infection.

This strategy is very successful where pathogens naturally elicit immune responses which are protective against any subsequent exposure, should the individual survive acute infection. However, where pathogens have evolved to evade natural immunity, or where variants rapidly escape under immune selection pressure, the biological problems facing vaccine development are considerable.

The impact of immunization

Immunization programmes have had spectacular success. In 1980, the World Health Organization announced the global eradication of smallpox and marked the end of a sustained, world-wide vaccination campaign in 1982. The western hemisphere has been declared free of wild-type polio, and most western industrialized countries have eradicated measles. The global eradication of measles and polio is achievable with existing vaccines, and a recently revised target of 2005 has been set for polio by the WHO. In 1994, Finland announced the eradication of measles, mumps, and rubella, 12 years after introducing the two dose combined MMR programme.[1]

The impact of pathogen-specific vaccines in the prevention and control of infectious diseases was evident in the abrupt fall in incidence rates of diphtheria, polio, tetanus, pertussis, measles, and more recently, haemophilus B infection, hepatitis B, and yellow fever, following the introduction of immunization.

While improved general health, nutrition, and living standards have contributed to the reduction of vaccine-preventable diseases in developed countries, they do not account for its dramatic association with routine immunization in countries where high vaccine uptake was achieved rapidly. Reduction of invasive Haemophilus influenzae B diseases in affluent Western countries followed inclusion of the vaccine in the childhood immunization schedule, and underscored the susceptibility of otherwise healthy infants to virulent pathogens, if they lacked specific immunity. It is nevertheless true that the impact of routine immunization is most evident where the burden of disease is high, as it is in developing countries with poor living standards, inadequate nutrition and high levels of co-morbidity.

Outbreaks of infection occur when vaccine uptake falls precipitously. In the 1970s, the uptake of pertussis vaccine fell because of fears of a causal link with brain damage, and led to an upsurge in notified cases of pertussis. This declined again in the wake of restored confidence and increased vaccine uptake. Where routine vaccine uptake remains low in defined groups (e.g. the Amish, or in travelling communities) localized outbreaks of highly communicable diseases such as measles occur. In Ireland, in 2000, when uptake fell to 76 per cent, a serious outbreak with two fatalities occurred. In developing countries where routine immunizations are not yet adequately deployed, the burden of vaccine-preventable infection remains very high.

Cost-effectiveness of immunization programmes

Immunization against measles, polio, tetanus, diphtheria, and pertussis are among the most cost-effective public health measures known. The ability to immunize against many infections simultaneously and the availability of safe, effective combination vaccines have enhanced the uptake and speed of acquisition of immunity, and dramatically increased the cost-effectiveness of childhood immunizations.

It is much more expensive to give routine immunizations outside the infant schedule: BCG is ~40 times more so in developing countries.[2] A similar inflation of cost is seen when other vaccines are given out of schedule, and this is a critical factor for countries with scant resources, whose ability to deliver childhood immunization routinely is contingent on maximizing cost-effectiveness, or otherwise relying on outside aid.

Requirements for successful immunization programmes

If a vaccination programme is to succeed as a preventive health intervention, the benefits of protection must outweigh the risks at individual and population level. Three elements are needed for this to happen: (i) safe, effective vaccines (and when indicated, immunoglobulins for passive immunization); (ii) appropriately designed immunization programmes, accessible and acceptable to the target population; and (iii) continuing surveillance to monitor the uptake and impact of immunization and to detect unexpected side-effects or declining efficacy of vaccines.

The many successes of immunization programmes have been due to the effectiveness and high uptake of vaccines, across genetically diverse human populations. The relative genetic stability of target organisms has contributed to vaccine efficacy, and allowed the components of many routine immunizations to remain essentially unchanged. High uptake has been possible in developed countries because of infrastructure for delivering immunization and, until recently, the widespread public motivation for vaccine-prevention of life-threatening or disabling infections. In addition, most developed countries have comprehensive monitoring of vaccine uptake and adverse reactions, which have allow planned responses to evidence of falling vaccine uptake, and rapid withdrawal of vaccines associated with significant adverse reactions.

Challenges to immunization in the twenty-first century

For a while in the twentieth century, there was optimism that infectious diseases might become a thing of the past, eliminated by existing methods

Table 1 Vaccine-preventable infections

Disease	Routine (R)/ special (S) ([a] in other populations)	Vaccine types (intramuscular or deep subcutaneous, unless stated)	Comments
Adenovirus	S	Live attenuated virus, oral	USA military
Anthrax	S	Inactivated	Occupational; bioterrorism
Tetanus	R	Toxoid	
(Cholera)	N/A	Inactivated	Withdrawn: poor efficacy
Diphtheria	R	Toxoid	Non-toxigenic strains appearing
Haemophilus influenzae B	R (S)	Conjugated capsular poly	
Hepatitis A	S	Recombinant surface Ag	Travel to endemic areas
Hepatitis B	S[b] (R[a])	Recombinant surface Ag	Contact/exposure to contaminated body fluids
Influenza virus A and B	S	Inactivated; sub-unit	Need to annually uptake; at risk groups: elderly; chronic disease, immunosuppressed
Japanese encephalitis	(R[a])		Risk of anaphylaxis
Leprosy	(R[a])	Live BCG	
Measles	R	Live attenuated virus	
Meningococcal C *Meningococcal A* Meningococcal Y *Meningococcal W135*	R (S) S ? S S	Conjugated capsular poly Capsular polysaccharide	At risk of invasive bacterial infection A/Y/W135 important in pilgrims to Saudi Arabia
Mumps	R	Live attenuated virus	
Pertussis	R	Inactivated whole cell; acellular	
Polio	R	OPV: live, attenuated virus, oral IPV: inactivated	
Pneumococcal	S	Capsular polysaccharide	Asplenics, and other groups at risk of invasive capsulated bacterial infection
	S (R[a])	Conjugated-polysaccharide	Introduced into USA recently
Q fever (Coxsiella burnetti)	S	Inactivated	Lab, vet, and abbatoir workers in endemic areas
Rabies	S	Inactivated	Post-exposure prophylaxis works
(Smallpox)	Not in use	Live; highly attenuated	? Bioterrorism[c]
Tick-borne encephalitis	S (R[a])	Inactivated (unlicensed in UK)	Walkers/campers in Eastern Europe and Scandinavia
Typhoid	S	Capsular polysaccharide; live, attenuated, oral	Travel to endemic area
Tuberculosis	S[b]	Live BCG	
Varicella-zoster	R	Live viral	Introduced into USA recently
Yellow Fever	S (R[a])	Live viral	Travel to endemic area
Yersinia (plague)	S	Inactivated	Laboratory and field workers

[a] May be routine in other countries/populations.

[b] But included in the routine childhood immunizations (see below) for at risk neonates in the UK.

[c] May be indicated for special use if bioterrorism expands the threat; otherwise not in use.

Note: Vaccines commonly given in the UK by 'special indication', to individuals or groups at enhanced risk of exposure or complications of disease, are printed in italics.

of immunization, effective antimicrobial treatment, or environmental and vector control. The last 20 years has revealed this view to be naïve, and there are essentially three main challenges for the prevention and control of infectious disease, each of which has already produced an intense response from disciplines involved in the development, delivery, and presentation of immunization.

Firstly, the burden of vaccine-preventable infections is still carried predominantly by developing countries who are too poor to implement routine childhood immunizations. The challenges are primarily economic, political and organizational, and implementation in many developing countries depends on outside resources and agencies working with local personnel. The Expanded Programme of Immunization (EPI, see below) was designed by the WHO to address the epidemiological needs of prevention in Sub-Saharan Africa and the Indian subcontinent. It involves modifications to both the contents and the schedules normally used in the developed world. Many countries have now updated the EPI as resources gradually become available to address additional disease burdens.

Secondly, the elimination of vaccine-preventable infections such as measles, polio, and diphtheria from some parts of the world, given their persistence in others, is inherently unstable. The link between falling vaccine uptake and outbreaks of infection have been referred to. When population immunity to highly communicable infections drifts below critical levels, isolated outbreaks which would have been 'fire-walled' by pre-existing immunity can spread exponentially. Maintaining vaccine uptake in developed countries is increasingly difficult. As disease incidence declines, public memory of their severity fades and concerns about rare, often unfounded, vaccine side-effects cause a sharp fall in uptake and with it renewed threats of disease outbreak. This is a major challenge to the acceptability of existing programmes, vaccines, and schedules. In many ways, it is the challenge most closely identifiable with the business of primary care in the developed world.

Thirdly, there is an enormous challenge to traditional vaccinology from the escalating burden of non-vaccine preventable infections, many of which are caused by genetically unstable organisms amongst which rising anti-microbial and vector resistance threatens effective treatment or secondary control.

The astonishing genetic mutability and diversity of pathogens has led to the emergence of major new viral infections, the most significant of which is HIV, and to the re-emergence of multidrug resistant malaria and tuberculosis. These are now the leading infectious causes of death world-wide. There are as yet no licensed vaccines against HIV or plasmodium malariae, and the efficacy of existing BCG vaccine against TB varies unpredictably between populations, suggesting that human genetic polymorphisms may be important to consider in the design of new vaccines.

Influenza is such a virulent infection for clinically vulnerable groups that it is cost-effective to annually tune the antigenic composition of vaccines to match predicted circulating strains and keep pace with minor genetic drift. However, vaccines capable of longer term protection against a wide range of sub-types would be a major breakthrough. At present, the threat of an influenza pandemic requires constant global surveillance and continual updating of international contingency plans for a rapid response to an outbreak with a potentially lethal new sub-type, requiring a totally new vaccine.

These rapidly mutating pathogens and many other infectious agents still exact a heavy toll of death and disease world-wide. Respiratory syncytial virus, rotaviruses, bacteria which colonize mucosal surfaces (gonorrhoea, chlamydia, cholera) and parasitic infections (trypanosomes, schistosomes, filaria, and helminths) have resisted the development of effective, safe vaccines. They have evolved to successfully escape, evade or subvert a range of natural host defences including adaptive, antigen-specific immune responses and pose many similar problems for traditional approaches to vaccine development.

Compounding all these challenges are the rapid human and environmental changes which continue to drive the dynamic evolution of pathogens. Whether currently or potentially vaccine-preventable, the speed and scale of infectious disease transmission is facilitated by air travel and the forced migration of individuals and population groups due to economic, political, military, and climatic disaster. Fewer and fewer ecological niches remain stable enclosures for the 'natural' containment of infection.

As this chapter is being written, the risk of biological warfare has suddenly become a reality, and the spectre of terrorist re-introduction of smallpox, and the release of anthrax or bubonic plague, are being seriously evaluated by the WHO and governmental public health departments.

Understanding the anatomy of existing vaccines and programmes aids appreciation of the modifications already made for different epidemiological situations, and the need for novel vaccines against emergent and established infections which are not yet preventable by active immunization.

Effective, safe immunization

Active immunization

Vaccination induces long-term immunity and depends on an adequately functioning immune system. Vaccines are broadly divided into 'live' products which replicate following immunization (attenuated strains of viruses or bacteria) and 'inactive' products which do not, but provide a fixed 'bolus' of antigenic material (whole inactivated viruses or bacteria, antigenic components, or sub-units of pathogens, or toxoids). In the absence of contraindications, licensed vaccination is the safest, most cost-effective method of inducing individual, long-term immunity to a wide range of bacterial and viral infections. Passive immunization, providing short-term protection, is discussed later.

Effective, safe vaccines

All new vaccines are rigorously tested before licensing and continually monitored afterwards for unexpected side-effects or loss of function. No vaccine is 100 per cent safe or effective, however, and known factors which might enhance individual risk should always be discussed and excluded at the point of delivery (see Table 2).

Correlates of protection

Currently licensed vaccines, with the exception of BCG, generate pathogen-specific antibodies which neutralize infectivity or toxicity. Antibodies recognize three-dimensional features of molecules in their natural conformation, and can 'intercept' intact pathogens or their products in the extra-cellular phase, preventing their invasion of cells or toxic effects on tissues.

Vaccine efficacy depends on several factors. Firstly, antibodies generated must lead to the elimination of the pathogen following contact, without causing severe immune-mediated disease in the process. This has not been the case with all vaccines developed. In the 1970s, inactivated RSV vaccines caused an unexpected increase in the severity of bronchiolitis following subsequent exposure to the virus, leading to vaccine withdrawal at an early stage. Recently, a highly effective vaccine against rotaviruses was withdrawn shortly after licensing because of a rare but causal association with intussception. The protection associated with BCG against tuberculosis, which is variable, is cell mediated and antibodies generated do not lead to elimination of the pathogen.

Secondly, vaccine antigens must remain cross-reactive with the pathogen if immune responses are to remain protective. This has been true for many vaccines, but for rapidly mutating pathogen it may not be the case. Rapid genetic drift of influenza viruses leads to successive replacement of strains under antibody selection pressure. There have been occasional reports of antibody-resistant hepatitis B viruses in SE Asia, and non-toxigenic diphtheria strains have emerged in some populations, although they are not very virulent.

Thirdly, immunity must last as long as required to provide protection, if necessary, for life. Antibodies must be present in adequate concentration in body compartments appropriate to the pathogenesis of infection and mode of spread of the agent and, if necessary, their concentration must rapidly increase to match the dose of infecting pathogen. Vaccination addresses these requirements by inducing pathogen-specific immunological memory. When memory is successfully induced, secondary exposure to the antigen, whether a booster vaccine dose or contact with the pathogen, leads to accelerated, amplified antibody responses of enhanced efficiency. Such secondary exposure helps maintain immune memory and when due to contact with the pathogen, leads to its rapid elimination.

Where virulence depends on blood-stream spread systemic antibodies are required and protection is closely linked to levels of circulating pathogen-specific IgG, the predominant serum antibody. Pathogens whose portal of entry is the respiratory, digestive, or uro-genital tract may be neutralized by IgA present in secretions, and local mucosal immunity is an important additional protection against invasive disease. It is also important for population immunity, by reducing the carriage and transmission of pathogens which colonize these surfaces.

Induction of antibody-mediated protection: cellular and molecular mechanisms

Vaccine antigens, whether individually selected in inactivated sub-unit or component vaccines, or unselected as in whole inactivated or live

Table 2 Summary of contra-indications to immunization[a]

	Contra-indications	Comments
All immunizations[b]	Acute illness	Minor coughs/colds without fever or systemic upset not contra-indications
	Definite severe reaction to preceding dose	Severe systemic: fever ≥39.5 within 48 h; anaphylaxis; bronchospasm; laryngeal oedema; generalized collapse; prolonged unresponsiveness; prolonged inconsolable or high pitched crying >4 h; convulsions or encephalopathy within 72 h Severe local: indurated redness/swelling over most of antero-lateral thigh or circumference of arm
	Evolving neurological illness	Not stable epilepsy, stable neurological deficit, febrile convulsions (but advise on fever prevention/control) or FH of epilepsy
	Definite allergy to antibacterials contained in some viral vaccines	e.g. neomycin, polymyxin B
	Definite egg allergy	Influenza and yellow fever contra-indicated MMR not contra-indicated
Live immunizations[c]	Pregnancy	Balance risks of exposure to yellow fever, polio; benefits to woman may outweigh risks
	Avoid within 3/12 of NHIG[d]	Except yellow fever vaccine
BCG, yellow fever, oral typhoid	Immunosuppression: all causes	AVOID in HIV infected even if clinically well Avoid for 3/12 after stopping corticosteroids; 6/12 after stopping chemotherapy
OPV[e], measles, mumps, rubella	Immunosuppressed:	GIVE to HIV infected unless severely symptomatic; consider NHIG, if HIV+ is exposed to measles/varicella-zoster
	AVOID for 3/12 after corticosteroids; 6/12 after chemotherapy	OPV virus excreted for longer by HIV+'s; wash hands after changing nappies; HIV+ contacts at greater risk of acquisition of OPV virus from nappies. If HIV + symptomatic, consider IPV protection

[a] General guide: consult local and national guidelines and product literature. Above based on UK guides.

[b] Avoid i.m. route if bleeding disorder (haemophilia, thrombocytopaenia).

[c] Multiple live vaccines: give simultaneously at separate sites (unless in combined vaccine), or leave 3-week intervals between.

[d] Normal human immunoglobulins.

[e] Oral poliomyelitis vaccine.

Note: The following are NOT contra-indications to immunization: family history of adverse vaccine reaction; previous history of pertussis, measles, rubella, mumps; prematurity: do not postpone vaccinations; stable neurological conditions; contact with infectious disease; asthma, eczema, hayfever, 'snuffles'; antibiotics, local steroids; child's mother pregnant; breast-fed infant; neonatal jaundice; low weight; over recommended age; 'replacement' corticosteroids.

attenuated vaccines, determine the pathogen specificity and protection afforded by immunization. Induction of antibody-mediated immunological memory requires activation of the cellular immune system, in particular CD4+ helper T-lymphocytes, which regulate many aspects of immune induction. CD8+ cytotoxic T-lymphocytes (CTL) are necessary for safe immunization with live vaccines which replicate intracellularly.

Unlike antibodies, T-lymphocytes do not recognize cell-free antigens in their natural conformation, but human cell-surface molecules (histocompatibility antigens) which have been rendered 'foreign' by binding to short peptides derived from the degradation of foreign proteins inside the cell. Efficient T-cell antigens are therefore protein-based.

Peptides derived from the intracellular pathway of lysosomal digestion, into which antigens from inactivated vaccines and released by live vaccines are taken up, bind to Class II histocompatibility antigens (MHC Class II). Helper T-cells specific for these complexes are activated on recognition, releasing cytokines which facilitate: (i) the expansion and differentiation of pathogen-specific B-cell memory clones, which constitute the source of antibody-mediated memory, and (ii) the 'switch' from early IgM secretion to IgG, the predominant serum antibody and, in appropriate locations of induction, secretory IgA associated with mucosal immunity.

Naturally occuring protein-based antigens can provide both B-cell stimulation (in their native conformation) and stimulation of helper T-cells (via their degraded peptides), but it is not necessary that the same antigen provides both signals. Non-protein antigens can be artificially linked (conjugated) to unrelated 'carrier' proteins which can serve the same purpose of eliciting T-cell help.

The technology of conjugating non-protein based antigens such as bacterial polysaccharides to carrier proteins has led to a new generation of vaccines against invasive, virulent capsulated bacteria. These are effective in infants under 18 months, in contrast to plain polysaccharide vaccines. This has allowed the expansion of routine infant immunization programmes to include immunization against Haemophilus influenzae B in the 1980s, and more recently against Meningococcus C in the United Kingdom. Polyvalent conjugated vaccines against multiple, virulent pneumococcal strains have already been introduced into the United States, and are likely to be introduced more generally into the infant schedule as individual countries assess their public health priorities and resources. They are expected to have a major impact on invasive pneumococcal disease in infancy.

Pathogen-specific CTL are crucial for terminating the replication and hence limiting the spread of attenuated live vaccines, and are normally induced following such vaccination. However, in the absence of cellular immunity immunization with live vaccines which cause intracellular infections (all live viral vaccines, BCG, live typhoid vaccines) is unsafe and contra-indicated (see Table 2). CTL recognize complexes of Class I histocompatibility antigens with short foreign peptides, which are generated by a different intracellular pathway, into which samples of newly synthesized proteins from replicating intracellular parasites are directed. Class I histocompatibility antigens are expressed on almost all cell types, allowing CTL specific for the complex to recognize and selectively destroy cells from a wide range of tissues which are infected with replicating intracellular parasites, predominantly viruses but also intracellular bacteria (mycobacteria, typhoid) and protozoa (malaria sporozoites).

Location and duration of antibody-mediated protection: role of vaccine type, dosing schedule and route of administration

Live attenuated vaccine strains replicate in tissues relevant to natural infection and mucosal replication reliably leads to local as well as systemic immunity. Inactivated vaccines differ in their capacity to induce mucosal immunity, and are more sensitive to route of administration. Inactivated polio vaccine does not induce gastrointestinal immunity, and unlike oral polio vaccine is not effective in reducing the carriage or transmission of polio. Current influenza vaccines given parenterally do not reliably induce IgA in respiratory secretions and the extent to which they inhibit transmission is unclear. Nasal administration of inactivated or live attenuated influenza vaccines does induce specific IgA, and may reduce transmission more effectively.

The steady release of antigen during replication of a single dose of live, attenuated vaccine given parenterally may be sufficient to induce solid immunological memory in most recipients. Two doses of the combined MMR vaccine are given because 10 per cent of recipients do not sero-convert initially, and population coverage is less than 100 per cent with the first dose, jeopardizing population immunity. Oral live vaccines and most inactivated vaccines require three separate doses to establish primary immune memory because a single dose of sufficient strength would be too toxic. Inactivated vaccines may be adsorbed onto mineral adjuvants such as alum, to enhance their immunogenicity and reduce reactogenicity. Depending on the vaccine, the age at presentation and the risks of individual exposure, booster doses of vaccine may be needed to maintain individual and population immunity.

The combination of 'like' types of vaccine, where sets of different live strains, or sets of different inactivated antigens, are combined into a single multivalent vaccine, has not been associated with any reduction of immunogenicity or increase in adverse reactions compared with single agent vaccines. The possible exception of a reduction in Hib antibody responses in quadrivalent DaPT-Hib vaccines which use the acellular rather than the whole cell pertussis component is under review, but is likely to be a technical rather than a 'biological' problem, and relatively easy to overcome. Single antigen vaccines are available where clinically indicated or where the epidemiology makes this appropriate (e.g. the use of single antigen measles in some developing countries), but are not recommended on safety or efficacy grounds otherwise.

Unwanted effects of vaccines

Vaccine associated risks are usefully considered as two dimensional: with a 'real' and a 'perceived' component. 'Real' risks are measurable but extremely small. Perceived risks can be very large in their effect, and cause an immediate and sustained drop in vaccine uptake. Perceptions are generated by isolated cases or individual studies which claim that severe complications are causally associated with vaccination simply because of their temporal occurrence, which may be coincidental. Anxiety can persist even in the face of evidence that goes directly against a causal link, as has happened recently with the MMR vaccine. Anxiety is much more readily sown when there is no public memory of the severity of the target diseases, and to this extent vaccination can become a victim of its own success.

Unwanted vaccine effects which are rare but measurable can be broadly divided into: (i) quality control problems; and (ii) intrinsic adverse vaccine reactions. The latter may either be related to the presence of individual factors of predictable risk which are not accounted for prior to immunization (see Table 2), or alternatively, to risks which are unpredictable individually but predictable in the population based on cumulative epidemiological reports.

Quality control problems

These cover all aspects of the commercial mass production of biological products including contamination, levels of additives such as preservatives (e.g. thiomersal) and antibiotics. It also includes the quality of the cold chain from production through to delivery and local storage. This is an important area which can only be touched on. Batch testing of all vaccines is mandatory, in addition to the various regular statutory reviews of vaccine safety and efficacy post-licensing, ongoing epidemiological monitoring of the impact of vaccination and the reporting and investigation of adverse reactions. Some points are topical, however.

Levels of thiomersal, a mercury-containing preservative, are higher in the US infant schedule than most European schedules, including the United Kingdom, because a greater number of separate vaccine injections are cumulatively received. There have been no cases of harm reported in the United States or elsewhere, but efforts are already being made to find alternative preservatives, which are not associated with the theoretical risk of mercury containing additives. Traces of antibiotics are declared where relevant, and routine contraindications exclude individuals with known sensitivity. Genuine, unexpected antibiotic sensitivity revealed by vaccine reaction is extremely rare.

Bacterial and fungal contamination should be excluded by batch testing and by discarding and reporting at the point of use any individual product which on direct inspection appears turbid. However, recent theoretical concerns about contamination by infectious agents for which routine screening is unavailable, such as prions or unknown viruses, presents a situation where the only guarantees are the strict adherence to protocols and reagents which are not known to be associated with risk. Failure to observe such protocols can lead to disciplinary action and the immediate withdrawal of suspect products: as occurred with some polio vaccines in 2000 in the United Kingdom, prepared using potentially BSE contaminated bovine media.

Intrinsic adverse vaccine reactions

Severe reactions (see Table 2) following immunization are extremely rare with licensed, modern vaccines, and occur with a frequency of ~1 in 10^5 overall. They are always thoroughly investigated. It is the duty of health professionals delivering vaccination to exclude predictable risk factors, including severe local or general reactions to previous immunization.

Immunization is intended to produce an immune response! Sometimes, the cytokines released cause perceptible inflammatory or febrile reactions which are mild and transient, and about which individuals or their parents should be warned, in order that appropriate measures such as fever reduction can be taken promptly. This is important if there is a history of infantile febrile convulsions. Mild to moderate local reactions can be minimized by careful injection technique appropriate to the vaccine, and the use of needles of sufficient length and bore to achieve deep subcutaneous or intramuscular delivery if appropriate. Confident handling of infants and their parents reduces the immediate distress of injections, and should be routine to health professionals involved in immunization.

Live vaccines sometimes cause milder versions of the natural infection, after the typical incubation period. Rash, fever, or parotid swelling may occur after MMR immunization, reflecting the vaccine components. Severe complications following live viral vaccines are rare, but more common where immunity is significantly depressed (a contra-indication to live vaccination). OPV-related paralysis is 1000 times less common (1 in 1 000 000) than following natural infection (1 in 1000). Severe complications following MMR immunization are equivalent to that which would be expected from the individual components given separately, as shown in Table 3, which also emphasizes the benefits of MMR vaccination.

Table 3 Risks of complications from natural disease with the risks of first dose MMR[a]

Condition	Rate after natural disease	Rate after first dose of MMR
Convulsions	1 in 200	1 in 1000
Meningitis/encephalitis	1 in 200 to 1 in 5000	Less than 1 in 1 000 000
Thrombocytopaenia	1 in 3000	1 in 24 000
Severe allergic reaction (anaphylaxis)	—	1 in 100 000
Deaths	1 in 2500 to 1 in 5000, depending on age and population	0

[a] Taken from Health Promotion England (2001). Crown Copyright.

Separated, single antigen vaccination against measles, mumps and rubella increases the cumulative risk of mild–moderate reactions, rather than enhancing overall safety, and is not recommended.

Once a pathogen has been eradicated from a population the risks of live vaccination, though tiny, may outweigh the risk of natural disease. Where safe, effective inactivated alternatives are available, these may partially or completely replace live vaccines for individual protection. Increasingly, developed countries are replacing exclusive use of OPV with IPV for some or all doses of the infant schedule. The United Kingdom retains OPV because the number of cases of vaccine-paralysis is only one to two cases per year, and the risk of polio introduction from areas where it is still endemic is considered too high to abandon the greater benefits of population immunity associated with OPV. This evaluation may change with changing epidemiology.

Inactivated vaccines are safe in the immunocompromised, although the immune responses generated may be sub-optimal. There is a tendency for inactivated vaccines to be more reactogenic. Improvements in vaccine design have significantly reduced, but not abolished, this risk.

In the 1970s, an association between early whole cell pertussis vaccines (wP) and severe irreversible brain damage was suggested on the basis of anecdotal reports. Intensive independent investigation failed to prove an association but it was not disproved, and anxiety has lingered. Failure to disprove a link, coupled with a small, but more common association of severe systemic and local reactions with the wP component (compared with other components of tri- and quadrivalent vaccines) has had three consequences.

Firstly, prolonged inconsolable crying associated with wP vaccination is considered a serious systemic reaction. Secondly, a variety of less reactogenic acellular pertussis vaccines (aP) have been developed, which differ in the number of individual antigens selected. Thirdly, if serious reactions including inconsolable crying occur following wP containing vaccines, pertussis immunization should be completed with single antigen aP, if necessary under medical supervision. Unfortunately, the efficacy of aP vaccines varies with the number of component antigens, and only the pentavalent products have equal efficacy to the wP vaccine. For this reason, the United Kingdom continues to initiate pertussis immunization with wP.

Excessive dosing may increase the reactogenicity of some inactivated vaccines such as tetanus toxoid and plain polysaccharide vaccines. Routine ATT boosters every 10 years are no longer recommended in the absence of clinical indications, and plain polysaccharides vaccines should not be repeated within 5 years. The safe dose of diphtheria toxoid is lower for adults and older children than for infants. The problem of unavoidable extra doses associated with the use of combination vaccines, to complete schedules started in different countries or in patients with unknown vaccination histories, has to be balanced against the benefits of ensuring full immune protection.

It has been suggested that even routine schedules of childhood vaccination, which include a core use of inactivated vaccines, is associated in some individuals with subsequent development of atopy, through the excessive stimulation of sub-types of helper T-cells associated with the development of IgE-based allergic reactions. The extent to which this may be true is unclear, but if so it is an invitation to research for improvements in vaccine design, rather than an indication to discard the overwhelming benefits of vaccination that epidemiological evidence has accumulated.

Repeat doses of live viral vaccines does not appear to enhance adverse effects. The second dose of MMR is associated with fewer adverse reactions. In many developing countries where National Immunization Days (NIDs) are organized to cover the whole population, irrespective of immunization history, millions of people have received extra doses of OPV without adverse outcome.

Passive immunization

Immediate, short-term protection against some infections and toxins can be provided by passive immunization with pre-formed donor antibodies (see Table 4). This bypasses the need for a functioning immune system or the time required for active induction of immunity. This may be important where urgent pre- or post-exposure prophylaxis is needed, or where active immunization is contra-indicated.

Table 4 Passive immunization products[a]

Type of passive immunization	Indications
Normal human immunoglobulins (NHIG):	
Intravenous NHIG	Prophylaxis of neonatal infections
Intramuscular NHIG	Prophylaxis of infections following exposure, particularly measles[b] and hepatitis A
Hyperimmune serum globulin (human):	
Hepatitis B (HBIG)	Prophylaxis following exposure
Varicella-Zoster (VZIG or ZIG)	Prophylaxis of immunocompromised
Rabies (RIG)	Prophylaxis following dogbite
Cytomegalovirus (CMV-IVIG)	Prophylaxis and treatment following infection
Tetanus (TIG)	Prophylaxis of major wounds if not adequately immunized. Treatment of tetanus
Animal sera	
Rabies antiserum (EARS) (equine)	When RIG unavailable
Tetanus antitoxin (TAT) (equine)	When TIG unavailable
Diphtheria antitoxin (DAT) (equine)	Prevention of diphtheria if not adequately immunized; treatment of diphtheria
Botulism antitoxin (equine)	Treatment of botulism
Snake, fish, scorpion, tick, jelly-fish, and spider antivenoms (equine or ovine)	Various antivenoms, mono- or polyspecific, for treatment of bites and stings

[a] Based on *Table of Passive Immunizations* by D. Isaacs and E.R. Moxon, *Oxford Textbook of Medicine*.

[b] If within incubation period of exposure to measles, and no contra-indication to live immunization, then active measles immunization can be undertaken.

Globally, the most important form of passive immunization is natural, associated with the transfer of transplacental IgG to the foetus. This is exploited in the Expanded Immunization Programme, by actively immunizing pregnant women with Tetanus Toxoid, to reduce the incidence of neonatal disease. Breast-feeding is hugely important in passively providing secretory antibodies to a range of gastrointestinal pathogens, and in devoloping countries this benefit typically outweighs the risk of transferring HIV by this route.

The duration of passive protection is dependent on the half-life of donor antibodies in the recipient and is a few weeks at most. Long-term protection against common infections would require regular systemic antibody infusions, and for reasons of efficacy, safety, acceptability, cost-effectiveness, and product supply is inappropriate except in rare individuals with severe immunodeficiency.

Population immune protection

The infectiousness of a disease is estimated by the number of secondary cases a single infected case generates in a non-immune population. This is referred to as Ro, or the basic reproductive rate of infection. Epidemics occur when more than one secondary case is generated, that is, when Ro is greater than unity, and to prevent an epidemic Ro must be reduced to less than one. Increasing the proportion of immune, non-infectious individuals causes an exponential decline in the spread of infection. The critical level of population immunity required to drive Ro less than 1 provides a minimum estimate of the proportion of individuals who must be immunized to prevent an epidemic.

When vaccine uptake sustains population immunity well above this critical level, epidemic spread is blocked and endemic infection will eventually die out. This is a prerequisite for eradication of transmissible pathogens and was the basis of the global eradication of smallpox and the elimination of measles and polio from most developed countries in the western hemisphere.

Measles, pertussis, mumps, and polio are so infectious however, with Ros in excess of 15 in some populations, that vaccine uptake in excess of 95 per cent of the population is required to maintain adequate population immunity. The 'local' population immunity provided by immunized parents, sibs, and older contacts is vital to protect infants against measles during their first year of life. Measles is highly virulent in this age group, and after maternal antibodies have decayed, infants are susceptible until actively immunized. Where population immunity can be sustained, it is true that a residual, tiny proportion of non-immunized people will be indirectly protected by the absence of endemic circulation and the inability of an epidemic to spread from an isolated case introduced into the population.

Unfortunately, the level of vaccine uptake can change very quickly, for example in response to public anxiety, and population immunity cannot be relied upon indefinitely for individual protection. It is therefore extremely important for health professionals to encourage and explain the importance of immunizing every child without contra-indications. Until eradicable pathogens are finally driven to extinction by sustained global population immunity, fluctuating sub-optimal levels of vaccine uptake will permit conditions for epidemic spread and every non-immune child will therefore be at risk. In the United Kingdom in recent months, uptake of the MMR vaccine has dropped to 88 per cent creating conditions where this is very possible.

The impact of infant immunization programmes which reduce transmission is particularly sensitive to vaccine uptake when the complications of natural infection increase with age or at critical periods of later life. Mathematical models have an important role in simulating the impact of immunization at different levels of vaccine uptake, as they can model events on a scale and under conditions which would be unethical in human trials.[(4)] They show that for infections with age-related complications, it is critical to take account of the average age of infection prior to infant immunization in order to determine whether vaccination should be introduced.

The propensity for sub-optimal vaccine uptake to cause an upward shift in the average age of infection of a communicable disease is a critical factor in the public health decision to introduce infant rubella immunization. In countries where the average age of infection is already infancy or early childhood, poor uptake could lead to an absolute increase in the number of cases of congenital rubella syndrome. This would be predicted for a developing country such as the Gambia, and has been observed in Greece.[(5)]

Population immunity is powerful. It can be used 'acutely' within a community where an outbreak has already occurred. The rapid deployment of immunization to 'ring-fence' an isolated case of smallpox was highly effective in 'mopping -up' the residual reservoirs of the pathogen in the final stages of eradication. The occurrence of a single case of wild-type polio represents an epidemic, as the pathogen is highly infectious with an infection: case rate of about 100 : 1. 'Ring-fencing' strategies of immunization are therefore vital in bringing potentially explosive epidemics of polio, or measles, under rapid control.

Immunization programmes

Immunization programmes are highly organized public health strategies for delivering vaccination to those at risk. The decision to introduce an immunization programme is based on a full evaluation of its potential impact on the population, and an appraisal of the resources available to implement the programme safely and effectively and to make it accessible and acceptable to the target population.

Routine immunization is required when all the population is at risk of exposure or complications, or where comprehensive population immunity is required to eradicate or control disease. Special immunizations are indicated, and may be more cost-effective, where individuals or groups are at particular risk of exposure to serious pathogens through travel, occupation or lifestyle, or at enhanced risk of complications because of co-morbidity.

Organization of routine immunizations

Long-term routine immunization programmes requires meticulous organization to coordinate: (i) vaccine delivery; (ii) maintenance of the cold chain; (iii) call and recall systems suitable for accessing the target populations; (iv) reliable records and returns for monitoring vaccine uptake; (v) public health surveillance for tracking epidemiological patterns and adverse effects; (vi) provision of training for all health professionals involved in the administration and implementation of immunization; and (vii) ongoing public health education and information.

Public and primary health care must be closely integrated to maximize vaccine uptake and this depends on a minimum level of economic and political stability. The effects of breakdown of a previously efficient system are evident in countries of the former USSR, where decentralization has led to a decline in organized distribution of immunization resulting in outbreaks of diphtheria.

The style of organization depends on the infrastructure available for delivering health care. Reliable and sustainable mechanisms must be in place to ensure continuing high vaccine uptake. As the incidence of vaccine-preventable disease falls in developed countries, public memory fades and motivation to be immunized (and perhaps to immunize) may wane. In stable societies, accessibility to immunization relies on the coordination of demographic data with call–recall systems to track and target children at scheduled times. This is kick-started by the birth of a child. Core schedules are guided by vaccine requirements, but additional devices to tie in scheduled times with routine child health surveillance or 'life-events' (birth, starting school, leaving school, etc.) assist access and uptake.

In developing countries, where the infrastructure cannot be guaranteed, international aid may need to be made available if requested, either for the introduction or for the temporary support of routine immunization programmes. Such aid may need to be deployed very rapidly where dense populations of highly susceptible people are acutely congregated, for example in refugee camps. Wherever possible in these circumstances, programmes should be implemented by local personnel who can discuss concerns, provide information, and give advice in the most familiar spoken language.

Immunization schedules

Primary courses of routine immunizations are offered in infancy and childhood to maximize benefit and cost-effectiveness. The basic schedule for developed countries is illustrated in Table 5, using that current for the United Kingdom. Additional immunizations are included in primary schedules according to public health priorities of individual countries, and some of these differences are also indicated in the table. Some vaccinations given within the infant schedule, for example neonatal BCG and Hepatitis B, may be routine in some countries but reserved for special indication in others.

Immunization is started as early as is compatible with vaccine efficacy and safety. The accelerated primary schedule at 2, 3, and 4 months of age (rather than 3, 5, and 7) has now been formally validated for the UK population.[(6)] All children should be offered the full course of immunizations unless specific contra-indications develop (see Table 2) or parents withhold consent. Schedules can be resumed or started at other times if immune protection is incomplete, and details of 'catch-up' schedules will vary according to the vaccine and the age at presentation.

The disproportionately high burden of vaccine-preventable diseases borne by developing countries led to the WHO sponsored Extended Programme of Immunization (EPI), illustrated in Table 6. A significant difference is the neonatal commencement of oral polio vaccination, and the introduction of measles vaccination at 9 months of age. This reflects the increased risk of both these diseases given the high incidence and case-morbidity/mortality rates which prevail, because of low population immunity, poor nutrition and co-existing disease, particularly HIV. Although the efficiency of immunization against measles is lower at 9 than

Table 5 Example schedule of routine immunizations in developed countries: based on UK schedule 2001[a] (includes important vaccines given on special indication if timed into infant schedule)

Disease	Route	Age	Comments
Tuberculosis[b] (BCG)[b]	i.d.; s.c.	Neonatal	If at high risk. BCG protects more consistently against infant/childhood TB than adult forms
Hepatitis B[b]	i.m.	Neonatal, 1 month, and 6 months 5-yearly boosters if still at risk	Determine risk individually. If a mother who is HbsAg+ is HbeAg+ but lacks e markers, or has had acute hepatitis during pregnancy, neonate may need HBIG in addition to active immunization
Diphtheria/tetanus/ pertussis/Haemophilus influenzae type B (DTwP-Hib)	i.m.	2 months 3 months 4 months	Primary course (three doses, a month between each)
Polio (OPV)	Oral	4 months	Note: the whole cell pertussis vaccine currently used for primary course, unless severe reaction (see text)
Meningococcal type C (men C)	i.m.	4 months	
Measles/mumps/ rubella (MMR)	i.m.	12–15 months	First dose (can be given at any age over 12 months)
Diphtheria/tetanus/ pertussis (DtaP)		3–5 years (3 years after completion of primary course)	Booster dose Note: the acellular pertussis component has been introduced into the UK schedule from November 2001, in response to evidence of waning pertussis immunity by adulthood
Polio (OPV)		3–5 years (3 years after completion of primary course)	Booster dose
MMR		3–5 years	Second dose
Tetanus/low dose diphtheria (Td)		13–18 years	Booster dose
Polio (OPV)		13–18 years	Booster dose
Tuberculosis[b] (BCG)		10–14 years	Regional variation in use. Not routine. Not if tuberculin positive. No immunizations to be given in same arm for 3 months: risk of regional lymphadenitis

[a] Based on PHLS and DOH UK information.

[b] Vaccines given by special indication during routine schedule.

Note: In all cases, it is crucial to consult current local and national guidelines about correct dose for age, route and site of administration, and exact schedule. The US and some other developed countries routinely immunize against hepatitis B neonatally. The US has also introduced the conjugated pneumococcal vaccine to the infant schedule, and the live attenuated varicella-zoster vaccine against chickenpox, in view of the severity of the adult disease.

Table 6 Schedule of expanded programme of immunization (EPI) for developing countries, recommended by WHO, with updates included by some countries shown in parentheses[a]

Age	Vaccines	Comments
Birth	BCG; OPV; (Hep B)[b]	
6–8 weeks[b]	DPT; OPV; (Hib)[b]; (Hep B)[b]	
10–12 weeks	DPT; OPV; (Hib)[b]	
14–16 weeks	DPT; OPV; (Hib)[b]; (Hep B)[b]	
9 months	Measles; (Yellow fever)	YF, where endemic
Women of childbearing age	Tetanus toxoid	Exploits route of natural transplacental passive immunization, to reduce neonatal tetanus

[a] See under WHO website (www.WHO.int) for current schedules of individual countries.

[b] Many developing countries use: (i) DPT vaccination schedule at 2, 3, and 4 months; (ii) include the Hib vaccine at 2, 3, and 4 months; (iii) include Hepatitis B vaccine at birth, 2 and 4 months, with boosters as indicated; (iv) where epidemiology indicates, yellow fever vaccination at 9 months (simultaneously with measles vaccination).

BCG, Bacille–Calmette–Guerin; DPT, diphtheria–pertussis–tetanus; OPV, oral polio vaccine.

at 13 months, immune protection generated is sufficient to make a major impact on disease burden.

The schedules shown here are indicative but not definitive, and it is vital for practitioners to consult current national guidelines for details of immunizations,[7,8] which vary considerably between countries and over time, both in the developed and the developing world.

Acceptability and informed consent

The United Kingdom and many other countries use informed consent as the basis for immunization, and would not wish to see a return to legal enforcement. Where routine immunization is a legal requirement for school entry, there are usually extensive 'opt-out' clauses for conscientious objectors.

Parents are motivated to protect their children, and anxieties and concerns which they may have about the efficacy or safety of immunizations can and should be carefully addressed. The importance of attentive, non-patronizing and friendly discussion with parents cannot be over-emphasized. Clear, consistent information about the overwhelming benefits of routine immunization and the risk to their children of not being immunized are central to any discussion.[9]

It is also important to give parents the information they need to confidently manage vaccine reactions that might occur: the majority are mild and transient. The very small risk of more serious reactions needs careful explanation, with clear guidelines about any immediate action which may be necessary should they occur.

Some affluent countries have a vaccine compensation scheme, which acknowledges that while the benefits of immunization to the individual and to the population are overwhelming, no vaccine is 100 per cent safe, and very occasionally individuals have, or cannot be proved *not* to have had, a serious vaccine reaction. Such schemes are designed to help retain public confidence in the accountability of immunization as a preventive health intervention.

When consent is obtained, it should be clearly recorded. When parents remain ambivalent but there is no rejection of the benefit–risk evaluation or cultural or religious objections to immunization, the possibility of 'injection-anxiety' needs consideration. Some parents may simply be unable to witness or physically cooperate with parenteral immunization of their child, and this situation needs sensitive handling. Usually, acceptable solutions can be found by confident, trained primary care staff, in particular health visitors (in the United Kingdom) and nurses who are the key professionals discussing and delivering routine immunization.

Where consent for immunization is withheld, parents should be reassured that this will not affect their medical care or that of their children. It is important to try to remain in dialogue, as parents, or in later life their children, may wish to commence or complete missed immunizations. Nevertheless, when private choice leads to opting increasing numbers of children out of routine immunizations, not only are they left individually unprotected, but population immunity falls catastrophically.

The 'MMR scare'

The single most damaging perception about immunization safety in recent years has been focused on the combined MMR vaccine. Unsubstantiated fears about an association between the vaccine and the onset of infant autism and inflammatory bowel disease have resulted in vaccine uptake declining to 88 per cent of the susceptible population in some parts of the United Kingdom. This is low enough for epidemic spread of measles to be inevitable, should an isolated outbreak occur.

In essence, a study published in 1998[10] claimed an association, based on parental recall, between environmental triggers and the onset of autism and inflammatory bowel disorder in a small group of children admitted to hospital. Media coverage pointed to MMR vaccination as the most commonly recalled trigger. This study, and subsequent immuno-histological and retrospective epidemiological studies from the same group, were technically and analytically flawed but were widely reported in the media as evidence against the safety of the MMR vaccine.

Unfortunately, during the initial years of the vaccine 'scare', the beliefs, attitudes and advice of primary health professionals suggested a similar spectrum of anxiety. Furthermore, such professional attitudes correlated with highly variable, often inadequate, knowledge about the benefits and risks of immunization, suggesting inconsistent and poor advice from primary care was compounding the problem.[11]

No independent evidence has confirmed an association between MMR and these conditions. Most importantly, independent epidemiological data[12] and time trend analyses of MMR uptake and the incidence of autism[13,14] have shown that while there has indeed been an increase in the reported incidence of autism, which is unexplained, the uptake of MMR remained static throughout, which strongly argues against a causal link. Major independent reviews[15] have concluded: (i) there is no evidence of an association of MMR vaccine with either of the two infant disorders; and (ii) no evidence in favour of giving measles, mumps and rubella immunization separately. In fact, the reverse is true, as infants will remain susceptible to infection for a longer period of time, and will have the increased cumulative risks and distress of six, rather than two, separate injections.

Despite convincing epidemiological evidence for the safety and efficacy of the combined MMR vaccine, there are increasing demands for the option of separate, single antigen vaccines. This signifies a deepening mistrust of the veracity of evidence used by the medical profession and government organizations. It is critically important to try to understand the complex causes of this mistrust, to know how best to address it.

It is apparent that while many people have uncertainties which can be addressed by further studies, which are planned[16] and educational outreach[17] which has already commenced, for others the issues are more properly debated in the arena of beliefs about the nature of health, disease, and individual freedom. Much of this debate is currently taking place informally, in individual discussions between health care providers and between health care providers and parents themselves. However, there are major issues of moral, legal, and political significance which impact directly on the tension between personal choice and public health outcome.[18] This cannot be resolved solely in the medical arena.

Special immunization programmes

Immunizations indicated for special use in the United Kingdom are listed in Table 1. The indications are summarized but local guidelines and should be consulted.

Influenza vaccination is cost-effective to prevent severe acute infection in: (i) the elderly (>65 years) in developed countries; (ii) those with chronic diseases which enhance susceptibility to acute infection: diabetes, chronic cardiac conditions, respiratory diseases including asthma, chronic renal failure, immunosuppression; and (iii) those in long-stay nursing and residential homes. Studies in UK primary care indicate that influenza vaccination is more likely to be taken up if recommended by a doctor or a nurse, and having had influenza vaccination previously is a strong predictor of subsequent uptake.

Protection against invasive, capsulated bacteria (pneumococcal strains, meningococcal strain C where, indicated by the epidemiology, and Haemophilus influenzae B) is recommended for people with functional or actual asplenism, or with the above chronic conditions. The newer conjugated vaccines against pneumococcal and meningococcal infections are likely to replace plain polysaccharide products for special as well as routine use as they become more widely available. At present however, older children and adults travelling to the meningitis belt of Sub-Saharan Africa still need to have AC, or ACYW135 combined protection, still only available as plain polysachharide products.

Indications for special vaccination against Hepatitis B cover situations of increased exposure to Hepatitis B positive body fluids, whether through i.v. drug use, sexual contact, occupational exposure (particularly health care workers and morticians), close family contacts of carriers, prisoners, and travellers to areas of high endemicity who may put themselves at risk. These are not exhaustive categories, and individual risk assessmentis essential, especially in neonates borne to mothers infected with the virus.

It is important to note that post-exposure prophylaxis works against rabies, and should not be delayed if contact is suspected on the history. Further details about special indications for the other vaccines listed in Table 1 can be found in national and international guidelines, but may be modified by local public health policies and recommendations, whose advice should also be sought. Individual risk is not always easy to assess, and for travellers to areas of endemic infection, much depends on the precise details of itinerary, personal choice, and behaviour.

Monitoring and surveillance and population catch-up strategies

When models simulating epidemic spread are combined with sero-epidemiological data marking the level of population immunity, advance warnings can be given of the risk of disease outbreak given observed trends in vaccine uptake and population immunity. In 1994 in the United Kingdom such models predicted a measles epidemic in the cohort of school age children aged over 9, many of whom had not received MMR in infancy and 10 per cent of whom would not have sero-converted with a single dose.

A national, school-based catch-up programme with MMR was successfully undertaken irrespective of immunization history, and a measles epidemic averted. At the time of going to press, a rise in the rate of Hib diseases in the United Kingdom has led to plans for a catch-up programme for infants aged 6 months to 4 years.

Where epidemiological surveillance indicates the persistence of vaccine-preventable disease, for example polio or measles, and routine schedules consistently fail to reach large sections of the susceptible population, some countries organize National Immunization Days (NIDs), where irrespective of previous immunization history, vaccination is undertaken. These 'catch-up' policies are extremely important in accessing people who may find it impossible to link in with routine schedules or standard clinic opening times.

Future vaccine developments

Future vaccine development will proceed in many directions. Existing technology may still be effective against some pathogens which have genetically stable antigens associated with protective antibody responses.

Better methods of inducing mucosal immunity are likely to lead to a greater range of oral and nasal products against gastrointestinal and respiratory pathogens. Vaginal and urethral routes of delivery could be exploited for vaccines against sexually transmitted diseases. Plant vaccines could provide cheap, mass-produced, painless antigen delivery, which could revolutionize immunization programmes in developing countries. Unfortunately, they are likely to meet considerable public resistance as genetically modified products. All these methods would avoid or minimize the number of injections given to infants, saving their distress and much parental anxiety.

Both live and current inactivated vaccines have limitations. Concern about the potential for reversion of attenuated live strains to wild type makes such prototypes unlikely candidates for HIV or Hepatitis C prevention. Not all pathogens can be safely attenuated: for example, respiratory syncytial virus. The enhanced risk of disseminated disease in the immunosuppressed is a limiting contra-indication to the use of routine live vaccines. The theoretical risk, for which there is no direct evidence, of unsuspected viral or prion-like agents contaminating live vaccines is minute, but impossible to exclude. The development of 'pseudo-live' DNA vaccines is a rapidly expanding field, aimed at safely delivering encoded rather than expressed vaccine antigens. However, much work remains to be done to ensure that DNA–vaccine integration into the genome of the host cell does not occur, or if it does, it is not deleterious. However, the human genome already contains a significant amount of 'ancient' genetic material derived from retroviral-like agents. The interchange of genetic material between microorganism and human may not always be disadvantageous.

One of the key biological problems to overcome however is antigen escape, under the immune selection pressure of antibodies. Attempts to keep pace with influenza virus drift have been described. The inclusion of successively more antigens, as in the plain and conjugated pneumococcal vaccines, aims to match as many virulent, co-circulating strains as possible. However, the diversity and speed of immune escape of HIV makes such an approach futile. Complex parasites such as malaria pose similar problems. Although there is in principle an almost infinite repertoire of different, antigen-specific antibodies and T-cell receptors, in practice the range of T-cell receptor/antigen complexes which can be recognized is restricted by the histo-compatibility loci which, with other genes, regulate the immune response. Each allele of the highly polymorphic human MHC loci has a direct restricting effect on recognition of antigens by T-lymphocytes and indirectly therefore on the induction of T-cell dependent antibody-mediated immune memory, because each MHC molecule has a preference for binding to a peptide of characteristic amino acid sequence.

However, in the case of rapidly mutating intracellular parasites, particularly viruses such as HIV and protozoa such as malaria, the attraction of searching for antigens which are more stable leads inexorably towards T-cell antigens, and CTL antigens in particular. This is because many of the pathogen-specific peptide antigens recognized by CTL are not from external, structural proteins, but those internal to the pathogen, or regulatory enzymes expressed exclusively during the intracellular phase of replication. Where these peptide sequences are crucial to the function or replication of the pathogen, they may have less freedom to mutate without significant survival disadvantage.

Vaccines currently under development against HIV, malaria, tuberculosis, and RSV infection are exploiting the potential of CTL-mediated immunity. Schedules using a range of prototype recombinant vaccines, using the highly attenuated vaccinia-virus 'backbones' (deployed in the latter stages of the smallpox eradication programme) into which HIV, malaria or tuberculosis-specific genes are recombined, are already at advanced stages of development.

Acknowledgements

I am grateful to David Mant for contributing to proof reading and corrections, and to Richard Moxon and Dave Isaacs for allowing me to use and adapt their Table of Passive Immunisation Products.

References

1. **Peltola, H., Heinonen, O., Valle, M.** et al. (1994). The elimination of indigenous measles, mumps and rubella from Finland by a 12 year, two-dose vaccination programme. *New England Journal of Medicine* **331**, 1397–402.
2. **Jamison, D.T.** (1993). An overview. In *Disease Control Priorities in Developing Countries* (ed. R. Detels, J. McEwen, and G. Omenn), p.13. Oxford: Oxford Medical Publications, Oxford University Press.
3. **Isaacs, D. and Moxon, E.R.** (1996). Immunisations. In *Oxford Textbook of Medicine* Vol. 1 (ed. D. Weatherall, D.A. Warrell, and J.G. Ledingham), p. 317. Oxford: Oxford Medical Publications, Oxford University Press.
4. **Anderson, R.M.** (1998). Mathematical models of transmission and control. In *Oxford Textbook of Public Health* (ed. R. Detels, J. McEwen, and G. Omenn), pp. 689–719. Oxford: Oxford Medical Publications, Oxford Univeristy Press.
5. **Panagiotopoulos, T., Antiomiadon, I., and Valassi-Adam, E.** (1999). Increase in congential rubella occurrence after immunization in Greece: retrospective survey and systematic review. *British Medical Journal* **319**, 1462–6.
6. **Fleming, P., Blair, P., Platt, M.** et al. (2001). The UK accelerated immunization programme and sudden unexpected death in infancy: case-control study. *British Medical Journal* **322**, 822–5.
7. **Department of Health.** *Immunizations Against Infectious Disease (with updates).* London: HMSO, 1996.
8. **British Medical Association and Royal Pharmaceutical Society of Great Britain.** *British National Formulary*, Vol. 41. London: BMJ Books, 2001.
9. **Harnden, A. and Shakespeare, J.** (2001). 10-minute consultation: MMR immunization. *British Medical Journal* **323**, p. 32.
10. **Wakefield, A., Murch, S., Anthony, A.** et al. (1998). Ileal-lymphoid-nodular hyperplasia, non-specific colitis and pervasive developmental disorder in children. *Lancet* **351**, 637–41.
11. **Petrovic, M., Roberts, R., and Ramsay, M.** et al. (2001). Second dose of measles, mumps and rubella vaccine: questionnaire survey of health professional attitudes. *British Medical Journal* **322**, 82–5.
12. **Taylor, B., Miller, E., Farrington, C.** et al. (1999). Autism and measles, mumps and rubella vaccine: no epidemiological evidence for a causal association. *Lancet* **353**, 2026–9.
13. **Kaye, J., del Mar Merero Montes, M., and Jick, H.** (2001). MMR vaccine and the incidence of autism recorded by general practioners: a time trend analysis. *British Medical Journal* **322**, 1–2.
14. **Farrington, C., Miller, E., and Taylor, B.** (2001). MMR and autism: further evidence against a causal association. *Vaccine* **19**, 3632–5.
15. **Halsey, N. and Hyman, S.** (2000). Measles-mumps-rubella vaccine and autistic spectrum disorder: Report from the New Challenges in Childhood Immunizations Conference convened in Oak Brook, Illinois, June 12–13. *Pediatrics* **107** (5), 1–23.

16. **Smeeth, L., Hall, A., Fombonne, E.** et al. (2001). A case-control study of autisim and MMR vaccination using the general practice research database: design and methodolgy. *British Medical Council Public Health* **1**, 1–2.
17. **Health Promotion England**. London: Department of Health, 2001.
18. **Heller, T.** (2001). Vaccination against mumps, measles and rubella: is there a case for deepening the debate. *British Medical Journal* **323**, 838.

Websites for immunization information on MMR

www.immunisation.org.uk/immprof.html
American Academy of Pediatrics: www.aap.org (search under MMR)
Institute of Medicine: www.nap.edu/books/0309074479/html
Medical Research Council: www.mrc.ac.uk (search under Autism)
WHO (2001): www.who.int/vaccines-diseases/safety/hottop/mmrstatement.shtml

General immunizations

WHO: www.who.int/vaccines-diseases
Health Promotion England: www.immunisation.org.uk
Department of Health: www.doh.gov.uk
Public Health laboratory Service: www.phls.org.uk
American Academy of Pediatrics: www.aap.org
American Institute of Medicine: www.aiom.org

11.3 Screening

Peter Burke

Introduction

A stitch in time saves nine—Proverb.
It is hard to make someone who feels well, feel better—Osler.

In this chapter, I hope to discuss the principles of population screening. While what follows is written from a UK primary care perspective, a great deal of it can be applied in other settings. However, some caution is needed, as there are wide international variations both in the prevalence of disease and in the social and political context of screening.

What is screening?

Screening aims to improve health or life-expectation.[1] One definition is 'organised periodic procedures performed on large groups of people for the purpose of detecting disease'. The UK National Screening Committee[2] defines screening as 'a public health service in which members of a defined population, who do not necessarily perceive they are at risk of, or are already affected by a disease or its complications, are asked a question or offered a test, to identify those individuals who are more likely to be helped than harmed by further tests or treatment to reduce the risk of a disease or its complications'. The emphasis, in this more specific definition, is on the welfare of the individual rather than the community as a whole.

The terms *case-finding* and *opportunistic screening* are sometimes applied to a screening activity in which a professional offers a test as a result of contact first made by the patient. *Surveillance* is a broader term encompassing a wide range of preventive health activities, including screening but also the active observation of people with established problems or risk factors (see Chapter 10.3).

A brief history

Systematic programmes of screening for ill-health started in the late nineteenth century. Screening of recruits during the Boer War famously unmasked much real and potential illness in an apparently healthy community—the so-called 'iceberg of ill-health'.

Multiphasic screening, or the 'periodic health examination' started in the United States with Gould in 1900. Among milestones in its development were the start of the Peckham project in 1926, the Kaiser Permanente Organization, active in the United States since the 1940s, and the South-East London Group, established in 1967.[3] More recently in the United Kingdom, the Oxcheck study[4] and the Family Heart Study[5] described targeted interventions in a primary care context, and found measurable if not overwhelming gains in health outcomes.

The development of specific screening programmes has gone hand in hand with that of investigational techniques and effective therapies. Radiographic screening for tuberculosis had its heyday following World War II. Cervical cytology was made possible by the work of Papanicolaou in 1943. Screening mammography was proposed in 1960, and was applied systematically in the United Kingdom in 1993, following the Forrest Report.[6] Over the last decade there has been increasing interest in early detection of tumours of the intestine, prostate, and ovary.

Often, the evolution of screening programmes is driven by public opinion, only some of it well informed. The death of a celebrity, such as that of American actress Gilda Radner from ovarian cancer, can act as a major stimulus. To promote consistent evidence-based planning, several countries have established advisory bodies. Examples are the National Screening Committee[2] set up in the United Kingdom in 1996, the Canadian Task Force on Preventive Health Care,[7] and the United States Preventive Services Task Force. Their task is advising on the case for implementing new screening programmes and modifying or withdrawing existing ones. Simultaneously, there have been many highly publicized episodes in which screening programmes—particularly cervical cytology—were perceived as falling short of the required standard, and the need for quality control has been highlighted.[8]

Since 1998, Health Authorities in the United Kingdom have been under an obligation to develop Health Implementation Plans and the introduction of National Service Frameworks brought with it a renewed emphasis on prevention in primary care. The NHS Cancer Plan[9] in 2000 made a specific commitment to expansion in cancer screening programmes, with reduction in regional inequalities of access.

Gains and penalties

Why screen? The short answer is because of the promise that early detection of a disorder or risk factor will lead to greater health or longer life.

A screening test may have two desirable outcomes. Firstly, that confident reassurance can be given that a significant condition has been excluded. Secondly, that a clinically significant condition has been identified and effective treatment started. Sometimes, however, the outcome falls into neither of these categories. There may be an equivocal result. False reassurance may be given.[10] A condition may be detected for which there is no treatment. The treatment instituted following the test may subsequently prove to be unnecessary, ineffective, or even deleterious. Furthermore, a potential problem may be identified, which, while not treatable, disadvantages the patient in terms of employment or insurability. Here the true beneficiary is not the patient but a third party. Screening to identify risk for such purposes (*mandated* screening) is legitimate, but the patient must enter upon it aware of the implications.

The problems do not end there. There is evidence, perhaps contrary to expectations, that even following a negative test the individual may show a decline in self-perceived health status.[11] Finally, there is the 'certificate of health effect'—a person found to be screen-negative could consider this to be carte blanche to continue with an unhealthy lifestyle.

All this has ethical and medico-legal implications, particularly where the patient has been invited for testing with a promise of benefit. Consumers of health care can make autonomous, informed choices about their treatment. Many people will make an informed choice not to be screened, and are entitled to have this respected, whatever we as professionals may feel. Counselling is about decision support as well as information giving.[12]

Money and resources

Screening tests may be paid for by the person being screened, by an insurance plan or other third party, or by the taxpayer. In planning screening programmes, purchasers of health care must achieve value for money. Every pound spent on screening has an *opportunity cost*, that is, it is no longer available for other health care purchases. Indeed, in setting priorities the cost of the screening programme may have to compete for funds with care of the condition screened for.

The costs of a screening programme can be considered under several headings:

1. the costs of the test;
2. the cost of administering the programme, for example, call–recall systems;
3. the costs of further investigations required for the assessment of test-positive patients;
4. the costs of treatment carried out on those who require it;
5. the costs of offering adequate pre- and post-test counselling (this in particular is easily neglected).

In the UK context, it is worth recalling that while items 1 and 2 may be funded from outside the NHS, items 3–5 are very likely to be borne by the taxpayer.

It is possible to divide the number of people screened by the number benefiting: this gives the number needed to screen.[13] One needs also to take account of the size and duration of any benefit. Economists often do this in terms of QUALYs (Quality-Adjusted Life Years). A 'cure' achieved at age 40, with 40 years of expected lifespan ahead, would thus yield significantly more QUALYs than a similar result at age 75, or a postponement of death at a younger age. An example: an economic evaluation was done of the Oxcheck study—a nurse-based one-off cardiovascular risk screen of middle-aged individuals. The cost per discounted life-year gained (at 1996 prices) comes to £900 if we postulate that the benefit lasts 20 years. It rises to up to £30 000 per life year gained if the benefit lasts only 1 year.[14]

Evaluating a screening programme

Wilson and Jungner[15] in 1966 proposed a set of criteria that are still often quoted as the gold standard for a screening test. They have been variously modified over the years, most recently by the UK National Screening Committee (Table 1).

Table 1 Criteria for a screening programme proposed by the UK National Screening Committee

All of the following criteria should be met before screening for a condition is initiated:

The condition

1. The condition should be an important health problem
2. The epidemiology and natural history of the condition, including development from latent to declared disease, should be adequately understood and there should be a detectable risk factor, or disease marker and a latent period or early symptomatic stage
3. All the cost-effective primary prevention interventions should have been implemented as far as practicable

The test

4. There should be a simple, safe, precise, and validated screening test
5. The distribution of test values in the target population should be known and a suitable cut-off level defined and agreed
6. The test should be acceptable to the population
7. There should be an agreed policy on the further diagnostic investigation of individuals with a positive test result and on the choices available to those individuals

The treatment

8. There should be an effective treatment or intervention for patients identified through early detection, with evidence of early treatment leading to better outcomes than late treatment
9. There should be agreed evidence-based policies covering which individuals should be offered treatment and the appropriate treatment to be offered
10. Clinical management of the condition and patient outcomes should be optimized by all health care providers prior to participation in a screening programme

The screening programme

11. There must be evidence from high-quality randomized controlled trials that the screening programme is effective in reducing mortality or morbidity. Where screening is aimed solely at providing information to allow the person being screened to make an 'informed choice' (e.g. Down syndrome, cystic fibrosis carrier screening), there must be evidence from high-quality trials that the test accurately measures risk. The information that is provided about the test and its outcome must be of value and readily understood by the individual being screened
12. There should be evidence that the complete screening programme (test, diagnostic procedures, treatment/ intervention) is clinically, socially, and ethically acceptable to health professionals and the public
13. The benefit from the screening programme should outweigh the physical and psychological harm (caused by the test, diagnostic procedures, and treatment)
14. The opportunity cost of the screening programme (including testing, diagnosis, treatment, administration, training, and quality assurance) should be economically balanced in relation to expenditure on medical care as a whole (i.e. value for money)
15. There must be a plan for managing and monitoring the screening programme and an agreed set of quality assurance standards
16. Adequate staffing and facilities for testing, diagnosis, treatment, and programme management should be made available prior to the commencement of the screening programme
17. All other options for managing the condition should have been considered (e.g. improving treatment, providing other services), to ensure that no more cost-effective intervention could be introduced or current interventions increased within the resources available
18. Evidence-based information, explaining the consequences of testing, investigation, and treatment, should be made available to potential participants to assist them in making an informed choice
19. Public pressure for widening the eligibility criteria for reducing the screening interval, and for increasing the sensitivity of the testing process, should be anticipated. Decisions about these parameters should be scientifically justifiable to the public

Although these criteria are quoted as the sine qua non of an acceptable screening programme, it is extremely difficult to meet them all. I would like to discuss some of the criteria listed in a little more detail.

The condition

An 'important health problem' (Table 1, point 1) must have an impact on health and be reasonably common in the community. For example, oesophageal carcinoma may possibly warrant screening in an Oriental population and sickle cell anaemia among those of African origin, but not the reverse. There must be a sufficiently long pre-symptomatic phase during which a test can be applied (point 2). Thus, cervical cytology is a useful intervention while screening for testicular cancer is not.

The test

A *test* is something done by a professional to try to separate those affected by a condition from those not affected. It is not confined to laboratory or radiological investigations, but includes clinical examinations, questionnaires, or even simply the asking of a question. It may also refer to a combination of tests, for example, rectal examination plus PSA measurement (Table 2).

The *yield* of a test is the number of people correctly identified by the test as suffering from a condition, as a percentage of the population as a whole.

The *sensitivity* of the test is its ability correctly to identify 'cases', that is, it is the ratio between true positives and total affected. The denominator is defined by a gold-standard test, for example, biopsy, or by subsequent events, for example, development of cancer within a specified period.

Specificity is the ability to correctly identify those free of disease, that is, the ratio between true negatives and total disease-free.

The *pre-test probability* refers to the likelihood of a condition being present before any test is done. It is equal to the *prevalence*. The *post-test probability* is the likelihood of the condition once the result of the test is known. It is also called the *predictive value*.

The *likelihood ratio* is the ratio between the likelihood of the condition being present if the test is positive, and its likelihood if the test is negative. In other words, it tells us about how powerful the test is in determining outcome.

A good test has high sensitivity and specificity, but also high predictive value and likelihood ratio. However, this is not enough: it must also be validated and acceptable (Table 1, point 4), and that there should be an agreed policy on further investigation (Table 1, point 7).

Assessing a test would be straightforward if what it measured were a *categorical* variable, for example, present/absent, dead/alive. Very little of what is sought in screening falls into this category. Most of the variables we measure are *continuous*, for example, height, blood pressure, haemoglobin, uric acid, bone mineral density, and prostate-specific antigen.

Table 2 Calculations of operating characteristics of a screening test

	Condition present	Condition absent
Test positive	A	B
Test negative	C	D

Prevalence = (A + C)/(A + B + C + D).

Yield = A/(A + B + C + D).

Sensitivity = A/(A + C).

Specificity = D/(B + D).

Positive predictive value (PPV) = A/(A + B).

Negative predictive value (NPV) = D/(C + D).

Misclassification rate = (B + C)/(A + B + C + D).

Likelihood ratio = Sens/(1 − spec) = A(B + D)/B(A + C).

See Table 4 for an example.

An ideal test—which is rare—would divide the population into two distinct groups, those who are disease-free and those who are affected (Fig. 1a). In practice most test results have a continuous distribution in which affected and unaffected individuals overlap (Fig. 1b).

Pickering put it well:

> Essential hypertension is a type of disease not hitherto recognised in medicine in which the defect is quantitative not qualitative. It is difficult for doctors to understand because it is a departure from the ordinary process of binary thought to which they are brought up. Medicine in its present state can count up to two but not beyond.[16]

In establishing a screening policy, we have to decide upon a cut-off point (Table 1, point 5) above which we will carry out further assessment, and below which we will declare the test negative. By moving the cut-off point to the left, we ensure that a larger proportion of people is classified as potentially abnormal: we therefore reduce the false-negative rate but increase the false positives, with attendant costs and anxiety for the participants. By moving it to the right, we increase the risk of missing significant disease and giving false reassurance. It is possible, by assigning a utility to each of the possible outcomes, to determine an optimal cut-off point. It is not, however, easy. Although convention may define the population normal range as that which includes 95 per cent of readings, this is a purely statistical definition.

Receiver operator characteristic (ROC) curves: An ROC curve plots sensitivity, or true-positive rate (TPR) against false-positive rate (FPR) for a given test. As the cut-off point of the test is altered, both rates rise, but to different degrees. A good test (Test a in Fig. 2) is one in which a significant rise in true positives can be achieved without the penalty of a high FPR. Conversely, in the case of a poor test (Test b) the relationship is more nearly linear, that is, there is no cut-off point at which many true positives and few false positives can be achieved. The area under the ROC curve (range 0.5–1.0) is a shorthand way of expressing the efficacy of the test.

Screening tests are intended to be predictive rather than diagnostic. Any GP who has had to communicate the implications of a 'positive' triple test to a pregnant woman will realize the importance of this distinction. By the same token, a programme that set out to identify the top 5 per cent of the population in terms of serum cholesterol would correctly label a small group at especially high risk of cardiovascular mortality, but would ignore a larger number in which the majority of cardiovascular events occur. The implication of this is that a high-risk strategy of this nature can never

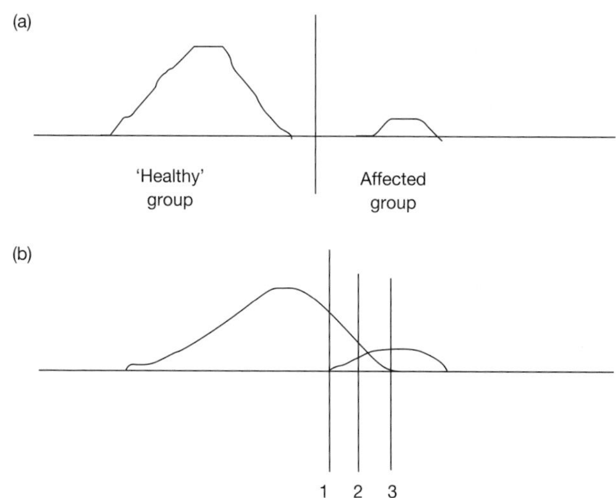
(a)
'Healthy' group
Affected group
(b)
1 2 3
1. Low threshold: high sensitivity, low specificity, many false positives.
2. Optimal threshold.
3. High threshold: high specificity, low sensitivity, many false negatives.

Fig. 1 Tests to separate those affected by a condition from those who are disease free. (a) An ideal test. (b) An actual test.

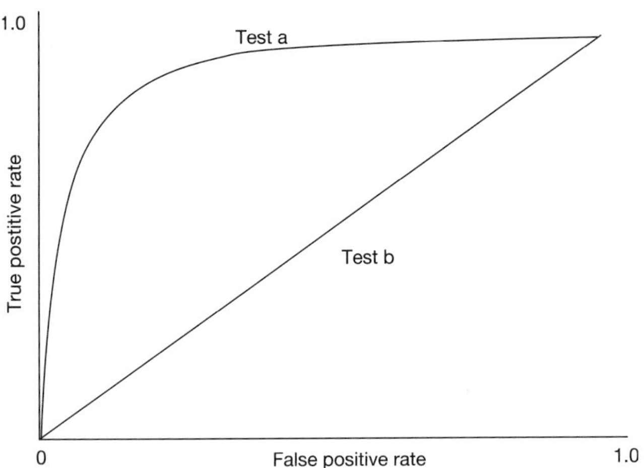

Fig. 2 Receiver operator characteristic curves showing a good test (Test a) and a poor test (Test b).

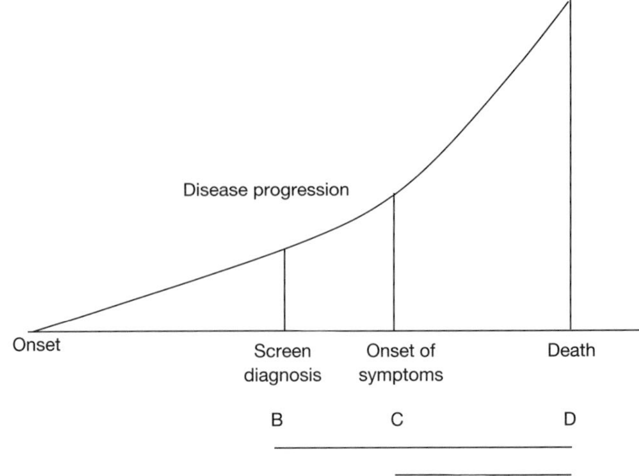

Fig. 3 The phenomenon of lead-time bias.

prevent all adverse outcomes, and is no substitute for population-based strategies (e.g. primary prevention in the form of smoking cessation, dietary advice, etc.).

The performance of a test depends crucially on the prevalence of the condition screened for. Thus, if the condition is common, a positive test is more likely to be a true positive, that is, the positive predictive value rises. It does not do so in a linear fashion, but according to a mathematical principle known as *Bayes' theorem*. Where the condition is uncommon, even an apparently accurate test can yield a high proportion of false positives.

The treatment

If a screening programme detects conditions for which treatment is unavailable or ineffective, then it is unlikely to be satisfactory. Similarly, if the treatment is one that the patient considers unacceptable, then it might have been preferable not to carry out the test in the first instance. Hence, the importance of good pre-test counselling.

The screening programme

The criteria recommend (Table 1, point 11) that there is good evidence of effectiveness from randomized controlled trials. The reason is that it is all too easy to overestimate the benefits of screening. The importance of such evidence is highlighted in the next section.

Bias

There are many conditions for which screening is available, and may indeed be accurate, but for which the interventions are as yet not shown to improve outcome. In such circumstances, the test leads to more patients being diagnosed earlier, and to a longer period between diagnosis and survival. This can be misinterpreted as improved outcome. This phenomenon is *lead-time bias.* (See Fig. 3.)

Length bias is illustrated in Fig. 4. The term describes the phenomenon whereby slow-growing lesions, particularly tumours, are more likely by their nature to be detected by a screening test, whereas more rapidly growing ones are more likely to be *interval cancers*, that is, presenting with symptoms between screens. The result is that screen-detected lesions are more likely to behave benignly, and be associated with longer survival.

Misclassification bias refers to a more extreme instance of length bias. Many lesions are detected by screening, are treated, and never recur—however, an unknown percentage of these would never have developed into invasive cancer. They have, in effect, the same impact as false positives.

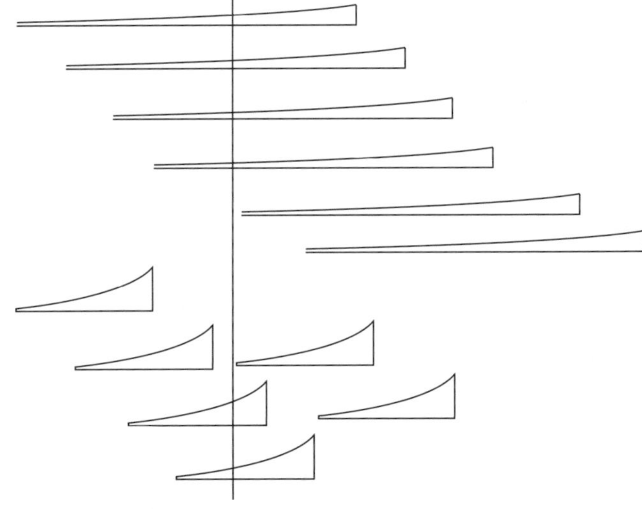

Fig. 4 The effect of length bias. Tumours may be slowly progressive (top of figure) or rapidly progressive (bottom). Because they are available to be detected for a longer period, the slowly progressive tumours are more likely to be detected on screening, while the rapidly progressive group are more likely to present with symptoms. The result is that screen-detected tumours by their nature have a longer survival.

Two further factors need to be remembered in looking at the results of screening trials. Such trials are done by enthusiasts with high input and often a higher uptake than can be achieved in the outside world. Secondly, screening a 'naive' population for the first time (the *prevalence* screen) will inevitably have a higher yield than will be found on later re-screens, because the first screen is in effect trawling a long-standing backlog. Attempts to replicate the early results of pilots can, therefore, end in disappointment.

There is no substitute for prospective long-term studies that examine hard outcomes such as mortality.

Uptake

The inverse care law was first described by Tudor Hart.[17] Those most likely to benefit from a medical service are also those least likely to receive it. Early attenders at screening programmes tend to be the affluent, while heart disease and most cancers (breast cancer being a notable exception) are commonest among the deprived. Therefore, yield is often disappointing, especially when uptake is low. In more successful programmes, as uptake approaches 100 per cent, the yield and effort required per person screened both increase. The inverse care law helps explain why screening has sometimes produced a higher yield when done opportunistically than systematically: the high-risk populations are more likely than average to attend the surgery for unrelated problems.

Frequency of screens

A negative screen offers a degree of reassurance. As time passes this reassurance wanes, and the time comes to repeat the test. Shortening the screening interval can increase the yield, but is subject to the law of diminishing returns. Optimal interval depends on the natural history of the condition. In cervical cytology, for example, a move from 3-yearly to 1-yearly screening would make a smaller impact than even a modest reduction in the number who have never once been screened.

Patient choice

Screening should address the needs of the individual patient. The emphasis should be on invitation rather than recruitment, with the patient making an informed choice to take part, with full knowledge of the possible outcomes and limitations of the test.

Screening for different diseases

How do screening programmes compare? Various backlists and whitelists have been produced, in which some programmes can be embraced and some dismissed, but very many fall into the intermediate area of 'insufficient evidence'. Table 3—from the Canadian Task Force—is an example.

A number of screening programmes are targeted at specific age groups and are discussed in more detail in other parts of this book. These include cervical cytology,[18] breast screening, ovarian cancer screening,[19] hypertension, and cardiovascular disease as well as generic screening for disease in the elderly. However, it is worth considering in detail a number of specific examples not covered in depth elsewhere both as exemplars and because they are contentious.

Prostatic cancer

Prostate cancer is currently the subject of heated debate. In several respects it is an attractive target for screening enthusiasts. It is common: it causes about 3 per cent of male deaths in the United Kingdom. Prevalence at post-mortem is about 15 per cent by age 60 and 34 per cent by age 80. It has a long pre-symptomatic phase during which it grows slowly (cell doubling time about a year). There are fairly simple and acceptable screening tests: digital rectal examination and PSA (prostate specific antigen). Of the two, PSA is the more sensitive—above 70 per cent.[20] A positive test seems to antedate clinical diagnosis by a long period. In one study of male physicians,[21] stored blood samples were tested for PSA. Among men who developed prostatic cancer, PSA measured 4 years earlier would have been raised (above 4 ng/ml) in as many as 73 per cent. Had the tests been read at the time the diagnosis would have been brought forward by several years. The proportion of prostate cancers diagnosed before becoming metastatic is higher in screened than unscreened populations (70 versus 35 per cent). Advocates of screening argue that such evidence points to the possibility of lives being saved.

However, there are several problems about this view:[22]

1. Positive predictive value of PSA is low. It rises with the PSA threshold chosen, but so does false-negative rate. Studies tend to show an area under the ROC curve of the order of 70 per cent. Taking a threshold of 4–10 ng/ml, PPV is between 8 and 33 per cent. Table 4 gives a typical picture.[23]
2. There is no easy gold standard test for further assessment of those who are screen positive. Trans-rectal ultrasound guided biopsy is unpleasant and complicated by bleeding or infection in about 1 per cent.
3. There is lack of consensus about the indications for, and the benefits of, treatment. Both surgery and radiotherapy can be complicated by impotence or incontinence.
4. Whether treated or not, the majority of men who have prostate cancer die with their tumour rather than of it. Indeed, even without treatment, patients with grade 1 cancers have virtually the same prognosis as those who are disease-free.[24]

The need for further investigation may possibly be avoided in some borderline patients by the use of additional tests, particularly the free PSA to PSA ratio. However the role of testing remains unclear. The European Randomised Study of Screening for Prostate Cancer and the American PLCO study, now in progress, may help.

Pending the results of trials, there is at least some consensus that screening is difficult to justify unless the person screened has a life expectancy of 10 years or more. In the United States, screening is already widely practised, while in the United Kingdom it is not.[25] The National Screening Committee in 1996 argued strongly against the introduction of a national screening programme. More recently, the emphasis has moved towards informed choice: that is, the test should not be withheld from those requesting it; however, it should not be performed until adequate counselling has been offered. An information sheet has been provided for the purpose (http://www.nsc.nhs.uk/pdfs/prostate_cancer.pdf).

Lung cancer

Lung cancer causes more deaths than any other, and occurs in a clearly defined risk group, smokers. It should thus, in principle, be worth diagnosing early. However, the value of screening remains unproven. In an often-quoted study[26] from the Mayo clinic, about 9000 smokers were randomized: half were screened for lung cancer by chest X-ray and sputum cytology. Patients were seen 4-monthly for 6 years. A significantly larger proportion of screened patients were diagnosed early with lung cancers, and cancers diagnosed early were more likely to be at an early stage and had a longer 5-year survival from diagnosis. That this excess was solely accounted for by length and lead-time bias becomes clear when we see that the overall mortality from lung cancer was identical in both groups (Table 5). However, this may not be the last word. Adherence to the protocol was only 75 per cent in the study group and 50 per cent in controls. There was contamination, with 50 per cent of controls having a chest X-ray. Several other trials have been equally negative. The only studies showing benefit have been non-randomized.

More recently, with advances in technology the issue is once again being debated.[27] The ELCAP study has shown that spiral computerized tomography (CT) is much more sensitive than radiography for detecting stage 1 malignant nodules (yield 2.3 versus 0.4 per cent in smokers aged over 60). If biopsy was restricted to lesions showing progression, biopsy rate was 27 per 1000 and PPV was as high as 97 per cent. Unfortunately, we still do not know whether this would translate into improved survival. Most importantly, the costs of this technology are high. In the United Kingdom, the figure for investigational costs alone has been put at £50–250 million for the first round of screening. In a resource-hungry service it is unlikely that this will be considered money well spent until more compelling evidence is available.

Colorectal cancer

There is now significant trial evidence that faecal occult blood screening is associated with improved outcome of colonic cancers. Among the many studies, Hardcastle et al.[28] is a good example. In a large prospective trial

Table 3 An example of a classification of screening programmes based on strength of evidence

The following are extracts from the current recommendations (1997) of the Canadian Task Force on Preventive Health Care. This body has set out to classify preventive procedures according to the strength of evidence in their favour. The table includes only selected screening activities relating to adults, and excludes those which solely concern high-risk groups

'A' recommendations—good evidence to include in periodic health examination
Breast cancer—mammography and clinical exam in women aged 50–69 years
Dental caries and periodontal disease
Hypertension (young adults and high-risk elderly)
Tobacco-caused disease

'B' recommendations—fair evidence to include in periodic health examination
Cervical cancer—Papanicolaou smear
Diminished visual acuity in the elderly
Hearing impairment in the elderly
Hypertension in the elderly
Problem drinking

'C' recommendations—when evidence is inconclusive
Abdominal aortic aneurysm by palpation or abdominal ultrasound in general population
Age-related macular degeneration by fundoscopy in the elderly
Screening mammography in women aged 40–49 years at average risk of breast cancer
Cognitive impairment—mental status screening in the elderly
Colorectal cancer—faecal occult blood testing, sigmoidoscopy, or colonoscopy
Measurement of blood total cholesterol level in general population with case-finding for males 30–59 years
Voluntary HIV antibody screening in general population including pregnant women
Hypertension in adults aged less than 21 years, isolated systolic hypertension, some elderly subgroups
Lead exposure—universal screening (blood lead level or questionnaire) in general population
Obesity—BMI measurement in general population
Ovarian cancer—pelvic exam, transvaginal ultrasound, CA 125 or combination in pre- and post-menopausal women or family history first-degree relative
Prostate cancer—digital rectal examination in males above 50 years
Skin cancer—physical examination in general population
Testicular cancer—physical exam or self-examination in adolescent or adult males
Thyroid cancer—neck palpation in adult population
Thyroid disorders—TSH in perimenopausal women
Tobacco-caused disease
Urinary infection—urine dipstick or culture in elderly ambulatory women

'D' recommendations—fair evidence to exclude from periodic health examination
Bladder cancer—urine dipstick or cytology in general population
Breast cancer—by breast self-examination in women aged 40–49 and 50–59 years
Carotid disease/stroke—neck auscultation or carotid endarterectomy in general population
Cervical cancer—use of human papillomavirus screening in women
Chlamydial infection—smear, culture, or analysis in general population
Cystic fibrosis—DNA analysis for carrier status, or sweat test in the general population
Depression by General Health Questionnaire in the general population
Diabetes mellitus—fasting blood glucose, in non-pregnant general population
Gonorrhoea—gram stain/culture of cervical or urethral smear in the general population
Lung cancer—chest radiography in general population
Oral cancer—population screening by clinical examination in general population
Osteoporotic fractures—bone mineral density screening in women
Ovarian cancer—pelvic exam, transvaginal ultrasound, CA 125 or combination in pre- and post-menopausal women
Pancreatic cancer—abdominal palpation, ultrasound, or serologic tumour markers in general population
Progressive renal disease—urine dipstick in general population
Prostate cancer—prostate specific antigen in males above 50 years
Prostate cancer—transrectal ultrasound in males above 50 years
Testicular cancer—tumour markers in adolescent and adult males
Urinary infection—urine dipstick or culture in elderly, ambulatory men

'E' recommendations—good evidence to exclude from periodic health examination
Lung cancer—sputum cytology in general population
Tuberculosis—Mantoux test in general population

(150 000 patients) in the age range 45–74, mortality from colonic cancer during the period of observation was reduced by 15 per cent, from 0.7 to 0.6 per 1000 person-years. This translates into a number-needed-to-screen of 10 000 to save one life over 1 year. The predictive value of a single test was only 10 per cent. However, many of the false negatives were in fact adenomas, a proportion of which would have progressed if left alone. Initial uptake in the trial was 53 per cent and some of the refusers were later recruited. Strikingly, the yield of cancer among the latter group was over double that in the population as a whole—a good example of the inverse care law.

Table 4 PSA performance (cut off point 4 ng/ml) combined with digital rectal examination (see also Table 2)

	Cancer present	Cancer absent	Total
Test positive	A = 197	B = 1169	1366
Test negative	C = 29	D = 5828	5857
Total	226	6997	7223

Prevalence = (A + C)/(A + B + C + D), 226/7223 = 3.1%.

Yield = A/(A + B + C + D), 197/7223 = 2.7%.

Sensitivity = A/(A + C), 197/226 = 87%.

Specificity = D/(B + D), 5828/6997 = 83%.

Positive predictive value (PPV) = A/(A + B), 197/1366 = 14%.

Negative predictive value (NPV) = D/(C + D), 5828/5857 = 99%.

Misclassification rate = (1169 + 29)/7223 = 16%.

Likelihood ratio = A(B + D)/B/(A + C) = (197 × 6997)/(1169 × 226) = 5.2.

Table 5 The Mayo Lung Project

	Screened (n = 4618)	Controls (n = 4593)
Cases detected	206	160
Early stage (operable)	46%	32%
Five-year survival	33%	15%
Eleven-year cumulative lung cancer mortality	122 (3.2 per thousand person-years)	115 (3 per thousand person-years)

At present, the result of a community-based pilot study is awaited before a decision is made to implement a full-scale screening programme in the United Kingdom.[29] However, it seems likely that this will eventually occur.

Conclusion

General practice has moved away from a reactive model of care to one in which prevention is an integral part. While it is not possible in a few words to give a blueprint for a practice screening programme, Fry et al.[30] provide valuable guidance that can be paraphrased as follows:

- Opportunistic screening and systematic screening are both necessary.
- Screening needs to address a defined group within the population.
- Every member of the team should share in the ownership of the screening programme, understand its objectives, and contribute to its planning.
- Because of the inverse care law, one needs to identify non-attenders and send reminders. On the other hand, patients staying at home are exercising a valid right and should not be stigmatized.
- Invitations to screening need to be positive, friendly, and personal. Invitations can achieve a higher uptake if they specify a fixed date and time.
- Accessibility, convenience of timing, and good communication can help improve uptake.
- Taking the opportunity to address lifestyle issues, for example, smoking, alcohol, diet, and exercise, may be just as valuable as the search for physical disease.
- Computers are invaluable in identifying the target population, auditing care, and providing prompts for opportunistic screening. However, we need to remember the dictum 'garbage in, garbage out'. Thus, registers need to be accurate and up to date.

However, no guidance on screening can be everlasting. Change is inevitable. Diseases and treatments come and go. At least as importantly, public attitudes evolve. Developments such as the rise of HIV infection bring in their train dilemmas as to who should be tested and when. Genetic testing opens new doors almost daily. It has benefits for individuals but it may prove even more attractive to third parties, such as the insurance industry. So caution is required.

Many screening activities, which are currently seen as of doubtful value, will earn their place as the evidence comes in and as test performance improves. Others will be found wanting and rejected. Only an optimist can feel certain that all screening will be evidence-based. Growth in private screening, both mainstream and complementary, is unlikely to abate. We need to be ready to defend an evidence-based approach to screening, and make it clear that this is not motivated solely by professional self-interest.

There is no doubt that a more sophisticated and demanding public will come to expect an active role in deciding what screening is done. Information technology is already seeing to it that the patient frequently enters the consulting room better informed than the professional. We find ourselves having to share the evidence and justify our recommendations. As doctors we do not need to see this as a threat. It is, rather, an opportunity to reinvent the relationship between those who provide and those who use the service, as one of partnership and cooperation.

References

1. **Hart, C.** (1992). Theory and its application. In *Screening and Surveillance in General Practice* (ed. C. Hart and P. Burke), London: Churchill Livingstone.
2. **National Screening Committee.** *Second Report of the UK National Screening Committee.* London: Health Departments of the United Kingdom, 2000 (http://www.nsc.nhs.uk/).
3. **The South East London Study Group** (1977). A controlled trial of multiphasic screening in middle age—results of the South East London Screening Study. *International Journal of Epidemiology* **6**, 357–63.
4. **Imperial Cancer Research Fund. Oxcheck study** (1995). Effectiveness of health checks conducted by nurses in primary care: final results of the Oxcheck study. *British Medical Journal* **310**, 1099–104.
5. **Family Heart Study Group** (1994). Randomised controlled trial evaluating cardiovascular screening and intervention in general practice: principal results of British family heart study. *British Medical Journal* **308**, 313–20.
6. **Forrest, P.** *Breast Cancer Screening: Report to the Health Ministers of England, Wales, Scotland and Northern Ireland.* London: HMSO, 1986.
7. **Canadian Task Force on Preventive Health Care:** http://www.ctfphc.org/
8. **Nuffield Institute for Health.** *Quality Management for Screening: Report to the National Screening Committee*, 2000.
9. **NHS Cancer Plan.** September 2000 (http://www.doh.gov.uk/cancer).
10. **Petticrew, M.P., Sowden, A.J., Lister-Sharp, D., and Wright, K.** (2000). False-negative results in screening programmes: systematic review of impact and implications. *Health Technology Assessment* **4** (5), 1–120.
11. **Stoate, H.** (1989). Can health screening damage your health? *Journal of the Royal College of General Practioners* **39**, 193–5.
12. **O'Connor, A.** et al. (1999). Decision aids for patients facing health treatment or screening decisions: systematic review. *British Medical Journal* **319**, 731–4.
13. **Rembold, C.** (1998). Number needed to screen: development of a statistic for disease screening. *British Medical Journal* **317**, 307–12.
14. **Wonderling, D.** et al. (1996). What can be concluded from the Oxcheck and British family heart studies: commentary on cost-effectiveness analyses. *British Medical Journal* **312**, 1274–8.
15. **Wilson, J.M.G. and Jungner, G.** *Principles and Practice of Screening for Disease.* Geneva: WHO (Public Health Paper), 1968.
16. **Pickering, G.W.** *High Blood Pressure* 2nd edn. London: Churchill, 1968.
17. **Hart, J.T.** (1971). The inverse care law. *Lancet* **i**, 405–12.
18. *Informing Choice in Cervical Screening.* Cervical Screening Programme Annual Review 2001. London: HMSO, 2001.
19. **Bell, R., Petticrew, M., Luengo, S., and Sheldon, T.A.** (1998). Screening for ovarian cancer: a systematic review. *Health Technology Assessment* **2** (2), 1–84.
20. **Goldstein, M.M. and Messing, E.M.** (1998). Prostate and bladder cancer screening. *Journal of the American College of Surgery* **186**, 63–74.

21. **Gann, P.H., Hennekens, C.H., and Stampfer, M.J.** (1995). A prospective evaluation of plasma prostate specific antigen for detection of prostatic cancer. *Journal of the American Medical Association* **123**, 19.
22. **Austoker, J.** (1994). Cancer prevention in primary care: screening for ovarian, prostatic and testicular cancers. *British Medical Journal* **309**, 315–20.
23. **Meyer, F. and Fradet, Y.** (1998). Prostate cancer: 4. Screening. *Journal of Canadian Medical Association* **159**, 968–72.
24. **Lu-Yao, G.L. and Yao, S.-L.** (1997). Population based study of long-term survival in patients with clinically localised prostate cancer. *The Lancet* **349**, 906–10.
25. **Dearnaley, D.P., Kirby, R.S., Kirk, D., Malone, P., Simpson, R.J., and Williams, G.** (1999). Diagnosis and management of early prostate cancer. Report of a British Association of Urological Surgeons Working Party. *British Journal of Urology* **83**, 18–33.
26. **Fontana, R.S.** (2000). The Mayo Lung Project: a perspective. *Cancer* **89** (11 Suppl.), 2352–5.
27. **Ellis, J.R.C. and Gleeson, F.V.** (2001). Lung cancer screening. *British Journal of Radiology* **74**, 478–85.
28. **Hardcastle, J.D., Chamberlain, J.O., Robinson, M.H.E., Moss, S.M., Amar, S.S., Balfour, T.W., James, P.D., and Mangham, C.M.** (1996). Randomised controlled trial of faecal-occult-blood screening for colorectal cancer. *The Lancet* **348**, 1472–6.
29. **Steele, R.J.C., Parker, R., Patnick, J., Warner, J., Fraser, C., Mowat, N.A.G., Wilson, J., Alexander, F.E., and Paterson, J.G.** (2001). A demonstration pilot trial for colorectal cancer screening in the United Kingdom: a new concept in the introduction of healthcare strategies. *Journal of Medical Screening* **8**, 197–203.
30. **Fry, J., Jeffree, P., and Scott, K.** (1990). *The Screening Handbook.* London: Kluwer, 1990.

Useful websites

The National Electronic Library for Screening: http://www.nelh.nhs.uk/screening/

UK National Screening Committee: http://www.nsc.nhs.uk/

CancerBacup Screening Pages: http://www.cancerbacup.org.uk/reports/screening-mac.htm

The National Coordinating Centre for Health Technology Assessment: http://www.ncchta.org

National Office of the NHS Cancer Screening Programmes: http://www. cancerscreening.nhs.uk/

US Preventive Services Task Force (USPSTF): http://www.ahrq.gov/clinic/uspstfix.htm

Institute of Cancer Research Cancer Screening Evaluation Unit: http://www.icr.ac.uk/cseu/

Canadian Task Force on Preventive Health Care: http://www.ctfphc.org/

Journal of Medical Screening: http://jms.bmjjournals.com/

11.4 Changing behaviour: smoking

Tim Lancaster

Why do people smoke?

Most smoking behaviour is sustained by psycho-pharmacological addiction to nicotine. Nicotine probably acts through neurobiological reward pathways in the brain, particularly the dopamine system. Cigarette smokers typically increase their smoking, either in quantity or intensity, to maintain serum levels of nicotine. Nicotine dependence in turn leads to physical and psychological symptoms of withdrawal when cigarettes are stopped. There is continued debate about whether nicotine itself is a pleasurable stimulus, or whether its benefits result from relief of withdrawal symptoms. Either way, people who smoke usually say that cigarettes provide pleasure, decreasing stress and improving concentration.

An interaction of social, psychological, and biological factors determines why some people take up smoking and continue to smoke. Twin studies suggest that genetic factors predispose to tobacco addiction. Molecular genetic studies have found differences in allele frequency at certain dopamine loci, suggesting a possible pathway for genetic susceptibility. Differences in the cytochrome P450 genes involved in metabolizing nicotine may also play a role, and there are likely to be multiple gene–gene interactions influencing susceptibility to smoking.[(1)]

As with other behaviours, whether an individual smokes reflects the interaction of genetic factors with environmental factors. It is important to avoid naïve, deterministic concepts of genetic susceptibility. Indeed, the changing patterns of cigarette smoking over the past 30 years suggest that its prevalence is, increasingly, determined by social factors. In the United Kingdom, for example, the overall prevalence of smoking has fallen substantially in the past 20 years in response to an array of tobacco control strategies and changing social norms. Between 1973 and 1996 it fell from 53 to 29 per cent in men and from 42 to 28 per cent in women.[(2)] However, these encouraging data hide a widening disparity between different social classes. While rates among the most affluent have fallen by more than 50 per cent, they have not decreased at all among the most disadvantaged. In the United Kingdom, the likelihood that an individual will smoke is greater among lower occupational class groups, the unemployed, those of lower educational attainment, those living in rented housing and overcrowded accommodation, and those without access to a car. The risk of smoking is also increased in those who are divorced, separated, or lone parents. It is particularly high in people who are homeless, heavy users of alcohol, or mentally ill.[(2)] Among the most disadvantaged sectors of British society over 80 per cent of adults smoke. The most plausible explanation for this finding is that individuals use smoking as a form of 'self-medication' to allow them to cope with the stress of their social situation.

The social gradient is similar in many other countries in which the tobacco epidemic is mature. Meanwhile, in many less affluent countries, historically low rates of smoking are increasing across the social spectrum. Exploitation of changing social values by tobacco manufacturers seeking new markets has led to huge increases in smoking prevalence in countries such as China, where the health consequences in the next century will be catastrophic. These disparities are an important cause of widening inequalities in health status both within and between nations.

What are the health benefits of stopping smoking?

About half of those who start smoking before they are 20 and continue beyond middle age will die early from a smoking-related cause. Of the death and disability caused by smoking, the commonest causes are vascular disease, lung cancer, and respiratory disease.[(3)] The relative importance of these varies in different countries. For example, chronic lung disease causes relatively more deaths in China than in Western Hemisphere countries.[(4,5)] Smoking contributes to the risk of other cancers, particularly of the oropharynx and oesophagus. Smoking also increases morbidity. For example, children exposed to passive smoking have an increased risk of respiratory tract infections, otitis media, asthma, and the sudden infant death syndrome. Continuation of worldwide consumption at current levels will cause about 450 million premature deaths in the next 50 years. An increasing proportion of these deaths will occur in societies where life expectancy is already reduced by other poverty-related diseases of nutrition and infection.

How can mortality from smoking be reduced?

The increased risk of death from smoking on health occurs many years after initiation of the habit. This means that measures to stop children from starting to smoke will have no effect on mortality for at least 50 years.[6] Smokers who give up before middle age shed almost all their excess risk of premature death. Those who quit after middle age continue to have a higher risk of death than lifelong non-smokers, but reduce their risk compared to continued smokers.[7] Quitting by current smokers is therefore the only way in which tobacco-related mortality can be reduced in the medium term. Peto and Lopez estimate that a reduction of 50 per cent in the number of current smokers would avoid about 20–30 million premature deaths in the first quarter of the century and about 150 million in the second quarter.[6] If this could be achieved, it would save more adults from premature death than any other available health care intervention.

Is smoking a clinical issue or a social problem?

The class gradient in smoking prevalence suggests that the long-term solution to the tobacco problem will be social rather than medical. Public health strategies to control tobacco include bans on advertising, fiscal policies, restrictions on smoking in public places, and retailer restraint. They have proved their value in decreasing prevalence in both developed and some developing countries. However, their main effect is usually to reduce smoking among the more affluent. A more equitable reduction in smoking will only be achieved with social policies that improve the quality of life of the less well off.

Does it make sense then to treat smoking as a clinical problem? Historically, the majority of successful quitters reported that they gave up without formal help. Sceptics have used this as an argument for keeping smoking out of the clinical arena. But this now seems to be an outdated notion. In more recent surveys, almost half of successful quitters report that they have used some form of treatment.[8] Every society that has successfully reduced prevalence of smoking has given attention to cessation. Randomized trials show that appropriate advice and treatment can help people to stop smoking, even if the absolute effects are small. As the epidemiology of smoking changes, those who continue to smoke may be those with the highest levels of nicotine dependence. Socially disadvantaged groups appear to have particularly high dependence levels.[2] There is thus a strong argument for increasing facilities for clinical treatment of nicotine dependence. Indeed, this may be the only short-term way of reducing social inequalities in tobacco-related mortality.

Which treatments are available?

The available treatments include 'talking treatments', drugs, and complementary therapies. Talking treatments range from simple advice to intensive counselling driven by psychological theory. Drug treatments may reduce withdrawal symptoms. Many have been tested, but there is most evidence of effectiveness for nicotine replacement and antidepressants. Each form of treatment has a different rationale and most strategies include more than one modality. For example, psychological treatments that promote and sustain motivation combine logically with drug treatments to reduce the physical and psychological symptoms of nicotine withdrawal.

What can primary care do to help people stop?

Ask and advise

The simplest way for health workers to help people to give up smoking is to offer them advice. In order to advise, they need to ask and record whether their patients smoke. A systematic review showed that simple advice during routine clinical care consistently increases the number of people who stopping, by about one and half to two times[9] probably by motivating a quit attempt.[10] The absolute rates are of course small. The background quit rate is about 1 per cent a year, so doubling that would mean just one more non-smoker from 100 advised. However, provided consistently, this simple intervention can make a substantial contribution over time.

Assess motivation and nicotine dependence

Advice and treatment should be tailored to the individual. A practical approach is to link advice to an assessment of each individual's motivation and readiness to change.[11] Someone who has no active interest in quitting, needs only brief advice and a promise of future support. For the smaller number ready to stop, primary care workers should make a fuller assessment including reasons for smoking, barriers to quitting, and level of nicotine dependence. They can then help the patient to draw up a plan for quitting that may include further support and pharmacological treatment for nicotine dependence.

Direct motivated individuals to sources of further support

More intensive psychological interventions provide support and may help motivated smokers to deal with the consequences of nicotine withdrawal. Such treatments can be delivered one-to-one, or in a group. They can be provided in primary care, or in specialist clinics. Compared to brief advice or usual care, individual counselling increases the likelihood of quitting about one and a half times.[12] Group therapy is more effective than self-help materials, but not consistently better than other interventions involving personal contact.[13] Direct comparisons have not shown any difference in effectiveness between groups and individual counselling. Groups are theoretically more cost-effective, but their usefulness is limited by difficulties in recruiting and retaining participants. Individual counselling, provided by doctors, nurses, or pscyhologists, is a more practical way of providing support in primary care.

Behavioural interventions aim to equip smokers with the motivation, skills, knowledge, and support for quitting and avoiding relapse. Counsellors can provide general support through encouragement, information, and empathy. They may also draw on a variety of cognitive and behavioural techniques such as problem solving and skills training, relaxation techniques, contracts based on rewards and punishments, social support, and cognitive restructuring. Counselling can help individuals to recognize and deal with 'danger situations' likely to increase the risk of smoking. General lifestyle changes, particularly diet and exercise, are important as they may reduce the post-cessation weight gain that many smokers find unacceptable. Because most studies of behavioural treatments have included multiple elements, there is little evidence about which components are the most important. Many of the principles can be incorporated into brief advice strategies even if specialized counselling is not available.

Aversion therapy is a particular form of treatment that pairs smoking with an unpleasant stimulus, with the aim of extinguishing the urge to smoke. Aversion can be produced pharmacologically (e.g., with the drug silver acetate) or by methods such as smoking cigarettes at a fixed, rapid rate to produce unpleasant physiological symptoms. Controlled trials of aversion therapy have given conflicting results, and these treatments are not now widely used.

One way of reaching out to more people is to deliver the content of behavioural interventions as self-help materials. These are available in many forms including brief leaflets, complex manuals, audiotapes, videotapes, and computer programs. They may be given to support personal contact or on their own. A systematic review of randomized trials found that self-help materials had no additional benefit over brief personal advice. However, in 12 trials with no face-to-face contact, there was a statistically significant effect of self-help materials, increasing quit rates by about 25 per cent compared to no intervention.[13] More recent approaches have concentrated on ways of making self-help materials appropriate for the needs of individual smokers. Rather than providing generic materials, individually tailored materials are prepared taking into account such factors as level of addiction, motivation to quit, and readiness to change.[14] In eight randomized trials comparing personalized materials to standard materials, there was a significant increase of about 40 per cent in those quitting. There was no evidence that materials tailored solely to group characteristics (such as age, gender, or race) were better than standard materials. Reinforcing self-help with personal contact by telephone can increase the quit rates achieved with self-help materials.

Consider specific treatment for nicotine dependence

Withdrawal from nicotine causes a number of unpleasant symptoms, including restlessness, difficulty concentrating, irritability, anxiety, craving for nicotine, and change in appetite. These symptoms improve when a cigarette is smoked. Nicotine dependence can be assessed with a couple of simple questions. Smoking the first cigarette within an hour of waking and being a heavier smoker (more than about 15 per day) suggest that the patient is dependent and may be helped by drug treatment.

Nicotine replacement therapy (NRT)

The aim of NRT is to reduce withdrawal symptoms by replacing the nicotine from cigarettes. The usual aim is to break the smoking habit and then wean the patient from NRT. However, there is increasing interest in continued use of NRT to reduce the number of cigarettes smoked, a concept of harm reduction borrowed from drug treatments.[15] Not all smokers are nicotine dependent, and NRT is unlikely to be helpful when it is absent.

NRT is available as chewing gum, transdermal patch, nasal spray, inhaler, sub-lingual tablet, and lozenge. A systematic review of over 90 trials found that NRT helps people to stop smoking, increasing the chances of quitting about one and a half to two times.[16] The quit rate was higher in both placebo and NRT arms of trials that included intensive support, so the effect of NRT seems to be to increase the rate from whatever baseline is set by other interventions. Since all the trials of NRT reported so far have included at least some form of brief advice, this is the minimum that should be offered in order to ensure its effectiveness. It is likely, of course, that more people will succeed when NRT is combined with behavioural support, but there is observational evidence that it is effective even in minimal contact settings, such as purchase over the counter from a pharmacist.[17]

There is little evidence that any NRT product is more effective than another. One study that directly compared four products found no difference in short-term abstinence rates or withdrawal symptoms.[18] Thus, the decision about which to use should be made according to individual characteristics and preferences. The nicotine patch delivers a steady level of nicotine throughout the day, and can be worn unobtrusively. The main side-effect is skin irritation, and it is unsuitable for individuals with widespread skin conditions such as psoriasis. Wearing the patch only during waking hours (16 h/day) is as effective as wearing it for 24 h/day. Eight weeks of patch therapy is as effective as longer courses and there is no evidence that tapered therapy is better than abrupt withdrawal. Nicotine gum is unsuitable for individuals with dentures, and many find its taste unpleasant. The nicotine inhaler resembles a cigarette and may be useful for individuals who want a substitute for the act of smoking. The nasal spray delivers nicotine more rapidly and may be suitable for satisfying surges of craving. It tends to cause sneezing and irritation in the nose.

Some clinicians recommend combinations of nicotine products (e.g. providing a background nicotine level with patches, and controlling cravings with faster acting preparations such as gum or spray). There have been too few trials to provide clear evidence about the effectiveness of patch and gum combinations.[19,20] In one trial, the combination of nasal spray and patch was better than patch alone.[21]

Antidepressants

Antidepressants are the newest form of commercially available drug treatment for nicotine dependence. Observations that some patients entered in drug trials for depression seemed to find it easier to give up smoking led to formal trials of several types of antidepressant. The slow release form of the atypical antidepressant bupropion (Zyban) is licensed for smoking cessation in many countries. It probably inhibits neuronal uptake of noradrenaline and dopamine. In two published trials, there was a significant increase in quitting in patients taking bupropion compared to placebo. Bupropion increased the quit rate about two and half to three times.[22,23] These trials recruited heavier smokers who were also offered behavioural support. In one trial bupropion alone or combined with a nicotine patch was more effective than nicotine patch alone.[22] Bupropion can cause dry mouth and insomnia. Some patients develop allergic reactions such as urticaria. There are also reports of rarer, more serious serum-sickness type reactions. The manufacturers report a risk of seizures of 1 in 1000 users from sustained-release bupropion up to 300 mg/day. The drug should not be used when there is a history of epilepsy or risk factors for fits such as a brain tumour or prior head injury. Bupropion also inhibits cytochrome P4502D6, and may therefore interfere with the metabolism of certain drugs including metoprolol, flecainide, paroxetine, and risperidone. On the limited evidence, bupropion may be more effective than NRT. However, many clinicians consider NRT to be the first line drug treatment for nicotine dependence because of its excellent safety profile.

Other antidepressants may also help smoking cessation. In two placebo-controlled trials, the tricyclic antidepressant nortriptyline had a similar effect to bupropion, increasing quit rates almost threefold, but with the usual side-effects of this class of drugs.[24,25] One abstract reported that fluoxetine, a selective serotonin re-uptake inhibitor, increased quit rates, but the results of other studies of this drug have not yet been published.[26] These results raise the possibility that antidepressants as a class may be effective, rather than specific drugs. In the trials the drugs were effective whether depression was present or not, so their effect appears to be independent of antidepressant activity.

Other pharmacological therapies

Licensed primarily as an antihypertensive, clonidine shares some pharmacological effects with bupropion and tricyclic antidepressants. A systematic review of six clinical trials showed evidence that it has an effect, but its usefulness is limited by sedation and postural hypotension.[27] The nicotine antagonist mecamylamine has been investigated as a cessation aid in combination with nicotine replacement. It is not licensed for this use. Two studies suggest an effect of mecamylamine, started pre-cessation and continued post-cessation, in aiding smoking cessation.[28] The studies also suggest that the combination of mecamylamine with nicotine replacement, started before cessation, may increase the rates of cessation beyond those achieved with nicotine alone. Studies of anxiolytics and narcotic antagonists have failed to show that they help stop smoking.

Complementary therapies

Randomized trials of acupuncture and hypnotherapy have failed to show specific effects of these treatments on smoking behaviour.[29,30] However, individuals may well benefit from the non-specific effects and general support involved with these treatments.

Conclusions

Giving up smoking is a difficult task that usually requires a number of attempts. Social and economic factors interact with personal susceptibility in determining whether individuals are successful in quitting smoking. Primary care health workers can provide motivation, support, and treatment for people seeking to quit. At a minimum, they should find out whether their patients smoke and offer them advice if they do. For motivated individuals with evidence of nicotine dependence, they should advise about NRT or antidepressants to reduce withdrawal symptoms. If resources permit, primary care teams should give continued support and behavioural counselling. In addition, primary care practitioners have an important part to play in broader tobacco control strategies. They are ideally placed to support social and public health strategies through role modelling, advocacy and links to community initiatives.

References

1. **Bergen, A.W. and Caporaso, N.** (1999). Cigarette smoking. *Journal of the National Cancer Institute* **91**, 1365–75.
2. **Jarvis, M.J. and Wardle, J.** (1999). Social patterning of individual behaviours: the case of cigarette smoking. In *Social Determinants of Health* (ed. M.G. Marmot and R.G. Wilkinson), pp. 240–56. Oxford: Oxford University Press.
3. **Peto, R., Lopez, A.D., Boreham, J., Thun, M., and Heath, C.** (1992). Mortality from tobacco in developed countries: indirect estimation from national vital statistics. *The Lancet* **339**, 1268–78.
4. **Liu, B.Q.** et al. (1998). Emerging tobacco hazards in China: 1. Retrospective proportional mortality study of one million deaths. *British Medical Journal* **317**, 1411–22.
5. **Niu, S.R.** et al. (1998). Emerging tobacco hazards in China: 2. Early mortality results from a prospective study . *British Medical Journal* **317**, 1423–4.
6. **Peto, R. and Lopez, A.D.** (2000). The future worldwide health effects of current smoking patterns. In *Critical Issues in Global Health* (ed. C. Everett Koop, C.E. Pearson, and M. Roy Schwarz), New York: Jossey-Bass.
7. **Doll, R., Peto, R., Wheatley, K., Gray, R., and Sutherland, I.** (1994). Mortality in relation to smoking: 40 years' observations on male British doctors. *British Medical Journal* **309**, 901–11.
8. **Hughes, J.R.** (1999). Four beliefs that may impede progress in the treatment of smoking. *Tobacco Control* **8**, 323–6.
9. **Silagy, C.** (2001). Physician advice for smoking cessation (Cochrane Review). In *The Cochrane Library* Issue 1. Oxford: Update Software.
10. **Hughes, J.R., Goldstein, M.G., Hurt, R.D., and Shiffman, S.** (1999). Recent advances in the pharmacotherapy of smoking. *Journal of the American Medical Association* **281**, 72–6.
11. **Prochaska, J.O.** (2000). Stages of change model for smoking prevention and cessation in schools—authors applied adult dose for smoking to adolescents when smoking behaviour is different in the two. *British Medical Journal* **320**, 447.
12. **Lancaster, T. and Stead, L.F.** (2001). Individual behavioural counselling for smoking cessation (Cochrane Review). In *The Cochrane Library* Issue 1. Oxford: Update Software.
13. **Stead, L.F. and Lancaster, T.** (2001). Group behaviour therapy programmes for smoking cessation (Cochrane Review). In *The Cochrane Library* Issue 1. Oxford: Update Software.
14. **Prochaska, J.O. and Velicer, W.F.** (1997). The transtheoretical model of health behavior change. *American Journal of Health Promotion* **12**, 38–48.
15. **Hughes, J.R.** (1996). The future of smoking cessation therapy in the United States. *Addiction* **91**, 1797–802.
16. **Silagy, C., Mant, D., Fowler, G., and Lancaster, T.** Nicotine replacement therapy for smoking cessation (Cochrane Review). In *The Cochrane Library* Issue 1. Oxford: Update Software.
17. **Shiffman, S., Gitchell, J., Pinney, J.M., Burton, S.L., Kemper, K.E., and Lara, E.A.** (1997). Public health benefit of over-the-counter nicotine medications. *Tobacco Control* **6** (4), 306–10.
18. **Hajek, P., West, R., Foulds, J., Nilsson, F., Burrows, S., and Meadow, A.** (1999). Randomized comparative trial of nicotine polacrilex, a transdermal patch, nasal spray, and an inhaler. *Archives of Internal Medicine* **159**, 2033–8.
19. **Puska, P., Korhonen, H.J., Vartiainen, E., Urjanheimo, E.L., Gustavsson, G., and Westin, A.** (1995). Combined use of nicotine patch and gum compared with gum alone in smoking cessation: a clinical trial in North Karelia. *Tobacco Control* **4**, 231–5.
20. **Kornitzer, M., Boutsen, M., Dramaix, M., Thijs, J., and Gustavsson, G.** (1995). Combined use of nicotine patch and gum in smoking cessation: a placebo-controlled clinical trial. *Preventive Medicine* **24**, 41–7.
21. **Blondal, T., Gudmundsson, L.J., Olafsdottir, I., Gustavsson, G., Westin, A.** (1999). Nicotine nasal spray with nicotine patch for smoking cessation: randomised trial with six year follow up. *British Medical Journal* **318**, 285–8.
22. **Jorenby, D.E.** et al. (1999). A controlled trial of sustained-release bupropion, a nicotine patch, or both for smoking cessation. *New England Journal of Medicine* **340**, 685–91.
23. **Hurt, R.D., Glover, E.D., Sachs, D.P.L., Dale, L.C., and Schroeder, D.R.** (1996). Bupropion for smoking cessation: a double-blind, placebo-controlled dose response trial. *Journal of Addictive Diseases* **15**, 137 (Abstract).
24. **Prochazka, A.V., Weaver, M.J., Keller, R.T., Fryer, G.E., Licari, P.A., and Lofaso, D.** (1998). A randomized trial of nortriptyline for smoking cessation. *Archives of Internal Medicine* **158**, 2035–9.
25. **Hall, S.M.** et al. (1998). Nortriptyline and cognitive-behavioral therapy in the treatment of cigarette smoking. *Archives of General Psychiatry* **55**, 683–90.
26. **Niaura, R.** et al. (1997). Fluoxetine for smoking cessation: a multicenter randomized double blind dose response study. *Annals of Behavioral Medicine* **19**, S042 (Abstract).
27. **Gourlay, S.G., Stead, L.F., and Benowitz, N.L.** (2001). Clonidine for smoking cessation (Cochrane Review). In *The Cochrane Library* Issue 1. Oxford: Update Software.
28. **Lancaster, T. and Stead, L.F.** (2001). Mecamylamine (a nicotine antagonist) for smoking cessation (Cochrane Review). In *The Cochrane Library* Issue 1. Oxford: Update Software.
29. **White, A.R., Rampes, H., and Ernst, E.** (2001). Acupuncture for smoking cessation (Cochrane Review). In *The Cochrane Library* Issue 1. Oxford: Update Software.
30. **Abbot, N.C., Stead, L.F., White, A.R., Barnes, J., and Ernst, E.** (2001). Hypnotherapy for smoking cessation (Cochrane Review). In *The Cochrane Library* Issue 1. Oxford: Update Software.

11.5 Changing behaviour: diet and exercise

Chris van Weel and Jaap J. van Binsbergen

Introduction

The potential benefits of advice to 'stop smoking, take more exercise, and keep to a healthy diet' are scientifically proven and well known. Nevertheless, the recommendations are in general poorly followed.[1,2] Reasons why this is the case are many, but an important factor is the need for the individual to change his or her behaviour (lifestyle)—and for benefits that might only become perceptible in the long-term. A healthy diet, exercise, and avoidance of smoking are generic health-promoting factors. Accomplishment of lifestyle changes depends more on the patient than on the disease avoided.

General practitioners (GPs) are in a good position to identify and treat patients who are at an increased risk of disease.[3,4] For this group, in particular, lifestyle interventions can be valuable, but there are many barriers to changing lifestyles that greatly reduce the effects of advice. In addition, the GP who addresses lifestyles in his preventive counselling lacks validated tools to assess dietary intake or physical activity,[5] hampering reliable baseline measurement.

Effectiveness of general practice interventions

The population strategy in industrialized societies is clear: more physical exercise and healthy food (i.e. less saturated fat, more vegetables, fruit, and fish). But the advantage for the individual patient may be small.[6] This is the so-called prevention paradox: small changes in population behaviour have great consequences for the health of the population as a whole but will have minimal effect on the health status of that individual. On the other hand, obtaining behavioural changes in the small number with the poorest health may benefit the individual, but have little impact on the health of the population. The GP's role in advising on nutrition and exercise brings the prevention paradox into the consulting room and causes tension. This is particularly reinforced by the lack of convincing evidence.

Placebo-controlled double-blind intervention studies with hard clinical endpoints are scarce. The difficulty of standardizing the study population and adequately defining exercise and nutritional interventions make randomized control trials difficult to perform.[7] The best trial evidence on the effect of nutritional advice is in relation to cholesterol reduction and is summarized in a number of reviews.[8–10] Reviews of the effectiveness of advice to increase physical activity are equivocal,[11,12] even in relation to smoking cessation.[13] Recommendations are, therefore, based to a large extent on theoretical concepts of behaviour change, the known effects of exercise or diet on intermediate endpoints, and on observational studies showing the potential for change. However, practitioners can be supported in their interventions by simple validated self-assessment tools to measure exercise or food habits.[14–17]

Lifestyle changes: the challenge

The challenge of lifestyle is to obtain lasting changes over time. Three factors at least play a role: (a) the disease (risk) for which the advice is part of the management plan; (b) the individual who is to be counselled; and (c) the socio-cultural environment in which the advice is to be put into effect. The risk of the disease can be large or small but just as important is the patients' perception of that risk and the advantages of behavioural changes—which depend on knowledge and information.[18] But the trust and the interaction with the care provider who gives the advice is also important, as has been demonstrated in nutritional counselling.[19–21]

Individual norms and values of sport and leisure, of food and nutrition are encompassed in that individual's social environment—in particular, the family and the peer group. This may facilitate or impede to a large extent individual susceptibility to advice and guidance to change behaviour. The interactions of disease, individual, and social environment form the complexity in which lifestyle changes in general practice have to take place.

The role of the primary care professional

GPs and their primary care teams are involved in lifestyle advice for a number of reasons. Lifestyle changes are—potentially—important interventions for many health problems encountered in general practice. GPs are in regular contact with those who could benefit most from changing their diet or inactivity and patients regard their GP as the most reliable and trustworthy professional in the field. For nutrition guidance at least there is convincing evidence in this respect,[19,22] but this positive role stands in contrast to most GPs' self-perception of their effectiveness.

GPs claim scepticism of the effects of dietary intervention on health, show a lack of specific knowledge,[23] and doubt patients' motivation to change their habits. The strong cultural value attached to eating, drinking, and leisure makes GPs apprehensive to intervene: intervention is seen as taking away pleasure, without guaranteed health gains. This is particularly true for those who are well, the domain of primary prevention, where lifestyle changes are an important message, but the 'numbers needed to change behaviour' are large. Under these circumstances, GPs hesitate to intrude upon the patients' privacy.[24] Nevertheless, there are enough arguments to motivate primary care staff to increase their involvement,[25] and this chapter analyses the way GPs could cope successfully with the challenges of changing patients' lifestyles, and reviews the strengths and weaknesses of the personal doctor.

Objective of lifestyle interventions in general practice

Despite the reservations of GPs, it is difficult to escape the fact that a large amount of patient care *is* related to behavioural changes. For patients with diabetes mellitus, obesity, hypertension, cardiovascular disease, asthma, and obstructive airways disease, state-of-the-art management includes physical activities, refraining from smoking, and a healthy diet. Achieving compliance with prescribed drugs and regular medical reviews, often necessitating a change in the patient's behaviour, is part of the nuts and bolts of diagnosis and treatment. Here, lifestyle changes are part of regular patient care, the core business of general practice. A second group for whom GPs should aim lifestyle changes are patients with an identified, substantially elevated risk of disease. GPs possess important clinical information about their patients and families to identify individual risks, and the personal bond between patient and GP often enhances the effectiveness to modify individual high risk. GPs should concentrate on behaviour changes in the context of state-of-the-art treatment and individual secondary prevention activities and make sure that what is done is done well. Whether GPs involve themselves in population-directed lifestyle changes for better primary prevention remains dependent on local circumstances.

Health problems involved

The GP faces a lot of lifestyle-related health problems in daily practice:[26] in approximately 16 per cent of the presented episodes of illness, nutrition and diet must be considered an essential part of treatment.[27] Physical activity will play a role in at least the same proportion. Table 1 summarizes the annual number of new and already known cases of top 10 chronic diseases in general practice,[28] those marked in bold are 'lifestyle-sensitive'.

Diabetes mellitus, obesity, hyperlipidaemia, cardiovascular diseases, asthma/obstructive airways disease, and arthritis can be found is this list and lifestyle advice is often of a 'proactive' nature—the GP will advise diet and/or physical activity, irrespective of the patient explicitly asking for it. Deficiency in activity as well as nutritional status is common in elderly and those admitted to hospital. There is growing awareness of the risk of falls in those poorly trained and the hazards of under-nutrition in the chronically ill.

Table 1 Ten most common diagnosed chronic diseases in general practice (1989–1993)—those amenable to nutritional intervention in bold print[28]

Disease	Incidence	Prevalence
Hypertension	**3**	**54**
Obesity	**2**	**42**
Chronic ischaemic heart disease	**5**	**37**
Arthritis of hip or knee	**5**	**33**
Obstructive airways diseases	**5**	**32**
Eczema	5	23
Diabetes mellitus	**2**	**21**
Hay fever	5	18
Hyperlipidaemia	**4**	**17**
Psoriasis	2	13

Incidence: number of new diagnoses per year per 1000.

Prevalence: total number of cases (new and already diagnosed) per year per 1000.

On the other hand, there are a number of health problems where diet or physical activity present themselves in a very specific way. A team approach, including a physiotherapist and a dietician, would enable adequate support to help fielding awkward questions. Sport-related questions may focus on the (non)sense of exercise or rest, and for nutrition these are the issues of perceived food allergy, food and gastrointestinal problems, or infant feeding problems. Moreover, GPs are often consulted about possible food-related problems but fibre, sugar, fat, salt, and starch were the most relevant issues requiring guidance from the general public's perspective.(21) In other words, nutrition guidance is first and foremost concerned with healthy food rather than exotic dietary regulations.

Models of success

An important precondition of successfully changing lifestyles is consistency in information. It is generally agreed that a preventive population strategy is doomed to fail unless it is supported by the professionals in the curative field. For that reason alone GPs should give advice on physical activity and nutrition, even when they do not claim a role in primary preventive work.(29) In addition, patients present with nutritional questions and regard the GP as the most valued expert in this field,(20) and the same applies to physical activity.

In defining their role, GPs should realize that changing these lifestyles is a part of routine care. As perceived lack of knowledge is, however, common,(23) there is a need for more instructions during vocational training.(30,31) One of the strongest motivators for GPs and the primary care team is evidence from practice-based research under usual care conditions, which clarifies effective strategies to change patients' lifestyles.(5,6,25) Another way to strengthen the role of the GP is a knowledge-based critical attitude to cope with the many claims of patients or the food and leisure industry.(19,32) This is becoming particularly important when the industry increasingly promotes foods as having therapeutic effects.

Living up to promises?

Patients think that GPs should be interested in their lifestyle behaviours,(33) so doctors should be able to reduce lifestyle-associated diseases. It is widely argued that the influence of the GP in modifying lifestyle is far-reaching,(34) but reliable evidence from GP-based lifestyle interventions is lacking. Primary care prevention, particularly targeted to high-risk patients, is effective in decreasing cardiovascular risk levels,(35) but poor discrimination between high- and low-risk patients may lead to sub-optimal preventive care.(36) It is also clear that if general practice-based health promotion is effective, a greater number of GPs will need to become involved than currently occurs.(8) Since quite a number of patients are unaware of their unhealthy lifestyle,(15) active anticipation is needed to, for instance, obtain permanent reduction of dietary saturated fat and partial replacement by unsaturates.(37) The short-term reduction of lipid levels achieved by a dietician is better than the effect achieved by physicians,(38) but in other trials dieticians have been no better than self-help groups.(10) More trials are needed to investigate the effectiveness of dietary interventions on patients with the high risk of familial hypercholesterolaemia.(39) However, in general, it appears that dietary intervention in general practice can be efficient(40) and cost-effective, particular in conjunction with a dietician.(41) Additionally, in the case of community-based diabetic care, computerized recall with prompting for patients and their family doctors can achieve high standards of care.(42)

Another major lifestyle-related problem is the increasing number of overweight patients in the general practice, adults as well as children. To achieve long-term weight reduction, a comprehensive approach involving nutritional intervention and regular physical activity is needed.(43) A mix of behavioural change methods including goal-setting and self-monitoring over a longer period may be best.(44) The effect of reducing body weight on obesity-related co-morbidity seems to be proven for hypertension(45) and diabetes mellitus.(46)

Besides an unbalanced eating pattern, lack of physical activity is a major lifestyle risk factor in developing chronic degenerative diseases in the industrialized world. The benefits of physical activity are proven: there is an inverse dose–response relationship with mortality risk,(47,48) particularly for obesity(49) and cardiorespiratory fitness.(50) Despite this, only a minority of physicians advise their patients about physical activity.(51) This reflects the fact that routine primary care consultations are not always the right place to give advice about physical activity.(52) It is also argued that providing tailored advice on exercise is more difficult than on nutrition,(53) perhaps because GPs are seldom well informed about the existing levels of exercise taken by their patients.(54,55)

A strategy that works under primary care conditions

Guidance of planned changes in nutrition and activity pattern over time can be found in models like the 'Stages of Change'.(56) This model is based on the empirical observation that individuals, when changing their behaviour or lifestyle, progress through successive phases—moving from a phase when the medically undesired behaviour or lifestyle is accepted by the patient, through considering and planning change, to taking action to effect change. Once this last stage is reached, it is important that the healthy behaviour can be continued: 'maintaining changed behaviour'.

The initial intervention for each individual consists of the 'diagnostic' assessment of the phase in which the individual is at that moment. Further management follows from this. For example, information and health education are relevant for those in whom no change or behaviour is considered; but for those who already are aware or have changed their lifestyle, health education and information is not the first priority. Instead, the GP should concentrate his/her limited time to discuss ways to actually change behaviour or lifestyle and offer supportive care for those considering change, and provide encouragement and support for those actually making changes.

When focused on nutrition and physical activity, specific interventions can be defined for each of these stages of change. The feasibility of this model must be related to a key aspect of general practice—continuity of care. As can be concluded from Table 1, GPs not only encounter a lot of nutrition-related morbidity, but these encounters take place with the same patients over time. In defining nutrition guidance in the format of healthy food, and in focusing guidance to changing individual behaviour, continuity of general practice care provides a valuable framework in implementing individual changes in lifestyle improvements in general and nutrition habits in particular.

Tool kits for the consultation and the practice

Continuity of care is essential in bringing individuals to change their lifestyle, and recording the advice and counselling helps to structure the next contact. The proactive approach that is usually the basis of lifestyle changes makes active involvement of the patient a crucial first step. Information gathering of the components of the diet or level of physical activities is the staring point.(1) A simple diary will suffice to give the GP and, more importantly, the patient the necessary self insight.(17) For nutritional counselling, simple self-assessment tools that include an assessment of food groups are available.(16)

In addition, many guidelines and protocols for general practice provide practical information for advice and counselling of patients. Some general practice computer software includes primary care guidelines, and this offers an ideal setting to standardize health education material for patients—for example, the set based on the guidelines of the Dutch College of General Practitioners illustrates their potential.(57) This leaves open the possibility to refer complicated cases like diabetes mellitus, heart failure, or malnourished patients with cancer to a nutrition specialist.(58)

Teamwork

Changing lifestyles is complex and more in-depth expertise is available to support the GP. For nutrition, the expert in primary care is the dietician who is trained in translating dietary advice from the drawing table to the dining table. For physical activities this expertise is less clarified in professional terms. Physiotherapists can play an important role, but so can peer groups and clubs. It is of utmost importance in motivating patients to bear in mind the possibilities and especially the impossibilities. Encouraging a 55-year-old housewife to live a more active life requires a different form of support than that needed to bring an isolated 17-year-old asthmatic into the arena of regular recreational sport. In the same way, advice to an old lady to improve the daily intake of fruit and vegetables is completely different from the advice one might give to a lorry driver to avoid fatty food.[59] For that reason building a professional network in the community and knowing about local facilities is important. This will help increase the skills and self-assurance in coping with lifestyle-related problems of the primary care team as a whole.[1]

Conclusions

The main conclusion is that guidance on nutrition and physical activity is necessarily a substantial part of the workload in general practice. A key to the potential success of the GP is his/her role as a personal doctor, and from this it follows that GPs should direct their guidance to individual behaviour. However, the interface between individual behaviour and the norms and values in the community imply that coordination with public health can enforce the effectiveness of individual counselling. In the primary care team, the dietician and physiotherapist are obvious partners.

A large number of the many episodes of illness presented to the GP include lifestyle issues as part of good routine management and, together with assessment of individual health risks, provide a potential opportunity for individual guidance. Individual needs are proposed as the focus in anchoring nutrition and activity guidance although presenting health problems may present a critical opportunity to encourage nutritional changes.

Nutrition guidance should be concerned with promoting healthy food, with individual needs determining the emphasis on specific aspects (like salt, fibre, or starch). This allows a more generic form of guidance avoiding mystifying disease-specific details. General guidelines and more specific disease-related protocols should contain clear guidance on non-pharmacological interventions.

As nutritional guidance aims at changing behaviour, it is mandatory to build it into a model that enables change. Concepts like the Stages of Change provide such a model and can be linked to the GP's continuity of care over time and presents a framework for promoting individual nutrition guidance. It must be based on the individual needs for change and the potential to change in relation to the family's circumstance, the society's norms, and cultural values. From this individual assessment, health problems presented over time can be used as critical incidents to motivate nutritional change and activity pattern, initiating and preserving new lifestyle behaviour. However, the motivation of the GP, underpinned by sound evidence-based knowledge, is crucial.

References

1. **Backett, K., Davison, C., and Mullen, K.** (1994). Lay evaluation of health lifestyles: evidence from three studies. *British Journal of General Practice* **44**, 277–80.
2. **Leese, B. and Bosasnquet, N.** (1995). Family doctors and change in practice strategy since 1986. *British Medical Journal* **310**, 705–8.
3. **van Weel, C.** (1999). Nutritional guidance in general practice—a conceptual framework. *European Journal of Clinical Nutrition* **53** (Suppl. 2), S108–11.
4. **Peirera Gray, D.** (1999). Dietary advice in British General Practice. *European Journal of Clinical Nutrition* **53**, S3–8.
5. **Little, P. and Margetts, B.** (1996). The importance of diet and physical activity in the treatment of conditions managed in general practice. *British Journal of General Practice* **46**, 187–92.
6. **Little, P. and Margetts, B.** (1996). Dietary and exercise assessment in general practice. *Family Practice* **13**, 477–82.
7. **Truswell, A.S.** (1999). What nutrition knowledge and skills do primary care physicians need to have, and how should this be communicated? *European Journal of Clinical Nutrition* **53** (Suppl. 2), S67–71.
8. **Ashenden, R., Silagy, C., and Weller, D.** (1997). A systematic review of the effectiveness of promoting lifestyle change in general practice. *Family Practice* **14**, 160–76.
9. **Tang, J., Armitage, J., Lancaster, T., Silagy, C., Fowler, G., and Neil, H.** (1998). Systematic review of dietary intervention trials to lower blood cholesterol in free living subjects. *British Medical Journal* **316**, 1213–20.
10. **Thomson, R.L., Summerbell, C.D., Hooper, L., Higgins, J.P.T., Little, P.S., Talbot, D., and Ebrahim, S.** (2001). Dietary advice given by a dietitian versus other health professionals or self-help resources to reduce blood cholesterol (Cochrane review). In *The Cochrane Library* Issue 1. Oxford: Update Software.
11. **Eakin, E.G., Glasgow, R.E., and Riley, K.M.** (2000). Review of primary care-based physical activity intervention studies. *Journal of Family Practice* **49**, 158–68.
12. **Wee, C.C.** (2001). Physical activity counseling in primary care: the challenge of effecting behavioural change. *Journal of the American Medical Association* **286**, 717–19.
13. **Ussher, M.H., West, R., Taylor, A.H., and McEwen, A.** (2001). Exercise interventions for smoking cessation (Cochrane review). In *The Cochrane Library* Issue 4. Oxford: Update Software.
14. **Little, P., Barnett, J., Margetts, B., Kinmonth, A.L., Gabbay, J., Thompson, R., Warm, D., Warnick, H., and Wooton, S.** (1999). The validity of dietary assessment in general practice. *Journal of Epidemiology and Community Health* **53**, 165–72.
15. **Little, P., Slocock, L., Griffin, S., and Pillinger, J.** (1999). Who is targeted for lifestyle advice? A cross-sectional survey in two general practices. *British Journal of General Practice* **49**, 806–10.
16. **Little, P., Barnett, J., Kinmonth, A.L., Margetts, B., Gabbay, J., Thompson, R., Warm, D., and Wooton, S.** (2000). Can dietary assessment in general practice target patients with unhealthy diets? *British Journal of General Practice* **50**, 43–5.
17. **Calfas, K.J., Zabinski, M.F., and Rupp, J.** (2000). Practical nutrition assessment in primary care settings: a review. *American Journal of Preventive Medicine* **18**, 289–99.
18. **Vaandrager, H.W. and Koelen, M.A.** (1997). Consumer involvement in nutritional issues: the role of information. *American Journal of Clinical Nutrition* **65** (Suppl.), 1980s–4s.
19. **van Woerkom, C.M.J.** (1997). Media choice in nutrition education of general practitioners. *American Journal of Clinical Nutrition* **65** (Suppl.), 2013s–15s.
20. **Hiddink, G.J., Hautvast, J.G.A.J., van Woerkom, C.M.J., Fieren, C.J., and van't Hoff, M.A.** (1997). Consumers' expectations about nutrition guidance: the importance of primary care physicians. *American Journal of Clinical Nutrition* **65** (Suppl.), 1974s–9s.
21. **Buttriss, J.L.** (1997). Food and nutrition: attitudes, beliefs and knowledge in the United Kingdom. *American Journal of Clinical Nutrition* **65** (Suppl.), 1985s–95s.
22. **Hiddink, G.J., Hautvast, J.G.A.J., Van Woerkum, C.M.J., Fieren, C.J., and van't Hoff, M.A.** (1997). Nutrition guidance by primary-care physicians: LISREL-analysis improves understanding. *Preventive Medicine* **26**, 29–36.
23. **Feldman, E.B.** (1995). Nutrition concepts for the primary care/generalist physician. *Southern Medical Journal* **88**, 204–16.
24. **Truswell, A.S.** (2000). Family physicians and patients: is effective nutrition interaction possible? *European Journal of Clinical Nutrition* **71**, 6–12.
25. **Moore, H., Adamson, A.J., Gill, T., and Waine, C.** (2000). Nutrition and health care agenda: a primary care perspective. *Family Practice* **17**, 197–202.

26. **van Binsbergen, J.J.** (1997). Nutritional factors in Dutch family medicine: an inventory. *American Journal of Clinical Nutrition* **65** (Suppl.), 1967s–73s.
27. **van Weel, C.** (1997). Morbidity in family medicine: the potential for individual nutritional counseling, an analysis from the Nijmegen Continuous Morbidity Registration. *American Journal of Clinical Nutrition* **65** (Suppl.), 1928s–32s.
28. **van Weel, C.** (1996). Chronic diseases in general practice—the longitudinal dimension. *European Journal of General Practice* **2**, 17–21.
29. **Worsley, A.** (1999). How to improve the impact of nutrition guidance by general physicians: Public health versus individual patient? *European Journal of Clinical Nutrition* **53** (Suppl. 2), S101–7.
30. **Kolasa, K.M.** (1999). Developments and challenges in family practice nutrition education for residents and practicing physicians: an overview of the North American experience. *European Journal of Clinical Nutrition* **53** (Suppl. 2), S89–96.
31. **Maiburg, H.J.S., Hiddink, G.J., van't Hoff, M.A. Rethans, J.J., and van Ree, J.J.** (1999). The NECTAR-Study: development of nutrition modules for general practice vocational training; determinants of nutrition guidance practice of GP-trainees. *European Journal of Clinical Nutrition* **53** (Suppl. 2), S83–8.
32. **van Woerkum, C.M.J.** (1999). Nutrition guidance by primary care physicians: models and circumstances. *European Journal of Clinical Nutrition* **53** (Suppl. 2), S19–21.
33. **Richmond, R., Kehoe, L., Heather, N., Wodak, A., and Webster, I.** (1996). General practitioners' promotion of healthy life style: what patients think *Australian and New Zealand Journal of Public Health* **20**, 195–200.
34. **Kerse, N.M., Flicker, L., Jolly, D., Arroll, B., and Young, D.** (1999). Improving the helath behaviours of elderly people: randomised controlled trial of a general practice education programme. *British Medical Journal* **320**, 683–7.
35. **Ketola, E., Makela, M., and Klockars, M.** (2001). Individualised multifactorial lifestyle intervention trial for high-risk cardiovascular patients in primary care. *British Journal of General Practice* **51**, 291–4.
36. **Thomsen, T.F., Jorgensen, T., Ibsen, H., and Borch-Johnsen, K.** (2001). Assessment of coronary risk in general practice in relation to the use of guidelines: a survey in Denmark. *Preventive Medicine* **33**, 300–4.
37. **Hooper, L., Summerbell, C.D., Higgins, J.P.T., Thompson, R.L., Clements, G., Capps, N., Davey Smith, G., Riemersma, R.A., and Ebrahim, S.** (2001). Reduced or modified dietary fat for preventing cardiovascular disease (Cochrane review). In *The Cochrane Library* Issue 4. Oxford: Update Software.
38. **Henkin, Y., Shai, I., Zulk, R., Brickner, D., Zuilli, I., Neumann, L., and Shany, S.** (2000). Dietary treatment of hypercholesterolemia: do dietitians do it better? A randomized, controlled trial. *American Journal of Medicine* **109**, 549–55.
39. **Poustie, V.J. and Rutherford, P.** (2001). Dietary treatment for familial hypercholesterolaemia (Cochrane review). In *The Cochrane Library* Issue 2. Oxford: Update Software.
40. **Traeden, U.I., Holm, L., Sandstrom, B., Andersen, P.K., and Jarden, M.** (1998). Effectiveness of a dietary intervention strategy in general practice: effects on blood lipids, health and well-being. *Public Health Nutrition* **1**, 273–81.
41. **Pritchard, D.A., Hyndman, J., and Taba, F.** (1999). Nutrition counselling in general practice: a cost effective analysis. *Journal of Epidemiology and Community Health* **53**, 311–16.
42. **Griffin, S. and Kinmonth, A.L.** (2001). Systems for routine surveillance for people with diabetes mellitus (Cochrane review). In *The Cochrane Library* Issue 4. Oxford: Update Software.
43. **Lyznicki, J.M., Young, D.C., Riggs, J.A., and Davis, R.M.** (2001). Council on Scientific Affairs, American Medical Association. Obesity: assessment and management in primary care. *American Family Physician* **63**, 2185–96.
44. **Hardeman, W., Griffin, S., Johnston, M., Kinmonth, A.L., and Wareham, N.J.** (2000). Interventions to prevent weight gain: a systematic review of psychological models and behaviour change methods. *International Journal of Obesity and Related Metabolic Disorders* **24**, 131–43.
45. **Mulrow, C.D., Chiquette, E., Angel, L., Cornell, J., Summerbell, C., Anagnotelis, B., Brand, M., and Grimm, R. Jr.** (2001). Dieting to reduce body weight for controlling hypertension in adults (Cochrane review). In *The Cochrane Library* Issue 4. Oxford: Update Software.
46. **Anonymous** (2001). Cochrane Protocol diabetes. Weight reduction for reducing mortality in obesity and overweight (Cochrane review). In *The Cochrane Library* Issue 4. Oxford: Update Software.
47. **Blair, S.N.** et al. (1989). Physical fitness and all-cause mortality: a prospective study of healthy men and women. *Journal of the American Medical Association* **262**, 2395–401.
48. **Kujala, U.M., Kaprio, J., Sarna, S., and Koskenvuo, M.** (1998). Relationship of leisure-time physical activity and mortality: the Finnish twin cohort. *Journal of the American Medical Association* **270**, 440–4.
49. **Ross, R.** et al. (2000). Reduction in obesity and related comorbid conditions after diet-induced weight loss or exercise-induced weight loss in men: a randomized controlled trial. *Annals of Internal Medicine* **133**, 92–103.
50. **Dunn, A.L.** et al. (1999). Comparison of lifestyle and structured interventions to increase physical activity and cardiorespiratory fitness: a randomized controlled trial. *Journal of the American Medical Association* **281**, 327–34.
51. **Wee, C.C., McCarthy, E.P., Davis, R.B., and Phillips, R.S.** (1999). Physician counseling about exercise. *Journal of the American Medical Association* **282**, 1583–8.
52. **Lawlor, D.A. and Hanratty, B.** (2001). The effect of physical activity advice given in routine primary care consultations: a systematic review. *Journal of Public Health Medicine* **3**, 219–26.
53. **Bull, F.C., Jamrozik, K., and Blanksby, B.A.** (1999). Tailored advice on exercise—does it make a difference? *American Journal of Preventive Medicine* **16**, 230–9.
54. **Dupen, F., Bauman, A.E., and Lin, R.** (1999). The sources of risk factor information for general practitioners: is physical activity under-recognised? *Medical Journal of Australia* **171**, 601–3.
55. **Podl, T.R., Goodwin, M.A., Kikano, G.E., and Stange, K.C.** (1991). Direct observation of exercise counseling in community family practice. *American Journal of Preventive Medicine* **17**, 207–10.
56. **McConnaughy, E.A., DiClemente, C.C., Prochaska, J.O., and Velicer, W.F.** (1989). Stages of change in psychotherapy: a follow-up report. *Psychotherapy* **26**, 494–503.
57. **van Binsbergen, J.J. and Drenthen, A.J.M.** (1999). ICPC-code approach of nutritional questions in general practice: a look at the future. *European Journal of Clinical Nutrition* **53** (Suppl. 2), S22–4.
58. **Lazarus, K.** (1997). Nutrition practices of family physicians after education by a physician nutrition specialist. *American Journal of Clinical Nutrition* **65** (Suppl.), 2007S–9S.
59. **Buttriss, J.** *Nutrition in General Practice. Promoting Health and Preventing Disease.* London: The Royal College of General Practitioners, 1995.

11.6 Changing behaviour: promoting sexual health

Helen Ward

Introduction

Forty million people are living with HIV/AIDS, including nearly 3 million children under the age of 16.[1] In 2001 alone, 5 million people were newly infected with HIV, and 3 million people died. The overwhelming majority of cases are transmitted through sexual contact, reason enough to explore health promotion in the field of sexual behaviour. HIV is only one of the potential adverse outcomes of sexual contact: the World Health Organization estimates that 340 million new cases of curable, bacterial sexually transmitted infections occurred worldwide in 1999.[2] A further 20 million women are thought to undergo unsafe abortions each year, of whom 78 000 will die and many more will suffer complications such as sepsis, haemorrhage, and permanent damage to the genital tract.[3]

For these and other reasons, promoting safety in sexual behaviour is now a recognized target of health services. The concept of sexual health is relatively recent, and variously defined. It has been broadly defined as 'the enjoyment of sexual activity of one's choice without causing or suffering physical or mental harm'.[4] This has been expanded by the UK Department of Health:

> Sexual health is an important part of physical and mental health. It is a key part of our identity as human beings together with the fundamental human rights to privacy, a family life and living free from discrimination. Essential elements of good sexual health are equitable relationships and sexual fulfilment with access to information and services to avoid the risk of unintended pregnancy, illness or disease.[5]

Sexual health has not always been so high on the agenda, indeed until the world began to get devastated by HIV disease in the mid-1980s there was little interest in the topic outside of the marginalized specialties of genitourinary medicine and family planning. Sexual dysfunction, another peripheral topic, has now been found to be extremely common and demand for effective services far outstrips provision.

In this chapter, I will outline the relationship between sexual behaviour and health, including what is known about trends, briefly consider those factors that are known to influence sexual behaviour, and then look at the evidence of effective interventions, ending with a discussion of the role of primary care and other front-line services in promoting sexual health.

The relationship between sexual behaviour and health

There is no doubt that sexual activity has a major impact on health. Positive health outcomes relate to both the enjoyment and satisfaction of sexual contact, and to reproduction: for many people the ability to have a family is a major factor in the sense of well-being that underpins health. Adverse outcomes can be grouped into the following broad areas: reproductive, infectious, social, and psychological or physical trauma.

Heterosexual intercourse can lead to pregnancy, which can be both a negative or a positive outcome in terms of health. On the positive side the ability to plan, conceive, and produce a healthy child is a major source of well-being and satisfaction for many people, while problems in reproducing cause stress to millions of couples. Pregnancy is a challenge to the health of a woman, involving increased risk of thrombo-embolic disease, hypertension, and pre-eclampsia, and the exacerbation of existing pathology such as congenital heart disease and diabetes. The birth itself is a dangerous moment in a woman's life, with a risk of maternal death that remains alarmingly high in some populations, and persists, albeit at a much lower level, in others.

Unwanted pregnancy is a common outcome of sexual behaviour. Up to 50 per cent of all pregnancies in the United Kingdom are unplanned, and for teenagers this figure rises to 80 per cent. Unplanned does not equate with unwanted, but a large proportion of women choose to terminate pregnancy for social or medical reasons. In the United Kingdom, there were approximately 200 000 legal therapeutic abortions in 2001.[6] The physical risks of therapeutic termination are small, particularly where services are available to facilitate early referral followed by medical or surgical termination. But even a clinically straightforward termination can leave major psychological sequelae.

For couples using contraception, the risk of pregnancy is reduced, but replaced by other, considerably smaller, risks. Major, but rare, complications include thrombo-embolic disease from combined oral contraception, upper genital tract infection, and ectopic pregnancy from intrauterine devices; less serious but more common side-effects include mood and weight alterations and headaches with oral contraception.

Concern about reproduction has tended to focus on teenage pregnancy. Teenage mothers are likely to live in poverty without completing their education or finding employment. Their children are more likely themselves to become teenage parents, producing a cycle of poverty and social exclusion.[7] The rates are very uneven between countries, with Britain having the highest rate in Western Europe. Every year some 90 000 teenagers in England become pregnant, including 8000 who are under 16. Despite a concerted government campaign, conception rates for under-16s have remained steady in recent years at 8.3 per 1000 for England and Wales.

Infection

The second most obvious risk associated with sexual contact relates to sexually transmitted infection (STI). Global figures for HIV and STI have already been cited in the introduction.

Data from the network of genitourinary medicine clinics in the United Kingdom (excluding Scotland) showed for 2000, 66 000 cases of genital warts, 64 000 cases of chlamydia, 20 000 of gonorrhoea, 16 800 genital herpes, and over 300 cases of syphilis.[8] These are underestimates of the true levels of infection since they are based on diagnosed cases attending GUM services. Many others will remain undiagnosed, or unreported where they are treated in other settings. Recent data on the prevalence of chlamydia infection in unselected population samples shows that infection is widespread; in a UK study in 2000, *Chlamydia trachomatis* was found in 3 per cent of women aged 16–24 years.[9] In selected populations, there are much higher rates of chlamydial infection including 8 per cent of women seeking terminations and 16 per cent of women attending GUM clinics.[10]

In the early 1990s, it had been tempting to think that improved diagnosis and treatment, along with behaviour change in response to the AIDS epidemic, would lead to the continued decline and possible eradication of some of these common bacterial infections.[11,12] Such optimism proved premature. Recent trends in gonorrhoea infection in the United Kingdom show a doubling in number of cases since 1995, and outbreaks of syphilis have once again been seen in the United Kingdom.[8] In the United Kingdom, there were an estimated 24 000 people living with diagnosed HIV in 2000, and an additional 9400 (28 per cent) undiagnosed, the latter being mainly heterosexual men and women.[13]

There are many sequelae of STI, including chronic pelvic pain, tubal infertility, miscarriage, ectopic pregnancy, tertiary syphilis, and chronic hepatitis. Mother-to-child transmission is associated with neonatal conjunctivitis, congenital syphilis, and HIV infection. Viral STI such as genital herpes and genital warts can cause ongoing morbidity, and mortality linked to anogenital cancer, hepatocellular cancer, and HIV disease.

Adverse social and psychological impacts of sexual behaviour are also widespread. Society has always regulated sexual behaviour, surrounding it in legal and social conditions. While there is cultural variability, the most widespread social censure relates to sex outside of marriage, between people of the same sex, with young people, or as a commercial exchange.[14] In some cases, people who transgress are directly punished by law, in others they face social stigmatization and isolation. These inevitably have an impact on the health of individuals.

Sexual dysfunction is common, although precise estimates are lacking. In one large study in the United States, 35 per cent of men aged 40–70 reported moderate or complete impotence, with the prevalence three times higher for men in their 50s than men in their 20s.[15] A review of population-based studies suggests a much lower figure, with up to 5 per cent of men reporting erectile dysfunction, 5 per cent premature ejaculation, and 10 per cent of women reporting orgasmic disorder.[16] The overall prevalence of sexual dysfunction in women in the United States has been placed at 30–50 per cent.[17]

Finally, some sexual behaviour is directly abusive and violent to others, resulting in extensive physical and psychological damage to the victims.

Factors associated with poor sexual health

In common with almost all indices of ill-health, poor sexual health is fundamentally related to gender, ethnicity, residence, family background, social class, education, and occupation. The impact of social change on reproductive health can be shown by the dramatic increase in STI and HIV in countries undergoing social transition and disruption. In China and in the countries of the former USSR, for example, the 1990s saw epidemics of bacterial STI, with predictions that HIV will soon follow.[18–20]

Young people are at increased risk of poor sexual health outcomes, including unplanned pregnancy, infection, and abuse. Early coitarche, for example, is associated with an increased risk of cervical cancer, and teenage pregnancies have a higher risk of hypertensive complications, premature delivery, and low birth weight. There is a 50 per cent higher infant mortality rate, and teenage mothers have a threefold increase in rates of post-natal depression. At the other end of reproductive years, pregnancy and childbirth over the age of 35 years is linked to an increased risk of breast cancer, and to increased risks of congenital abnormalities.

General risks for STI include numbers of sexual partners, younger age, living in metropolitan areas, ethnicity (there are higher rates of gonorrhoea, e.g., in Black Caribbean men and women in the United Kingdom than in other ethnic groups) and sexual orientation. Specific risk factors vary by condition, but for cervical cancer, for example, include infection with Human papillomavirus (HPV, particularly types 16 and 18), *C. trachomatis*, early coitarche, unprotected vaginal intercourse with more sexual partners, poverty, oral contraceptive pill use, smoking, contact with a man with HPV or penile cancer.[21]

Transmission of pathogens varies, but in general anal or vaginal penetration carries highest risk (for receptive partner), orogenital contact lower, and non-penetrative lower still. Condoms are an effective way of reducing the transmission in penetrative sex, reducing the risk of HIV transmission by an estimated 80 per cent.[22]

There has been a secular trend in recent decades towards earlier age at first sexual intercourse and later age at first marriage, creating a norm of multiple partnerships in people in their teens and early 20s. Recent data for the United Kingdom suggest that the trend towards earlier first intercourse for women stopped in the mid-1990s.[23] In a population survey of 11 161 people, Wellings et al. also found a sustained increase in condom use and a decline in the proportion of men and women not using contraception when they first had sex. Of men and women aged 16–24 at time of interview, 80 per cent had used a condom for their first episode of intercourse, compared with just over 40 per cent of those aged 30–34 at time of interview (whose first sexual experience would have been some 10 years earlier). The same study identified risk factors for early first intercourse: not living with both parents until the age of 16 years, leaving school at 16 years, and not citing school as the main source of information on sexual matters. For women, being under 13 at menarche and having parents in manual occupations was also associated with early first sex. Motherhood, but not abortion, before the age of 18 was associated with low educational attainment.

The same study estimated the prevalence of risks for HIV and other STI, and compared them with similar data from 1990.[24] There has been an increase in many risk behaviours, including numbers of heterosexual partners, homosexual partnerships, concurrent partnerships, anal sex, and payment for sex. The authors also documented a considerable rise in consistent condom use, but not sufficient to outweigh the increased rate of partner change.[24,25] They postulate that this increase in risk behaviour underlies the recent upsurge in STI and HIV in the United Kingdom.

Objectives of interventions to improve sexual health

Unlike many health promotion programmes where the aim of the intervention is clear, for example, to reduce smoking rates, there are major disagreements over some of the objectives of interventions linked to sexual health. The ultimate aim is to reduce poor sexual health, but some programmes seek to achieve this through controls on sexual activity, for example, aiming to delay onset of sexual activity, reduce numbers of sexual partners, re-orientate homosexuals, re-educate men who buy sex and people who sell it. There has been considerable debate about whether health programmes for young people should advocate abstention until marriage, as is the case in many US school programmes. Such programmes would not, in my mind, be about promoting sexual health, but about controlling sexual behaviour and imposing one set of values on people, which is both inappropriate and impractical.[21] In line with some other health promotion programmes, for example, in relation to drug use, the primary aims should be to help people make healthy choices in relation to sex.

Measuring the effectiveness of interventions

Determining the effectiveness of sexual health promotion is complex. The key outcomes are indices of sexual health itself, such as unwanted pregnancy, STIs including HIV, cervical cancer, sub-fertility, psychosexual problems, and sexual dysfunction. In order to measure the impact of interventions on these major outcomes would require very large studies and long follow-up. A few have been carried out and will be cited later. However, most studies look for more proximate measures, primarily changes in knowledge, attitudes, sexual behaviour, and use of appropriate services.[26]

Knowledge has been widely studied, and most interventions can produce measurable increases in knowledge in, for example, modes of transmission of HIV infection. However, it is well established that increased knowledge and changed attitudes do not on their own correlate with changed behaviour.[27]

The second major outcome is sexual behaviour, or more precisely, reported sexual behaviour as it cannot be measured directly. Although there is concern about the validity of self-reported sexual behaviour, most studies show that with the correct settings, survey tools and training of researchers, behaviour can be reliably measured.[24,28] This reproducibility does not necessarily indicate validity: respondents may be consistent in, for example, under-reporting behaviours that are considered socially undesirable,[29] although some studies of couples indicate good validity in reported condom use.[30] This uncertainty underlines the important of additional objective measures, including incidence of infection and pregnancy.

Effective interventions

Social change

Given the strong association between social factors and sexual health, it is clear that major improvements in sexual health are difficult to achieve without tackling social exclusion and poverty. For example, educational and service-based programmes to reduce the numbers of pregnancies in young women may well be of limited use where young women have low expectations of work and other challenges in their lives. Reducing family poverty, improving housing, helping to keep children out of institutional care, and supporting continued education beyond 16 years are all likely to reduce teenage pregnancy and sexual ill-health.[7] A review of campaigns to reduce teenage pregnancy in the United States included programmes that targeted the non-sexual antecedents, including skills and confidence training, promoting education and job opportunities, and mentoring schemes. Some of the strongest evidence for reducing teenage pregnancy comes from these programmes, either alone or combined with sex education and condom distribution.[31]

School-based programmes

Interventions directed at young people are essential in promoting sexual health. Adolescence is a time when sexual activity starts for most people; ideally educational interventions should target school age children before this age. Debates have raged for many years on the values and risks of sex education in schools; opponents of sex education for young children argue that it is wrong to introduce children to the realities of sex, that it will lead to greater experimentation and risk. There is very good evidence to refute these claims, and indeed most studies show that early, well-designed sex education in schools tends to delay the onset of sexual intercourse and promote condom use and other contraception when the young person has sex.[32]

In a recent population survey in the United Kingdom, most adolescents reported obtaining information on sexual matters through schools, in contrast to two decades previously, when friends and other sources were more commonly cited.[23] This presents an important opportunity for effective school programmes, but all too often political rather than evidence-based considerations are used in design and implementation.[25]

The characteristics of effective school-based interventions have been outlined in many systematic reviews. Kirby's review of school-based interventions was based primarily on US studies,[31,33] but there is evidence from other quarters to support generalizing these results. He concludes that programmes including sexuality, sex, AIDS education, school-based clinics, and condom availability do not lead to an increase in sexual experimentation as some have feared, and that many lead to an increase in knowledge and a reduction in sexual risk taking: outcomes include delaying the onset of sexual activity, reducing numbers of partners and increasing condom use and other contraception. Evaluation of school-based or school-linked clinics have been less conclusive; they are often popular and a way of distributing condoms and other services, but studies have not found they lead to an overall reduction in sexual risks for the whole school population.

Kirby[31] identifies 10 characteristics of effective sex and HIV education programmes, which are summarized in Table 1.

There has been substantial debate on the importance of abstinence programmes for young people. In the United States, these programmes are given specific financial support and are strongly supported by lobbyists. However, there is no good evidence that these delay onset of sexual activity or reduce sexual activity, and some evidence that they may be counterproductive.[31,34,35]

General population

Aside from programmes for young people, sexual health promotion has been directed towards the general adult population, and specific subgroups. The mass media has been effectively used to raise knowledge and awareness. One indicator of the success of an HIV awareness programme is an increase in the number of people seeking testing. The United Kingdom was one of the first countries to have a mass media campaign targeting the whole population in an attempt to raise awareness of AIDS. The Don't Die of Ignorance campaign in 1986–1987 included television advertisements and leaflets to every household. Evaluation of media campaigns show that they are associated with increases in condom use, but ongoing and consistent information is required if the effect is to be sustained.[36] In Switzerland, there was a sustained campaign, Stop AIDS, whose main message was the promotion of condom use. The use of condoms by people aged 17–30 years with non-regular partners increased from 8 per cent in 1987 to 56 per cent in 1994.[37]

Other media, such as drama, performance art, and television soap operas, may be helpful in raising awareness of HIV and, in particular, combating discrimination.

Table 1 Characteristics of effective sex and HIV education programmes*

The curricula of the most effective sex and HIV education programmes share 10 common characteristics. These programmes

1. focus on reducing one or more sexual behaviours that lead to unintended pregnancy or HIV/STD infection
2. are based on theoretical approaches that have been demonstrated to influence other health-related behaviour and identify specific important sexual antecedents to be targeted
3. deliver and consistently reinforce a clear message about abstaining from sexual activity and/or using condoms or other forms of contraception. This appears to be one of the most important characteristics that distinguishes effective from ineffective programmes
4. provide basic, accurate information about the risks of teen sexual activity and about ways to avoid intercourse or use methods of protection against pregnancy and STDs
5. include activities that address social pressures that influence sexual behaviour
6. provide examples of and practice with communication, negotiation, and refusal skills
7. employ teaching methods designed to involve participants and have them personalize the information
8. incorporate behavioural goals, teaching methods, and materials that are appropriate to the age, sexual experience, and culture of the students.
9. last a sufficient length of time (i.e. more than a few hours)
10. select teachers or peer leaders who believe in the programme and then provide them with adequate training

Generally speaking, short-term curricula—whether abstinence only or sexuality education programmes—do not have measurable impact on the behaviour of teens

* Adapted from Kirby.[31]

More focused interventions have been conducted among groups at increased risk, for example, women in inner city neighbourhoods, men who have sex with men, sex workers, and drug users. There is a vast literature on these areas, usefully summarized by Kalichman[26] and Peterson and DiClemente.[38] In addition, the United Nations Programme on HIV/AIDS has produced a resource pack of case studies on innovative approaches to HIV Prevention, based largely on work in less industrialized countries.[39]

Shepherd et al.[21] considered interventions to promote sexual risk reduction behaviour among women. While the primary focus of the review was cervical cancer, the behaviour changes considered were common to most aspects of sexual health. The reviewers looked primarily at proximate outcomes as few studies have been able to measure the impact of interventions on the incidence of cervical cancer. Outcomes included condom use for vaginal intercourse, delayed first intercourse, sexual partner reduction, development of sexual negotiating skills, abstinence, and, in a few studies, incidence of STIs.

The interventions selected for review focused on improving sexual health through providing information on transmission and prevention of STI and HIV along with skill acquisition (for negotiating with sexual partners, or using condoms correctly). Interventions were usually with groups of women, for example sex workers, young inner city women, STD clinic attendees, and delivered by health care workers, social workers or trained peers in various settings (clinics, community centres, prisons).

All the controlled trials showed a positive effect of the intervention, including an increase in condom use and in skills. There was no consistent reduction in numbers of sexual partners or increase in abstinence. Only short-term follow-up was included, in the region of 3–6 months, and sustainability cannot be assumed. Programme evaluation has shown considerable attrition over time unless interventions are repeated and sustained.[40]

Another key form of intervention is based on outreach work, usually with specific target groups such as sex workers, gay men, and drug users. Outreach involves taking services or, in this case, prevention activities, out from health care settings into the areas where people live, work or meet socially. The content of outreach varies from a simple way of delivering health promotion material to a more integrated programme of support in the community including distribution of condoms, individual health advice, counselling on risk reduction, and working with peer educators. Outreach may take place on the street, on mobile units that include counselling, education and even clinical facilities, or in local venues such as bars, clubs, or workplaces. Given the wide range of interventions under the umbrella term of outreach, it is difficult to summarize effectiveness; very few interventions have been subject to controlled trials. It is difficult to distinguish individuals exposed to the outreach from those who were not, since there is likely to be a spreading out of information from those directly exposed. One major evaluation was the AIDS Evaluation of Street Outreach Projects (AESOP) in six US cities. The evaluation was based on serial surveys in the intervention areas, and showed reductions in self-reported risk behaviours (ref. 26, Chapter 6). Outreach has been extensively used with sex workers and the evidence, again largely based on observational rather than experimental studies, suggests that condom use and access to health care increases.[(41–43)]

Outreach and work with community leaders is linked to a more general approach to promoting sexual health, namely community mobilization. Many programmes have linked campaigns by health professionals with attempts to organize people in the community. Kelly, recognizing the importance of broad influences within population groups, developed the Social Influence Model, and applied this using local 'opinion leaders' to try and shift social norms. In a controlled trial in the United States, key men were identified in a series of gay bars, and were enrolled in the programme of training and skills. There was a reduction in risk behaviours in men attending the intervention bars, compared with control bars.[(44)]

Another example, the Mpowerment Project, trained a group of peers as part of an outreach and workshop based intervention for gay men in Oregon.[(45)] The intervention was difficult to evaluate; there was a reduction in individual risk behaviours compared with a control population, but the single site design did not permit a full assessment.[(46)]

In the field of sex work, structural obstacles to safety are well described and community mobilization, peer education, and work with managers and clients have all been linked to improvements in safer sex.[(47,48)] Again, evidence is observational rather than experimental.[(41)]

Interventions in clinical settings

The previous sections have hopefully shown the effectiveness of population, group and structural approaches to risk reduction, but they may leave the individual practitioner feeling impotent. In other areas, for example, smoking cessation, there is strong evidence for the effectiveness of individual counselling. For sexual health the results are less clear. HIV testing, combined with pre- and post-test counselling, has been widely implemented as a strategy not only for case finding, but also as part of risk reduction for those who test positive or negative.

The evidence for effectiveness in reducing HIV risk behaviours is unconvincing (ref. 26, Chapter 4). As Kalichman points out, it is not surprising that a single counselling session combined with testing does not lead to sustained change of such a complex set of behaviours. What is surprising is the large amount of resources directed to this approach.

There is much better evidence for the effectiveness of enhanced and sustained counselling associated with testing. For example, Project RESPECT was a large multicentre trial conducted in US STI clinics in the 1990s. HIV-negative individuals were randomly assigned to receive standard information and education, two risk reduction counselling sessions, or four enhanced counselling sessions based on theories of reasoned action and social cognitive theory (including steps towards risk reduction). The people in the two counselling groups showed reduced risk behaviours and lower rates of STI. The best results in terms of sustained increases in condom use were from the more intensive intervention. This suggests that more intensive interventions are needed than current guidelines would permit.[(26)]

The limitation of individual clinical consultations may be illustrated by a report from Churchill et al. on teenage pregnancy.[(49)] Pregnant women under 20 were interviewed, and 71 per cent reported that they had discussed contraception with a health professional within the previous year. Many of them had been prescribed the pill, suggesting many other obstacles to effective contraception than simple availabilty. Advice on how to use the pill needs to be provided along with attempts to overcome problems of stigma associated with young women's sexuality.

Sexual health in everyday practice

This short review of sexual health promotion describes some of the interventions at the social, community, group, and individual level that appear to work. There is less evidence for the effectiveness of interventions by individual health care practitioners in changing sexual behaviour. However, the current limited evidence does not mean that practitioners have no role to play in promoting sexual health.

Firstly, practitioners can be important advocates of social change. They can also identify those groups within the local population who are vulnerable to poor sexual health and press for interventions, including community outreach, education, and intensive counselling. Local practitioners can be a key part of the teams that provide the most effective interventions we have identified, namely sex education in schools.

Secondly, in the clinical setting practitioners play a key role in educating individual patients about risks and harm minimization; while knowledge on its own has not been sufficient to change behaviour, without it no progress can be made. This suggests that practitioners must be able to talk to their patients about sex and harm minimization, and refer those who may benefit to more specialist intervention services. Programmes to reduce the harmful impact of domestic violence and sexual abuse have found that victims are rarely asked about possible abuse by their doctors, but that most would welcome such enquiries and think they would be useful in helping them to reduce future vulnerability.

Finally, practitioners are key is in the provision of accessible local services for the improvement of sexual health, including contraception, HIV and STI screening and appropriate referral. Improved sexual health depends not only on changing sexual behaviour, but on identifying those at risk, diagnosing problems including infections, fertility problems and abuse, and ensuring effective management. This should include partner referral for people diagnosed with an infection is a key and effective part of infection control in the population.[(50,51)]

References

1. **Joint United Nations Programme on HIV/AIDS (UNAIDS) and World Health Organization.** *AIDS Epidemic Update, December 2001.* Geneva. UNAIDS.01.74E—WHO/CDS/CSR/NCS/2001, 2001.
2. **World Health Organization.** *Global Prevalence and Incidence of Selected Curable Sexually Transmitted Infections.* Geneva: WHO, 2001, p. 1.
3. **World Health Organization.** *Unsafe Abortion: Global and Regional Estimates of Incidence of a Mortality due to Unsafe Abortion with a Listing of Available Country Data* 3rd edn. Geneva Ref. WHO/RHT/MSM/97.16 (Chapter 4), 1997.
4. **Renton, A., Hawkes, S., Hickman, M., Ward, H., Claydon, E., and Taylor-Robinson, D.** (1997). Epidemiological based needs assessment: genitourinary medicine services. In *Health Care Needs Assessment. The Epidemiologically Based Needs Assessment Reviews* 2nd Series (ed. A. Stevens and J. Raftery), pp. 397–453. Oxford: Radcliffe Medical Press Ltd.

5. **Department of Health.** *National Strategy for Sexual Health and HIV.* London: Department of Health. Available at: www.doh.gov.uk/nshs/strategy.htm.

6. **Office of National Statistics.** *Terminations of Pregnancy Data 2001 for England and Wales, Scotland,* 2001.

7. **Social Exclusion Unit.** *Teenage Pregnancy: Report of the Social Exclusion Unit,* 1999.

8. **Communicable Disease Surveillance Centre.** *Trends in Sexually Transmitted Infections in the UK: New Episodes seen at Genitourinary Medicine Clinics, 1995–2000.* London: Public Health Laboratory Service, 2001.

9. **Fenton, K.A., Korovessis, C., Johnson, A.M., McCadden, A., McManus, S., Wellings, K., Mercer, C.H., Carder, C., Copas, A.J., Nanchahal, K., Macdowall, W., Ridgway, G., Field, J., and Erens, B.** (2001). Sexual behaviour in Britain: reported sexually transmitted infections and prevalent genital *Chlamydia trachomatis* infection. *Lancet* **358**, 1828–9.

10. **Chief Medical Officer.** *Main Report of the Chief Medical Officer's Expert Advisory Group on Chlamydia trachomatis.* London: Department of Health, 1998.

11. **Bignall, C.** (1994). The eradication of gonorrhoea can be achieved. *British Medical Journal* **309**, 1103–4.

12. **Cronberg, S.** (1993). The rise and fall of sexually transmitted diseases in Sweden. *Genitourinary Medicine* **3**, 184–6.

13. **Communicable Disease Surveillance Centre.** *CDR Weekly,* 31 January 2002.

14. **Weeks, J.** *Sex, Politics, and Society: The Regulation of Sexuality since 1800* 2nd edn. Essex: Longman, 1989.

15. **Morgentaler, A.** (1999). Male impotence. *Lancet* **354**, 1713–18.

16. **Symons, J.S. and Carey, M.P.** (2001). Prevalence of sexual dysfunctions: results from a decade of research. *Archives of Sexual Behaviour* **30**, 177–219.

17. **Berman, L.A., Berman, J.R., Chhabra, S, and Goldstein, I.** (2001). Novel approaches to female sexual dysfunction. *Expert Opinion on Investigational Drugs* **10**, 85–95.

18. **Atlani, L., Carael, M., Brunet, J.B., Frasca, T., and Chaika, N.** (2000). Social change and HIV in the former USSR: the making of a new epidemic. *Social Science and Medicine* **50**, 1547–56.

19. **Tichanova, L., Borisenko, K., Ward, H., Meheus, A., Gromyko, A., and Renton, A.** (1997). Epidemics of syphilis in the Russian Federation: trends, origins and priorities for control. *Lancet* **350**, 213–15.

20. **Chen, X.S., Gong, X.D., Liang, G.J., and Zhang, G.C.** (2000). Epidemiologic trends of sexually transmitted disease in China. *Sexually Transmitted Diseases* **27**, 138–42.

21. **Shepherd, J., Weston, R., Peersman, G., and Napuli, I.Z.** (2002). Interventions for encouraging sexual lifestyles and behaviours intended to prevent cervical cancer (Cochrane Review). In *The Cochrane Library* Issue 1. Oxford: Update Software.

22. **Weller, S. and Davis, K.** (2002). Condom effectiveness in reducing heterosexual HIV transmission (Cochrane Review). In *The Cochrane Library* Issue 1. Oxford: Update Software.

23. **Wellings, K., Nanchalal, K., Macdowall, W., McManus, S., Erens, B., Mercer, C.H., Johnson, A.M., Copas, A.J., Korovessis, C., Fenton, K., and Field, J.** (2001). Sexual behaviour in Britain: early heterosexual experience. *Lancet* **358**, 1843–50.

24. **Johnson, A.M.** et al. (2001). Effect of computer-assisted self interviews on reporting of sexual HIV risk behaviours in a general population sample: a methodological experiment. *AIDS* **15**, 111–15.

25. **DiClemente, R.J.** (2001). Development of programmes for enhancing sexual health. *Lancet* **358**, 1828–9.

26. **Kalichman, S.C.** *Preventing AIDS: A Sourcebook for Behavioural Interventions.* Mahwah NJ: Lawrence Earlbaum Associates, 1988.

27. **Prochaska, J.O., Redding, C.A., Harlow, L.L., Rossi, J.S., and Velicer, W.F.** (1994). The transtheoretical model of change and HIV prevention: a review. *Health Education Quarterly* **21**, 471–86.

28. **Coates, R., Soskolne, C., Calzavara, L., Read, S., Fanning, N., Shepherd, F., Klein, M., and Johnson, J.** (1986). The reliability of sexual histories in AIDS related research: evaluation of an interview administered questionnaire. *Canadian Journal of Public Health* **77**, 343–8.

29. **Brody, S.** (1995). Heterosexual transmission of HIV. *New England Journal of Medicine* **331**, 1718.

30. **Padian, N.S.** (1990). Sexual histories of heterosexual couples with one HIV infected partner. *American Journal of Public Health* **80**, 990–1.

31. **Kirby, D.** *Emerging Answers: Research Findings on Programs to Reduce Teenage Pregnancy* (Summary). Washington DC: National Campaign to Prevent Teen Pregnancy, 2001.

32. **Wellings, K., Wadsworth, J., Johnson, A.M., Field, J., Whittaker, L., and Field, B.** (1995). Provision of sex education and early sexual experience: the relation examined. *British Medical Journal* **311**, 417–20.

33. **Kirby, D.** (2000). School-based interventions to prevent unprotected sex and HIV among adolescents. In *Handbook of HIV Prevention* (ed. J.L. Peterson and R.J. DiClemente), pp. 96–7. New York: Kluwer Academic/Plenum Publishers.

34. **Roosa, M.W. and Christopher, F.S.** (1990). Evaluation of an abstinence-only adolescent pregnancy prevention program: a replication. *Family Relations* **39**, 363–7 (cited in ref. 21).

35. **Stammers, T. and Ingham, R.** (2000). For and against. Doctors should advise adolescents to abstain from sex. *British Medical Journal* **321**, 1520–2.

36. **Wellings, K. and Field, B.** *Stopping AIDS: AIDS/HIV Public Education and the Mass Media in Europe.* London: Addison-Wesley Longman, 1997.

37. **Rivers, K. and Aggleton, P.** (2000). HIV prevention in industrialised countries. In *Handbook of HIV Prevention* (ed. J.L. Peterson and R.J. DiClemente), p. 249. New York: Academic/Plenum Publishers.

38. **Peterson, J.L. and DiClemente, R.J.,** ed. *Handbook of HIV Prevention.* New York: Academic/Plenum Publishers, 2000.

39. **UNAIDS.** *Innovative Approaches to HIV Prevention: Selected Case Studies.* Geneva: UNAIDS/00.35E, 2000.

40. **Kilmarx, P.H., Palanuvej, T., Limmpakarnjanarat, K., Chitvarakorn, A., St Louis, M.W., and Mastro, T.D.** (1999). Seroprevalence of HIV among female sex workers in Bangkok: evidence of ongoing infection risk after the '100 per cent condom program' was implemented. *Journal of Acquired Immune Deficiency Syndromes* **21**, 313–16.

41. **Ward, H., Day, S., and Weber, J.N.** (1999). Risky business: health and safety in the sex industry over a nine year period. *Sexually Transmitted Infections* **75** (5), 340–3.

42. **Ward, H.** (1999). Evaluating outreach clinics—are we asking too much? *Sexually Transmitted Infections* **75**, 146–7 (editorial).

43. **Mac, R.** *EUROPAP: European Intervention Projects AIDS Prevention for Prostitutes.* Gent: Academia Press, 1996.

44. **Kelly, J.A.** et al. (1997). Outcomes of a randomized controlled community level HIV prevention intervention: effects on behaviour among at-risk gay men in small US cities. *Lancet* **350**, 1500–5.

45. **Kegeles, S.M., Hays, R.B., and Coates, T.J.** (1996). The Mpowerment Project: a community level HIV-prevention intervention for young gay men. *American Journal of Public Health* **86**, 1129–36.

46. **Fishbein, M.** (1996). Great expectations, or, do we ask too much from community-level interventions. *American Journal of Public Health* **86**, 1075–6.

47. **Day, S. and Ward, H.** (1997). Sex workers and the control of sexually transmitted disease. *Genitourinary Medicine* **73**, 161–8.

48. **European Network for HIV/STD Prevention in Prostitution.** *Hustling for Health: Developing Services for Sex Workers in Europe.* London: Imperial College, 1999.

49. **Churchill, R., Allen, J., Pringle, M., Hippisley-Cox, J., Ebdon, D., MacPherson, M., and Bradley, S.** (2000). Consultation patterns and provision of contraception in general practice before teenage pregnancy: case control study. *British Medical Journal* **321**, 486–9.

50. **Ward, H.** (2001). Partner notification and contact tracing. *Medicine* **29** (8), 81–2.

51. **Bell, G., Ward, H., Day, S., Ghani, A., Goan, U., Claydon, E., and Kinghorn, G.R.** (1998). Partner notification for gonorrhoea: a comparative study with a provincial and a metropolitan UK clinic. *Sexually Transmitted Infections* **74** (6), 409–14.

11.7 Anticipatory care of established illness: vascular disease

Carlos Brotons and Antonio Maiques

Introduction

Cardiovascular diseases are the main cause of death in middle-aged and older adults in most European countries.[1] In nearly all these countries, cardiovascular mortality represents around 40 per cent of all-causes mortality before the age of 74 years.

The overall objective of anticipatory care for established cardiovascular disease, also called secondary prevention of cardiovascular disease, is to reduce the risk of a second event, and thereby reduce premature disability and mortality, and prolong survival. Cardiovascular disease can be defined as those atherosclerotic diseases of the heart, cerebral or peripheral vessels leading to clinical events such as coronary heart disease (CHD), myocardial infarction (MI), angina, sudden death, stroke, and intermittent claudication.

Patients with established cardiovascular disease are the first priority in cardiovascular disease prevention. Primary care physicians should target this high-risk patient population, because the potential for prevention action is greater.

In this chapter, first, the evidence of lifestyle changes goals, of risk factor management, and of prophylactic treatment for patients with established cardiovascular diseases will be reviewed (Table 1). Second, results of surveys showing the implementation of recommendations on secondary prevention will be discussed. And third, results of effectiveness studies promoting secondary prevention of cardiovascular disease in primary care will be also reviewed and discussed. Finally, conclusions from these three parts will be drawn, and suggestions for future questions for research will be presented.

Review of the evidence

Lifestyle changes

Lifestyle changes are the first and more important step in anticipatory care of cardiovascular diseases, not only because they are risk factors by themselves, but also because they can influence the level of other risk factors—blood pressure, serum cholesterol, blood glucose—and indeed, reduce the risk of further non-fatal and fatal events.

Table 1 Goals for lifestyle changes, for management of risk factors and prophylactic treatment for patients with established cardiovascular disease

Lifestyle
Stop smoking, choose Mediterranean-style diet, practice exercise or be physically active and achieve ideal weight
Risk factors
Blood pressure <140/90 mmHg or <130/85 mmHg in diabetic subjects, total cholesterol <5.0 mmol/l (190 mg/dl), LDL-cholesterol <3.0 mmol/l (115 mg/dl)
Prophylactic treatment
Aspirin (at least 75 mg/dl)
β-Blockers in patients after MI
ACE inhibitors, especially those patients with signs or symptoms of heart failure after MI, or with low ejection fraction (<40%)
Anticoagulants in selected patients

Smoking

There are no randomized controlled trials (RCTs) of the effects of smoking cessation on cardiovascular events in people with cardiovascular diseases, probably for ethical reasons. However, many observational studies found that people with CHD, stroke, or intermittent claudication who stop smoking rapidly reduce their risk of cardiac death, MI, stroke, and critical limb ischaemia. In addition, there is good evidence that nicotine replacement therapy (NRT) in the form of nicotine patches, nicotine gum, nicotine inhaler, and nicotine nasal spray are effective, safe and without adverse events in patients with CHD and strong nicotine dependency.[2] Caution, however, is required for those patients in the immediate (within 2 weeks) post-myocardial infarction period, those with serious arrhythmias, and those with serious or worsening angina pectoris. It is imperative that patients should not smoke while using this therapy. More recently, it has been demonstrated that one antidepressant—sustained-release bupropion hydrochloride—is an efficacious smoking cessation treatment, generally well tolerated, and may be an alternative to NRT. Unlike NRT, patients should begin bupropion treatment 1–2 weeks before they stop smoking.

Diet

There is good evidence from RCTs indicating that Mediterranean-style diet (bread, vegetables, fruit, fish and olive oil) and the replacement of butter and cream with rapeseed margarine has a beneficial effect [adjusted relative risk reduction (RRR) of death of 70 per cent, number needed to be treated to avoid one event (NNT) of 25 over 2 years] in middle-aged people with a recent MI.[3] Conversely, there is no evidence for a beneficial effect of low-fat or high-fibre diets in reducing mortality from CHD in patients after MI.

For a patient with cardiovascular disease it is highly recommended to increase intake of fish, fresh fruits, cereals and vegetables, and to reduce total calorie intake when weight reduction is needed.

Physical activity

Evidence from three systematic reviews[4,5] has indicated that exercise and cardiac rehabilitation interventions after MI result in a reduction of the risk of cardiovascular deaths of approximately 20–25 per cent when compared with usual care. In addition, prospective studies evaluating the role of physical activity among survivors of a first MI have shown that those individuals who are physically active have a lower risk of a recurrent MI or death from all causes or CHD than do those who are sedentary. Exercise is widely held to be beneficial to patients with intermittent claudication—it improves the distance that patients could walk. European guidelines[7] recommend aerobic exercise (e.g. walking, swimming, or bicycling) for 20–30 min, four to five times a week.

Management of cardiovascular risk factors

Blood lipids

One systematic review[8] and subsequent large RCTs have found that lowering lipid concentrations in people with established ischaemic coronary events substantially reduces the risk of cardiovascular morbidity and mortality.[8–12] The review found that statins reduced CHD mortality (odds ratio, OR 0.71), cardiovascular mortality (OR 0.73), and all cause mortality (OR 0.77) compared with placebo. The absolute benefits increased as baseline risk increased, but they did not seem to be influenced by the individual's absolute cholesterol concentration.

The effect of lipid-lowering treatment on reduction of cardiovascular events based on results of several clinical trials is displayed in Table 2.

Lowering cholesterol concentration with lipid lowering drugs after atherosclerotic stroke, transient ischaemic attack, or intermittent claudication probably reduces recurrent events, but there is no direct evidence. Evidence from systematic reviews and RCTs in people with established CHD indirectly supports the notion that patients with cerebrovascular and peripheral vascular diseases can also benefit from lipid-lowering drugs.

According to European guidelines,[7] the blood cholesterol goals in patients with established cardiovascular disease are a total cholesterol

Table 2 Effect of lipid-lowering treatment on reduction of cardiovascular events based on the results of several clinical trials

Study	Cases/total placebo	Cases/total treatment	Relative risk	Absolute risk	NNT[a]
CHD reduction					
4S	622/2223	431/2221	32*	9	11
CARE	274/2078	212/2081	22.7*	3	33
LIPID	715/4502	557/4512	22.6*	3.6	28
VAHIT	275/1267	219/1264	20.2*	4.4	28
BIP	232/1542	211/1548	9.4	1.4	71
Stroke reduction					
4S	98/2223	70/2221	28.5*	1.25	78
CARE	78/2078	54/2081	30.8*	1.15	31
LIPID	204/4502	169/4512	17.3*	0.78	127
VAHIT	76/1267	58/1264	23.5	1.40	71
BIP	77/1542	72/1548	6.8	0.34	292
Coronary mortality					
4S	189/2223	111/2221	41.2*	3.50	28
CARE	119/207	96/2081	19.4	1.11	90
LIPID	373/4502	287/4512	23.2*	1.92	52
VAHIT	118/1267	93/1264	21.0	1.95	51
BIP	88/1542	95/1548	−7.5	−0.43	−233
Total mortality					
4S	256/2223	182/2221	28.84*	3.32	30
CARE	196/2078	180/2081	8.29	0.78	128
LIPID	633/4502	498/4512	29.34*	4.58	22
VAHIT	220/1267	198/1264	9.78	1.69	59
BIP	152/1542	161/1548	−5.5	−0.54	−184

[a] NNT = Number Needed to Treat.

* Statistically significant.

4S, Scandinavian Simvastatin Survival Study; CARE, Cholesterol and Recurrent Events (simvastatin); LIPID, Long-Term Intervention with Pravastatin in Ischaemic Disease (pravastatin); VAHIT, Veterans Affairs Cooperative Studies Program High-Density.

consistently below 5.0 mmol/l (190 mg/dl), and LDL cholesterol below 3.0 mmol/l (115 mg/dl). Preferences should be given to statins as this class of lipid lowering drugs have the strongest evidence in reducing cardiovascular events. Other drugs as fibrates may be useful when levels of triglycerids are elevated (>200 mg/dl) or when levels of HDL cholesterol are low (<40 mg/dl).

Blood pressure

No RCTs have been specifically designed to examine the effect of blood pressure reduction in patients with established CHD. However, observational studies and extrapolation from primary prevention trials [13–15] (in which people with pre-clinical coronary disease were probably included) support a beneficial effect of lowering blood pressure also in secondary prevention. Although some observational studies have found increased mortality among those patients with low diastolic blood pressure, there is no evidence from clinical trials of a J-shaped relation between blood pressure and death. Following MI, treatment preference for hypertension should be given for β-blockers as this drug class reduces the risk of all cause mortality, coronary mortality, recurrent non-fatal MI, and sudden death.[16] Angiotensin converting enzyme (ACE) inhibitors may also be used to reduce blood pressure particularly in those patients who have had an MI and have left ventricular dysfunction or heart failure.[17] Another alternative is long-acting calcium channel blockers that also have demonstrated a reduction of recurrent MI and refractory angina, but only for those people without signs or symptoms of heart failure.

The results of some clinical trials of antihypertensive treatment among patients with a history of cerebrovascular disease point to a probable benefit in the secondary prevention of stroke, although results of trials in progress will elucidate this further. Blood pressure goals in patients with established cardiovascular disease are the same as in those patients without the disease, that is, blood pressure consistently below 140/90 mmHg.

Table 3 'Action levels' for waist circumference in men and women[18]

	Non-obese	Action level 1 (alerting zone)	Action level 2 (professional advice needed)
Men	<94 cm	94–101 cm	≥102 cm
Women	<80 cm	80–87 cm	≥88 cm

Overweight and obesity

Although there is no evidence that weight loss in obese patients with CHD reduce mortality, body mass index (BMI) $\geq 30\,kg/m^2$ is associated with an increased risk in all-cause mortality and cardiovascular mortality in particular, and has adverse effect on cardiovascular risk factors such as blood pressure, plasma LDL-cholesterol, HDL-cholesterol, triglycerides, and glucose tolerance. BMI alone, however, is not a sufficient predictor of the detrimental effect of obesity. Central obesity (waist circumference ≥102 cm in males and ≥88 cm in females) provides a better estimation of abdominal fat, which is considered to be a chief determinant of metabolic complications associated with increased risk of cardiovascular disease. Action levels for waist circumference in men and women have been defined,[18] and they are shown in Table 3.

Diabetes

Good blood glucose control reduces the risk of microvascular disease and other diabetic complications in diabetic patients with CHD, although there is no evidence that it reduces the risk of recurrent cardiovascular disease. There is strong evidence that supports the effect of lowering blood pressure and total cholesterol in diabetic patients with established cardiovascular disease. One systematic review that included seven trials of secondary prevention in diabetic patients[19] found that ACE inhibitors and β-blockers reduced the risk of subsequent cardiac events in people with diabetes with previous MI, with or without hypertension. Several clinical trials have also found that aggressive control with target diastolic blood pressure of $\leq$85 mmHg reduces cardiovascular mortality compared with less tight control.[20–22] One RCT has also demonstrated that ACE inhibitors are beneficial in reducing cardiovascular events in patients with diabetes who had a previous cardiovascular event (about 70 per cent of the patients included in the trial) or at least one cardiovascular risk factor, and with mean baseline blood pressure of about 142/80 mmHg.[23] The recommended goals for blood pressure in diabetic patients with cardiovascular disease is 130/85 mmHg or less.

The available evidence for the effect of lowering blood cholesterol is based entirely on subgroup analysis of four secondary prevention trials involving people with diabetes.[8–12] The recommended goals[7] for adequate glucose control in patients with Type 1 diabetes are: fasting blood glucose 5.1–6.5 mmol/l (91–120 mg/dl); post-prandial glucose 7.6–9.0 mmol/l (136–160 mg/dl); HbA1C 6.2–7.5 per cent; and avoidance of serious hypoglycaemia. In patients with Type 2 diabetes, even lower goals can be safely achieved.

Prophylactic treatment

Various prophylactic drugs have been found to be effective in patients with established cardiovascular disease, and should also be considered either for most of the patients or for selected patients only.

Aspirin

One collaborative overview of aspirin and other antiplatelet treatment versus control, in various categories of patients with vascular disease,[24] provided convincing evidence of a significant reduction in all-cause mortality, vascular mortality, non-fatal reinfarction, and non-fatal stroke. It was found that aspirin 75 mg daily is as effective as higher doses. Patients who have had an MI, or who have stable angina, or with a history of a stroke or transient ischaemic attack should be treated with 75 mg of aspirin daily. There is insufficient evidence to support the use of prophylactic aspirin in patients with intermittent claudication but no additional indications of raised vascular risk. When aspirin is not tolerated there is good evidence that clopidogrel could be an effective alternative.[24]

β-Blockers

There is strong evidence[16] that β-blockers reduce the risk of all cause mortality (RRR 20 per cent, NNT 48), recurrent non-fatal MI (RRR 25 per cent, NNT 56), and sudden death (RRR 30 per cent, NNT 63) in people after MI. The highest absolute benefit was seen in sub-groups with the highest baseline risks.

Angiotensin converting enzyme (ACE) inhibitors

There is strong evidence that ACE inhibitors reduce rates of death (RRR 26 per cent, NNT 17), hospitalization for congestive heart failure (RRR 27 per cent, NNT 28), and recurrent non-fatal MI (RRR 20 per cent, NNT 43) in patients who have had an MI and have left ventricular dysfunction.[17] Additionally, further information on the beneficial effects of ACE inhibitors in patients with previous MI without impaired ventricular function or evidence of congestive heart failure has been discovered,[26] although this finding needs to be confirmed from other ongoing large clinical trials.

Oral anticoagulants

There is evidence from a systematic review[27] that oral anticoagulation in people with CHD reduce the odds of the combined outcome of death, MI or stroke compared with control (OR 43 per cent, NNT 10). However, the risk of serious bleeding is higher than antiplatelet therapy, and regular monitoring is required. The issue of whether adding oral anticoagulants to aspirin provides additional net benefit is still not resolved. It is recommended[7] that anticoagulation following MI should be given in selected patients at increased risk of thromboembolic events, including patients with large anterior MI, left ventricular aneurysm or thrombus, paroxysmal tachyarrhythmias, chronic heart failure, and those with a history of thromboembolic events. It is not clear how long this treatment should be continued for some of these conditions. There is no clear benefit from long-term anticoagulant therapy in people with non-embolic presumed ischaemic stroke or transient ischaemic attack.

Hormone replacement therapy (HRT)

Although many observational studies have found reduced rates of clinical events of CHD in postmenopausal women using HRT, including women with pre-existing CHD, one large RCT[28] that assessed the effects of oestrogens plus progestins on clinical outcomes in women with CHD, found no significant differences compared with placebo in rates of non-fatal MI or deaths caused by CHD, and in other secondary cardiovascular outcomes as well.

Table 1 summarizes the goals for lifestyle changes, for management of risk factors and for prophylactic treatment for secondary prevention of cardiovascular diseases.

Implementation of anticipatory care for cardiovascular diseases in clinical practice

It is true that there may be difficulties in incorporating results from large-scale trials into clinical practice because the benefits observed in trials often reflect a strictly defined population and do not necessarily apply to a wider selection of patients. However, there is still considerable potential to reduce the risk of a further ischaemic event or death, particularly in patients with established CHD.[29,30] A recent survey in the United Kingdom[31] has shown that even in well organized general practices, improvements are needed in the detection, recording, and intervention of major cardiovascular risk factors in patients with established coronary vascular disease: a quarter of patients still smoked, more than 35 per cent of the patients had blood pressure values higher than 160/90 mmHg, total cholesterol was never recorded in 42 per cent of the patients, and total cholesterol was higher than 5 mmol/l in 44 per cent of the patients.

Another survey carried out in 15 European countries[32] has shown a high prevalence of unhealthy lifestyles, modifiable risk factors and, inadequate use of prophylactic therapies (see Tables 4–6). These results are not very optimistic, although a considerable variation was found between European countries in patient lifestyles, especially for smoking (from a prevalence of 14.6 per cent in Slovenia to a prevalence of 30.1 per cent in Hungary), and also, in the use of some prophylactic drug therapies.

Another survey carried out in survivors of MI, stroke, or both in a nationally representative sample of US adults[33] also has found a high prevalence of inadequate secondary prevention, particularly in middle-aged persons, African Americans, and women.

Effectiveness studies promoting secondary prevention of cardiovascular disease in primary care

The last piece of information that it is important to know is how we can improve the performance of anticipatory care of cardiovascular disease in

Table 4 Reported lifestyle advice (%) given to 5556 CHD patients at least 6 months after hospitalization by diagnostic category

	CABG	PTCA	MI	Ischaemia
Stop smoking[a]	81.1	90.7	89.2	81.2
Lose weight[b]	61.1	57.0	55.2	54.1
Diet to lower blood cholesterol[c]	62.0	66.6	61.9	56.5
Exercise[d]	72.7	68.4	69.3	52.7
Cardiac rehabilitation	67.0	34.6	49.1	16.6

[a] For sub-group of smokers.

[b] For sub-group of overweight.

[c] For sub-group with hyperlipidaemia.

[d] For the total group.

CABG, coronary artery bypass graft; PTCA, percutaneous transluminal coronary angioplasty; MI, myocardial infarction.

Table 5 Prevalence (%) of coronary heart disease risk factors at interview by diagnostic category at least 6 months after hospitalization by diagnostic category

	CABG	PTCA	MI	Ischaemia
Current smoking[a]	16.2	22.6	25.7	19.4
Obesity[b]	29.6	29.7	30.3	37.1
Raised blood pressure[c]	54.0	46.4	46.5	56.8
Elevated TC[d]	56.4	55.9	56.4	66.7

[a] Self-reported and/or CO in breath >10 ppm.

[b] Body mass index $\geq$30 kg/m^2.

[c] Systolic blood pressure $\geq$140 mmHg and/or diastolic blood pressure $\geq$90 mmHg.

[d] Serum total cholesterol $\geq$5 mmol/l.

TC, total cholesterol; CABG, coronary artery bypass graft; PTCA, percutaneous transluminal coronary angioplasty; MI, myocardial infarction.

Table 6 Reported medication (%) at interview by diagnostic category at least 6 months after hospitalization by diagnostic category

	CABG	PTCA	MI	Ischaemia
Antiplatelets	88.0	92.1	86.5	73.6
β-Blockers	59.4	67.0	68.4	54.3
ACE inhibitors	37.8	36.2	45.1	31.5
Lipid-lowering drugs	64.8	68.4	60.4	45.5
Anticoagulants	7.8	4.9	8.4	5.0

CABG, coronary artery bypass graft; PTCA, percutaneous transluminal coronary angioplasty; MI, myocardial infarction.

primary care. To answer this question different methods have been tested in the primary care setting.

Health education

The value of a personalized health education programme for patients with angina in reducing risk factors for cardiovascular disease and lessening the effect of angina on everyday activities has been assessed.[(34)] It was found that at the end of 2 years, the intervention group reported more daily physical exercise and eating a healthier diet than the control group, and also less restriction by angina. However, the authors reported later[(35)] that 3 years after the implementation of the programme most of the benefits identified at the end of 2 years had worn off.

Specific health professionals

The value of specific health professionals selected to improve secondary prevention has been evaluated.

One study assessed the effects of secondary prevention clinics run by nurses in primary care as opposed to usual care by general practitioners.[(36)] Significant improvements were found in aspirin use, blood pressure and lipid management, physical activity and diet, and no effect was observed on smoking cessation.

Another study assessed the effectiveness of a liaison nurse leading a support programme in general practice for patients with CHD diagnosed in hospital, which sought to improve communication between hospital and general practice.[(37)] No significant differences were found between the intervention and the control groups in smoking, lipid concentrations, blood pressure, or fitness, although the programme was effective in promoting follow-up in general practice.

Prompts

Postal prompts to patients and to their general practitioners to see whether they improve the implementation of effective secondary prevention have been evaluated.[(38)] It was found that this method did not improve the prescribing of cholesterol-lowering drugs and β-blockers in the intervention group. The prompts did improve general practice recording of cardiovascular risk factors and lifestyle advice given to patients, but they made no difference to patients' reports of changes in lifestyle.

Audit, feedback and recall

The effectiveness of three different interventions for improving secondary preventive care at the level of general practice (audit and feedback; recall to a general practitioner; and recall to a nurse clinic) has been assessed.[(39)] It was observed that adequate assessment of all three risk factors was much more common in the nurse and general practitioner recall groups (85 and 76 per cent, respectively) than in the audit group (52 per cent), although the advantage of the nurse recall group was reduced after adjustment for baseline levels of risk factors. However, these differences in assessment were not reflected in clinical outcomes. Specifically, mean blood pressure, total cholesterol, and cotinine levels varied little between the nurse recall, general practitioner recall, and audit groups, respectively, as did prescribing of hypotensive and lipid-lowering drugs. The only significant treatment benefit observed was an improvement in the prescribing of antiplatelet drugs.

Conclusions

Patients with established cardiovascular disease are at high risk of subsequent vascular events and death that can be substantially reduced by changes in their lifestyles and risk factors, and by prescription of prophylactic treatment. However, we fall short in the implementation of evidence-based secondary prevention, at both hospital and primary care levels. Several strategies have been tested in primary care to see whether assessment of risk factors, follow-up visits and prescribing of prophylactic drugs improved over time, but the results have not identified a fundamental strategy that radically improves the implementation of secondary preventive recommendations.

There are some barriers to the implementation of anticipatory care that are not easy to overcome and these can differ between countries. Particularly, health care resources in some countries are scarce and this fact affects cardiovascular prevention as well as the management of other conditions. In other countries, regulations for drug reimbursement may also influence the effectiveness of care. These and other barriers might explain part of the gap between evidence-based recommendations and clinical practice.

How can we improve performance?

Hospital level

The process should start from the hospital before the patient is discharged. Different methods have demonstrated to be successful to ensure better results with regard to secondary prevention at the hospital, such as a system of case manager prompting and computer-assisted discharge planning. The information displayed on discharge documents is also of particular importance. As a minimum standard, all these documents should contain the risk factor history, risk factor measurements, risk factor goals, and drug therapies including actual and optimal doses.(32)

Interface of hospital specialists and general practitioners

The second important aspect is to ensure better communication among specialists and primary care physicians. The cardiologist who usually cares for the patient in the hospital during the acute episode often leaves the initiation of secondary prevention to the referring general practitioner. General practitioners, however, are strongly influenced by hospital recommendations, and may assume that the cardiologist, who is the expert, has already prescribed all necessary therapies even if they do not appear completely adequate, and make no further changes in the patient's treatment regimen. Hospital specialists and general practitioners need to coordinate their efforts and create an integrated strategy for prevention of cardiovascular diseases. Ignorance about the importance of secondary prevention could be another barrier, suggesting that scientific evidence does not always reach all practitioners in the hospital or in primary care.

Patient level

The third aspect is related to the patient. Some patients do not return for follow-up, and so, after discharge, no further treatment strategies may be initiated.

Others have poor compliance with their medication, and therefore, they do not achieve risk factor management goals. Better patient education with clear instructions at the hospital and primary care levels can help in overcoming this barrier. Patient empowerment through education could also be important in successful secondary prevention. If patients are more informed about their condition and asked to take responsibility for future checks or visits, they may improve their lifestyle goals and risk factor management as well.

Primary care level

The fourth important issue is how secondary prevention can improve at the primary care level. This is a question still not solved, and an effective strategy in one country or region could be ineffective in another one unless it is adapted to its particular health care system. It seems that nurses can play an important role in assessment of risk factors and in achieving lifestyle goals, and that patient education could also be useful.

References

1. **Sans, S., Kestellot, H., and Kromhout, D. on behalf of the Task Force** (1997). The burden of cardiovascular diseases mortality in Europe. Task Force of the European Society of Cardiology on Cardiovascular Mortality and Morbidity Statistics in Europe. *European Heart Journal* **18**, 1231–48.
2. **Fiore, M.C.** et al. *Treating Tobacco Use And Dependence: Clinical Practice Guideline.* Rockville MD: US Department of Health and Human Services. Public Health Service, 2000.
3. **de Lorgeril, M.** et al. (1994). Mediterranean alpha-linoleic acid-rich diet in secondary prevention of coronary heart disease. *Lancet* **343**, 1454–9.
4. **Oldridge, N.B., Guyatt, G.H., Fisher, M.S., and Rimm, A.A.** (1988). Cardiac rehabilitation after myocardial infarction: combined experience of randomised clinical trials. *Journal of the American Medical Association* **260**, 945–50.
5. **O'Connor, G.T.** et al. (1989). An overview of randomised trials of rehabilitation with exercise after myocardial infarction. *Circulation* **80**, 234–44.
6. **Berlin, J.A. and Colditz, G.A.** (1990). A meta-analysis of physical activity in the prevention of coronary heart disease. *American Journal of Epidemiology* **132**, 612–28.
7. **Wood, D., De Backer, G., Faergeman, O., Graham, I., Mancia, G., and Pyörälä, K.** (1998). Recommendations of the Second Joint Task Force of European and other Societies on Coronary Prevention. *European Heart Journal* **19**, 1434–503.
8. **LaRosa, J.C., He, J., and Vupputuri, S.** (1999). Effect of statins on risk of coronary disease: a meta-analysis of randomised controlled trials. *Journal of the American Medical Association* **282**, 2340–6.
9. **Scandinavian Simvastatin Survival Study Group** (1994). Randomised trial of cholesterol in 4444 patients with coronary heart disease: the Scandinavian Simvastatin Survival Study. *Lancet* **344**, 1383–9.
10. **Sacks, F., Pleiffer, M., Moye, L., Rouleau, J., and Cole, T.** (1996). The effect of pravastatin on coronary events after myocardial infarction in patients with average cholesterol events. *New England Journal of Medicine* **335**, 1001–9.
11. **The Long-term Intervention with Pravastatin in ischaemic Disease (LIPID) Study Group** (1998). Prevention of cardiovascular events and death with pravastatin in patients with coronary heart disease and a broad range of initial cholesterol levels. *New England Journal of Medicine* **339**, 1349–57.
12. **Hebert, P.R., Gaziano, J.M., Sau Chan, K., and Hennekens, C.** (1997). Cholesterol lowering with statin drugs, risk of stroke, and total mortality: an overview of randomised trials. *Journal of the American Medical Association* **278**, 313–21.
13. **Dahlof, B.** et al. (1991). Morbidity and mortality in the Swedish trial in old patients with hypertension (STOP-Hypertension). *Lancet* **33**, 1281–5.
14. **Medical Research Council Working Party** (1992). MRC trial on treatment of hypertension in older adults: principal results. *British Medical Journal* **304**, 405–12.
15. **Systolic Hypertension in Elderly Patients (SHEP) Cooperative Research Group** (1991). Prevention of stroke by antihypertensive treatment in older persons with isolated systolic hypertension. *Journal of the American Medical Association* **265**, 3255–64.
16. **Yusuf, S., Peto, R., Lewis, J., Collins, R., and Sleight, P.** (1985). Betablockade during and after myocardial infarction: an overview of the randomised trials. *Progress in Cardiovascular Diseases* **27**, 335–71.
17. **Flather, M., Kober, L., and Pfeffer, M.A.** (1997). Meta-analysis of individual patient data from trials of long term ACE-inhibitor treatment after acute myocardial infarction (SAVE, AIRE, and TRACE studies). *Circulation* **96** (Suppl. 1), 1–706.
18. **Han, T.S., van Leer, E.M., Seidell, J.C., and Lean, M.E.J.** (1995). Waist circumference action levels in the identification of cardiovascular risk factors: prevalence study in a random sample. *British Medical Journal* **311**, 1401–5.
19. **Fuller, J., Stevens, L.K., Chaturvedi, N., and Jolloway, J.F.** (1999). Antihypertensive therapy in diabetes mellitus. In *The Cochrane Library* Issue 4. Oxford: Update software.
20. **UK Prospective Diabetes Study Group** (1998). Tight blood pressure control and risk of macrovascular and microvascular complications in type 2 diabetes: UKPDS 38. *British Medical Journal* **317**, 703–13.
21. **UK Prospective Diabetes Study Group** (1998). Efficacy of atenolol and captopril in reducing risk of macrovascular and microvascular complications in type 2 diabetes: UKPDS 39. *British Medical Journal* **317**, 713–20.
22. **Hansson, L.** et al. (1998). Effects of intensive blood-pressure lowering and low-dose aspirin in patients with hypertension: principal results of the Hypertension Optimal Treatment (HOT) randomised trial. *Lancet* **351**, 1755–62.
23. **The Heart Outcomes Prevention Evaluation (HOPE) Study Investigators** (2000). Effects of ramipril on cardiovascular and microvascular outcomes in

people with diabetes mellitus: results of the HOPE study and the MICRO-HOPE study. *Lancet* **355**, 253–9.

24. **Antiplatelet Trialists' Collaboration** (1994). Collaborative overview of randomised trials of antiplatelet therapy. I. Prevention of death, myocardial infarction and stroke by prolonged antiplatelet therapy in various categories of patients. *British Medical Journal* **308**, 81–106.
25. **Caprie Steering Committee** (1996). A randomised, blinded trial of clopidogrel versus aspirin in patients at risk of of ischaemic events. *Lancet* **348**, 1329–39.
26. **The Heart Outcomes Prevention Evaluation (HOPE) Investigators** (2000). Effects of angiotensin-converting enzyme inhibitor, ramipril, on cardiovascular events in high risk patients. *New England Journal of Medicine* **342**, 145–53.
27. **Anand, S.S. and Yusuf, S.** (1999). Oral anticoagulant therapy in patients with coronary artery disease: a meta-analysis. *Journal of the American Medical Association* **282**, 2058–67.
28. **Hulley, S. et al.** (1998). Randomized trial of estrogen plus progestin for secondary prevention of coronary heart disease in postmenopausal women. *Journal of the American Medical Association* **280**, 605–13.
29. **Brotons, C., Calvo, F., Cascant, P., Ribera, A., Moral, I., and Pernanyer-Miralda, G.** (1998). Is prophylactic treatment after myocardial infarction evidence-based? *Family Practice* **15**, 457–61.
30. **Campbell, N.C., Thain, J., Deans, H.G., Ritchie, L.D., and Rawles, J.M.** (1998). Secondary prevention in coronary heart disease: baseline survey of provision in general practice. *British Medical Journal* **316**, 1430–4.
31. **Brady, A.J.B., Oliver, M.A., and Pittard, J.B.** (2001). Secondary prevention in 24431 patients with coronary heart disease: survey in primary care. *British Medical Journal* **322**, 1463.
32. **EUROASPIRE II Study Group** (2001). Lifestyle and risk factor management and use of drug therapies in coronary patients from 15 countries. Principal results from EUROASPIRE II Euro Heart Survey Programme. *European Heart Journal* **22**, 554–72.
33. **Qureshi, A.I., Suri, F.K., Guterman, L.R., and Hopkins, L.N.** (2001). Ineffective secondary prevention in survivors of cardiovascular events in the US population. *Archives of Internal Medicine* **161**, 1621–8.
34. **Cupples, M.E. and McKnight, A.** (1994). Randomised controlled trial of health promotion in general practice for patients at high cardiovascular risk. *British Medical Journal* **15**, 993–6.
35. **Cupples, M.E. and McKnight, A.** (1999). Five year follow up of patients at high risk cardiovascular risk who took part in randomised controlled trial of health promotion. *British Medical Journal* **319**, 687–8.
36. **Campbell, N.C., Ritchie, L.D., Thain, J., Deans, H.G., Rawles, J.M., and Squair, J.L.** (1998). Secondary prevention in coronary heart disease: a randomised trial of nurse led clinics in primary care. *Heart* **80**, 447–52.
37. **Jolly, K., Bradley, F., Sharp, S., Smith, H., Thompson, S., Kinmonth, A.-L., and Mant, D., for the SHIP Collaborative group** (1999). Randomised controlled trial of follow up care in general practice of patients with myocardial infarction and angina: final results of the Southampton heart integrated care project (SHIP). *British Medical Journal* **318**, 706–11.
38. **Feder, G., Griffiths, C., Eldridge, S., and Spence, M.** (1999). Effect of postal prompts to patients and general practitioners on the quality of primary care after a coronary event (POST): randomised controlled trial. *British Medical Journal* **318**, 1522–6.
39. **Moher, M., Yudkin, P., Wright, L., Turner, R., Fuller, A., Schfield, T., and Mant, D., for the Assessment of Implementation Strategies (ASSIST) Trial Collaborative Group** (2001). Cluster randomised controlled trial to compare three methods of promoting secondary prevention of coronary heart disease in primary care. *British Medical Journal* **322**, 1–7.

11.8 Anticipatory care of mental health problems

Tony Kendrick

Introduction

Mental health problems constitute a major threat to the public health. Major depressive disorder (see Vol. 2, Chapter 9.1) affects more than 10 per cent of adults each year and the lifetime prevalence is as high as 17 per cent. It is predicted by the World Health Organization to become the second leading world health problem after heart disease by 2020.[(1)] In addition, a significant proportion of the population suffer symptoms of mental ill-health which do not reach the threshold for categorical psychiatric disorder. The Office of Population Censuses and Surveys' community survey of psychiatric morbidity in Great Britain found that around 14 per cent of adults aged 16–64 had some sort of mental health problem, including 7 per cent with mixed anxiety and depression.[(2)] Mental health problems account for around 1 in 3 days lost from work due to ill-health.

Risk factors for mental health problems

Genetic factors are implicated in the development of mental health problems, although a positive family history is very common and family members of people with mental illness can be reassured that it is not a significant predictor in itself. Environmental factors are more important for most common mental health problems. These include childhood problems, such as the loss of parents at a young age, neglect, and child abuse. Social adversity including burdensome child care, unemployment, financial difficulties, bereavement, chronic physical ill-health, and a lack of social support, in particular, the lack of a confiding relationship,[(3)] have all been shown to predispose people to mental ill-health[(4)] (see Fig. 1). There is some evidence that the prevalence

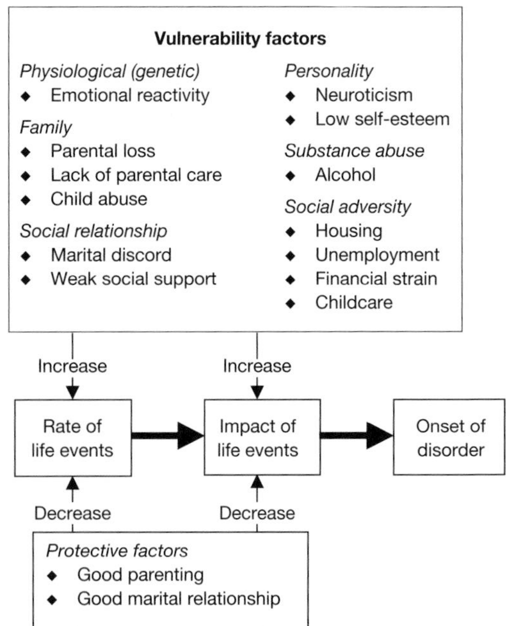

(Model adapted from Goldberg, D. and Huxley, P. *Common Mental Disorders. A Bio-Social Model.* London: Routledge, 1992).

Fig. 1 Genetic and environmental factors for mental health problems.

of mental health problems may have increased in the last 20 years in Western nations, which is thought to reflect increasing socio-economic inequality and increasing social fragmentation, with fewer extended families and poorer social networks, particularly in inner city areas.

The continuous distribution of common mental health problems

Given that common mental health problems are multifactorial in origin, it is no surprise that symptoms of mental illness are distributed continuously in the population. Figure 2 is a graph of the scores of patients on a self-report measure of depression, the Hospital Anxiety and Depression Scale (HADS). The depression (HAD-D) score is made up of seven items each of which is scored from 0 to 3, so the maximum score is 21. This graph shows HAD-D scores among more than 18 000 general practice attenders screened as part of the Hampshire Depression Project,[5] and is shown with the permission of Professor Chris Thompson of the University of Southampton School of Medicine. Note that the modal score is not zero, and that there is no obvious point of rarity or inflection in the distribution that separates a population of depressed individuals from the rest of us. In effect, at any one time nearly all of us are depressed to an extent. A similar continuous distribution is seen using any measure of mental health problems, such as the score on the General Health Questionnaire (GHQ),[6] which is the most extensively used measure.

Comparisons of different populations have demonstrated that the prevalence of above-threshold scores on the GHQ is highly correlated with the mean score for the measure in the population as a whole.[6] This means that the prevalence of mental health problems is strongly associated with the general characteristics of the population in which they arise, and that interventions aimed at reducing them are most likely to be effective if they affect the whole of the population (public health measures) rather than concentrating on the 'high-risk tail' (individual health and social care interventions). Anderson et al. argue that their findings indicate that 'the mental health of society is integral and reflects its social economic and political structure. At this point psychiatric epidemiology and prevention merge into social policy—they cannot exist apart'.[6]

Population versus high-risk approaches

It seems likely from the above that social deprivation and inequality need to be tackled on a grand scale to reduce the overall prevalence of mental health problems significantly.

Primary care professionals may, therefore, be forgiven for wondering what on earth they can do to help people who are depressed because they lack a job, help with child care, or decent housing. However, they do still have the responsibility of seeking to help their individual patients. One approach is to identify high-risk groups on which to concentrate preventive action.

Weich et al. have compared the potential impact of high-risk and population-based approaches to the prevention of psychiatric disorder in a representative sample of general practice attenders in South London.[7] They estimated that intervening among the individuals at high risk might reduce the prevalence of psychiatric disorder by around 10 per cent, compared with a reduction of twice as much if just one item of socio-economic adversity among the population as a whole were to be eliminated.

This suggests that, in fact, while population approaches would be preferable, nevertheless the potential gain from health service interventions is far from negligible. Black has pointed out that health education, prevention, more equal access to care, and an emphasis on the health of mothers and children have important contributions to make.[8]

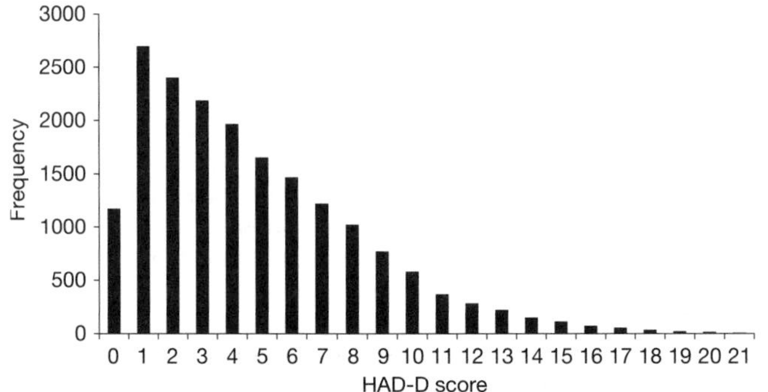

Fig. 2 HADS score of patients on a self-report measure of depression.

Primary, secondary, and tertiary prevention

In the following sections, I shall deal with preventive interventions using a framework of primary, secondary, and tertiary prevention. Primary prevention interventions aim to prevent the onset of health problems and include health education and the promotion of healthy behaviours. Secondary prevention means early diagnosis and prompt treatment, to prevent more serious impairment. Tertiary prevention in established illness includes attempts to limit consequent disability, and interventions that remove or reduce the likelihood of recurrence or relapse.

Primary prevention, or mental health promotion

There is a growing body of evidence that early intervention can be effective in preventing mental health problems developing in those at high risk. Successful interventions in such *'mental health promotion'* have been well summarized in an NHS Effective Health Care Bulletin.[9]

Primary care physicians, community nurses, health visitors, and family practice-based nurses have regular opportunities to identify people at risk of mental health problems, including new mothers, vulnerable children, the bereaved, and long-term carers (Box 1). Primary care teams must make themselves aware of effective interventions for such high-risk groups and of available local services in order to be able to refer people to sources of support and therapy. Where effective social interventions and mental health promotion services are not widely available, it behoves primary care professionals to attempt to increase access to such sources of support. This will usually mean active attempts to engage with local social and welfare services, and can be facilitated by combining health and social care budgets, as is planned in the United Kingdom.

Box 1 Risk factors for depression

- Recent unemployment, bereavement or divorce, financial difficulties, or housing problems
- Among women, recent childbirth, demanding child care, or menopausal symptoms
- Bereavement in the last 12 months, caring for a disabled relative, and living in residential care
- Recent myocardial infarction or cerebrovascular accident or malignancy
- Early dementia, Parkinson's disease, Huntington's disease, diabetes mellitus, chronic obstructive pulmonary disease, and chronic pain
- Multiple unexplained physical symptoms

Perinatal interventions

During pregnancy and the post-natal period, home visits and support from midwives and health visitors can improve the mental health of mothers and their children. In the United Kingdom health visitors have a statutory duty to visit all families 10 days after the delivery of a new baby. Health visitors have been shown to be effective in detecting depression in the post-natal period, by using the Edinburgh Postnatal Depression Scale (EPDS) screening instrument, and in treating depression with specific forms of counselling (see Vol. 2, Chapter 9.14).

Interventions with families with young children

Parents of a child with a 'difficult temperament' may be helped enormously by professional recognition of this as a constitutional problem in the child rather than blaming the child's behaviour on bad parenting. Around one in 10 children can be categorized as difficult, in terms of having unpredictable patterns of sleep, hunger, and bladder and bowel functions, of being resistant to change, slow to adapt to new situations, and in displaying emotions with high intensity. The prognosis for change in temperament is good, given consistent and positive handling, although the time-scale is over months or years rather than days. It is important to take every opportunity to congratulate a parent on their handling of a child with such a temperament.[10]

It is helpful for health professionals to recognize poor parenting and to consider referral for parent-training programmes, where they are available. Good parenting involves recognizing the child's immature status and setting limits, but in a justifiable and loving way. Poor parenting includes, on the one hand, over-permissiveness and disorganization, and on the other, punitive, affectionless handling. Pre-school parent-training programmes and support have been shown to improve the mental health of parents and their children in disadvantaged communities.[9] Parent training is based on a combination of behavioural techniques and attention to the parents' own emotional needs.

More serious than poor parenting is abuse, whether emotional, physical, or sexual, and this is more likely to lead to later psychiatric problems in the child. It is unclear whether abuse can be prevented by home visiting by health visitors and social workers—sometimes the only answer is to remove the child. Health professionals have a clear duty to identify abuse and refer families to the appropriate authorities.

A number of preventive programmes directed towards improved parenting have now been established for some years. In the United Kingdom, these include *Homestart* and *Newpin*, which are befriending schemes for mothers. *Newpin* is a voluntary organization specifically interested in the impact on their children of mentally ill parents. The befrienders have been through the scheme themselves and have, therefore, overcome similar problems. Professional support is provided through group meetings. Studies have shown that a high proportion of mothers entering *Newpin* can sustain their involvement, despite troubled childhoods and continuing psychiatric problems of their own. Improvements in the mother's psychiatric state may not occur for some months, so participants need to be encouraged to persist with the programme.

Early intervention programmes in the United States have shown that it is possible to counter the effects of environmental deprivation, with long-term benefits. High-quality pre-school and nursery education such as the *Headstart* and the *High/Scope Perry Preschool Program* have been shown to produce improvements in self-esteem, motivation, social behaviour, and other educational and social outcomes.[9] Follow-up of the *High/Scope Perry* project showed a more positive attitude to school, better grades, and less need for special education at 15 years of age. Follow-up at age 19 showed higher literacy, less learning disability, less unemployment, higher earnings, and fewer pregnancies among the girls.[10]

Parents may ask health professionals if young children are likely to suffer if the mother returns to work. Various studies have shown that the young children of working mothers are not at risk for mental health problems so long as the care provided is adequate, and the positive effect on the mother's self-esteem of working may be beneficial by protecting against depression.

Bereavement

Prospective studies have enabled the identification of high-risk groups for mental health problems following bereavement.

Higher risk follows:

- the death of a parent in early childhood or adolescence;
- the death of a child;
- sudden, unexpected, and untimely deaths particularly if the circumstances were horrific;
- deaths by suicide, manslaughter, or murder.

Vulnerable individuals include:

- those with previous mental health problems;
- those with poor social support;
- those with an ambivalent attitude towards the deceased relative.

Primary care professionals can help prepare relatives for bereavement by being honest and willing to talk about the prognosis where their patients develop terminal illnesses. Among bereaved patients at higher risk, individual counselling, and self-help groups, which increase contact between bereaved people, have both been demonstrated to be beneficial.[11]

Counselling may give the bereaved person 'permission to grieve' initially, and in the later stages advice to stop grieving and get on with life may be helpful. Counselling has been shown to be effective in reducing mental health problems, at least among bereaved relatives of patients dying in hospices, and among high-risk relatives of patients dying in hospitals. Findings from studies of palliative care bereavement services suggest that professional services and professionally supported volunteer and self-help services can reduce the risk of psychiatric disorders and the use of health services following bereavement. No large-scale trial of such support has been carried out in primary care for other bereaved groups, however. Advice to bereaved patients to refer themselves to self-help support agencies such as CRUSE may be beneficial, although there is no hard evidence to recommend such an approach routinely.

Long-term carers

Mental health problems among long-term carers can be prevented by respite care for their dependant relatives, and measures to increase social support.[9] It is particularly important for community health professionals, such as district nurses, physiotherapists, and podiatrists, to be aware of the risk of such problems and the potential benefits of respite and support.

Secondary prevention

Early detection of depression

Only around one-third to one-half of all cases of major depressive disorders are recognized by primary care practitioners.[12,13] Many patients consult with physical symptoms, which may explain why their depression goes unrecognized. While it is true that a proportion of the cases missed on a single occasion are subsequently recognized, and moreover that practitioners do recognize the large majority of patients with more severe depression; nevertheless, there is clearly significant under-recognition of treatable depression in primary care (see Vol. 2, Chapter 9.1).

In response to these findings, educational interventions have been proposed to improve the early recognition and treatment of depression, as well as campaigns to raise awareness among the public, such as the *Defeat Depression Campaign* run by the Royal Colleges of General Practitioners and Psychiatrists in the United Kingdom in the 1990s.

There is evidence that giving individual feedback on videotaped consultations can change interviewing behaviours and improve detection rates of mental health problems when compared to the findings of psychiatric diagnostic interviews, among small groups of family doctors, including those in vocational training in the United Kingdom, and among older, established practitioners in the United Kingdom and the United States. However, such interview skills training is time consuming and difficult to implement on a large scale using the postgraduate educational systems in place, even in countries like the United Kingdom where there is a well-established unified health service and associated funding for programmes of continuing professional development. The Hampshire Depression Project, a recent trial carried out in 60 group practices, of giving practice teams a few hours of guideline-based education about the detection and management of depression, which would be feasible to implement on a national scale, unfortunately showed no benefit in terms of detection rates or outcome for patients at 6 months.[5]

Changing practitioner behaviour takes more than simply giving information; it necessitates a consideration of how hard-pressed professionals might implement changes in their practice—not easy when the average consulting time is around 8 min as it is in the United Kingdom, most patients present more than one problem in that time, and often choose to present physical rather than psychological symptoms when they are depressed. Longer consultation times have been shown to be associated with more discussion of psycho-social problems, although it has not been demonstrated that lengthening the time between appointments leads to greater detection of mental health problems.

It has, therefore, been suggested that screening for depression should be carried out outside the consultation, either by postal survey, or more commonly among patients attending practices, through giving them questionnaires in the waiting room.

Screening and case-finding

There are a number of well-validated screening questionnaires in use, widely employed for the purposes of research. These questionnaires are acceptable to patients and reasonably sensitive and specific when compared with diagnostic psychiatric interviews.

However, before embarking on a screening programme, which may be expensive and which would expose those screened to some extra anxiety about the test and its meaning, it is necessary to understand the natural cause of the disorder and its response to treatment in order to be sure that we have something worthwhile to offer the patient who screens positive. Most sufferers of depression seem to recover within 6–12 months, often without any treatment. A poorer outcome is associated with persisting social difficulties and particular personality types. Unfortunately, neither initial recognition of the disorder by the primary care physician nor disclosure to the physician of the patient's score on a screening questionnaire has been shown to lead to a better outcome.[14] In light of these findings, screening programmes for depressions are not justifiable.

However, individual primary care professionals still have the responsibility to identify, among those people attending our practices, patients at higher risk on whom preventive efforts may be focused (opportunistic screening or case-finding).

High-risk groups

Primary care professionals should ask about and record the presence or absence of depression among patients they encounter with the following risk factors: recent unemployment, bereavement, or divorce; financial difficulties; housing problems; recent childbirth; and demanding child care (see Vol. 2, Chapter 9.1).

Among people aged 65 and over, we should enquire about depression in those who have been bereaved in the last 12 months, those who are caring for a disabled relative, and those who are living in residential care, where as many as one in two may be significantly depressed. We should also consider depression in those who are suffering from a recent myocardial infarction or cerebrovascular accident, malignancy, early dementia, Parkinson's disease, Huntington's disease, diabetes mellitus, chronic obstructive pulmonary disease, chronic pain, and multiple unexplained symptoms.

We should also be alert to the fact that sleep disturbance and fatigue are two symptoms with relatively high positive predictive value for the presence of depression, and any patient presenting with such symptoms should be asked about other symptoms of depression.

Towards earlier detection of other mental health problems in primary care

Although they have not been subject to evaluation in controlled trials, a number of suggestions are worth considering when thinking about early detection of mental health problems in primary care.

Eating disorders

Appointments for family planning and cervical smear tests provide opportunities to look for eating disorders among young women patients.[15] Eating disorders should also be considered among women complaining of menstrual problems or recurrent abdominal pains (see Vol. 2, Chapter 9.6). Child health surveillance consultations may reveal maladaptive attitudes towards eating, weight, and shape among young mothers.

If low weight is readily apparent, women should be asked

- whether they are dieting;
- how much exercise they do;
- whether they are happy with their weight;
- whether they fast for whole days at a time.

If concerns arise about possible bulimia, women should be asked

- whether they feel in control of their eating;
- whether they find they cannot stop eating when they want to.

If an eating disorder of either type is suspected, direct questions should be asked about

- vomiting;
- laxative use;
- menstrual abnormalities.

Alcohol misuse

Alcohol can affect nearly every organ and system in the body, but clinical signs such as tremor, liver enlargement, and bruising occur late and are, therefore, not of much use in early detection. All adult patients should be asked about their alcohol consumption routinely, and have it recorded in their medical record. Where alcohol misuse is suspected, the CAGE questionnaire may be used. Positive answers to two or more of the four questions below suggests problem drinking, with a sensitivity of around 50 per cent compared to longer interviews:

- Have you ever felt you should **C**ut down on your drinking?
- Have people ever **A**nnoyed you by criticizing your drinking?
- Have you ever felt bad or **G**uilty about your drinking?
- Have you ever had a drink first thing in the morning to steady your nerves or to get rid of a hangover (**E**ye-opener)?

Practitioners may wish to use more sensitive questionnaires to screen for alcohol problems, such as the Alcohol Use Disorders Identification Test (AUDIT), which has a sensitivity of more than 90 per cent for hazardous drinking, and a low false-positive rate of around 6 per cent (see Vol. 2, Chapter 9.5). Blood tests are not usually helpful—a raised gamma-glutamyl transferase level has a positive predictive value of only 25 per cent in a general practice population with a 10 per cent prevalence of drinking problems.[16]

Drug misuse

Requests for prescriptions for drugs with potential for abuse, including opiate analgesics and tranquilizers, may raise concerns about possible drug misuse, especially where these requests are made out of hours, and the doctor is not the person's usual medical attendant. Suggestive symptoms and signs include unexplained constipation or diarrhoea, marked constriction or dilatation of the pupil, puncture marks, and scars over injection sites. Behavioural clues include unaccountable drowsiness, elation, or restlessness, an apparent loss of interest in one's appearance or work, and a history of offences to obtain money.[16] Additional information should be sought from the patient's previous doctor where appropriate (see Vol. 2, Chapter 9.4).

Improved prescribing practice should reduce the number of people dependent on benzodiazepines. Patients on long-term benzodiazepine prescriptions should be reviewed by the family practitioner and a structured withdrawal programme considered where appropriate (see Vol. 2, Chapter 9.9).

Tertiary prevention

Prevention of relapse and recurrence in depression

Primary care professionals should recognize that depression is a relapsing and recurring life-long condition (see Vol. 2, Chapter 9.1). A past history of major depression should be recorded prominently in a patient's record. A patient with a past history should be taken seriously if they complain they feel they may be entering a new episode, even if their symptoms are few and of short duration. If such patients present for other problems, an enquiry should be made each time about possible symptoms of depression.

Many studies have shown that relapse rates in patients withdrawn early from antidepressants (around 40 per cent) are substantially reduced (to around 20 per cent) by continuing treatment for at least 6 months.[17] Therefore, the treatment of the acute episode should continue for at least 4 months after recovery. Some patients recover only incompletely from the first episode of major depression, and up to 25 per cent of patients become chronic sufferers in the long-term. Each episode conveys a 10–15 per cent risk of chronicity.[18] Therefore, we need to consider long-term therapy in a proportion of patients.

Patients should be considered for maintenance treatment if they have had three or more episodes of major depressive disorder, or two episodes of major depressive disorder and other circumstances that increase the risk of relapse (see Vol. 2, Chapter 9.1). A decision about maintenance treatment will also depend on the potential impact on a person's life and career, and the person's willingness to commit themselves to long-term treatment. A specialist psychiatric opinion may be valuable in making the decision about whether or not to continue treatment, and for how long.[17]

Primary care and the long-term management of schizophrenia

There is good evidence from a number of controlled trials that two measures significantly reduce the risk of relapse in schizophrenia. The first is maintenance treatment with antipsychotic drugs, either orally, or by depot injection for patients where concordance is improved through adopting this route of administration.[19] The second important intervention is work with family members to reduce expressed emotion (EE). EE includes hostile and critical remarks made about a sufferer by their immediate carers, but also emotional over-involvement and smothering. Most patients with chronic schizophrenia do best in an environment that is supportive but does not demand too much social interaction from them, and families can be helped to provide such an environment through education, either individually or in groups.[20]

Both these measures, drug treatment carefully matched to patients' needs, and education and long-term support for their families, are best accomplished by multidisciplinary specialist mental health teams. Specialist services are also best placed to help patients join programmes of sheltered employment or structured day-care, which can improve their quality of life and are also thought to reduce the risk of relapse. However, there is still a role for primary care, in maintaining contact with patients who are in remission, and referring them back to secondary care services when contact needs to be re-established because of relapse, or for intermittent specialist review of a person's long-term care.

Studies have shown consistently that 25–40 per cent of people with chronic schizophrenia lose contact with specialist psychiatric services over time. In the United Kingdom the health professional in most frequent

Side 1

Name:	DOB:
First diagnosed:	Hosp no:
Hospital admissions:	
Relatives/other carers:	
GP:	CPN:
Consultant:	SW:
Psychologist:	OT:
Pattern of relapse:	
Important notes:	

Side 2

Date				
Medication				
Anxiety				
Depression				
Hallucinations				
Delusions				
Appearance				
Behaviour				
Preventive				
Physical				
Housing				
Finance				
Daily activities				

Fig. 3 A general practice structured review card for patients with chronic psychotic illnesses.

contact with such patients is therefore usually their general practitioner, who sees them for physical health problems, repeat prescriptions, and sickness certification where appropriate. In addition, a significant proportion of patients established on depot injections receive them from the practice nurse, which means that general practitioners and practice nurses often have unique opportunities to review the care of patients with chronic schizophrenia and other psychotic illnesses.

However, there is evidence that general practitioners and practice nurses frequently just deal with the immediate physical complaint, or re-issue medication, or both, and fail to take the opportunity to review the patient's mental state and the suitability of their current treatment. This has led to trials of structured reviews of the care of such patients in primary care. Figure 3 shows a general practice structured review card for patients with chronic psychotic illnesses.

A controlled trial of teaching general practitioners to carry out such structured assessments of their disabled long-term mentally ill patients in routine surgery appointments, conducted in 16 group practices in and around south London, demonstrated improvements in the process of care, specifically increases in the proportion of patients referred back to psychiatrists and mental health nurses, and an increase in the numbers undergoing changes of treatment. Patient outcomes were not measured, however.[21]

A similar trial of teaching general practice nurses to carry out structured assessments of patients receiving depot antipsychotic medication in their treatment room sessions showed no differences in outcome for patients in terms of psychiatric symptoms or social functioning, which may have been because the nurses did not feel empowered to act on problems revealed by their assessments.[22] Further research is needed to evaluate joint approaches by general practitioners and practice nurses, in special clinic sessions for long-term mentally ill patients. Such clinics could be set up to serve the patients of a number of practices within a Primary Care Trust.

Conclusion

Education, mental health promotion, and preventive interventions offer significant prospects for improving the mental health of our patients. Reductions in consultations and treatment costs arising from preventing mental illness would directly benefit primary care service providers. Primary care professionals should consider their daily contacts with patients as opportunities to practise prevention, primary, secondary, and tertiary. However, any large improvement in the mental health of the population is likely to require governments to introduce public health measures.

References

1. **Murray, C. and Lopez, A.D.** (1997). Alternative projections of mortality and disability by cause 1990–2020: Global Burden of Disease Study. *Lancet* **349**, 1498–504.
2. **Meltzer, H., Gill, B., and Petticrew, M.** *The Prevalence of Psychiatric Morbidity Among Adults Aged 16–64, Living in Private Households, in Great Britain.* London: OPCS, 1994.
3. **Brown, G.W. and Harris, T.** *Social Origins of Depression: A Study of Psychiatric Disorder in Women.* London: Tavistock Publications, 1978.
4. **Weich, S.** (1997). Prevention of the common mental disorders: a public health perspective. *Psychological Medicine* **27**, 757–64.
5. **Thompson, C.** et al. (2000). Effects of a clinical practice guideline and practice based education on detection and outcome of depression in primary care: Hampshire Depression Project randomised controlled trial. *Lancet* **355**, 185–91.
6. **Anderson, J., Huppert, F., and Rose, G.** (1993). Normality, deviance and minor psychiatric morbidity in the community. *Psychological Medicine* **23**, 475–85.
7. **Weich, S., Lewis, G., Churchill, R., and Mann, A.** (1997). Strategies for the prevention of psychiatric disorder in primary care in south London. *Journal of Epidemiology and Community Health* **51**, 304–9.
8. **Black, D.** *A Doctor Looks at Health Economics.* London: Office of Health Economics, 1994.
9. **Effective Health Care Bulletin.** *Mental Health Promotion in High-Risk Groups.* York: NHS Centre for Reviews and Dissemination, 1997.
10. **Spender, Q. and Hill, P.** (1996). Primary prevention of childhood mental health problems. In *The Prevention of Mental Illness in Primary Care* (ed. T. Kendrick, A. Tylee, and P. Freeling), pp. 21–40. Cambridge: Cambridge University Press.
11. **Parkes, C.M.** (1996). Bereavement. In *The Prevention of Mental Illness in Primary Care* (ed. T. Kendrick, A. Tylee, and P. Freeling), pp. 74–87. Cambridge: Cambridge University Press.
12. **Freeling, P., Rao, B.M., Paykel, E.S., Sireling, L.I., and Burton, R.H.** (1985). Unrecognised depression in general practice. *British Medical Journal* **290**, 1880–3.
13. **AHCPR Depression Guideline Panel** (1993). Depression in primary care: Volume I. Detection and diagnosis. *Clinical Practice Guideline*, no. 5. Rockville MD: US Department of Health and Human Services, Public Health Service, Agency for Health Care Policy and Research.
14. **Dowrick, C. and Buchan, I.** (1995). Twelve month outcome of depression in general practice: does detection or disclosure make a difference? *British Medical Journal* **311**, 1274–6.
15. **Raphael, F.** (1996). The prevention of eating disorders. In *The Prevention of Mental Illness in Primary Care* (ed. T. Kendrick, A. Tylee, and P. Freeling), pp. 207–22. Cambridge: Cambridge University Press.
16. **Williams, H. and Ghodse, H.** (1996). The prevention of alcohol and drug misuse. In *The Prevention of Mental Illness in Primary Care* (ed. T. Kendrick, A. Tylee, and P. Freeling), pp. 223–45. Cambridge: Cambridge University Press.
17. **Paykel, E.** (1996). Tertiary prevention: longer-term drug treatment in depression. In *The Prevention of Mental Illness in Primary Care* (ed. T. Kendrick, A. Tylee, and P. Freeling), pp. 281–93. Cambridge: Cambridge University Press.
18. **Kupfer, D.J. and Frank, E.** (2001). The interaction of drug- and psychotherapy in the long-term treatment of depression. *Journal of Affective Disorders* **62**, 131–7.
19. **Burns, T. and Kendrick, T.** (1997). The primary care of patients with schizophrenia: a search for good practice. *British Journal of General Practice* **47**, 515–20.
20. **Leff, J., Kuipers, L., Berkowitz, R., and Sturgeon, D.** (1985). A controlled trial of social intervention in the families of schizophrenic patients: two-year follow-up. *British Journal of Psychiatry* **146**, 594–600.
21. **Kendrick, T., Burns, T., and Freeling, P.** (1995). Randomised controlled trial of teaching general practitioners to carry out structured assessments of their long-term mentally ill patients. *British Medical Journal* **311**, 93–8.
22. **Burns, T., Millar, E., Garland, C., Kendrick, T., Chisholm, B., and Ross, F.** (1998). Randomised controlled trial of teaching practice nurses to carry out structured assessments of patients receiving depot antipsychotic injections. *British Journal of General Practice* **48**, 1845–8.

Further reading

Effective Health Care Bulletin. *Mental Health Promotion in High-Risk Groups.* York: NHS Centre for Reviews and Dissemination, 1997.

Kendrick, T., Tylee, A., and Freeling, P., ed. *The Prevention of Mental Illness in Primary Care.* Cambridge: Cambridge University Press, 1996, pp. 21–40.

Newton, J. *Preventing Mental Illness.* London: Routledge, 1998.

Newton, J. *Preventing Mental Illness in Practice.* London: Tavistock/Routledge, 1992.

Weich, S. (1997). Prevention of the common mental disorders: a public health perspective. *Psychological Medicine* **27**, 757–64.

12

Practice management

12 Practice management

12.1 Practice structures

Mike Pringle and Sally Irvine

Introduction

This chapter examines the structures and characteristics that define primary care and, in particular, general practice, reflecting on the skills deployed, on the organization of those skills and the culture in which they develop. Both family and general medicine are key to primary care, and general practitioners are an important and enduring element in primary care services.

However, the way in which primary care is organized in a particular country determines the contribution that it makes to health care. The extent to which family doctors work collaboratively with other family doctors, the range and depth of their primary care teams, the extent of the right of referral and patient registration, the routes to accountability, payment methods and incentives, and the use of technologies all contribute to the special nature of family medicine, country to country. This chapter explores these issues.

How primary care doctors work together

Throughout Europe, the working practices of family physicians vary widely. The ratio of population to numbers of family doctors varies from less than 1000 to over 2000. In the British Isles, for example, the average numbers of patients registered with each general practitioner varies from 1859 in England to 1695 in Wales and 1441 in Scotland. Even within countries, the density of general practitioners varies. In many countries, family doctors are clustered in cities and more affluent areas, with deprived or remote areas less well served.[1]

The characteristics of family medicine are not, however, dictated by numbers. Roles, expectations, payment methods, and relationships all play a key part. The extent to which family doctors work in isolation or in groups, the nature of the groups where they exist, their contracts, and their arrangements for out-of-hours care all influence the nature of primary care and the working lives of family doctors, and we examine these in turn.

Single-handed family practice

In some countries, such as Italy,[2] family practice is overwhelmingly delivered by doctors working 'single-handed'. Although they may work in the same building as other general practitioners and may, therefore, share expenses, they usually see their own patients and keep their incomes separate. In other countries, such as Ireland, about half are single-handed. By contrast, in Britain only 10 per cent of all general practitioners now work single-handed, although in many deprived urban areas such as southeast London over 30 per cent work as sole practitioners. Nevertheless, the overall global trend is a gradual one away from single-handed practice to doctors working in groups.[3,4]

In the United Kingdom, this trend was enhanced by a deliberate policy decision to encourage group practice. In 1965, the General Practice Charter included a payment for those general practitioners entering partnership agreements. Subsequently, a complex debate has occurred. In summary, policy makers argue for the virtues of economies of scale, and the increased efficiency, management simplicity, and accountability of group practices and the profession argues that group practice offers a wider range of services, more consistent care, and better potential for teaching, research, and audit.

On the other hand, those working in small practices argue that single-handed practices offer personal care, innovation, and a better service.[5] They are satisfied with their sole status and do not yearn to join partnerships.[6] Patients in a range of countries agree that smaller practices offer better communication, personal care,[7] and availability. They are seen as providing better continuity of care and to be more accessible.[8] Smaller practices are, overall, preferred by patients[9] and they achieve higher levels of patient satisfaction.[10]

In Britain, the National Health Service (NHS) has special reasons to be grateful for single-handed doctors since they tend to work in areas of the greatest deprivation and need. Perversely, deprivation is associated with lower prevention uptake and higher referral rates, emergency admissions and patient consultation rates—all then used as evidence to demonstrate the 'problems' and limitations of small practices. Indeed, some studies have suggested that single-handed family doctors were less likely to address patients' somatic problems, less likely to follow clinical guidelines,[11] and were more likely to suffer from depression.[12] In contrast, in a recent study that adjusted in its analysis for deprivation, and the ethnicity and age of the practice population, the authors found no evidence that single-handed general practitioners were clinically under-performing.[13] The dichotomy between patient choice and political imperative will continue to be a global theme as societies decide whether single-handed family medicine offers an appropriate model for the future.

Family medicine in groups and partnerships

For family physicians, the main pressure towards group practice derives from a desire to share workload, especially out of hours, resources,[14] and costs. In many countries, for example, the Netherlands, doctors work in the same building, sharing some costs and covering each other's clinical work when absent or on holiday, but remaining financially and clinically independent. They may share education and quality assurance activity, but they are not committed to sharing protocols and clinical practice. In other circumstances, family physicians choose to enter a partnership in which workload, costs, income, and clinical policies are shared equally among the partners.

To an extent, the degree to which family physicians enter into collaboration depends on the contractual arrangements of the country and the political climate. However, it also depends on two other characteristics of the health service—registration and the right of referral.

If patients do not register with a family physician who is normally the source of their primary health care, then there is more open competition between primary care providers. A person may see a series of family physicians and complementary therapists, each unaware of the involvement of the others. In these circumstances, cooperation may lead patients to migrate to consulting a colleague who they see because their usual doctor is unavailable. Health care systems without registration place a high value on choice and competition while reducing emphasis on continuity of care, population approaches, and a lifelong medical record.

In countries in which there is a 'right of referral', the normal route into secondary care is through primary care and a formal referral. For emergency and urgent care this right of referral (as a barrier to entry to hospital care) does not apply, and it is suspended in special circumstances such as genito-urinary medicine. Patients prove adept at circumventing the system when they feel they need to. However, the right of referral does reinforce the position of the family physician as the central conductor of a patient's care, steering them through the labyrinths of the health care system. Societies again choose whether they value choice and freedom of access over cost-effectiveness and efficient use of the overall health care resource.

By and large, those countries with the right of referral and registration see greater incentives for group working, while those without see more advantages from single-handed and small group family practice.

Another key driver is the development of human and technological resources in primary care. In countries where the role of primary care and the extent of the primary care team have increased, the rationale for group practice has also grown. If there is no reimbursement or salary support for receptionists, practice nurses, practice managers, and so on, as in the United States, outside of Health Maintenance Organizations (HMOs), family medicine has remained an interaction between a doctor and the patient. Where staffing has burgeoned, economies of scale can be obtained through group practice. The rise in the cost of infrastructure—most recently and notably of information technology—has also acted as an incentive.

There are two other trends influencing the extent of group practice. The first is the increasing responsibility of family physicians for the overall costs of patient care. When a fixed or capped budget is available for clinical care, then the larger the population covered, within reason, the more predictability there can be within the system. As America has moved towards managed care, using HMOs as the holder of a fund to cover a defined population's care, these HMOs have had to employ family physicians to deliver the service.

In a similar vein, general practitioners in the United Kingdom found in the 1990s that the optional fundholding scheme (in which they managed a budget that covered many aspects of the health care of their population) was easier for large practices since they could distribute the risk and the administration costs over a larger population.

The second, and related, trend influencing practice size is the expansion of the role of general practice into what has traditionally been regarded as 'public health'. Rather than dealing with prevention and treatment solely in a medical paradigm, family practitioners are becoming concerned with wider causes of illness and reduced quality of life.

These new dimensions include deprivation, housing, the environment, inequalities, high-risk life choices, occupation (and unemployment), and diet. For example, it is only relatively recently that teenage pregnancy has been regarded as a key issue for family medicine. Early attempts to reduce the rate of such pregnancies focused on contraception and safe sex, including emergency contraception. Access to acceptable provision of services has been emphasized. Now, however, many are realizing that we must also address poverty, education, poor job prospects, the housing system, relationships, and social responsibility. General practitioners cannot achieve this alone—a partnership with a range of social agencies is needed—and will be able to act better if they are in groups with sufficient critical mass. If the changing agenda and organization of health care is working in the same direction as political forces, then group practice is likely to become more common throughout the world.

Contractual arrangements in primary care

It is no surprise, therefore, that other models of working have evolved. Both single-handed practice, cooperative groups, and partnerships have been predicated on the 'independent contractor status'—the most common way to deliver family medicine services throughout the world.

The independent contractor is usually paid by individual patients, an insurance company on behalf of patients or by a non-salary arrangement with the state. The implications of this contract are discussed below. However, increasing numbers of family physicians wish to have a more normal contractual arrangement, as is common in hospitals and community teams. They may be motivated to look for a salary because of a desire to limit risk and liability and to reduce non-patient care activities such as administration or paper work. Many want to work part time or wish to emphasize their personal needs alongside those of patients or the health service.

Many chose to be employed by other family physicians either as locums or on fixed term contracts (sometimes called 'non-principals'). However, the option of being salaried on a more normal basis to a health service organization is being increasingly taken up.

The model of the HMO is being duplicated elsewhere, especially in the provision of care to high deprivation communities. In England, the Personal Medical Services (PMS) contract (see below) has been created in order to allow flexible employment options, including a salaried contract, into general practice.

Unlike independent contractors with their open-ended contract, salaried doctors have a clear definition of the work for which they are responsible and the limits of the expectations that can be placed upon them. However, the consequent reduction in a doctor's responsibility is mirrored by a reduction in discretion (sometimes seen as freedom) and control. For many doctors, the autonomy of the independent contractor status remains a stronger attraction.

It is this autonomy that creates much of the concern felt by patients, health care providers, and governments. Before health care became organized in America, the market largely determined the services provided and their price. In many countries, for example, Australia, Germany, France, Belgium, Switzerland, and Canada, the predominant income source for family physicians is through fees for service. In addition to the constraint that the market place creates, the state and insurers keep the cost of each consultation under control through co-payment or reimbursement.

The idea of unrestrained primary care operating solely on the foundation of professional regulation with range of services, quality of services, and cost of services unregulated is now untenable. All societies have recognized that the ill are vulnerable and they need protection. In many countries, the public's role in health care decision-making and self-help has led to a robust attack and re-examination of the 'all-powerful doctor' role, the 'doctor knows best' culture. Most recognize the need to provide primary care services for the poor, the young, the elderly, and those with high cost or long-term illnesses. One way in which this is expressed is through the family physician contract.

If the two polar positions are expressed as a salaried contract and a fee-for-service contract, there are a number of ways in which within those poles payments can be made to family physicians (see Box 1).

In a report of an international conference on payment systems for family physicians,[15] delegates from most countries identified that their contracts used a mixture of these modalities. In the United Kingdom, all of these are part of the traditional general practitioner contract and its increasing complexity has resulted in a decision to negotiate a new, simpler contract, but in this the United Kingdom is not unique. Moves towards negotiating fundamentally new contracts appear to be a global phenomenon—similar discussions are occurring in countries as disparate as Australia, Belgium, Switzerland, and Holland.

Box 1 Types of payments for family physicians' services

- Salary for all services.
- A 'salary' payment as a part of income (either as a reimbursement of 'average expenses' or as a base on which other payments are made).
- Item of service per consultation.
- Item of service for specific activities (e.g. cervical cytology, out-of-hours consultation).
- Capitation for each registered patient (either fixed rate or graded by age group, gender, or overall list size).
- Target payments (for reaching performance indicator thresholds, e.g. 80% uptake of aspirin in secondary prevention of ischaemic heart disease).
- Reimbursements of expenses (for premises, staff, equipment, etc., and either total or partial).
- Payments for professional activities (such as continuing professional development, quality assurance, teaching, etc.).
- Quality and loyalty payments (including seniority and quality of care).
- Recruitment and retention payments (such as deprivation payments and schemes to delay retirement).

Another key difference between countries is the extent to which family physicians' pay is determined very locally (in the individual consultation or practice), locally, regionally, or nationally. In many instances, there is a national framework and local flexibility.

Out-of-hours care

Primary care is required 24 h a day, 365 days a year. In some countries, such as the United States, care out-of-office hours, especially in urban settings, is provided by a combination of ambulances and hospitals. Such primary care is delivered mainly in emergency rooms. Many people choose to attend accident departments rather than call their family doctor, even when a full primary care based out-of-hours service is available.

Junior doctors in hospital emergency departments are often inexperienced in primary care and they adopt the secondary care model. Rather than accepting uncertainty, dealing with risks on the basis of likelihood, and using time as a diagnostic tool, they tend to over-investigate, over-refer, and over-treat. It is, therefore, not surprising that when experienced general practitioners are employed in emergency units, the cost of care drops and patient outcomes improve.[16,17]

In some countries, such as Italy, the health service funds a separate service that takes over from general practitioners at night or weekends. However, in many countries the responsibility for organizing and providing 24-h cover is placed on the primary care service, often as a direct contractual responsibility of general practitioners themselves. A range of models for delivering this care has evolved.

The 'historical' model is for the family physician to be on call for his or her patients except when on holiday or away. Indeed, general practitioners who rely on a fee for service direct from patients often still adopt this very personal commitment. It is only viable when the demand for out-of-hours care is low and the doctor is prepared to make the remarkable commitment to the patient population, or is reimbursed sufficiently to make it attractive.

The model that usually took over from personal total cover was the out-of-hours rota, by which groups of family physicians, usually those collaborating in a group or partnership, share the out-of-hours work between them. The amount of time on call is still large for individual doctors—perhaps one night and weekend in three or four—but the workload is manageable.

In urban areas, deputizing services have often been a popular option, usually run commercially. In some countries, the doctor pays the deputizing service provider (usually paying more than the notional part of the GP salary for out-of-hours commitment), while in others, such as Australia, the patient pays the deputizing service for an out-of-hours consultation. However, deputizing services have been criticized for the poor quality of some of their staff and their response times.[18,19]

The fourth model, common now, for example, in Britain[20] and Denmark,[21] is the out-of-hours cooperative. Although the general practitioners still pay some of the cost, the state provides funds for a central facility, transport, and drivers. The general practitioners themselves provide the clinical service, with very many fewer shifts to work, but a much greater intensity of work when on call. However, there is an inevitable market value for this work, with some shifts covered by locum doctors or by general practitioners opting to work more shifts than allocated. The effect on doctors and their families has been positive.[22]

The primary health care team

Background

Throughout the world, the movement is now towards team-based primary care. Even the single-handed family physician works with community nurses and social services, albeit not perhaps as a recognizable team. The family physician is increasingly only one person in a complex network both within and outside the general practice. This section looks at the historical development of these primary care teams, their roles and functions, and alternative ways of delivering primary care.

The development of teams

The move towards teams is determined by the extent to which societies expect their primary care to offer services beyond those that are clinically reactive, and the extent to which services are to be effectively administered.

As soon as preventive and proactive care is placed within primary care, family physicians need to operate call and recall systems, to work to guidelines and best practice, and to record and audit their care. As the wider public health role expands, the range of skills required within the team expands. As demand outstrips the capacity of general practitioners to deliver all general practice consultations, the need for new skill mixes, especially with nurse triage and consultations, increases. The advent of appointments systems and repeat prescribing push family physicians first towards administrative staffing and then towards computerization. And lastly, responsibility for rationing and fund management for populations requires complex primary care management.

Patients increasingly want to see services integrated, with the minimum of dislocation and duplication when they move from one health professional to another. They expect team working, consistency, communication, and integration. They look for single sites to offer them a wide range of services without having to visit many locations.

These developments and expectations are pushing family physicians throughout the world to work with administrative and managerial support, to use information technology, and to work with a range of health professionals, especially primary care nurses, to offer a full clinical service. Box 2 shows the range of members that might be part of a primary care team in the twenty-first century.

Roles and skill mix

In essence, family physicians still undertake the same core clinical tasks that they have been doing for the past century. In many countries, they have, however, often shed many administrative and clinical roles to other

Box 2 The possible membership of a primary health care team

(a) In the general practice:
Family physicians
Practice nurses
Counsellors
Receptionists
Practice secretaries
Practice managers

(b) Based in the general practice:
Community nurses
Public health or prevention nurses (in Britain called 'health visitors')
Community midwives
School nurses
Nursing support staff
Physiotherapists

(c) In the local community:
Pharmacists
Dentists
Chiropodists
Optometrists
Complementary therapists

(d) Outreach from the hospital:
Psychiatric social workers
Dieticians
Diabetes specialist nurses
Stoma nurses
Palliative care nurses

members of the primary care team. The core roles for a family physician continue to be these:

Delivery of complex medical care

A family physician is presented with the full range of symptoms, signs, and histories in the physical, psychological, and social domains. Dealing with these needs high level knowledge, the ability to tolerate uncertainty, the skill to create a safe, effective but not unnecessarily complex management plan, and high-level communication skills. The complexity of this role, at the interface between perceived illness and disease, must not be underestimated.

Flexibility

This is a hallmark of the personal care delivered by family physicians. They reformulate their care to meet the needs of individual patients as they evolve, developing roles to suit the needs of patients.

Developing the use of health care

This results from family physicians empowering patients to take responsibility for their own care when appropriate, from identifying the right routes through the primary and secondary care services, and from taking increasing responsibility for complex patient care in the community setting.

Delivering continuity of care

People appreciate seeing a doctor who knows them and remembers key events in their life and that of their family, who will be there subsequently when required and who takes a longer term view of care and its outcomes. Continuity of care has been shown to reduce use of secondary care services and to improve patient satisfaction.

Population context and advocacy

In addition, a family physician must see care in the context of the individual, the family, the group, the community, and the population. Without this variety of perspectives, the family physician cannot be involved in health needs assessment, addressing health inequalities, prevention, and the commissioning of health services. This is linked to advocacy the family physician provides not only for individuals, but also for groups and entire communities.

Team working

The general practitioner fulfils a key role within the primary health care team. Every user of primary care needs to know that someone—their general practitioner—is taking clinical responsibility for the care they receive and can be held to account for that care, regardless of which team member they consult.

Leadership

In this egalitarian age, this concept may seem perverse, but the family physician has a clear leadership role in primary care and, increasingly, in the entirety of health care systems.

Practice nurses have gradually moved from traditional nursing tasks, such as dressings, into prevention and early detection,[23] taking over day-to-day responsibility for smoking advice,[24] diet and exercise advice, cervical cytology, immunizations, new patient registration checks, well person clinics, medicals for older people, and foreign travel advice.[25]

In the last two decades, their role has extended into monitoring of care in chronic diseases, contraception, menopausal interventions, and minor surgery.[26] They may be trained for these tasks 'in house' and start with protocols to follow under supervision. Increasingly, however, they are properly trained as nurse practitioners and take their own clinical responsibility for clinical decisions, but with the explicit support of the family physicians in the practice.

More and more nurses are caring for urgent problems, running open access clinics to assess and manage patients with self-limiting and minor illness, filtering out those with more significant problems who require a general practitioner consultation.[27] As people become accustomed to nurse advice on telephone lines, and to nurse follow-up for their chronic diseases, they will begin to accept and expect nurse assessment and advice for new and urgent problems.

Community nurses have important roles caring for people after discharge from hospital, especially after surgery, offering palliative care, continuing care for stomas and catheters, for wounds, infections and injuries, and for the frail or vulnerable person.

In addition to dispensing medicines, community pharmacists have traditionally fulfilled a key role in offering advice, filtering out those who need to consult a family physician, and supporting self-care. Many countries are exploring the increased use of pharmacists as members of the primary care team with expertise in prescribing and it seems likely that their roles will become more central to primary care internationally.

Many countries have 'public health nurses'—in Britain called health visitors—who have responsibility for the health of the population through lifestyle and general advice and interventions for young children and their families, the elderly, the vulnerable, and those with chronic illness. They may also play a key role in assessing health needs and commissioning to reduce health inequalities. They can be central to attempts to improve health promotion and healthy choices, and to the practice team's efforts to deliver effective primary and secondary prevention—especially given the evidence of geographic and gender inequalities in prevention.

In the last decades of the twentieth century, many health services increased access to counsellors or psychologists, including practice-based counsellors. Counsellors can offer a range of psychological supports, including cognitive behaviour therapy, and see people with anxiety, depression, relationship problems, and lifestyle issues. They do not usually manage major psychological or psychiatric illness, but they have an increasing role as team members in the management of eating disorders and chronic fatigue syndrome.

As general practices become more complex organizations, the requirement for professional managers increases. Some primary care managers are little more than secretaries or administrators, and the family physicians continue to undertake the more complex organizational and managerial tasks. Others are senior members of the team, even profit-sharing partners, who negotiate on behalf of the practice, and have delegated responsibility for employment issues, health and safety, risk management, systems of care, and legal issues.

As these key roles develop, the need for team coordination and team working will increase to prevent duplication and lack of coordination, and thus to make best use of thinly spread resources. In particular, team members need to share their expertise, strive for quality of care together, and seek education and continuing personal development as teams.

Alternative providers of primary care

In its widest definition, primary care is provided by hospital emergency centres (called Accident and Emergency in Britain), the ambulance service, complementary therapists, direct access hospital clinics, pharmacists, dentists, optometrists, and telephone advice services as well as the primary health care team in which the family physician works.

People seek advice from a variety of sources beyond even this wide list. They consult voluntary specialist organizations, friends, the newspapers and magazines, television and radio, books, and increasingly the Internet. They often attend as well-informed consumers of health care, seeking specific actions or advice. This is placing the concept of the family physician as the 'expert' under the spotlight.

There are two general responses. First, the family physician needs to be better informed. Desktop access to comprehensive databases and to decision support software is becoming a common feature of the primary care consulting room. The family physician must be at least as well informed as the patient, or be able to become fully informed.

The second response concerns modes of access to advice and health care. In many countries, including Canada, Australia, and now England (with Walk-in Centres), the need for fast, convenient, and impersonal care is met by clinics that offer low-grade assessment and treatment. These centres do not offer continuity or care for complex problems, but they meet a need when family physicians are not able or willing to offer an equivalent service. These centres particularly flourish in cities or in locations with transient populations.

Health services are also offering accredited advice through websites and telephone advice services. In England, for example, NHS Direct is a nurse-delivered telephone advice service that uses computer algorithms to offer best advice to callers. Early evidence suggests that it reduces attendance at Accident and Emergency but does not reduce use of general practice services.[(28)] In time it is likely that NHS Direct will become the common portal for access to out-of-hours care, including that provided by general practice cooperatives; and then perhaps to become a daytime route for urgent appointments at general practices.

External structures

Primary care in policy making

In almost every country, general practice started and often remains outside the main 'health service', and in countries such as Australia, the United States, and Canada family medicine is still politically peripheral to the health system. The paradigm is of hospital medicine heavily funded by the state or insurance, regulated, monitored, and managed, while general practice is regarded as a largely private exchange between the patient and the practitioner and is only lightly regulated, supervised, or managed. This situation is changing as awareness of the significance of primary care has risen throughout the world.

Politicians take note of primary care if they use the tax payers' money to fund it; if primary care is perceived to be a high-risk area either in patient care or political terms; or if primary care is seen, correctly, as the key to constraining health care costs while increasing patient outcomes. And, in addition, issues around quality and accountability have to be addressed.

From Barbara Starfield's seminal work on international comparisons[(29)] and work by Fry and Horder,[(30)] it is clear that the more primary care orientation there is in a health care system the higher is patient satisfaction with the health care system; the lower the overall expenditure on health care is, the better the population health indicators become, and fewer prescribed drugs are taken per head of population.

Once politicians become aware of this, the more they move primary care to the top of their priority list. Through innovations such as 'fundholding' in Britain—where family physicians were given a budget to purchase some aspects of hospital care—through to the Independent Provider Associations (IPAs) in New Zealand,[(31)] there have been attempts to empower family physicians within health care systems.

This search for primary care solutions to health service problems is replicated in other countries.[(32,33)] Although the American system has continued to be the free-market in the western world, even there the health insurance industry has attempted to cap costs through HMOs using family physicians.

Standard setting and monitoring

More aware consumers of health care and governments increasingly demand of primary care that is quality assured. Governments are faced with increased political risks from health care, soaring costs, and ever increasing expectations.

The move towards standard setting and monitoring in primary care has largely been founded on the work of Avedis Donebedian who set out the triad of structure, process, and outcome. In Britain and many other countries, this quantitative thread has been taken through into clinical auditing. Early audits looked at workload, prescribing patterns, morbidity, patient satisfaction, referral, and consultation rates. Advocates like Ian McWhinney began to espouse medical audit as a facet of continuing education: 'As an educational experience a good system of medical audit is worth any number of postgraduate courses'.[(34)] The link between clinical audit and continuing professional development, particularly in establishing educational needs and in vocational training, persists to this day.

A second type of quality assurance has been case-based auditing. This has its basis in the ward round, case conferences, and confidential enquiries. The development of case-based auditing came late to general practice where it is referred to as significant event auditing.[(35)] However, in a short period of time it has become established as a key component of risk management, quality markers such as Fellowship by Assessment and Membership by Assessment of the Royal College of General Practitioners, and the assessment of care in a range of countries.

These issues are addressed in more detail in Chapter 13.

Accountability

Together with quality assurance, there is concomitant accountability. The age-old reliance on the personal values of a professional as a bulwark against incompetence has been eroded as public confidence in doctors has declined. Registering and regulating bodies are increasingly expecting high standards on entry to the profession, continuing demonstration of those standards throughout a career, high levels of probity and personal behaviour, and protection for patients against doctors who themselves become ill.

In the United Kingdom, increasing accountability for practising doctors will be expressed through a new system of annual appraisal by peers and a 5-yearly submission of evidence of fitness to practice (called revalidation) to the licensing body. Additionally, local structures will be in place through the National Clinical Assessment Authority to respond to concerns of poor performance locally, and the state's clinical governance processes are designed to ensure clinical care is monitored, meets the expectations of the health service, and is cost-effective.

The increasing trend towards accountability of health professionals allied to an emphasis on delivering health services to meet the needs of patients will continue in all countries, and will continue to have a major impact upon the structure and organization of general practice.

References

1. **Cox, J.** *Rural General Practice in the UK.* Occasional Paper 71. London: Royal College of General Practitioners, 1995.
2. **Pringle, M.** (1991). General practice in Italy. *British Journal of General Practice* **41**, 472–4.
3. **Bass, M., McWhinney, I., Stewart, M., and Grindrod, A.** (1998). Changing face of family practice. *Canadian Family Physician* **44**, 2143–9.
4. **Friedman, E.** (1993). Changing the system: implications for physicians. *Journal of the American Medical Association* **269**, 2437–42.
5. **Green, J.** (1993). The views of single-handed general practitioners: a qualitative study. *British Medical Journal* **307**, 307.
6. **Lunt, N., Atkin, K., and Hirst, M.** (1997). Staying single in the 1990s: single-handed practitioners in the new National Health Service. *Social Science and Medicine* **45**, 341–9.
7. **Maguire, N. and Clarke, J.** (1996). Do Irish general practitioners know how often their patients consult? *Irish Medical Journal* **89**, 219.
8. **Campbell, J.** (1996). The reported availability of general practitioners and the influence of practice list size. *British Journal of General Practice* **46**, 465–8.
9. **Baker, R. and Streatfield, J.** (1995). What type of general practice do patients prefer? Exploration of practice characteristics influencing patient satisfaction. *British Journal of General Practice* **45**, 654–9.
10. **Baker, R.** (1996). Characteristics of practices, general practitioners and patients related to levels of patients' satisfaction with consultations. *British Journal of General Practice* **46**, 601–5.
11. **James, P., Cowan, T., Graham, R., and Majeroni, B.** (1997). Family physicians' attitudes about and use of clinical guidelines. *Journal of Family Practice* **45**, 341–7.
12. **Chambers, R. and Campbell, I.** (1996). Anxiety and depression in general practitioners: associations with type of practice, fundholding, gender and personal characteristics. *Family Practice* **13**, 170–3.
13. **Hippisley-Cox, J., Pringle, M., Coupland, C., Hammersley, V., and Wilson, A.** (2001). Processes and outcomes of care for patients registered with single-handed practices in Trent: cross sectional study. *British Medical Journal* **323**, 320–3.
14. **Tudor Hart, J.** *A New Kind of Doctor.* London: Merlin Press, 1988.
15. **Brown, S.** *Physician Funding and Health Care Systems—an International Perspective.* A summary of a conference hosted by the WHO, WONCA and RCGP at St John's College, Cambridge. London: Royal College of General Practitioners, 1999.
16. **Dale, J., Roberts, J., Green, J., and Glucksman, E.** (1996). Cost effectiveness of treating primary care patients in accident and emergency: a comparison between general practitioners, senior house officers and registrars. *British Medical Journal* **312**, 1340–4.
17. **Freeman, G., Meakin, R., Lawrenson, R., Leydon, G., and Craig, G.** (1999). Primary care units in A&E departments in North Thames in the 1990s: initial experience and future implications. *British Journal of General Practice* **49**, 107–10.
18. **Cragg, D., McKinley, R., Roland, M., Campbell, S., Van, F., Hastings, A., French, D., Manku-Scott, T., and Roberts, C.** (1997). Comparison of out of hours care provided by patients' own general practitioners and commercial deputising services: a randomised controlled trial. I: the process of care. *British Medical Journal* **314**, 187–9.
19. **McKinley, R., Cragg, D., Hastings, A., French, D., Manku-Scott, T., Campbell, S., Van, F., Roland, M., and Roberts, C.** (1997). Comparison of out of hours care provided by patients' own general practitioners and commercial deputising services: a randomised controlled trial. II: the outcome of care. *British Medical Journal* **314**, 190–3.
20. **Jessopp, L., Beck, I., Hollins, L., Shipman, C., Reynold, M., and Dale, J.** (1997). Changing the pattern of out of hours: a survey of general practice co-operatives. *British Medical Journal* **314**, 199–200.
21. **Christensen, M. and Olesen, F.** (1998). Out of hours service in Denmark: evaluation five years after reform. *British Medical Journal* **316**, 1502–5.
22. **Charles-Jones, H. and Houlker, M.** (1999). Out-of-hours work: the effect of setting up a general practitioner cooperative on GPs and their families. *British Journal of General Practice* **49**, 215–16.
23. **Calnan, M., Canr, S., Williams, S., and Killoran, A.** (1996). Involvement of the primary care team in coronary heart disease prevention. *British Journal of General Practice* **46**, 465–8.
24. **Lancaster, T., Dobbie, W., Vos, K., Yudkin, P., Murphy, M., and Fowler, G.** (1999). Randomised trial of nurse-assisted strategies for smoking cessation in primary care. *British Journal of General Practice* **49**, 191–4.
25. **Calnan, M., Canr, S., Williams, S., and Killoran, A.** (1994). Involvement of the primary care team in coronary heart disease prevention. *British Journal of General Practice* **44**, 224–8.
26. **Jefreys, L., Clark, A., and Koperski, M.** (1995). Practice nurses' workload and consultation patterns. *British Journal of General Practice* **45**, 415–18.
27. **Kinnersley, P., Anderson, E., Parry, K., Clemjkent, J., Archard, L., Turton, P., Stainthorpe, A., Fraser, A., Butler, C., and Rogers, C.** (2000). Randomised controlled trial of nurse practitioner versus general practitioner care for patients requesting 'same day' consultations in primary care. *British Medical Journal* **320**, 1043–8.
28. **Munro, J., Nicholl, J., O'Cathain, A., and Knowles, E.** (2000). Impact of NHS Direct on demand for immediate care: observational study. *British Medical Journal* **321**, 150–3.
29. **Starfield, B.** *Primary Care: Balancing Health Needs, Services and Technology.* New York: Oxford University Press, 1998.
30. **Fry, J. and Horder, J.** *Primary Health Care in an International Context.* London: Nuffield Provincial Hospitals Trust, 1995.
31. **Malcolm, L.** (1997). GP budget holding in New Zealand: lessons for Britain and elsewhere? *British Medical Journal* **316**, 1890–2.
32. **Gervas, J., Perez Fernandez, M., and Starfield, B.** (1994). Primary care, financing and gatekeeping in western Europe. *Family Practice* **11**, 307–17.
33. **Mason, A. and Morgan, K.** (1995). Purchaser–provider: the international dimension. *British Medical Journal* **31**, 231–5.
34. **McWhinney, I.** (1972). Medical audit in North America. *British Medical Journal* **2**, 277–9.
35. **Pringle, M., Bradley, C., Carmichael, C., Wallis, H., and Moore, A.** *Significant Event Auditing.* Occasional Paper 70. London: Royal College of General Practitioners, 1995.

12.2 Staff

Hilary Haman and Pieter van den Hombergh

Introduction

Effective management of people is a prerequisite for any service organization, whether in the private, public, or voluntary sector. People who deliver that service should be managed and developed in a way that ensures that the delivery of the services meets the standards set by the organization.

Health services, however they develop in the future, will always be dependent on people for the quality of the service provided. The standard of work performed by an organization's personnel is the single major factor which differentiates the excellent from the merely good business, and the good from the mediocre.[1] The needs of the people providing this service, whether they be doctors, nurses, receptionists, managers, administrators, clerks, or cleaners, must be met in a way that both satisfies realistic expectations and motivates them to fulfil their potential both in the delivery of care and in their own career development. The aim must be to develop primary care personnel in such a way that patient care is being provided at an optimum level by a fulfilled and stimulated team.

The challenge for any practice and every primary health care organization is to manage staff in an effective, sensitive, and confident manner, applying the skills of personnel management. This is sometimes poorly understood by general practitioners (GPs) in charge of a practice and often also by professional managers in general practice care.

The chapter finds its origin in the United Kingdom, where general practice care is delivered by larger organizations. Management is more explicit and these tasks are often handled by professionals. Therefore, attention has been given to making the chapter generally applicable even to the single-handed practitioner with only one member of staff.

Recruiting the right staff

One of the key functions of those responsible for staff—we refer to the GP, coordinator, or manager—is the recruitment and selection of staff. The purpose of an effective recruitment and selection process is to appoint a person with the appropriate mix of skills, knowledge, experiences, and attitudes to effectively perform the job on offer and to fit in with the rest of the team.

The process, at its most basic, involves describing the vacant post and its requirements, advertising the post, selecting applicants for interview and after interview, appointing a successful candidate.

Recruitment is a risky business and vulnerable to subjective and hastily made decisions. Appointing the wrong applicant can cause distress to the organization and the individual concerned. This is particularly true for small practices. In a single-handed practice, help from outside may offer some reduction of mistakes. Ensuring a process designed to realize the best possible assessment, would minimize these risks.

Although recruitment is commonly thought of in terms of the recruitment interview, the interview is only one of a number of stages in the recruitment process. These stages are now described.

The exit interview

If a vacancy has arisen because someone is leaving the organization, the first person to talk to is the leaver. This discussion could be called the 'exit interview' and leavers are a good source of valuable information. Talking through in detail the reasons why the person is leaving is vital. In this way their views of the job and the organization can provide insight into the requirements of the job, the type of person needed to fill the vacancy, or even to question whether the job needs to be done at all.

The job description and person specification

Once clear about the type of vacancy, preparatory work needs to be done on two important documents—the job description and the person specification. These documents are crucial in ensuring that as objective an assessment as possible is used in selecting the right candidate. The job description describes the main duties and responsibilities of the vacancy and must be written before the person specification, which describes the type of person needed to undertake those duties and responsibilities. This latter document translates the job description into a profile of the person required to do the job. This profile is expressed in terms of the qualities needed and whether such qualities are essential or merely desirable.

Advertising the post

The job description and personal specification inform the advertisement which should contain enough of the 'essential' factors to attract eligible candidates and deter unqualified ones. Allow ample time to select the right medium for advertising: local paper, professional journal, Internet, etc.

Applications

Applications need to be screened according to the person specification. This is where the time and effort invested designing and preparing this document reaps huge benefits in terms of objectivity and time. Applicants who do not meet the essential criteria can safely be rejected, leaving only those applicants which can then be assessed according to the 'desirable' criteria.

The interview

The purposes of a recruitment interview are to get as much information about the candidate in order to make a judgement of their suitability for the job. Similarly, it enables candidates to receive sufficient information in order to make a judgement about the job and the organization and for both parties to explore the potential match between the individual and the organization. It is a good idea to provide the candidate with sufficient information about the job to ensure minimal time is wasted on clarifying the exact content of the job during the interview. The candidate should always be asked if he/she has a clear idea about the job and what extra information he/she would like to get.

Decisions need to be made as to who in the organization will interview. Panels of more than four people may daunt interviewees and not allow sufficient time for in-depth questioning and probing of candidates.

Ideally, recruitment interviewing techniques should be known to the interviewers. Specific areas to explore should be allocated to interviewers and each interviewer should write down the opening and follow-up questions in his/her area of questioning. All questions should relate to the qualities sought as identified on the person specification and should not under any circumstances stray into such discriminatory areas as child care arrangements, family planning intentions, etc.

Haman and Irvine[2] have summarized the main points of successful interviewing:

Do	Don't
Plan the interview	Start the interview unprepared
Establish an easy and informal relationship	Plunge too quickly into demanding questions
Encourage the candidate to talk	Ask leading questions
Cover the ground as planned	Jump to conclusions on inadequate evidence
Probe where necessary	
Analyse career and interests to reveal strengths and weaknesses, patterns of behaviour	Pay too much attention to isolated strengths or weaknesses
Maintain control over the direction and time taken by the interview	Allow the candidate to gloss over important facts
	Talk too much

The preparatory work described above is essential in successfully recruiting and selecting the right person and should not be foreshortened when an internal candidate seems to be a likely appointee. All the main stages described above need to be followed as much for internal candidates as for external candidates.

Selecting the successful candidate

Selecting the successful candidate should be done only after all candidates have been interviewed and each has been assessed in relation to the job description and personal specification. The interview assessment form is extremely useful at this point in the process. It provides the objective record of the candidate's history and interview performance against which the personal specification is compared. The temptation, at this point, to compare candidates with each other must be resisted; if not, the best candidate may be appointed and the best may be the best of a bad or mediocre bunch and not the right candidate for the job. Previous or current employers' references may be available at the time of interview, but if not the job offer should only be made when satisfactory references have been received.

Documentation

The recruitment and selection of staff should be carefully documented. To help the interview, a record should be kept of each candidate's response by way of a simple assessment form. The advantages of using an assessment form are:

- minimizes the problem of interviewers confusing the candidates;
- ensures a record is being maintained throughout the interview;
- helps identify discrepancies which can be explored later in the interview;
- is in accordance with good organization in the elimination of illegal discrimination in employment;
- helps ensure that assessments made about a candidate are objective.

Accurate notes and the reasons for selecting and rejecting at each stage should be maintained for two main reasons: the applicants' rights to have access to personal data and possible allegation of illegal discrimination.

Agreeing to a suitable contract of employment

Once the successful candidate accepts the offer of employment and the terms and conditions on offer, a legal relationship has been formed between the employer and employee and the content forms the contract of employment. It is a common misconception that a contract does not exist if no written statement has been drawn up. In many countries, employees at common law are bound to their employers by individual contracts, even if there is nothing in writing. The absence of a written statement merely makes enforcing the agreed terms, or changing them, more difficult.

Any contract of employment comprises broadly five elements—written and agreed 'express' terms (those which are explicitly articulated), implied terms (those implicit but often unspoken), custom and practice, incorporated terms (derived from agreements with employees' bodies) and statutory terms defined by national and local law. These elements are now described more fully.

Express terms

In the European Union, employers are required to give written statements of the main terms and conditions of employment to their staff. Such terms can include job title, salary, hours of work, holiday entitlement, notice periods, etc. In addition to the main terms, employers should also include other terms of employment, which they wish to be contractually binding on both employer and employee. Examples of such additional terms include a retirement age and the right to give pay in lieu of notice. Be clear and explicit about those terms which are discretionary and not contractual.

It can save a lot of time, money, emotion, and adverse industrial relations if the major terms are put in writing and clearly expressed.

Implied terms

Many rights and obligations on either side are left unexpressed and unspecified. A good rule is that a term will be implied in a contract if it is necessary to give such a contract business efficacy, or if it is so obvious that it does not need expressing.

Terms commonly implied are the employees' duties of:

- fidelity;
- obedience;
- working with diligence and care;

and the employer's duties:

- to maintain a relationship of trust and confidence with the employee;
- to provide a safe system of work and a safe working environment;
- to provide wages, although there is no general duty to provide work;
- to act reasonably.

Custom and practice

Terms may be implied in employment contracts if they are regularly adopted in a particular trade or industry or in a particular locality. For instance, an organization which regularly, over a number of years, gives Christmas bonuses cannot withdraw this benefit without first gaining consent from staff to what is in effect a change to their contracts. Although such bonuses may not be written into the contract, the custom and practice of providing bonuses firmly establishes it as part of the contract. (Frisehars Ltd versus Taylor, 1979 EAT 386/79.)

Customs and practices are often quite quickly established in organizations and it is wise to be aware that where a particular practice is introduced it may, once consistently established, become part of the contract of employment.

Incorporated terms

These refer to the express incorporation of terms determined by national and/or local collective agreements struck with recognized trades unions representing the employees.

Statutory terms

These are the legal provisions relating to employment relationships. In EEC countries, the contract of employment will only override these if it exceeds statutory minimum employment rights of the employee.

In summary, a contract of employment involves more than the written terms. There will always be certain areas of relationships between employer and staff that cannot be codified but that nevertheless form an integral part of the total contract. They reflect good will and 'give and take', which cannot and should not be documented.

Providing a healthy and safe environment

One of the fundamental requirements of any employment relationship is the commitment needed by both parties to health and safety. It is clearly imperative that all those working in primary health care are role models of health and safety, promoting healthy working for its staff. Many people tend to think that 'common sense' and a health and safety policy, on their own, are all that is needed to meet health and safety requirements in the work place. Health and safety involves far more than this and requires managers to be proactive in its promotion.

A first step is to look at any applicable legislation in the country concerned. All workplaces have to abide by basic health and safety rules, for example, local regulations of the fire brigade. These regulations normally include having a health and safety policy which sets out the organization's commitment to health and safety, the procedures to be used to minimize risks (particularly of hazards) and what to do in an emergency, for example, evacuation drill in case of fire.

In addition to training everyone in the policy, someone should be made responsible for the following activities:

- Reviewing the work place, noting any hazards. These may not be confined to hazardous substances or dangerous equipment (e.g. is cleaning of instruments done with protective gloves?) but may also involve a risk of violence (Are measures taken to protect staff in case of threat; alarm, warning systems, escape routes?). Talking to staff and listening to their concerns in this area, is vital in gaining a comprehensive overview of potential risks in the work environment.
- Undertaking a formal risk assessment exercise on an annual basis. Hazards need to be identified and analysed for their risk potential, including identifying who may be at risk and how such a risk can arise. Ensuring that the current safety procedures are sufficient to reduce or eliminate a potential risk is the next step in this responsibility. A more general review should also be taken of such things as lighting, heating,

ventilation, noise levels and the general level of comfort for both staff and patients and any other visitors to the organization's premises.

- Staff training. An organization's best protection in breaches of health and safety lies in the awareness, and therefore vigilance, of its own staff. This awareness does not develop automatically but through training, reinforced by an organizational culture which takes health and safety seriously. All new staff require health and safety training as part of their induction programme. Regular refresher briefings are also required to reinforce the importance of health and safety and keep staff up to date as and when new legislation and regulations come into force.

Health and safety issues specific to primary health care include appropriate storing of vaccines and other medicines, contracting serious infections, particularly hepatitis B and associated with this, needle-stick injuries. Other areas of concern include theft/abuse of drugs on the premises and accidents involving dangerous or poisonous substances. In addition, primary health care shares with other sectors health and safety issues around office working and administration, particularly VDU screens, the use of keyboards and manual lifting, although it is not yet clear whether the awareness of repetitive strain injury (RSI) is heightened by the attention to these measures. The measures should therefore be routine and not the overkill after the first symptoms of RSI occur.

Often underestimated are psychological hazards such as stress caused by bullying and harassment. Larger organizations should have a prevention of harassment policy, in which all personnel are trained. But also in small practices this requires attention and staff may, for example, need support when abused by demanding patients.

Regularly updating the organization's health and safety policy will itself prompt a review of health and safety regulations. An analysis of any changes introduced into the work environment which may have a health and safety dimension.

The art of delegation

Once the new recruit has settled into the job, the GP together with the existing staff should be looking at ways of increasing interest in the job itself, maintaining motivation, and testing out the employee's potential. Delegation can play an important part in this and is vital to leading a team. Delegation of routine tasks such as immunization, specialized areas like computing, protocol-driven tasks like culling records, can all release time for GPs to do what they are good at. Moreover, done well, delegation enables everyone to develop their full potential (e.g. a nurse wishing to extend her diabetes-management skills), and to ensure job satisfaction and high morale.

Good delegation requires careful planning and an investment of time beforehand. Irvine[3] has summarized the rules for good delegation:

- Decide whether a task could be done by somebody else more effectively, or at another time, or whether it needs to be done at all.
- Always think about the purpose of the delegated task and share it with the delegatee.
- Use clear language, spell out the tasks involved, explain what is expected, and negotiate what constitutes good performance, together with the means of monitoring.
- Provide adequate resources, including training and/or experience.
- Take account of the impact on other parts of the delegatee's workload.
- Treat mistakes as learning opportunities for both delegator and delegatee.

Many people find it difficult to stop trying to do everything themselves and to recognize another person's skills and responsibilities. Doctors, in particular, can find delegation a problem because they are trained specifically to rely on themselves in the one-to-one relationship in the consulting room. As a result they can end up 'dumping' rather than delegating. Dumping unwelcome roles (e.g. getting the health centre manager to confront a doctor about his/her rude behaviour) and tedious tasks onto others simply through one's power relationship with them is self-centred and counter-productive. It makes people feel devalued and frequently fails to convey to them the purpose of the task. Without that and effective and negotiated authority to carry it out, the delegation is unlikely to succeed to anybody's satisfaction.

Effective appraisal

Many organizations recognize that the development of an individual can be best addressed by the use of an effective appraisal system, which in itself should be the central plank of any organization's quality control arrangements.[4] Regular developmental appraisal makes delegation more effective both in terms of identifying appropriate delegated tasks and supporting the delegatee.

Appraisal provides the opportunity of having protected time to consider, analyse and discuss one's own performance and development needs. There is evidence that it is highly beneficial to both the individual and the organization.[5]

The word appraisal can conjure up ideas of judgement and criticism and even the most self-confident will experience some form of anxiety. Managing this anxiety and ensuring that the outcome of the appraisal interview is constructive for the individuals concerned and the organization is not easy. Indeed it could be argued that an appraisal interview is probably one of the most sophisticated types of interviews managers have to conduct. A quiet, comfortable room free from interruptions will facilitate a constructive interview as well as the following strategies.

The first aim is to relax the appraisee as he/she must be able to make full use of this opportunity to reflect objectively upon successes and failures. The competence of the appraiser as a willing mentor is crucial to this process. Establishing rapport and allowing the appraisee to both reflect on past performance and express their hopes and plans for the future is fundamental to the interview's success. The appraisee may have been asked to provide a written self-assessment before the appraisal, and this will act as a guide to many of the points covered during the interview.

An appraisal interview should be not be focused on the appraiser telling but rather encouraging the appraisee to assess his/her own strengths and weaknesses and to come up with ideas on improving his/her performance and identifying development needs. An appraisal interview should also give the appraised person opportunities to give comments on the practice, its organization, strong and weak points and aspects in need of improvement. This criticism will need encouragement by the appraiser, who may feel very content about the organization and could be annoyed. He/she should appreciate his/her audacity to bring up such criticism for the benefit of the practice and the patients.

Appraisal interviews can be emotional minefields. Even so there is no excuse for not tackling areas of poor performance or fudging sensitive issues. Indeed failing to do so will adversely affect the credibility of the appraisal scheme. Appraisal is a skill. One can train to avoid destructive criticism and to approach problematic areas in a constructive manner, focusing on performance and not personality.

When nearing the end of an appraisal interview, concrete targets and objectives with time scales and follow-up dates should be agreed upon and documented. If appropriate the appraisee should be asked to summarize the main points of the interview. This can reinforce commitment to change and helps to ascertain the depth and accuracy of the appraisee's understanding of the issues discussed.

Whilst discussing training and development needs, it is important to ensure that false expectations are not raised. For instance, it is easy to imply that a person will receive training and education which may not be feasible. Any written material, summarizing the content and outcomes of the appraisal, should be read and agreed upon by the appraiser and appraisee before being finalized.

Individual and organizational performance will be enhanced if information and knowledge is available, assessed objectively, and discussed skilfully. Time spent attending to individual performance yields demonstrable benefits to the organization, the individual and the appraiser's management skills and competence.

Developing an effective team

An effective and robust appraisal scheme will help to develop genuine team work. Teams and team-building are needed to ensure consistency between individual members and the organization's goals. These overall objectives of health care may well be shared within a unit, but the methods by which such objectives can be achieved are likely to stimulate considerable disagreements between those who contribute to them. Indeed life is built on conflict and a manager's task must be directed at harmonizing that conflict, not adding to it.[5] Furthermore, the tensions between administrative and financial efficiency, and clinical efficacy, can create significant challenges for the multidisciplinary team. This risk of rivalry and a polarization of views is a major obstacle to the full development of teamwork in primary health care. The challenge is to make the orchestra (the team) play a well-tuned piece of music.

An environment that creates and encourages participation can turn existing tension and stimulus into a strength to handle the ranges of activities offered in a organization and make people work better together in a significant way. Teamwork needs to be based on agreed and explicit basic value systems. A clearly understood, shared and negotiated vision—what is it that everybody feels the team should be striving for—is a vital factor in team working. At the same time differing perspectives, personal goals, and views about the clinical directions should not be suppressed.

To achieve it, each member of each team needs a shared understanding of each others' potential contribution and actual function. It is vital that each member of the team understands what their role contributes to the roles of others. For instance patients coming into a health centre see their total experience on the basis of the ease with which they get appointments, get through on the telephone, how kind the nurse is, and so on. Each person with whom the patient comes into contact is contributing to the image of the organization.

GPs and managers have three interlocking functions:

- to get the task done (make the orchestra play);
- to take care of the needs of individuals who are working on the task;
- to maintain the cohesion, morale, and effectiveness of the working team.

A good manager is acutely aware of the nature of teamwork, of the impact it can have on individuals and of how to manage working teams so as to get the best out of them. When reviewing how effective a group of people are in working as a team, the box below lists some of the behaviours which indicate the presence or absence of team work.

Good team work	Poor team work
Openness, honesty, and respect for each other	Not sharing information
Taking responsibility and being able to influence decisions	Blaming others and passing on problems
A climate of excellence	Performing below expected standards
Having a shared view of the team's goal	Aggressive behaviour and point scoring
Safety in proposing new ideas and support	Paying lip service and passivity
Safety in challenging each other	Forming cliques or unexpected liaisons
Providing support to others	Losing interest in team's activities
Expecting support (though not necessarily agreement)	Using information as a source of power

In order to move a group of people from working poorly as a team to working well as a team, the leader should:

- have a clear vision of what he/she wants to achieve;
- be able to communicate that vision to others;
- shape the values and aspirations of the team;
- motivate and inspire team members;
- ensure that team members are able to achieve their potential;
- demonstrate interest in personal development of team members;
- take a proactive role in the team;
- be responsible for and exert control over team resources;
- maintain high standards of personal performance and behaviour, and demand the same from others;
- demonstrate flexibility of approach and use a wide range of leadership styles.

Leadership

Leadership is essential for proper staff management and is the spirit behind skills like appraisal, delegation, motivating people and cooperation. Covey[6] was the first to present a comprehensive theory to link the person of the manager—his/her values, beliefs, integrity, and personality—to the effectiveness and efficiency of an organization. His focus on integrity and on fairness and creating a win-win situation is attractive reading. The leader is responsible for his/her own motivation and inspiration, for it is the starting point for motivating others and for good cooperation. For example, if a GP who is heading the practice always turns up late while promising he will improve on his habits, this GP casts serious doubts on his trustworthiness or integrity concerning and may cast a shadow on his leadership and threaten the quality of cooperation with his staff.

Coase[7] asserts that leadership in organizations can provide a context for purpose-based conversation or bargaining instead of reliance on more costly, rights-based solutions. Reinertsen[8] describes the physician's role in providing this type of leadership and methods for executing those leadership responsibilities. Coase shows that lack of leadership can be costly. For example: if a practice would like to make an effort to have a midwife seeing patients and would need the physician's room during his absence, the latter could insist on his rights for that room. Leadership focusing on the benefit for patients could solve this problem by negotiating a solution.

Leadership fosters cooperation using five evidence-based methods[9] which

1. develop a shared purpose;
2. create an open and safe environment;
3. include all those who share the common purpose and encourage diverse viewpoints;
4. learn how to negotiate agreement; and
5. insist on fairness and equity in applying rules.

The shift in the meaning of leadership to being a central participant in a larger whole should strengthen its effectiveness. When Covey speaks of creating a win-win situation, he means exactly this. Always try to create a situation that the other or the whole team wins. Intuitive leaders do so by nature but one can develop the skill. Glorious leadership with followers is hopefully a thing of the past.

Berwick and Nolan point out that physicians work hard to become excellent professionals, but are not taught to pursue a better organization to increase their effectiveness in helping patients.[10] He focuses on four elements that actually lead to progress.

1. *Aim.* Capable improvers answer the question, What are we trying to accomplish?
2. *Measurement.* Capable improvers want to know whether a change is an improvement. They monitor costs and benefits.

3. *Good ideas for change.* Capable improvers are always eager to try what could result in improvement (as defined by aim and measurement) based on a thorough analysis of the status quo. They particularly embrace evidence-based strategies for change.
4. *Testing.* Capable improvers test real changes on a small scale and adjust. Focusing on relevant outcome they ask: Did it work?

For example, a GP would like to give his diabetic patients the best of care. Proper guidelines are available and make it possible to set realistic goals. Division of tasks with the staff makes realization of these goals a challenge. After selecting the best strategy in cooperation with his staff, the diabetic care in the practice is organized accordingly. The strategy is tested for relevant end points like attendance and blood sugar levels, as formulated in the goals of their plan. The plan is transparent and the success visible to all. Try to think of the above mentioned example without leadership and one knows why it is indispensable.

Training and education of staff

A paragraph on training and education cannot be omitted. It is the single most motivating activity for all participants, including the physicians. The habit of considering continuous education a privilege of academic professions is dangerous.

Training and education are part of any change and can either be organized outside the practice or as part of the practice activities. Regular training in the practice and reserving time for it gives GPs and other care providers an opportunity to facilitate changes and gain the respect and understanding that come with teaching and coaching. One of the most successful forms of education is peer review in GP-groups which has been proven to be effective in bringing about change.[(11)] Consequently, exchanging experiences, training/education, and/or peer review of staff is an opportunity to make their work more attractive. Other opportunities besides stimulating participation in training includes paying for membership of their professional organization.

It is the responsibility of the management or head of the practice to find out about the learning needs of the staff and how to fulfil them.

Dealing with disciplinary issues fairly and professionally

Even the best managed work places will, occasionally, meet problems with an individuals' behaviour which falls below accepted standards. The key issue is the ability of the organization to manage that behaviour constructively and professionally.

When standards do fall below what is acceptable, primary care organizations need to have the means to deal with such breaches quickly, fairly and effectively. The major tool in achieving this, is the organization's own disciplinary procedure.

When dealing with a disciplinary issue, four key stages need to be followed—investigation, disciplinary interview, disciplinary decision, and appeal.

Stage 1—the investigation

The first step should be a thorough investigation by a person who has not been implicated. This is necessary both to ensure fair play and to abide by the law. Such investigations must be thorough and a record made of the investigation. If, after this exercise, it is clear that some form of action needs to be taken, the employee is informed.

All disciplinary interviews should be characterized by reasonableness and respect for the employee. Other staff will be closely watching the manner in which the problem is handled.

An employee should be informed of any complaint against him/her and be given an opportunity to state his/her case before any decisions are reached. In order to ensure that the employee is able to defend him/herself the available evidence needs to be given to him/her prior to the interview. The purpose of the interview is not to 'prove' the allegations or to 'trip up' the employee, but to test out the evidence and provide the employee with the opportunity to defend him/herself including any mitigating circumstances. To prepare for the interview the employee should have sufficient time (at least 2–3 days). The employee should also be encouraged to be accompanied by a colleague of their choice or if applicable, by a trade union representative.

Stage 2—the disciplinary interview

Disciplinary interviews take place at various stages in the disciplinary procedure. They can take the form of either informal or formal meetings. Claims of unfair dismissal will often succeed or fail on the employer's conduct prior to and during the disciplinary interview.

If the disciplinary charge is not serious, the interview can be informal and can be the opportunity to counsel staff in improvements in conduct or performance. No matter how serious the issue or informal the interview, a careful written record of these encounters must be kept.

Personal problems often manifest themselves at work in a deterioration in performance or relations with colleagues. Verbal warnings should be recorded and the employee given a copy of the record which should contain the penalties for any further breaches. Warnings should have a specific life span and this too should be specified.

If the interview is likely to cause stress, arrange the time for late afternoon allowing the employee to go straight home.

Disciplinary procedures should indicate who should attend a disciplinary interview. This may include witnesses.

Stage 3—the decision

Once all the evidence has been heard, the interview should then be adjourned before announcing a decision. The time taken, however, should not be so long (1–2 days) as to cause undue stress to the employee.

Stage 4—the appeal

An employee should be given the right to appeal.

Although most day to day problems are solved informally, it is impossible to accurately predict and anticipate human behaviour. It is far better for relations if disciplinary rules and procedures are firmly established before, rather than after, an event which may occasion disciplinary action. The very fact that there are no established rules and procedures may make any subsequent dismissal unfair.

Conclusion

People are the most expensive part of any organization's budget in terms of money, time, environmental needs, and social and emotional demands. They are also the most valuable of any organization's assets. This combination makes the management of staff crucial to the delivery of quality patient care. Personnel management is often seen as simply a matter of common sense coupled with good intention. These are important but there is no substitute for expertise in managing people. This chapter has highlighted some ways toward gaining this expertise and developing leadership.

References

1. **Hunt, J.** *Managing People at Work* 2nd edn. London: McGraw Hill, 1990.
2. **Haman, H. and Irvine, S.** *Good People, Good Practice: A Practical Guide to Managing Personnel in the New Primary Care Organisation.* Oxford: Radcliffe Press, 2001.
3. **Irvine, S.** *Balancing Dreams and Discipline.* London: The Royal College of General Practitioners, 1992.

4. **Irvine, S. and Haman, H.** *Making Sense of Personnel Management* 2nd edn. Oxford: Radcliffe Medical Press, 1997.
5. **Kramer, H.** (1975). The philosophical foundation of management rediscovered. *Management International Review* **15**, 2–3.
6. **Covey, S.R.** *Principle Centered Leadership.* Gurteen, 1991.
7. **Coase, R.** (1960). The problem of social cost. *Journal of Law and Economics* **III**, 1–45.
8. **Reinertsen, J.L.** (1998). Physicians as leaders in the improvement of health care systems. *Annals of Internal Medicine* **128**, 833–8.
9. **Clemmer, P.T., Vicki, J., Spuhler, R.N., Berwick, D.M., and Nolan, T.W.** (1998). Cooperation: the foundation of improvement. *Annals of Internal Medicine* **128**, 1004–9.
10. **Berwick, D.M. and Nolan, W.N.** (1998). Physicians as leaders in improving health care: a new series in Annals of Internal Medicine. *Annals of Internal Medicine* **128**, 289–92.
11. **Grol, R.** (1994). Quality improvement by peer review in primary care: a practical guide. *Quality Health Care* **3**, 147–52.

12.3 Equipment and premises in general practice

Pieter van den Hombergh, H.J. Schers, F.W. Dijkers, and Roger Jones

Introduction

Good premises and equipment are a prerequisite for the provision of good primary care.[1] There is a growing consensus in some European countries on the care that general practice can and should provide[2] and on the consequent practice requirements[3] that might contribute to optimal patient care, but these can be different in different health systems. The practice ideally should have the diagnostic and therapeutic facilities to address up to 90 per cent of patients' problems presented to them. Proper equipment can allow general practitioners (GPs) to treat more patients without referral and, more importantly, can contribute to increasing quality of care. For example, when a glucometer is available in the practice, the GP may be more inclined to check the blood sugar concentration in a thirsty obese lady, rather than when she has to be referred to a distant laboratory. This would also be true, in the same way, for possession of an ear-thermometer when a child presents with lower abdominal pain, and a proctoscope in a patient presenting with rectal bleeding.

In the future, health care insurance companies as well as general practice professional organizations are likely to set standards for facilities in general practice, and recommendations of this kind have already proved effective in the improvement of premises and equipment in practices in Australia,[3] New Zealand,[4] and Estonia.[5] However, few countries have issued firm recommendations or guidelines on diagnostic and therapeutic equipment for primary care. The lack of a generally accepted systematic framework for practice management contributes to the variation between countries, although there are likely to be considerable differences in the appropriateness of guidelines in the developed and developing countries.

In preparing this chapter, we searched for national guidelines on equipment in general practice, and found five of these in Australia,[4] New Zealand,[5] Estonia,[6] United Kingdom,[6] and the Netherlands.[7,8] We have compared the recommendations contained in these guidelines, and in Table 1 have summarized recommendations made for basic equipment contained in all or most of the guidelines, including recommendations for equipment to be carried in an emergency bag. In Table 2, we have provided a comprehensive list of all the equipment mentioned in all of the guidelines in order to document the range of equipment that GPs may wish to be considered in setting up their practice. Clearly, the distinction between basic and optional equipment will vary greatly from country to country; a cardiac defibrillator is likely to be a basic tool in remote Australia, but it may be less relevant in urban Belgium. A hospital laboratory may be essential in a remote primary care facility, but almost superfluous in a general practice setting close to a large hospital laboratory. At present, there appears to be a high demand for the use of the electrocardiogram (ECG) in primary care in eastern Europe, where access to secondary care diagnostic services is difficult, but in other settings, where hospital access is better and ambulance and paramedic personnel are able to interpret ECGs, the use of the ECG in general practice is less widespread.

Table 1 Basic equipment needed for practice in New Zealand, Australia, the United Kingdom, Estonia, and the Netherlands (Bag means they are also listed for the doctor's bag)

1.	Stethoscope	Bag	14. Band aid	Bag
2.	Auroscope or otoscope	Bag	15. Gauzes	Bag
3.	Ophthalmoscope		16. Cotton wool	Bag
4.	Sphygmomanometer	Bag	17. Disposable gloves	Bag
5.	Adult weight scales		18. Thermometer	Bag
6.	Visual acuity card[a]		19. Tourniquet	Bag
7.	Investigation bench		20. Needles and syringes	Bag
8.	Inspection light		21. Vial container	Bag
9.	Vaginal specula		22. Sterilization equipment	
10.	Reflex hammer	Bag	23. Kidney shaped basins	
11.	Spatulae	Bag	24. Blood glucose meter	
12.	Pocket light	Bag	25. Urinary test strips	
13.	Wound dressings	Bag	24. Peak flow meter (adult)	

[a] Schnellen card, Landholt rings card.

In this chapter, we provide a concise inventory of the premises and equipment required for general practice, touching on the variation in these recommendations appropriate to various countries, and give some indications for their use and relevance for good clinical practice. We also discuss issues of maintenance of systems and equipment and problems faced in everyday practice. Very basic equipment such as stethoscopes and auroscopes, are not discussed, because they are generally accepted to be essential (for these 'essentials' see Table 1). We only briefly address office and stationary items and computer hardware and software; the use of the computer in general practice is discussed elsewhere in this book (Chapter 5.7), and for laboratory equipment the reader is referred to Chapter 12.4.

Premises

The practice should, ideally, be situated at a place accessible for public and private transport, and for handicapped people and an ambulance trolley. The services provided by the practice, including times of clinics, a list of staff, and arrangements for out-of-hours contacts, should be clearly visible outside the practice. The entrance should, as far as possible, be welcoming and provide clear directions for the patient, including, perhaps, a map of the area with other important care facilities. To prevent draughts and sometimes for safety reasons, an entrance with inner and outer doors may be advisable. The intervening space can then be used for facilities that are available for 24 hours a day, such as a box for repeat prescriptions and an electronic entry system. The waiting room should be arranged so that it is visible from the reception desk, also so that conversations at the reception desk are not audible to others in the waiting room. It should preferably contain soft chairs, a table with reading material and patient information, and a children's playing area. Entrances and exits to the consulting rooms should be clearly marked and secured.

Table 2 Recommendations on equipment for the practice in publications and assessment manuals from NZ (New Zealand),[9] Aus (Australia),[13] UK (United Kingdom),[6] Est (Estonia), and Neth (the Netherlands)[7,8] (x = should be present in the practice; b = specific guideline for the doctor's bag)

	Country				
	NZ	Aus	UK	Est	Neth
Premises and special furniture					
One consultation room per doctor	x	x	x		
Screened area allowing patient to (un)dress unobserved			x		
Examination couch attached to each consultation room		x	x		
Toilet and hand washing facilities		x	x		x
Separate room for the practice assistant in the practice	x		x		x
Separate space for meetings in the practice	x				x
Privacy for patients in distress		x			
Access for invalids, appropriate physical access	x	x			x
Draft sluice in the entrance					x
Parking space for staff and patients	x				
Table for instruments on wheels					x
Tabouret or stool on wheels					x
Head phone for hands-free calling					x
Paper shredder					x
Pedal bucket					x
Sanitary pads in investigation room					x
Disposable diaper in investigation room					x
Towel machine or paper towel dispenser					x
Bucket or basin for used instruments					x
Shoehorn (long) in investigation room					x
Tissues on the bureau					x
Ear thermometer in the surgery					x
Visible clock in the surgery					x
Mirror in investigation room					x
Toys in playing corner for children in the surgery					x
Computer and printer for each GP/back-up with tapes		x		x	x
Fax		x			x
Modem and internet connection					x
Tel. answering machine, call diversion, paging system		x			
24-h repeat prescription telephone line					
Emergency telephone line					x
Dictaphone	x				x
Visible sign outside practice with information (after hours)		x			x
Fire extinguisher					x
(Yellow) container for disposal of sharps		x			x
Leak-proof container for infectious/hazardous waste		x			
Fridge with Celsius min/max thermometer	x		x		x
Protective equipment when dealing with blood/fluids		x			
Practice information sheet		x	x		x
Practice instruction form for assistant (lab, procedures)		x			x
Diagnostic equipment					
Tuning fork(s)	x		x	x	x
Measuring tape	x		x	x	x, b
Height measure	x		x	x	x

Continued

Table 2 Continued

	Country				
	NZ	Aus	UK	Est	Neth
Baby scales	x	x		x	x
Cervical smear equipment (brush, Ayre spatula)	x			x	
Rectal thermometer	x				x, b
Proctoscope	x		x		x
Sigmoidoscope	x				
Nasal speculum (large and small)	x			x	x
Headlamp, mirror	x				
Indirect laryngoscopy mirrors	x				x
Peak flow meter (paediatric)			x		
Footboards of 1/2, 1, 2 cm for assessing posture					x
Monofilaments (Semmes Weinstein) for sensitivity					x
Jobson Horne probe	x				
Magnifying loupe	x				x
ECG or service within 10 min	x		x	x	x
Doppler			x		x
Audiometer	x				x
Spirometer	x				x
Ultrasound	x				
Monoauricular stethoscope				x	x
Glucometer	x			x	x, b
Eye equipment					
Visual acuity card for short sighted visual impairment					x
Light chamber behind the visual acuity card					x
Binocular magnifying device (loupe)					x
Eye drill					x
Slit lamp	x				x
Stenopeic aperture					x
Amsler card					x
Colour vision charts	x	x		x	
Eye local anaesthetic	x				x
Fluorescein dye for eyes	x				x
Blue/fluorescent light source					x
20-D magnifying glass for fundoscopy					x
Equipment for treatment					
Ear syringe and/or suction	x			x	x
Cerumen hook or loop					
Quire or Buck to remove FB from ear					x
Splinter tweezers or pincer					x
Heavy duty nail scissors					
Nail remover plier					x
Comedone squeezer					x
Nebulizer, large spacer device	x	x			
Various pessaries for testing					x
IUD insertion set					x
Male and female urinary catheters and lubricant	x			x	x
Haemorrhoid ligator for Barron rings					x
Suture equipment	x		x	x	x

Table 2 Continued

	Country				
	NZ	**Aus**	**UK**	**Est**	**Neth**
Surgical instruments (forceps, scissors, etc.)	x			x	x
Vaccinostyle					x
Tape material					x
Nitrogen container for long-term use (>4 weeks)	x				x
Hyfrecator, Electrocauter (Surgitron)	x				x
Instruments for an enema				x	
Emergency treatment					
Tampon or plug to stop epistaxis					x, b
Caustic (e.g. TCA) to treat epistaxis					x
Mayo tubes (adult/child)	x				x, b
Oxygen	x				
Laryngoscope and endotracheal tubes	x				
Emergency IV-drip set	x			x	x
Defibrillator	x				
Set to treat anaphylactic shock (adrenalin, antihist, cortico)					x
Suction device for freeing airway	x			x	x
Glue for small wounds					x
Steri-strips or butterfly band aids					x, b
Ring removal device					x
Finger splints					x
Splints				x	
Instruments for gastric lavage				x	
Good adjustable light source			x		x
Sterilizer or autoclave	x		x		x
Plaster of Paris					x
Laboratory equipment					
Urine testing sticks			x	x	x, b
Blood sugar testing strips			x	x	x, b
Haemoglobin meter				x	x
Urine culture equipment					x
ESR equipment					x
Microscope	x				x
Intracutaneous allergy testing set					x
Patient instructions and leaflets					
Filing system for the various patient leaflets		x			x
Small library of relevant books for patients					x
Illustrations to demonstrate various topics					x
Models for demonstration of anatomy or IUD, spacers, etc.					x
Social card system (addresses of other care providers)					x
Emergency kit equipment/doctor's bag					
Airways—varied sizing from 00 to adult	x, b	x, b			x
Ambubags—paediatric, adult volume, oxygen masks	x, b	x, b			
IV equipment—canulae, butterflies	x, b	x, b		x	x
Saline, Haemacel/other plasma expander	x, b			x	x
Tourniquet	x, b			x	x, b
Oxygen	x, b				

Continued

Table 2 Continued

	Country				
	NZ	Aus	UK	Est	Neth
Pocket breezer					b
Defibrillator if not available in a 10 min. radius or rural	x, b				
Torch	x	x, b			b
Stationary (letterhead), forms, pocket formulary of drugs		x, b			x, b
List with important phone numbers/social map					x, b
Drugs available in the practice/doctor's bag					
Adrenalin i.m./s.c. (1 ml)	x				x, b
Atropine i.m./i.v. (1 ml)	x				x, b
Butylscopolamine i.v. (1 ml)					x, b
Clonazepam i.v. (1 ml)					x, b
Corticosteroid inj. (dexamethasone) (1 ml)	x				x, b
Glucose 50% (10 ml)/Glucagon (1 ml)	x				x, b
Haloperidol i.m./i.v. (1 ml)					x, b
Morphine s.c./Fentanyl i.v. (1 ml)					x, b
Antihistamine inj. (Clemastine) (2 ml)	x				x, b
Diazepam (inj./rectal) (2 ml)	x				x, b
NSAID (Diclofenac) (3 ml)					x, b
Diuretic (Furosemide) (4 ml)					x, b
Ergotamine or Syntometrine	x				
Naloxone inj.	x				
Local anaesthetic inj.	x				x, b
Penicillin inj.	x				
B-sympathicomimetic spray and chamber	x				x, b
Nitroglycerin spray	x				x, b
Aspirin	x				x, b

Whilst funding considerations are likely to affect the design and contents of primary care premises, there is an increasing interest in the relationship between health and the environment. Evidence is now accumulating to support the common-sense view that aesthetically pleasing, informal surroundings are likely to create less anxious and more satisfied patients than traditional, institutional architecture. Attention also needs to be paid to the working conditions of the medical and non-medical staff in primary care, and dedicated space for meetings and relaxation over coffee and meals are also important. An adequate security system is essential, because primary care premises contain substantial amounts of computer equipment, as well as drugs. Attention must be paid to health and safety regulations, including the provision of adequate fire exits and fire extinguishing equipment.

The consultation and examination room

Ideally, this should be a single unit, with a separate space for examining the patient. A curtain or a screen is a fairly primitive solution, but may be necessary when space is at a premium. The consultation room should have a personal touch and not appear too 'clinical', to put patients, and particularly children, at ease. In the consultation room, the GP needs ready access to information, including books, instruction material, patient leaflets, and a computer; a telephone with a hands-free headset to facilitate computer use is also desirable. These items should be situated on the side of the consultation desk away from the entrance to the room, so that welcoming patients and guiding them to their seats is facilitated. Natural light should be used whenever possible. A separate laboratory room or a special corner with a corrosion-free slab facilitates on-site laboratory investigations. A small playing corner, with toys, is a welcome distraction for children. Basic equipment in the consulting room should include an auroscope, ear thermometer, measuring tape, tuning fork, magnifying glass, throat spatulae, a tendon reflex hammer, weighing scales, and height measuring equipment; some of these items, including a sphygmomanometer, can usefully be duplicated, and often wall-mounted, in the examination area.

The treatment room

Whilst basic diagnostic and therapeutic procedures can be undertaken in the examination room, the treatment room is required for more complex procedures and those requiring a more hygienic environment. Adequate space should be available for patients to dress and undress comfortably; thus, items such as hanging space for clothes, shoe horn, wall mirror, sanitary pads, and disposable diapers should be made available. Again, wall-mounted instruments provide easy access and avoid clutter. A comfortable examination and procedures couch should be provided. If the couch can be lowered and raised electrically it is possible to do without a step-up arrangement to help infirm patients on to the couch, which can be hazardous. Such high/low couches are now affordable, facilitate optimal comfort, especially for the doctor, and are usually more stable. Adequate lighting, preferably from a ceiling-mounted light source, is important. A bucket for used instruments, disposable towels, a container for used needles and sharp objects, and waste containers for contaminated material should also be provided; maintenance routines for replenishing these items and for maintaining hygiene should be instituted. All practices carrying out surgical and invasive procedures should have an adequate surgical sterilizer. The autoclave is the sterilizer of choice and affordable models are available for general practice. It will usually be situated in the treatment room, so that re-usable items such as speculae and minor operating equipment can be effectively sterilized.

In many primary care premises, the treatment room is principally used by a practice nurse, or practice assistant, depending on local arrangements. Additional uses will then include procedures such as suturing and removal of sutures, dressings for wounds and ulcers, injections for a variety of purposes including vaccinations, travel, vitamin B12 replacement, and psychotropic depot therapy. Other procedures including cervical cytology, taking microbiological swabs, ear syringing, and diagnostic procedures such as electrocardiography and spirometry may also be carried out in this room, with further implications for the provision of equipment. A computer terminal or PC is recommended for the various functions. The treatment room may also be the most appropriate site for a locked drug cupboard in which to store opiates and other registered drugs, and supplies of injectable and other medications required for routine and emergency use. Once again a regular system for stock-taking and replenishment of these items needs to be established.

The laboratory

Facilities within and outside the practice will determine the appropriateness of establishing a small laboratory on primary care premises, the use of such a laboratory, and the equipment that it should contain, is discussed in detail in Chapter 12.4. Whether a dedicated laboratory area, separate from the consulting rooms, is used, or whether simple investigations are performed in the consulting room, basic equipment should include solid-phase chemistry stick testing for urinary abnormalities, equipment for taking microbiological swabs and urine and stool samples, and blood-taking equipment for samples to be transported to the central laboratory.

Many practices now regard a blood glucose meter as essential equipment, and many will also have facilities for basic haematological testing, including haemoglobin and erythrocyte sedimentation rate. Keeping a store of materials for faecal occult blood testing should also be considered.

Diagnostic and therapeutic instruments

Medical emergencies are not uncommon in primary care premises, particularly in larger, well-equipped group practices, which patients may attend in preference to a hospital emergency department. The most serious of these include cardiac arrest, myocardial infarction, epileptic seizures, acute severe asthma, anaphylactic shock, acute abdominal emergencies, and acute gastrointestinal and vaginal haemorrhage. The practice needs to be able to deal appropriately with all of these, and this has implications for training of all staff working at the practice, as well as for the provision of appropriate equipment.

Full resuscitation facilities should be readily available. These include oxygen, either piped or via a portable oxygen cylinder, a laryngeal face mask, facilities for endotracheal intubation, drugs commonly used in cardiopulmonary resuscitation, particularly intravenous adrenaline, lignocaine, and atropine, and a portable automatic cardiac defibrillator, although the use of defibrillators in primary care is not widespread. Other essential drugs that should be readily available include systemic steroids (hydrocortisone and dexamethasone), systemic antihistamines, glucagon, diazepam (systemic and rectal), and oxytocin. Appropriate intravenous cannulae, fluids, and giving sets must also be easily available to allow administration of drugs in the emergency situation. Finally, an electric nebulizer to treat acute severe asthma, along with supplies of appropriate drugs for nebulization, is essential.

Equipment is also required to deal with the minor emergencies often encountered in general practice. Finger splints and dressings to support finger and limb fractures should be available. Instruments to remove foreign bodies from ears and nose are frequently required (adjustable hook, e.g. Quire or Buck) and self-absorbing nose tampons (e.g. Merocell) for the treatment of acute epistaxis should be available. Nasal specula, for adults and children, should be available to allow adequate inspection of the nose and facilitate the removal of foreign bodies. A silver nitrate stick is also useful for dealing with minor epistaxis when the bleeding vessels are easily visualized. Bladder catheters for men with acute urinary retention, with a lubricant and local anaesthetic, and a short catheter for women are useful; equipment to remove foreign bodies from the eye, including a strong eye magnet, can also be extremely useful. Fluorescein strips and a blue light source are necessary to detect conjunctival and corneal lesions. A full set of suturing equipment, with appropriate closure materials and local anaesthetic for injection, should be available for dealing with lacerations that are within the capabilities of the primary care team; in practices undertaking minor surgical procedures this equipment will already be available. For acute wounds in children, Dermabond glue is an asset, and is superior to normal suturing. For the removal of ear wax an ear syringe is required. A large syringe may be difficult to handle in small hands and one should look for a smaller size, preferably with an automatic refill device. Some practices use a dental water tooth pick with an intermittent jet stream. This may fail in stubborn otitis external with mixed cerumen clots. A cerumen hook is useful to mobilize or remove the clot. Timely ear irrigation with water or oil (arranged by telephone on making the appointment) or a polyalcohol eardrop administered in the practice may save the patient an extra trip to the practice.

The emergency bag

Some of the basic items of the emergency bag are listed in Table 1, and this list could be extended to include items taken from the practice to the patient's home, as described above, including catheters, a nebulizer, nose plug, urinalysis sticks, blood glucose meter, suction device, Mayo tubes, band aids, and sterístrips. Doctors visiting patients at home for medical emergencies should have appropriate information about hospital admission arrangements and essential telephone numbers and addresses, laboratory and X-ray forms, patient information material, and practice-headed notepaper and envelopes for hospital referral.

Most of the parenteral medications listed above should be available for use in the emergency bag, to which could be added low-dose aspirin (75–300 mg), simple analgesia (paracetamol and a non-steroidal anti-inflammatory), a nitroglycerine spray, oral sedatives such as diazepam, and starter packs of tablets or sachets of antibiotics and antipyretic analgesics for adults or children with acute infections.

Diagnostic instruments

Ear, nose, and throat

Basic ear, nose, and throat practice equipment includes an auroscope with an adequate light source and a range of speculae, ear syringing equipment (manual or water jet), a tuning fork, a nasal speculum, and spatulae and swabs for inspecting the throat and taking samples.

More advanced practice equipment, not essential but likely to optimize care in certain patients, includes an audiometer to confirm and characterize hearing loss in adults and children over the age of 5, and a tympanometer for the detection and confirmation of chronic secretory otitis media in children, facilitating selection of cases for specialist referral.

Eyes

Basic equipment for ophthalmological diagnosis includes an ophthalmoscope with an adequate light source, a Snellen chart or other method for measuring visual acuity and Ishihara charts to detect colour vision deficiences. The Snellen chart or a card with Landalt rings or other optotypes, including one for children, should be illuminated by at least 200 W from two light sources on the card. An alternative arrangement is to have a light source in a box behind a transparent card. If the size of the room is not sufficient, a mirror can make up for the required viewing distance of 5 m.

An ophthalmoscope is required for direct fundoscopy or a 20 D lens for indirect fundoscopy. The stenopeic aperture differentiates between a refraction problem or a macular disorder.

More advanced ophthalmological equipment might include an Amsler card to detect astigmatism and visual field loss, a tonometer to detect high intraocular pressure (rather unusual in general practice at present), and a slit lamp for use by GPs trained in this technique, to provide more accurate diagnosis of eye problems and to improve selection of patients for specialist ophthalmological or optometric referral.

Cardiovascular and pulmonary diagnosis

Basic equipment in primary care includes an electrocardiograph (ECG) which contributes to the diagnosis of conditions such as myocardial infarction, cardiac arrhythmias, and left ventricular hypertrophy, and a peak flow meter, important in managing asthma and obstructive airways disease and, when used as part of a beta-agonist reversibility test, in the diagnosis of asthma.

More advanced equipment includes a spirometer, essential in making accurate diagnoses of lung disease in primary care, and providing important information to guide therapy in patients with asthma, chronic obstructive pulmonary disease, and restrictive pulmonary problems, such as in interstitial lung disease and fibrosing alveolitis. Spirometry is also capable of picking up relatively subtle changes indicative of respiratory dysfunction. Many of these procedures can effectively be delegated to practice nurses and practice assistants, and carried out in the treatment room.

Doppler ultrasonography is another, relatively advanced, technology which is finding its way into primary care. It is used in antenatal care, where the sound of the baby's heart often provides welcome reassurance to the mother. With a different probe, it is also used to diagnose and monitor peripheral vascular disease. It is a cheap and easy way to establish or exclude peripheral arterial obstruction, and has been piloted as a method of identifying abdominal aortic aneurysms. Some large practices have invested in cardiac ultrasound equipment, so that the diagnosis of heart failure can be established in primary care and treatment guided accordingly.

Gastrointestinal diagnosis

Proctoscopy with a Kelly metal proctoscope (22–27 mm and length 50 mm), also available in a disposable form, should be a routine procedure, and rigid sigmoidoscopy is well suited to larger practices, when an assistant is available to help the GP undertake the procedure. Both are useful in the differential diagnoses of painful anal complaints, including external and internal haemorrhoids, fistulae, proctitis, and rectal neoplasia. Some practices now have the facilities to treat external haemorrhoids by banding (Barron rings), using a special ring ligator and a haemorrhoid grip plier. This procedure is safe in expert hands, and is the treatment of choice for internal haemorrhoids.

Endoscopic techniques are now finding their way into primary care. Although very expensive, a flexible sigmoidoscope provides an effective and acceptable means of assessing patients presenting with rectal bleeding and other lower bowel symptoms, and may soon prove to be the screening modality of choice for colorectal cancer. In some large practices, upper gastrointestinal endoscopy and even colonoscopy are conducted in specially equipped rooms.

Gynaecological equipment

Apart from standard speculae, spatulae, and cyto brushes for pelvic examination and cervical cytology, facilities should be available in large practices for the insertion of intra-uterine contraceptive devices and the newly introduced progesterone coils. Gynaecological leg strirrups may occasionally be useful for difficult pelvic examinations. Facilities for the insertion of contraceptive diaphragms and ring pessaries should also be available, and these include test pessaries of various sizes and demonstration models.

Therapeutic equipment

Apart from minor surgical facilities for the excision and biopsy of skin lesions, a number of other technologies are available for dealing with skin abnormalities. Liquid nitrogen, either provided in thermos containers or stored in a larger thermos barrel, in which the nitrogen can be stored for up to 3 months, can be used to remove a number of skin lesions. Other equipment, such as a hyfrecator and a surgitron, can be used for the removal of benign skin lesions. The surgitron results in less burning and allows more useful pathological examination of excised tissue. Paraphimosis can be relieved without distress after applying EMLA cream. Curettes are useful for removing seborrhoeic keratoses, warts, and mollusca, and EMLA cream is also useful in this context, and in the treatment of condylomata with the hyfrecator. Ingrowing toenails can be treated by application of phenol to prevent recurrence, and this has proven to be the treatment of choice over wedge excision, which should be reserved for recurrent infections. A tourniquet is required to provide a local anaesthetic ring block and a bloodless field. Heavy scissors are useful in all procedures involving toenails.

Dressing of various kinds, absorbing, protecting, fixing, and supporting should be available, not only to deal with sprains, strains, and operative injuries, but also to provide compression therapy for venous ulceration of the leg.

Maintenance

Turning a blind eye on maintenance does not visibly result in inferior patient care, but unless adequate systems are in place for testing, maintaining, and replenishing equipment and supplies, the use and safety of the procedures described in this chapter will be compromised. Clear delegation of tasks and visual reminders are likely to be helpful in ensuring that these routines are carried out, and Lefley and colleagues have published details of a successful system of this kind, developed in the United Kingdom.[10]

Equipment maintenance, usually performed annually, is essential for the weighing scale, height measuring equipment, peak flow meters and spirometer, ECG machine, sterilizer, sphygmomanometers, glucometer, haemoglobin meter, and other laboratory equipment. Dated tags should be attached to these machines, and checked regularly. Maintenance also extends to taking care of premises, ensuring that the contents of the emergency bag and drug cupboards are replenished, including checking expiry dates of medication, and ensuring that waste disposal and cleaning procedures are monitored.

Conclusion

Investment in adequate equipment is likely to pay off and it is penny wise but pound foolish for a practice to become under-equipped and understaffed, particularly in an entrepreneurial primary care environment. In a salaried system, on the other hand, with a fixed budget for equipment and staff, GPs may experience less ownership of their premises and have less flexibility in their ability to develop new services.

Standards and guidelines are likely to help only if they take into account the interests of all parties in a given health care system.

There is limited research on the possession and use of diagnostic and therapeutic equipment in general practice at present,[11,12] and further investigations are needed to determine the sources of variation and the opportunities that exist to address these. We hope that the information provided in this chapter will stimulate GPs and their teams to consider the acquisition of equipment to provide new and better services for their patients.

References

1. **van den Hombergh, P., Grol, R., van den Hoogen, H.J.M., and van den Bosch, W.J.H.M.** (1997). De uitrusting van de huisartspraktijk. (The equipment of general practices in the Netherlands.) *Huisarts Wet* **40** (1), 9–13.
2. **Baker, R.** (2000). Reforming primary care in England—again. Plans for improving the quality of care. *Scandinavian Journal of Primary Health Care* **18** (2), 72–4.
3. **Royal Australian College of General Practitioners.** *Entry Standards for General Practices.* Sydney: RACGP, 1996.
4. **The Royal New Zealand College of General Practitioners.** *Aiming for Excellence in General Practice; Standards for General Practice.* New Zealand, 2000 (ISBN: 0-9582176-0-2).
5. **Kalda, R. and Lember, M.** (2000). Setting national standards for practice equipment. Presence of equipment in Estonian practices before and after introduction of guidelines with feedback. *International Journal for Quality in Health Care* **12** (1), 59–63.
6. **Anonymous.** *Quality Practice Award.* RCGP: North East Scotland Faculty, November 1997.
7. **Dijkers, F.** *The Equipment of the GP Out of Office.* Utrecht: Dutch College of General Practice, 1993.
8. **Dutch College of General Practice.** *The Equipment of the Practice.* Utrecht: NHG, 1989.
9. **Anonymous.** *Quality Assurance Programme Reference Manual.* RNZCGP, May 1993.
10. **Lefley, P., Yardley, A., Sutton, J., and Willmott, A.P.** *Outline of Quality systems.* Hinckley, 1992.
11. **Baker, R.** (1992). General practice in Gloucestershire, Avon and Somerset: explaining variations in standards. *British Journal of General Practice* **42**, 415–18.
12. **van den Hombergh, P., Grol, R., van den Bosch, W.J.H.M., and van den Hoogen, H.J.M.** (1998). Assessment of management in general practice: validation of a practice visit method. *British Journal of General Practice* **48**, 1743–50.

12.4 The office laboratory

Sverre Sandberg, Geir Thue, and Per Hjortdahl

Introduction

Laboratory tests are essential in the diagnosis and monitoring of many diseases. Tests requested by general practitioners (GPs) may either be performed at the office laboratory or be sent to a larger laboratory. In general, it is difficult to specify the tests that should be analysed in the general practice office laboratory and which should be sent off to a larger laboratory, because conditions differ from country to country. In many countries, near patient testing represents a vast 'laboratory' with a great number of tests performed annually. Office laboratory equipment has seen significant technological improvement and is heavily marketed in some parts of the world. In addition, laboratory tests are a cornerstone of monitoring and assessing a number of clinical conditions in the primary care setting. However, office testing varies considerably from country to country; it is much more widespread in Germany than in the United Kingdom, and much more common in the United States than in Canada.

This chapter begins with an account of the arguments for analysing samples in the office laboratory rather then sending them (or the patient) to a larger laboratory. Suggestions for a reasonable primary care office laboratory repertoire are offered, before stating some essentials necessary for running a small laboratory. The chapter concludes with a brief description of factors that should be taken into account when interpreting laboratory results. A further discussion of near-patient and office-based tests is provided in Chapter 6.5.

To have or not to have an office laboratory

Deciding whether or not to have an office laboratory and which tests to perform is an important task. Points that should be taken into consideration can be summarized in the following two questions:

- Is there an advantage of getting the laboratory results during a consultation in terms of clinical decision making or saving of time?
- What are the costs in terms of workload and money compared to the alternatives?

The most important argument for analysing samples in the office is to have the results available during the consultation. For patients consulting for a chronic disease such as diabetes or when on anticoagulation therapy, samples can be drawn just before the patient sees the doctor and actions taken during the ensuing consultation. The alternative could be to have the samples drawn and analysed at a central laboratory a few days before the consultation for the results to be available to the clinician at the time of the appointment. In other cases, the samples can be drawn just after the consultation, and the patient waits for the results so that actions may be taken before the patient leaves the office. Even analysing the samples later the same day might be sensible, since the doctor can inform the patient that he will contact him later if 'something is wrong with the result'. Laboratory results are seldom needed in the immediate management of the patient in general practice, although every now and then detection of severe hypoglycaemia, hyperglycaemia, or anaemia is critically important.

Whether or not doing the laboratory analyses in the office increases or reduces the workload and cost is uncertain. Less work is generated related to requesting and sending tests to a central laboratory, and the test may result in an economic gain through reimbursement systems. In some countries, the results from the central laboratories can be transferred electronically directly from the larger laboratory into the patient record. This will reduce the workload related to handling of reports from external laboratories, as well as make the laboratory results available sooner. In addition, the running costs per test are usually less in hospitals, because incorporating primary care tests in many instances causes only a marginal increase in workload and little need for extra equipment.

Choosing a repertoire

If it is decided that an office laboratory should be established, it is wise to contact a clinical chemist or pathologist for advice, especially with regard to whether suitable equipment is available. When determining whether a certain test should be taken into use or not, and supposing that the medical and economical criteria are met, two important questions have to be answered:

- Is the analytical quality of the test good enough in the setting in which it will be used?
- Is it possible to perform internal and external quality control of the test procedures?

Overall, analytical quality should be as good in the office laboratory as in hospital laboratories. This is not always possible, and the GP should be aware that, for example, glucose results produced in the office laboratory are suitable for monitoring diabetes, but are not good enough for diagnostic purposes. Furthermore, some test constituents are not stable in transport for more than 6–12 h. It may thus be an advantage to analyse these in the office; examples are mean corpuscular volume (MCV), and the differential white blood cell count. Independent studies of instrument and test kit performance both in laboratory settings and in primary care are undertaken by organizations such as The National Coordinating Centre for Health Technology Assessment in the United Kingdom and the Scandinavian evaluation of laboratory equipment for primary care (SKUP). Such data are crucial to be able to choose instruments that are robust and suitable for primary care use. It is important that both internal and external quality controls are feasible, especially since analytical quality needs documentation. This aspect could well have legal consequences. Advice should be sought on these matters from a large laboratory or from organizers of external quality assurance schemes (EQAS).

The list below contains suggestions which may be more relevant in developed countries. The reader must carefully evaluate what is needed in the office laboratory in his/her environment. We have divided the list into two sections—first a basic repertoire, requiring only small instruments or test kits, and then a larger repertoire, probably suitable for larger practices, or in circumstances where service from a hospital laboratory is sub-optimal or the primary care centre is remote from the base hospital. In addition, all office laboratories should have equipment for drawing and sending samples to larger laboratories of clinical chemistry, microbiology, and pathology.

The basic laboratory repertoire

Haemoglobin

The analytical quality of haemoglobin on office instruments is close to what is usually obtained in the hospital laboratory. It is important to be aware that many of the instruments will give falsely elevated results in the presence of hyperlipaemia or leukocyte counts above 50×10^9 per litre. Such problems should be stated in the manual of the instrument.

Glucose

Glucose measurements are important for physicians dealing with diabetic patients, and perhaps most important in countries where self-measurement of glucose by patients is not generally in use. The quality of the test is generally poorer in primary care than when performed in the hospital, and most instruments are therefore only suitable for monitoring diabetic patients, and not in diagnosing new cases. In principle, the instruments should report the results from the same material as the nearest hospital. In most cases, instruments reporting plasma results should be preferred.

C-reactive protein (CRP)

This test will often be used in the differential diagnosis between viral and bacterial infections, in monitoring patients with inflammatory rheumatic diseases, and to differentiate between upper and lower urinary tract infections. It is important to be aware that results from different analytic methods should be interpreted differently. There are semi-quantitative methods with less than optimal precision making it difficult to monitor small changes in the patients' condition, whereas quantitative methods are usually better in this regard. For the semi-quantitative methods precision will result in a 'diagnostic paralytic range' of about ±25 mg/l around the decision level. This means that if the 'decision level' for bacterial versus viral infection is at 50 mg/l, the interval of uncertainty is from 25 to 75 mg/l.

Erythrocyte sedimentation rate (ESR)

The ESR is an old test, and is probably overused in clinical medicine. It should not be used in screening situations, such as health check-ups, and when it comes to diagnostic value regarding most inflammatory diseases, CRP has replaced it. Still, it confers some help in situations with vague symptoms, and in the differential diagnosis of some rheumatic diseases. 'Closed' systems for analysis are in use, but it is important to be aware that vibrating centrifuges, high temperatures, and tilted tubes increase the ESR considerably.

Tests for mononucleosis

Rapid tests for mononucleosis are based on the detection of heterophilic antibodies. Some patients, however, do not develop such antibodies, resulting in a false negative mononucleosis test. This is often the case for children below 5 years. In such cases, it may be better to send samples to a larger laboratory to be analysed for specific antibodies against Epstein–Barr virus.

Urine strips (haemoglobin, leucocytes, nitrites, protein, and glucose)

Urine strips should seldom be used in a screening situation, and if so, only tests with as few fields as possible should be used. The fields for leukocyte esterase and nitrites can replace urine microscopy in the diagnosis of urinary tract infection. The haemoglobin field will give a positive result in 3–5 per cent of a normal population. The fields are semi-quantitative, and one should be aware that the actual concentrations of the constituent may vary between the different manufacturers and even within one manufacturer; that is '++' or '2' may reflect different concentrations depending on the strips used. Readings based on instruments offer no advantages compared to visual readings.

Human chorionic gonadotrophin (hcg) in urine (pregnancy test)

Several test kits are available, and most are good quality tests, giving a positive result if the concentration of hCG in the urine exceeds 25 IU/l. This means that the test will stay positive some time after an abortion, and that the test may not be positive in the early stages of ectopic pregnancy. When ectopic pregnancy is suspected, a hCG test using serum is recommended.

Tests for occult faecal bleeding

Most are chemical tests for haemoglobin, but immunological tests for human haemoglobin are also marketed. The usefulness of these tests in screening is being debated.

Tests for streptococcus A antigen

Several immunological tests kits are available, and most of these are of good quality. Correct sampling technique is important to obtain bacteria or bacterial degradation products. Good clinical algorithms exist as to when this test is indicated.

The extended repertoire

Microscopy

Use of the microscope has a long tradition, but skill and regular practice is needed to get the most out of this procedure. It is mostly used for detecting urinary tract infections, but in this respect has largely been replaced by strips. Other diseases with urine microscopy findings are rare. Findings of trichomonas and candida in vaginitis by microscopy may be useful, as is detection of fungi in dermatological disease. Blood smear analysis is largely used to diagnose infectious mononucleosis and malignant blood diseases and examination of a thick film is important in diagnosing malaria. Manual cell counting (white blood cells and platelets) is imprecise compared to using automated cell counters. Certainly, microscopy is important in detecting certain tropical diseases, such as malaria.

Urine culture

Specialized media for growing uropathogens are available, and diagnosis of *Escherichia coli*, or distinction of Gram positive from Gram negative bacteria as the cause of a urinary tract infection is possible. This information is only useful when patterns of antibiotic resistance are readily available, although the detection of significant amounts of bacteria may be important even if the strain of bacteria is not identified.

Micro-albumin

Detection of very small concentrations of albumin in the urine is possible using relatively simple instruments or strips. Instruments yielding the albumin/creatinine ratio should probably be preferred, since they correct for the degree of dilution of the urine.

Haemoglobin A1C, glycosylated haemoglobin (HbA1c)

HbA1c is important in monitoring diabetic patients, but is still not recommended for diagnostic purposes. Several small instruments yielding good quality results are available for use in general practice.

Prothrombin time

The prothrombin time analysis is available using small instruments. Methodological problems exist so that analysis on small instruments may yield results that differ from results from a more complex instrument, and advice should be sought from a larger laboratory.

Clinical chemistry

These analyses in general involve more expensive and complex instruments, some of which have quite large analytic repertoires. We recommend using just a few tests that may be needed with some frequency in many clinical situations. We thus recommend ALT and gamma-GT, cholesterol, creatinine, and potassium.

Haematology

Cell counters are available for the general practice office laboratory. We recommend such instruments primarily for white blood cell and platelet counts. Measurement of MCV is useful in the diagnosis of anaemia (and this measurement is not stable after transportation).

Running the office laboratory

Some GPs are directly involved in doing office laboratory work, but most are not. Usually it is left to ancillary staff, for example, nurses, technicians, or even lay-persons educated in the practice. In most circumstances, however, the GP is responsible for all that is done in the practice laboratory, thus in a sense functioning as a 'laboratory director'. This is an important function, and its role should not be underestimated.

In larger practices, the task of running the office laboratory can be delegated to one staff member and one doctor. This small team should have the responsibility of ensuring that all staff involved in laboratory work are familiar with routines, that instruments are maintained, and stocks kept at a sensible size to avoid the use of outdated reagents and kits. Also, they should oversee the repertoire of tests at regular intervals.

Training

What kind of education or training is necessary to work in the practice laboratory? There is no easy answer, as test repertoire and the complexity of performing the different analyses vary. Also, education should be focused and adjusted to needs, that is, both regarding repertoire and regulations in the form of certification. Some test kits for single use are simple with built-in controls to ensure correct function of the kit, and could probably be carried out by personnel educated in the practice. But handling of instruments, and adherence to hygiene and quality control routines (see below), implies that some formal education is necessary. The GP must ensure that employees have an understanding of test principles and routines, and will have to upgrade his own knowledge about the subject matter regularly.

Safety

Routines to protect both staff and patients from infectious diseases through handling of biological materials must be established. These include dividing the laboratory into contaminated (drawing and handling of samples) and clean zones (telephone, data processing). Plastic-coated paper should be used on all surfaces used for handling of test material. Personal hygiene is important, that is, removal of rings, bracelets, and wristwatches during working hours, and frequent hand washing. Non-latex gloves for single use should be used when handling test material, and when obtaining capillary blood samples, but is not necessary for ordinary venepuncture using 'closed' systems (see later). Secure techniques for handling and disposing of needles are important, suitable working clothes should be provided, and drinking (even coffee), eating, and smoking is prohibited in the office laboratory. Vaccination against hepatitis B could be considered, but in this context offers only a limited protection, since more serious diseases may also be present (HIV, hepatitis C). Good routines are therefore paramount, since all biological materials should be considered contagious.

Drawing, preparing, and sending blood samples

Even though some tests are performed in the office laboratory, nearly all practices will have to draw and prepare blood samples to be analysed in larger laboratories. All patients should be identified properly before samples are drawn.

Blood samples can be obtained either as capillary samples or by venepuncture. Capillary samples should usually be obtained from a finger (not ear). In children younger than 3–6 months, capillary samples should be obtained from the heel (need for special equipment and skill). If prothrombin time is to be analysed, this should be done in the first drop of blood. Cellular constituents should not be analysed in the first drop. The random error when using capillary samples is larger for cellular constituents compared to venous samples so that haemoglobin results vary more using this technique.

Tubes with or without added anticoagulants (EDTA, heparin, or citrate) are used in venepuncture. Tubes must be labelled accurately, and material from patients with certain contagious diseases (e.g. hepatitis C) should receive a special labelling. In most instances so-called 'gel' tubes are convenient alternatives to ordinary tubes, as serum will be separated from the blood cells by the gel material. If analysis can be done within 48 h, the gel tube can be transported without further preparation. Haemolysis during preparation of serum or plasma samples can cause elevated values of potassium, LD, AST, ALT, and CK whereas glucose values will decrease.

Most constituents are stable for 1–2 days for transport to a laboratory. Stability will be dependent on both the constituents and the method by which it is analysed. This is especially pronounced for prothrombin-time, leucocytes, platelets, reticulocytes, and MCV. Contact your local laboratory for further information. Bilirubin and porphyrins are photodegraded when exposed to light.

Principles of quality assurance

It is important for the physician to be able to document the analytical quality of the devices used. This is done by securing reproducibility (precision) by internal quality control, and agreement with a true value (trueness) by external quality assurance.

Internal quality control

Internal quality control implies the analysis of a control sample at least once a day whenever patient samples for that constituent is analysed. A control sample is usually a commercially available test material that should be as similar to patient samples as possible. Preferentially, this analysis should be done in the morning before patient samples are analysed. Results for patient samples should not be issued until it is clear that no change in the measuring method has occurred. The result of the internal quality control material should be compared with the limits for acceptable deviation from the mean of the previous results. Thus, internal control is established to secure 'stable' measurements in the laboratory.

Limits for acceptable performance should be set for each constituent by the office laboratory in cooperation with the local hospital, or with medical technologists especially educated to deal with the laboratory in primary health care. Limits given by the manufacturer of the control material should not be used as limits for acceptable performance once the mean for the office results has been obtained. An example of an internal quality control scheme for haemoglobin is shown in Fig. 1.

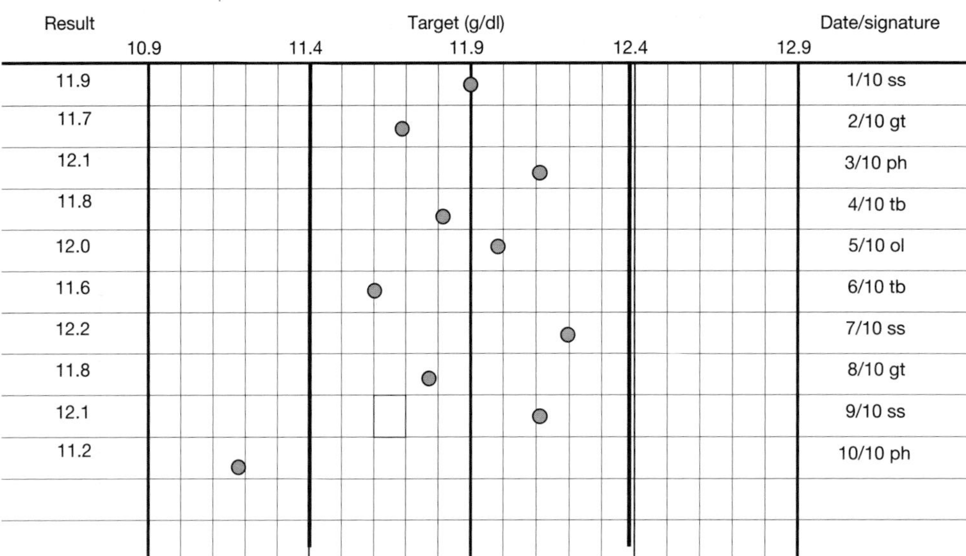

Fig. 1 Scheme for monitoring the internal quality control. One sheet for each month is used. In principle, the target value is established by analysing the sample at least 10 times. The acceptability limits are established in cooperation with the local hospital using the obtained precision. In the case shown here, the target for haemoglobin is 11.9 g/dl. The CV (see 'imprecision') was 2, and the limits are 11.9 ± 0.5 g/dl (2 × CV × 11.9/100). The control is analysed at the start of the day: On Oct 10th, the control is outside the limits and measures must be taken to examine the cause (first, the sample is re-analysed).

The use of internal quality control in primary health care must be performed with some pragmatism. Thus, it is important to evaluate the benefit of the control procedures, such as how often do results fall outside acceptability limits due to problems with the instrument or with reagents? If this is a rare occurrence, the frequency of controls can be reduced or the limits should be re-evaluated. Your local hospital laboratory should be able to give you advice on this. For test kits, internal quality control is often an integrated part of the kit, and the use of other internal control material in these cases is not necessary.

External quality assurance (EQA)

External quality assurance is a way of maintaining and improving the analytical quality methods so that they yield similar results, that is, that haemoglobin values do not vary too much between different office laboratories. It consists of the following features:

- samples (e.g. blood, urine, plasma) are distributed to the participants;
- samples are analysed for the given constituent and the results are reported back to the organizer of the scheme;
- results are processed;
- feedback reports with explicit statements regarding analytical quality are returned to the participants;
- mechanisms for follow-up of unsatisfactory performance should be established (e.g. through an advice service).

EQA schemes for primary health care laboratories should be designed locally in each country or county. Often laboratories in primary health care participate in schemes designed for larger laboratories. This may be unsatisfactory as these schemes usually are designed in a more complicated way with too many samples distributed.

The information from a feedback report depends on the samples circulated. If samples are native blood samples, target values common for all methods (e.g. all instruments analysing haemoglobin) can be established by reference methods. In this case information concerning both the performance of the participant and the different instrument groups used by the participants can be given. If processed samples are used, information is often limited to the performance of participants in relation to others using similar instruments. Example of a feedback report for haemoglobin is shown in Fig. 2.

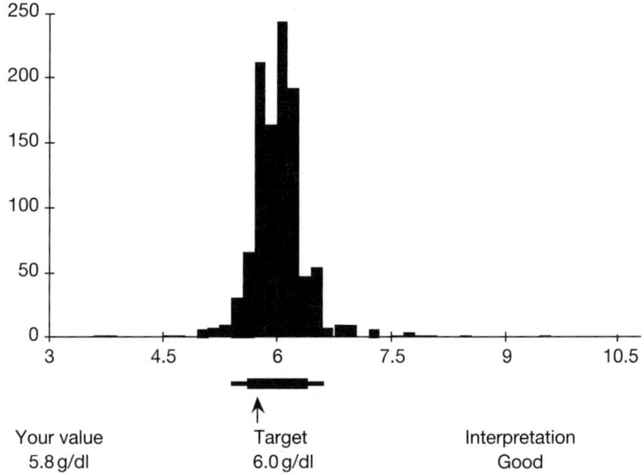

Fig. 2 Feedback report from an external quality control organization. In this external quality control scheme (from NOKLUS, Norway), fresh EDTA blood was sent from the organizers of the scheme to the office laboratory and haemoglobin was analysed twice. Results were returned to the organizers of the scheme. The target value was determined by the reference method. In the feedback report, the distribution represents the results from all the participants. The thick line represents the interval for 'good' results, the thin line represents the interval for 'acceptable' results. Results outside these limits are 'poor'. The arrow indicates the mean of the two results from the office laboratory.

Interpretation of laboratory results

We will describe pre-analytical variation, proper use of the reference interval, and sources of variation that should be taken into account when interpreting laboratory results.

Pre-analytical variation

Position of the body

If a person changes position from lying to standing, the blood volume will decrease about 500–700 ml. The new equilibrium will take place after about

10 min, and all cellular or protein bound constituents (e.g. leucocytes, haemoglobin, cholesterol) will increase about 10 per cent. This effect will be exaggerated if the patient has oedema. Standard sampling means obtaining samples from a patient who has been sitting for at least 15 min.

Drugs

Drugs can change the results of certain constituents either with an *in vivo* effect (e.g. intramuscular injections will increase creatine kinase) or *in vitro* by interfering with the measurements method. Contact the local laboratory if you think that drugs may be the cause of unexpected results.

Food

Glucose, triglycerides, and alkaline phosphatase may increase after eating. Samples should generally be drawn more than 4 h after a fat-containing meal since lipids interfere with some analytical methods.

Physical activity

Strenuous activity will cause elevated values (variable from person to person) of CK, ALAT, ASAT, and creatinine. Haemoconcentration may also occur.

The reference interval

For a certain constituent, the reference interval encompasses 95 per cent of results obtained from a population presumed to be healthy. The limits of the interval are usually determined as the 2.5 and 97.5 percentile. If the results have a Gaussian distribution, the limits will be within ±2 standard deviations (SD) of the mean. For a given test result, we can infer the probability that the result may stem from a healthy person by its distance from the mean of the population, but we cannot tell that person's probability of actually having a disease. To do so, we must know the distribution of test results from patients with the disease in question. If 'n' tests are requested, the probability is $100 \times (1 - 0.95n)$ per cent that at least one of the constituents will have a result outside the reference interval, for example, amounting to 40 per cent probability if 10 tests are requested. Most reference intervals are sex and age dependent, and may differ between various ethnic populations.

Action limits

An action limit is the limit where the result generates some actions by the doctor in relation to the patient (such as repeating the test, or starting treatment). The action limit may be similar to the reference limit or different (e.g. the upper reference limit for cholesterol is 7.8 mmol/l, but the action limit implying treatment may be 6.0 mmol/l). Usually, results of a certain test in the healthy population will overlap with results obtained in the patient population. In these cases some healthy people will be classified as sick (false positives) and some sick people will be classified as healthy (false negatives). The proportion of persons with a false classification will depend on the value of the action limit, and in general, limits should be set depending on which mistake makes least harm. This is dependent on both professional and economical conditions. In general practice, action limits should be set higher than in hospitals as the prevalence of disease is less in general practice.

Analytical variation

These are errors that are due to the measurement method. Principally, two different kinds of errors can be recognized: random error (imprecision) or systematic error (bias) (see Fig. 3).

Random error/imprecision

The degree of imprecision reflects the ability to reproduce results from a single test sample. The imprecision is usually given as a coefficient of variation (CV), which is simply the standard deviation of the distribution of results as a percentage of the mean of the measurements. Common reasons

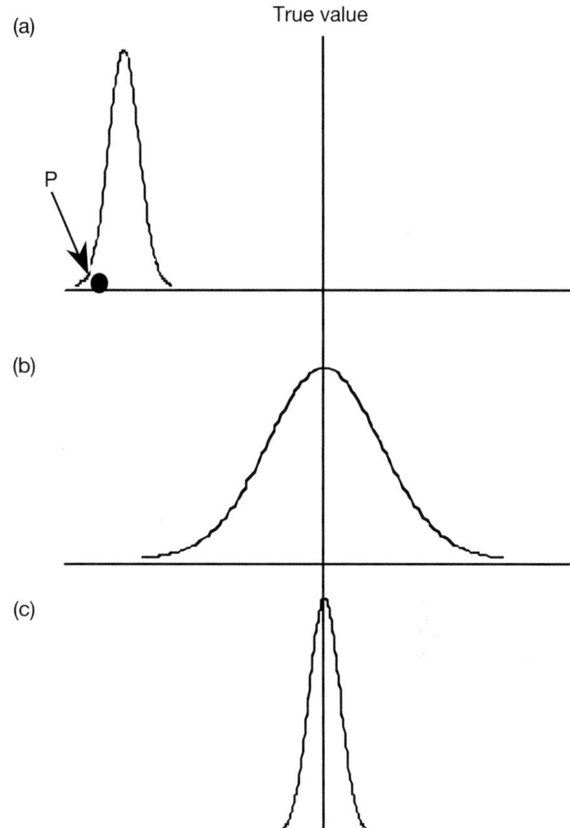

Fig. 3 Different kinds of measurement errors. Random error (imprecision): the distribution of independent results of measurements. Systematic error (bias): the difference between the mean of a large number of measurements and a true value. (a) Small random error (the curve represents independent results of measurements) and a large systematic error. The difference between one of the results termed 'P' and the true value is entitled '*deviation*'. (b) Large random error, but no systematic error (no bias). (c) Small random error and no systematic error.

for imprecision are instrument dependent random errors concerning the pre-analytical phase, for example, sample drawing, problems with pipetting of samples, or involving different members of staff in doing the laboratory work.

Systematic error/bias/deviation

Systematic errors occur when measurements are 'off target', and may be detected when performing external quality control. The difference between the mean of several measurements and the true value obtained by strict methods (so-called reference methods) is named *bias* whereas the difference between a single result and the true value is named *deviation* (see Fig. 3). In external quality control, several measurements of control samples are requested to establish the bias of your office instrument. Usual reasons for bias are problems with calibration of the instrument, or use of new batches of reagents or test strips.

Biological variation

This is the variation caused by the changes in the levels of constituents *in vivo*. The interindividual or between-subject variation is the basis for establishing the reference interval. The intraindividual or within-subject variation is the changes in the levels within one person. The within-subject variation is a variation around a homeostatic set point for the constituent. This variation is different from person to person. For cholesterol, the within-subject variation measured as CV can vary from 1 to 20 per cent with a mean CV of 6 per cent.

Difference between two results

When monitoring patients, for example, assessing changes in HbA1c or in haemoglobin, it is important to know how large a difference between two results must be before it is of clinical importance. Assuming that no systematic error has occurred between the two measurements, only random variation has to be taken into consideration, that is the pre-analytical, analytical, and biological variation.

When samples are obtained by venepuncture, the pre-analytical variation is usually small, and only the analytical and biological variations need consideration. These sources of variation differ considerably, see Table 1.

What difference between two test results should be considered of importance? This will depend on the clinical situation, that is, how certain you need to be that a real change has occurred. For most purposes, about 90–95 per cent certainty is acceptable. This means that the probability that the difference between two cholesterol results is due to analytical and biological variation is 5–10 per cent. To calculate this 'critical difference', the CV total is multiplied by a constant signifying the probability. For most practical purposes, doubling the CV total signifies a real change, with 95 per cent probability (meaning that the constant is set to be 2). For cholesterol, this means that the change must be greater than 13 per cent (Table 1); that is, if the first result was 8 mmol/l, the next must be below 6.9 mmol/l. For haemoglobin, the change is smaller, about 6.5 per cent. For capillary samples with a rather large pre-analytical variation due to sampling technique, the change in haemoglobin value must be about 10 per cent to be considered real, and not only a consequence of analytical and biological variation.

Table 1 Biological (within-subject) variation, analytical variation, and critical differences

Constituent	Within-subject variation (CVi)	Analytical variation (CVa)	Critical difference (%)
ALAT	14	4	29
Albumin	3	2	7
Alkaline phosphatase	8	4	9
Bilirubin	18	3	36
Calcium	2	1	4
Cholesterol	6	3	14
Creatine kinase	23	3	46
Creatinine	6	2	24
Ferritin	10	4	22
Gamma-GT	10	2	20
Glucose	7	3	15
Haemoglobin	3	1	6
HbA1c	5	3	11
Iron	23	3	46
Lactate dehydrogenase	9	3	19
Leucocytes	12	3	25
Platelets	10	6	23
Potassium	4	2	9
Prothrombin time	10	4	21
Protein	3	2	7
Sodium	1	0.5	2
Triglycerides	22	2	44
Urate	11	2	22

The analytical variation is obtained from a typical hospital laboratory. In a primary care setting, these numbers may be a little higher. The critical difference, i.e. the difference that must be present between two results to be sure that a real change has taken place, is calculated using the formula

$CV_{total} = \sqrt{CV^2_{intraindividual} + CV^2_{analytical} + CV^2_{pre\text{-}analytical}}$.

Often the pre-analytical variation is set like zero. The critical difference is about $2 \times CV_{total}$.

Conclusion

In many practices, the establishment of an office laboratory can be considered. The repertoire of the laboratory should be assembled to take into account whether there is a medical reason for performing the test, whether the analytical quality is good enough, whether internal and external controls can be performed, and whether the costs are acceptable. We suggest a basic repertoire and an extended repertoire of tests.

When running the laboratory it is important to evaluate the training necessary for employees to be able to take care of safety and analytical aspects in the laboratory. Knowledge about how to perform and interpret internal and external quality control is essential.

To be able to interpret laboratory results in a sensible way, it is important to have information about the analytical and biological variation of the constituent in question, and the pre-analytical factors that can influence the test result. When monitoring patients, this information is important when estimating how large the difference must be between two results before it is of clinical importance. Action limits for a constituent should be set according to clinical needs and not necessarily be based on the limits of the reference interval.

Further reading

Guder, W.G., Narayanan, S., Wisser, H., and Zawta, B., ed. *Samples: From the Patient to the Laboratory.* Darmstadt: GIT Verlag Gmbh, 1996.

Hobbs, F., Delaney, B.C., Fitzmaurice, D.A., Wilson, S., Hyde, C.J., Thorpe, G.H, Earl-Slater, A.S.M., Jowett, S., and Tobias, R., ed. *A Review of Near Patient Testing in Primary Care.* Southampton: National Coordinating Centre for Health Technology Assessment, 1997.

Sox, H., Blatt, M.A., Higgins, M.C., and Marton, K.I., ed. *Medical Decision Making.* Boston MA: Butterworth-Heinemann, 1988.

Speicher, C.E., ed. *The Right Test—A Physicians Guide to Laboratory Medicine.* Philadelphia PA: WB Saunders Company, 1989.

Tietz, N.W., ed. *Clinical Guide to Laboratory Tests.* Philadephia PA: WB Saunders Company, 1995.

Young, D.S., ed. *Effects of Preanalytical Variables on Clinical Laboratory Tests.* Washington DC: AACC Press, 1997.

Young, D.S. and Friedman, R.B., ed. *Effects of Disease on Clinical Laboratory Tests.* Washington DC: AACC Press, 2001.

12.5 Organization of services

John L. Campbell and Sandra Gower

Introduction

The provision of high-quality primary care services depends on a number of important practical and theoretical issues including the control of access, the availability of clinician time both in and out of hours, and decisions on who should actually see the patient. Nursing staff are key members of the primary health care team, and the organization and distribution of their time, along with the organization of other staff, is important. Of increasing importance is the role of patient input to informing the development and delivery of primary care services.

The accessibility of primary medical care

Although some health care systems address the issue of provider 'availability' (e.g. defining this in terms of weeks and hours in the year during which a health professional is 'available' to patients), an important distinction has been recognized by a number of authors in differentiating between 'availability' and 'accessibility' of care.[1–3] The supply of a service (availability) has been identified as a prerequisite for accessibility, which, in these terms, is then of secondary importance. The availability of primary medical care is subject to professional and political constraints and will, at least in part, be determined by the policies of governments and health care planners.

The accessibility of a service is probably of more direct relevance to the consumer. Thus, a child-screening service may be made available through the general practitioner, but if that service is located in geographically distant areas from the target potential users, or provided at times during which the users are unlikely to avail themselves of the service, then accessibility becomes a real problem. Penchansky and Thomas[2] identified five dimensions of access following a survey of General Motors employees in North America (see Box 1).

Components considered as contributing to the accessibility of primary care services include the geographical elements of distance, travel time, and transport. Important issues relating to the design of premises and the siting of facilities relative to the population distribution also need consideration. Despite this, studies from Holland have identified that organizational issues and issues determining accessibility of care were reported as of less importance to patients with long-term health problems than those relating to professional competence and relational aspects of care.[4] International comparative studies have highlighted the consistency in expectation between countries of the importance of getting enough time during the consultation, quick services in case of emergencies, and confidentiality of information on patients. Although patients in different cultures and health care systems may have different views on some aspects of care, many common views are shared, particularly as far as doctor–patient communication and accessibility of services are concerned.[5]

Box 1 Five dimensions of access—the fit between the patient and health care system

1. Availability—volume and type of services
2. Accessibility—locational considerations
3. Accommodation—organizational resources
4. Affordability—financial constraints
5. Acceptability—attitudinal factors

Researchers have often concentrated on service utilization and patient satisfaction as proxy measures of accessibility. Distance from a service may relate to the rate of utilization of that service—the so-called distance decay effect.[6,7] One study from Edinburgh has highlighted transport availability as an important restricting factor in the accessibility of local medical services.[8] Research from North America has shown that transport availability may be an important influence in service-usage patterns amongst children and their families.[9]

Organization of services: the National Health Service in the United Kingdom

The UK National Health Service (NHS) is the largest employer in Europe. Despite this, most of the provision of primary health care services comes from relatively small business organizations of general practitioner partnerships. The trend is towards multi-partner practices. More than one-fourth of all UK general practitioners are now working in groups of six or more doctors.

The concept of a 'primary health care team' in which professionals work together as an interdisciplinary unit, facilitating co-ordination and mutual support in the planning and delivery of care, and replacing the isolated functioning of a lone medical practitioner, was introduced in many western European countries in the early 1970s.[10] In recent years, an increasing emphasis on health promotion and disease prevention activities has seen the emergence of new skills and management arrangements for evolving primary care teams. The number of staff working in primary care rose by 20 per cent between 1995 and 2000, with nurses being the highest number of health professionals working in this setting.

In the United Kingdom, 100 000 doctors provide care to 52 million members of the population. Of these, 26 700 are general practitioners providing general medical services. Over the years, there has been a downward trend in the number of patients cared for by each general practitioner (Fig. 1). Doctors initially regarded an average list of around 2000 as the ideal, but as this has been achieved, there has been a recognition that the move to a community-based, primary care-led NHS has resulted in an increased demand on community services, and this has been paralleled by calls for a reduction in average list sizes to 1700 patients per general practitioner. The Italian health service has an average list size of 1030 patients per general practitioner (with regional variations of 871 to 1756), whilst in Portugal, average lists are in the order of 1500 patients per general practitioner. For most countries, care is organized to provide a ratio of one primary care practitioner for every 1000–3000 of the population. Doctors looking after smaller average list sizes have been reported to have longer average consultation lengths, both in the United Kingdom and elsewhere.

In the United Kingdom, the numbers and distribution of general practitioners are regulated by the Medical Practices Committee, brought into

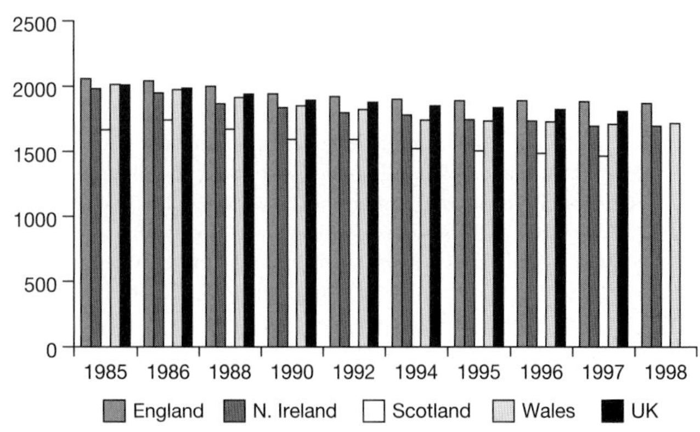

Fig. 1 Average practice list size in UK countries 1985–1998.

being at the start of the National Health Service to ensure that the number of medical practitioners working in defined areas was adequate. The Medical Practices Committee cannot direct doctors to work in a given area, and its effect is largely mediated through its negative controlling power in restricting the number of general practitioners operating in areas that may be classified as 'over-doctored'.

The numbers of general practitioners working at any one time relates to elements of both supply and demand. Medicine has not been exempt from the widespread social changes resulting in moves towards a shorter working week, a desire for earlier retirement, and a wish to protect or increase leisure time—such preferences bring pressure to bear on medical workforce planners, including those planning the supply of general practitioners. These factors also underlie the changing popularity of general practice as a postgraduate medical career choice.[11]

Appointments systems in general practice

From 2 per cent of UK practices operating appointments systems in 1951, the years to 1965 saw a burgeoning in the use of appointments systems. Ritchie's study of access[12] reported that 27 per cent of patients were from practices with no appointments system and that 65 per cent of the sample reported having appointment-only arrangements. Ten years later, in a survey from northwest England of 793 randomly selected patients from a large number of practices,[13] 72 per cent reported they always needed an appointment when consulting. Appointments systems may be seen not only as a means of organizing work, but also as one of the non-economic means of controlling patient access to medical care, with one study reporting that 21 per cent of younger patients had put off seeing the doctor because of the need for an appointment.[14] The 'approachability' of family practice consultations has been investigated as a function of the ability to make an appointment, as well as the openness and approachability of the general practitioner. Making an appointment is a complex social process in which reception staff have an important role, and where the social characteristics of patients may be of importance in the legitimization of appointment requests.

Booking arrangements

Smith[15] has described three appointment booking systems, and the use of modified block scheduling has been explored in non-primary care settings.[16] Practices may combine approaches, this being recommended as an ideal by some researchers.[13] Much of the work carried out examining appointments systems in general practice has been observational in nature, examining the effects of adjustments in appointment operation in only one practice, or even on some doctors or some consulting sessions within a practice. It is known that different doctors will initiate return appointments in a widely disparate manner. Such an approach may be used by doctors to 'buy time' in the midst of busy schedules, and practices with longer appointments have been reported to have fewer return visits, whether initiated by doctors or patients. Luthra and Marshall[17] have reported the wide spectrum of arrangements observed amongst 79 practices in one area in their management systems for responding to requests for same-day consultations.

To aid discussion on the introduction of an appointments system in one inner city practice, Fallon et al.[18] undertook two surveys of patients and staff, first regarding attitudes to appointments systems and secondly in relation to the operation of the system already in place. Nearly three-fourths of the patients surveyed reported not favouring appointments systems and 24 per cent reported that they would consider leaving the practice should such a system be introduced. This contrasted with the views expressed by staff in the practice—appointments systems were seen as giving staff more control over consulting but as less flexible for the patient. This issue of 'whose needs count?' is raised, with a recognition in health policy in recent years of the primacy of patients' views. Hays et al.[19] have noted the negative impact of difficulty in obtaining appointments on patients' ratings of care.

Overall provision

Fundamental to an examination of the impact of appointments systems on the accessibility of primary medical care is a recognition of the relationship between the supply of, and demand for, consulting time in a practice. Expressed need is (in this context) converted to a demand for a consultation whilst unexpressed need (from the health professionals' point of view) may be managed by the patient using a number of alternative pathways. Hannay[20] described the iceberg of disease, but it is not clear which are the important variables in determining the proportion of the iceberg above water. In particular, the effect of modifying the supply of consultation time on subsequent patterns of demand remains to be defined. The UK Royal College of General Practitioners has proposed guidelines for general practitioner accessibility using practice based and auditable criteria (Box 2).

The availability of clinician time

Wide variations exist between countries in the amount of time primary care doctors spend in direct consultations with patients. In the United Kingdom, the current contract determining general practitioners working arrangements allows for full-time general practitioners to provide services over 42 weeks in any year, and to be available for not less than 26 h over 5 days in any such week—that availability being at times likely to be convenient to patients. Working patterns in other countries are discussed in Chapter 12.7 (use of time).

A number of factors are known to influence average consultation length (Box 3). Doctors with longer consultations have been shown to be more likely to recognize and deal with long-term health problems and psychosocial problems when compared with doctors with shorter consultation lengths.[22] Longer consultations are 'better' than shorter consultations as judged on a number of criteria, independent of the attitude of the doctor to their work and the nature of care they deliver, or to their speed of consulting. Howie et al. have suggested that 'the advantages of longer consultations do not simply lie in more services being provided but in a larger proportion of the needs which have been recognised being followed up by the doctor'.

In North America, the number of patients seen per hour was identified as an independent predictor of prescribing volume.[23] Camasso and

Box 2 UK Royal College of General Practitioners guidelines on general practitioner accessibility[21]

- The doctor is available at specified times for surgery consultations and telephone advice.
- The system for monitoring appointments can identify and correct significant delays.
- For urgent matters the patient is able to see their own doctor, partner, or deputy at the next surgery, or speak to the duty doctor.
- For routine matters the patient is usually offered the opportunity to see the doctor of their choice within a period set by the practice and published to the patients.

Box 3 Some determinants of consultation length (see text)

Longer consultations:
For example, United States, New Zealand, Canada, Sweden
Women patients
Presentation of new problems
Consultations with psychological component
Higher social class of patients
Smaller numbers of patients cared for per doctor

Camasso[24] have suggested a critical demarcation point of three consultations per hour, above which comprehensiveness of medical history taking and female preventive care activity were observed to decline. Such findings are in keeping with those of Morrell[25] who found that at consulting sessions booked at 5-min intervals, compared with 7.5- or 10-min intervals, doctors spent less time with the patients and identified fewer problems, and the patients were less satisfied with the consultation. Ridsdale[26] has reported that patients allocated non-systematically to longer appointments received longer consultations in which they asked and received answers to more questions regarding their problem.

Alternative proxy measures of consultation length have also been adopted. Baker[27] reported that booking fewer patients per hour was associated with higher levels of patient satisfaction than more intense appointment booking patterns. This approach has been validated by Campbell and Howie[28] who noted that, as in other studies, it appeared that the potential time advantage of longer appointment intervals was not passed on in full to consulting patients.

Whilst consultation length has attracted considerable research interest, in-practice waiting times have received less attention although a recent survey in the United Kingdom[29] found that nearly 30 per cent of patients reported waiting more than 30 min at their last practice attendance. Research from North America and elsewhere has highlighted that practice waiting times are related to the appointment scheduling system used as well as the tendency of doctors to start consulting sessions late.

New roles for nurses

Triage is a process by which management of a group of patients is prioritized or sorted according to their need for care. In the context of primary care, the term has often been applied to a specific role undertaken by some primary care nurses, and may be seen as a means of managing workload. Triage may involve the allocation of the management of minor illnesses or patients requesting same-day appointments to nurses. There is also an increasing role for nurses in primary care in chronic disease management programmes and in health promotion. In Scandinavia, it is not uncommon for nurses to have a role in managing practice appointment systems, and to undertake the 'physician assistant role', which includes performing venepunctures, laboratory analyses, and other procedures.

Research in this area has tended to focus on the diversion to nurse management of patient problems that traditionally might have been seen by the general practitioner. Shum et al.[30] examined the role of practice nurses in the management of minor illnesses in a multi-centred randomized control trial of five London practices. These authors concluded that practice nurses offered an effective service for patients with minor illness who requested same-day appointments in primary care. Over a 6-month period, 86 per cent of 696 cases managed by trained nurses required no subsequent contact with doctors, 79 per cent did not reconsult on account of the same problem, and 50 per cent of patients received only advice on self-care. Recent work by Kinnersley et al.[31] examined the role of nurse practitioners in primary care. Patients randomized to receive nurse practitioner care received longer consultations, were given more information, and were generally more satisfied than those seeing general practitioners, and the authors suggested that the study supports the extension of the role of nurse practitioners to include seeing patients requesting same-day consultations.

Telephone consultations

Although 90 per cent of British households now have access to a telephone,[32] British general practitioners, in contrast to their Danish counterparts,[33] have no contractual obligation to provide telephone accessibility to their patients. Research, however, has suggested that an increase in the availability of such consultations would be welcomed by patients, and that the single most important step in improving the accessibility of and satisfaction with primary medical care would be the increased availability of telephone medical advice.[13]

Receptionists have a central role in controlling the telephone accessibility of doctors to patients, and it would appear that, in the United Kingdom at least, most have received little or no training for this aspect of their work.[34] Telephone consultations between British general practitioners and their patients currently remain uncommon events. An extensive study from the north of England reported that 60 per cent of 1500 general practitioners surveyed reported having less than four such patient contacts per day.[35] The introduction of a dedicated telephone advice service in one large general practice resulted in only three telephone consultations per day for the 14 000 patients of the practice;[36] in contrast, Swedish general practitioners handle three telephone consultations per year for each member of the population,[37] and in North America, one call was made or received for every 2.6 surgery consultations.[38]

Maximizing the opportunities for access by telephone consultations is best achieved through dedicated telephone consulting sessions that are advertised.[35,39] Such arrangements are in demand by patients,[13] although the fear of additional workload may have led some doctors not to publicize their service.[35] Nagle et al.[36] found that telephone contact with the doctor resulted in patients who were reassured, and who reported (in 75 per cent of cases) that the contact had obviated the need for an appointment. Brown and Armstrong[39] reported similar findings following the review of an established 'phone-in clinic', which had resulted in an estimated saving of 15 face-to-face consultations and three home visits per week for each doctor. It is of some interest that there was no difference between cases using telephone consultations and age–sex matched controls with regard to the availability of transport—supporting the suggestion of Allen et al.[13] that telephone accessibility was not being used as an alternative by patients simply on account of specific problems of the geographical accessibility of practice premises.

Bhopal[40] and Hallam[35] have considered the problems of scheduling telephone consulting sessions in the midst of a busy reception. An audit of telephone accessibility[41] identified that 57 per cent of first calls to the practice were met with an engaged tone. Following the study, the authors' proposal to purchase alternative telephone equipment would be usefully informed by Hallam's recommended standard[42] of one incoming telephone line per 2500 patients. Detailed guidelines have also been proposed for the use of answering machines where direct telephone access may not be possible.[43]

Whilst the quality of care in telephone consultations has been questioned,[44] and the drawbacks of being unable to examine the patient and of interrupted consultations identified,[45] no follow-up studies have been reported allowing for a comparison using agreed outcomes of telephone and face-to-face consultations. A Swedish study[46] has reported high levels of concordance between information obtained and management plans formulated during a telephone consultation with a nurse, and a follow-up visit to the surgery for a consultation with the same nurse, or a doctor. Telephone consultations were concluded to be complementary to surgery consultations—in contrast to work reporting the value of telephone consultations as a substitute for routine clinic follow-up in a wide variety of hospital-based clinical situations.[47,48]

A further area where telephone advice has been examined relates to the delivery of primary care outside normal working hours. A large cooperative of doctors providing out-of-hours care for patients across southeast London manage about 65 per cent of 72 000 annual contacts on the telephone[49] and NHS Direct, a nurse-led telephone health advice service, has recently been established in the United Kingdom with an objective of providing a single call one-stop gateway to out-of-hours health care by 2004.[50] Early studies have found that patients receiving telephone advice following an out-of-hours contact were less satisfied with their care and reported increased information needs and help-seeking during the following week when compared with patients who received a face-to-face consultation at the primary care centre.[51]

Box 4 Improving accessibility in primary care

- Adequate numbers of telephone lines staffed by individuals trained to give advice.
- Planned services accounting for patient's time constraints, local geography, and local transport arrangements.
- Optimal use of primary care skills base.
- Smaller numbers of patients per doctor.
- Appropriate gender mix of health professionals.
- Quality control and monitored targets for accessibility.
- Flexible appointments systems, sensitive to the needs of patients.
- Health professionals with excellent communication skills.

User involvement

Although some national health care systems now have a statutory duty to involve and consult the public on the planning and delivery of local health services,[52] involving patients in this activity is not new. In 1978, the Alma Ata declaration stated: 'the people have the right and duty to participate individually and collectively in the planning and implementation of care', and recent reports from the World Health Organization have stated that health care systems should be 'responsive'—the outcome achieved when institutions and institutional relationships are designed in such a way that they are cognisant and respond appropriately to the universally legitimate expectations of individuals.[53]

Patient participation groups are one means whereby health care organizations may obtain the views of users. The benefits of such groups include those relating to learning, with an improved understanding of 'how the other side works' and trust and confidence between patients and the primary care team. Furthermore, contributions maybe made to improvement in the services through effective partnership working resulting in new services to meet identified patient needs such as a citizens advice centre operating from practice premises.[54]

More complex mechanisms for obtaining user input to service planning have been described. The 'Citizens' Jury' is distinguished from other models of citizen participation as combining information, time, independence, and scrutiny.[55] However, simple measures often work better than the more complex systems in primary care such as suggestion boxes for patients to contribute suggestions. For a fuller description of this subject see Chapter 13.7.

Box 4 lists some measures for improving accessibility in primary care.

References

1. **Joseph, A.E. and Phillips, D.R.** *Accessibility and Utilisation: Geographical Perspectives on Health Care Delivery.* New York: Harper and Row, 1984.
2. **Penchansky, R. and Thomas, J.W.** (1981). The concept of access: definition and relationship to consumer satisfaction. *Medical Care* **19** (2), 127–40.
3. **Aday, L.A. and Andersen, R.** (1974). A framework for the study of access to medical care. *Health Services Research* **9** (3), 208–20.
4. **Wensing, M.** Patients evaluate general practice. MD thesis, University of Nijmegen, 1997.
5. **Grol, R.** et al. (1999). Patients' priorities with respect to general practice care: an international comparison. European Task Force on Patient Evaluations of General Practice (EUROPEP). *Family Practice* **16** (1), 4–11.
6. **Shannon, G.W. and Dever, G.E.A.** *Health Care Delivery: Spatial Perspectives.* New York: McGraw-Hill, 1974.
7. **Acton, J.P.** *The Demand for Health Care When Time Prices Vary More Than Money Prices.* Santa Monica CA: Rand Corporation, 1973.
8. **Murray, S.A., Tapson, J., Turnbull, L., McCallum, J., and Little, A.** (1994). Listening to local voices: adapting rapid appraisal to assess health and social needs in general practice. *British Medical Journal* **308** (6930), 698–700.
9. **Margolis, P.A., Carey, T., Lannon, C.M., Earp, J.L., and Leininger, L.** (1995). The rest of the access-to-care puzzle. Addressing structural and personal barriers to health care for socially disadvantaged children. *Archives of Pediatrics & Adolescent Medicine* **149** (5), 541–5.
10. **Annual Report of the Department of Health and Social Security.** London: DHSS, 1974.
11. **Lambert, T.W., Goldacre, M.J., and Parkhouse, J.** (1997). Intentions of newly qualified doctors to practise in the United Kingdom. *British Medical Journal* **314**, 1591–2.
12. **Ritchie, J., Jacob, A., and Bone, M.** *Access to Primary Health Care.* London: OPCS, 1981.
13. **Allen, D., Leavey, R., and Marks, B.** (1988). Survey of patients' satisfaction with access to general practitioners. *Journal of the Royal College of General Practitioners* **38**, 163–5.
14. **Cartwright, A. and Anderson, R.** *General Practice Revisited: A Second Study of Patients and their Doctors.* London: Tavistock, 1981.
15. **Ridsdill Smith, R.M.** (1983). Out-of-hours calls. *Update* 274–7.
16. **Popa, K.** (1993). Modified block scheduling: an approach to the efficient use of procedure time. *Gastroenterology Nursing* **16**, 27–9.
17. **Luthra, M. and Marshall, M.N.** (2001). How do general practices manage requests from patients for 'same-day' appointments? A questionnaire survey. *British Journal of General Practice* **51** (462), 39–40.
18. **Fallon, C.W., Hamilton, I., Bhopal, J.S., Gilmour, H.W., and Bhopal, R.S.** (1990). Introduction of an appointment system in a general practice: surveys of patients and staff. *Health Bulletin* **48**, 232–7.
19. **Hays, R.D., Brown, J.A., Spritzer, K.L., Dixon, W.J., and Brook, R.H.** (1998). Member ratings of health care provided by 48 physician groups. *Archives of Internal Medicine* **158** (7), 785–90.
20. **Hannay, D.R.** *The Symptom Iceberg—A Study of Community Health.* London: Routledge and Kegan Paul, 1979.
21. **Royal College of General Practitioners** (1987). In *Fellowship by Assessment.* (ed. D.J. Pereira Gray). Exeter: Royal College of General Practitioners. Occasional Papers of the RCGP.
22. **Howie, J.G.R., Porter, A.M., Heaney, D.J., and Hopton, J.L.** (1991). Long to short consultation ratio: a proxy measure of quality of care for general practice. *British Journal of General Practice* **41**, 48–54.
23. **Hartzema, A.G. and Christensen, D.B.** (1983). Nonmedical factors associated with the prescribing volume among family practitioners in an HMO. *Medical Care* **21** (10), 990–1000.
24. **Camasso, M.J. and Camasso, A.E.** (1994). Practitioner productivity and the product content of medical care in publicly supported health centers. *Social Science and Medicine* **38** (5), 733–48.
25. **Morrell, D.C. and Kasap, H.S.** (1972). The effect of an appointment system on demand for medical care. *International Journal of Epidemiology* **1** (2), 143–51.
26. **Ridsdale, L., Carruthers, M., Morris, R., and Ridsdale, J.** (1989). Study of the effect of time availability on the consultation. *British Journal of General Practice* **39**, 488–91.
27. **Baker, R.** (1996). Characteristics of practices, general practitioners and patients related to levels of patients' satisfaction with consultations. *British Journal of General Practice* **46** (411), 601–5.
28. **Campbell, J.L. and Howie, J.G.R.** (1992). Changes resulting from increasing appointment length: practical and theoretical issues. *British Journal of General Practice* **42**, 276–8.
29. **Airey, C., Brewster, S., Erens, B., Lilley, S., Pickering, K., and Pitson, L.** *National Surveys of NHS Patients. General Practice.* London: NHS Executive, 1998.
30. **Shum, C., Humphreys, A., Wheeler, D., Cochrane, M.A., Skoda, S., and Clement, S.** (2000). Nurse management of patients with minor illnesses in general practice: multicentre, randomised controlled trial. *British Medical Journal* **320** (7241), 1038–43.
31. **Kinnersley, P.** et al. (2000). Randomised controlled trial of nurse practitioner versus general practitioner care for patients requesting 'same day' consultations in primary care. *British Medical Journal* **320** (7241), 1043–8.

32. **Rao, J.N.** (1994). Follow up by telephone. *British Medical Journal* **309**, 152–3.
33. **Hallam, L.** (1992). Patient access to general practitioners by telephone: the doctor's view. *British Journal of General Practice* **42** (358), 186–9.
34. **Copeman, J.P. and Van Zwanenberg, T.D.** (1998). Practice receptionists—poorly trained and taken for granted. *Journal of the Royal College of General Practitioners* **38**, 14–16.
35. **Hallam, L.** (1991). Organisation of telephone services and patients' access to doctors by telephone in general practice. *British Medical Journal* **302** (6777), 629–32.
36. **Nagle, J.P., McMahon, K., Barbour, M., and Allen, D.** (1992). Evaluation of the use and usefulness of telephone consultations in one general practice. *British Journal of General Practice* **42** (358), 190–3.
37. **Marklund, B. and Bengtsson, C.** (1989). Medical advice by telephone at Swedish health centres: who calls and what are the problems? *Family Practice* **6**, 42–6.
38. **Greenlick, M.R., Freeborn, D.K., Gambill, G.L., and Pope, C.R.** (1973). Determinants of medical care utilisation: the use of the telephone in total medical care. *Medical Care* **11**, 121–34.
39. **Brown, A. and Armstrong, D.** (1995). Telephone consultations in general practice: an additional or alternative service? *British Journal of General Practice* **45**, 673–5.
40. **Bhopal, R.** (1994). Telephone access in general practice. *British Journal of General Practice* **44** (379), 95.
41. **Marshall, M.N.** (1993). Telephone access in general practice. *British Journal of General Practice* **43**, 535–6.
42. **Hallam, L.** (1993). Access to general practice and general practitioners by telephone: the patient's view. *British Journal of General Practice* **43** (373), 331–5.
43. **Benett, I.J.** (1992). Prerecorded answerphone messages—influence on patients feelings and behavior in out of hours requests for visits. *British Journal of General Practice* **42**, 373–6.
44. **Virji, A.N.** (1992). Usefulness of telephone consultations in general practice. *British Journal of General Practice* **42** (358), 179–80.
45. **Dearden, A., Smithers, M., and Thapar, A.** (1996). Interruptions during general-practice consultations—the patients view. *Family Practice* **13**, 166–9.
46. **Marklund, B., Koritz, P., Bjorkander, E., and Bengtsson, C.** (1991). How well do nurse-run telephone consultations and consultations in the surgery agree—experience in Swedish primary health-care. *British Journal of General Practice* **41**, 462–5.
47. **Wasson, J., Gaudette, C., Whaley, F., Sauvigne A., Baribeau, P., and Welch, H.G.** (1992). Telephone care as a substitute for routine clinic follow-up. *Journal of the American Medical Association* **267**, 1788–93.
48. **Tutty, S., Simon, G., and Ludman, E.** (2000). Telephone counseling as an adjunct to antidepressant treatment in the primary care system. A pilot study (see comments). *Effective Clinical Practice* **3** (4), 170–8.
49. **Cade, J.** *Primary Care Activity Audit. Winter Planning 2000/2001.* London: GKT School of Medicine Immediate Access Project, 2001.
50. **NHS Executive.** *The NHS Plan.* London: HMSO, 2000.
51. **Shipman, C., Payne, F., Hooper, R., and Dale, J.** (2000). Patient satisfaction with out-of-hours services; how do GP co-operatives compare with deputizing and practice-based arrangements? *Journal of Public Health Medicine* **22** (2), 149–54.
52. **Department of Health.** *Primary Care, General Practice and the NHS Plan.* London: Department of Health, 2001.
53. **De Silva**, A. *A Framework for Measuring Responsiveness.* Geneva: WHO. GPE Discussion Papers Series No. 32, 2002.
54. **Gower, S.** (1999). A beacon of co-operation. *Health Management*, October 23.
55. **McIver, S.** *Obtaining the Views of Black Users of Health Services.* London: Kings Fund, 1994.

12.6 The medical record

Job F.M. Metsemakers and Danny Tayar

Introduction

The medical record (MR) can be considered as the information that exists about a patient in a medical service. It can be a paper or electronic record. With the fast developing computing and communication systems, a wider definition of the future Medical Record can be considered as: all the relevant biopsychosocial information about a patient available at any given time, regardless of where or how it is stored. Although the terms 'record-keeping' and 'registration' are often used interchangeably, they actually mean two different things. Records are written accounts of what has been discussed or what has occurred. Notes jotted down on a patient's record card or status sheet or entered into a computer are all examples of records. The information is sorted and reduced, of course, as not everything can be recorded, but also because doctors are focused and selective in their observations. Registration, on the other hand, means keeping track of certain specific matters which have the doctor's or medical researcher's particular interest. Registered data can be used in calculations: they can be added, subtracted, used to compute percentages, etc. Such data might concern a patient's health problems, proposed diagnoses, medication that has been prescribed or referrals to other types of assistance. To ensure that registered data are properly organized, doctors use classifications, systems in which similar data are grouped into classes, for example, diagnoses.

This chapter will primarily deal with the content and structure of MR, although in one paragraph attention will be given to registration and classification.

Basically, the MR contains non-medical data (such as personal demographic details and background information) and medical data. These can be divided in four different categories: problem list; (progress) notes/journal; medication list; basic medical data/(diagnostic) archive.

Objectives of record-keeping and registration

The main reason to take notes on consultations with patients is that the GP can re-read these notes before the next consultation. This is the *memory function* of record-keeping in *patient care* (see Table 1).

No doctor can expect to remember everything about every single patient. The primary purpose of record-keeping, then, is to refresh the doctor's memory. To provide optimal care, it is necessary to take the patient's biopsychosocial history into account. Proper record-keeping helps the doctor to review the past while evaluating the present, and hence to take more effective decisions and avoid repetition; in short, to enhance the quality and efficiency of services provided.

Records have a *communication function* when more than one care provider are involved in the management of the same patient, for example, because one of them works part-time or has been replaced for various reasons. Records are also a means of communication when a patient moves practice. Provided that they are clear and comprehensible, they enable a new practice to tailor care provision to the patient's needs.

Table 1 Functions of record-keeping and registration

	Memory	Communication	Analysis
Patient care	***	***	*
Evaluation of quality of care	**	**	***
Medical research	**	*	**

* Of lesser importance; ** important; *** highly important.

When different doctors work together, records are both a memory refresher and a means of communication. After all, a doctor will need to consult the records in order to write a referral or respond to a colleague's questions. The record can also tell about patients' investigations and treatment in the past. This *analysis* is simpler when records have been computerized than when they are hand-written. Data from records facilitate practice management. If certain pieces of information contained in a record have been collected for medical research purposes, then such data are usually assigned a classification code and are regarded as registered.

Record-keeping also plays an important role in assessing the *quality of care*. In case of peer review, the doctor's level of performance as reflected in the records, can be evaluated and compared with agreed protocols, guidelines or standards. When the quality of care is being assessed by an external party, for example, a health inspector or medical disciplinary board, a failure on the part of a doctor to keep proper records is often regarded as a serious shortcoming. Medical disciplinary boards issue warnings and reprimands to doctors who fail to keep proper records or to update them adequately. Nevertheless, the main purpose of record-keeping is to assist the doctor in his or her work. The legal aspects are merely derived from this primary purpose. Nevertheless in many countries it is mandatory by law to keep some kind of medical record.

At times, physicians are asked to record information on the effects of treatments or medication according to pre-determined protocols for *medical research* purposes. The government, medical insurers, and researchers are naturally interested in what happens in the health care sector. Hence, records are to keep track of epidemiological statistics such as: how many patients are admitted with particular diseases, or how many patients visit a clinic. Different registration networks have evolved in general practice; in such networks, GPs often work together with a university. Each network emphasizes a different qualitative or quantitative aspect of registration. Many can be regarded as morbidity registrations: some focus on chronic illnesses such as diabetes, asthma, and COPD; others concentrate more on contacts, the number of referrals made, and prescriptions written.

Requirements for records

The requirements that records should meet concern their form and content, but both of these take second place to the requirement of availability (Box 1). Records must, first of all, be available relatively *quickly for the easy entering and retrieval of information*. The use of computers in health care will enhance the availability of records, as it becomes possible to access patient records regardless of it's place. In general practice, all the information ideally is stored in a single database, but that is not always the case. Sometimes some of the data have been computerized, other information is stored in a file along with letters from specialists, while the patient's previous history is still in the 'old' hand-written file. In hospitals there is the problem that diagnostic results are usually available for every attending physician, but the records kept by the internist, for example, cannot always be inspected by the orthopaedist and vice versa. Such new devices as the patient-specific data card, a smart card with a chip that contains a patient's most relevant medical information (problem list, allergies, medication), may perhaps contribute to reduce this problem, until a better interchangeable data system is available.

Of course, the comments and notes must be *legible* for others. Illegible hand-writing will be less of a problem as more and more records are computerized. The requirement of *comprehensiveness* is a difficult one to meet. Too much information would make the record unreadable and messy. Nevertheless, doctors must make an effort to record the highlights of each consultation: what the patient says, important aspects of the history and the examinations performed, an evaluation in the form of a (differential) diagnosis or definition of the problem, how the doctor intends to proceed, including his advice, and explanations to the patient.

The information documented in the record must be *reliable*, not only for such measurements as blood pressure or Hb level, but also for the history and the physical examination. The record should provide an accurate reflection of reality and never be ambiguous in meaning.

Finally, the contents must be clearly formulated and the information is presented in such a way that the doctor's underlying thought process is clear and *comprehensible*.

The requirement of *conciseness* appears to contradict that of comprehensiveness. Conciseness, however, refers to the way in which the relevant information is worded, with unnecessary words being cut out. This does not, however, mean that the doctor should write in abbreviations, as this would make the information less reliable. 'Lungs: none' noted on the patient record card of a 70-year-old says very little. It might mean that the doctor has performed a physical diagnostic examination of the lungs as stipulated and heard nothing unusual either during auscultation or percussion, nor felt anything out of the ordinary when eliciting vocal fremitus. That is all fine and well if other doctors reading his report are aware of this. If they are not, however, then 'Lungs: none' is not a clear and concise abbreviation; in fact, it may be regarded as a careless notation. Usually a more detailed comment is required which specifically states the results of auscultation and percussion.

The requirement of *accessibility* concerns whether specific information can be easily found in the record, and is closely related to the *structure* of the record. A well-structured record will allow the doctor to easily locate and retrieve the information he or she is seeking.

Medical records should be kept in a *secured* place and must be dealt with in a *confidential* manner, preventing access of unauthorized person.

Specialists who treat a patient in a clinic tend to keep records that are geared to their particular discipline and which cover a limited time span, at least when treatment can be concluded. A GP's records, on the other hand, are more ongoing in nature because they contain data recorded over the course of several years. These data are furthermore supplemented by relevant information provided by specialists, physiotherapists, nutritionists, etc. When patients are hospitalized, a great deal of information about them is collected and recorded in a short period of time; this is frequently referred to as the patient's status. Every time the patient is re-admitted, all the information is collected again and in detail, as if the hospital had no prior data on the patient. Specialists do this in order to have all the material they need available for differential diagnostic purposes.

> It is important to determine a set of national and international standards, to assure the possibility of exchanging information between different recording systems of different providers of care.

Box 1 Requirements for records

- Quickly and readily available for *easy entering and retrieval of information*
- *Content:* legible, comprehensive, reliable, and comprehensible
- *Form:* concise, accessible and well structured
- Confidential and secure

The structure of records

The structure of a record indicates, first of all, where the non-medical and medical data can be found.

Non-medical data (such as demographic data and background information) are required not only for administrative purposes; they also give the doctor some idea of the patient's circumstances, which can be important in determining the course of treatment or preventive measures (Box 2). The information concerned consists, for example, of the patient's name, date of birth, address, gender, telephone number, insurance type, national health service number. Then there is the background information: marital status, home situation, educational background, occupation, religion, nationality.

Box 2 Examples of relevant background information

- *Jehovah's Witness:* will refuse blood transfusions for religious reasons
- *Butcher:* increased chance of pyodermias; prohibited to work if suffering from *Salmonella* infection

The *medical data* can be divided into four different categories.

- The problem list
- (Progress) notes/journal
- Medication list
- Basic medical data/(diagnostic) archive

The problem list

The pivot for a doctor's thoughts and actions when considering a course of treatment is an outline of all the patient's health-related problems, both past and present. One very common and highly suitable type of outline is the '*The problem list*'. The list only contains problems which have had a long-term or significant impact on the patient's functional condition or on his or her prognosis.

Such problems might consist of:

- diagnoses, for example, diabetes mellitus, bronchus carcinoma;
- patterns of illnesses, for example, chronic back pain;
- abnormal test or examination results, for example, Pap smear class IV;
- risk factors, for example, drug abuse, predisposition in family history;
- other problems, for example, an allergic reaction to amoxicillin.

The outline in Box 3 clearly shows which health problems still require attention: smoking and endometriosis. The other health problems are no longer active. Some will remain highly relevant throughout the patient's life, even when no longer active, for example, the appendectomy. Other events, such as a miscarriage, will become less relevant after the patient passes through the menopause.

(Progress) notes/journal

Any contact between the doctor and the patient is recorded in (*progress*) *notes/journal.* For each contact, the doctor should record at least the date, the place (i.e. doctor's office/house call), the problem or request for help, the examinations or tests performed, the diagnosis and how the doctor proposes to proceed. What emerges is a chronological outline of all contacts between the doctor and patient.

(Progress) notes/journal were often not structured in the past and depending on the doctor's habit just consisted of a short description of the patients complaints, diagnosis and treatment. Sometimes only the prescription was recorded. Nowadays there is a fixed set of information that should be collected and recorded for a number of specific health problems; such information is usually defined in guidelines or standards for the relevant illness and is therefore generally accepted (Box 4). Computerized 'disease-management systems' are being developed for specific chronic conditions.

Notes taken on a doctor–patient consultation are recorded under various letters that together form the acronym SOAP.

SOAP structure of (progress) notes/journal

The S stands for subjective data, for example, the patient's reason for encounter, problems, requests for assistance and the history of the presented complaint(s). The O standards for objective data, that is, the results of the physical examination, the laboratory tests, or X-rays, etc.

The information classified under S and O can be very clear and its interpretation is sometimes quite simple. In such cases, the diagnosis will be briefly and clearly noted under the A for assessment.

Box 3 Problem list, Ms Peters

Ms Peters, born 30/8/1962

Active	*Problem*	*Inactive*
12/08/1974	Acute appendicitis—appendectomy	12/08/1974
01/01/1980	Smokes: 15 cigarettes a day	
09/07/1984	Spontaneous abortion	13/07/1984
06/12/1984	Spontaneous abortion—curettage	08/12/1984
13/04/1986	Marital problems—divorce	12/06/1988
07/02/1990	Lateral meniscus tear—meniscectomy	14/10/1990
19/06/1993	Endometriosis	

Box 4 Record of full annual review of diabetes mellitus Type 2

History

- General well-being
- Hypoglycaemia
- Compliance with nutritional advice/medication
- Vision problems
- Angina
- Claudication
- Cardiac decompensation
- Sensory impairment, pain, tingling in legs
- Sexual dysfunction
- Weight
- Physical movement
- Smoking
- Consumption of alcohol

Examination

- Weight
- Foot examination
- Pulsation of foot arteries
- Blood pressure
- Examination of sensation by monofilament
- Blood glucose
- Creatinine
- GlyHb
- Total cholesterol level (if necessary, total lipid spectrum)
- Patients under the age of 50: albumin/creatinine ratio in early morning urine

Source: Guidelines for diabetes mellitus Type 2, Dutch College Family Physicians 1999.

If the available information does not lead to an easy diagnosis, then the doctor will have to define the problem as specific as possible and record his or her thought process as concisely as possible at that point. During the next visit, the GP will be able to review his or her train of thought and offer a more specific diagnosis and further solutions based on new information.

The A is the point of departure for the plan, which is represented by the P. The plan consists of: (a) further diagnostic procedures; (b) treatment; (c) information; and (d) the doctor's proposed policy. It will, for example, include agreements made with the patient for follow-up visits.

To prevent the (progress) notes/journal from becoming a long, disjointed summary of patient consultations, doctors should try to link together those consultations that focus on a particular illness. They can then link up corresponding doctor–patient consultations in the records as well, in what is known as *episode registration*. An episode in this sense is regarded as a series of consultations all having to do with a single health problem, from the first time the problem is presented to the GP to the final contact registered for that particular illness or problem.

Medication

The advantage of maintaining a specific record of the patient's medication separate from the (progress) notes/journal is that it gives the GP a better picture of the type of medication the patient is taking or has used in the past. A separate overview also makes communication with other care providers easier. The overview should, at the very least, state the medication (preferably the generic name), the dosage, the number of doses per day/week, the duration of treatment, and the date it was prescribed or changed.

Basic medical data/(diagnostic) archive

When a GP sends a patient for laboratory imaging or function tests, he or she must decide in advance where to record the results. Sometimes they will be recorded in the (progress) notes/journal, with a direct reference to the consultation, so that any reader will understand the doctor's policy. However, grouping results by type and in chronological order, for example all imaging or all laboratory test results together, may make the data more accessible, comprehensible to others and easier to follow in time.

GPs might consider to include the results of tests ordered by other doctors in this archive. This will help to avoid repeating tests, which can be irksome for patients and increase costs.

Computerization of records

Paper records are gradually being replaced by computerized records. GPs are increasingly making use of Electronic Health Care Records (EHCR), which also include an Electronic Patient Record (EPR). The various components of a record as reviewed above must form part of every EPR, although the actual design differs from one EHCR to the next. Fully computerized records offer opportunities impossible with written records, such as statistics reports for the individual patient or for the practice/community. It is, for example, not difficult in an EPR to review all the medication used by a certain patient in the past 2 years. The computer warns the GP if he or she has prescribed medicines that can lead to undesirable interactions or allergic reaction. It can be programmed to remind the GP when and what preventive activities to perform. Referral letters can include all the stored information; for example, the problem list and medication overview can be included.

> The great advantage that computer systems offer is the possibility to communicate, transfer, and share information between different providers of care, within and outside the practice, provided that the different software can 'speak to each other'.

Of course, there are also disadvantages to computerized record-keeping. To begin, using a computerized record-keeping system requires some typing skill. The EPR furthermore offers so many options that it can be difficult for GPs to remember how to record certain types of information most efficiently. Programs are becoming more user-friendly, but they are naturally much more restricting than writing a few lines down on a patient record card in freehand. The GP who does not enter information consistently and carefully cannot expect the computer program to impose more of a structure in the data than performed originally.

The biggest fear, of course, is that the computer will crash owing to a power failure or hardware/software problem. The GP loses his memory and only then realizes how important the memory function of record-keeping is. Fortunately, there are ways to minimize the risk of losing the entire EPR, but GPs using computerized records are more vulnerable than their more old-fashioned colleagues in this respect.

Registration and classification

Before data can be entered, they must be classified. It is important to remember that you will lose some information in this process. After all, it is possible to express subtle nuances in records, while in classifications a choice has to be made between various similar classes.

Like lawyers, architects, and carpenters, doctors have their own language, their medical nomenclature. This language makes it easier for them to communicate with each other. The nomenclature used is generally fine for everyday use; when doctors consult each other about a patient, their use of certain terms generally does not lead to major misunderstandings.

When it comes to medical research, health care policy, or even refresher training and peer evaluation, the terms used must be defined as precisely as possible and organized into a classification system. In scientific studies involving patients with diabetes mellitus Type 2, the diabetics belonging to Type 1 and those belonging to Type 2 must be described in detail. The same holds for the term hypertension. Are hypertension sufferers all those people who are being treated with antihypertensive drugs, or do they include people who have a systolic pressure of more than 140 mmHg and/or a diastolic pressure of more than 90 mmHg?

A classification is a system in which the nomenclature used is organized hierarchically, so that the terms are mutually exclusive. The rules are drawn up in such a way that a specific diagnosis: (a) is unique; (b) can only be made in a single manner; and (c) can only be entered into the system in a single way. Before a diagnosis can be made, the rules of inclusion must be met. The International Classification of Primary Care (ICPC), for example, requires the user to satisfy two conditions before coding the diagnosis of depression: there must be no psychosis and at least three out of six symptoms must have been observed. The first condition—the lack of psychosis—is an example of the hierarchy referred to. If psychosis is observed, then psychosis must be registered, and not depression.

One of the advantages of using a classification system is that it forces GPs to define explicitly what the patient's problem is. That leads to discussions amongst themselves and provides them with instruments for mutual evaluation. We should also be aware that some distortion always arises when classification systems are used. At present, there are three major classification systems for illnesses:

1. The International Classification of Diseases (ICD);
2. The International Classification of Primary Care (ICPC);*
3. The Diagnostic and Statistical Manual of Mental Disorders (DSM).

Every classification has its own unique characteristics that are related to the occupational group that uses it. General practitioners cover the entire field of health care, but they use only a small proportion of the over 9000 known diagnoses regularly. They therefore do not require a highly specific classification which allows them to code many rare diseases separately.

Specialists, on the other hand, cover only a narrow part of the health care field and see rarer diseases with some regularity. As a result the specificity of the classification is much more important to them. The ICD, for example, differentiates between 14 different types of pneumonia, and even divides some classes into further categories. These 14 classes are divided into four chapters. The ICPC only lists one type of pneumonia, which is described in

* See also the chapter on the International Classification of Primary Care by Henk Lamberts.

the chapter 'Respiratory System'. In recent years, much attention has been given to Clinical Terminologies defined lists of clinical terms or phrases, often with codes attached, whose purpose is to create a clinical record. Examples are Read Codes and SNOMED Clinical Terms. Although Clinical Terminologies are not primarily intended for registration of data they can be used as such. Work is undertaken to relate the different classifications with the Clinical Terminologies in such a way that conversion will be possible. Classification systems are discussed in detail in Chapter 4.3.

Legal aspects of record-keeping

Every country will have laws and guidelines concerning patients rights and the management and sharing of patient data. Although of course different in detail most have common directives. Doctors must exercise great care when noting down their actions involving patients. Law usually does not indicate which data should be recorded, nor does it specify how this information is to be structured. It is up to doctors themselves to decide what should be recorded in the interests of 'providing the patient with proper care'. Some court rulings have made it clear that dossiers are expected to contain diagnoses, treatments commenced, the effects of such treatments, reports on further diagnostic tests, and the course of the illness.

Records should be kept for a statutory period of 10 years, commencing on the date that the information is recorded. Doctors must, however, keep such records for longer than 10 years if such 'is reasonable in the interests of providing proper assistance'. As record-keeping plays an important role in ensuring continuity of care, only certain elements of medical records can be destroyed or not be kept. Obviously, any information on which a doctor has based a diagnosis and is still administering treatment must not be destroyed. Depending on the law, patients have the right to have some or all of their records destroyed; doctors must comply with this wish, unless doing so is contrary to statutory rules or other legal or medical interests.

Patients are also entitled to inspect their records and obtain a copy, unless their doing so would infringe the privacy of others. The latter would be the case if the doctor's notes report something that the patient's partner or a family member said without the patient being informed. The doctor's personal working notes are also exempt from the patient's right to inspect or obtain a copy of his or her records. It is difficult to say precisely what personal working notes are, but in actual fact they consist of jottings that the doctor makes of his own ideas on the patient's case. The history and the results of the examination come from the patient himself/herself and may hence be inspected. The doctor's reflections on the patient's disorder can be regarded as personal working notes. The diagnosis, once it has been made, may however be inspected by the patient.

Physicians are bound by the principle of professional secrecy and may not provide others with information on patients. They may only do so with the patient's explicit consent. If another care provider is involved in the treatment, it is understood that the doctor does not have to request such consent. If, however, an organization such as an insurance company requests information from the doctor's records, for example, to ensure that tests are not being repeated, then the doctor may provide this information only with the patient's written consent. The doctor must then refrain from any interpretation. He or she may only provide factual information. There is also the question of to whom the record belongs, especially in he case of a GP who is an employee of an ensurer, or an HMO, for example.

Audit of the medical record

Data from the MR are often used for the evaluation of quality of care. In assessing the quality of diabetes care, for instance, glycated-Hb levels derived from the record can be used. When one uses MRs in this way the quality of the MR needs to be studied too.

An audit of the MR can be performed at several levels. A very simple way would be to see whether the record follows the given structural guidelines. That however, will tell nothing about it's actual use. A more elaborate way is to use a set of quality indicators which specify very precisely what should be assessed. As an example, quality indicators for the problem list would be:

- major and significant biopsychosocial health issues;
- based on data, facts;
- as specific as possible;
- dated;
- coded;
- allocated with a problem number.

Such an extensive audit can only be performed if clear guidelines have been provided for using the record forms.

An example of quality criteria of the MR is included in the Appendix. It will provide a good assessment of the use of the MR.

Conclusions

The MR can serve several functions but the most important one is the *memory and communication function* in patient care. In order to fulfil this task several requirements have to be met. Firstly: quick availability, easy recording, and retrieving information. Furthermore, the record should have a well organized structure, whether on paper or computerized.

Non-medical and *medical data* can be distinguished, while the latter can be divided into four different categories [problem list; (progress) notes/journal; medication list; basic medical data/(diagnostic) archive].

Paper records are being replaced by computerized records which have a number of advantages. But not all programs are user-friendly yet, requiring special skills from the GP.

If the MR is to be used for research purposes, part of the data will have to be coded.

Legal aspects will differ in various countries but in general doctors must exercise great care when noting down their actions involving patients. Privacy aspects have to be considered too, including rules on authorized access.

A set of quality criteria for the MR is defined and can be used to assess the quality of the MR.

Appendix

Quality-criteria of the Medical Record (MR)

1. How many of the following demographic data can be found in the MR:
   Date of birth (1 Pt)
   Telephone number (1 Pt)
   Gender (1 Pt)
   Full address (1 Pt)
   Occupation (1 Pt) **(1 Pt each, maximum 5)** **Score:** ❑❑
2. Do all the major problem/diagnosis, made in the past 5 years, appear on the Problem-List.
   —No major problem found in the record, that does not appear on the Problem-List = **10 Pts**
   —One major problem found in the record, that does not appear on the Problem-List = **5 Pts**
   —Two or more major problems found in the records, which do not appear on the Problem-List = **0 Pts** **Score:** ❑❑
3. Is there any comment (positive or negative) about allergies/sensitivities in the MR? (If there are no allergies known, it should be mentioned in the MR.)
   —The name of the substances and the clinical expression, or 'no allergies' = **10 Pts**
   —Only the name of the substances = **5 Pts**
   —No comment about allergies/sensivities = **0 Pts** **Score:** ❑❑

4. Is the smoking status clearly noted? (maximum 10 Pts)
   —'Non-smoker' or no. of cigarettes/cigars/pipes smoked a day and for how long = **10 Pts**
   —Only 'smoker' = **5 Pts**
   —No comment on smoking status = **0 Pts** **Score:** ❑❑
5. In how many of the last five encounters, the patient's complaints or reasons for visit are in the record? (stated as such!)
   (1 Pt. each, maximum 5) **Score:** ❑❑
6. How many of the last five encounters include a defined problem/ diagnosis?
   (1 Pt. each, maximum 5) **Score:** ❑❑
7. In how many of the last five encounters, the problem/diagnosis is supported by the recorded data?
   (1 Pt. each, maximum 5) **Score:** ❑❑
8. How many of the last five encounters include a plan? (treatment, investigations, referrals, recommendations . . .)
   (1 Pt. each, maximum 5) **Score:** ❑❑
9. How many of the last five encounters include a note of what the patient was told?
   (1 Pt. each, maximum 5) **Score:** ❑❑
10. In how many of the last five encounters, the Physician responsible for the visit, can be identified?
    (1 Pt. each, maximum 5) **Score:** ❑❑
11. In what percentage of recommendation for oral medication, given in the past 2 years, the duration of treatment is specified?
    —In >90% the duration of treatment is noted = **5 Pts**
    —In 75–90% the duration of treatment is noted = **3 Pts**
    —In <75% the duration of treatment is noted = **0 Pts**
    Score: ❑❑
12. Are the imaging results stored in a chronological order?
    —>90% stored in a chronological order, or no imaging results found = **10 Pts**
    —75–90% stored in a chronological order = **5 Pts**
    —<75% stored in a chronological section = **0 Pts** **Score:** ❑❑
13. Are laboratory test results recorded in a specific section of the MR?
    —>90% stored in a specific section, or no test results found = **10 Pts**
    —75–90% stored in a specific section = **5 Pts**
    —<75% stored in a specific section = **0 Pts** **Score:** ❑❑
14. Is the MR safe from unauthorized access? (maximun 10 Pts)
    —Absolutely safe = **10 Pts;** **Score:** ❑❑
    —Not safe = **0 Pts** **Total:** ❑❑❑

Maximum possible score: 100 Pts

Further reading

Easton, R.E. *Problem-Oriented Medical Records Concept.* New York: Appleton Century Crofts, 1974.

Hurst, J.W. and Walker, H.K. *The Problem Oriented Systems.* New York: MEDCOM Press, 1970.

Lang, G.S. and Dickie, K.J. *The Practice-Oriented Medical Record.* Germantown MD: Aspens Systems Corporation, 1977.

Margolis, C.Z. *The Pediatric Problem Oriented Record. A Manual for Implementation.* Pleasantville NY: Docent Corporation, 1977. (Niet verkrijgbaar in Nederland.)

McIntyre, N. (1974). Obtaining information from medical records. *Journal of the Royal College of Physicians,* **8** (3), 267–75.

Petrie, J.C. and McIntyre, N. *The Problem Orientated Medical Record.* Edinburgh: Churchill Livingstone, 1979.

Tayar, D., Azzopardi, A., Benes, V., Doumenc, M., Gottardi, G., Karotsis, A., Kersnik, J., Mixa, O., Murphy, D., Passerini, G., Petric, D., Samuelson, M., Spenser, T., and Szecsenyi, J. Comprehensive set of quality indicators for the improvement of the personal Medical Record. EQuiP Medical Record Project Team, http://www.equip.ch.

Walker, H.K., Hurst, J.W., and Woody, M.E. *Applying the Problem-Oriented System.* New York: MEDCOM Press, 1973.

Weed, L.L. (1964). Medical records, patient care and medical education. *Irish Journal of Medical Science* **6**, 271–82.

Weed, L.L. (1968). Medical records that guide and teach. *New England Journal of Medicine* **278**, 593–652.

Weed, L.L. *Medical Records, Medical Education and Patient Care.* Cleveland OH: Case-Western Reserve University Press, 1969.

12.7 General practitioners' use of time and time management

Peter P. Groenewegen, Wienke G.W. Boerma, and Brenda Sawyer

Introduction

Time is scarce and there are always competing ways of spending it. We all must make choices about the allocation of our time to private, social, and professional activities, and this is no less true of general practitioners (GPs). For most of us, the proportion of our time reserved for professional activities, and the flexibility to expand this proportion occasionally, is limited, and depends on the constraints of other personal and social obligations. In general practice, the process of clarifying our patients' problems, making accurate diagnoses and providing effective management, and giving information and reassurance to patients all need time. GPs frequently complain about lack of time and time pressures, recognizing that this may threaten the quality of care that can be provided to patients, and is likely to adversely affect their own health.(1)

The problem of the use of time in general practice has its roots in both the demand side and the supply side of health care. The problems presented to GPs tend to be increasingly complex, and patients' demands and expectations are high. Changes in other parts of health care, such as shorter hospital stays, more community-based care, longer waiting lists and a shift in the focus of care from secondary to primary care, all affect demand and the increasing range of tasks presented to primary physicians.(2) In many countries, these developments are taking place against the background of a rapidly growing proportion of female and part-time GPs, with mixed professional portfolios, and in societies with ever shortening working weeks. In seeking solutions to the conflict between workload and available time, we need to recognize that the workload of GPs consists not only of the demands of direct patient care, provided both in the surgery and in patients' homes and which may be difficult to predict and manage, but also includes essential financial and administrative duties and activities aimed at keeping up-to-date, including continuing education and professional development. GPs vary widely in the time they are able to allocate to these various professional activities, and this chapter aims to clarify the sources of this variation, which are rooted both in the characteristics of the individual GP and also in the characteristics and organization of the practice. In examining international comparisons between GPs, the influences of different health care systems are also important.

In this chapter, we present evidence on the ways in which GPs use time in a number of European countries and relate variation in the use of time to these three dimensions: characteristics of the GP, the practice population, and the health care system. Data were collected in a Europe-wide survey in 1993–1994, the European study of task profiles of GPs.[3,4] In 32 countries, 8183 GPs completed and returned uniform questionnaires in their own language, with a response rate of almost 50 per cent. We also provide practical suggestions to help GPs manage their time and organize their work, arising from the experience of one of the authors (B.S.) as a professional advisor of GPs in this area.

Sources of variation in use of time

Higher patient demand requires more time to be spent in clinical care by GPs, but this patient-related workload is not related simply to the number of patients cared for, but also to the type of patients. The old and the very young have more frequent contacts with the GP, and consultations with older patients usually take more time. Less educated patients and those living in disadvantaged areas have higher needs, but the evidence about actual utilization of services is mixed. The clinical case mix also has an important effect on workload.

GPs differ in their response to a high patient demand. Some are able to avoid being over-stretched by efficiently managing both their time and their work, often by delegating tasks and creating new skill-mixes within the primary care team. This variation is often related to the personal characteristics of the GP. Another source of variation in GPs' use of time is related to the health care system in which they work. In some countries, GPs work 55 h or more, while in others GPs follow the usual working week of 36 h of public sector employees. These differences are related to the structure of the health care system and probably to more general cultural traits, such as patterns of work and leisure time in society in general. These influences and the groups of activities which make up the primary care workload are summarized in Fig. 1.

Practice organization, and to a lesser extent, the personal working style of GPs offer the best opportunities for controlling time and workload, while other factors are more difficult to change. The appropriateness of strategies to cope with pressures of time depend on whether the pressure is temporary or long-standing. One option is simply to expand the total working time, but if this is not possible the GP is likely to compensate for an expansion of time in one task area by reduction of time devoted to other tasks. Clearly, this strategy may be harmful to the quality of the services provided by GPs. A third, superior, approach is to use the available time more efficiently. There are many strategies by which surgery hours, home visiting rates, administrative tasks, and other commitments can be better

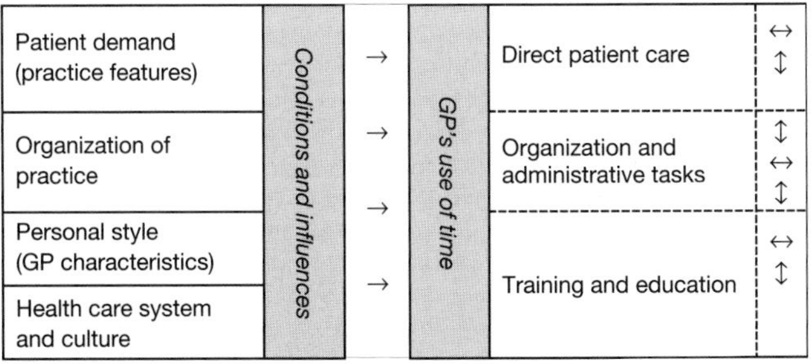

Fig. 1 Influences on the general practitioners' use of time.

organized, by restructuring roles within the team or by acquiring more time-efficient working habits.

Patient demand: consultations and home visits

Larger practice sizes generate more patient contacts, and this requires more time from the GP.[5–7] However, practice size alone is not the only influence on the number of patient contacts, but as described earlier the demographic characteristics of the practice populations are important. In some health care systems, GPs or practices serve a defined, registered practice population (e.g. the list system in the United Kingdom and Norway), whilst in other systems patients are free to consult a physician of their choice. Studies in systems where patients are listed with a GP or a specific practice show that the relationship between list size and the time needed for direct patient care is not linear.[8] The average length of consultations is negatively related to list size; in other words, GPs caring for larger practice populations spend less time per consultation. Furthermore, if a distinction is made between patient-initiated and doctor-initiated consultations, patient-initiated contact rates tend to be lower in larger practices, suggesting less accessibility or some form of substitution, for instance, by practice staff.[9]

According to the European Study,[3] variation in the total working time of GPs appears to be more related to direct patient care than to administration and education. Individual GPs and health care systems vary considerably in the number of total working hours of general practitioners, and the number of hours spent on direct patient care. For non-patient-related activities, however, the variation is much smaller. So it seems, therefore, that non-patient-related activities require a more or less fixed amount of time, irrespective of the size of the practice and the local situation.

Another influence on demand in general practice, and consequently on the time that needs to be spent, are the GPs' contractual obligations concerning availability outside normal office hours. Working hours will be lower if demand outside the normal office hours is diverted to special services. Recent years have seen a move away from a personal commitment of GPs to the provision of out-of-hours care to the use of deputizing services and GPs' cooperatives.

Managing patient demand: practice organization

General practice has been described as demand-led,[5] meaning that aspects of demand are the main determinants of how GPs use their time. This relationship was confirmed in the European Study,[3] which showed that only a very small part of the variation in GPs' use of time is related to the organization of practice, while a much larger part was related to aspects of demand. However, GPs may cope with their workload by adopting various time-saving habits and by organizing their practices efficiently.[10] Using an appointment system instead of an open surgery system with an unplanned flow of patients is one effective way of managing workload.[11] In appointment systems, GPs have to fix booking intervals. Booking intervals are at the same time a reflection of past experience and a constraint on the actual length of consultations. There is evidence that longer consultations give more room to patients to present their problems, especially if these are of a psychosocial nature.[12,13]

In some countries, appointment systems are predominant, sometimes in combination with a short open surgery early in the morning, while in others this is much less common. Practices offering an open surgery system spend more time in direct patient care and less time in other activities than those with an appointment system (Table 1).[9]

More patients visit the practice when no appointment needs to be made. Making an appointment, even for the following day, presumably serves as a modulator of patient demand. The management of telephone calls from patients is also important, and Marsh has shown that by allocating a slot of

Table 1 Number of working hours per week (total, patient-related, and non-patient-related) and deviations by the influence of aspects of practice organization

	Working hours per week and deviations		
	Total	Patient-related	Non-patient-related
Overall average number of hours	51	45	6
Having an appointment system	−0.5	−1.2	+0.7
Working with other GPs	−2.9	−2.3	−0.6
Keeping patient records	+2.7	+1.6	+1.1
Using a computer	+0.2	−0.6	+0.8

time to reply to non-urgent calls from patients, time lost through interruptions of consultations can be reduced.[10] The use of intrapractice e-mail as an internal communication system is increasingly popular. Messages displayed on the computer screen give the doctor more control over time and ways of responding to demand. In the future it is possible that telephone consultations will be replaced by e-mail consultations between patients and doctors.[14]

GPs who share accommodation in health centres with other GPs tend to work fewer hours. This may point to different ideas and preferences of those working in certain teams, but it is possible that teams can also provide better opportunities for time management, for example, by levelling out peaks in workload. Additionally, the availability of ancillary staff in the practice creates the opportunity to delegate administrative or patient-related tasks, to cope better with a given workload and to keep working hours within limits. The involvement of practice nurses in acute and chronic care can permit economies in general practitioners' consultations and, in larger teams, the employment of a practice manager has been shown to improve overall efficiency of the use of time and resources.[15,16] However, the beneficial effects of employing ancillary staff may be neutralized if new services are provided in addition to tasks already delegated from GPs.[17] This probably explains why the European Study did not find an effect of the numbers of employed ancillary staff on patterns of the use of time.

Restructuring of roles within a team

- Computers saving administrative time for receptionists.
- Receptionists being trained in phlebotomy and simple clinical measurements previously undertaken by nurses.
- Nurses trained to undertake triage and allocating patients to appropriate health professionals or advising themselves.
- Nurses trained up to Nurse Practitioner level and taking more complex cases.
- GPs transferring some work to the GP specialist, and being relieved of some cases that will be dealt with by nurses.

This should free up the GPs to re-schedule time to suit their needs.

Medical record-keeping is usually seen as an important tool for providing continuity of care. But, in the European Study, comprehensive record keeping was found not to be common practice. In southern Europe especially substantial numbers of GPs do not keep comprehensive records (see Chapter 12.6). GPs who reported keeping routine records also reported to work more hours, particularly in administrative duties.

The use of computers is often seen as an opportunity to rationalize the use of resources and time and the European Study showed that using a computer in the practice had an effect on the use of time. GPs who used a computer spent, in absolute and relative terms, more time in activities unrelated to patient care, perhaps reflecting an individual choice in which the computer is used for other tasks, such as research and audit, that are also time-consuming. The efficient use of information technology may well prove only to be a time-saving strategy when it is fully integrated into the consulting process, and when applications go beyond administrative and financial issues.[1] The differences found in the European Study are likely to reflect differences between GPs in their familiarity with the use of this technology. The use of mobile telephones, laptop, and hand-held computers may provide further assistance in the efficient use of time in general practice, particularly when GPs are travelling or waiting for appointments.

Time savers

- Just say 'No'
- Important things first
- Right first time
- Stop when it's good enough
- Think, read, and decide faster (rapid reading course)
- Master information technology skills yourself
- Delegate maximally
- Communicate with brevity
- Strategy saves time in the long-term
- Carry a small pocket notebook at all times

Time wasters

- Unpunctuality
- Meetings and overlong communications
- Paperwork
- Underestimating time required
- Procrastination
- Unpreparedness

Individual variation: personal characteristics

Irrespective of other influences, the age and gender of GPs are related to the variations in the way time is used. Older GPs tend to work less hours, and to be less involved in providing the services from which they can opt out, such as out-of-hours care and preventive surveillance clinics for young children. On the other hand, there is still evidence that older GPs make more home visits, which is likely to be more time-consuming. The gender of the GP is also a discriminating factor with respect to working hours; female GPs consistently work fewer hours than male colleagues, approximately 4 h less each week, taking differences in health system, demand, and organization into account. This smaller number of hours is equally divided between patient-related and other practice activities. Female GPs, who are sometimes more constrained by the traditional division of labour in families, often prefer a part-time work with activities which are easier to plan. They make fewer home visits than their male colleagues, when differences in age and part-time working are controlled. Conversely, they tend to be more involved in child surveillance clinics, which can easily be scheduled.

Other personal characteristics may be important. Some people are at their brightest in the morning and others at night. Early risers do best by arranging to undertake complicated tasks in the morning, when their thought processes and actions are likely to be quicker and more effective. Conversely, the night owls work better at night. Using quality time for important issues is an essential aspect of time management. Personal characteristics should be taken into account or used efficiently, but efficiency can also be acquired by the GP, for instance, when writing a referral letter to a specialist. This can be done efficiently by dictating or typing the letter into the computer at the time of consultation. When appropriate, this may be done in the presence of the patient, thus keeping the patient fully informed. To undertake this task immediately may lengthen the consultation, but is likely to save time over all.

The country dimension: systems and cultures

Data from the European Study showed marked differences in patient loads between countries. The number of contacts that GPs have with patients was high in Germany, Austria, Hungary, and the Czech Republic, with around 50 office contacts per day on average. The lowest averages, around 15 per day, were found in the Baltic States, France, Sweden, Iceland, and Belgium. In Belgium, this low number is partly compensated for by an extremely high number of home visits (averaging 44 per week per GP*). High numbers of home visits were also made in Germany, Austria, France, and Hungary, with five or fewer visits weekly in Portugal, Sweden, Finland, Iceland, and Israel. Home visits are time-consuming, and are not always remunerated, explaining at least in part why this service has been reduced over the last decade by GPs under pressure of time and the need to work more efficiently. In countries with relatively low GP densities and where competition is low, GPs can more easily resist the patients' pressure to make unnecessary home visits.[18]

Data from a workload diary, kept over one working week, disclosed considerable differences in working hours. On average very long working weeks of 60 h or more were reported by GPs in Austria, Belgium, France, Germany, Ireland, Luxembourg, Switzerland, and the United Kingdom, with relatively short working weeks (40 h or less) in Latvia, Lithuania, and Sweden (see Fig. 2).

As mentioned earlier, countries differ in whether or not GPs use an appointment system, but when they do and use fixed booking intervals we are also able to look at the average length of the booking intervals (Table 2).

Countries with over 80 per cent of GPs using fixed booking intervals are to be found in the northwest of Europe. The United Kingdom and the

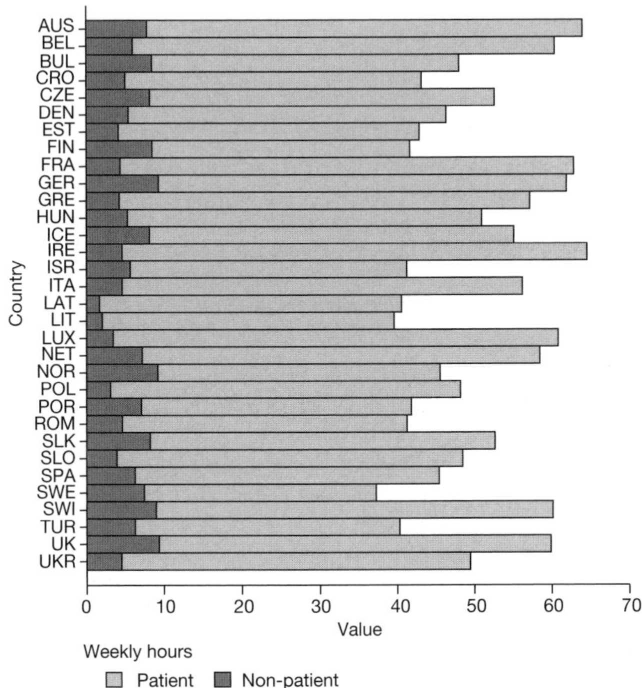

Fig. 2 Number of working hours (total and patient-related and non-patient-related) by country.

* Home visits are not always equally distributed over the days, so this was asked per week.

Table 2 Percentage of GPs having an appointment system with fixed intervals and average length of booking intervals by country

Country	% of GPs using fixed intervals	Length (min)
Austria	34	15
Belgium	63	19
Bulgaria	29	13
Croatia	15	12
Czech Republic	19	18
Denmark	92	13
Estonia	27	16
Finland	89	18
France	69	20
Germany	66	13
Greece	15	21
Hungary	9	14
Iceland	90	17
Ireland	50	14
Israel	63	11
Italy	20	22
Latvia	14	21
Lithuania	27	17
Luxembourg	61	18
Netherlands	93	10
Norway	82	19
Poland	22	21
Portugal	58	16
Romania	23	19
Slovak Republic	28	7
Slovenia	21	13
Spain	54	10
Sweden	71	24
Switzerland	78	15
Turkey	4	19
United Kingdom	85	8
Ukraine	9	15

Netherlands are countries with a high prevalence of fixed booking intervals and a short length of the intervals.

The variation in the number of working hours is not only related to individual and practice characteristics, but also to the health system or culture; more than one quarter of the total variation is related to this system level. Here, the influence of the GP's employment status, the position as a gate keeper, and the distinction between Eastern and Western Europe needs to be considered.

The employment status of GPs in a country has an important relation with time use. In countries where GPs are mainly self-employed, they work more hours in total and in patient-related activities, but not in other professional activities. Gate-keeping GPs, who usually have a defined population to care for, work fewer hours, when demand differences are taken into account. This might partly be related to efficiency; these GPs tend to know their patients better and are likely to have more complete records on them, so that their consultations are likely to be more efficient. It may also be related to more restricted opportunities for patients to switch between GPs if they are not satisfied with service provided to them.[19]

There appears to be an 'East–West' distinction in the use of time by GPs. In the former Eastern Bloc countries, GPs spent less time in activities unrelated to direct patient care but this only holds true when other influences on the use of time, such as practice organization, are not taken into account. Many GPs in Central and Eastern Europe still work in large polyclinics, where they are not involved in most administrative duties.

Conclusions

The relevance of the use of time and time management lies in the way that they are related to professional, patient, and personal outcomes.[20] Time is an important asset in general practice; the length of consultations can be related to whether or not psychosocial aspects of people's health problems are identified and acted on. The use of time is related both to the content and to the quality of care.[7,12,13,21] However, the relationship is not undebated and the relationship between consultation length and uptake of, for example, psychosocial problems could also be the other way around.[22] Time use and time management might also be related to personal consequences, such as burn-out.[23]

The evidence presented in this chapter shows that demand-related variables are important in determining the use of time, and are much more important than variables related to the organization and type of practice. This provides an important message about the characteristics of general practice. There are large differences between countries in the number of consultations people have and in the opportunities GPs have to manage this demand. In the 'Eastern' European health care culture doctors generally have a low professional status and are not in a position to say 'no'. They receive little support from health care managers and patients have high demands. In Western European countries, patients increasingly adopt a consumerist approach, which may be difficult for some doctors to deal with, particularly in countries with a high density of doctors, where there is competition to provide patient care.

Appointment systems have been shown to be helpful in managing demand and workload. Time management techniques and organizational solutions to cope with patients' demand should, however, not reduce the accessibility of the practice to patients. Delegation of tasks from GPs to nursing and allied health personnel is seen as one solution to dealing with an increased demand for care.[24] An expansion of nursing roles in general practice is altering the skill mix and distribution of time allocated to patients between team members. Two important developments include nurse triage systems and the development of nurse practitioners. In triage, a nurse makes a needs assessment with patients requesting to see a GP on the same day and, in many cases, patients' fears can readily be allayed. Triage may result in the patient seeing the GP on the same day, but in many cases advice can be given which obviates the need for an immediate consultation.

Nurse practitioners undertake a higher level of decision-making and cover more comprehensive health treatments than practice nurses. In the United Kingdom, nurse practitioners spend on average 12 min face to face with patients, compared with less than 8 min spent by doctors.[25] These initiatives may save doctors' time and help to cope with increasing patient demand.

Another development affecting the allocation of time in practice is the introduction of GP specialists. Although in its infancy, this development could result in more complex cases being directed to a GP within the team who possesses expertise in a specific field. Indeed, this may save time, but could also lead to de-skilling of GPs; this subject is discussed in more detail in Chapter 8.4.

The survey that produced much of the evidence on which this chapter is based was undertaken in 1994. There is no empirical information available for more recent years on a Europe-wide scale. Since 1994, there have been further significant changes throughout general practice. The countries of Central and Eastern Europe were then at the beginning of a lengthy process of reform, moving towards independent practice with self-employed GPs. For these GPs, the need for practice management and efficient use of time have become more and more important. In other countries, new tasks and changing patient demands have induced GPs to pay more attention to the efficient use of time. The need for adaptation to these new circumstances has been reflected, during recent years, in growing feelings of frustration and lack of morale among GPs in many countries. Although it has been conjectured that GPs are working less hours and having more time to see patients,[14] their subjective experience seems at odds with that trend. It is unlikely that some of the relationships discussed in this chapter, such as those between demand and the use of time, have changed significantly during the past decade, but changes may have occurred in GPs' expectations and the ways in which they cope with pressure of time and competing obligations. Although subjective factors, such as workload and personal coping mechanisms, play major roles in burn-out, these can be influenced indirectly by controlling the size of the practice and the number of working hours, and the organization of other duties, such as out-of-hours care.[26]

References

1. **Morrison, I. and Smith, R.** (2000). Hamster health care: time to stop running faster and redesign health care. *British Medical Journal* **321**, 1541–2.
2. **Scott, A. and Vale, L.** (1998). Increased general practice workload due to a primary care led National Health Service: the need for evidence to support rhetoric. *British Journal of General Practice* **48**, 1085–8.
3. **Boerma, W.G.W., Van der Zee, J., and Fleming, D.M.** (1997). Service profiles of general practitioners in Europe. *British Journal of General Practice* **47**, 481–6.
4. **Boerma, W.G.W. and Fleming, D.M.** *The Role of General Practice in Systems of Health Care*. London: The Stationery Office/WHO, 1998.
5. **Calnan, M. and Butler, J.R.** (1988). The economy of time in general practice: an assessment of the influence of list size. *Social Science and Medicine* **26**, 435–41.
6. **Groenewegen, P.P., Hutten, J.B.F., and Van der Velden, K.** (1992). List size, composition of practice and general practitioners' workload in the Netherlands. *Social Science and Medicine* **34**, 263–70.
7. **Hutten, J.B.F.** *Workload and Provision of Care in General Practice: An Empirical Study of the Relation Between the Workload of Dutch General Practitioners and the Content and Quality of their Care*. Thesis, Utrecht: Nivel, 1998.
8. **Calnan, M., Groenewegen, P.P., and Hutten, J.B.F.** (1992). Professional reimbursement and management of time in general practice: an international comparison. *Social Science and Medicine* **35**, 209–16.
9. **Groenewegen, P.P. and Hutten, J.B.F.** (1995). The influence of supply-related characteristics on general practitioner workload. *Social Science and Medicine* **40**, 349–58.

10. **Marsh, G.N.** *Efficient Care in General Practice. Or: How to Look after Even More Patients.* Oxford: Oxford University Press, 1991.
11. **Gallagher, M., Pearson, P., and Drinkwater, C.** (2001). Managing patient demand: a qualitative study of appointment making in general practice. *British Journal of General Practice* **51**, 280–5.
12. **Howie, J.G.R., Porter, A.M., Heaney, D.J., and Hopton, J.L.** (1991). Long to short consultation ratio: a proxy measure of quality of care for general practice. *British Journal of General Practice* **41**, 48–54.
13. **Campbell, S.M., Hann, M., Hacker, J., Burns, C., Oliver, D., Thapar, A., Mead, N., Gelb Safran, D., and Roland, M.O.** (2001). Identifying predictors of high quality care in English general practice: observational study. *British Medical Journal* **323**, 784.
14. **Mechanic, D.** (2001). How should hamsters run? Some observations about sufficient time in primary care. *British Medical Journal* **323**, 266–8.
15. **Bolden, K., Lewis, A., and Sawyer, B.** *Practice Management.* Oxford: Blackwell, 1992.
16. **Whynes, D. and Baines, D.** (1996). Predicting activity and workload in general practice from the demographic structure of the practice population. *Journal of Health Services Research and Policy* **1**, 128–34.
17. **Richardson, G., Maynard, A., Cullum, N., and Kindig, D.** (1998). Skill mix changes: substitution or service development? *Health Policy* **45**, 119–32.
18. **Boerma, W.G.W. and Groenewegen, P.P.** (2001). GP home visiting in 18 European countries. Adding the role of health system features. *European Journal of General Practice* **7**, 132–7.
19. **Grol, R.** et al. (2000). Patients in Europe evaluate general practice care: an international comparison. *British Journal of General Practice* **50**, 882–7.
20. **Mechanic, D.** (1970). Correlates of frustration among British general practitioners. *Journal of Health and Social Behaviour* **11**, 87–104.
21. **Howie, J.G.R., Heany, D.J., Maxwell, M., Walker, J.J., Freeman, G.K., and Rai, H.** (1999). Quality at general practice consultations: cross sectional survey. *British Medical Journal* **319**, 738–43.
22. **Carr-Hill, R., Jenkins-Clarke, S., Dixon, P., and Pringle, M.** (1998). Do minutes count? Consultation lengths in general practice. *Journal of Health Services Research and Policy* **3**, 207–13.
23. **Appleton, K., House, A., and Dowell, A.** (1998). A survey of job satisfaction, sources of stress and psychological symptoms among general practitioners in Leeds. *British Journal of General Practice* **48**, 1059–63.
24. **Iliffe, S.** (2000). Nursing and the future of primary care: handmaidens or agent for managed care. *British Medical Journal* **320**, 1020–1.
25. **Venning, P., Durie, A., Roland, M., Roberts, C., and Leese, B.** (2000). Randomised controlled trial comparing cost effectiveness of general practitioners and nurse practitioners in primary care. *British Medical Journal* **320**, 1048–53.
26. **van Dierendonck, D., Groenewegen, P.P., and Sixma, H.** *Opgebrand. Een inventariserend onderzoek naar gevoelens van motivatie en demotivatie bij huisartsen.* (Burned out. An inventory of feelings of motivation and demotivation with GPs.) Utrecht: Nivel, 1992.

13

Quality improvement

13 Quality improvement

13.1 Principles and models for quality improvement

Richard Baker and Richard Grol

Introduction

The policy makers, patients, and professionals of the health care systems in the majority of developed and developing countries have come to regard quality improvement as a priority. The principal reasons are pervasive concerns about cost and the growth in expectations among the users of services. In consequence, professionals working in primary medical care must understand the general principles of quality improvement and be able to take part in quality improvement projects. Some professionals will also have particular responsibility for leading quality improvement and they will require a more detailed understanding of the methods. In this section of the textbook, this chapter describes the principles and models for quality improvement, Chapter 13.2 considers measuring and monitoring for quality improvement, Chapter 13.3 addresses evidence-based medicine as a tool in quality improvement, Chapter 13.4 considers guideline development and use, Chapter 13.5 outlines tools for quality improvement and changing practice, Chapter 13.6 discusses total quality management and continuous quality improvement, and Chapter 13.7 considers the important role of patients in improving quality.

Of course, a wide range of activities will influence or improve the quality of care, including the initial and continuing education of clinicians, practice organization, and the level of funding available. However, these activities have a variety of aims and methods, and should not, therefore, be regarded as typical examples of quality improvement techniques. Quality improvement may be defined as a process of planned activities that have the aim of improving care.[1] It involves the specification of desired performance, the review of actual performance, the implementation of changes in care if necessary, followed by further review of performance to check the impact of the changes. The process is frequently depicted as a cycle (Fig. 1), but although the cycle conveys the general framework for quality improvement, it is deceptively simple. In the rest of this chapter, we address the basic principles underlying the cycle and the various models in which it is employed.

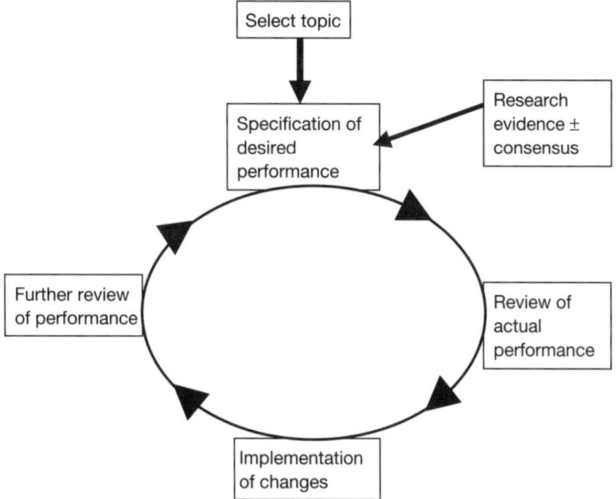

Fig. 1 The quality improvement cycle.

What is quality?

The most widely used definition of quality of care is that of the Institute of Medicine—the degree to which health services for individuals and populations increase the likelihood of desired health outcomes and are consistent with current professional knowledge.[2] Numerous other definitions have been proposed, each emphasizing different aspects, for example, costs, equity or the availability of care. However, if health outcomes and current professional knowledge are interpreted as including a broad range of issues, it is possible to argue that the Institute's definition does incorporate most other definitions. Nevertheless, one issue is overlooked. In determining which health outcomes are desirable, the values of different individuals, groups, and parties in health care become important, and it is the difference between these values that creates the continuing debate about the meaning of 'quality of care'.

One of Donabedian's less familiar definitions of quality suggested that it was a property of, and a judgement upon, an element of care.[3] He placed the judges of quality into three broad groups—health professionals who are most likely to take the technical aspects of care into account; patients, who will place more weight on the interpersonal aspects; and managers or policy makers, who may be more interested in efficiency and costs. Of course, the three groups are arbitrary, and they may have more views that are the same than ones that are at variance, but the underlying principle is helpful. We must conclude that there is no completely unified view of what constitutes quality of care, and that quality improvement must, therefore, be recognized as an attempt to improve aspects of care regarded by some people (but not others) as being important for quality.

The different values of professionals and patients are an example of the tensions that can arise about the meaning of quality. Professionals may regard high rates of infant immunization as an indicator of quality, and the policy makers may set targets for immunization linked to remuneration. But patients may take a different view, and place greater weight on being given sufficient information for them to make their own informed decision. An individual patient may demand penicillin for their sore throat, but the doctor may refuse on the grounds of evidence cited in a good-quality guideline or on professional consensus. Patients may expect quick access to medical care for minor complaints, but professionals may regard this as inappropriate, and potentially putting the care of people with serious illnesses at risk. The imposition of strict care protocols through the implementation of evidence-based guidelines could be regarded as another example of the professional or health service view of quality overriding the patient's view. It should not go unremarked that different parties also hold different views about the most appropriate methods for improving quality, professionals preferring education and best evidence, but managers may prefer accreditation or external assessments.

Since conflict between the alternative views of quality is inevitable, a mechanism is needed to ensure a reasonable balance. All health care systems have such mechanisms, and they consist of various legal, professional, and social codes that govern the practise of clinicians. These codes set boundaries around the roles of patients and professionals, and give authority to their judgements about quality. Many codes are explicit, for example, those contained in the rules that govern the certification and discipline of doctors, or the policies governing the operation of health care organizations. A breach of these codes may be followed by appeal to the courts or to complaints procedures. Some codes require doctors to resist the requests of some patients for inappropriate treatments, and others set limits to the power of doctors to treat patients in their best clinical interests without consent. Problems arise, however, when the codes are implicit, and not clearly expressed in legislation or regulation. In these circumstances, professionals and patients may have different views, and the subsequent confusion can lead to patients losing trust in their doctors.

It should also be noted that individual primary care professionals will have different values that influence their views on quality. Some professionals regard technical outcome as paramount, and emphasize the role of evidence-based medicine and illness prevention. Others regard the personal relationship between professional and patient as critical, and argue that the most important aspects of care cannot be measured. Thus, there is no single absolute view on the quality of care. Therefore, the views of different parties have to be included in any concept or model of quality improvement. A comprehensive approach is needed that includes different views and approaches. It is within such a comprehensive model that the quality improvement cycle becomes an important tool.

The quality improvement cycle

Having discussed what is meant by quality in health care, we now outline the steps in the quality improvement cycle (Fig. 1). In many countries, this cycle has become familiar to professionals in primary care, and teaching about the methods is now commonly included in training. Therefore, we have not provided a detailed description, but comprehensive practical manuals are readily available in other publications.[4,5] In the description that follows, we emphasize the principles that apply to quality improvement projects undertaken by small local groups or individuals, and to large multicentre projects.

Selecting topics

Before the first stage of the cycle can begin, a quality improvement topic must be selected. A variety of factors may lead to the selection of a topic: an identified problem or error in care; the introduction of a new procedure or treatment; agreement of local or national priorities for health care; the needs of a particular patient group; a complaint from a patient. In primary care organizations that have relatively limited experience of quality improvement, topics are often selected because they are simple to undertake, change in care is easy to achieve, and, therefore, they offer an excellent introduction. Particular individuals may also suggest topics based on their own interests, but in the longer term, as the practice or organization develops experience in quality improvement, a more systematic approach will be required to ensure that the issues of greatest importance are addressed. These include those that have the greatest impact on health (severity of disease, numbers of patients), are allocated priority in the health care service, or are of concern to patients. Furthermore, the selection of topics can give expression to the views of different parties on good-quality care. The discussion of the meaning of quality makes clear that in an organization with a fully developed quality improvement programme, the concerns of patients would have a key role in the selection of topics for quality improvement. The practice or organization, therefore, requires a structure for consulting patients or patient representatives.

Specifying desired performance

The general views about what constitutes quality must be developed into specific, measurable aspects of care. Two broad approaches can be applied, either together or separately.

Outcomes

Since the aim of health care is to prolong healthy life, it is natural that the impact of care on outcomes should be a key interest (Table 1). However, despite the importance of outcome, it is relatively unusual for it to be included in quality improvement. Some outcomes are delayed following care for months or even many years. In primary care, this applies particularly to mortality and the measurement of mortality in primary care quality improvement projects is rare. The limited information systems available in primary care present difficulties in the collection of data about adverse outcomes, and in any case deaths and serious adverse outcomes are relatively infrequent and it can be unwise to draw firm conclusions from a small number of cases. The administration of quality of life scales in quality improvement is likewise uncommon. Such instruments can require expertise to interpret and relatively large numbers of patients to ensure meaningful conclusions. The use of patient surveys to assess satisfaction or patient reports of their care is more common. For example, a standardized instrument is now being widely used in Europe.[6] Qualitative methods are also occasionally used to enquire into patients' experiences of care, but this method could be used more frequently, although the skill to conduct and analyse interviews is difficult to acquire. Information about the use of resources is generally more simple to collect; indeed, in many health care systems the collection of information about prescribing, investigation, and referral rates and/or costs has become routine.

A key problem in the use of outcomes is the impact of patient factors or case-mix. Primary care teams each have unique patient populations with their own social, economic, and health characteristics that influence the level of resources required to provide health care to the population, and the potential impact of care on health outcomes. Therefore, the comparison of outcomes between doctors, health care teams, or organizations can give rise to misleading conclusions. One response to this difficulty is to compare only like with like—to select patient populations that are similar in socio-economic and health terms. Another approach is to use statistical techniques to adjust for the effects of case-mix. The use of these techniques is as yet relatively unusual in primary health care, although is more common in acute specialities.

The determination of the level of outcome to expect also requires consideration, for example, how does a primary care organization judge how many people with diabetes would be likely to suffer a major adverse event such as sight loss or amputation if care was optimum? In one approach, the

Table 1 Types of outcomes

Age and sex adjusted mortality rates
Incidence of adverse outcomes (e.g. sight loss in diabetes)
Quality of life or functional abilities assessed by use of valid scales
Use of resources (e.g. costs of prescribing, investigations, referrals)
Patients' views (e.g. satisfaction surveys, complaints)
Patient behaviour (e.g. smoking quit rates, patient initiated changes of provider)

primary care organization would seek published evidence from research reporting on the levels of performance achieved by others or in the confines of carefully conducted clinical trials. Benchmarking offers another approach, although at present this is more commonly used in secondary than primary care. Benchmarking requires the collection of performance data about the outcomes (or processes) of care from a number of teams or organizations. The top performers are identified as the benchmarks, and the methods they use to attain their high performance are emulated. In summary, outcomes are often not included in quality improvement projects in primary care. However, the aim of health care is to improve outcome, and techniques are being developed for enabling judgements about quality from outcome data, and a greater role for outcome assessment in quality improvement is becoming possible.

Process

Assessment of the process of care is more common in quality improvement than assessment of outcome. Process concerns what health professionals and services do for patients and, therefore, the findings of process assessment provide direct information about what needs to change. Furthermore, it is generally easier to collect information about process than about outcome. In assessing the process of care, the elements of care that are appropriate must be specified. Whereas for outcome the level of desired performance is specified by reference to what has been achieved in the ideal circumstances of research studies or through benchmarking, for process research findings, evidence-based guidelines and/or expert opinion are used. The principal yardstick for judging the appropriateness of elements of process is the extent to which an element of process influences the outcome of care, but patient preferences should also be taken into account. When research evidence is limited or conflicting, the opinion of professionals may be used.

Since the identification of evidence from numerous research studies can be laborious, it is increasingly common to turn to up-to-date summaries of evidence in systematic reviews or good-quality clinical practice guidelines (see Chapters 13.3 and 13.4). Indeed, a relatively recent development in quality improvement has been the interest in the implementation of guidelines. The recommendations in guidelines or findings of systematic reviews must be expressed in terms—or review criteria—that facilitate the assessment of care. Review criteria are defined as 'systematically developed statements that can be used to assess the appropriateness of specific health care decisions and outcomes'. In undertaking a quality improvement project, the criteria specify in precise and measurable terms what care is desirable, and also determine what data are to be collected.

When convincing research evidence is not available, the group developing a quality improvement project must decide whether to develop criteria, and if so, how they will reach consensus. The eventual criteria will be influenced by the constitution of the group and the methods they use to reach agreement. Thus, a group that consists only of health professionals is unlikely to produce criteria that fully reflect the concerns of patients or funders. Methods of reaching agreement may be limited to informal discussion, in which case the views of the most influential person are most likely to predominate. Alternatively, formal methods such as the nominal group or Delphi techniques are available and can produce greater consensus.

Assessing care

The sources of information for assessing the appropriateness of quality of care include clinical records, registers of procedures or investigations, specially developed encounter sheets, and direct observation of professional/patient interactions that can include audio or video recording (Table 2). Each method has advantages and disadvantages.[7]

The main factors to be taken into account in selecting a source of information are the completeness of the information, its accuracy, and the feasibility of collecting it. In responding to these issues, the source of information should be selected to ensure that information can be obtained about the aspects of care that are of interest, and consideration should be given to using more than one data source.

Table 2 Sources of information about the process of care

Clinical records	General practitioners' records, nurses' records, patient-held records, hospital records etc.
Registers	Disease registers, appointment books, procedure registers
Observation	Directly, video tape, audio tape
Encounter sheets	The professional records information at the consultation on a specifically designed form
Patient reports	Patients are asked to report, on paper or in an interview, on what exactly took place in the contact with a professional or service

Completeness has two elements: (a) the extent to which the information source records full details about the process of care; and (b) the extent to which the information is completely recorded. Different information sources record information about different aspects of care. For example, video records of consultations between a professional and a patient potentially contain a complete record of the verbal exchange in the consultation, although aspects of the consultation may be excluded, such as a clinical examination. Records, on the other hand, may contain notes about the key findings on examination, prescribing and referral, but not the information given by the professional to the patient. However, factors other than the characteristics of the source can influence the completeness of the information. In the case of video tape, technical problems can lead to poor recording of sound. In the case of clinical records, different professionals have different habits in recording aspects of care, rendering the comparison of performance between such professionals impossible to interpret.

Problems with accuracy most commonly occur with registers of cases for diagnoses or procedures, for example, errors in coding diagnoses may have occurred. A pilot investigation to check the proportion of cases with such errors may be advisable. In extracting information from records, different data extractors may have placed slightly different interpretations on record entries and, therefore, careful training of data extractors is required to ensure a standardized approach. Although direct observation of consultations can provide complete information about verbal communication between professional and patient, the method would not be feasible for use with a very large number of professionals and patients. Similarly, the collection of information from a large number of records is costly in time and resources. Since the quality improvement cycle requires that data be collected more than once to check that improvements have been achieved (if required), the data collection systems must be efficient as well as sufficiently accurate.

Finally, the number of cases to be included should be adequate to ensure that confidence can be placed in the findings. Data relating to only a small number of selected patients will almost certainly give a misleading impression about the quality of care.

Changing performance

The key task of quality improvement is to change clinical practice when necessary. This issue is considered from different viewpoints in Chapters 13.4–13.6, and only a few salient points are made here. There is no method of implementing change that can be relied upon to be effective in all settings and circumstances, and the challenge facing those undertaking quality improvement is to match the chosen change strategies to the circumstances. A useful five-stage framework has been suggested by Grol[8] (see Table 3).

In the first stage, the change proposal, for example, a clinical guideline or review criterion, is developed and presented in an accessible and engaging format. In the second stage, an investigation of the obstacles to change is undertaken. These may be different for different professional groups or individuals, and may relate to the organization of the stage in the change process. In the third stage, the interventions to overcome the obstacles are selected. In the fourth stage, an explicit plan is developed for delivering the interventions, and in the fifth stage, the plan is carried out and evaluation

Table 3 A framework for implementing change

1. *Develop a change proposal* Crucial elements well defined Based on evidence and consensus Tested in practice, adapted to local needs Low complexity, compatible with existing routines Attractive, accessible format Credible source
2. *Identify obstacles to change* Obstacles related to clinician, social context of care provision, or organizational context Obstacles related to stage in change process (dissemination, adoption, implementation, continuation) Segmentation of target group
3. *Link interventions to obstacles* Dissemination: improve interest and understanding Adoption: improve attitude and intention to change Implementation: improve actual use Continuation: fixed habit
4. *Develop a plan* Combination of strategies Define intermediate and long-term aims Arrange procedures and tasks Set a time schedule
5. *Carry out the plan and evaluate progress* Carry out different steps and continuously evaluate progress

Reproduced with permission from Grol, R. (1997). *British Medical Journal* **315**, 418–21.

undertaken. This process can be related to theories of behaviour change, including educational, organizational, and marketing approaches, and also to evidence about the effectiveness of different implementation strategies in health care settings.[9,10]

It is essential to emphasize the final point. Information must be collected to monitor the success of attempts to improve care. Since no strategy can be relied on to be effective, monitoring is required to guide the use of additional methods when the degree of improvement is unsatisfactory. And once change has been achieved, there is always a risk that performance will deteriorate to earlier levels, and ideally, therefore, performance should be monitored at further intervals. If the topic is truly important in terms of patient health, arrangement for continuous monitoring should be considered. This is the stage at which the quality improvement cycle (Fig. 1) is completed by a further assessment of performance to determine whether changes have been successful.

Models of quality improvement

Quality improvement is a relatively recent innovation in health services and as yet no single model has emerged as the most effective. At intervals new approaches have been put forward, building on the experience of past approaches, but no predominant model has gained general acceptance. Most of the innovations have been evaluated first in secondary care settings, and progress in primary care has tended to adapt these models rather than develop new models for its own use.

The rational versus complex models

The rational model of quality improvement is based on the premise that individuals and health care teams are essentially rational, and if they are presented with information to show that their performance should be improved, they will take effective action. Thus, feedback of information about performance indicating lower standards in comparison with peers would be followed by appropriate change; likewise, education about better methods of delivering care would prompt change. In past years, most quality improvement activities have rested on the assumptions of the rational model. Of course, in view of the limited achievements of the model, the assumptions are now easy to regard as naive, but available research evidence does include examples in which substantial changes followed feedback or education alone. Therefore, professionals do sometimes behave in a rational way, but often other largely unknown factors operate to prevent rational behaviour.

The idea that quality improvement is a complex process has led to several models that are not mutually exclusive but form the foundation to various approaches to quality improvement. Exploration of the role of the individual professional has led to the emergence of the concept of the reflective practitioner.[11] Reflection on experience is used by the professional to devise and experiment with new and potentially more effective ways of working. This approach would suggest that the provision of feedback or education cannot be expected to produce change unless the professional has the opportunity to reflect. Theories about human behaviour change have been proposed as aids to increasing the impact of quality improvement efforts, including both psychological theories such as the transtheoretical model or social influence theory,[12] or the theories relating to marketing that underpin educational outreach.[13] The association of such theories with statistical techniques for monitoring performance gave rise to the method of total quality management that has been widely used in commercial settings.[14] In health care, the principles have been adapted and are often referred to as continuous quality improvement[15] (see Chapter 13.6). This approach firmly acknowledges that professional behaviour is human and not always rational, and emphasizes the need for functional teams, leadership, a focus on systems of care rather than individuals, and a culture that promotes learning from error rather than blame. Rapid cycles of data collection and adjustment of systems of care maintain motivation and promote continued incremental improvement.

Interest in the impact of the health care organization on quality of care is the most recent example of the complex model superceding the rational one. Theories of organizational behaviour seek to explain how the structure, processes, and culture of organizations influence their performance. Leadership within organizations is critical in ensuring that organizational behaviour is matched to the task the organization performs, but to regard organizations as being large human groups that follow a leader would be an over-simplification. Health care is a complex process, involving numerous important decisions each day for professionals. Innovations arise in rapid succession, and have to be evaluated and brought into routine practice if appropriate. Patients are infinitely diverse in conditions and preferences, and central leadership, however skilled and inspirational, cannot possibly ensure that the innumerable daily decisions are all appropriate. These considerations have led to a view of health care organizations as complex adaptive systems[16] in which leadership is required throughout all levels—including that of teams within primary health care—and is empowered to make decisions. It follows that primary health care teams need flexible leadership, empowerment to make decisions, and training in these skills.

Although the complex model of quality improvement is replacing the rational one in most fields, it has yet to have major impact on the training, continuing education, and organization of health professionals. The concept of the reflective practitioner is widely accepted and informs education, but the implications of recognizing that the decision-making and personal development of professionals is complex rather than rational have not been fully explored or implemented. The concept of the 'complex professional' and the methods needed to support and develop such an individual have yet to emerge.

The professional and organization models

A second set of contrasting models is related to the focus of quality improvement—who undertakes it, and who controls it? In the professional model, it is regarded as being an activity undertaken by health professionals. The activity is viewed as self-regulatory, confidential to professionals with data being protected from review by the public or authorities, the topics are

Table 4 Aspects of the role of the primary care organization in quality improvement

Setting objectives in the light of national priorities
Developing information systems
Training professionals in quality improvement methods
Creating a culture that promotes quality improvement and learning from error
Liaison with patients and local citizens on health care quality issues
Allocating resources (including time) for quality improvement activities
Making quality an overriding issue for the organization
Acting on the findings of quality improvement projects
Recognizing the achievements of teams and individuals in making improvements
Being accountable to the public and the health service

chosen by professionals, participation is voluntary, and the process is regarded as essentially educational. In some countries, quality improvement in primary care has largely grown from systems for continuing education. There are clear advantages in this model. It creates confidence among health professionals and encourages them to take part. It does not threaten professional status, and may even increase professional standing and self-esteem. It also enables professionals to learn the methods of quality improvement and develop positive attitudes towards their responsibility for maintaining quality.

The model also has inherent disadvantages. Since participation is voluntary, some professionals will not take part, and it is conceivable that those who most need to improve performance would be those least likely to participate. The methods of implementing change are likely to be limited in range and effectiveness. Education and feedback may have some impact, but changes that require the reallocation of resources or design of new systems of care may well demand the involvement of other disciplines, managers, and funders. Professionals are likely to concentrate their activities on topics of greatest concern to them, and indeed quality improvement systems should enable professionals to address such issues. But there is a risk that topics of importance to patients or those that are given local or national priority would be given less attention.

Some of these criticisms have been addressed by developments of the professional model. For example, in the Netherlands the model has been incorporated within a comprehensive system for assuring and improving quality. In the United Kingdom, medical audit for doctors was replaced by multiprofessional clinical audit in which teams of health professionals were encouraged to take part. However, the alternative to the professional model, or developments of it, is only gradually being introduced. The organization model of quality improvement is founded on the assumption that the organization has the major responsibility for motivating staff to undertake quality improvement, for providing resources and leadership, and for acting on the findings using a wide range of methods for changing performance. It is the organization, therefore, that is ultimately accountable for the quality of care. This development has taken place at the same time as the complex model of quality improvement has become more accepted.

The organization has many potential roles, and some of these are indicated in Table 4. In general terms, the organization should make quality an important issue, and provide the resources and leadership to enable all staff in the organization to contribute to making improvements. Given the range of functions that organizations can have, it is not surprising that in many countries this model is slowly being adopted, although the pace of change is slower in general practice where the professional model is still dominant. However, the long-term success of quality improvement systems may well rest on the extent to which the professional and organizational models are allowed to operate in harmony.

A key role of organizations should be liaison with patients and the local community to ensure that they both have a full role in quality improvement. This issue is discussed in detail in Chapter 13.7 and is not considered in detail here.

Table 5 Activities at the level of the health care system related to quality improvement

Leadership	The importance of quality and quality improvement; promoting an appropriate culture
Policy making	Legislation, resources, health service policy, national priorities for topics
Clinical guidance	National guidelines, guidance statements, national standards of care
Contracts	Methods of reimbursing staff, incentives and sanctions, fee-for-service or capitation payments
Regulation	Certification, revalidation, disciplinary procedures
Inspection	Inspection of health care organizations, including assessment of their quality improvement activities
The public	Listening and responding to concerns, managing expectations
Education	Policies on education for professionals, in association with professional bodies

The political/legal model

The final model to consider is at the level of the health care system. Different countries have different legislative and managerial frameworks for promoting quality and quality improvement. To some extent these reflect the different structures of heath care systems, but also reflect different political views about the role of the state in society, and the legal and other codes that govern the national definition of quality of health care. Nevertheless, it is possible to identify a set of functions that relate to the health care system at national level, and a trend towards greater involvement at this level in activities related to quality improvement in most countries, including the United States, although such involvement is not necessarily governmental. Table 5 lists some of these activities.

The political/legal model argues that the policies of the health care system influence quality improvement activities, and that the role of policy makers and the system they create is to promote quality improvement and to account to the public for the quality of care achieved. For the most part, the activities in themselves do not constitute quality improvement. However, they do create the framework for quality improvement in health care settings, and encourage it to take place.

An assumption that appears to underlie many of the activities at the health system level is that a greater degree of control or involvement from the national level is likely to increase quality improvement activity and ultimately the quality of care. However, it is difficult to identify from the various activities those that will sustain the dedication and motivation of health professionals in their working lives. The political/legal model does not yet incorporate activities to nurture these fundamental qualities of people who care for the sick. Indeed, it is possible that as the influence of the political/legal model extends, the role of the professional model will contract. This would be to the eventual detriment of the quality of care, but as this process becomes clear, we must hope that the political/legal model will evolve in a way that corrects this deficiency.

Conclusions

In this chapter, we have outlined some of the key principles for quality improvement. The meaning of quality has been discussed, the perspective of different groups being emphasized. The quality cycle has been discussed and a framework for implementing change outlined. Finally, the general models underlying specific approaches to quality improvement have been discussed. Since quality improvement is a relatively new activity in health care, evidence and experience about its impact is limited. Nevertheless, there is increasing recognition of the importance of complex factors that include the behaviour of professionals, organizations, and health care systems. The following chapters consider in more detail particular aspects of quality improvement methods.

References

1. **Marwick, J., Grol, R., and Borgiel, A.** *Quality Assurance for Family Doctors.* Report of the Quality Assurance Working Party of the World Organization of Family Doctors. Jolimont: WONCA, 1992.
2. **Institute of Medicine.** *Medicare: A Strategy for Quality Assurance* Vol. II. Washington DC: National Academy Press, 1990.
3. **Donabedian, A.** *Explorations in Quality Assessment and Monitoring. The Definition of Quality and Approaches to its Assessment* Vol. 1. Ann Arbor: Health Administration Press, 1980.
4. **Grol, R. and Lawrence, M.** *Quality Improvement by Peer Review.* Oxford General Practice Series. Oxford: Oxford University Press, 1995.
5. **Fraser, R.C., Lakhani, M.K., and Baker, R.H.** *Evidence-Based Audit in General Practice.* Oxford: Butterworth-Heinemann, 1998.
6. **Grol, R., Wensing, M., Mainz, J., Ferreira, P., Hearnshaw, H., Hjortdahl, P., Olesen, F., Ribacke, M., Spenser, T., and Szecsenyi, J.** (1999). Patients' priorities with respect to general practice care: an international comparison. *Family Practice* **16**, 4–11.
7. **Rethans, J.J., Westin, S., and Hays, R.** (1996). Methods for quality assessment in general practice. *Family Practice* **13**, 468–76.
8. **Grol, R.** (1997). Personal paper: beliefs and evidence in changing clinical practice. *British Medical Journal* **315**, 418–21.
9. **Grol, R. and Grimshaw, J.** (1999). Evidence-based implementation of evidence-based medicine. *Journal on Quality Improvement* **25**, 503–13.
10. **Baker, R., Stevenson, K., Shaw, E., Redsell, S., Morrell, C., and Scrivener, R.** *Best Practice in Clinical Audit: Review of the Evidence.* National Institute for Clinical Excellence. Abingdon: Radcliffe Medical Press, 2002.
11. **Schon, D.A.** *The Reflective Practitioner. How Professionals Think in Action.* London: Maurice Temple Smith Ltd, 1983.
12. **Robertson, N., Baker, R., and Hearnshaw, H.** (1996). Changing the clinical behaviour of doctors—a psychological framework. *Quality in Health Care* **5**, 51–4.
13. **Mittman, B., Tonesk, X., and Jacobson, P.** (1992). Implementing clinical practice guidelines: social influence strategies and practitioner behavior change. *Quality Review Bulletin* **18**, 413–22.
14. **Oakland, J.S.** *Total Quality Management* 2nd edn. Oxford: Butterworth-Heinemann, 1993.
15. **Berwick, D.M.** (1992). Heal thyself or heal thy system: can doctors help to improve medical care? *Quality in Health Care* **1** (Suppl.), s2–8.
16. **Institute of Medicine.** *Crossing the Quality Chasm: A New Health System for the 21st Century.* Washington DC: National Academy Press, 2001.

13.2 Measuring the quality of primary medical care

Martin Roland and Martin Marshall

Introduction

The last decade of the twentieth century has seen an enormous increase in interest in measuring and monitoring the quality of medical care. There are two main reasons for this; first the importance of measurement for improving quality and secondly the need for greater explicit accountability of health professionals and health systems. For many branches of medicine, primary care included, this focus on measurement was new. In this chapter, we describe some of the key issues around measurement in family practice. We start by highlighting some of the political, societal, and professional reasons for focusing on measurement. We then provide a framework for measuring quality in family practice and explore the development and role of quality indicators in this process. We describe some of the ways in which indicators can be used and ways in which we believe they should not be used. Finally, we emphasize the need to move beyond what is easily measured in order to truly reflect the nature and role of general practice.

Why should quality of primary care be measured?

The first reason for measuring quality of care was the recognition of how much variation existed in the quality of care provided. Initially, researchers focused on technical issues, for example, demonstrating large geographic variation in rates for surgical procedures. More sophisticated methods were then developed to assess the appropriateness of these procedures.[1] These showed that a substantial proportion of procedures carried out on patients did not need to be done, while other patients who would benefit from the procedures did not receive them.[2] Inappropriate over-use, under-use, and misuse of medical procedures appeared to co-exist, and this could be found wherever the issue was studied.[3–5] Although this research was initially done in relation to specialist practice, considerable gaps are also found between the care that primary care physicians aim to give, and the care which they actually deliver.[6]

Recognition of the phenomenon of variation is not new. Over 2000 years ago, Hippocrates commented that:

> In acute diseases, practitioners differ so much among themselves that those things which one administers thinking the best that can be given, another holds to be bad . . . and similar differences are to be found in the examination of entrails.
>
> Hippocrates, 460–377 BC

Variation in medical practice is not of itself a bad thing. However, it may be a bad thing where variation is associated with demonstrable deficiencies in quality of care. The demonstration of variation in medical practice led in the late 1990s to the widespread realization that some aspects of medical care were frankly unacceptable. In several countries, there have been high-profile health scandals and medical error is now recognized as an important cause of harm to patients.[7,8]

In the public's mind there has been some confusion between the research showing widespread variation in medical practice and the presence of the very small number of doctors whose practice is totally unacceptable. Nevertheless, both of these issues have combined to produce demands for greater accountability from the medical profession. Doctors needed to be able to assure the public that the quality of medical care they provided was of a high standard. This was in line with other societal changes where citizens expected demonstrable high standards from both public services and private industry. The medical profession has not been immune from these expectations.

Some of the drivers for change have been doctors themselves. The rise of evidence-based practice has given doctors the means to examine their own care. Their own professional ethic of doing as well as they can for their patients has been to a large extent been behind the widespread move in the last decade of the twentieth century for doctors to participate in medical audit and quality circles, most often within their own practices or medical groups.

The relative influence of these various factors has played out differently in different countries. In the Netherlands, there has been a strong professional movement to develop national clinical guidelines, and to encourage professional development activities around these guidelines. This has been a 'bottom up' approach, led by the doctors themselves. In the United Kingdom, on the other hand, government has taken a much more 'top down' central role in attempting to introduce a national system of mandatory quality reporting and assessment. In the United States, the link between quality improvement and cost containment has become blurred, with the public regarding attempts to reduce the inappropriate over-provision of care (e.g. by strengthening the gate-keeper role of the primary care physician) as depriving them of choice and a reduction in quality.

The impact of these international societal changes on the medical profession has been profound, and doctors struggle with changes in the way society views them. The old English adage 'Trust me, I'm a doctor' now rings hollow, and doctors wonder what their new place in society will be. It is clear that a new type of professionalism is emerging, which Irvine defines as:

- Clear professional values compatible with public expectations.
- The use of explicit standards.
- The adoption of collective as well as personal responsibility for observing standards of practice.
- Systematic process for showing that doctors are up to date and perform well.
- Effective local medical regulation, including swift and effective machinery for dealing with dysfunctional doctors.

Derived from Irvine[9]

Given this background, there are a number of reasons for measuring quality of care. The main ones relate either to improving quality, or to providing external accountability. Another important reason is to provide consumers or payers (e.g. employers) with information to give them choice about the health care they seek.

Where quality of care is demonstrably deficient, the response of most professionals will be to try to improve it. Thus, for example, clinical audit is an activity undertaken by professionals in order to assess the quality of care they are providing, and, if necessary, to improve it. This is an activity that takes place entirely within the practice or workplace of the individual doctor or group of doctors. Improving quality of care is the first reason for measuring quality of care, and it is the one that is likely to be uppermost in the minds of doctors. Measuring quality is an essential prerequisite to improving care:[10] improvements are unlikely to take place unless data are available on what is already being achieved.

The second reason for assessing quality of care is to demonstrate to the public that acceptable standards of care are being provided—public accountability. This is a driver that is most likely to be given prominence by governments and payers for health care who are looking for value for money and want to be able to demonstrate to the population that their health service is delivering a high quality of care.

What aspects of care should be measured?

The first section of this chapter outlined the political, societal, and professional forces behind the drive to measure the quality of medical care. What then should be measured?

This question is a particularly taxing one for primary care. For some branches of medicine, there are fairly clear outcomes. In cardiac surgery, for example, communication with the patient and quality of the hospital food might both be measured, but the assessment of case-mix adjusted success rate, complication rate, and mortality are of prime importance. Most effort will, appropriately, go into assessing these latter aspects of care.

Primary care is different. The work of primary care is diffuse, and addresses a wide range of patients' needs. Quality in primary care is multifaceted and cannot be assessed in terms of a single or simple outcome. Assessment of quality, therefore, needs to be multifaceted in order to avoid an inappropriate focus on narrow areas and to prevent perverse incentives for improvement.

Box 1 What patients want from primary care[11,12]

- Availability and accessibility, including availability of appointments, waiting times, physical access, and telephone access.
- Technical competence, including the doctor's knowledge and skills, and the effectiveness of his or her treatments.
- Communication skills, including providing time, exploring patients' needs, listening, explaining, giving information, and sharing decisions.
- Interpersonal attributes, including humaneness, caring, supporting, and trust.
- Organization of care, including continuity of care, coordination of care, and availability of onsite services.

Box 2 Domains of quality in primary care[14,15]

Quality of care for individuals is determined by
- Access
- Effectiveness of care
  - Technical care
  - Interpersonal care
- Organization of care

Quality of care for populations is additionally determined by
- Equity
- Efficiency

In thinking about what aspects of primary care should be measured and monitored, it is appropriate to start with what patients want most from their primary care physicians. This is summarized in Box 1.

There are a number of ways in which the domains of quality of care can be classified. The central domains are access and effectiveness—can patients get to health care and is it any good when they get there? From a general practice perspective, it is important to recognize that effectiveness includes both effective clinical care and effective interpersonal care in order to reflect the prominence of interpersonal care in what patients want. Both clinical care and interpersonal care have technical elements that can be taught and learned, and neither is sufficient on its own. Providing good clinical care is not sufficient to be a good general practitioner,[13] and good interpersonal skills cannot be a substitute for poor clinical skills. Providing good access and providing effective care cannot be delivered without there being good organization of care, and assessing practice organization and management may be an important part of the equation.

For populations, there are two other elements that are important—equity and efficiency. Efficiency is an important marker of quality of care for populations as inefficient care (e.g. prescribing expensive but ineffective drugs) may have opportunity costs for the care that can be provided to other patients. These domains of quality are summarized in Box 2.

Any approach to assessing the quality of primary medical care needs to be aware of these domains of care. To focus on one risks devaluing other aspects of care. For example, doctors taking part in a major quality improvement scheme focusing on the quality of chronic disease management noted that access and interpersonal aspects of care sometimes suffered as a result.[16]

How can quality of care be assessed?

Following a description of the domains of quality that are important to primary medical care, the next question is how these should be measured. A wide range of methods are available.[17] To date, much quality assessment has been carried out entirely within practices—doctors have set out to find out about aspects of their care that could be better, and used this as a starting point for improving quality.[18] Medical audit[19] requires that the doctors of the practice set standards and review their own practice against those standards.

However, there is an increasing focus on using methods that more readily allow information to be shared outside the practice. They may focus on assessing competence (what a doctor is capable of doing) or performance (what he or she actually does). Consultations may be observed directly or on videotape (a requirement for gaining a licence as a general practitioner in the United Kingdom) or assessed indirectly from patient questionnaires (now a routine part of much US practice). The doctor's work can be examined by reviewing medical records (a regular part of peer assessment visits in the Netherlands) or by data provided for payers (a method used routinely in the United States). Sometimes, specific payments are tied to information about quality of care, for example, the attainment of specified levels of cervical cytology or immunization coverage in the United Kingdom.

When quality assessment is required for external review, it is most frequently measured by applying quality indicators. A quality indicator relates to a specific measurable aspect of care that is sensitive to change and can be applied retrospectively to assess quality of care.[20] Quality indicators also need to represent aspects of care that are under the control of the practitioner. Quality indicators highlight areas of performance that may require further investigation: they do not make definitive judgements about quality. Indicators are different from guidelines, targets, and standards (Box 3). In many cases, it is not appropriate to set targets for quality indicators—minimum standards may be set locally if appropriate but the onus for the majority of practices should be to show sustained improvement over time. This is more important than absolute levels of achievement, since some practices will have greater difficulty achieving specific targets, often for reasons outside their control (e.g. patient characteristics or lack of resources).

Quality indicators can assess structure, process, or outcomes of care. In practice, outcomes are rarely suitable as quality indicators for primary care—they often occur long after the care given by the primary care physician, and may be confounded by factors outside his or her control. So, for example, ensuring that blood pressure is monitored and controlled is a more appropriate quality indicator for primary care of diabetes than the incidence of stroke or renal failure.

In practice, few indicators satisfy all the criteria for a good quality indicator, and many look more like guidelines–that is, they are more suitable for prospective guidance than retrospective assessment. In the appendix to this chapter, some examples are provided of quality indicators that could be applied to primary medical practice. These are mapped to the domains of care outlined in Box 2. In addition to these indicators, others are available relating to clinical care for some of the most common conditions seen in general practice.[21]

Apart from quality indicators, there are other established ways of approaching quality assessment in primary care. Colleges and Associations of family physicians have been among the leaders of promoting quality assurance systems for primary care. Available measures of quality in primary care include:

United Kingdom: The Royal College of General Practitioners. This has a number of schemes, including Membership by Assessment of Performance, Fellowship by Assessment, the Quality Practice Award, and Quality Team Development. These are described at www.rcgp.org.uk. The UK College is the only English-speaking college that published full details of all quality criteria and methods of assessment on its website. A range of quality indicators for the problems seen most commonly in British general practice are also available.[21] In future, general practitioners' remuneration in the United Kingdom is likely to depend on their performance against a broad set of quality indicators.

Australia: The Royal Australian College of General Practitioners publishes standards for general practice that can be ordered from its website. The website also contains downloadable guidelines for an 'enhanced primary care program' and details of its practice accreditation scheme. These are available at www.racgp.org.au.

United States: The American Association of Family Practice website contains a limited number of clinical policy statements, relating especially to childhood disorders and immunization, www.aafp.org. The HEDIS measures, which are widely used in the United States are described in outline at www.ncqa.org and can be ordered from the National Committee for Quality Assurance website at www.ncqa.org. The US government also maintains a national guideline clearing house at http://www.guideline.gov/index.asp. Quality indicators relevant to primary care have also been developed by the RAND Corporation.[22–24]

Netherlands: The Dutch College of General Practitioners has been among the most active in taking a systematic approach to developing clinical guidelines for general practitioners, and disseminating them among its membership. They are published in two books,[25,26] and are currently available in English on the website of the college, www.artsennet.nl/nhg. From 60 of these guidelines about 140 indicators have been produced and are currently being validated in Dutch general practices.

Both the College of Family Physicians of Canada, www.cfpc.ca, and the Royal New Zealand College of General Practitioners, www.rnzcgp.org.nz, currently publish a small selection of web based guidelines.

In other cases, academic groups have led efforts to develop sets of quality indicators that could be used on a widespread basis, either based around interpersonal aspects of the consultation,[27] or by applying the principles of evidence-based practice.[28] Other resources relevant to the development of quality indicators, for example, availability of information on evidence-based practice, are described in more detail in Chapter 13.3.

Patient evaluation is an important part of quality assessment, especially for interpersonal aspects of care and assessment of patients' access to primary care. A number of instruments are available for assessing patients' views. Those available in the public domain include:

The Primary Care Assessment Survey[29,30] (PCAS) has been used widely in the United States, and has evidence of both predictive validity and sensitivity to change.[31,32]

The General Practice Assessment Survey[33,34] (GPAS) was developed from the American PCAS for use in the United Kingdom. Its website (www.gpas.co.uk) contains the instrument, manual, national benchmarks, and software for analysis using both Excel and SPSS.

EUROPEP (www.equip.ch/groups/pep/europep.pdf) takes a similar approach to GPAS, and is available in 15 European languages.

Box 3 Examples of guidelines, indicators, and targets or standards

Guideline: Eligible women are offered routine cervical screening.

Indicator: The proportion of eligible women who have had cervical screening carried out within the recommended period.

Target or standard: The proportion of eligible women who have had cervical screening carried out within the recommended period should exceed 80 per cent.

Methods of developing quality indicators

In the past, quality indicators have most frequently been developed by experts meeting and forming a consensus about what care should be given and how it should be assessed. Sometimes, this can lead to strikingly inappropriate results, for example, when a group dominated by specialists produces measures for use in primary care. This process can be improved by deriving indicators directly from clinical guidelines. This method has been used extensively in the Netherlands where detailed guidelines have been produced from research evidence and professional consensus. The emergence of evidence-based practice offered an opportunity to introduce new rigour into the indicator development process, and some groups have explicitly concentrated on evidence in producing quality indicators.[25] However, the evidence base, certainly in terms of randomized controlled trials, is weak for much of the medicine which primary care physicians practice. So, methods are needed to combine both what is known from the literature (including but by no means exclusively trials) and professional opinion from appropriate sources—for example, primary care practitioners with particular expertise in an area. These approaches can be combined systematically to develop quality indicators for primary care. The importance of making use of both evidence and professional opinion is well demonstrated by the finding that of a set of quality indicators produced for asthma, angina, and diabetes management in primary care, only 26 per cent were judged by the panelists to have a strong evidence base.[35] Furthermore, some important aspects of care may simply be unmeasurable with methods currently available—it is, therefore, important to recognize the extent to which any set of quality indicators can only offer a partial window on quality of care.

When quality indicators are developed, it is important that the details of the method used should be explicit. There should be a description of how evidence was collected from the literature, when the literature was searched (quality indicators may change as new evidence accumulates), who assessed the evidence, and how they developed indicators from the information they had available. There is no perfect method, and the way in which the process is carried out can have a substantial impact on the end result.

The need for caution when using quality indicators

While there may be some benefits to measuring quality of care, there are also substantial potential drawbacks. Before thinking about using any quality indicators, there are some very important issues to bear in mind:

- Any set of quality indicators for primary care that sets out to be comprehensive needs to reflect the many and varied functions fulfilled by primary care. This will prevent an inappropriate focus on narrow areas of activity. However, if indicators attempt to be comprehensive, they will almost certainly be too cumbersome for practical use.
- There may be substantial data collection costs associated with measuring the quality of primary care without any clear benefit in terms of quality improvement. Measuring quality on its own does not improve care. Therefore, there is little point in setting out to assess quality unless there is some sort of infrastructure to ensure that the data are used.
- Some indicators will inevitably be more 'evidence based'. Even for disorders like angina, diabetes, and asthma, the proportion of quality indicators that can truly be evidence based is quite small. However, all indicators should have face validity, for example, reflecting professional consensus in medical practice.
- The data available for assessing quality, for example, clinical data in medical records may vary greatly between physicians and practices. This can make it very difficult to compare data between sites.
- Practices vary considerably in the ways in which they are organized and how they provide services for their patients. A number of the indicators may not be appropriate for every practice, or for practice in every country.
- Within localities, it can still be difficult to interpret apparent differences between the performance of physicians or practices or to know what, if any, action needs to be taken.
- It is important to remember that these are *indicators* of quality, not definitive judgements. As such, caution is required when making comparisons between practices or over time. The great strength of indicators is in promoting discussion about the possible reasons for any differences found and ways of improving the quality of care provided.
- Quality indicators will always be subject to gaming or mis-representation by some individuals or organizations. This is a particular risk when indicators are used inappropriately to make judgements, rather than to encourage engagement with a quality improvement process. The risk of gaming should be recognized and minimized where possible but it should be clear that there is more to be gained than to be lost by trusting primary care professionals to use quality indicators honestly.

What information is routinely available for assessing quality care?

Most health care systems have had little or no information available on quality of care until quite recently. The United States has been most active in developing systems for providing information on clinical activity that can be used to assess quality of care. Although the United States is relatively data rich in terms of what goes on in primary care, such data have in the past been almost exclusively collected for the purposes of billing. Information collected for financial reasons is unlikely to be well designed for quality assessment, but in recent years, systems have been developed (e.g. HEDIS, discussed earlier) which allow individual health plans to be compared by those purchasing health care (mainly employers) or those who use them (the patients). Report cards that describe the quality of care given by health plans are now widely available in the United States, though their validity and reliability are uncertain.[36]

The UK government has also taken a lead in disseminating information on quality of care. Unfortunately, the first attempts were based entirely on routinely available data. Since these data were not collected with quality in mind, it was hardly surprising that they were a very poor reflection of quality of care—with one commentary regarding 'the remedy as worse than the malady'.[37] These indicators included aggregates of hospital admission rates for conditions where good primary care might be expected, in theory at least, to prevent admission (e.g. diabetes, epilepsy, and heart failure), and a number of prescribing indicators. Where routine data for payment do relate to quality of care, then such data may allow widespread comparisons to be made validly. Also in the United Kingdom, target payments have been made to primary care practitioners for some years for meeting cervical cytology and immunization targets—measures that have broad acceptance as being at least partial measures of quality of care in those clinical domains, albeit crude ones.

Where this field moves in future remains to be seen. If payers for medical care (e.g. insurance companies or governments) are serious about wishing to assess quality of care on a routine basis, then information systems could certainly be designed to provide such information.[38] Whether the benefits in terms of quality improvement would be worth the data collection costs remains to be seen.

One further source of information on quality of care relates to the licencing of individual doctors. For reasons outlined earlier in this chapter, many developed countries are developing systems for accrediting or revalidating their doctors.[39] While re-certification has been practiced in the United States for some years, systems are now being introduced in the United Kingdom, the Netherlands, Australia, Canada, and New Zealand. The United States is the only country to rely heavily on external testing. The other countries are developing systems that rely more on the demonstration of planned professional development (e.g. developing and following a personal learning plan), and demonstration of standards achieved (e.g. clinical audit). In the Netherlands and Australia, this is combined with peer assessment carried out through a series of practice visits.[40] As with other aspects of quality assessment, it remains to be seen what mixture will provide the best balance in terms of assuring the quality of medical care at an acceptable cost.

To whom should information on quality of care be available?

Given the increasing moves towards measuring quality of care, there has been considerable debate about who the information should be made available to. The United States has led on making information available to the general public. This is ostensibly to provide external accountability, and to give the public information so that they can take quality into account when choosing where to get their medical care. However, even in this most consumerist of societies, the public has actually taken little notice of information on quality of care. Moreover, doctors have been highly mistrustful of the quality of data provided. Thus, from either the doctor or the patient end, making information on quality of care publicly available appears to have little impact at present. However, providing this information to management in health care organizations (e.g. health plans) appears to have had greater effect, and it is perhaps at this level that information will have its greatest impact.(41)

The United Kingdom is also moving down the road of making information on quality of care routinely available outside the individual practice. In 2000, 50 per cent of primary care groups and trusts were making or planning to make comparative information on quality of care available in identified form to the practices within their group, and 9 per cent were planning to make such information available to the public.(42) However, patients may differ from professionals in the aspects of care that they consider important for quality and the benefits of making such information available,(43) either in terms of improved quality or in terms of public confidence in medical care remain to be seen. Both public and doctors are at present suspicious of the motives and value of making such information available.(44)

Conclusion

Primary care physicians cannot escape the current trend to want to measure quality. For the reasons outlined in this chapter, it is desirable that general practitioners engage with and influence the measurement process. Nevertheless, the trend towards explicit measurement poses considerable problems for a discipline such as general practice. Much of what general practitioners do is diverse and difficult to define. Good communication, attention to interpersonal care, integration of care, and coordination of care are all important aspects of what general practitioners do. Yet, they are much more difficult to measure than more mechanical tasks such as compliance with chronic disease management protocols. Furthermore, reducing general practice to identifiable component parts risks misunderstanding the patient focus of general practice care(45) and hence missing the benefits of a comprehensive generalist service.

The measurement culture, therefore, creates a dilemma for general practice. Will the things that are measured simply be those that can be measured easily? If so, any accountability based on quality indicators will be a very partial activity. Will the unmeasured parts then be forgotten and devalued? Alternatively, should general practice develop measures of some of its fundamental and defining features? In doing so, there is a risk that this will simply perpetuate the reductionist environment in which health services throughout the world increasingly operate. We believe that crucial aspects of what general practitioners do, such as providing high-quality interpersonal care, must be included in future performance indicators for primary care. This would do much to preserve their importance at a time when many fear that traditional values are being lost from general practice. In rapidly changing times, general practitioners need to keep sight of their core values that will ensure that the contribution of general practice to patient care is appropriately valued and rewarded.

Appendix

Examples of quality indicators for family practice

1. Access to care

- For urgent matters, patients should be able to see or speak to a doctor or nurse on the day of the request.
- Routine appointments with doctors and nurses should be booked at intervals of no less than 10 min.

2. Effectiveness of care: clinical care

- The childhood immunization rate should be over 90 per cent, or if below, efforts should be made to improve the rate year on year.
- Patients with coronary artery disease should be advised to take 75–150 mg aspirin per day indefinitely unless contraindicated.
- HbA1c levels should be checked at least every 14 months as part of an annual check in all diabetic patients.
- Drug therapy should be offered to all patients with sustained blood pressure of more than 160/100, if non-pharmacological measures have been applied.

3. Effectiveness of care: interpersonal care

- Practices should seek information about patient/carer experience at least once every 3 years, using a recognized technique, and the results should be made available to the practice population.
- A report of the number and type of complaints made to the practice, and of the response of the practice should be available for scrutiny.

4. Organization of care

- Practices should be organized so that members of the primary care team have an opportunity to meet at regular intervals, appropriate to the team needs.
- Patient records should be in chronological order, with a clear summary of key conditions and medication.
- Practices should have a written management guideline for conditions identified as priorities, for example, diabetes, enduring mental health problems, coronary artery disease, hypertension and these guidelines should be updated as required.
- Practices should have and use a prescribing formulary (developed within or outside the practice).

5. Efficiency

- The generic prescribing rate of individual doctors should be known and monitored.
- The rates of admission and referral to specialists should be known and discussed.

6. Equity

- Practices should accept all patients living within their practice area or be able to provide an acceptable explanation for refusal to do so: practices should not systematically refuse to register particular categories of patient, for example, the homeless, the severely mentally ill, or those with problems of substance or alcohol misuse.

References

1. **Kahan, J.P.** et al. (1994). Measuring the necessity of medical procedures. *Medical Care* **32**, 357–65.
2. **Shuster, M.A., McGlynn, E.A., and Brook, R.H.** (1998). How good is the quality of health care in the United States? *Milbank Quarterly* **76**, 517–63.
3. **McGlynn, E.A.** et al. (1994). Comparison of the appropriateness of coronary angiography and coronary artery bypass surgery between Canada and New York State. *Journal of the American Medical Association* **272**, 934–40.
4. **Meijler, A.P., Rigter, H., Bernstein, S.J., Schloma, J.K., McDonnell, J., Breeman, A., Kosekoff, J.B., and Brook, R.H.** (1997). The appropriateness of intention to treat decisions for invasive therapy in coronary artery disease in the Netherlands. *Heart* **77**, 219–24.
5. **Bernstein, S.J., Kosecoff, J., Gray, D., Hampton, J.R., and Brook, R.H.** (1993). The appropriateness of the use of cardiovascular procedures. British versus US perspectives. *International Journal of Technology Assessment in Health Care* **9**, 3–10.
6. **Seddon, M.E., Marshall, M.N., Campbell, S.M., and Roland, M.O.** (2001). A systematic review of the quality of clinical care provided in general practice in the United Kingdom, Australia and New Zealand. *Quality in Health Care* **10**, 152–8.
7. **Kohn, L.H., Corrigan, J., and Donaldson, M.S.**, ed. *To Err is Human.* Washington DC: National Academy Press, 2000.
8. **Department of Health.** *An Organisation With a Memory.* London: Department of Health, 2000.
9. **Irvine, D.** (1999). The performance of doctors: the new professionalism. *Lancet* **353**, 1174–7.

10. **Deming, W.E.** *Out of Crisis*. Cambridge MA: Massachussets Institute of Technology, 1986.
11. **Buetow, S.** (1995). What do general practitioners and their patients want from general practice and are they receiving it: a framework. *Social Science and Medicine* **40**, 213–21.
12. **Wensing, M., Jung, H.P., Mainz, J., Olesen, F., and Grol, R.** (1998). A systematic review of the literature on patient priorities for general practice. Part 1: description of the research domain. *Social Science and Medicine* **47**, 1573–88.
13. **McWhinney, I.R.** (1988). Core values in a changing world. *British Medical Journal* **316**, 1807–9.
14. **Roland, M.O.** (1999). Quality and efficiency: enemies or partners? *British Journal of General Practice* **49**, 140–3.
15. **Campbell, S., Roland, M., and Buetow, S.** (2000). Defining quality of care. *Social Science and Medicine* **51**, 1611–25.
16. **Spooner, A., Chapple, A., and Roland, M.** (2001). What makes doctors take part a major quality improvement initiative? A qualitative study of the reasons for professional behaviour change. *Journal of Health Services Research and Policy* **6**, 145–50.
17. **Rethans, J.-J., Westin, S., and Hays, R.** (1996). Methods for quality assessment in general practice. *Family Practice* **13**, 468–76.
18. **Grol, R. and Lawrence, M.** *Quality Improvement by Peer Review*. Oxford: Oxford University Press, 1995.
19. **Lawrence, M. and Schofield, T.** *Medical Audit in Primary Health Care*. Oxford: Oxford University Press, 1993.
20. **Lawrence, M. and Olesen, F.** (1997). Indicators of quality in health care. *European Journal of General Practice* **3**, 103–8.
21. **Marshall, M., Campbell, S., Roland, M., and Hacker, J.** *Quality Indicators for Common General Practice Problems*. Royal Society of Medicine Press, 2001.
22. **Kerr, E.A., Asch, S., Hamilton, E.G., and McGlynn, E.A.** *Quality of Care for General Medical Conditions: A Review of the Literature and Quality Indicators*. Santa Monica CA: RAND Health Program, 1998.
23. **Kerr, E.A., Asch, S., Hamilton, E.G., and McGlynn, E.A.** *Quality of Care for Cardio-Pulmonary Conditions: A Review of the Literature and Quality Indicators*. Santa Monica CA: RAND Health Program, 1998.
24. **McGlynn, E.A., Kerr, E.A., Damberg, C., and Asch, S.** *Quality of Care for Women: A Review of Selected Clinical Conditions and Quality Indicators*. Santa Monica CA: RAND Health Program, 1997.
25. **Geijer, R.M.M., Burgers, J.S., van der Laan, J.R., Wiersma, T.J., Rosmalen, C.F.H., and Thomas, S.**, ed. *NHG-Standaarden voor de huisarts 1. Maarsen*. The Netherlands: Elsevier/Bunge, 1999.
26. **Thomas, S., Geijer, R.M.M., van der Laan, J.R., and Wiersma, T.J.**, ed. *NHG-Standaarden voor de huisarts 2. Maarsen*. The Netherlands: Elsevier/Bunge, 1999.
27. **Howie, J.R.G., Heaney, D.J., Maxwell, M., Walker, J.J., and Freeman, G.K.** (2000). Developing a 'consultation quality index' (CQI) for use in general practice. *Family Practice* **17**, 455–61.
28. **McColl, A., Roderick, P., Smith, H., Wilkinson, E., Moore, M., Exworthy, M., and Gabbay, J.** (2000). Clinical governance in primary care groups: the feasibility of deriving evidence based performance indicators. *Quality in Health Care* **9**, 90–7.
29. **Safran, D.G.** et al. (1998). The Primary Care Assessment Survey: tests of data quality and measurement performance. *Medical Care* **36**, 728–39.
30. **Murray, A. and Safran, D.G.** (2000). The Primary Care Assessment Survey: a tool for measuring, monitoring and improving primary care. In *Handbook of Psychological Assessment in Primary Care Settings* (ed. M.E. Maruish), pp. 623–65. Mahwah NJ: Lawrence Erlbaum Associates Inc.
31. **Gelb Safran, D.G., Montgomery, J.E., Chang, H., Murphy, J., and Rogers, W.** (2001). Switching doctors: predictors of voluntary disenrollment from a primary physician's practice. *Journal of Family Practice* **50**, 130–6.
32. **Murphy, J., Chang, H., Montgomery, J.E., Rogers, W.H., and Safran, D.G.** (2001). The quality of physician-patient relationships: patients' experiences 1996–1999. *Journal of Family Practice* **50**, 123–9.
33. **Ramsay, J., Campbell, J., Schroter, S., Green, J., and Roland, M.** (2000). The General Practice Assessment Survey (GPAS): tests of data quality and measurement properties. *Family Practice* **15**, 272–9.
34. **Campbell, J.L., Ramsay, J., and Green, J.** (2001). Age, gender, socio-economic and ethnic differences in patients' assessment of primary health care. *Quality in Health Care* **10**, 90–5.
35. **Campbell, S.M., Roland, M.O., Shekelle, P.G., Cantrill, J.A., Buetow, S.A., and Cragg, D.K.** (1999). The development of review criteria for assessing the quality of management of stable angina, adult asthma and non insulin dependent diabetes mellitus in general practice. *Quality in Health Care* **8**, 6–15.
36. **Hofer, T.P., Hayward, R.A., Greenfield, S., Wagner, E.H., Kaplan, S.H., and Manning, W.G.** (1999). The unreliability of individual physician report cards for assessing the costs and quality of a chronic disease. *Journal of the American Medical Association* **291**, 2098–105.
37. **Davies, H.T.O. and Lampel, J.** (1998). Trust in performance indicators? *Quality in Health Care* **7**, 159–62.
38. **Shekelle, P. and Roland, M.** (1998). Measuring quality in the NHS: lessons from across the Atlantic. *Lancet* **352**, 163–4.
39. **Peck, C., McCall, M., McLaren, B., and Rotem, T.** (2000). Continuing medical education and continuing professional development: international comparisons. *British Medical Journal* **320**, 432–5.
40. **van den Hombergh, P., Grol, R., van den Hoogen, H.J.M., and van den Bosch, W.J.H.M.** (1999). Practice visits as a tool in quality improvement: acceptance and feasibility. *Quality in Health Care* **8**, 167–71.
41. **Marshall, M.N., Shekelle, P.G., Leatherman, S., and Brook, R.H.** (2000). The public release of performance data: what do we expect to gain? A review of the evidence. *Journal of the American Medical Association* **283**, 1866–74.
42. **Campbell, S., Roland, M., and Wilkin, D.** (2001). Primary care groups: improving the quality of care through clinical governance. *British Medical Journal* **322**, 1580–2.
43. **Wensing, M., Grol, R., van Montfort, P., and Smits, A.** (1996). Indicators of the quality of general practice care of patients with chronic illness: a step towards the real involvement of patients in the assessment of quality. *Quality in Health Care* **5**, 73–80.
44. **Marshall, M.N., Hiscock, J., and Sibbald, B.** (2002). Attitudes to the public release of comparative information on the quality of general practice care: qualitative study. *British Medical Journal* **325**, 1278–81.
45. **Stewart, M.** (2001). Towards a global definition of patient centered care. The patient should be the judge of patient centered care. *British Medical Journal* **322**, 444–5.

13.3 Evidence-based medicine as a tool in quality improvement

Trisha Greenhalgh and Anna Donald

What is evidence-based medicine?

Evidence-based medicine (EBM) is a problem-solving process that helps health professionals, patients, and their families make decisions about their health and health care. There are many definitions of EBM. These reflect (among other things) the different uses for its techniques.[1,2] For busy primary care clinicians, one way to think about EBM would be 'the enhancement of a clinician's skills in diagnosis, treatment and prevention through the framing of relevant and answerable questions, the systematic search for robust research evidence, and the appropriate use of estimates of probability and risk in clinical decision-making'.

This chapter covers a lot of ground, and if you are new to the subject of EBM, you may find some of the sections daunting. It is not essential to read (or understand) everything in this chapter to gain a feel for how the techniques can be used in quality improvement. We recommend that for a general overview, you should study the section that follows, along with Fig. 1, and consider the examples in the Boxes 1–3. In this chapter, more details on the quantitative and qualitative techniques of EBM are provided. A guide to database searching is provided and some electronic resources are listed in Table 3. Figure 2 gives a summary algorithm for critical appraisal. Finally, some barriers to implementing EBM in practice are considered.

What can evidence-based medicine contribute to quality improvement?

Most commonly, EBM helps to establish quality standards by providing the likelihood that certain outcomes will result from different courses of action, such as prevention programmes, diagnostic tests, and various treatments. Such estimates give different decision-makers a common, objective reference point from which they can make further decisions.

In this way, EBM is both practical and political—that is, it helps the individual practitioner make decisions in the clinic, and it also provides the tools for separating facts from values when discussing policy. By hastening agreement about common standards, EBM enables conversations about quality improvement to develop more quickly rather than getting sunk early by disagreements over baseline facts.

Specifically, EBM helps to establish both the size of effect expected from a certain course of action, as well as the likelihood of its occurring, such as the likelihood that the measles, mumps, and rubella (MMR) vaccine causes autism, inflammatory bowel disease, and so forth.

Typically, EBM helps to ask and to answer questions that start with 'What is the chance that . . . certain outcomes will result from certain courses of action in defined groups of people?'; for example, 'What is the chance that the MMR vaccine is just as safe and just as effective as individual vaccines in children aged 2–6 months?'. Such questions are usually answered with quantitative research, which gives answers in the form of probability estimates, such as 'one half', or '70 per cent as likely', or '2 per cent more likely'.

Evidence-based medicine helps decision makers both by clarifying questions and by providing decision makers with the few, best-quality research findings available—no small task, given the millions of studies, most of poor quality, currently available in research databases such as MEDLINE. Box 1 describes a real example of how accessible summaries of online evidence allow the busy practitioner to make evidence-based decisions at the bedside and in the clinic with very little additional time investment. The creation and use of these summaries is described further below.

Evidence-based medicine clarifies questions by turning fuzzy 'What should we do next?' questions into more precise, answerable questions, such as 'What is the chance that we will have fewer deaths and dependency from strokes if we establish a specialist stroke unit in this hospital?'. It answers questions with good research by providing well-validated search, evaluation, and synthesis methods, developed from the principles of statistics and epidemiology, which enable decision makers and those assisting them to find the most relevant, reliable evidence on any particular question.

That EBM draws so heavily on quantitative research is not surprising, coming as it does from the fields of epidemiology and statistics. It can, however, for the same reasons, also help people make better use of good-quality qualitative research. Just as it can clarify the components of 'What is the chance that' questions, EBM also helps to clarify the components of the 'How' and 'Why' questions that require qualitative and basic science research for answers. For example, 'Why is the sky blue?' 'How do men feel about retirement?' 'How does endothelium work?' Table 1 shows examples of both quantitative and qualitative questions that might prompt the development of evidence-based quality standards in primary care, while Fig. 1 illustrates how EBM contributes to the development of clinical quality standards.

Box 2 describes a clinical case that might well prompt a practice team to review the preventive care they offer and to consider changing the information and education they provide to patients about acute chest pain. In this example, it is the practice nurse who decides to search the literature following a critical event, but once evidence is found and confirmed to be valid and relevant, it must be shared with the wider primary health care team who should address its implementation at both clinical and organizational level as described in the other chapters in this section.

Box 1 EBM in everyday clinical practice

A 73-year-old man consults Dr Fernando with night cramps, asking for quinine. Dr Fernando has a vague memory that quinine has never been shown to be effective for this condition, but he decides to check. He has access to the Internet so consults the online version of *Clinical Evidence* (www.clinicalevidence.com) and enters the search term 'leg cramps'. He quickly learns that the latest systematic review found that quinine significantly reduced the frequency of nocturnal leg cramps compared to placebo. The time taken to gain this information was only 90 s, and Dr Fernando now feels confident in prescribing the drug.

More details on quantitative evidence: frequency and probability

Asking answerable questions

The literature on medicine, nursing, health sciences, and health service organization contains some 25 million articles.[12] One of the commonest mistakes people make when approaching this literature is to start searching with only a vague idea of what information they want. Vague questions generally produce too many articles, most of which are irrelevant.

In order to address complex or ill-defined clinical problems through clinical research studies, these problems must first be broken down into a series of more precise questions, each of which should be expressed in a structured and linear format ('If we do A, will B result?') similar to an experimental hypothesis. Hence, rather than asking 'What should I do about leg ulcers in my practice?', the research-oriented clinician might ask, 'In non-diabetic patients aged 60 and over with uncomplicated venous leg ulcers, what is the relative effectiveness of compression bandaging compared to simple daily dressings in terms of time taken to heal?'.

The general format of the hypothesis-driven question is represented by the acronym PICOT (Patient-Intervention-Comparison-Outcome-Time) and is illustrated in Table 2. Note that if the question relates to a question about prognosis (i.e. having the general format 'What is the chance that a person with condition A [or who has been exposed to agent B] will meet outcome C in time period D?', the four-part question is better expressed as PECOT [Patient-Exposure (or risk factor)-Comparison (no exposure or no risk factor)-Outcome-Time]).[13]

Choosing the right research design to address the question

Clinical epidemiology classifies quantitative research into a number of distinct categories, which are listed below.

- *Benefit.* Research studies about the benefits of drugs and medicines (and, similarly, about the benefits of surgical operations, psychological support, educational interventions, diets, exercise programmes, diagnostic tests, or entire screening programmes) provide numerical estimates in response to the general question type 'What is the chance that this drug/operation/therapy/intervention/test/screening programme leads to a beneficial outcome of some kind?' The preferred research design for

Table 1 Examples of quantitative and qualitative research questions

Clinical field	Example of a quantitative research question	Example of a qualitative research question
Acute myocardial infarction	'What is the chance that prompt thrombolytic therapy improves survival in acute myocardial infarction compared with survival in those not receiving this therapy?'	'Why do some patients delay seeking help when they have acute central chest pain?'[3]
Cervical screening	'What is the chance that a woman with a history of genital warts will have a pre-cancerous cervical smear, compared to the chance in a woman without such a history?'	'When a woman is told her smear is "mildly abnormal", what does she think is happening?'[4]
Smoking cessation	'What is the chance that a smoker will give up when advised to do so by a doctor?'	'What sort of smoker responds to advice to quit, and how to improve the success rate with other smokers?'[5]
Acute febrile illness in young children	'What features of acute febrile illness predict serious disease such as bacterial meningitis?'	'What worries parents when their preschool children are acutely ill, and why?'[6]

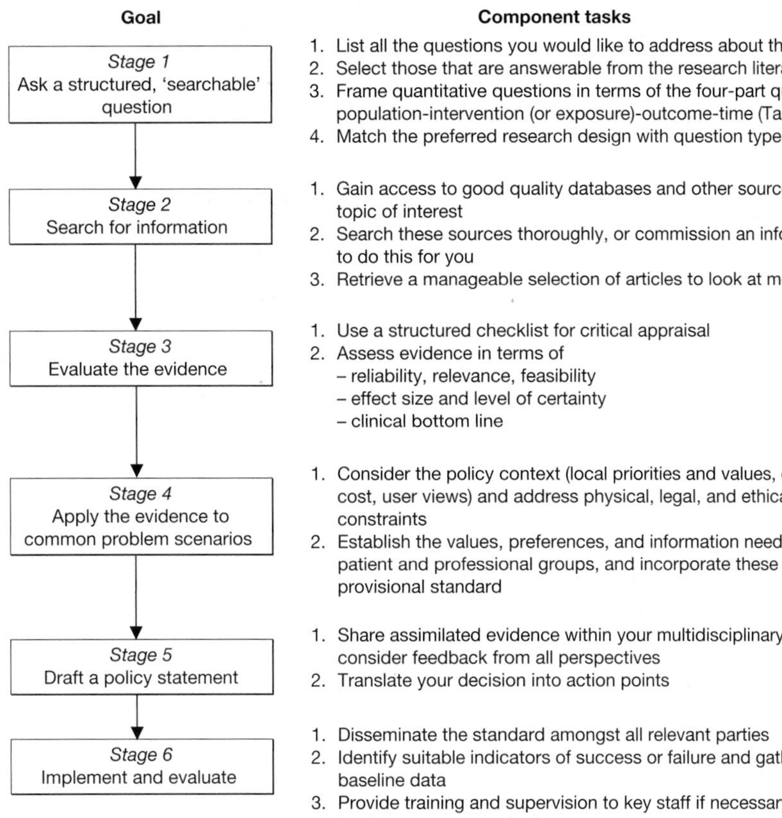
Goal
Component tasks
Stage 1
Ask a structured, 'searchable' question
1. List all the questions you would like to address about this problem
2. Select those that are answerable from the research literature
3. Frame quantitative questions in terms of the four-part question population-intervention (or exposure)-outcome-time (Table 3)
4. Match the preferred research design with question type
Stage 2
Search for information
1. Gain access to good quality databases and other sources on your topic of interest
2. Search these sources thoroughly, or commission an informaticist to do this for you
3. Retrieve a manageable selection of articles to look at more closely
Stage 3
Evaluate the evidence
1. Use a structured checklist for critical appraisal
2. Assess evidence in terms of
– reliability, relevance, feasibility
– effect size and level of certainty
– clinical bottom line
Stage 4
Apply the evidence to common problem scenarios
1. Consider the policy context (local priorities and values, opportunity cost, user views) and address physical, legal, and ethical constraints
2. Establish the values, preferences, and information needs of local patient and professional groups, and incorporate these into a provisional standard
Stage 5
Draft a policy statement
1. Share assimilated evidence within your multidisciplinary team and consider feedback from all perspectives
2. Translate your decision into action points
Stage 6
Implement and evaluate
1. Disseminate the standard amongst all relevant parties
2. Identify suitable indicators of success or failure and gather baseline data
3. Provide training and supervision to key staff if necessary to help implement new standard
4. Set a date for review

Fig. 1 Stages of EBM applied to the setting of quality standards.

such questions is the *systematic review of randomized controlled trials* or, if no systematic review is available, a high quality and adequately sized randomized controlled trial.

- *Harm.* Questions about the potential harm caused by drugs, operations, other therapeutic interventions, diagnostic tests, screening programmes, or risk factors provide estimates in response to the general question type 'What is the chance that the drug/operation/intervention/test/screening programme/risk factor/environmental factor leads to a harmful outcome of some kind?'. The preferred research design for such questions is a prospective cohort study.
- *Incidence.* Research studies on incidence address the general question 'What is the chance that someone in a defined population will newly develop a particular condition within a set period of time?'. The preferred research design for such questions is a prospective study design that allows researchers to track new events as they occur.
- *Prevalence.* Research studies on prevalence address the general question 'What is the chance that someone in a defined population already has a particular condition at a set point in time?'. The preferred research design for such questions is a cross-sectional survey.
- *Prognosis.* Research studies on prognosis address the general question 'What is the chance that a person who already has a particular condition or risk factor will develop a particular outcome (e.g. death) within a particular time period?'. The preferred research design for such questions is a prospective cohort study.

Box 2 EBM and local policy development

Mrs Gough makes an urgent appointment to see her practice nurse, Rena Patel. She is distraught because her 54-year-old husband died of a heart attack last night after developing mild 'indigestion' 2 days earlier. He had only contacted the doctor when the pain became severe, some 24 h after its onset. Mr Gough had had a company medical last month and had been told that his cholesterol level was 6.8 mmol/l and his blood pressure was 150/100—both of which were described as 'mildly raised'. He had been given a summary of these tests to give to his GP but had not got round to it because of pressure at work. Rena offers her condolences to Mrs Gough, but later she decides to use this tragic case to address a general 'quality' issue within the practice.

The first step in EBM is to generate focused questions that can be answered from the research literature (see Fig. 1). For example:

1. The question 'Could we have known that Mr Gough was heading for a heart attack?' prompts the more general question 'What is the chance that a 54-year-old White smoker who takes no regular exercise and has "mildly raised" cholesterol and blood pressure will develop heart attack over the next 5 years?' (an example of a question on prognosis). Using the PubMed Clinical Queries facility, the librarian retrieves a recent meta-analysis of studies that have addressed prognosis (most usually through the control arms of randomized controlled trials), which includes a link to a risk score website. Rena enters Mr Gough's details and calculates that his 5-year risk of death was only 3.6% but that he was certainly in a high-risk group for his age.[7]
2. The question 'What could we have done to prevent Mr Gough's heart attack?' prompts the more general question 'What drugs or lifestyle interventions reduce the risk of acute coronary syndromes in middle-aged smokers, and by how much?'. This broad question can be broken down into a series of more specific ones such as, 'What impact would therapy to reduce blood pressure from 100 diastolic to 90 diastolic have on the risk of heart attack?' (an example of a question on therapy). The librarian helps Rena find a meta-analysis on hypertension management.[8]
3. Another important question is 'Even though his risk factors were "mildly raised", perhaps should we have treated him more aggressively given that he had several risk factors—but which risk factor should we focus on first?'. A search of MEDLINE for review articles on hypertension management produces an evidence-based overview of how to incorporate individual cardiovascular risk into decisions on the management of patients with hypertension.[9]
4. The question 'Could we have helped Mr Gough stop smoking, and if so, how?' leads, of course, to a question about the comparative efficacy of different strategies. A recent Cochrane review is not hard to identify.[10]
5. The question 'Why didn't Mr Gough call the doctor when he got chest pain?' prompts the more general question 'Why do people with acute chest pain delay seeking help?' (an example of a question for which qualitative research is needed). Using the MeSH term 'Myocardial infarction', and the text terms 'delay' and 'qualitative research', Rena finds a paper describing in-depth interviews with survivors of acute chest pain.[3]

Using a critical appraisal checklist, Rena concludes that whilst these papers all have some limitations, their conclusions are broadly transferable to her own practice. She calls a meeting of the practice team to discuss how they might be used to improve standards of care.

The first paper suggests that many heart attacks occur in people who lie outside the 'high-risk' category and suggest that there is no simple

Box 2 Continued

route to targeted primary prevention strategies.[7] Nevertheless, the paper supports a more systematic approach to the recording and management of risk factors, along the lines of the National Service Framework for Coronary Heart Disease.[11] The second paper suggests a disappointing impact of antihypertensive therapy alone in middle-aged men with multiple risk factors,[8] and the third—an evidence-based overview—strongly suggests that the greatest impact on outcome in patients like Mr Gough would be obtained from giving up smoking.[9] Lancaster's systematic review shows that a range of interventions including brief advice, generic antismoking literature, individual and group counselling, and pharmacological treatments such as nicotine replacement therapy, all produce significant benefit at relatively modest cost.[10] The final paper suggests that patients who delay seeking help may have a somewhat stereotyped view of a heart attack, with the victim collapsing to the ground in immediate agony, whereas in reality symptoms can build up gradually and be confused with indigestion or other minor ailments.[3]

Rena and her team discuss these papers and consider the local context. The practice is in a stable, lower middle class area, with a high proportion of office workers and teachers. Since most patients attend the surgery at least once a year, opportunistic recording of smoking status, blood pressure, and cholesterol level (if indicated) should be commenced. Furthermore, active antismoking advice, leaflets, counselling, or medication should be offered where appropriate and recorded in the notes. Priority will be given to patients with established cardiovascular disease.[11] The team agrees on a baseline audit of existing data capture and plan to review the situation in 6 months.

It is also agreed that a simple, low-cost intervention that could save lives is an amendment of the practice leaflet and the very popular practice website. The sentence 'If you develop any new chest pain, even if it does not seem very severe, call the doctor immediately; do not wait for morning or to see if it gets better' is added to both in a prominent place. Another readily implemented change is a training session for all reception staff, in which they are reminded never to reassure or defer a patient who telephones with chest pain. Finally, Rena obtains some educational posters to flag up the same message in the waiting room.

- *Diagnostic tests.* There are two sorts of question pertaining to this type of research:
  - Questions about the *interpretation of a particular test result* ('What is the chance that this test accurately predicts disease in this person?') Such questions need a formal, independent validation of the new test against an established gold standard in a representative cohort of study participants.
  - Questions about the *reliability of a diagnostic test* for an individual or group of people ('What is the chance that this test works better overall than that test [or than no test]?') Such questions require a randomized controlled trial of one test option against the other.
- Questions about the *cost-effectiveness or economic value* of a treatment, test, or risk factor ('How do the costs of two interventions compare, weighted by their different levels of effectiveness [or harm]?'). Such questions require good-quality economic analyses, themselves based upon high-quality epidemiological studies that give a reliable estimate of the chance of outcomes occurring.

The detailed description of different study designs is covered in Section 14 (Research).

Table 2 The four-part clinical question

Element	Suggestions to help	Example
1 Patient or problem	'How would I succinctly describe a group of patients similar to this one?'	In children under 12 years with eczema ...
2a Intervention (i.e. test, treatment, process of care)	'What is the main action I am considering?'	Would adding tiger balm ointment to their existing therapy of 1% hydrocortisone cream ...
2b Comparison (where relevant)	'What are the alternative option(s)?'	... compared to continuing with hydrocortisone cream alone ...
3 Outcome	'What do I/the patient want to happen/not happen?'	... improve symptom control without increasing the risk of adverse events ...
4 Time	'Over what period of time should the outcomes be evaluated?'	... over the subsequent 3 months?

Qualitative evidence

How and why questions

Qualitative studies address questions that tend to begin with 'How ...', 'Why ...?', or 'In what way does ...?'. As with quantitative studies, however, good qualitative studies usually require defined research questions from the outset (e.g. 'Why do parents of young children telephone the emergency services out of hours?'), although, using some research models, these may be modified as the research progresses (e.g. leading to the second-round question: 'What aspects of the child's condition make parents think there is a life-threatening illness?').

The characteristics of a good qualitative research question are:

- It includes an unambiguous statement of whom the research relates to (in the example above, the research relates to parents of young children)—this is known also as the 'target population'.
- It gives a clear statement of the setting and context of the research.
- It is not designed to confirm particular beliefs or prejudices of the researcher—that is, it is protected as much as possible from researcher bias.

Qualitative research designs

Unlike quantitative research, for which there are a limited number of well-known study designs, qualitative research employs a wide range of techniques. Valid techniques all minimize the introduction of unacceptable levels of bias, confounding, and poor measurement validity, which would render the study's results meaningless to the original question asked.

Well-known techniques used in qualitative research are described in detail elsewhere but include:[(14)]

- In-depth individual interviews, which are generally semi-structured—that is, they include a list of open-ended questions but allow scope for the participant to answer the question in their own words and include what is important to them.
- Focus groups—meetings in which a trained facilitator uses the group interaction to test the extent to which views expressed by one individual are shared or contested by others.
- Observation of events (e.g. sitting in on consultations or group meetings).
- Analysis of contemporaneous material (such as letters, e-mails, minutes of meetings, diagrams, flip chart paper, etc.).

Qualitative research undoubtedly contributes crucially to the quality improvement agenda. Indeed, it is the *only* way to address any question beginning 'How' or 'Why'! For example, the question 'Why do patients delay seeking help when they have acute chest pain?' was the basis of an in-depth interview study of survivors of acute coronary events and provided considerable insight into reasons for delayed 'pain to needle time'.[(3)]

Such qualitative insights can prompt both biomedical as well as non-biomedical interventions, including organizational changes such as an extended out-of-hours telephone service, inclusion of brief advice on the practice leaflet, or an education programme for high-risk patients and their relatives. What the study cited above did not (and could not) answer was the quantitative question 'What is the chance that a person with chest pain will delay seeking help for more than 4 hours?'—which, of course, requires a quantitative study.

Finding evidence—approaching electronic databases

Most clinicians, if asked their preferred source of evidence, cite a favourite textbook or even the name of an esteemed specialist colleague, neither of whom can be relied upon to contain the very latest evidence on all topics! If pressed, doctors will probably suggest the MEDLINE database, and nurses might know of the equivalent CINAHL (Citation Index of Nursing and Allied Health—effectively a subset of the Medline database with some additional nursing journals). These and other databases are now available online.

Evaluating evidence: the science of critical appraisal

Critical appraisal means reading a research paper carefully, using a structured checklist to help address two key questions:

- Can I trust this paper?
- Is it relevant to the question I need to answer and the patient(s) I plan to treat?

Figure 2 presents a flowchart for evaluating the quality and relevance of published studies. This chart includes both quantitative and qualitative papers, since the underlying question sequence is similar. For both types of research, the two main issues that determine whether a published paper is trustworthy are bias (including confounding, which is perhaps more appropriately known as 'left out variable bias') and internal validity.

Bias can be defined as 'any factor arising from the design and conduct of a study that skews the data in one particular direction, either away from or towards the "true" value that is being estimated with the study'. Examples of bias in quantitative research include selection bias (e.g. when sicker patients are allocated to active treatment and less sick ones to placebo); observer bias (when an assessor knows that a patient had the 'real' procedure or active drug and subconsciously assesses improvement as greater than it really is); withdrawal bias (when a high proportion of participants withdraw from a study before it is completed, especially if they differ systematically from those who continue); measurement bias (caused by systematic errors in instruments used to assess outcomes); and publication bias (authors and editors keener to publish 'positive' results).

One of the commonest forms of bias is confounding, or 'left out variable bias' in which the relationship between two measured variables (such as

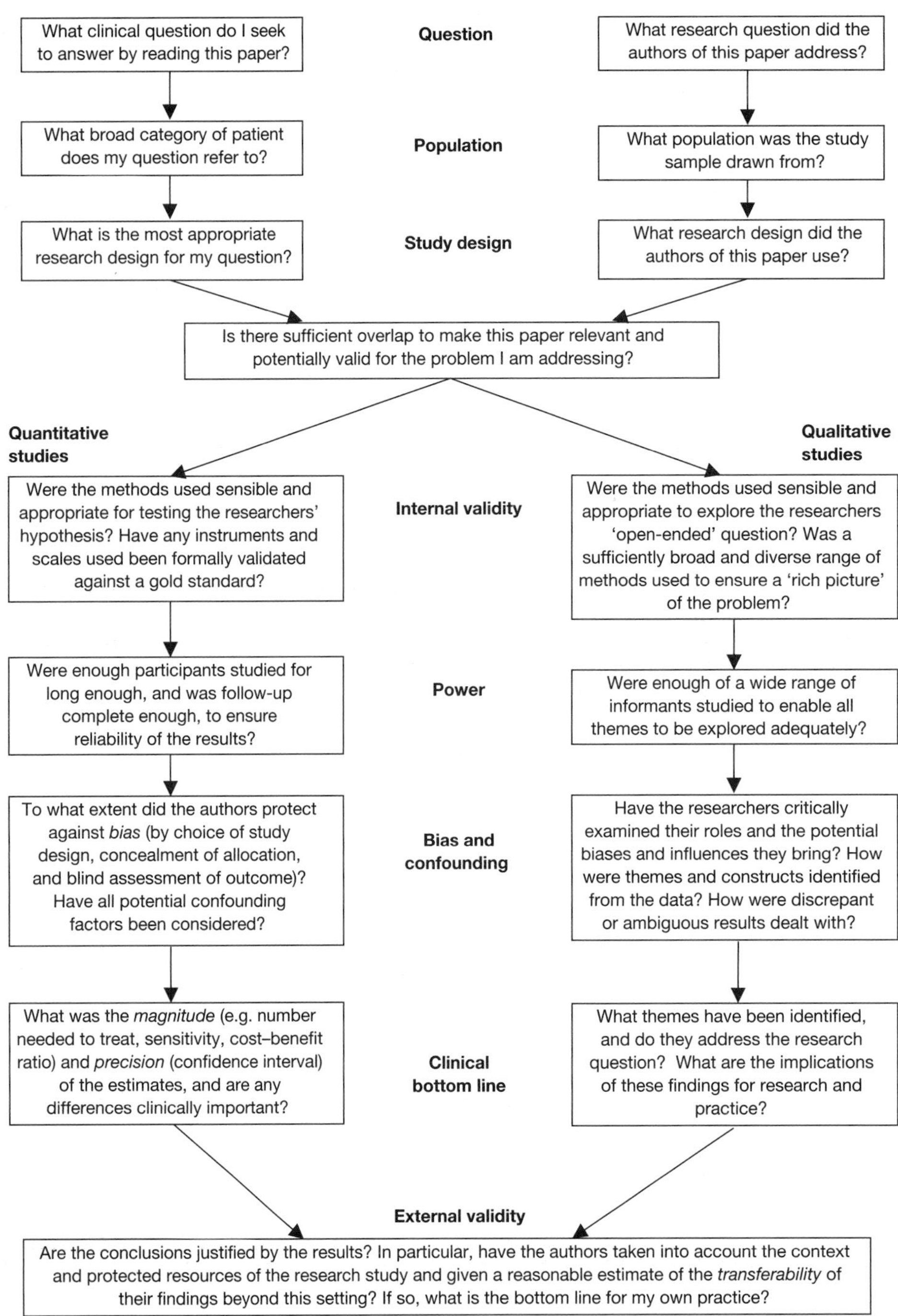

Fig. 2 Critical appraisal flowchart for assessing the quality and relevance of a research paper.

smoking and heart disease) is mediated via a third, unmeasured variable (such as social class).

In qualitative research, just as in quantitative research, researcher bias occurs when researchers do not critically examine their own perspective and the influence that they themselves might have had on the results. An obvious example is the GP or nurse who asks a sample of patients what they think about conventional and alternative forms of hormone replacement therapy, but who does not sufficiently consider that their own position as an authority figure in conventional medicine might prejudice the interviewees' responses.

Internal measurement validity is the relevance of the actual measures used—either equipment (e.g. sphygmomanometers), questionnaire scales (e.g. the SF-36 as a measure of overall health status[(15)]), or the various techniques adopted by the qualitative researcher to develop a 'rich picture' of a problem—to the aspects of health or illness that the researchers claimed they wanted to measure. Poor internal measurement validity arises when the measurements used do not accurately measure (or are irrelevant to) the outcomes and exposures of interest. One of the most widely cited examples of poor internal validity is the gap between what GPs *say* they do and what they *actually* do in clinical practice—suggesting that sending GPs a questionnaire asking how they treat condition X is not a valid way of establishing what goes on.[16]

External validity is another term for relevance. The findings of a study undertaken in another country, another region, or even a general practice down the road may not be directly transferable to one's own practice. Figures for the prevalence of teenage pregnancy in Tunbridge Wells (an affluent middle-class UK town with a stable, mainly white population) may not be transferable to Tottenham (an inner London district with a highly mobile population and diverse ethnicity), or to the population of Rome, Lisbon, or Harlem.

A more detailed discussion of bias, confounding, and validity, as well as a full set of critical appraisal checklists is available in specialized EBM textbooks.[17,18] But even if you were confident in the finer points of epidemiology and highly skilled at critical appraisal, time would not be on your side. The *Clinical Evidence* team (see below) have found that it takes up to 500 h to complete a short review of the literature to answer a common clinical question, and that such a review must be updated frequently to stay on top of new literature. Although critical appraisal is intellectually satisfying, and its basic principles important for everyone, it has proved to be a specialist skill that is impractical for daily use by most health practitioners.[19,20]

Processed information with 'bottom-line' evidence-based summaries and guides to practice are accumulating rapidly and they make evidence-based practice increasingly time-efficient. The most popular sources of secondary evidence are shown in Table 3. These publications, along with more specialized secondary sources (guidelines, protocols, decision support systems[21]) and EBM 'facilitators' (such as 'evidence-based on-call' and informaticist services[22]) are an important option for the busy or less confident practitioner, who should invest time in identifying such support services locally or via the Internet.

Barriers to evidence-based quality improvement

As the title of this chapter suggests, EBM is a tool, not a formula. Anyone—professionals, patients, politicians, and policy makers—can approach the medical literature systematically and incorporate research evidence into their quality agenda. Published examples of primary health care teams (or, more commonly, enthusiasts within those teams) who set out to use EBM as a lever for change suggest that the road to implementing best evidence is by no means smooth.[23,24]

The barriers can be divided into four main groups: the evidence itself; human factors (educational and motivational); organizational factors (practical and structural); and external factors (political, economic, technological, and social).

The evidence itself

It is often said that there is little or no good evidence on key clinical topics, especially in primary care. But good evidence is now accumulating (and being competently summarized) at a phenomenal rate.[12,25–27] In 1997, the Cochrane library contained less than 50 systematic reviews. Today, it has over 1200, and a growing proportion of these is on topics relevant to primary care.

It can also be frustrating to discover that the evidence suggests one course of action one year, but by next year, recommendations have changed to incorporate evidence from new research! Research evidence is, and probably always will be, incomplete and dynamic. Furthermore, it is important to note that EBM is not about setting facts in stone. It is about

Table 3 Electronic databases and other sources of evidence available online

Name	Description	Internet address
Bandolier[a]	Clearly presented summary journal with refreshingly down-to-earth editorial style. Includes a range of commissioned review topics for the UK NHS Research and Development Directorate	http://www.jr2.ox.ac.uk/Bandolier/
Cochrane Collaboration[a]	Website giving details of both the Cochrane Collaboration and the Cochrane Library. Subscribers may access full text of systematic reviews from this site	www.nelh.nhs.uk/cochrane.asp (free login for UK NHS staff), www.update-software.com/cochrane/ (for individual subscribers and those outside the UK)
Effective Health Care Bulletins[a]	Full text (with downloadable reports) of a bi-monthly bulletin for decision-makers which examines the effectiveness of health care interventions	http://www.york.ac.uk/inst/crd/ehcb.htm
National Guideline Clearinghouse (US)[a]	A comprehensive database of evidence-based clinical practice guidelines and related documents produced by the Agency for Health Care Policy and Research (AHCPR), in partnership with the American Medical Association (AMA) and the American Association of Health Plans (AAHP)	http://www.guidelines.gov/index.asp
NHS Economic Evaluation Database[a]	Public access database with quality assessed structured abstracts of clinical trials that include an economic evaluation	http://nhscrd.york.ac.uk/nhsdhp.htm
NHS Health Technology Assessment Database[a]	Public access database with quality assessed structured abstracts of clinical trials that include an evaluation of health technology	http://nhscrd.york.ac.uk/htahp.htm
National Institute of Clinical Excellence[a]	Website of the UK's advisory body on the effectiveness and cost-effectiveness of interventions. Includes downloadable guidance on cost-effectiveness of drugs, medical devices, and health care programmes. NICE also has a clinical guidelines section classified by clinical topic	http://www.nice.org.uk
PubMed	Free, fast, and up-to-date version of MEDLINE from the US National Library of Medicine, with built-in search filters	http://www4.ncbi.nlm.nih.gov/PubMed/

[a] Secondary sources of evidence (i.e. derived from quality-assessed and summarized primary evidence).

defining what we need to know; agreeing on ways of knowing (i.e. on what counts as best evidence); and establishing what is known (and with what degree of confidence). Change is inherent to medical progress, which is why EBM focuses on process (how to find out) rather than content (what you might find on any particular day). To dismiss EBM because 'the facts are not all there yet' is a misguided approach.

Even when there is good evidence on a particular topic, experts (and, even more so, non-experts) often disagree about what it means. But experts have always disagreed—partly because some so-called experts are actually nothing of the sort, but mainly because of the interpretive dimension of research evidence. EBM generally diminishes the magnitude of disagreement between experts. And when disagreement still occurs, EBM allows decision makers to identify the nature of the disagreement: whether it is in the evidence itself, the inferences made from the evidence, or differences in values or preferences.

Human factors

Applying the tools of EBM properly requires considerable skill, organization, and technical resources, as well as time and confidence, and most clinicians in primary care do not possess all these in sufficient measure.[12,28,29] One important reason why it took a generation or more for even innovative and highly motivated clinicians to adopt an evidence-based approach to practice was the lack of adequate training in database searching, clinical epidemiology, basic statistics, and critical appraisal. However, the situation is changing rapidly. Medical and nursing students, and health professionals in training, are acquiring these sophisticated skills as part of the core curriculum for undergraduate and postgraduate training.[30] Courses for more experienced clinicians are also available—though a recent review criticized them for emphasizing critical appraisal at the expense of the wider skills needed for EBM (see Fig. 1).[31]

It would be naive, however, to assume that human barriers to the use of EBM are all to do with training and time. At least as important are motivation and values. The issue of resistance to EBM is considered in other chapters, notably Chapter 13.5.

Organizational factors

Barriers to the practice of EBM at organizational level often focus on, but are rarely confined to, the availability of information technology. That the practice computers are old-fashioned, confined to the doctors' desks, and used only for a fraction of their potential is, of course, a technological issue, but the fact that the practice repeatedly fails to allocate a budget for upgrading the machines or training staff is probably an issue of organizational culture, leadership (or lack of it), and the personal ideology of key decision makers. Other chapters in this book address the general problem of change management in primary health care (Chapters 13.5 and 13.6).

Various research studies have attempted to identify the different organizational factors that influence the adoption of evidence-based practice, which are covered in more detail in Chapter 13.5.[32]

External factors

Management textbooks often suggest four dimensions of external constraints that should be taken into account when trying to implement change within an organization: political, economic, sociological, and technological. Technological progress has been crucial to the emergence of evidence-based practice. Until recently, ordinary computers were simply not powerful enough to run large databases like the Cochrane Library or MEDLINE (see Table 3) on people's desks. Many organizations, especially primary care teams, are still getting used to the idea that it is now possible to 'pipe in' research and statistical information to the clinician's desktop. Another major 'technological' breakthrough has been the work of librarians and informaticists in developing epidemiological 'filters' to sift out poor-quality studies—for example, when the searcher is looking for studies on therapy, the filter will only provide papers that describe randomized controlled trials. These filters did not exist outside the expert arena until the late 1990s, but they are now available free of charge on the Internet (Table 3).

This chapter is not the place for a detailed analysis of the changing social context or political fortunes of EBM. However, it is undoubtedly true that its rise to prominence in many countries including the United Kingdom, United States, Canada, the Netherlands, and Australia was accelerated (and even occasionally imposed) by its mainstream position in government policy documents[33–38] and that the underpinning values of the EBM movement (to offer the best available treatment to patients in all situations and contexts) align well with the rising interest in quality, accountability, and 'the new professionalism' described by Irvine[39] (see Chapter 13.2).[40–43]

Economic constraints on the implementation of research evidence are often a major issue both locally and nationally. Indeed, the academic skill of critical appraisal is arguably of little use if there are insufficient funds for the recommended technology or service.

Evidence-based medicine is not, of course, designed to resolve issues about ethics (whether society 'should' fund particular expensive treatments) or values (the extent to which a particular benefit such as a 3-week extension of life in terminal cancer is considered 'worth it'); and it cannot take the politics out of policy-making (e.g. it cannot generate resources when insufficient funds have been allocated). But the tools and methods of EBM can supplement decisions about values; inform decisions about economic priorities; and help define, in objective terms, the gap between what is desirable and what is available or affordable.

Conclusion: EBM in the real world

This chapter has attempted to provide an overview of the tools and methods of EBM (essentially, those of clinical epidemiology for quantitative research and a range of in-depth, exploratory methods for qualitative research). As the other chapters in this section show, EBM should not be thought of as one isolated (and optional) alternative in the approach to quality improvement, but as a benchmark for the appropriateness, completeness, and rigour of the data gathered or used in a variety of approaches including user consultation, clinical audit, guidelines development, and the development of appropriate administrative and management infrastructures for the delivery of care.

References

1. **Sackett, D.L., Rosenberg, W.C., and Gray, J.A.M.** (1996). Evidence based medicine: what it is and what it isn't. *British Medical Journal* **312**, 71–2.
2. **McMaster University EBM Website:** http://www.hiru.mcmaster.ca/ebm, 2001.
3. **Ruston, A., Clayton, J., and Calnan, M.** (1998). Patients' action during their cardiac event: qualitative study exploring differences and modifiable factors (see comments). *British Medical Journal* **316**, 1060–4.
4. **Kavanagh, A.M. and Broom, D.H.** (1997). Women's understanding of abnormal cervical smear test results: a qualitative interview study. *British Medical Journal* **314**, 1388–91.
5. **Butler, C.C., Pill, R., and Stott, N.C.** (1998). Qualitative study of patients' perceptions of doctors' advice to quit smoking: implications for opportunistic health promotion (see comments). *British Medical Journal* **316**, 1878–81.
6. **Kai, J.** (1996). What worries parents when their preschool children are acutely ill, and why: a qualitative study (see comments). *British Medical Journal* **313**, 983–6.
7. **Pocock, S.J., McCormack, V., Gueyffier, F., Boutitie, F., Fagard, R.H., and Boissel, J.P.** (2001). A score for predicting risk of death from cardiovascular disease in adults with raised blood pressure, based on individual patient data from randomised controlled trials. *British Medical Journal* **323**, 75–81.
8. **Gueyffier, F., Froment, A., and Gouton, M.** (1996). New meta-analysis of treatment trials of hypertension: improving the estimate of therapeutic benefit. *Journal of Human Hypertension* **10**, 1–8.

9. **Pignone, M. and Mulrow, C.D.** (2001). Evidence based management of hypertension: using cardiovascular risk profiles to individualise hypertensive treatment. *British Medical Journal* **322**, 1164–6.
10. **Lancaster, T., Stead, L., Silagy, C., and Sowden, A.** (2000). Effectiveness of interventions to help people stop smoking: findings from the Cochrane Library. *British Medical Journal* **321**, 355–8.
11. **Department of Health.** *National Service Framework for Coronary Artery Disease: Modern Standards and Service Models.* London: HMSO, 2001.
12. **Wyatt, J.C.** (2000). Reading journals and monitoring the published work. *Journal of the Royal Society of Medicine* **93**, 423–7.
13. **Sackett, D.L., Haynes, R.B., Guyatt, G.H., and Tugwell, P.** *Clinical Epidemiology. A Basic Science for Clinical Medicine.* Boston: Little Brown & Company, 1991.
14. **Denzin, M. and Lincoln, P.** *Handbook of Qualitative Research.* London: SAGE, 1994.
15. **Anderson, R.T., Aaronson, N.K., and Wilkin, D.** (1993). Critical review of the international assessments of health-related quality of life. *Quality of Life Research* **2**, 369–95.
16. **Adams, A.S., Soumerai, S.B., Lomas, J., and Ross-Degnan, D.** (1999). Evidence of self-report bias in assessing adherence to guidelines. *International Journal of Quality in Health Care* **11**, 187–92.
17. **Donald, A. and Greenhalgh, T.** *A Hands-On Guide to Evidence Based Health Care.* Oxford: Blackwell, 2002.
18. **Sackett, D.L., Richardson, W.S., Rosenberg, W.M.C., and Haynes, R.B.** *Evidence-Based Medicine: How to Practice and Teach* EBM. London: Churchill-Livingstone, 2000.
19. **Donald, A.** *The Front Line EBM Project.* Final report. London: Department of Health, 1998.
20. **Guyatt, G.H., Meade, M.O., Jaeschke, R.Z., Cook, D.J., and Haynes, R.B.** (2000). Practitioners of evidence based care. Not all clinicians need to appraise evidence from scratch but all need some skills (see comments). *British Medical Journal* **320**, 954–5.
21. **Wyatt, J.C.** (2000). Practice guidelines and other support for clinical innovation. *Journal of the Royal Society of Medicine* **93**, 299–304.
22. **Greenhalgh, T., Hughes, J., Rogers, S., Humphrey, C., Swinglehurst, D., and Martin, P.** (2002). A comparative case study of two models of a clinical informaticist service. *British Medical Journal* **324**, 524–9.
23. **Lipman, T. and Price, D.** (2000). Decision making, evidence, audit, and education: case study of antibiotic prescribing in general practice. *British Medical Journal* **320**, 1114–18.
24. **Greenhalgh, T.** (2000). What can we learn from narratives of implementing evidence? *British Medical Journal* **320**, 1118.
25. **Wyatt, J.C.** (2000). Keeping up: continuing education or lifelong learning? *Journal of the Royal Society of Medicine* **93**, 369–72.
26. **Wyatt, J.C. and Anagnostelis, B.** (2000). Reference material: books and multimedia packages. *Journal of the Royal Society of Medicine* **93**, 244–6.
27. **Wyatt, J.C.** (2000). Clinical questions and information needs. *Journal of the Royal Society of Medicine* **93**, 168–71.
28. **McColl, A., Smith, H., White, P., and Field, J.** (1998). General practitioners' perceptions of the route to evidence based medicine: a questionnaire survey. *British Medical Journal* **316**, 361–5.
29. **Greenhalgh, T. and Douglas, H.-R.** (1999). Experiences of general practitioners and practice nurses of training courses in evidence-based health care: a qualitative study. *British Journal of General Practice* **49**, 536–40.
30. **Green, M.L.** (2000). Evidence-based medicine training in graduate medical education: past, present and future. *Journal of Evaluation in Clinical Practice* **6**, 121–38.
31. **Green, M.L.** (1999). Graduate medical education training in clinical epidemiology, critical appraisal, and evidence-based medicine: a critical review of curricula (Review). *Academic Medicine* **74**, 686–94.
32. **Greenhalgh, T.** (2000). Implementing research findings. In *How to Read a Paper: The Basics of Evidence Based Medicine* (ed. T. Greenhalgh), pp. 179–99. London: BMJ Publications.
33. **Department of Health.** *Promoting Clinical Effectiveness: A Framework for Action in and Through the NHS.* Leeds: NHS Management Executive, 1996.
34. **Mulrow, C.D. and Lohr, K.N.** (2001). Proof and policy from medical research evidence (Review). *Journal of Health Politics, Policy & Law* **26**, 249–66.
35. **Department of Health.** *Research and Development for a First Class Service—R&D Funding in the New NHS.* London: Department of Health, 2000.
36. **Department of Health.** *Information for Health: An Information Strategy for the Modern NHS 1998–2005.* London: NHS Executive, 1998.
37. **Department of Health.** *The NHS Plan.* London: NHS Executive, 2001.
38. **NHS Executive UoS.** *Promoting Clinical Effectiveness in Education and Training.* Bristol: NHS Executive South West, 1998.
39. **Irvine, D.** (1999). The performance of doctors: the new professionalism. *Lancet* **353**, 1174–7.
40. **Eriksson, C.** (2000). Learning and knowledge-production for public health: a review of approaches to evidence-based public health (see comments) (Review). *Scandinavian Journal of Public Health* **28**, 298–308.
41. **Bedregal, P. and Ferlie, E.** (2001). Evidence based primary care? A multi-tier, multiple stakeholder perspective from Chile. *International Journal of Health Planning & Management* **16**, 47–60.
42. **Perleth, M., Jakubowski, E., and Busse, R.** (2001). What is 'best practice' in health care? State of the art and perspectives in improving the effectiveness and efficiency of the European health care systems. *Health Policy* **56**, 235–50.
43. **Murray, C. and Frenk, J.** (2001). World Health Report 2000: a step towards evidence-based health policy (see comments). *Lancet* **357**, 1698–700.

13.4 Using and developing clinical guidelines

Paula Whitty, Martin Eccles, Steven H. Woolf, Jeremy Grimshaw, Brian Hurwitz, James Mason, and Paul Shekelle

Introduction

Aim of this chapter

The chapter offers a description of why and how to use guidelines and provides readers with an understanding of how guidelines should be developed.

What is a guideline and do they work?

Terminology in this field is bedevilled by overlapping meanings. The term 'guideline' is often used interchangeably with 'protocol', 'care pathway', or 'practice policy'. The US Institute of Medicine defines guidelines as:

> Systematically developed statements to assist practitioner and patient decisions about appropriate health care for specific clinical circumstances.(1)

Guidelines can be categorized by method of development and also by topic (disease or condition), intervention (e.g. 'screening guidelines'), or setting (primary care, hospice, etc.). There is an increasing international trend to move towards 'evidence-based guidelines', developed from a systematic assessment of the relevant effectiveness evidence, which explicitly links guideline recommendations to the supporting evidence. Rigorous evaluations have shown that guidelines can improve the process and outcome of care.(2)

Background

Interest in clinical guidelines has its origin in issues common to all health care systems: rising health care costs, increased demand for care, more expensive technologies, and an ageing population; variations in service delivery between providers, hospitals, and geographic regions and the presumption that at least some of this variation stems from inappropriate care, either over- or under-use of services; and the intrinsic desire of health care professionals to offer better care. Clinicians, policy makers, and managers see guidelines as a tool for promoting more consistent and efficient care, for closing gaps between what clinicians do and what scientific evidence supports.

The history of guideline development has been summarized in a recent survey of the United States, Canada, Australia, New Zealand, and nine European countries.[3] The United States led the development of consensus statements on biomedical issues in the late 1970s. In 1982, the Netherlands adopted this approach to develop multidisciplinary consensus statements to support health care providers in hospitals. In 1989, the Dutch College of General Practitioners started to publish guidelines for primary care. The US governmental Agency for Health Care Research and Policy (now the Agency for Health Care Research and Quality) began in 1990 with setting multidisciplinary, evidence-based guidelines, while a US programme to produce guidelines for preventive services had already commenced. Technology assessment programmes were also starting to develop and the first guideline clearinghouse was set up in Germany in 1992. In the early 1990s, cancer guideline programmes were created in France and Canada, and the Scottish Intercollegiate Guidelines Network (SIGN) in Scotland and the Agence Nationale d'Accréditation et d'Evaluation en Santé (ANAES, before 1997 ANDEM) in France started guideline development on a large scale. In the past few years, a growing number of industrial countries have set up national guideline programmes (including the establishment of the National Institute for Clinical Excellence in England and Wales).

When to use a guideline?

Clinical guidelines make sense when practitioners are unclear about appropriate practice and when scientific evidence can provide an answer; they are less useful in other situations. Too often, advocates view guidelines as 'magic bullets' for health care problems and ignore more effective solutions. When attempting to improve the quality of care, the initial step is to identify the problem to be tackled and then to choose an appropriate 'tool' to address it. Guidelines are only one such tool, and a full description of the 'toolbox' of ways to translate evidence into practice and improve the quality of care is given in Chapter 13.5.

How might guidelines be used?

Guidelines can be useful to clinicians and health systems in three broad areas (Box 1). Firstly, as an information resource, valid clinical guidelines provide an up-to-date broad overview of the supporting evidence regarding the management of a condition or the use of an intervention. In this context, guidelines have potential advantages over systematic reviews, with a broader scope and application of evidence to actual clinical problems in real-world settings.

Secondly, clinicians may refer to specific sections of guidelines to answer focused clinical questions arising out of their day-to-day practice, such as the correct dose of a drug or the proper immunization schedule for a childhood vaccine.

Thirdly, health care organizations may use guidelines as tools for quality assurance activities. In this context, the broad integrated scope of guidelines has advantages over other evidence reviews. The explicit recommendations they provide can be used to develop care pathways, reminder systems, standing orders, performance indicators, review criteria, and audits, to facilitate guideline implementation and evaluation.[2] Guidelines can also assist health services in setting priorities by calling attention to under-recognized health problems, clinical services, and preventive interventions and to neglected patient populations and high-risk groups.

Box 1 When guidelines might be useful

- Information resource for management of a condition or use of an intervention.
- Answering focused questions arising from everyday clinical practice.
- Tools for quality assurance activities—to support development of:
  - care pathways;
  - reminder systems;
  - standing orders;
  - performance indicators;
  - audits.
- Identifying research priorities from gaps in evidence.
- Help health services to set priorities.

Guidelines are useful to audiences other than clinicians and health systems. The research community often benefits from the ability of evidence-based guidelines to focus attention on gaps in evidence that are of importance in assessing the appropriateness of interventions. Noting there is inadequate evidence to support a treatment or technology is often an impetus for further research to address such uncertainty.

What are the 'pros and cons' of guidelines?

Pros

For patients (and almost everyone else in health care), the greatest benefit that could be achieved by guidelines is to improve the quality of care that patients receive. Guidelines that promote interventions of proven benefit and discourage ineffective ones have the potential to improve morbidity, mortality, and quality of life, at least for some conditions. Guidelines can improve the consistency of care. Guidelines aim to empower patients to make more informed health care choices and to consider their personal needs and preferences in selecting the best option.[4] Finally, clinical guidelines can help patients by influencing public policy.

Cons

The most important limitation of guidelines lies in the possibility of their recommendations being wrong (or at least wrong for individual patients).

Firstly, scientific evidence about what to recommend is often lacking, misleading, or misinterpreted. Only a small subset of what is done in medicine has been tested in appropriate, well-designed studies. Where studies do exist, the findings may be misleading because of design flaws, which contribute to bias or poor generalizability.

Secondly, recommendations are influenced by the opinions, clinical experience, and composition of the guideline development group. Tests and treatments that experts *believe* are good for patients may, in practice, be inferior to other options, ineffective, or even harmful. The beliefs to which experts ascribe, often in the face of conflicting data, can fall victim to misconceptions, faulty recollections, and misunderstanding of population norms.[5]

Thirdly, patients' needs may not be the only priority in making recommendations. Practices that are suboptimal from the patient's perspective may be recommended to help control costs, serve societal needs, or protect special interests (e.g. physicians, risk managers, politicians). Inflexible guidelines can harm by leaving insufficient room for clinicians to tailor care to patients' personal circumstances and medical history ('cookbook medicine'[6]). Blanket recommendations, rather than a menu of options or recommendations for shared decision-making, ignore patient preferences in situations where, on the basis of the evidence, choices are available to them.[7]

Guidelines have an important role in addressing variation in health care standards, especially where there is strong evidence for effective treatment and there is little valid justification for significant departures. But it is mistaken to maintain that clinical guidelines are required whenever there is practice variation. Inherent uncertainties, lack of evidence, poor consensus, and differences in patient choices and expectations can make uniform policies improper. Indeed, where substantial uncertainty exists, it may not be appropriate or safe to ask clinicians to deviate from their norms to unfamiliar patterns of care without clear evidence for change. The frequently touted benefit of clinical guidelines—more consistent practice patterns and reduced variation—may be gained at the expense of reducing individualized care for patients with special needs.

How to use a guideline

Having decided that a guideline is the best way to address a clinical problem, the following questions arise:

- How can we find evidence-based guidelines?
- How do we know if a guideline is valid and useful?
- Having identified a relevant, valid guideline, how do we implement it in our practice or wider primary care environment?

Where to find existing evidence-based guidelines

Identifying clinical guidelines in a systematic and thorough manner can be difficult for two reasons. Firstly, many guidelines are not published in journals and, therefore, not indexed in the commonly available bibliographic databases. Secondly, even when guidelines are published in indexed journals, optimal search strategies to locate them have not yet been developed. The US National Library of Medicine has developed an index that allows practice guidelines to be identified under a variety of headings including: *guideline* (publication type), *practice guideline* (publication type), *practice guidelines* (MeSH heading), *Consensus Development Conference* (publication type), and *Consensus Development Conference, NIH* (publication type). *Guideline* (publication type) is probably the most sensitive and specific individual search term. Fortunately, there are a number of Internet sites that catalogue clinical guidelines (e.g. the National Guidelines Clearinghouse http://www.guideline.gov/; for other examples, see Box 2), and many organizations that develop guidelines provide full-text versions or abstracts on their websites. In the future, it is likely that such sites will become the best source for identifying guidelines.

How do we know if a guideline is valid and useful?

When a clinician or practice has identified relevant guidelines, it is important to appraise their validity before deciding whether to adopt their recommendations.

A number of checklists for guideline appraisal have been proposed. A collaboration of several European countries with Canada, New Zealand, and the United States has produced a validated critical appraisal tool for guidelines (Box 3) (the Appraisal of Guidelines for Research and Evaluation in Europe—AGREE—tool[8]); other appraisal criteria are also available.[9] We suggest that health care organizations promote guidelines that report development methods explicitly by including a methods section within the guideline or supporting papers.[10,11] Although using such a filter would exclude many guidelines, without such information it is impossible to appraise the extent to which recommendations are based on good evidence and valid rationales.

Box 2 Identifying guidelines

Search terms for common bibliographic databases

Medline and Healthstar—*guideline* (publication type) and *consensus development conference* (publication type) (*Note:* Healthstar includes non-Medline referenced journals and grey literature, e.g. government agency guidelines)

CINAHL—*practice guidelines* (publication type) (*Note:* includes full text version of some guidelines)

EMBASE—*practice guidelines* (subject heading) (*Note:* this is used for both articles about and which contain practice guidelines; furthermore, the term was only introduced in 1994)

Useful websites

National Institute for Clinical Excellence (NICE)—www.nice.org.uk

Scottish Intercollegiate Guidelines Network—full text versions of guidelines and quick reference guides (www.sign.ac.uk)

US National Guideline Clearinghouse—http://www.guideline.gov/

Canadian Medical Association Clinical Practice Guidelines Infobase—index of clinical practice guidelines includes downloadable full text versions or abstracts for most guidelines (http://www.cma.ca/cpgs/index.html)

German Guideline Clearing House—http://www.leitlinien.de

Box 3 Summary of dimensions from the AGREE instrument[12] for critically appraising guidelines

Twenty-three questions covering six dimensions scored on a scale of 'strongly agree to strongly disagree':

Scope and purpose

1. The overall objective(s) of the guideline is (are) specifically described.
2. The clinical question(s) covered by the guideline is (are) specifically described.
3. The patients to whom the guideline is meant to apply are specifically described.

Stakeholder involvement

4. The guideline development group includes individuals from all the relevant professional groups.
5. The patients' views and preferences have been sought.
6. The target users of the guideline are clearly defined.
7. The guideline has been piloted among end users.

Rigour of development

8. Systematic methods were used to search for evidence.
9. The criteria for selecting the evidence are clearly described.
10. The methods used for formulating the recommendations are clearly described.
11. The health benefits, side-effects, and risks have been considered in formulating the recommendations.
12. There is an explicit link between the recommendations and the supporting evidence.
13. The guideline has been externally reviewed by experts prior to its publication.
14. A procedure for updating the guideline is provided.

Continued

Box 3 Continued

Clarity and presentation

15. The recommendations are specific and unambiguous.
16. The different options for management of the condition are clearly presented.
17. Key recommendations are easily identifiable.
18. The guideline is supported with tools for application.

Applicability

19. The potential organizational barriers in applying the recommendations have been discussed.
20. The potential cost implications of applying the recommendations have been considered.
21. The guideline presents key review criteria for monitoring and/or audit purposes.

Editorial independence

22. The guideline is editorially independent from the funding body.
23. Conflicts of interest of guideline development members have been recorded.

How to implement a valid and relevant guideline in a general practice or wider primary care setting

Adaptation of valid guidelines

Once guidelines of acceptable quality have been identified, they may need to be adapted for use within the relevant health care setting. The amount of work required to do this depends on their complexity and clinicians' general agreement with the guidelines' recommendations at the outset. For example, a small general practice identifying a valid but non-controversial guideline for managing hypertension may need little more than a meeting with relevant members of the primary care team to agree to move forward with implementation. In a wider administrative area, on the other hand, where the guideline has implications for primary, secondary, and tertiary care, for prescribing and other budgets, and for other factors, a more formal guidelines adaptation process may be needed.

Where a formal adaptation process is required, the first step is to set up an appropriate multidisciplinary group. For most clinical conditions good health care involves a multidisciplinary team, and in these situations guideline implementation requires planning within a multidisciplinary perspective. Patient representation is also important. The task of such a group is to gain acceptance of the recommendations and then to plan presentation, use, and evaluation of it within the local setting. The development of evaluation tools requires reformatting its recommendations in terms of measurable criteria and targets for quality improvement.(13)

Two factors influence whether and how a local group adopts or adapts a guideline: the strength of recommendations within the guidelines and local circumstances. Because the interpretation of evidence is inherently subjective, there is always the potential for a different group to re-interpret evidence and derive different recommendations. An example of this was the difference in recommended age for beginning mammography screening in the United States (40 versus 50 years old) from different national expert bodies, all reviewing the same body of evidence.(14–16) Deciding whether or not to derive different recommendations should be based, in large part, on the nature of the supporting evidence, either published evidence about effectiveness or local evidence about epidemiology, complication rates, or other parameters that differ from assumed rates in the generic guideline. Local adaptation groups should be wary of changing recommendations that are based upon good evidence but may feel more sanguine about changing those based upon weak(er) evidence. Where recommendations based on good evidence are changed, the rationale for this should be explicitly stated.

Adaptation may be needed to address local circumstances; local adaptation of a guideline on the management of heart failure, for example, should be influenced by whether open access echocardiography facilities are available or whether access to this investigation is by referral to a cardiologist.(17)

Legal issues to consider when using guidelines

Clinicians seem to fear that the proliferation of guidelines will increase their medico-legal exposure.(18) The only published study of the use of guidelines in litigation reviewed 259 US claims (both open and closed). It found 17 cases (6.6 per cent) in which guidelines had played 'a relevant or pivotal role in the proof of negligence', 12 in favour of the claimant, and four for the defendant.(19) Nevertheless, regulatory bodies now advise clinical teams to practise in accordance with guidelines(20) and it may seem wise to note down in medical records any rationale for deviation from authoritative, evidence-linked guidelines.(21)

In both common law and civil law jurisdictions, the legally required standard of medical care a doctor generally owes a patient is based upon notions of due care and 'reasonableness'.(22) How a 'reasonable standard' becomes represented in a legal test varies from country to country; in common law countries, case law generally adopts conformity with a body of responsible medical opinion as the appropriate test in matters of diagnosis and treatment.

In the United Kingdom, doctors can successfully defend a charge of negligence if they can show they have acted in accordance with the practice of a body of responsible medical practitioners.(23) In the words of the judge of this case, 'the test is the standard of the ordinary skilled man exercising and professing to have that special skill'.(23) Expert testimony helps the courts ascertain what is accepted as proper practice in specific cases, recognizing that there may be more than one acceptable approach to medical treatment. Professionally generated clinical standards are thereby applied, legally, rather than standards derived from elsewhere (e.g. from guidelines).(24)

Hitherto, one justification for judicial reliance upon these 'customary care' standards has been the belief that medical matters are beyond the understanding of judges and lay people; the courts, therefore, require to hear evidence of appropriate standards from 'medical experts'. Because guidelines now offer doctors, patients, and managers explicit examples of detailed, evidence-linked standards of care for use in specific clinical circumstances, they could remove the need for expert testimony in court regarding relevant customary care standards.(25)

In attempting to retain medical staff in high-risk liability specialties and to cut down reliance on defensive practices, some US jurisdictions have tried replacing the court testimony of expert witnesses with standards determined according to clinical guidelines.(26) Such guidelines can be used only if 50 per cent or more of physicians in the relevant specialty formally accept them, and these guidelines are available only for use by the case for the defendant (not for the claimant). One of the schemes (in Maine) has not been extended beyond its statutory experimental period although other US states continue to explore the value of guidelines in defining legal standards.(27)

In the United Kingdom, clinical guidelines have not been credited by the courts with special 'self-evident' status. Even where guidelines have been found in court proceedings to embody the appropriate legal standard of care,(28) guidelines generally have a subservient place in the legal process to that accorded to the expert witness. A leading barrister has concluded that guidelines 'are not evidence themselves as to good or any practice. Procedurally they must be produced by an expert. If that expert relies on the protocol as summing up good practice, the expert will have to say so and say why he says it. There cannot procedurally be mere trials by protocol'.(29) This remains the position in most common law countries.

Although clinical guidelines undoubtedly are becoming more influential in the way health care is practised, and in the manner in which doctors are held accountable,(24) legally they function as indicators of what good care is, rather than as legal standards themselves.

Developing guidelines

The aim of this section is to introduce the reader to the process of evidence-based guideline development, which should illuminate the criteria for appraisal of guidelines referred to earlier (Box 3).

Background

There is an increasing international trend to develop formal, evidence-based guidelines. These have the advantages of both systematic review and of setting out the evidence, such as it is, with explicit linkages to guideline recommendations.

There are five steps in the initial development of an evidence-based guideline:[30]

- identifying and refining the subject area of a guideline;
- convening and running guideline development groups;
- obtaining and assessing the evidence about the clinical question or condition;
- translating the evidence into a clinical practice guideline;
- external review of the guideline.

Identifying and refining the subject area of a guideline

Guidelines can be developed for a wide range of subjects. Clinical questions can be concerned with conditions (diabetes, coronary artery disease) or procedures (hysterectomy, coronary artery bypass surgery). Given the large number of potential areas, some form of prioritization is needed to select a particular topic for guideline development. Potential areas for practice guideline development can emerge from an assessment of the major causes of morbidity and mortality for a given population, uncertainty about the appropriateness of health care processes, or the evidence that they are effective at improving patient outcomes, or the need to conserve resources in providing care.

Convening and running guideline development groups

The tasks that need to be undertaken include the identification, synthesis, and interpretation of relevant evidence, and the production of the resulting guidelines. These may be carried out by the guideline development group members, by support staff, or by a combination of the two.

Guideline group members need to be competent to examine the evidence objectively. Whilst for primary care guidelines the majority of group members will be primary care clinicians, involvement of content area (often secondary care) experts is valuable, as they will understand the evidence and its clinical implications, and assist the wider professional ownership of the guideline. A balance of disciplines is also advantageous to counteract the potential for biased assessment of the evidence. When presented with the same evidence, a single specialty group will reach different conclusions than a multidisciplinary group, with the former being more likely to be in favour of performing procedures in which the specialty has a vested interest.[31,32] For example, the conclusions of a group of vascular surgeons favoured the use of carotid endarterectomy more than did a mixed group of surgeons and medical specialists.[33] There are good theoretical reasons to believe that individual biases are better balanced in multidisciplinary groups and that such balance will produce more valid guidelines.

It is very important that patient representatives are involved at this stage, although the best way to achieve this is an ongoing research issue.[34]

Identifying and assessing the evidence

Identifying and assessing the evidence is best done by a systematic review of the available evidence.[35] The purpose of a systematic review is to collect all available evidence, assess its potential applicability to the clinical question under consideration, inspect the evidence for susceptibility to bias, extract and summarize the findings.

The first step in gathering the evidence is to see if an authoritative and recent systematic review has already been published. The Cochrane Library includes the Cochrane trials register, database of systematic reviews, and the database of abstracts of reviews of effectiveness (see website http://www.cochrane.org). Relevant Cochrane review groups should also be contacted to see if a review is in progress. However, there are limitations to incorporating published systematic reviews within guidelines.[36]

If a current systematic review is unavailable, a computerized search of databases, such as MEDLINE and EMBASE, for original studies is the usual starting point, using search strategies that have been previously shown to be sensitive for detecting the types of studies one is looking for (though these have only been validated for randomized controlled trials [37]). For example, randomized controlled trials provide the best evidence to answer questions about the effectiveness of treatments whereas prospective cohort studies provide the best evidence for questions about risk. The Cochrane trials register contains references to over 290 000 clinical trials that have been identified though database and hand-searching, and represents the best initial source of such studies. As such it should be examined early on in any review process. It is helpful to check the references of all the articles identified for additional relevant articles not identified by the computerized search. Computerized searches have been shown to retrieve only a subset of all relevant studies.[37] Having experts in the field to examine the list of articles helps ensure there are no obvious omissions. Additional search strategies, including searches for articles published in languages other than English,[38–40] computerized searches of specialized databases, hand-searching relevant journals, and searching for unpublished material, will, in many cases, yield additional studies. Pragmatism requires that the scope of the search strategy is matched to the available resources.

Assessing studies for relevance and validity

The studies identified are then assessed for their relevance to the clinical questions of interest, their susceptibility to bias, and other judgements on validity. This is usually a two-step process, ideally using explicit criteria. The initial screen or sift for relevance (often possible by reading the abstract) narrows the set to those needing a more detailed assessment of validity.

Summarizing evidence

In the last step, data are extracted from the relevant studies on the benefits, harms, and, where applicable, costs of the interventions being considered. These are usually presented in a form that facilitates easy comparison of the designs and results of studies. Where appropriate, meta-analysis can be used to summarize results of similar studies.

Categorizing evidence

Summarized evidence should be categorized to reflect its underlying susceptibility to bias (which is dependent on study design, e.g. randomized controlled trials are by design less susceptible to bias than case series studies in assessing the efficacy of interventions). This is a short-hand method of conveying to a guideline reader specific aspects of the evidence. A number of such 'strength of evidence' classification schemes exist but empirical supporting evidence only exists for those categorizing effectiveness studies.[41,42] An example of a simple scheme is shown in Box 4.

There is controversy about whether and how to incorporate economic data (if available) with different countries exploring different approaches. Possibilities include a separate economic presentation alongside recommendations based solely on clinical effectiveness or recommendations that incorporate both cost and benefit domains. Williams[43] argues that guidelines based on effectiveness issues and then costed afterwards may differ substantially and may be less efficient than guidelines based on cost-effectiveness issues. Internationally, there is no widely accepted successful way to incorporate economic considerations into guidelines. Furthermore, given the prominence paid to systematic reviewing and evidence-based guideline

Box 4 Classification scheme to grade the category of evidence supporting practice guideline statements and the strength of recommendations

Category of evidence

Ia: evidence from meta-analysis of randomized controlled trials.

Ib: evidence from at least one randomized controlled trial.

IIa: evidence from at least one controlled study without randomization.

IIb: evidence from at least one other type of quasi-experimental study.

III: evidence from non-experimental descriptive studies, such as comparative studies, correlation studies, and case–control studies.

IV: evidence from expert committee reports or opinions and/or clinical experience of respected authorities.

Strength of recommendation

A: directly based on category I evidence.

B: directly based on category II evidence or extrapolated recommendation from category I evidence.

C: directly based on category III evidence or extrapolated recommendation from category I or II evidence.

D: directly based on category IV evidence or extrapolated recommendation from category I, II, or III evidence.

construction,[44] commentators have remarked that it is unclear how 'evidence' from the methodology of health economics, with its reliance on modelling, will sit alongside 'evidence' derived from the rigour of systematic review.

However, the incorporation of economic information will begin to change the nature of the decision-making process within guideline groups. A key issue is whether the group members tend to show an individual patient orientation or a utilitarian perspective. In the development of a guideline for the use of first-line antidepressants for the treatment of depression in UK primary care, the guideline development group had available a range of evidence about the two major drug groups.[45] The evidence showed no demonstrable difference in efficacy, no clinical (although a small statistical) difference in tolerability, large differences in drug acquisition costs, and large differences of the effects of toxicity in overdose. The guideline development group found their decision being made not on considerations of efficacy, but on the cost consequences of avoiding drug overdose related deaths.

The handling of economic issues in this and a series of other guidelines are described in a recent monograph,[30] and together feature a common approach. The various attributes (including costs), good and bad, of treatment alternatives are expressed as a profile. These are used as the basis of initial group discussion and for subsequent simple cost-effectiveness or cost-consequence presentations to help the guideline group in its deliberations—a process well received by group members.

It remains uncertain how the incorporation of economic considerations will affect the use of guidelines with individual patients. It may encourage a more explicit consideration of cost and consequences, in determining available treatment options within a health care system and within consultations where a guideline is used. However, the absence of economic data from guidelines may limit their usefulness to policy makers, clinicians, and patients in the long-term.

Translating evidence into a recommendation

Evidence alone is not sufficient to form a recommendation—the evidence needs to be interpreted and its application explored in the context of real health care settings. Some guidelines programmes have recently described their methods.[46] Since conclusive evidence exists for few health care procedures, deriving recommendations solely in areas of strong evidence would lead to a guideline of limited scope or applicability.[47] In certain limited circumstances, this could be sufficient if, for example, the guideline is to recommend the most strongly supported treatments for a given illness. More commonly, the guideline development group needs to interpret evidence where the trade off between benefits and harms is not so clear cut, and where patient preferences need to be taken into account.[47]

Box 5 Situations that might require clinical guidelines to be updated

1. Changes in the evidence on the existing benefits and harms of interventions.
2. Changes in the outcomes considered important.
3. Changes in the available interventions.
4. Changes in the evidence that current practice is optimal.
5. Changes in the values placed on outcomes.
6. Changes in the resources available for health care.

Resource implications and feasibility

In addition to scientific evidence and the opinions of expert clinicians within the guideline development group, practice guidelines must often take account of the feasibility of interventions. Feasibility issues worthy of consideration include the time, skills, personnel, and equipment necessary for the provider to carry out the recommendations and the ability of patients and systems of care to implement them.

Grading recommendations

It is common to grade each guideline recommendation. Such information provides the user with an indication of an amalgam of (a) the quality of the evidence, (b) the magnitude of benefits and harms to patients, and (c) weighing up the trade offs. While a number of 'strength of recommendation' classification schemes exist (e.g. Box 4), from simple to complex, no classification scheme has been shown to be superior. However, strong evidence does not always produce a strong recommendation and the classification should allow for this.

Prior to finalizing the guideline, it is important to have external review of the guideline for content validity, clarity, and applicability.

Updating clinical guidelines

While considerable resources are expended on the development of clinical guidelines, less attention has been paid to the process for assessing when guidelines should be updated and empirical descriptions of the process are few.[48] The most common advice is for guidelines to include a scheduled review date. However, this could result in wasted resources if a full update is undertaken prematurely within a slowly evolving field, or in guidelines in a rapidly evolving field becoming out-of-date before the scheduled review. Some guidelines state that they should be updated when new information becomes available; however, it is unclear how these should be operationalized. The situations that might require clinical guidelines to be updated are shown in Box 5.

The values placed on outcomes reflect clinical or societal norms: measuring these values and how these change over time is complex. When changes occur in the availability of resources for health care or the costs of interventions, a generic policy of updating is unlikely to be helpful, because policy makers in disparate health care systems consider different factors in deciding whether services remain affordable. A suggested model for updating focuses on defining when new information about interventions, outcomes, and performance justifies updating guidelines.[49] This process includes two stages: (a) identifying significant new evidence; and (b) assessing whether the new evidence warrants updating the guidance. This model has been applied to a set of national North American guidelines.[50]

Summary and key points

- *Definition of clinical guidelines:* 'Systematically developed statements to assist practitioner and patient decisions about appropriate health care for specific clinical circumstances'.
- Guidelines are only one option for improving the quality of health care. They are useful when clinicians are unclear about appropriate practice and when scientific evidence can provide an answer.
- If it is decided that using a guideline is the best strategy, identify rigorously developed guidelines from elsewhere and adapt them for local use.
- There are five steps that may be identified when an evidence-based guideline has been rigorously developed:
  - identifying and refining the subject area;
  - convening and running the guideline development groups;
  - obtaining and assessing the evidence about the clinical question or condition;
  - translating the evidence into a clinical practice guideline;
  - external review of the guideline.
- The range of treatment effects and costs of alternative patterns of care may be explored by a guideline group using a profiling approach, augmented by simple cost-effectiveness models.
- Guidelines also need updating at appropriate intervals.

References

1. **Field, M.J. and Lohr, K.N.**, ed. *Clinical Practice Guidelines: Directions for a New Program.* Institute of Medicine, Committee to Advise the Public Health Service on Clinical Practice Guidelines. Washington DC: National Academy Press, 1990.
2. **Centre for Reviews and Dissemination and Nuffield Institute for Health** (1994). Implementing clinical practice guidelines: can guidelines be used to improve clinical practice. *Effective Health Care* **1**, 1–12.
3. **Burgers, J.S., Grol, R., Klazinga, N.S., Mäkelä, M., and Zaat, J., for the AGREE Collaboration** (2003). Towards evidence-based clinical practice: an international survey of 18 clinical guideline programmes. *International Journal for Quality in Health Care* (in press).
4. **Holmes-Rovner, M., Llewellyn-Thomas, H., Entwistle, V., Coulter, A., O'Connor, A., and Rovner, D.R.** (2001). Patient choice modules for summaries of clinical effectiveness: a proposal. *British Medical Journal* **322**, 664–7.
5. **Kane, R.L.** (1995). Creating practice guidelines: the dangers of over-reliance on expert judgment. *Journal of Law and Medical Ethics* **23**, 62–4.
6. **Grimley Evans, J.** (1995). Evidence-based and evidence-biased medicine. *Age and Ageing* **24**, 461–3.
7. **Woolf, S.H.** (1997). Shared decision-making: the case for letting patients decide which choice is best. *Journal of Family Practice* **45**, 205–8.
8. **The AGREE Collaboration** (2000). Guideline development in Europe: an international comparison. *International Journal for Technology Assessment in Health Care* **16** (4), 1036–46.
9. **Hayward, R.S.A., Wilson, M.C., Tunis, S.R., Bass, E.B., and Guyatt, G.** (1995). Users' guides to the medical literature. VII. How to use clinical practice guidelines. Are the recommendations valid? *Journal of the American Medical Association* **274**, 570–4.
10. **Eccles, M.P., Clapp, Z., Grimshaw, J.M., Adams, P.C., Higgins, B., Purves, I., and Russell, I.T.** (1996). North of England evidence based guideline development project: methods of guideline development. *British Medical Journal* **312**, 760–1.
11. **Eccles, M., Freemantle, N., and Mason, J.** (1998). Methods of developing guidelines for efficient drug use in primary care: North of England Evidence Based Guidelines Development Project. *British Medical Journal* **316**, 1232–5.
12. **The AGREE Collaboration** (2001). Appraisal of Guidelines for Research and Evaluation (AGREE) Instrument (www.agreecollaboration.org).
13. **Grimshaw, J. and Eccles, M.** (1998). Clinical practice guidelines. In *Evidence Based Practice in Primary Care* (ed. C. Silagy and A. Haines), pp. 120–34. London: BMJ Publishing Group.
14. **Fletcher, S.W.** (1997). Whether scientific deliberation in health policy recommendations? Alice in the wonderland of breast-cancer screening. *New England Journal of Medicine* **336**, 1180–3.
15. **Ernster, V.L.** (1997). Mammography screening for women aged 40 through 49—a guidelines saga and a clarion call for informed decision making. *American Journal of Public Health* **87**, 1103–6.
16. **Woolf, S.H. and Dickey, L.L.** (1999). Differing perspectives on preventive care guidelines: a new look at the mammography controversy. *American Journal of Preventive Medicine* **17**, 260–8.
17. **Eccles, M., Freemantle, N., and Mason, J., for the North of England ACE-inhibitor Guideline Development Group** (1998). North of England Evidence-based Guideline Development Project: evidence-based guideline for the use of ACE-inhibitors in the primary care management of adults with symptomatic heart failure. *British Medical Journal* **316**, 1369–75.
18. **Newton, J., Knight, D., and Woolhead, G.** (1996). General practitioners and clinical guidelines: a survey of knowledge, use and beliefs. *British Journal of General Practice* **46**, 513–17.
19. **Hyams, A.L., Brandenburg, J.A., Lipsitz, S.R., Shapiro, D.W., and Brennan, T.A.** (1995). Practice guidelines and malpractice litigation: a two way street. *Annals of Internal Medicine* **122**, 450–5.
20. **General Medical Council.** *Maintaining Good Medical Practice.* London: General Medical Council, 1998.
21. **Jones, J.** (1999). Influenza drug to undergo 'fast track' assessment by NICE. *British Medical Journal* **319**, 400.
22. **Giesen, D.** *International Medical Malpractice Law.* Tubingen: JCR Mohr/Paul Siebeck, 1988.
23. **Bolam v Friern Hospital Management Committee.** All England Reports, 1957, pp. 118–28.
24. **Hurwitz, B.** *Clinical Guidelines and the Law.* Abingdon: Radcliffe Medical Press, 1998.
25. **Stern, K.** (1995). Clinical guidelines and negligence liability. In *Clinical Effectiveness: from Guidelines to Cost Effective Practice* (ed. M. Deighan and S. Hitch), pp. 127–35. Brentwood: Earlybrave Publications Ltd.
26. **Smith, G.H.** (1993). A case study in progress: practice guidelines and the affirmative defense in Maine. *Journal of Quality Improvement* **19**, 355–62.
27. **Solomon, R.P.** (2002). Clinical guidelines in the United States: perspectives on law and litigation. In *Clinical Guidelines: Law Policy & Practice* (ed. J. Tingle and C. Foster), pp. 137–59. London: Cavendish Publishing Ltd.
28. **Airedale NHS Trust v Bland.** All England Reports, 1993, pp. 821–96.
29. **Foster, C.** (2002). Civil procedure, trial issues and clinical guidelines. In *Clinical Guidelines: Law Policy & Practice* (ed. J. Tingle and C. Foster), pp. 111–20. London: Cavendish Publishing Ltd.
30. **Eccles, M. and Mason, J.** (2001). How to develop cost-conscious guidelines. *Health Technology Assessment* **5** (16), 1–69.
31. **Kahan, J.P.** et al. (1996). Variations by specialty in physician ratings of the appropriateness and necessity of indications for procedures. *Medical Care* **34** (6), 512–23.
32. **Coulter, I., Adams, A., and Shekelle, P.** (1995). Impact of varying panel membership on ratings of appropriateness in consensus panels—a comparison of a multi- and single-disciplinary panel. *Health Services Research* **30** (4), 577–91.
33. **Leape, L.L., Park, R.E., Kahan, J.P., and Brook, R.H.** (1992). Group judgements of appropriateness: the effect of panel composition. *Quality Assurance in Health Care* **4** (2), 151–9.
34. **van Wersch, A. and Eccles, M.** (2001). Involvement of consumers in the development of evidence based clinical guidelines: practical experiences from the North of England Evidence based guideline development programme. *Quality in Health Care* **10**, 10–16.
35. **Egger, M., Davey Smith, D., and Altman, D.G.**, ed. *Systematic Reviews in Health Care: Meta-analysis in Context* 2nd edn. London: BMJ Publishing Group, 2001.

36. **Eccles, M., Freemantle, N., and Mason, J.** (2001). Using systematic reviews in clinical guideline development. In *Systematic Reviews in Health Care: Meta-analysis in Context* 2nd edn. (ed. M. Egger, D. Davey Smith, and D.G. Altman), pp. 400–9. London: BMJ Publishing Group.
37. **Cochrane Reviewer's Handbook (updated July 1999)** (1999). In *The Cochrane Library* (database on disk and CD-ROM). The Cochrane Collaboration. Oxford: Update Software.
38. **Dickersin, K., Scherer, R., and Lefebvre, C.** (1994). Identifying relevant studies for systematic reviews. *British Medical Journal* **309**, 1286.
39. **Gregoire, G., Derderian, F., and Le Lorier, J.** (1995). Selecting the language of the publications included in a meta-analysis: is there a Tower of Babel bias? *Journal of Clinical Epidemiology* **48** (1), 159–63.
40. **Egger, M., Zellweger-Zähner, T., Schneider, M., Junker, C., Lengeler, C., and Antes, G.** (1997). Language bias in randomised controlled trials published in English and German. *Lancet* **350**, 326–9.
41. **Schulz, K.F., Chalmers, I., Hayes, R.J., and Altman, D.G.** (1995). Empirical evidence of bias: dimensions of methodological quality associated with estimates of treatment effects in controlled trials. *Journal of the American Medical Association* **273** (5), 408–12.
42. **Moher, D., Jones, A., Cook, D., Jadad, A.R., Moher, M., Tugwell, P., and Klassen, T.P.** (1998). Does quality of reports of randomised trials affect estimates of intervention efficacy reported in meta-analyses? *Lancet* **352**, 609–13.
43. **Williams, A.** (1995). How should information on cost effectiveness influence clinical practice? In *Outcomes into Clinical Practice* 1st edn. (ed. T. Delamothe), pp. 99–107. London: BMJ Publishing Group.
44. **Grimshaw, J., Eccles, M., and Russell, I.** (1995). Developing clinically valid practice guidelines. *Journal of Evaluation in Clinical Practice* **1**, 37–48.
45. **Eccles, M., Freemantle, N., and Mason, J.M.** (1999). The choice of antidepressants for depression in primary care. *Family Practice* **16**, 103–11.
46. **Harbour, R. and Miller, J.** (2001). A new system for grading recommendations in evidence based guidelines. *British Medical Journal* **323**, 334–6.
47. **Shekelle, P.G., Chassin, M.R., and Park, R.E.** (1998). Assessing the predictive validity of the RAND/UCLA appropriateness method criteria for performing carotid endarterectomy. *International Journal of Technology Assessment in Health Care* **14**, 707–27.
48. **Eccles, M., Rousseau, N., and Freemantle, N.** Updating evidence based guidelines. *Journal of Health Services Research & Policy* **7** (2), 98–103.
49. **Shekelle, P., Eccles, M.P., Grimshaw, J.M., and Woolf, S.H.** (2001). When should clinical guidelines be updated? *British Medical Journal* **323**, 155–7.
50. **Shekelle, P.G., Ortiz, E., Rhodes, S., Morton, S., Eccles, M.P., Grimshaw, J.M., and Woolf, S.** (2001). The validity of the agency for healthcare research and quality clinical practice guidelines: how quickly do guidelines go out of date? *Journal of the American Medical Association* **286** (12), 1461–7.

13.5 Tools for quality improvement and change in practice

Marjukka Mäkelä, Signe Flottorp, and Jeremy Grimshaw

Primary medical care is practised in a variety of settings and the ways of providing it are constantly changing. To suit different needs and resources, many practical approaches are used to change work processes, with the ultimate aim of improving the health outcomes reached. This chapter presents various tools for quality improvement (QI) and discusses the benefits and drawbacks of these methods. Educational approaches as such and the use of guidelines are not discussed here, as they are presented more extensively in other chapters.

The effectiveness of tools used daily in primary care QI is thinly studied. Most studies are descriptive, without comparative data from units that have not implemented QI methods. Shortell et al.[1] identified 56 studies assessing the impact of continuous quality improvement (CQI) on clinical practice. Fifty-three of these studies were uncontrolled and these suggested that CQI was effective, while no effect was seen in any of the randomized studies. The authors concluded that it was difficult to attribute the observed effects to CQI. As most studies (43 out of 56) also were done in single sites, their generalizability is limited.

Yano et al.[2] identified a number of successes in improving specific aspects of primary care but noted that there remain 'significant gaps in our knowledge'. For example, computer reminders and interventions using social influence promoted preventive care. However, they found few studies evaluating interventions to improve primary care goals such as access to care, continuity of care, comprehensiveness of care, aspects of patient outcome, or shift in care from inpatient to outpatient settings.

The individuals and teams studied have often been early adopters of quality improvement, with plenty of enthusiasm and typically also extra funding to apply the tools in their practices. The cost-effectiveness of the various methods has seldom been studied. Cost can vary greatly depending on the country and the setting, so that results are seldom transferable across borders.

Despite the relative lack of effectiveness data, many QI tools are widely spread and in active daily use. In the European Association on Quality in Primary Care (EQuiP), representatives from nearly 30 European countries have for 10 years discussed the different ways of promoting quality. The tools that this international group considered most useful were collected and published in a book.[3] In this EQuiP book, QI tools were classified according to the steps in the quality cycle: tools for choosing QI topics, tools for collecting performance data, tools for reflecting on the results by comparison or otherwise, and tools for changing actual work processes. All the tools had been used in one or more countries, so they had withstood the iron test of everyday practice. Most were very simple, requiring little extra resources except time.

This chapter presents in more detail six approaches for quality improvement in primary care:

- reminder systems;
- feedback of performance data;
- outreach visits;
- mutual practice visiting;
- quality cycle; and
- quality circles.

The first three methods are basically passive and depend on external support. The last three require active input from participants. All can be used by both single-handed professionals and teams. These methods usually need time for preparation, and they function best as an integral part of practice management. Many can be combined with other QI methods and incorporated in the development of more permanent quality management systems.

The terminology in this chapter follows the WONCA Classification Committee glossary,[4] which is slightly different from the concepts used in, for example, the Cochrane reviews on effective practice and organization of care. We have clarified each approach in a box at the beginning of the relevant section.

Clarify targets before selecting tools

Regardless of what method is used, a basic requirement for success is that the quality problem to be solved must be important to those who work with it. Most health professionals, teams, and patients can easily list a number

Table 1 Quality criteria to evaluate the management of benign prostatic hypertrophy[5]

Individual criteria	Population criteria
Change in symptom score (DAN-PSS-1)	Number of basic investigations
Change in residual urine volume	Number of detailed diagnostic procedures
Urine flow time (first 100 ml)	Proportions of patients treated with each method
Infections	Waiting times
Change in creatinine levels	Repeat operations
Complications	Complications

of areas or topics where practice performance could be improved. Everyday problems, such as diabetes, upper respiratory tract infections, and vaccinations, give plentiful ideas for change. It is difficult for physicians, however, to identify areas where change is needed most. When physicians are asked to choose a medical topic in which they wish to improve their knowledge, they frequently want to learn more about an area they already are interested in—and often also quite familiar with—while tending to disregard their real knowledge gaps.

The need for better care can be identified using simple tools such as brainstorming, complaint systems, or critical incident reports. In more systematic practice management, problems can be identified with patient satisfaction questionnaires or disease statistics. Useful criteria for prioritization of topics are, for example, the frequency or seriousness of the problem, identified gaps between current practice and available best evidence, and perceived ease of making changes. Regardless of the source of ideas, all suggestions need to be discussed openly among the members of the health team and prioritized by them. Change happens through motivated people.

'We would like to take better care of our asthma patients' is a good general direction of action. In order to create real and lasting change, however, the aim must be defined in detail. Care targets need to be based on high-quality evidence, and they must also be quantified. Any approach toward quality improvement needs to be based on valid measurement, as discussed in Chapter 13.2. Well-made guidelines can be a useful source of QI targets; at best, they provide a set of quality indicators ready to apply to practice populations. Otherwise quality criteria can be created by using the essential recommendations from a guideline, selecting indicators that are already available from statistics, or using generic measures of patient satisfaction. Table 1 gives an example of quality targets for treating benign prostatic hypertrophy from the Finnish evidence-based Current Care guideline.[5]

Reminder systems

Repeatedly occurring complicated decisions, such as combining medicines for several diseases or providing team care in chronic health problems, are common in primary care. Patients typically present with multiple problems and the general practitioner (GP) has to make several decisions in a short consultation. This presents a risk of omitting a necessary task or combining treatments in an adverse manner. Information overload is an enormous and ever increasing problem in medicine, and especially in primary care. GPs are expected to deliver evidence-based care for a wide range of conditions. It is impossible to keep updated in all fields, and it is even more difficult to remember and use the information when needed. There is not much time to reflect and search for information during the consultation.

Reminders are intended to help clinicians overcome these problems by prompting the doctor to recall information that they already know or would be expected to know, by presenting this information in an accessible and relevant format at a particularly appropriate time . For decades, GPs have used paper devices to combat this problem: problem-oriented sheets for diabetes or asthma patients, colour-coded tags in patient records for allergies, or simply notes in practice calendars.

Reminder systems

Reminder systems help clinicians to recall information that they already are aware of at an appropriate time in their decision-making process.

With practice computers, a whole new world of methods to support decision-making opens up. Machines are better than human beings in tasks that involve noticing and combining separate pieces of information from different sources. Computerized reminders are therefore expected to provide much help in the future—and also to prevent much trouble. Any tasks and decisions linked to functions already classified by the patient record system are suitable for reminder functions. These include tasks related to, for example:

- patient's age (vaccinations, periodic health checks);
- time of the year (pollen allergies, student teaching cases);
- medicines (interactions, drug dosage, need for laboratory tests);
- laboratory tests (appropriate use, pathological results);
- monitoring chronic conditions (yearly check-ups, warning for abnormal findings);
- social insurance systems (sick leaves);
- preventive care (screening programmes).

Reminders can also use guidelines as part of the decision support they provide. A reminder system may, for example, notice that a blood pressure reading recorded by a health visitor is in the intermediate–high area set for hypertensive patients. It then goes on to check the individual patient data. This patient's blood pressure levels are above the limits individually set for him for the third time within 3 months. The computer program then retrieves data on the patient's age, present and previous medication, renal function tests, and possible adverse reactions.

When the general practitioner next sees this patient—or even at the point when she goes to the general information section of her patient population—the computer has provided a message suggesting a change of medication. The computer may even have selected the least expensive product from the group of drugs recommended in the guideline for the treatment of this type of patient. Reminder functions rest on everyday logic, and as such they should be simple to include in any patient record system. Unfortunately, this is seldom achieved in practice. Software developers would be wise to collaborate with professionals in incorporating basic reminder functions into their programs.

Reminders can be combined with other QI tools, for instance feedback. The results of laboratory tests can be given with feedback about the requested tests, and with reminders about appropriate test use. The message given can be on paper or on screen, generic or patient-specific.[6,7] Some reminder systems require a response, others do not.

Factors that might influence the effect of the reminder include the type of targeted behaviour,[8] the source of the reminder and the involvement of target clinicians in the development of the reminder[9] and the involvement of patients or colleagues in the delivery of the reminder.[10] Information about the long-term effects of computer-based reminder systems is mixed: the benefits may remain constant or deteriorate over time.

Reminders to health care professionals can be effective in promoting practice change across a variety of clinical areas and settings.[11,12] Reminders have typically been evaluated as a part of a wide range of interventions aimed at improving professional practice[9,13] so that their independent effect is difficult to isolate. The use of computer-based decision support systems can lead to improvements in decisions on drug dosage, the provision of preventive care, and other aspects of medical care, but not convincingly in diagnostic decisions.[8]

Only few computerized reminder systems are available for use in daily practice in primary care, so it is natural that these systems have mostly been tested in specific projects only.[14] For example, the use of computer assistance in determining drug dosage has been studied in 15 trials, all for acute conditions in hospital settings. A systematic review of these trials[15] concludes that although the results are promising, further trials are necessary to determine whether the benefits seen in specialist applications can be realized in general use.

Feedback of performance

Seeing one's own patterns of practice is a sobering experience to most health care professionals. When someone else tells you what you have done, this can alter your behaviour and help you in adjusting to your peers, to standards, etc. Naturally occurring feedback is surprisingly often lacking even in group practices. The ability to reflect on practice and ask critical questions varies widely among GPs. It is difficult for each of us to identify our own 'blind spots' in knowledge and practice without help. As a GP, a good way to develop one's skills in selecting targets and using quality tools is within a peer group.[16]

Natural variation of health care practices is surprisingly wide (Fig. 1). Quality management does not aim at having all professionals or organizations provide care in exactly the same manner or at avoiding all errors. Instead, high quality performance means doing the right things in a continuously better manner.

Feedback of performance

> Feedback of performance provides the practitioner or the team with numerical data on their own patterns of practice. It can be combined with comparative results from colleagues; these are usually presented anonymously.

Receiving data not only on one's own practice but also on others' work gives a useful possibility for comparing with colleagues. Although audit with feedback has been widely studied[17] and shown to be moderately effective especially for changes in prescribing and diagnostic test ordering, there are few data on feedback alone. The social influence model suggests that feedback involving peer comparison is a more powerful tool for change than individual feedback alone, but this hypothesis has not been adequately tested. In all feedback involving several professionals, comparative data should be presented anonymously unless all participants have given their permission to be identified. The protection of individual patient data is a natural requirement in all comparative exercises.

Merely providing information to health care practitioners, however, is seldom enough to accomplish appropriate changes in practice.[18,19] Persons whose results are much higher or lower than others' may in the next observation period have moved slightly toward the mean value, but this does not necessarily signify improvement. Professionals who are outliers can also dismiss the data or rationalize their performance by asserting 'my patients are different'.

Information feedback is most likely to influence clinical practice if provided as part of a strategy targeting professionals who have agreed to review their practice.[20] The effect becomes clearer if the information is presented close to the time of decision-making. Short messages are more likely to be read, understood, and acted upon than long and complicated ones, so feedback should concentrate on essentials. The message, the provider of the feedback, its timeliness and the vehicle can all have influence on how well the feedback is received.[21] The questions of the optimum format, timing, layout, and quantity of information remain unanswered for the time being.

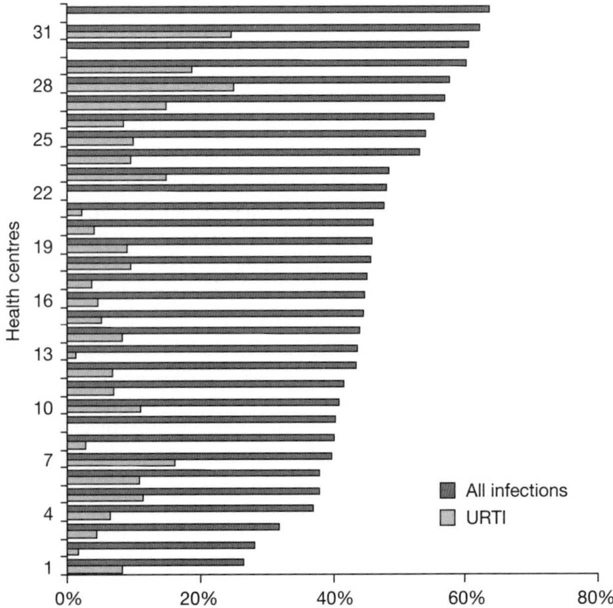

Fig. 1 Practice variation in the treatment of common infections in Finnish health centres: percentage of patients receiving antibiotic therapy for any infection and for upper respiratory tract infection (URTI). Courtesy of the Mikstra project (www.mikstra.fi).

Outreach visits

Trained facilitators can be used to help professionals incorporate a new working pattern, for example to implement a new guideline, in their practice. The facilitator can assist in updating patient files, provide training for practice personnel, teach the use of screening devices, etc. The traditional use of this method is the single visit by the medical industry (social marketing), and its effectiveness has been shown best for changing patterns of prescribing.[19,22] At the other extreme, the facilitator can provide a more sustained contact and support of practices over longer periods of time (facilitation model). Outreach visits can stimulate changes without demanding that the initiative comes from the busy practice itself. Well-conducted facilitation through outreach visits can root changes in a systematic fashion.

Outreach visits

> An outreach visit takes place at the workplace of a health care professional. It is a personal call by a trained person (facilitator) to a health provider in his or her own setting. The visitor provides various types of information, which may include feedback of performance or comparative data, in a one-to-one setting. Such visits can be single events (academic detailing) or repeated events over a period of time (facilitation model).

Pharmaceutical companies continue to spend large sums of money on this approach, which is one form of evidence for the effectiveness of these travelling salespersons. With more than a 100 years of sales experience, company representatives know they can influence prescribing patterns. Drug detailing can result in changing awareness and preferences as well as an increase of prescribing costs. This can be mediated through irrational prescribing, rapid prescribing of new drugs at the cost of older ones, and decreased prescribing of generic drugs.[23] Despite the fact that detailers shape prescribing behaviour so strongly, there is little published scientific evidence about the techniques or approaches of these representatives, so that we do not know how they might be used to reduce inappropriate prescribing.

A number of theories and principles of communication and behaviour change underlie the success of pharmaceutical companies in influencing prescribing practices. Based on these theories and several field trials, it is possible to design methods to improve physicians' clinical decision making so that the quality and cost-effectiveness of care are enhanced. According to Soumerai et al.,[24] some of the most important techniques of educational outreach visits include:

- familiarity with current prescribing patterns;
- focusing programmes on specific categories of physicians, including opinion leaders;
- defining clear educational and behavioural objectives;
- establishing credibility;
- stimulating active physician participation in educational interactions;
- using concise graphic educational material;
- highlighting and repeating the essential messages; and
- providing positive reinforcement of improved practices in follow-up visits.

Current prescribing patterns can be examined by using databases, but it is also necessary to conduct interviews to investigate the baseline knowledge and motivation of those to be approached by facilitators. Preliminary interviews before outreach visits can also help by identifying barriers to change. Facilitators might be especially useful when there are organizational or structural barriers for implementing the new mode of working. Credibility can be established through having a respected organizational identity as the source of information, by referencing authoritative and unbiased sources of information, and by presenting both sides of controversial issues.

Evidence supports the use of educational outreach visits combined with additional interventions to reduce inappropriate prescribing by physicians. The effects are small to moderate, but potentially of practical importance. The cost-effectiveness of this approach in different circumstances is unclear.[19]

Mutual practice visiting

General practitioners, primary care nurses, health visitors, or other primary care professionals can visit each other singly or in teams to observe practice facilities, management, and organizational patterns. They can also sit in on each other's consultations. This is typically done reciprocally. The visits can be supported with checklists; the doctor being observed can fill part of these before the visit. In Belgium, GPs have developed a manual to structure mutual visits and to provide a basis for written assessment (Fig. 2).

Practice visiting

Practice visiting is a mutual, structured peer observation of professionals' daily work. It is based on trust and change is facilitated by constructive feedback.

Practice visiting may help to spot problems that can be corrected almost immediately. Physicians often report that they benefit equally from observing

Visiting each other's practice

HOST: Name, address, telephone — VISITOR: Name, address, telephone

Make your choices of topics to cover:

I FACILITIES			
1. Reception			
2. Waiting room:	a. Furniture d. Child centredness	b. Reading materials, leaflets etc. e. Posters	c. Radio/TV
3. Toilet facilities			
4. Surgery:	a. Size	b. Dressing room	c. Dressing mat. etc.
5. Equipment:	a. ECG-equipment	b. X-rays	c. Minor surgery equipment etc.
6. Hardware and software			
II Management, organization			
7. Filing system:	a. System d. Correspondence	b. Problem oriented medical records e. X-rays etc.	c. Occupational accidents
9. Group practice:	a. Teamwork	b. Team management	
10. Appointment system			
12. Availability:	a. Out of hours services	b. Vacation services	c. Telephone system
13. Collaboration with:	a. Colleagues d. Pharmaceutical representatives	b. Specialists	c. Other health professionals
17. Professional/private life			
III Consultation			
20. Practice guidelines			
21. Continuing care:	a. Prescription behaviour	b. Referral: when, how	c. Follow-up
22. Physician-patient relationship			
24. Body language			
27. Coping with time pressure			
28. Telephone consultations			
IV Meta level			
31. Personal values and motivation			
32. Family life values			
33. Community involvement			
34. Discussion:	a. GP tasks & functions d. Patient profiles	b. GP satisfaction e. Personal limits	c. Patient satisfaction f. Professional growth

Fig. 2 Menu for structuring practice visits in Belgium (slightly abridged). (*From:* Seuntjens, L. and Remmen, R. (1998). Practice visiting. In *Tools and Methods for Quality Improvement in General Practice* (ed V. Alles et al.), pp. 35–6. Jyväskylä: EQuiP and Stakes.)

Table 2 Giving and receiving feedback

Guidelines for giving constructive feedback	Guidelines for receiving feedback
1. Give feedback only when asked to do so or when your offer of feedback is accepted	1. Listen to feedback
2. Give feedback as soon after the event as possible	2. Assume that feedback is constructive
3. Focus on the positive. You reinforce what you talk about. When possible, give positive feedback *first* and *last*	3. Consider only constructive elements of the feedback, and consider them carefully
4. Be descriptive, not evaluative	4. Pause and think before responding
5. Talk about specific behaviour and give an example where possible	5. Ask for repetition if you have not heard clearly
6. Where feedback is negative, suggest alternatives where appropriate	6. Ask for clarification or examples if statements are unclear or unsupported
7. Ask yourself: 'Why am I giving this feedback? For myself—or to help the other person?'	7. Receive both negative and positive feedback positively for consideration, instead of protecting yourself by dismissing it
8. Remember feedback says at least as much about the giver as the receiver	8. Ask for suggestions of how you might modify or change your behaviour
9. Negative feedback is useful only when given about things that can be changed	9. Respect the persons giving feedback and thank them

someone else's practice and from being observed. The time needed to prepare for the visit and to cover the practice in a structured manner is at least 4–6 h per visit, which can be an obstacle for single-handed GPs. This form of QI has also been used in large group practices, where different members of the team make a collective visit, each guided by their colleagues.

The use of indicators has been validated for use,[25] but otherwise we have not identified any studies evaluating this method of quality improvement. It is probably important that the aims of the visits are clearly defined. An essential condition for a constructive practice visit is that the process is based on trust. Areas of difference are always identified, as there is huge variation in practice for many conditions. We often take our own routines for granted. Visiting other practices that use other ways of organizing daily work and delivering care for specific conditions can be a rich source for reflection. Hopefully, the participating practitioners also can search for and find evidence for best practice, and not only discuss the pros and cons of their respective models of work.

Practice visits could be combined with other QI methods, for instance feedback. The practitioner receiving a visitor should remain open-minded and receptive, whilst the observing practitioner should aim at a positive and constructive approach, remembering that feedback can be threatening. Guidelines for giving and receiving feedback are helpful for both parties (Table 2).

Quality cycle

With a 'quality cycle' we mean a systematic use of medical audit and feedback, combined with changes and follow-up. Medical audit has been defined as 'systematic, critical analysis of the quality of medical care, including the procedures used for diagnosis and treatment, the use of resources, and the resulting outcome and quality of life for the patient'.[26] The WONCA glossary[4] describes medical audit as 'a professional activity where structure, process or outcome is analysed and compared with a gold standard, to see to what degree the professional performance reaches the criteria which the profession has defined as good or optimal'. Similar definitions are used for clinical audit, with the term 'medical care' replaced by 'clinical care'. Clinical audit is often interpreted as audit for clinical professions other than medicine. It can also be handled as multidisciplinary audit, involving a wide range of clinical professionals or the whole health team.

Quality cycle

The full quality cycle includes collecting performance data about the selected topic for QI, evaluating the results against others' performance or some type of standards or guidelines, identifying the most suitable modes for changing work processes, and evaluating the performance again after changes have been rooted.

Audits or quality cycles can be used within one practice or as a joint effort by several professionals or practices. In many countries, audit organizations give support to practices by providing data collecting sheets, comparative results and training. For example, the Danish Audit Project Odense (APO) has been providing such support for GPs for more than 10 years, facilitating prospective data collection by providing simple, structured sheets (Fig. 3).

Both single-handed professionals and group practices use the APO tools on a variety of topics. The idea has spread outside Denmark into Sweden, Norway, and Finland. Changes of practice have over the years been demonstrated in several topics and in different geographical areas. A typical project would be on the use of antibiotics in upper respiratory tract diseases, aiming at a reduction in overall antibiotic use and in the use of broad-spectrum antibiotics. The production of national guidelines has also been supported by the APO audit activity. A well-motivated peer group greatly supports the completion of a full audit cycle even when the APO tool is being used.

Evaluation of entire programmes of medical audit is difficult, because many studies do not explicitly state clear objectives. 'To improve the quality of care doctors provide for their patients' is a goal one cannot disagree with, but as in all QI activities, it is more difficult to find a common definition of quality. Almost all medical audit studies focus on the more easily measurable medical outcome aspects of quality, rather than issues of equity or patient satisfaction. A study of 448 audits identified 60 000 criteria, and found that only 3 per cent related to psychosocial aspects and 4 per cent to communication with patients.[27] The interpersonal aspect of health care, although clearly essential for patients, has rarely been investigated.

Quality circles

A quality circle regularly brings together professionals from different practices to discuss quality. Such groups can also plan and complete QI projects.[16] Depending on the tradition of the country, quality circles can vary in size and mode of action. They can be used for fairly unstructured discussion of problem cases, or be regular monthly arrangements that take on a new QI topic once or twice a year. Groups can be profession-based or include members from various specialities; in some circles, patient representatives or colleagues from other specialities are included.[3] Quality circles are typically self-regulating, but in several countries, centralized support for this type of QI is arranged on a regular basis. Quality circles are also an example of using the social influences model.

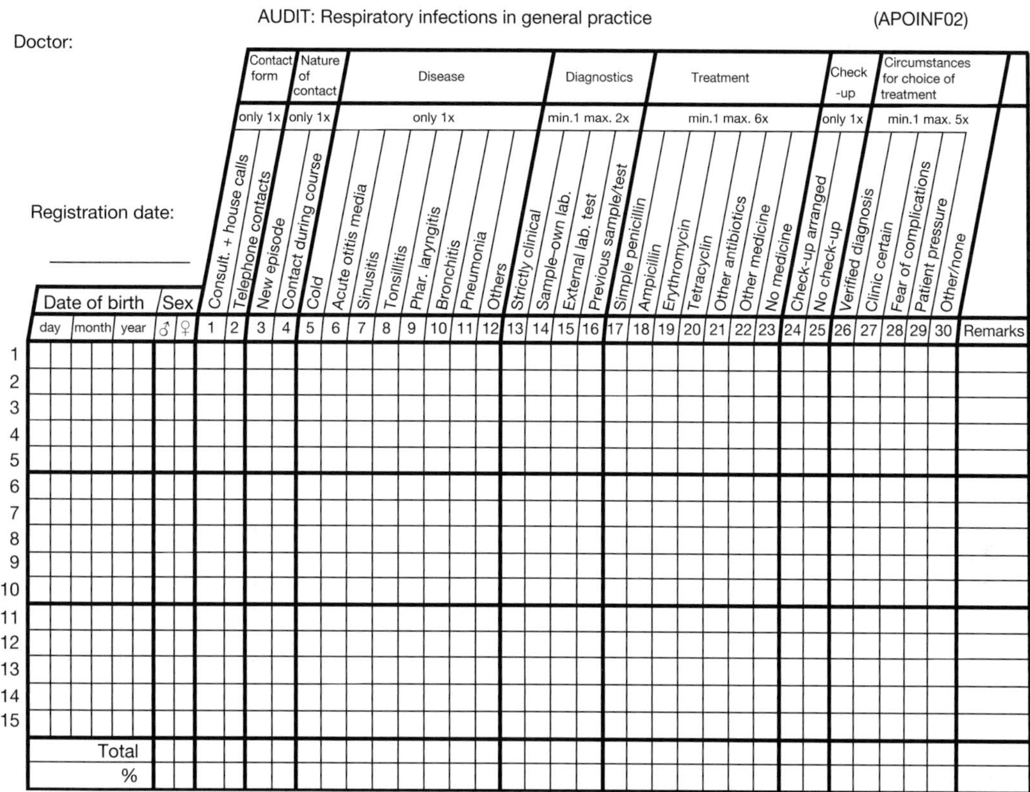
AUDIT: Respiratory infections in general practice (APOINF02)

Doctor:

Registration date: ____________

Contact form (only 1x)		Nature of contact (only 1x)		Disease (only 1x)								Diagnostics (min.1 max. 2x)				Treatment (min.1 max. 6x)							Check-up (only 1x)		Circumstances for choice of treatment (min.1 max. 5x)					
Consult. + house calls	Telephone contacts	New episode	Contact during course	Cold	Acute otitis media	Sinusitis	Tonsillitis	Phar. laryngitis	Bronchitis	Pneumonia	Others	Strictly clinical	Sample–own lab.	External lab. test	Previous sample/test	Simple penicillin	Ampicillin	Erythromycin	Tetracyclin	Other antibiotics	Other medicine	No medicine	Check-up arranged	No check-up	Verified diagnosis	Clinic certain	Fear of complications	Patient pressure	Other/none	
1	2	3	4	5	6	7	8	9	10	11	12	13	14	15	16	17	18	19	20	21	22	23	24	25	26	27	28	29	30	Remarks

Date of birth: day / month / year; Sex: ♂ ♀

Rows: 1, 2, 3, 4, 5, 6, 7, 8, 9, 10, 11, 12, 13, 14, 15; Total; %

Fig. 3 Audit sheet for respiratory infections in general practice from the APO project. (*From:* Munck, A. (1998). Audit Project Odense. In *Tools and Methods for Quality Improvement in General Practice* (ed. V. Alles et al.), pp. 70–2. Jyväskylä: EQuiP and Stakes.)

Quality circles

A quality circle is a group of professional peers meeting regularly to discuss practical quality issues, compare experiences, and practice data. People outside the practice team (e.g., other specialists, patients, or other care providers) can also participate.

The practitioners usually arrange quality circles themselves and participation is entirely voluntary. This tool is often used in countries where GPs work single-handed. The members of the group decide on the topics that they want to discuss or collect data about, and select the QI methods they want to use. Meetings can be arranged around case reports, video documents, or simple exchange of experiences on an agreed topic. Many quality circles have projects where all participants together go through the full quality cycle. Evaluations show high uptake and good acceptance of this method of QI among primary care workers. Improved self-awareness and changes in practice routines are obvious, but the impact on patient outcomes needs further research.[28]

Conclusions

Traditionally, the medical culture has focused on individual errors. The responsibility for mistakes—and for quality—is more often linked to persons than to the organization of daily work. In a culture of blaming, outcome measurement and feedback is often perceived as potentially dangerous, thus feared and avoided. When quality improvement provides the cultural framework, errors and deviations are seen as potential sources for learning activities. We are not aiming at perfect or error-free practitioners. On the contrary: it is important to admit that the art and science of medicine is rich in uncertainties and practised by people who will continue to make mistakes even in the best of health care systems.

There are many simple tools for quality improvement that can be used without much previous experience, and with little outside support. Very few quality tools, however, can engage those professionals who are uninterested or unwilling to observe their own work and discuss it critically.

References

1. **Shortell, S.M., Bennett, C.L., and Byck, G.R.** (1998). Assessing the impact of continuous quality improvement on clinical practice: what it will take to accelerate progress. *Milbank Memorial Quarterly* **76**, 1–37.
2. **Yano, E.M.** et al. (1995). Helping practices reach primary care goals. Lessons from the literature. *Archives of Internal Medicine* **155**, 146–56.
3. **Alles, V.** et al., ed. *Tools and Methods for Quality Improvement in General Practice.* Jyväskylä: EQuiP and Stakes, 1998.
4. **WONCA Classification Committee** (1995). An international glossary for general/family practice. *Family Practice* **12** (3), 341–69.
5. **Suomen urologiyhdistys ry.** Käypä hoito—suositus: Eturauhasen hyvänlaatuinen liikakasvu. (Current Care guideline: Benign prostatic hypertrophy. In Finnish.) October 2001 (http://www.duodecim.fi/kh/).
6. **Gordon, R.B.** et al. (2002). On-screen computer reminders: effects on professional practice and health care outcomes (Protocol for a Cochrane Review). In *The Cochrane Library* Issue 3. Oxford: Update Software.
7. **Gorman, P.N.** et al. (2002). Computer-generated paper reminders: effects on professional practice and health care outcomes (Protocol for a Cochrane Review). In *The Cochrane Library* Issue 3. Oxford: Update Software.
8. **Hunt, D.L.** et al. (1998). Effects of computer-based clinical decision support systems on physician performance and patient outcomes: a systematic review. *Journal of the American Medical Association* **280** (15), 1339–46.

9. **Grimshaw, J.** et al. (1995). Developing and implementing clinical practice guidelines. *Quality in Health Care* **4**, 55–64.
10. **Cohen, S.J., Halvorson, H.W., and Gosselink, C.A.** (1994). Changing physician behavior to improve disease prevention. *Preventive Medicine* **23** (3), 284–91.
11. **Buntinx, F.** et al. (1993). Influencing diagnostic and preventive performance in ambulatory care by feedback and reminders. A review. *Family Practice* **10**, 219–28.
12. **Wensing, M. and Grol, R.** (1994). Single and combined strategies for implementing changes in primary care: a literature review. *International Journal of Quality in Health Care* **6**, 115–32.
13. **Davis, D.A.** et al. (1995). Changing physician performance. A systematic review of the effect of continuing medical education strategies. *Journal of the American Medical Association* **274**, 700–5.
14. **Wyatt, J.** (1999). Computer-based clinical decision support systems can enhance physician performance but have been insufficiently studied with regard to patient outcomes. *Evidence-based Healthcare* **3**, 39.
15. **Walton, R.T.** et al. (2002). Computerised advice on drug dosage to improve prescribing practice (Cochrane Review). In *The Cochrane Library* Issue 3. Oxford: Update Software.
16. **Grol, R. and Lawrence, M.** *Quality Improvement by Peer Review*. Oxford: Oxford University Press, 1995.
17. **Thomson O'Brien, M.A.** et al. (2002). Audit and feedback versus alternative strategies: effects on professional practice and health care outcomes (Cochrane Review). In *The Cochrane Library* Issue 3. Oxford: Update Software.
18. **Grimshaw, J.M.** et al. (2001). Changing provider behavior: an overview of systematic reviews of interventions. *Medical Care* **39** (8 Suppl. 2), 112–45.
19. **Thomson O'Brien, M.A.** et al. (2002). Educational outreach visits: effects on professional practice and health care outcomes (Cochrane Review). In *The Cochrane Library* Issue 3. Oxford: Update Software.
20. **Mugford, M., Banfield, P., and O'Hanlon, M.** (1991). Effects of feedback of information on clinical practice: a review. *British Medical Journal* **303**, 398–402.
21. **Axt-Adam, P., van der Wouden, J.C., and van der Does, E.** (1993). Influencing behavior of physicians ordering laboratory tests: a literature study. *Medical Care* **31** (9), 784–94.
22. **Hulscher, M.E.J.L.** Implementing prevention in general practice: a study of cardiovascular disease. Thesis, Nijmegen, The Netherlands, 1998.
23. **Wazana, A.** (2000). Physicians and the pharmaceutical industry: is a gift ever just a gift? *Journal of the American Medical Association* **283**, 373–80.
24. **Soumerai, S.B.** et al. (1993). Improving choice of prescribed antibiotics through concurrent reminders in an educational order form. *Medical Care* **31**, 552–8.
25. **van den Hombergh, P.** et al. (1998). Assessment of management in general practice: validation of a practice visit method. *British Journal of General Practice* **48**, 1743–50.
26. **Department of Health.** *Medical Audit*. Working paper no. 6. London: HMSO, 1989.
27. **Berg, J.K. and Kelly, J.T.** (1981). Evaluation of psychosocial health care in quality assurance activities. *Medical Care* **19**, 24–9.
28. **Gerlach, F.M. and Beyer, M.** (1998). New concept for continuous documentation of development of quality circles in ambulatory care: initial results from an information system in Germany. *Quality in Health Care* **7** (1), 55–61.

13.6 Total quality management and continuous quality improvement

Paul E. Plsek, Leif I. Solberg, and Richard Grol

Introduction

The technological breakthroughs of modern medicine have also created a growing unease about quality, especially in primary care. It is hard to understand why a profession that can transplant hearts cannot provide higher rates of preventive services or control more hypertension. Consequently, interest in applying the concepts and tools of Total Quality Management (TQM) and Continuous Quality Improvement (CQI), adapted from industry, has grown rapidly in health care.

The terms TQM and CQI are used here interchangeably and refer to a comprehensive, organization-wide, systematic effort to coordinate, monitor and improve quality, with a focus that includes patient satisfaction, cost reduction, process efficiency, clinical outcomes, and (in some public health settings) societal impact.[1–3] While individual improvement projects begin and end, TQM/CQI is an ongoing effort to improve the whole organization. It is related to the discipline of systems thinking[4] in that it is holistic in its approach, recognizing that for an organization to be truly effective, each part of it must work properly together. The World Association of Family Doctors (WONCA) recently concluded 'Quality work in health care is increasingly heading towards quality systems'.[5]

Despite the seeming logic of this approach and many anecdotal reports of success, TQM/CQI has not yet demonstrated effectiveness in randomized trials in health care.[6,7] We will describe the somewhat disappointing current evidence for TQM/CQI and suggest that this experience is due primarily to the challenge associated with the effort required to actually implement a total quality system. Next, we will provide a description of basic principles and models, followed by a brief description of what is needed to adapt these principles to primary care. Since TQM requires that primary care practices understand the organizational aspects of quality that have traditionally not been a part of clinical training, we will then describe this critical new way of thinking. Finally, we will describe some encouraging trends and conclude that TQM/CQI does hold promise for dramatic improvements in primary care, provided that leaders rise to the challenge its implementation presents. (Note: we will simply use the term TQM to refer to TQM/CQI.)

Disappointing evidence for TQM in primary care

Total quality management efforts in primary care began in the mid-1990s with a number of observational and before/after studies suggesting that this methodology was likely to be effective.[8–14] However, each of these studies only partially addressed the issue of the general effectiveness of TQM.

For example, Carlin et al.[8] provided a case report of 19 clinics in the United States using QI teams to improve 2-year-old immunization rates from 53.5 to 86.5 per cent. Many similar reports describe improvement in a single topic area. While these are certainly a benefit to the patients and clinics involved, it is not the comprehensive, organization-wide effort envisioned by true TQM, and the changes may not persist without such an effort. Goebers et al.[12] describe a study involving 20 small practices in the Netherlands who were provided with trained TQM facilitators, and then compared to 19 control practices after 18 months. While all practices accepted the TQM model, and 33 projects on a variety of topics were completed during the study period, this did not result in sustainable changes in practice and physician performance. Hearnshaw et al.[14] describe an observational study of primary care teams in England participating in education on organization-wide TQM in which follow-up evaluations indicated that changes were still in place 3 years after the education. Unfortunately, this was true for only three of the six teams who participated in the education, and these six were self-selected from among 147 teams that were invited.

The first scientific trials of TQM in health care took place in primary care. Goldberg et al. describe an effort to implement guidelines for depression and hypertension that involved 15 teams in four clinics, with five teams randomized to add TQM to academic detailing.[15] The net impact on care of this addition was no greater than in control teams.

A second, larger trial involving 44 private primary care clinics was designed to test whether systems changes could improve the delivery of a broad range of important preventive services in the half of the clinics randomly assigned to a TQM-based training and facilitation intervention.[16] Each intervention clinic identified an internal team, whose leader and facilitator were then trained in both systems content and change management through a collaborative multisession process that was contiguous with their teams' actions. Most of the teams were enthusiastic, worked hard, and most (but not all) eventually implemented a common system to more consistently provide for mammography, Pap smears, immunizations, and screening for smoking, hypertension, and hypercholesterolaemia in adults. Optimism was fuelled by anecdotes of clinic change efforts and by early studies showing a doubling of system elements in the intervention clinics only.[17] Unfortunately, when the results of patient surveys and chart audits were finally analysed, only one preventive service had a small statistically significantly greater change in the intervention clinics over the course of 2 years.[18] The investigators suggested that there were multiple causes for this failure, including 'inadequate tension for change, limited organizational change experience, mixed leadership support, a sub-optimal CQI improvement model, inadequate content, enormous environmental turmoil, inexperienced team leadership, and insufficient time pressures and calendar time'.[19]

Since these problems seemed potentially solvable, the principal investigator went on to test a revised approach for depression management.[20] This time, three primary care clinics whose leaders had chosen to work on this problem used more modern 'rapid cycle' methods in a combined CQI team with an experienced leader and facilitator facing a 7-month deadline. An explicit goal was set by clinic leaders to improve follow-up care of depressed patients by creating a nurse care-manager role with systems support to provide periodic phone calls. Unfortunately, despite similar team enthusiasm and hard work, no overall changes could be demonstrated in either the process or outcome of care as compared to six matched control clinics in the same medical group. The principal cause for this failure appeared to be inadequate perceived necessity for change and a related lack of leadership pressure to truly implement the change in care processes.

Secondary care has a similar disappointing story to tell with regard to randomized trials of TQM in that many early efforts tended to view quality improvement in terms of specific projects rather than in its organizational context. However, since secondary care typically occurs in large institutions with clearer administrative leadership and systems, these shortcomings were recognized more quickly.

These remain the only scientific trials of TQM methods in primary care and they force the thoughtful practitioner embarking on such efforts to pay more attention to the organizational aspects of change. We remain convinced that some version of this approach to quality improvement is essential and will work; the anecdotal, observational, and before/after evidence is highly suggestive. What the above examples illustrate is that TQM is more than tools and individual projects; it requires truly committed effective leadership and the right mix of contextual and organizational factors.

TQM principles and models

While tools and projects are the place to start in any effort to improve quality in a primary care setting, successful implementation of TQM in primary care must be built upon a realization of what is meant by a comprehensive, organization-wide effort to improve quality. Various authors, both in general industry and health care, and various national and international bodies, have described the basic principles of TQM.[1,2,21–24] Typically cited principles include the following.

Understanding of processes and systems: All work involves the execution of processes. An organization effectively practicing TQM explicitly defines its processes in order to continuously redesign them to improve output and service, while reducing waste and unnecessary complexity.[25] For example, a practice might follow the flow of a laboratory order and then eliminate several transcription and handling steps by redesigning the order form and having it printed on paper that automatically produces multiple copies as the order is written. Organizations practicing TQM also understand that processes are further embedded within one another and linked in complex ways.

Patient- (or customer-) centred focus: Processes and systems exist to produce outputs and services that provide a benefit to, or meet the needs of, patients, families, and society.[26] These customers can be external to the organization (e.g. the patient is the customer of the drug prescribing system) or internal (e.g. the lab technician is a customer of the physician who writes the order for a test). It follows, therefore, that if an organization is going to carry out a process, it should seek to provide the greatest benefit to the customers of that process. TQM encourages such 'customer thinking' throughout the organization.

Understanding of variation: The outcomes of processes and systems are naturally variable.[27] For example, patients will not always take their medications as prescribed, and physicians will not always provide all of the preventive services that are needed by individual patients. This variation in outcome is due to both the intended and unintended variation in the people, machines, materials, methods, and measurements that make up the process.[2] Some of this variation is desirable, and some is undesirable or harmful. TQM tries to remove the undesirable variation while preserving what is needed to best meet the needs of individuals and situations.

Pursuit of continuous improvement: Organizations that implement TQM seek to push the performance of systems beyond existing standards and norms. The goal is to achieve and maintain a never-before-achieved level of performance. An effective total quality system should facilitate continuous improvements and redesigns by encouraging alternating cycles of change, followed by relative stability, followed by more change.[28]

Management by facts and continuous learning: Fundamental to TQM is the commitment to use data and a logical process to build knowledge, make decisions, and promote ongoing learning.[29] Systematic building of knowledge through disciplined data collection, evidence-based practice, and deliberate experimentation lies at the foundation of all effective TQM efforts.

Positive view of people: While some see people as the ultimate cause of all problems and inefficiencies, TQM views the people who work in the process as the ultimate source of knowledge about how to improve it.[30,31] TQM seeks to engage the people who actually do the work in efforts designed to improve that work. In keeping with an understanding of processes and systems, this also typically requires an unprecedented level of multidisciplinary teamwork.

Key role of leadership: The need for effective and visionary leadership is a central theme in TQM.[2,12,31] Without strong leadership and an organizational infrastructure to support quality efforts, improvement may not happen; or, if it does happen, may quickly dissipate because of neglect and lack of integration with other activities in the organization.

To facilitate attention to these principles, several 'frameworks' for TQM have emerged. These frameworks are all simply formalizations of the principles described above; often captured in the form of questions that can be used to plan for and assess the quality system in an organization.

For example, The Baldrige Award in the United States provides a seven-element framework of what constitutes a total quality management system (see Box 1).[23] Note that while individual quality improvement efforts in primary care answer somewhat narrower questions—Did the care match the relevant guidelines? or How can we lower HbA1c values in persons with diabetes?—the Baldrige framework for TQM pertains to much larger, more

Box 1 USA Malcolm Baldrige Award framework

1. *Leadership:* How do senior leaders address values, performance expectations, a focus on patients and other key customers and stakeholders, empowerment, innovation, learning, organizational direction, and responsibility to the public?
2. *Strategic planning:* What is the organization's strategic development process? By what means does it set, deploy, and track strategic objectives, action plans, and related financial and staffing plans?
3. *Focus on patients, other customers, and communities:* How does the organization determine the requirements and expectations of patients, other customers and the community in which it is embedded? How does it build ongoing relationships and determine satisfaction?
4. *Information and analysis:* What is the organization's performance measures system and how does it analyse and act upon information?
5. *Staff focus:* What does the organization do to enable all staff to develop and utilize their full potential, in a way that is aligned with the organization's objectives? How does it build and constantly improve the work environment and staff support climate to make it conducive to performance excellence, full participation, and personal and organizational growth?
6. *Process management:* How does the organization design and deliver processes that are aligned with customer expectations and waste-free? How does it work to involve suppliers and staff in all departments to produce smooth-flowing systems of work?
7. *Organizational performance results management:* How does the organization measure and feed back into the system its results on clinical outcomes; satisfaction of patients, staff, and public financial performance; and operational performance? How does the organization compare itself to other organizations?

all-encompassing questions about how the organization runs in general. McFarland et al. report on their use of the Baldrige framework in a community mental health facility in the United States with 120 staff and 1300 outpatients.[32] However, their report describes plans and early efforts only; no specific results.

The European Framework for Quality Management (EFQM) is another high-level model for a total quality system based on the principles described above. It has been used to assess a primary health care centre in Spain.[33] Further initiatives to make the EFQM model applicable in primary care are underway in the Netherlands. Similarly, the International Standards Organization ISO-9000 framework forms the basis for the total quality management systems in Finnish primary care and social services centres in Espoonlahti, Finland (population of 41 000). Results cited in the Finnish case include winning local awards for quality, easing a merger, building cooperation, improving service orientation, and enhancing patient focus; but no quantitative outcomes have been reported.[34]

Adapting TQM to primary care

Understanding the general principles and frameworks for TQM gives insight into why there is simultaneously good evidence of success in individual improvement projects in organizations that are internally compelled to improve, and little evidence of success when one attempts to implement comprehensive TQM in a randomly selected primary care organization. The work required to implement TQM is broad, deep, and time-consuming; not every organization will be up to it. In addition, the nature of general or family practice lends additional challenges. Many practices have structures in which the doctor is simultaneously an owner, manager, and worker. Many also have small staff that may lack the time, knowledge, and skills needed for formal quality improvement activities.[13] Nevertheless, case reports suggest that the basic concepts can be, and have been, adapted to primary care.

For example, Goebers et al.[22] describe a quality system model for primary care based on four core principles: leading role of management, actions based on factual data, a systematic approach, and close collaboration in quality improvement among all those who are involved in the care processes. Their quality system model includes: (i) involving all staff; (ii) setting targets for improvement; (iii) establishing priorities for subjects that especially need improvement; (iv) doing small and easy to handle improvement projects; and (v) using the quality cycle and easy to use tools and techniques. They describe favourable changes in participating practices, such as: having regular practice meetings on quality improvement with all staff, enhancing leadership by designating a quality coordinator role, making annual plans on improvement, and making annual reports on quality improvement activities and results.

This work illustrates that the principles and systems of TQM can be adapted conceptually to small, primary care practices. It should also be clear, however, that making the adaptation requires a considerable amount of effort on the part of the practice and represents nothing short of a transformation in thinking and action.

Organizational aspects of TQM

In order to be successful in adopting TQM, the practitioner needs to take advantage of the thinking and experiences of other industries, and the related fields of change management and organizational development, who have dealt with improvement and change far longer than has medical care.[35]

Unfortunately, the scientific studies on quality improvement through guideline implementation are virtually bereft of any recognition of the role of systems or organizational factors and have drawn little from current thinking in management theory and from the experiences of other industries.[36,37] The fields of change management and organizational development are summarized in an excellent overview by Weber and Joshi, the key points of which are outlined in Box 2.[38] The literature in these fields should be read early and re-read periodically by those wishing to implement TQM in a primary care setting.

The lessons learned in other fields and industries are that the context and culture of the organization matters a great deal when implementing TQM. Randomly selected organizations may not be prepared to implement TQM in its fullest sense.[39] Studies of the use of guidelines and evidence-based practice note that improvement efforts are sensitive to local differences in organizations, personnel, and disease condition that are poorly understood.[15,40] Øvretveit summarizes it best in his review of quality improvement work in Europe when he states:

> Transferring a method or approach that works in one organization to another organization, or changing the organization in a particular way, may not produce the same effect. The result in one setting is an effect of the method or approach working within that system, not just an effect of the method or approach alone.[41]

The experience in primary care teaches some simple but critical lessons for effective quality improvement that the thoughtful practitioner wishing to implement TQM would be wise to heed:

- Unless the leaders of the organization are strongly committed to change, improvement teams are likely to have only limited success with the improvement concepts and tools described in other chapters in this section.
- Leaders must be capable of leading the change. This is as true of a two-doctor practice as it is of one with 500 physicians; whether the 'leaders' are physicians or managers.
- It is unlikely that the organizational leaders will be sufficiently committed to the change unless they perceive that the external environment requires it and will reward those who achieve it.

Box 2 Key strategies for change (as summarized by Weber and Joshi[38])

The literature and experience on change in health care organizations points to eight crucial strategies:

1. Develop a long-term vision for change, but start with things that can be accomplished in a relatively short period of time in order to build momentum.
2. Focus on the change process itself; the 'how' of change is just as important as the 'what' of change.
3. Think carefully about which individuals and opinion leaders in the organization must respond to the change and what barrier may exist for these individuals.
4. Build constructive partnerships between physicians and administration.
5. Create a culture of continuous commitment to change where learning is always taking place.
6. Ensure that change begins with leadership; leaders should not expect others to change if they themselves are not role models for change.
7. Ensure that change is well communicated, through multiple channels, and in ways that create a positive 'buzz' throughout the organization.
8. Build in expectations, accountabilities, and rewards for change.

The practical advice then is to start with leadership and build a case for why a concerted and long-term effort to systematically improve quality is needed. Questions such as: Why is TQM important for *our* patients? What will TQM mean to *us*? and How do *we* intend to incorporate the principles of TQM in *our* practice? must be answered uniquely by every organization that pursues TQM. Unless these questions are clearly addressed by leaders, it will be difficult for the organization to move much beyond simply doing a few improvement projects.

In order to better understand what organizational factors are important for successful improvement (in this case for implementation of clinical guidelines), Solberg et al. collected the thinking of people responsible for managing change in medical practices of all sizes.[42] Participants were not top organizational leaders, but rather physicians, nurses, and administrators who had extensive experience (at least 5 years) with leading quality improvement efforts within their medical groups. Participants were asked to suggest important factors, and then to vote on which factors were the most important. The top five factors identified by this group (out of 87 possibilities) were:

1. the pre-existing presence of organized systems in the clinic;
2. commitment to the change by clinic leadership;
3. leadership of the change process by enthusiastic volunteers;
4. internal clinician champions for the clinical content of the change;
5. clinic priority for quality over finance.

The need for the active engagement of both clinical and administrative leaders clearly runs through these five factors. This theme is further evidenced in an evaluation of the Primary Care Clinical Effectiveness Project (PRICCE) in the United Kingdom.[43] The evaluators there found that leadership and teamwork were fundamental to success. Importantly, they also found that these improved with participation; indicating that there is some value in 'getting on with it' and not waiting until leadership and teamwork are perfected. In the end, we suggest a balanced approach that involves clear attention to leadership and organizational culture, with initial action informed by critical thinking rather than naivety.

Systems and systems thinking (the first factor in the list above) are probably the most important prerequisite for successful change management and improvement in care.[4,44] Recently, this field has further expanded beyond classic systems thinking based on mechanical metaphors to embrace new findings from the field of complex adaptive systems science based on biological metaphors.[45–48] Leaders who use mechanical systems thinking for guiding changes (e.g. developing detailed specifications for new behaviour) are likely to come away thinking that the clinic personnel are simply resistant to change. Complex adaptive systems thinking leads to an approach to change in which the leader is more like a farmer than an engineer (i.e. working to create the best conditions for participation and creative thinking by all, rather than trying to construct the desired result with detailed plans and specifications). Plsek and Kilo[49] report how quickly primary care practice personnel become flexible facilitators of change when leaders adopt these complexity-inspired approaches. Miller et al.[45] similarly report how these approaches help explain changes that succeeded and failed at two primary care practices.

Encouraging trends for TQM in primary care

The lessons of the organizational development literature are receiving more notice in recent large-scale efforts to establish TQM in primary care organizations. While we must await formal evaluations, the depth of the approach in these newer efforts clearly exceeds that of the past, and initial case reports are encouraging.

Clinical Governance Programme

Halligan and Donaldson describe clinical governance in the United Kingdom as '... the systematic joining up of initiatives to improve quality'.[50] The concept is applied to both primary and scondary care and includes elements addressing: (a) effective leadership; (b) planning of quality; (c) being truly patient-centred; (d) information, analysis, and insight; (e) staff development; (f) redesign of services and processes; and (g) demonstrated success. These seven elements closely mirror the Baldrige TQM framework described previously in Box 1.

The work is supported by a Clinical Governance Support Team that provides expertise and advice, and runs training and development programmes. The process begins at the Board level to stress the importance of the most senior leadership taking it upon themselves to develop an organizational culture that supports improvement, whole systems thinking, multidisciplinary teamwork, and ongoing development for all staff. The start-up process includes a large-scale review of current services and processes, along with comparisons to best practice. Multidisciplinary leadership teams from participating organizations attend a series of five workshops, punctuated by 8-week action periods spread over 9 months. As of mid-2001, 250 organizations (including primary care, specialty care, acute care, and other services) had committed to the effort.

The fact that leadership and organizational development are explicitly addressed in such a health system-wide, centrally funded and supported effort is encouraging relative to the observed shortcomings of past efforts. Primary care organizations working to establish TQM would seem to have a much higher likelihood of success in the presence of these enabling factors.

Case reports from the efforts in primary care settings describe radical redesign to provide family-centred care for children with complex needs, better detection and improved care for women with postnatal depression, and improved care and referrals processes for adolescents needing mental health services. Further examples of results are available through a regularly updated Internet website (www.cgsupport.org).

National Primary Care Collaborative (UK)

As of mid-2001, some 20 per cent of English primary care practices, covering a total patient population of 3 million people, are engaged in comprehensive quality improvement efforts through the work of the National Primary Care Development Team, under the auspices of the Modernization Agency. Multidisciplinary teams from enrolled practices meet periodically for learning workshops and have active project management help to implement changes in such areas as coronary heart disease (CHD), appointment access, and demand management. The teams learn TQM tools such as process mapping, understanding the patients' perspective, and rapid-cycle improvement, and are provided with ideas for change from recognized experts. The goal is to eventually ensure the systematic transfer of the learning from the project to all practices in England.(51)

Measurement is formalized in the project and results have been encouraging.(52) Practices in the effort report having the percentage of patients with diabetes who have had their eyes examined rise from 65 to 85 per cent, and those having their HbA1c levels measured rise from 47 to 80 per cent. The percentage of practices prescribing aspirin for over 80 per cent of their patients with CHD increased from 23 to 50 per cent in 10 months and continued to show a positive trajectory upward. A group of seven practices reduced the average number of days patients had to wait for a new appointment from 8 to 2 days in just 5 months. Formal evaluation of the overall effort is pending.

The Idealized Design of Clinical Office Practice Project

The most extensive efforts at a deep and comprehensive approach to quality in primary care are those being taken by participating organizations working in the Idealized Design of Clinical Office Practice Project (IDCOP), led by the Institute for Healthcare Improvement (IHI, Boston, USA).

The IDCOP project was born from observations about transformational change with regard to quality in the automotive industry.(53) The project began with an expert design team comprised of researchers and practitioners from around the United States and Europe who were asked to develop new design concepts that would result in office practices with fundamentally different performance characteristics from prevailing ones. These design concepts were then tested by over 30 prototype sites, ranging in size from a single-handed practice to groups of 200 or more doctors in a site.

Incorporating ideas from complex adaptive systems thinking,(46) the project is organized around statements of purpose in the form of simple rules. The goal is to have patients and staff say of a practice: 'They give me exactly the help I want and need, exactly when I want and need it, while maintaining and improving a joyful work environment and a financially viable organization'.

The redesign work is further organized around fundamental changes in four theme areas:

- *Access:* The goal is to offer patients appointments, with the provider they wish to see, on the day they call. A further goal is to provide access to health information around the clock through, for example, the Internet.
- *Interaction:* The goal is to individualize care to match the patient's preferences regarding such things as the communication of information, control over decisions, self-care options, involvement of family and friends, and cultural values.
- *Reliability:* The goal is to match actions to the best available knowledge and evidence, and to strive for a defect-free system of care.
- *Vitality:* The goal is to sustain the new design through structures and leadership actions that assure on-going financial viability and the constant adaptability inherent in a learning organization.(4)

This is clearly a comprehensive and deep change effort that touches every aspect of how the organization functions. Smith(52) cites leadership as the core ingredient behind the project; noting that it is 'hard work' and that some sites have 'fallen by the wayside'.

Case reports of initial results are impressive. ThedaCare, a 21-site primary care system in the United States covering 160 000 people, reports substantial improvement in diabetic care and estimates that annual hospital costs are reduced by $250 000 as a result of such efforts. La Clinica Campesina, a safety-net community health provider in the US reports that the percentage of patients with diabetes who were engaged in self-care methods rose from fewer than 5 to 60 per cent, and the percentage of patients with good control of blood sugar levels increased from fewer than 15 to 70 per cent. Sixteen primary care sites in a health system in the United States reduced the average number of days for a new appointment from 4.3 to 1.8. Participants in the project in the United States, United Kingdom, and Sweden also report other wide-ranging improvements involving the use of e-mail and Internet sites for interaction with patients, the establishment of locally derived care guidelines, better flow of patients and information, better interaction with specialists and acute care organizations, and higher levels of staff satisfaction. Formal evaluations of IDCOP are underway and should produce peer-reviewed publications in the early years of this decade.

Conclusions

The understanding of TQM in other industries is that it is an all-encompassing, leadership- and systems-intensive effort to improve everything that an organization does. It is much more than the establishment of a few improvement teams and projects.

The breadth and depth of organizational effort required to implement TQM was not fully appreciated in early efforts in primary care. Leadership and organizational culture are fundamentally important determinants of success in such efforts, but these attributes vary widely. Because primary care organizations are not homogeneous on these critical attributes, the use of simple randomized controlled trial designs to evaluate the effectiveness of TQM is questionable.(39) We do not believe that randomly selected health care organizations will respond in similar ways to an 'intervention' of TQM. More sophisticated designs and hypotheses are needed. Case reports and before–after comparisons in more recent efforts to utilize TQM in primary care are encouraging and do demonstrate that these methods from general industry can be usefully adapted to health care.

Leaders in primary care interested in adopting TQM should reflect carefully before embarking on the effort. Experience suggests that unless a significant proportion of key clinical and managerial leaders and staff feel an intense need for fundamental change, and are willing to support the change effort through the commitment of time and resources, comprehensive TQM efforts will likely stall.

This does not mean that leaders who are committed to individual quality improvement projects are forced to do nothing. It is possible to complete many such projects using the tools and concepts covered in other chapters in this section. Each project will have to stand on its own in terms of generating tension for change and securing resources for that change; but each project completed will provide some benefit to patients and staff. Leaders may also need to take special steps to maintain the gains over time from each improvement project, as the culture of the organization may not provide natural support systems.

Having stated these cautions, we encourage thoughtful practitioners to begin now the efforts to build TQM into primary care organizations. The first steps should involve assembling leaders for a reflective and honest dialogue about the extent to which the principles of TQM are currently practised or lacking in the organization, along with an honest assessment of the patients' experiences of care. The leadership team should engage in studying the lessons learned in health care and other industries about organizational culture, organizational development, systems thinking and change management. The leadership team should also build the case for TQM in a way that reflects the unique needs of the organization's patients, staff, and situation. Building on this foundation, the next steps would involve an assessment of its systems for demonstrating leadership, setting goals, building teamwork, redesigning processes, and measuring progress in order to begin the long-term effort to continuously improve these systems.

References

1. **Oakland, J.S.** *Total Quality Management.* Oxford: Heinemann Publishing, 1989.
2. **Ishikawa, K.** *What is Total Quality Control: The Japanese Way.* Translated by David J. Lu. Englewood Cliffs NJ: Prentice-Hall, 1985.
3. **Wu, A.W. and Johansen, K.S.** (1999). Lessons from Europe on quality improvement: report on the Velen Castle WHO meeting. *The Joint Commission Journal on Quality Improvement* **25** (6), 316–29.
4. **Senge, P.M.** *The Fifth Discipline: The Art and Practice of the Learning Organization.* New York: Doubleday, 1990.
5. **Alles, V., Makela, M., Persson, L., and Seuntjens, L.**, ed. *Tools and Methods for Quality Improvement in General Practice.* Jyväskylä, Finland: Gummerus Printing, 1998.
6. **Grol, R. and Grimshaw, J.** (1999). Evidence-based implementation of evidence-based practice. *The Joint Commission Journal on Quality Improvement* **25** (10), 503–13.
7. **Shortell, S.M., Bennett, C.L., and Byck, G.R.** (1998). Assessing the impact of continuous quality improvement on clinical practice: what it will take to accelerate progress. *The Milbank Quarterly* **76** (4), 593–624.
8. **Carlin, E., Carlson, R., and Nordin, J.** (1996). Using continuous quality improvement tools to improve pediatric immunization rates. *The Joint Commission Journal on Quality Improvement* **22** (4), 277–88.
9. **O'Conner, P.J., Quiter, E.S., Rush, W.A., Wiest, M., Meland, J.T., and Ryu, S.** Impact of hypertension guideline implementation on blood pressure control and drug use in primary care clinics. *The Joint Commission Journal on Quality Improvement* **25** (2), 68–80.
10. **Ketola, E., Sipila, R., Makela, M., and Klockars, M.** (2000). Quality improvement programme for cardiovascular disease risk factor recording in primary care. *Quality in Health Care* **9**, 175–80.
11. **Cox, S., Wilcock, P., and Young, J.** (1999). Improving the repeat prescribing process in a busy general practice: a study using continuous quality improvement methodology. *Quality in Health Care* **8**, 119–25.
12. **Goebers, H., van der Horst, M., Mokkkink, H., van Montfort, P., van den Bosch, W., van den Hoogen, H., and Grol, R.** (1999). Setting up improvement projects in small scale primary care practices: feasibility of a model for continuous quality improvement. *Quality in Health Care* **8**, 36–42.
13. **Lawrence, M. and Packwood, T.** (1996). Adapting total quality management in general practice: evaluation of a programme. *Quality in Health Care* **5**, 151–8.
14. **Hearnshaw, H., Reddish, S., Carlyle, D., Baker, R., and Robertson, N.** (1998). Introducing a quality improvement programme to primary healthcare teams. *Quality in Health Care* **7**, 200–8.
15. **Goldberg, H.I. et al.** (1998). A randomized controlled trial of CQI teams and academic detailing: can they alter compliance with guidelines? *The Joint Commission Journal on Quality Improvement* **24** (3), 130–42.
16. **Solberg, L.I., Kottke, T.E., Brekke, M.L., Calomeni, C.A., Conn, S.A., and Davidson, G.** (1996). Using continuous quality improvement to increase preventive services in clinical practice—going beyond guidelines. *Preventive Medicine* **25** (3), 259–67.
17. **Solberg, L.I., Kottke, T.E., and Brekke, M.L.** (1998). Will primary care clinics organize themselves to improve the delivery of preventive services? A randomized controlled trial. *Preventive Medicine* **27** (4), 623–31.
18. **Solberg, L.I.** et al. (2000). Failure of a trial of Continuous Quality Improvement and systems intervention to increase the delivery of clinical preventive services. *Effective Clinical Practice* **3**, 105–15.
19. **Solberg, L.I., Kottke, T.E., Brekke, M.L., and Magnan, S.** (2000). Improving prevention is difficult. *Effective Clinical Practice* **3** 153–5.
20. **Solberg, L.I., Fischer, L.R., Wei, F., Rush, W.A., Conboy, K.S., Davis T.F., and Heinrich, R.L.** (2001). A CQI intervention to change the care of depression: a controlled study. *Effective Clinical Practice* **4** (6), 239–49.
21. **Plsek, P.E.** (1993). Quality improvement models. *Quality Management in Health Care* **1** (2), 69–81.
22. **Goebers, H., Grol, R., van den Bosch, W., van den Hoogen, H., Mokkkink, H., van Montfort, P., and Oltheten, H.** (1999). A model for continuous quality improvement in small practices. *Quality in Health Care* **8**, 43–8.
23. **Goebers, H., Grol, R., van den Bosch, W., van den Hoogen, H., Mokkkink, H., van Montfort, P., and Oltheten, H.** *2000 Baldrige National Quality Program: Health Care Criteria for Performance Excellence.* Gaithersburg MD: National Institute of Standards and Technology, 2000. http://www.quality.nist.gov.
24. **Goebers, H., Grol, R., van den Bosch, W., van den Hoogen, H., Mokkkink, H., van Montfort, P., and Oltheten, H.** *Quality Management in Social Welfare and Health Care for the 21st Century: National Recommendations.* Saarijarvi, Finland: Gummerus Printing, 1999.
25. **Plsek, P.E.** (1997). The systematic design of health care processes. *Quality in Health Care* **6** (1), 40–8.
26. **Jung, H.P.** *Quality of Care in General Practice: The Patient Perspective.* Nijmegen, The Netherlands: Ponsen and Looijen, 1999.
27. **Berwick, D.M.** (1989). Continuous improvement as an ideal in health care. *New England Journal of Medicine* **320**, 53–6.
28. **Juran, J.M.** *Managerial Breakthrough.* New York: McGraw-Hill, 1964.
29. **Berwick, D.M.** (1996). Harvesting knowledge from improvement. *Journal of the American Medical Association* **275** (11), 877–8.
30. **McLaughlin, C.P. and Kaluzny, A.D.** (1990). Total quality management in health: making it all work. *Health Care Management Review* **15** (3), 7–14.
31. **Melum, M.M.** (1990). Total quality management: steps to success. *Hospitals* **64**, 42–4.
32. **McFarland, D., Harmann, L., Lhotak, C., and Wieselthier, V.F.** (1996). The quest for TQM in a community mental health center: using the Baldrige criteria as a framework. *The Joint Commission Journal on Quality Improvement* **22** (1), 37–47.
33. **Gene-Badia, J., Jodar-Sola, G., Peguero-Rodriguez, E., Contel-Segura, J.C., and Moliner-Molins, C.** (2001). The EFQM excellence model is useful for primary care health teams. *Family Practice* **18** (4), 407–9.
34. **Brommels, M., Outinen, M., Kupiainen, O., Stahlberg, M.R., Taipale, E., and Alanko, A.** (1997). Local heroes beat national champions: quality improvement in Finnish health care. *The Joint Commission Journal on Quality Improvement* **23** (1), 23–31.
35. **Garside, P.** (1999). Organisational context for quality: lessons from the fields of organisational development and change management. *Quality in Health Care* **7** (Suppl.), S8–15.
36. **Solberg, L.I.** (2000). Guideline implementation: what the literature doesn't tell us. *The Joint Commission Journal on Quality Improvement* **26** (9), 525–37.
37. **Koeck, C.** (1998). Time for organisational development in healthcare organisations: improving quality for patients means changing the organisation. *British Medical Journal* **317**, 1267–8.
38. **Weber, V. and Joshi, M.S.** (2000). Effecting and leading change in healthcare organizations. *The Joint Commission Journal on Quality Improvement* **26** (7), 388–99.
39. **Rogers, S., Humphrey, C., Nazareth, I., Lister, S., Tomlin, Z., and Haines, A.** (2000). Designing trials of interventions to change professional practice in primary care: lessons from an exploratory study of two change strategies. *British Medical Journal* **320**, 1580–3.
40. **Kitson, A., Harvey, G., and McCormack, B.** (1998). Enabling the implementation of evidence based practice: a conceptual framework. *Quality in Health Care* **7**, 149–58.
41. **Øvretveit, J.** (1997). Would it work for us? Learning from quality improvement in Europe and beyond. *The Joint Commission Journal on Quality Improvement* **23** (1), 7–22.
42. **Solberg, L.I.** et al. (2000). Lessons from experienced guideline implementers: attend to many factors and use multiple strategies. *The Joint Commission Journal on Quality Improvement* **26** (4), 171–88.
43. **Spooner, A., Chapple, A., and Roland, M.** *The PRICCE Project (Primary Care Clinical Effectiveness Project).* Report from the National Primary Care Research and Development Centre, University of Manchester, March 2000.
44. **Kotter, J.P.** *Leading Change.* Boston MA: Harvard Business School Press, 1996.
45. **Miller, W.L., Crabtree, B.F., McDaniel, R., and Stange, K.C.** (1998). Understanding change in primary care practice using complexity theory. *Journal of Family Practice* **46** (5), 369–76.
46. **Plsek, P.E. and Greenhalgh, T.** (2000). The challenge of complexity in health care. *British Medical Journal* **323**, 625–8.

47. **Axelrod, R. and Cohen, M.D.** *Harnessing Complexity: Organizational Implications of a Scientific Frontier.* New York: The Free Press, 1999.
48. **Zimmerman, B.J., Lindberg, C., and Plsek, P.E.** *Edgeware: Insights from Complexity Science for Health Care Leaders.* Dallas TX: VHA Publishing, 1998.
49. **Plsek, P.E. and Kilo, C.M.** (1999). From resistance to attraction: a different approach to change. *Physician Executive* **25** (6), 40–6.
50. **Halligan, A. and Donaldson, L.** (2001). Implementing clinical governance: turning vision into reality. *British Medical Journal* **322**, 1413–17.
51. **National Primary Care Development Team.** www.doh.gov.uk/about/nhsplan/who/modagency01.html.
52. **Smith, J.** (2001). Redesigning health care: radical redesign is a way to radically improve. *British Medical Journal* **322**, 1257–8.
53. **Womack, J.P., Jones, D.T., and Roos, D.** *The Machine That Changed the World: The Story of Lean Production.* New York: Rawson, 1990.

13.7 The patient's role in improving quality

Michel Wensing and Richard Grol

Introduction

Primary medical care has a long tradition of patient-centredness[1] and this chapter builds on that tradition. It describes a range of specific methods for integrating patients' views in primary medical care and its improvement. Examples are needs assessment questionnaires completed by patients before the consultation, procedures to involve patients in the development of clinical guidelines, and surveys among patients to provide feedback to care providers. Such methods can point out aspects of care that would otherwise remain unnoticed by the care providers, managers, and policy makers. Many countries have laws and professional regulations that prescribe that patients' voices are included in clinical decision-making, quality improvement, and health care planning. In some countries, efforts are made to create health care services around the preferences of the patient. The value of the methods for patient involvement should be assessed in terms of their effectiveness and feasibilitiy. This chapter aims to provide an overview of a range of methods for patient involvement and to describe the research evidence related to their use.

We use the term 'patient' to refer to a person who uses professional health care and the term 'individual' to a person who is a potential user. Involving patients in primary medical care and its improvement has different aims. Firstly, it is an ethical and legal rule that individuals and patients should be involved in the decisions concerning health care. Many patients wish to be involved, at least to some extent, and it is important to fulfil this need. Secondly, involvement may result in a better process and outcome of care. It helps care providers to reflect on patients' needs and preferences; it may contribute to implementation of evidence-based practice; and it can result in better self-management, health status, and satisfaction with care. Patients can be seen as co-producers of their health care, as their decisions and behaviour influence process and outcome of health care. Patient involvement may have the political objective of legitimizing the national view on what constitutes quality of care. In health care systems that promote competition between providers, patient involvement may offer providers competitive advantage.

Table 1 Overview of methods

	Increased involvement in actual care	**Increased involvement in quality improvement**
Individuals who seek health care		
Health education	×	
Internet communication	×	
Public reports	×	× (assessment)
Patients in episodes of care		
Needs assessment	×	× (priority setting)
Tailored patient education	×	
Shared decision-making	×	
Patient-held records	×	× (assessment)
Patients' feedback on medical care		
Surveys		× (assessment)
Complaint procedures		× (assessment)
Patient participation groups		× (priority setting, improvement)
Patient involvement in health care planning		
Community participation		× (priority setting, improvement)
Involvement in guidelines		× (improvement)
Patient organizations		× (priority setting, assessment)

The first section of this chapter discusses different types of information delivery to support individuals in their self-management of health problems and decisions to seek medical care. The second section focuses on tools which can be used by the individual patient and the clinician before, within or after the consultation. While these sections mainly focus on involving patients and individuals in their actual care, the remaining sections focus on involving patients and individuals in the improvement of the quality of care. Quality improvement includes priority setting regarding quality initiatives, assessment of current practice, and focused activities to improve the quality of care. The third section describes tools for identifying and providing feedback on patients' views on the primary medical care received. The fourth section discusses methods for community participation and involvement of patients in the planning of health care services. Table 1 lists the methods and indicates when these may be most appropriate.

Individuals who seek health care

This first section focuses on methods which are used to help individuals to make better decisions about self-management of health problems and the use of health care.

Health education

Health education may enhance the appropriateness of the decision to seek health care and stimulate self-management of the health problem. For instance, written information on common diseases, such as sore throat and sinusitus, distributed among parents of young children could lead to better use of health care. A campaign in the mass media on when to seek emergency care for different health problems could influence individuals' use of emergency care. The role of individuals is often limited to being the receiver of the information, but in an increasing number of cases an attempt is made to tailor the information according to their needs and preferences.

In general, information on health problems and their treatment is highly valued by individuals. It is of course crucial that the information is valid, based on evidence, and understandable to lay persons. Specific instruments are available to assess the quality of the information.[2] Health education can effectively change behaviour, particularly if the theme is relevant for the target group, the programme is adapted to individual needs, and the programme integrates feedback, rewards, and facilitation that promote the desired behaviour.[3] Mass media programmes have been proven to influence the use of health care services.[4] The effect on individuals appears to be influenced by the way the information is presented, for instance, positively or negatively framed, absolute or relative risk reductions. A more appropriate use of health care contributes to evidence-based practice, but a danger is that people perceive a reduced accessibility to health care providers if they are discouraged to attend a physician.

Internet communication

Internet is one of the media which can be used to provide health education, but internet may be unique in it possibilities to facilitate interactive types of communication. A large number of activities have been launched. Some general practices or primary health care centres have a website for patients and an increasing number of national websites provide information on health problems. Internet can be used to make patients into a valuable source of information for other patients with the same condition, by facilitating communication between patients.[5] There may be increasing demands for providers to communicate electronically with their patients and to provide recommendations for websites.[5]

Interactive communication on health issues through the internet is rapidly increasing, but poorly evaluated.[6] Like written information, its quality should be considered, and preliminary studies suggest that the validity of the information on many websites is yet poor. Many individuals value communication through the internet, but research on the effects on their health behaviour and their use of health care is limited. A study showed however that a weight loss programme delivered through the Internet could influence health status[7] (Box 1). Internet is likely to become an ever more important source of information on health and illness.

Public reports

The choice of a care provider is an opportunity of the individual to express his or her wishes and preferences regarding primary medical care. Providing information on the range of services, quality, costs, and health outcomes may help the individual in making choices between different care providers. Report cards describe the performance of different care providers on several indicators, such as types of services offered and organization of health care. Assessment of the quality of care by patients, such as patient satisfaction figures, may be included in the public reports. These cards have been used in the United States, where individuals and their employers can chose between competing managed care organizations. So far, their use was mainly related to hospital care.

The information provided should be valid, up-to-date, and corrected for variations in patient case-mix between different care providers. A review showed that individuals find it difficult to understand the information, that they distrust the information and use is rarely in their choice of care provider.[8] Physicians are sceptical about the information and they may respond defensively. A few studies, all in hospital settings, showed favourable effects on outcomes of care. Although individuals may lack the willingness or opportunity to choose actively between different care providers, public reports could influence the quality of care, as care providers may respond to the reports despite the limited effects on choice of care provider on the side of the public.

Box 1 Using internet technology to deliver a behavioural weight loss programme[7]

A randomized trial compared a structured Internet behavioural weight loss programme with weight loss education website. Ninety-one healthy, overweight adult hospital employees participated in this study. Their body mass index varied between 25 and 36 kg/m^2. The behaviour programme comprised 24 weekly lessons via e-mail, weekly online submission of self-monitoring diaries with individualized therapist feedback via e-mail, and an online bulletin board. The behaviour therapy group lost a mean (SD) of 4.0 (2.8) kg by 3 months and 4.1 (2.8) kg by 6 months. Weight loss in the education group was 1.7 (2.7) kg at 3 months and 1.6 (3.3) by 6 months. The differences were statistically significant ($p = 0.005$).

Patients in episodes of care

This section focuses on tools that can be used to involve individual patients in their actual care.

Needs assessment

The patient-centred approach to consultations emphasizes that the meaning of illness for the patient should be explored. Specific tools can be used to achieve this aim. The patient can write down health problems, symptoms, and needs for care before the consultation and introduce the list in the consultation. In its simplest form, this is a sort of a 'questions list' which is presented to the practitioner. Some forms are made for unselected patient populations, for instance to assess depressive symptoms or functional limitations in older patients. Other forms are for specific patient groups, for instance to assess the needs for advice on lifestyle changes in diabetes patients. A similar method used a separate session with an assistent, shortly before the consultation with the primary care provider, to help identify needs for care and motivate the patient to take an active role.

These tools aim to help patients and care providers to pay attention to specific problems and issues, which otherwise may remain unrecognized. Care providers do not always recognize patients' expectations in the consultation. Research evidence suggests that methods for needs assessment can indeed result in better recognition of health problems, particularly psychological problems, and higher patient satisfaction with care.[9] There is, however, little evidence to suggest their use substantially changed patient management or improved patient outcomes.[9] A study showed that a separate session with an assistant to prepare the patient for the consultation can lead to improved blood glucose levels in diabetes patients.[10] Questionnaires completed before the consultation seem to be acceptable to patients, but the feasibility for care providers is a challenge. A survey with 156 GPs and 115 practice nurses showed that 48 per cent of the GPs and 46 per cent of the practice nurses were unclear about how to use health outcomes data.[11]

Tailored patient education

If the provision of information and advice to patients in the consultation is interactive, it can be tailored to patients' individual needs and questions. The GP can be trained to address patients' needs for information and provide information as wished. Or the GP can hand out written summaries of the information which he/she has provided in the consultation. Alternatively, shortly before or after a consultation with the care provider, another professional, such as a nurse, can provide tailored information in a separate session. Other tools are interactive videotapes and CD-ROMs, shown at the practice, which provide information that is tailored to age and gender.

As described before, patients highly value information on their health problem and its treatment. Tools that require additional persons, materials, or programmes are often expensive. In general, patient education has a small but positive effect on compliance with treatment and advice.[12,13] It is unclear whether tailored education is more effective than non-tailored approaches. Patient education which is consistent with clinical guidelines can support their implementation. Although not all information materials meet criteria for high quality (Box 2),[14] patient information is indispensable from health care delivery.

Shared decision-making

Shared decision-making is a communication strategy between clinicians and patients that implies explicit recognition of patients' needs for health care, provision of information on treatment options and explanation of their benefits and risks, discussion about patients' preferences and choice between the options.[15] It has been proposed for complex clinical decisions, such as treatment choices for lower urinary tract symptoms in men, hormone replacement therapy in women, and atrial fibrillation. Decision aids can support shared decision-making; these are information tools that support an informed choice in the situation where more than one treatment alternative is available.[16] These decision aids differ from patient education programmes which aim to provide information, advice, and support with regard to already prescribed treatments.

Implementation of shared decision-making and decision aids in primary medical care is a challenge, because few doctors have the skills required for their application and many patients do not want to be involved in clinical decision-making.[15] The feasibility and acceptability of many decision aids was good according to patients who actually used them.[16] The effectiveness of patient participation in clinical decision-making is poorly understood. A review with 24 randomized trials showed that decision aids can indeed improve patients' knowledge and stimulate patients to be active in decision-making.[17] They had little effect on anxiety or satisfaction with the decision-making process, or satisfaction with the decision.

Patient-held records

Information and counselling can be used to motivate and enable the patient to take responsibility for treatment and monitoring of the health problem during an episode of care. For instance, the care provider can discuss barriers for adherence to treatment and strategies to overcome those barriers. Furthermore, special cards or books can be used to help the patient register clinical symptoms during an episode of care. Examples are patient-held personal health summaries with information on health promotion activities and sharing medical records with the patient.

Patient-held mini-records can indeed improve preventive screening and vaccination. They allocate control of preventive procedures to patients. A review with seven studies showed that it improves patients' adherence to management plans.[18] Although several studies showed that patients and practitioners received these records well, there is a danger that they feel unhappy with such a tool because of the changed control. The time and effort required of providers and patients are also potential barriers to the implementation of patient-held records.[18]

Box 2 Checklist for content of patient information materials[14]

1. Use patients' questions as the starting point.
2. Ensure that common concerns and misconceptions are addressed.
3. Refer to all relevant treatment or management options.
4. Include honest information about benefits and risks.
5. Include quantitative information where possible.
6. Include checklists and questions to ask the doctor.
7. Include sources of further information.
8. Use non-alarmist, non-patronizing language in active rather than passive voice.
9. Design should be structured and concise with good illustrations.
10. Be explicit about authorship and sponsorship.
11. Include reference to sources and strength of evidence.
12. Include the publication date.

Patients' feedback on medical care

After patients have received medical care, they can look back and evaluate its quality from their perspective. This section focuses on tools that can be used to receive feedback from patients.

Surveys

A patient satisfaction survey is probably the most well-known method to collect patients' evaluations and report them to care providers and others. Patient satisfaction surveys use structured or semi-structured questionnaires, which are filled in by patients in the practice or at home, or which is answered in a oral or telephone interview.[19] Alternatively, patients can complete pre-structured diaries during episodes of care. The survey and the feedback to care providers may focus on a broad range of aspects of care or on a specific domain of clinical practice, such as preventive care or the waiting room. The feedback can provide summaries of answers to open-ended questions or figures based on the questions with answering scales. For comparison, figures from previous surveys in the same setting or from surveys among patients from other primary care providers can be added.

A large number of patient satisfaction questionnaires has been developed and used, but only a small number of questionnaires and data collection procedures have been well validated.[19] Expectations and preferences probably influence patient evaluations of care, but the exact mechanism is not clear. Getting patients to contribute to the choice of aspects of care included in the questionnaire is crucial to making sure that it is their priorities that the questionnaire reflects. If patient satisfaction is compared across different care providers, adjustments for the composition of patient populations are needed.[19] Care providers are expected to reflect on the results of a survey and consider how they can make improvements. This is not an easy task. A controlled trial showed that the survey and feedback to medical residents influenced patients' evaluations positively.[19] A randomized trial with 55 GPs showed that feedback on patient satisfaction did not affect patients' evaluations of care, but that practitioners reported a number of changes in their routines (Box 3).[21]

Complaint procedures

Every health system should have adequate procedures for handling complaints expressed by patients. Complaints are negative evaluations of health care provision, which can signal aspects of care that need to be improved. Most patient complaints remain unnoticed, but some are expressed and handled by formal or informal complaint procedures. Formal procedures include the use of legislation and the courts. Many health care institutions have created informal opportunities to express complaints. This may be a special person or department who handles the complaints. Another method is the collection of complaints and comments that are expressed in open questions in patient satisfaction surveys, letters, or conversations with patients.

Box 3 Feeding back patients' evaluations of care[21]

A randomized trial was performed to determine the effect of feeding back patients' evaluations of care to general practitioners. Fifty-five GPs and samples of 3691 and 3595 adult patients, before and after the intervention, respectively, participated. GPs in the intervention group obtained an individualized, structured feedback report concerning evaluations of care provided by their own patients. Reference figures referring to other GPs were added as well as suggestions for interpretation of this feedback, an evidence-based overview of factors determining patients' evaluations of care and methods to discuss and plan improvements. Providing feedback on patients' evaluations of care to GPs did not result in changes in patients' evaluations of care. This conclusion challenges the relevance of feedback on patients' evaluations of care for quality improvement.

Some practitioners have strong emotional reactions to patients' complaints, including the feeling of loss of control over their professional performance and conflicts about their professional identity. Nevertheless, clinicians should try to learn from the complaint.[22] Many complaints are about bad communication rather than technical performance; and bad communication after a medical error has happened influences whether it will result in a complaint.[23] Complaints are not necessarily representative of patients' experiences with health care and not all complaints indicate physician negligence.[23] Nevertheless, each complaint should be seen as an opportunity to learn and improve professional practice.

Patient participation groups

Patient participation groups are groups of patients or former patients, linked to a specific general practice or regional service, which can develop standards for good practice, provide feedback on health care delivered and influence local quality improvement programmes. This method differs from the survey methods, because patients discuss their experiences and views with each other so that they can get a more comprehensive picture than individuals. So the method is somewhat similar to qualitative group interviews. Some would argue that care providers should be part of the group; it has been suggested that patients should not be in clinical relationships with them.[24] Particularly, groups at regional and national level may also include patient advocates, which are people with a general knowledge of the views and interests of patients and patient groups but who are not necessarily patients or former patients themselves.[24]

Research evidence on patient participation groups is limited and tends to focus on the experiences of the groups rather than their effectiveness. Some groups stop functioning after a short period, but other groups exist for many years. GPs involved in groups linked to a specific general practice suggested a number of reasons for stopping, such as the experience that all relevant problems had been discussed, a lack of patient interest, the feeling that a changing practice population cannot be represented well, and the idea that the lower class patient population is not used to have control of their lives.[25] Patient participation groups may have a positive influence on the quality of care, but research evidence to support this claim is lacking.

Patient involvement in health care planning

This final section deals with tools to involve patients and individuals' in quality improvement programmes and health care planning.

Community participation

Community participation may include the use of research tools, such as surveys and group methods, or the use of ways to involve the public directly, such as patient panels or advisory groups.[26] An example of a research approach is a study among patients from one health centre in the United Kingdom who were asked to imagine that they were to choose a new clinician and to indicate their criteria in this choice.[27] Another example is a postal survey to assess whether people felt unsure about where to get help and actual health care received for a range of health problems, including long-term illness, minor symptoms or signs, and psychological difficulties.[28] Ways to involve the public directly are for instance patient councils, health forums, and public meetings (NHS). The priorities and needs may be used for planning and improvement of health care services, for instance for the development of services in underserved areas or groups.

Some issues related to patient priorities and needs should be kept in mind. Individuals' priorities and needs may change over time, if new information or new health problems becomes available or if individuals' health status change.[28] Minority groups may be neglected if too much emphasis is placed on giving everyone an equal say.[28] Although it is difficult to determine the effectiveness, information on patient priorities and needs is useful as input for quality improvement and health care planning to counter-balance professional and managerial perspectives in the process of planning health care services.

Involvement in clinical guidelines

Clinical guidelines provide specific recommendations for clinical management of specific conditions and health problems. These are based clinical research evidence and professionals' expertise and considerations. Involving patients in the development of clinical guidelines is another approach to patient involvement. The contribution of patients could be an assessment of outcomes, burden of treatments, side-effects; and identification of relevant items for patient education and counselling. Different methods have been proposed, including involvement of individual patients in guideline development groups, assessment of patients' views by focus group interviews or surveys, and use of research literature describing people's experiences.

A British study compared four models of involving individual patients.[29] In all models, patients focused on the sections related to patient education and their contributions did not always influence the content of guidelines. Involving individual patients in guideline development groups or a 'one off' meeting with patients showed that patients had problems with the use of technical language. In a series of workshops it was possible to explain the technical elements of the guideline, but this was time-consuming. Involving a patient advocate in the guideline development group did not have these problems, but personal involvement with an illness is however different for a patient than for a patient advocate.[29]

Patient organizations

Patient organizations derive from different strands: local geographical interest groups, groups of people sharing the same health condition or experience of being harmed, groups to protest against particular developments on an ideological basis, groups with a shared identity such as ethnicity, and generic patient organizations which are also active outside health care.[30] Patient organizations can contribute to agenda setting for clinical audit, research and development, clinical guidelines, health care planning, and policy-making. They can identify what they consider to be acceptable and ideal levels of care; ensure that process and outcome measures reflect factors that patients consider important; contribute to patient education materials, continuing education of professionals and other improvement programmes; and report back on the extent to which expected standards are achieved.[31]

It is argued that patient organizations have indeed played a role in establishing patients' rights; putting previously unrecognized health issues on agenda's, such as sudden infant death syndrome and Alzheimers' disease and achieving public health goals, such as restricting the spread of HIV/AIDS in many countries.[30] On the other hand, an evaluation of lay involvement in primary care groups in the United Kingdom suggested that the lay voice was only faintly heard in the first 6 months of the operation of these groups.[32] It is uncertain whether patients with acute illness are well presented by patient organizations, as many organizations mainly include patients with chronic illness. There is little research evidence related to patient organizations, but representation of the views of patients and the public in committees in health care should contribute to increased focus on patient needs and priorities.

Conclusions

This chapter described a range of methods to involve patients in primary medical care and its quality improvement. Patients' views are relevant when they seek health care, during episodes of care, when they look back on the care received, and in the planning of health care services. Specific methods are available, for each of these areas, to facilitate, stimulate, and support individuals and patients to take an active role. Involvement of patients and the public is needed to counter-balance the power of professionals and managers. More research evidence is needed to determine the effectiveness of different methods, but there is evidence for the positive effects of at least some methods on process and outcomes of care.

With respect to individuals who seek health care, it can be concluded that tools for needs assessment, such as scoring lists completed before a consultation, can be helpful. Shared decision-making is a promising approach which has been developed more recently. However, the feasibility of both needs assessment and shared decision-making should to be improved. Education tailored to patients' individual needs, perhaps delivered outside the consultation, may help to overcome some of the problems. Patient-held records are probably useful in specific sub-groups of patients, such as patients with chronic illness.

After patients have received medical care, they can look back on their experiences. Patient satisfaction surveys have often been used to receive feedback on patients' views from larger groups of patients. This feedback can stimulate practitioners' reflection on the quality of care, if they receive such feedback for instance every few years. Patient participation groups are another approach to receive feedback from patients. Particularly, one-off focus groups may be cost-effective compared to patient surveys. Patients' satisfaction can also be reported in public reports, but the effectiveness of such reports is uncertain. A health care system should of course have opportunities for patients to put forward comments and complaints.

Community participation and patient organizations may raise awareness of aspects of care, which would otherwise remain unnoticed. It is unclear whether it is realistic to expect specific effects on professional practice and organization of care. There is little experience with the involvement of patients or patient representatives in guideline development, but it appears a promising approach to patient involvement, because guidelines are related to the actual process of care delivery.

A randomized trial on low back pain showed that 80 per cent would have chosen radiography if available, but that patients who received radiography more often experienced pain at 3 months compared to the control group but were nevertheless more satisfied with the care provided.[33] A balance should be found between the perspectives of health care professionals and patients/individuals, and between external incentives for improvement (from patients) and improvement driven by a desire for professional development.

References

1. **McWhinney, I.R.** (1998). Core values in a changing world. *British Medical Journal* **316**, 1807–9.
2. **Charnock, D., Shepperd, S., Needham, G., and Gann, R.** (1997). DISCERN: an instrument for judging the quality of written consumer health information on treatment choices. *Journal of Epidemiology and Community Health* **53**, 105–11.
3. **Kok, G., Van den Borne, B., and Mullen, P.D.** (1997). Effectiveness of health education and health promotion: meta-analyses of effect studies and determinants of effectiveness. *Patient Education and Counseling* **30**, 19–27.
4. **Grilli, R.** et al. (1998). Impact of mass media on health services utilization. In *The Cochrane Library* Issue 3. Oxford: Update Software.
5. **Ferguson, T.** (2000). Online patient-helpers and physicians working together: a new partnership for high quality care. *British Medical Journal* **321**, 1129–32.
6. **Robinson, T.N., Patrick, K., Eng, T.R., and Gustafson, D.** (1998). An evidence-based approach to interactive health communication. A challenge to medicine in the information age. *Journal of the American Medical Association* **280**, 1264–9.
7. **Tate, D.F., Wing, R.R., and Winett, R.A.** (2001). Using internet technology to deliver a behavioral weight loss program. *Journal of the American Medical Association* **285**, 1172–7.
8. **Marshall, M.** et al. (2000). The public release of performance data. *Journal of the American Medical Association* **283**, 1866–74.
9. **Greenhalgh, J. and Meadows, K.** (1999). The effectiveness of the use of patient-based measures of health in routine practice in improving the process and outcomes of patient care: a literature review. *Journal of Evaluation in Clinical Practice* **5**, 401–16.
10. **Greenfield, S., Kaplan, S.H., Ware, J.E., Yano, E.M., and Frank, H.J.L.** (1998). Patients' participation in medical care: effects on blood sugar control and quality of life in diabetes. *Journal of General Internal Medicine* **3**, 448–57.
11. **Meadows, K.A., Rogers, D., and Greene, T.** (1998). Attitudes to the use of health outcome questionnaires in the routine care of patients with diabetes: a survey of general practitioners and practice nurses. *British Journal of General Practice* **48**, 1555–9.
12. **Ashenden, R., Silary, C., and Weller, D.** (1997). A systematic review of the effectiveness of promoting life style change in general practice. *Family Practice* **14**, 160–76.
13. **Haynes, R.B., Montague, P., Oliver, T., McKibbon, K.A., Brouwers, M.C., and Kanani, R.** (1999). Interventions for helping patients to follow prescriptions for medications. In *The Cochrane Library* Issue 1. Oxford: Update Software.
14. **Coulter, A., Entwistle, V., and Gilbert, D.** (1999). Sharing decisions with patients: is the information good enough? *British Medical Journal* **318**, 318–22.
15. **Elwyn, G., Edwards, A., and Kinnersley, P.** (2000). Shared decision-making in primary care: the neglected second half of the consultations. *British Journal of General Practice* **49**, 477–82.
16. **Molenaar, S., Sprangers, M.A.G., Postma-Schuit, F.C.E., Rutgers, E.J.T., Noorlander, J., Hendriks, J., and De Haes, H.C.J.M.** (2000). Feasibility and effects of decision aids. *Medical Decision Making* **20**, 112–27.
17. **O'Connor, A.M., Stacey, D., Rovner, D., Holmes-Rovner, M., Tetroe, J., Llewellynn-Thomas, H., Entwistle, V., Rostom, A., Fiset, V., Barry, M., and Jones, J.** (2001). Decision aids for people facing health treatment or screening decisions (Cochrane Review). In *The Cochrane Library* Issue 3. Oxford: Update Software.
18. **Dickey, L.L.** (1993). Promoting preventive care with patient-held minirecords: a review. *Patient Education and Counseling* **20**, 37–47.
19. **Wensing, M., Grol, R., and Smits, A.** (1994). Quality judgements by patients on general practice care: a literature analysis. *Social Science and Medicine* **38**, 45–53.
20. **Cope, D.W.** et al. (1986). Modification of residents' behavior by preceptor feedback of patient satisfaction. *Journal of General Internal Medicine* **1**, 394–8.
21. **Vingerhoets, E., Wensing, M., and Grol, R.** (2001). Feeding back patients' evaluations of care: a randomised trial. *Quality in Health Care* **10**, 224–8.
22. **Jain, A. and Ogden, J.** (1999). General practitioners' experiences of patients' complaints: qualitative study. *British Medical Journal* **318**, 1596–9.
23. **Kravitz, R.L., Rolph, J.E., and McGuigan, K.** (1991). Malpractice claims data as a quality improvement tool. 1. Epidemiology of error in four specialties. *Journal of the American Medical Association* **266**, 2087–92.
24. **Williamson, C.** (1998). The rise of doctor–patient working groups. *British Medical Journal* **317**, 1374–7.
25. **Mann, R.G.** (1985). Why patient participation groups stop functioning: general practitioners' viewpoint. *British Medical Journal* **290**, 209–11.
26. **NHS Primary Care Groups** (2001). Public Engagement Toolkit. www.doh.gov.uk/pub/docs/doh/toolkit1/pdf.
27. **Al-Bashir, M.N. and Armstrong, D.** (1991). Preferences of healthy and ill patients for style of general practitioner care: implications for workload and financial incentives under the new contract. *British Journal of General Practice* **41**, 6–8.
28. **Hopton, J.L. and Dlugolecka, M.** (1995). Need and demand for primary health care: a comparative survey approach. *British Medical Journal* **310**, 1369–73.
29. **Van Wersch, A. and Eccles, M.** (2001). Involvement of consumers in the development of evidence based clinical guidelines: practice experiences from the North of England evidence based guideline development programme. *Quality in Health Care* **10**, 10–16.
30. **Bastian, H.** (1998). Speaking up for ourselves. The evolution of consumer advocacy in healthcare. *International Journal of Technology Assessment in Health Care* **14**, 3–23.
31. **Kelson, M.** (2001). Patient involvement in clinical governance. In *Advancing Clinical Governance* (ed. M. Lugon and J. Secker-Walker), pp. 5–18. London: Royal Society of Medicine.
32. **Pickard, S. and Smith, K.** (2001). A 'Third Way' for lay involvement: what evidence so far? *Health Expectations* **4**, 170–9.
33. **Kendrick, D., Fielding, K., Bentley, E., Kerslake, R., Miller, P., and Pringle, M.** (2001). Radiography of the lumbar spine in primary care patients with low back pain: randomised trial. *British Medical Journal* **322**, 400–5.

14

Research

14 Research

14.1 History and structure

Yvonne H. Carter and Glyn Elwyn

Introduction

Primary care is first contact, continuous, comprehensive, and coordinated care for individuals and populations undifferentiated by age, gender, disease, or organ system.[1] As an academic discipline, primary care has achieved a remarkable position in the international health care scene during the past 50 years. It is still, however, widely regarded as a newcomer by many researchers from other disciplines while those within it are seeing signs of a 'middle-age crisis'. This chapter explores how these two views can co-exist. Academic general practice and primary care (or its synonym family medicine) is a product of the 1950s: part of the fundamental re-evaluation of society that took place as the post-war generation challenged their surrounding world. In this era, the voice of the clinical generalist was heard as a reaction against the biomedical culture of the more traditional medical 'gaze'. The new thinking was exemplified by the systems thinking of von Bertalanffy[2] and the biopsychosocial view of medical practice promoted by Engel.[3] These ideas in turn shaped the development of one of the most fundamental concepts underpinning family practice: patient centredness.

Research in primary care was pioneered and developed in those countries that built their health care systems on the principles of generalist-based access to more specialized levels of health care. Countries where family practitioners work in parallel with other specialists found that primary care research was more difficult to initiate and develop. Nevertheless, significant investments are being made in such contexts as they recognize the potential research contribution of primary care.[4] Yet, despite the variation between health care systems, it was during the late 1960s and early 1970s that academic general practice found its feet as developed countries grappled with the need to establish a university-based niche for the main health care provider.[5] As Culpepper described it: the intellectual development of family medicine in the United States began with the unrest of the 1960s, which led to the creation of the specialty.[6] The early priorities in Northern Europe were centred on developing a teaching base and it is only after that foothold had been secured that the research agenda was given headroom. Similar patterns have been reported in other countries.[7–9]

Pioneers in primary care research

Although the 'academic' discipline of primary care research emerged during the 1960s, there had, of course, been pioneers who had made important contributions from the tradition of generalist care. Jenner found that inoculation of patients with cowpox provided protection against smallpox; Budd traced the spread of typhoid fever to water.[10] Finlay made the link between yellow fever and the mosquito, allowing a logical approach to control and prevention.[11] Descriptive research requires careful systematic observation and Mackenzie, Pickles, and Fry all worked in this way. Mackenzie noted in 1916 that there was no expectation in the minds of either the public or the profession that generalists could or should do research. He went on, however, to establish an international reputation for his pioneering research in the field of cardiology.[12] Pickles, the first President of the UK Royal College of General Practitioners, demonstrated that world-class research could be done entirely outside the hospital environment[13] by tracing the spread of infectious diseases in his practice population. Fry highlighted the important role of family doctors in the continuity of patient care and made research in the setting of ordinary every day practice a reality. He is particularly known for describing the profiles of disease[14] and his description of general practitioner researcher types still holds true today: those working alone, those working with others, those gathering information from others, and those willing to develop and test research methods in their own practices.

The growth of organizational support for primary care research

This section notes how a system of organized support for primary care researchers has been established. The pattern is one of initial development within professional Colleges of General Practice, followed by the establishment of academic departments, but more recently the development of even wider, and more diverse, networks. Founded in 1952, the UK College of General Practitioners was the first to stimulate a research agenda. Officers at that time noted three key obstacles: professional isolation; lack of research skills and experience; and a failure of general practice to penetrate the universities. The Research Committee was one of only four committees formed in 1953. Despite the lack of resources and tradition, all five members held a Doctorate in Medicine. There was a clear intent to promote quality and high standards and this led to the generation of a newsletter, a research register and the first steps towards a national morbidity survey.

Exactly when general practice or family medicine achieved the status of a discipline remains open to debate but 1961 marks a watershed when the College Journal in the United Kingdom was recognized by Index Medicus. In 1967, a Royal Charter was achieved. Based on this foundation, many similar professional Colleges of General Practice have been established, and many of them have had similar successful research programmes and outputs. The impact factors of the *British Journal of General Practice* and the US-based *Journal of Family Practice* are comparable to many other high-quality disciplinary publications and a sign of the respect and importance given to the research outputs from primary care.

The UK RCGP also led the way in the establishment of primary care based epidemiological Research Units[11] such as the Birmingham Unit and

Table 1 Trends in academic primary care

	1970s	2000s
Academic departments	Small departments in a handful of universities	Consolidated departments in most universities and establishment of primary care research units in other contexts (e.g. postgraduate medicine)
Clinical teaching	Negligible contribution to undergraduate teaching in medical schools	Substantial contribution to undergraduate curricula with trend to teach in community settings (clinical and communication skills)
Research	Based on pioneering work of committed individuals with no identified funding streams	Multidisciplinary research teams with integration of qualitative and quantitative methods, with interfaces with humanities (communication studies), epidemiology (population approaches), and health service research (programme evaluation and implementation research)
Links to service provision	Clinician-researchers providing direct care	Development of research practices and research networks with collaboration on project design and data collection
Information technology	Nil	Increasing convergence on electronic medical record as the basis for practice and some progress towards a globally agreed coding system

Manchester Units. The model provided by the RCGP has served as a template for the establishment of The World Organization of Family Doctors (WONCA) and other national Colleges. Early examples included the Dutch College of General Practitioners, founded in 1956, and the Australian College of General Practitioners formed in 1958, later becoming The Royal Australian College of General Practitioners (RACGP) in 1969. Similar colleges have been set up throughout the world, and international conferences organized by WONCA provide important platforms for the dissemination of research work in primary care. The WONCA-supported networks for research are an added layer of organizational support. There are extensive European networks devoted to quality (EQUIP), prevention (EUROPREV), and rural care (EURIPA). At the same time, Departments of General Practice have set up associations, such as the UK-based Society for Academic Primary Care (SAPC). This organization changed its name and constitution in 2001, having to recognize the wider membership implied by primary care and the fact that research in this area is also occurring outside traditional academic departments. Other examples of the open house approach are encapsulated by the European General Practice Research Workshop (EGPRW) and the North American Primary Care Research Group (NAPCRG). NAPCRG describes itself as: 'a multidisciplinary organization for primary care researchers in the United States, Canada, and throughout the world'.

Emergence of academic departments

Although there has been a tradition of teaching medical students in the setting of general practice, which dates back more than 200 years, before the 1950s there were no primary care lecturers on the staff of universities nor a single Chair of General Practice in a university department anywhere in the world. There were, therefore, precious few role models to inspire a new generation of researchers in primary care. The first independent University Department of General Practice and first Chair of General Practice were established in Edinburgh in 1957 and 1963, respectively. The recipient, Scott, had previously been appointed to the staff of the University of Edinburgh in 1956 through the support of social medicine (public health). Other medical schools were slow to follow Edinburgh's lead. When the Dutch College of General Practitioners was formed in 1956, one of the aims was to promote a more general practice oriented medical education. The consequence of the introduction of vocational training for GPs was that between 1966 and 1970 each Dutch Medical Faculty founded a Chair in General Practice. The Departments of General Practice were by origin very strongly education-oriented.(15) Byrne was not appointed to the first Chair in England at Manchester until 1972, and the 1970s then saw a gradual acceleration of this process. Every undergraduate medical school in the United Kingdom now has an academic Department and at least one chair in General Practice or Primary Care and this pattern has continued around the world. The possibility that general practice might be more than simply a teaching facility for a medical school has finally been acknowledged.

The development of general practice as a university discipline in the United Kingdom has mirrored that of departments in many other countries. The Mackenzie review in 1986(16) was significant in that it led to a number of organizational reforms. Although the pace of development of university departments of general practice or family medicine has been reasonable, the support for them has often been unsatisfactory as exemplified by shortages of accommodation, support personnel, and the lack of tenured posts for academic staff. Initially, the trend was to appoint single individuals or small groups. More recently, the general pattern has been to grow into large interdisciplinary teams working with colleagues across community health sciences. Working in partnership with networks of teaching and research active practices, a multiprofessional approach is illustrated by the variety of disciplines currently working within academic departments of general practice/primary care. These may include doctors, nurses, managers, social scientists, anthropologists, statisticians, psychologists, and others.

Senior appointments are being differentiated increasingly into either research or educational positions but, even so, progress towards an established career structure within academic general practice has been slow. In 1999, Wallace described the need to develop the academic agenda in family medicine in Europe and examined mechanisms to promote linkage between clinical work, research, and education(17) (see Table 1).

Research practices

Several types of primary care organization are now more actively involved in research, including health maintenance organizations in the United States. Along with the research potential of primary care groups or co-operatives of individual practices and the growth in primary care research networks (see Chapter 14.4), Kernick et al.(18) identified research practices as key to developing increased capacity. The first 'dedicated' research practice in the United Kingdom was appointed by the RCGP in 1994, which also provided limited financial support. Since this time the scheme has been evaluated(19) and there have been similar developments through regional and national research and development offices.(20) The development of research practices allows individual primary care teams to become more involved in research at a variety of levels.

In 1998, the RCGP developed a pilot scheme to accredit UK general practices undertaking primary care research and development. The Assessment Schedule included two levels: a Collaborative Research Practice with little direct experience of gaining project or infrastructure funding; or an Established Research Practice with more experience of research funding and activity and a sound infrastructure to allow for growth in capacity. The process for assessment involved the review of written documentation and an assessment visit by a multidisciplinary team. In 2001, recommendations were made to launch the scheme, renamed Primary Care Research Team Assessment (PCRTA), formally. The role of primary care research networks has been highlighted in relation to support and mentoring for research practices undergoing assessment. The new assessment scheme will help primary care trusts and individual practices to prepare and demonstrate their approach to research governance in a systematic way.[21]

Research themes

A balanced portfolio of research *in* and *on* primary care is essential if the discipline is to make progress at clinical and organizational levels. Research in primary care provides the clinical generalist (and scientist) with the means to test and improve clinical practice and to question population data. Research on primary care provides the means to improve the organization of services and to question beliefs or behaviours. The generalist clinician stands at one of the most complex intersections in society, as science, represented by psychological, physiological, and pharmaceutical interventions, and the humanities, as represented by the social contexts, beliefs, narratives, and shared mythologies, intermingle in consultations to formulate, on the one hand, interventions and their resultant outcomes and, on the other, extended stories that serve to embellish lives with hopes and fears. It is no wonder that research in primary care has, in distinction to other realms of medicine that largely embrace positivistic perspectives, uses the most diverse set of research methods. Generalists view the entire canvas of medicine, and are adept at taking ideas and investigative approaches from a wide range of disciplines, such as epidemiology, anthropology, sociology, and philosophy. More recently, and in tune with a post-modern condition, sociolinguistics, narrative,[22] chaos and complexity theories,[23] are examples of other ways of examining the weave of technical and social components that make up family medicine.

There are many ways in which primary care research activities could be categorized. One approach is to use the patient as an anchoring point. At the level of the individual patient, it is the *consultation* that has defined a major interest, and it is a field where family medicine has dominated the research effort, although, as is becoming apparent from disciplines such as psychology and linguistics, often without sufficient rigour.

Interestingly, work on the consultation did not start within a positivist paradigm. Balint's insights into the nature of the relationship between patients and clinicians was a trigger for an extensive research tradition that vigorously continues to examine the interpersonal interactions within clinical consultations, and their effect.[24] Byrne and Long were pioneers in the 'coding' tradition and attempted to quantify aspects of the consultation, as soon as it was feasible to introduce the tape-recorder into a clinical context.[25] These code-categorization studies have continued and diversified. Nevertheless, the plethora of research instruments in this field have not been rigorously developed in terms of their validity (fitness for purpose) or reliability.[26] The underlying assumptions of being able to make valid statements about the 'meaning' within interactions by aggregating coded segments of talk has also been questioned.[27] There is no standardized evaluation tool to assess the acquisition of communication skills by undergraduates and, therefore, no comparative work available. As revalidation and reaccreditation requirements arrive to drive the continuing professional development agenda, interest is also developing in the assessment of communication skills in the postgraduate years.[28]

Stott and Davies devised a doctor-based consultation framework,[29] where attendance to acute and chronic problems, and the modification of health seeking and promotion behaviour, could be visualized as being at odds with the patient-centred approach that others were beginning to promulgate.[30] Their divided box framework reflected an emerging view in the early 1970s that general practitioners had an implicit responsibility to a wider societal interest in the organization of their work, and inherently exhibits a tension between an *individual* or *population* focus in primary medical care.

Adopting a population perspective in primary care has been another major research activity and has underpinned the majority of studies (see Chapter 14.3). The use of practice and population data have seen quantum leaps in the availability of coded data as the potential of electronic clinical databases are being widely recognized.[31] A large number of coding systems exist, and although there are claims that episodes of care can be mapped across different frameworks, making data comparative and meaningful is still a significant challenge. Nevertheless, the potential power of this patient-level information, held in the multiple clinical databases, is being gradually realized, especially when morbidity and prescribing information can be linked and longitudinally related to other epidemiological data sources such as hospital admissions and discharges.[32]

Many studies in primary care have attempted to modify patterns of care, using the assumptions that self-limiting illnesses are over-presented and, consequently, over-treated and that chronic illnesses are, under-managed. Definitions of disease patterns are, however, difficult and variably applied with the consequence that the validity of aggregating broad categories such as 'acute bronchitis' as a single phenomenon is being questioned.[33] Studies undertaken at practice level have often been underpowered and it is only during the late 1990s that the impact of clustering within practitioners and organizations are being systematically addressed by appropriate statistical techniques.[34] The increasing interest on the effectiveness of health services has led to an emphasis on an appropriate assessment of complex interventions[35] and a corresponding interest in outcome measures, both generic (such as quality of life scales) and disease-specific measures.[36] Measuring 'quality of life' indices was only proposed in the mid-1980s but is now an area of active inquiry in primary care.[37] This field is widely known as health service research and it is no accident that many departments of general practice have been the originators and are likely to remain the main protagonists in the future.[38]

Primary care is also a good experimental field for implementation research and the early work on guideline development demonstrated how little effect passive dissemination has on professional practice.[39] This area is evolving into a field where area-wide interventions are provided and where practitioner- or patient-level outcome measures are collected using a mixture of routine data collection and specific measures. This so-called 'implementation' research will generate debates whether this is research conducted 'in' or 'on' general practice. Interest is also increasing in the applied behavioural science of organizational development and the managerial schools of thought that argue for process re-design as a way of improving health care outcomes.[40] Researchers in this field tend to use participatory-type methods (action research paradigms).

Research in general practice initially encompassed the consultation and the practice population. Interest in population effects increased and there are more multi-practice studies. There is an increasing realization over the last few decades of the importance of integrating both qualitative and quantitative research. van Weel[41] has suggested an explicit international exchange and comparison of general practice research:

- to transfer experience and expertise;
- to develop research methodology and techniques;
- to promote the exchange of translation research and implementation;
- to promote joint research on the contextual aspects of medical care.

The next developments in research will be about the amalgamation of large datasets to enable wide area benchmarking and the refinement of outcome measurement to evaluate the effects of complex interventions. As an underlying motivation for the research effort, the fundamental unresolved dilemma of health care remains as true today as it did in Hart's working context.[42] Poor communities get the lowest intensity and quality of health care services, across the globe. International developments with more emphasis on family practice present opportunities for national and international networks of primary care researchers to address this issue.

Career opportunities

Over the last decade, family physicians around the world and their attached staff have been increasingly recognized as being in an ideal position to address the health needs of their patients, to create a critical mass of research activity, and to bid for specific funding for primary care based research. However, training for family doctors and primary and community nurses usually provides little experience in research methods. Lack of protected time, resources, and infrastructure have been persistent barriers to progression.

In 1997, the Report of an Independent Task Force on Clinical Academic Careers(43) in the United Kingdom noted the difficulty in recruiting academic staff in general practice. It acknowledged that some significant improvements in the overall conditions of service for GP academics would be needed for the profession to prosper. The last few years has seen a flurry of policy publications relevant to the further development of the discipline.(44,45) The reports identified an urgent need to expand the research capacity in primary care from its historical low base, where research was poorly funded yet fundamental to raising the quality of patient care. Recommendations include the need to: increase the recruitment, development, and retention of R&D leaders in primary care; to increase the number of clinical staff with R&D expertise; to increase the involvement of staff in non-clinical disciplines; and to achieve an evidence-based culture in primary care. The recommendations of these reports have international significance.

New posts are being created for GP registrars/family medicine trainees and young family doctors with protected time for personal development and research. Flexible posts with linked clinical and protected academic sessions can aid recruitment and retention of family doctors in inner city practice. These posts may be linked to a taught masters programme in research methods. Young primary care practitioners are particularly expecting flexibility with a choice of entry routes into academia and established career pathways. A number of opportunities exist that enable junior academics to develop their research skills, under the personal supervision of a senior academic, whilst undertaking a research project related to general practice.(46) In nearly all countries in Europe, a research doctorate (MD or PhD) is a condition for an academic career leading to a professorship of general practice.(47) This can be interpreted as strengthening the academic base of primary health care.

Summary and conclusions

The history of research in general practice is a progression from exceptional individuals to multidisciplinary academic departments that balance the need to keep in touch with the grassroots of clinical practice whilst competing in academic environments. Although essentially still fighting for their recognition within university settings, these departments are also witnessing internal mid-life problems. Teaching and research are struggling to remain bedfellows, as community-based teaching becomes a major commitment and as researchers are driven to publish and increase research quality. Success also brings other challenges. Generalists, by their nature, turn their hands to many things, often with great enthusiasm. The discipline paradoxically encompasses multidisciplinary primary care using an ever-increasing range of research methods. As the academic world adapts to the fragmented face of primary care delivery in newly organized health care contexts,(48) a sense of questioning the meaning of it all is occasionally voiced, and as in most mid-life situations, it seems there are significant changes ahead

A key challenge for university-based departments is the decision to stay focused on clinical general practice or to develop wider expertise in health service research. The quality of the research versus teaching load also needs to be carefully considered. Will there only be a few research-based departments and will they have to have a full quota of expertise in qualitative methods, epidemiology, economics, and statistics to be successful in gaining grants from the prestigious research charities? Arguments of critical mass come into play here. Does this mean integrating primary care research with health services research and public health? This is becoming a global problem. The tension here is between research that is generalizable and of international stature and the development of a wider base of research-ready clinicians.

The next major challenge involves links to services and the purpose of networks. Are they really about high-quality research that is generalizable? Or are they training and capacity building networks? Would they be better considered as sampling frames (patients and electronic data) with shared standards? The same problem applies to research practices—what are their aims? The increasing inroads made by commercial/pharmaceutical companies into 'clinical trials' in primary care is an added complicating factor.

Opportunities to engage in research and development in primary care are growing and the scope for those wishing to become involved is finally widening. Infrastructure funding for research-active practices and the evolution of primary care research networks has helped to improve the research capacity and blur some of the boundaries between academic departments and clinical practice. We are beginning to see an increase in primary care based research, which is in turn leading to an increase in an evidence base for decision-making by family doctors and other disciplines working in primary care.

Acknowledgements

Our thanks to the many researchers who contributed to our literature search. These include Wolfgang Himmel and Michael Kochen (Germany), Richard Hays (Australia), Michel Wensing (Netherlands), Marjukka Makela (Finland), Donatella Sghedoni (Italy), Christopher Butler (Canada), and Martin Ryt-Hansen (Denmark).

References

1. **Starfield, B.** (1994). Is primary care essential? *Lancet* **344**, 1129–33.
2. **von Bertalanffy, L.** *General System Theory.* New York: Braziller, 1968.
3. **Engel, G.L.** (1960). A unified concept of health and disease. *Perspective in Biology and Medicine* **3**, 459–85.
4. **Kochen, M.M.** (1992). Forschung in der Allgemeindedizin. In *Allgemein und Familienmedizin (Duale Reihe)* (ed. M.M. Kochen), Stuttgart: Hippokrates.
5. **McWhinney, I.R.** (1966). General practice as an academic discipline: reflection after a visit to the United States. *Family Medicine* **23**, 11–15.
6. **Culpepper, L.** (1991). Family medicine research. *Family Medicine* **23**, 10–14.
7. **Gene-Badia, J., Jimenez-Villa, J., and Martin-Zurro, A.** (1993). Family practice research in Spain. *Family Practice Research Journal* **13**, 7–14.
8. **Backer, P.** (1993). National and international research in the future in general practice. *Scandinavian Journal of Primary Health Care* **11** (Suppl. 2), 4–6.
9. **Richards, J.G.** (1980). General practice research in New Zealand. *The Journal of Family Practice* **10**, 1097–9.
10. **Budd, W.** *Typhoid fever: its nature, mode of spreading and prevention.* London: Longmans Green and Co.
11. **Royal College of General Practitioners.** *Forty Years On. The Story of the First Forty Years of the Royal College of General Practitioners.* London: RCGP, 1992.
12. **Mackenzie, J.** (1883). A case of hemiparaplegia spinalis; with remarks on muscular sense. *Lancet* **1** (995–7), 1040–104.
13. **Pickles, W.** *Epidemiology in Country Practice.* Bristol: John Wright, 1939.
14. **Fry, J.** *Profiles of Disease. A Study in the Natural History of Common Diseases.* Edinburgh: E & S Livingstone, 1966.
15. **van Es, J.C., de Melker, R.A., and Goosmann, F.C.L.** *Characteristics of the General Practitioner.* Revised report on educational objectives of the Department of General Practice of the University of Utrecht. Utrecht: University of Utrecht, 1983.
16. **Howie, J.G.R., Hannay, D.R., and Stevenson, J.S.K.** *The Mackenzie Report. General practice in the Medical Schools of the United Kingdom 1986.* Edinburgh: University of Edinburgh, 1986.
17. **Wallace, P.** (1999). Building bridges: integrating research and undergraduate education into general practice/family medicine. *European Journal of General Practice* **5**, 116–19.
18. **Kernick, D., Stead, J., and Dixon, M.** (1999). Moving the research agenda to where it matters. *British Medical Journal* **319**, 206–7.
19. **Sibbald, B. and Dowell, J.** *Research Practices: an Evaluation.* Manchester: National Primary Care Research and Development Centre, 1998.

20. **Smith, L.F.P.** (1997). Research general practices: what, who and why? *British Journal of General Practice* **47**, 83–6.
21. **Carter, Y. and Shaw, A.** *Accreditation of Research and Development in UK General Practice.* Final Report. London: Royal College of General Practitioners, 2000.
22. **Greenhalgh, T. and Hurwitz, B.**, ed. *Narrative Based Medicine.* London: BMJ Publishing, 1998.
23. **Griffiths, F. and Byrne, D.** (1998). General practice and the new science emerging from the theories of 'chaos' and complexity. *British Journal of General Practice* **48**, 1697–9.
24. **Balint, M.** *The Doctor, the Patient and his illness.* London: Pitman, 1957.
25. **Byrne, P.S. and Long, B.E.L.** *Doctors Talking to Patients.* London: HMSO, 1976.
26. **Boon, H. and Stewart, M.** (1998). Patient–physician communication assessment instruments: 1986 to 1996 in review. *Patient Education and Counseling* **35**, 161–76.
27. **Inui, T.S. and Carter, W.B.** (1985). Problems and prospects for health service research on provider–patient communication. *Medical Care* **23**, 521–38.
28. **Elwyn, G., Edwards, A., and Riley, C.** (1999). Managing revalidation in general practice. *Clinician in Management* **8**, 193–7.
29. **Stott, N.C.H. and Davies, R.H.** (1979). The exceptional potential of the consultation in primary care. *Journal of the Royal College of General Practioners* **29**, 201–5.
30. **Levenstein, J.H.** (1984). The patient-centred general practice consultation. *South African Family Practice* **5**, 276–82.
31. **Pringle, M. and Hobbs, R.** (1991). Large computer databases in general practice. *British Medical Journal* **311**, 313–15.
32. **Pearson, N., O Brien, J., Thomas, H., Ewings, P., Gallier, L., and Bussey, A.** (1996). Collecting morbidity data in general practice: the Somerset morbidity project. *British Medical Journal* **312**, 1517–20.
33. **Arroll, B. and Kenealy, T.** (2001). Antibiotics for acute bronchitis. *British Medical Journal* **322**, 939–40.
34. **Campbell, M.K., Mollison, J., Steen, N., Grimshaw, J.M., and Eccles, M.** (2000). Analysis of cluster randomized trials in primary care: a practical approach. *Family Practice* **17**, 192–6.
35. **Campbell, M., Fitzpatrick, R., Haines, A., Kinmonth, A.L., Sandercock, P., Spiegelhalter, D., and Tyrer, P.** (2000). Framework for design and evaluation of complex interventions to improve health. *British Medical Journal* **321** (7262), 694–6.
36. **Fitzpatrick, R., Davey, C., Buxton, M.J., and Jones, D.R.** *Evaluating Patient-Based Outcome Measures.* Southampton: Health Technology Assessment, 1998.
37. **Muldoon, M.F., Barger, S.D., Flory, J.D., and Manuck, S.B.** (1998). What are quality of life measurements measuring? *British Medical Journal* **316**, 542–5.
38. **Guyatt, G., Walter, S., and Norman, G.** (1987). Measuring change over time: assessing the usefulness of evaluative instruments. *Journal of Chronic Diseases* **40**, 171–8.
39. **Grimshaw, J.M. and Russell, I.T.** (1993). Effect of clinical guidelines on medical practice: a systematic review of rigorous evaluations. *Lancet* **342**, 1317–22.
40. **Koeck, C.** (1999). Time for organisational development in healthcare organisations. *British Medical Journal* **317**, 1267–8.
41. **van Weel, C.** (1999). International research and the discipline of family medicine. *European Journal of General Practice* **5**, 110–15.
42. **Hart, J.T.** (1991). The inverse care law. *Lancet* **1**, 405–12.
43. **Committee of Vice Chancellors and Principals.** *Clinical Academic Careers: Report of an Independent Task Force.* London: CVCP, 1997.
44. **Mant, D.** *R&D in Primary Care: National Working Group Report.* Leeds: Department of Health, 1997.
45. **Medical Research Council.** *MRC Topic Review: Primary Health Care.* London: Medical Research Council, 1997.
46. **Hilton, S. and Carter, Y.H.** (2000). Academic careers in general practice and primary care. *Medical Education* **34**, 910–15.
47. **Kochen, M.M. and Himmel, W.** (2000). Academic careers in general practice: scientific requirements in Europe. *European Journal of General Practice* **6**, 62–7.
48. **Pollock, A.M., Player, S., and Godden, S.** (2001). How private finance is moving primary care into corporate ownership. *British Medical Journal* **322** (7292), 960–3.

14.2 Methods: qualitative

Benjamin F. Crabtree and William L. Miller

Introduction

'Everything feels stuck!' These are the frustrated words of patients, clinicians, families, practices, health services delivery systems, and even primary care researchers. This chapter describes the basics of qualitative research methods in primary care and suggests steps towards relief. Let us start with the story.

> Ms Wolfson slumps into a chair in the corner of the consultation room. As the nurse quickly exits, the husband deftly reaches into his briefcase and pulls out a little black book. Several minutes later, Dr Brown enters, looks around, settles his gaze on Ms Wolfson, and asks, 'How many seizures are you having?' This is the 12th visit in two years for this 36 year old woman with complicated chronic concerns of abdominal complaints, seizures, premenstrual problems and depression. She has seen many specialists without relief and, even though she remains on an anticonvulsant, the physicians, after extensive investigation, conclude the seizures are 'fake'. Ms Wolfson looks up, but her husband immediately holds out the open black book and explicates the exact times, situations, and descriptions of recent 'seizures'. The doctor briefly peruses the book, hands it back, and goes on to ask about her other concerns. Mr Wolfson tries to interrupt by noting that his wife is 'quite different' since her last seizure, but Dr Brown continues with questions about other physical complaints. Near the end of the encounter, Dr Brown inquires about depression, but hears only more physical concerns. Ms Wolfson leaves with a repeat prescription, another referral, and a return appointment. A chart audit reveals that the patient has received no preventive health services in over five years despite this being known as an exemplary practice for delivering such services. Everyone looks unhappy about what is happening. 'Everything feels stuck.'

What questions arise from this story? How can primary care research inform and help these stuck relationships? What are the qualitative research methods that can answer these questions?

The complexities and ambiguities of primary care require a multiplicity of research methods. The quantitative tools of epidemiology and randomized controlled trials (RCTs) are well known and described elsewhere. They help us to know how many, how much, the measurable associations between variables, if A, then B, and whether X is more effective than Y. But they are inadequate for seeking an understanding about what is important and why, what variations exist, what lived experiences mean to individuals and groups, and what patterns exist. These questions are the domain of qualitative methods such as depth interviews, focus groups, participant observation, and document analysis. The Generalist Wheel of Knowledge (Fig. 1) depicts the kinds of knowledge necessary for generalist clinicians and for primary care and health services researchers.[1] Four quadrants of knowledge and their appropriate methods can be differentiated within the wheel. The upper left corner (Quadrant I) represents clinician self-knowledge. The lower left corner (Quadrant II) is about the knowledge of patients, families, and communities, while the lower right corner (Quadrant III) represents the knowing about systems and organizations. The upper right corner (Quadrant IV) represents the knowledge of disease and illness processes. At the intersection of the four quadrants is the integrative function of primary care, informed by the different ways of knowing. Let us return with this wheel to the story of the Wolfsons and Dr Brown and explore the role of qualitative research methods in each of the quadrants.

What kind of encounter was this? What was Dr Brown's theory-in-action—his implicit thought process? These are questions of mindfulness,[2] Quadrant I questions concerning the clinician's own stories of this experience. This is the stuff of the reflective practitioner. Qualitative research using clinician diaries and action science tools is especially suited

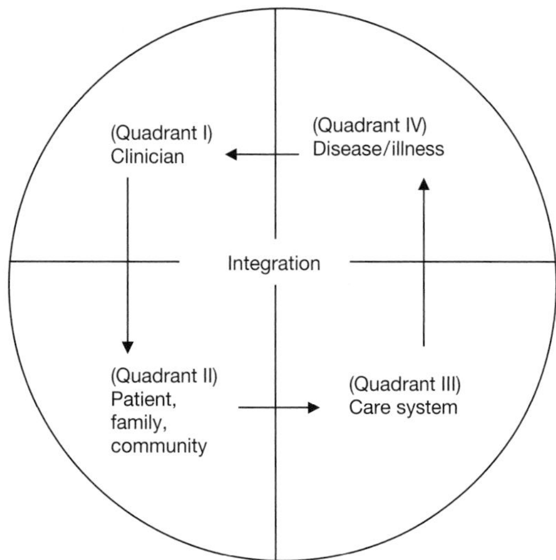

Fig. 1 Generalist Wheel of Knowledge.

for these questions. Malterud, studying her own clinical encounters with women who had 'undefined disorders', discovered how simple 'key questions' such as, 'What worries you the most about that?' opened a window towards better understanding.[3] Miller, using participant observation and key informant interviews, identified different kinds of encounters—routines, ceremonies, and dramas.[4] In the Wolfsons' story, we see a 'hopeless' maintenance ceremony being enacted despite the patient's readiness to embark on a new drama.

What works for helping frequent attenders, the heartsink patients like Ms Wolfson? These are questions of disease and illness evidence, Quadrant IV questions for epidemiology and RCTs. This is the stuff of information mastery, the POEMs (patient oriented evidence that matters) that inform and guide 'best practice'.[5] For the presenting concerns in the story, there is a paucity of evidence-based guidelines. The problem is not necessarily because of a lack of trials, but that we are never told about the experiences or expectations of the trial subjects, or about the context of the research setting and how it influenced the trial. A qualitative component in most RCTs would help, as suggested by two recent studies, one addressing how patients in dyspepsia treatment trials perceive their ability to influence their condition[6] and another on how women make sense of their own menstrual symptoms.[7]

What is Ms Wolfson's experience of her problems, of this visit, of her doctor? What's happening in this family? How are we to understand the husband's accountings? These are narrative questions, the Quadrant II questions of patient, family, and community stories. This is the stuff of pathography (patients' own accounts of their illnesses) and family systems. In the story, we see a patient struggling with her physician relationships. Could this be a parallel to struggles for control and attention within her own family of origin and with her husband? We need qualitative studies of these unfolding stories. These could include individual depth interviews or perhaps focus group interviews of family members, document analysis of patient and family diaries (even the 'little black book'), and life history interviews of patients.

How did the practice setting help or hinder the delivery of preventive health services for this patient? These are questions about health systems and the context of care, the Quadrant III questions of practice organization and health services. This is the stuff about error, variation, disparity, and quality of care. In the story, we see the chaos and competing demands of this patient's world overwhelm the systems of care. Qualitative studies of these contexts could include direct observation of activities in different settings, key informant interviews with participants, and the analysis of existing documents.[8] In fact, the Wolfson's story comes from a series of multimethod comparative case studies investigating the culture and operations of family practices.[9]

What would healing look like in this story? What was happening in the doctor–patient relationship? These are questions about healing and wellness, the 'Integration' questions about the craft of primary care. This is the stuff of diagnosis, relationship, communication, decision-making, and finding common ground. Qualitative methods have been used to reveal the dance of psychosocial explanation for physical complaints performed by patient and doctor,[10] a dance we see enacted in our story. Another qualitative study demonstrates the physician and patient points of view concerning irritable bowel syndrome and how they affect the relationship.[11] Participatory action research is particularly well suited for these questions about craft.[12]

Doing qualitative research closely parallels the process of clinical primary care. Primary care clinicians develop and test multiple hypotheses (diagnoses) through an iterative series of interview (history) and observation (exam and diagnostic testing) using purposeful, information rich, selective sampling. Interpretations and suggestions for care are then clarified and negotiated with the patient. The rest of this chapter explains these terms and how to do it.

Qualitative research process

In qualitative research, the investigators usually start with a problem or issue that emerges from a story, some experiential context. These problems and issues give rise to research questions. Designs and methods are then selected or created to best address these questions. What distinguishes qualitative research from quantitative approaches is that it seeks to inductively search for understanding and meaning. An additional distinguishing feature is the iterative process of gathering and interpreting data that usually occur concurrently. That is, analysis of early data often changes the sampling and data collection strategies because the investigators have gained insights they did not have at the beginning of the study. If one wants to understand how patients and clinicians experience depression, how patients respond when being informed that their cholesterol level is high, or how clinicians perceive the latest guidelines, then some form of qualitative research is the likely choice.

The term qualitative research conjures up different meanings to different people. Some biomedical researchers and epidemiologists consider survey research to be qualitative and routinely use the terms to refer to quantitative analyses of categorical or ordinal data. The qualitative research we are talking about in this chapter has evolved primarily from anthropology, sociology, psychology, education, social work, communication, history, and organizational studies.[13] Excellent overviews of the traditions and theoretical issues can be found in the *Handbook of Qualitative Research*[13] and in a review carried out by Health Technology Assessment,[14] which can be accessed on their website (http://www.ncchta.org). In this chapter, we take a more pragmatic approach in the hopes that the methods will be accessible to clinicians and a diversity of primary care researchers who are not steeped in the jargon of the different qualitative traditions.

The qualitative research methods most commonly used in health care research have roots in numerous social science disciplines and traditions, particularly sociology and anthropology.[13,15] An overview written for primary care researchers can be found in a series of 10 *British Medical Journal* articles published in 1995 and 2000 under the editorial guidance of Catherine Pope and Nicholas Mays. The series includes an introduction to qualitative methods in health and health services research,[16] as well as articles about different data collection and analysis approaches. Much of this work is available as part of an edited volume, now in its second edition.[17] Pope and Mays describe the goal of qualitative research as 'the development of concepts which help us to understand social phenomena in natural (rather than experimental) settings, giving due emphasis to the meanings, experiences, and views of all the participants'.[16]

In the following sections, we provide an overview of some of the more widely used design strategies. This is followed by sections describing data collection methods, sampling strategies, interpretation strategies, and some thoughts on rigour.

Qualitative traditions

There are a number of established strategies within the traditions of qualitative research that are widely recognized, for example ethnography, grounded theory, and phenomenology. Some researchers maintain methodological purity and stay within the precepts of their particular disciplinary training, while others prefer to borrow from the different disciplines. John Creswell provides an overview of qualitative traditions that have been used by different authors from different disciplines and fields.[18] He selected five of these traditions for detailed elucidation: biographical life history; phenomenology, grounded theory, ethnography, and case study.[18] We feel this is a good list and provide a brief overview of each, but add a sixth, clinical research,[19] that is particularly focused on clinical settings.[13] Other traditions include hermeneutics, human ethology, ecological psychology, heuristic research, ethnomethodology, symbolic interactionism, ethnoscience, and sociolinguistics, to name a few.

Ethnography is the trademark of anthropology. Multiple methods, particularly participant observation and key informant interviews, are used by the researcher to capture a holistic account of a defined group's daily life or culture. The researcher spends a prolonged time with those being studied, and often participates in activities in order to better understand the day-to-day lives of those being studied. The investigator generally identifies one or more key informants, people with special knowledge, and interviews them on a recurring basis to clarify observations. For example, Muller used an ethnographic approach to understand strategies used by internal medicine residents to cope with resuscitation.[20]

One of the most widely recognized qualitative traditions is that of *grounded theory* that emerged in the 1960s from the work of sociologists Barney Glaser and Anselm Strauss. Grounded theory seeks to identify the core social processes within a given context in order to build theory that is grounded in the reality of those being studied. Researchers using grounded theory generally employ the same interviewing and observational approaches used by ethnographers; however, the well-defined process of constantly and recursively coding the data, the 'constant comparative method', is the hallmark of grounded theory. For example, in an exploratory study of maternal concerns surrounding neonatal jaundice, Hannon et al. analysed audiotaped interviews of mothers of otherwise healthy infants to identify persisting misconceptions that clinicians should address.[21]

Phenomenology has its roots in the philosophical writings of Edmund Husserl (1859–1938) and seeks to understand the lived experience of the individual and their intentions. Researchers using a phenomenological perspective generally rely on in-depth interviews and use an interpretive process that 'brackets' their own preconceptions as they try to enter into the others' lifeworld. For example, McWilliam et al. collected indepth interviews and used a phenomenological approach to explore how women with breast cancer experienced communication with their physicians.[22]

Life history, diaries, and biographical methods focus on the individual's experience as told to the researcher or as found in existing documents. They are retrospective accounts of a person's life, or part of their life, that have been preserved in analysable text. These life histories provide rich portraits of an individual's story from which the research can identify turning points and core themes. This method was used by Stensland and Malterud to identify a patient's internal dialogues of illness and coping so it could be used to shape the medical conversation.[23]

Case study designs utilize multiple methods to intensively investigate a particular bounded system with a goal to describe and understand that system as an integrated whole. Case studies can be traced back to early ethnography, but really gained prominence as a tool used by sociologists to study urban environments. Educational and organizational researchers have especially promoted the use of case study designs. In primary care, Borkan used a comparative case study approach to understand how family practices cope with rapid changes in health care delivery.[24]

While not included as a separate tradition in most texts, the *Handbook of Qualitative Research*[13] includes *clinical research* as a separate qualitative tradition.[19] In fact, qualitative clinical research is more of a transdisciplinary philosophy than a tradition. Investigators are encouraged to mix and match methods and theoretical perspectives that best match the research question. Thus, it is multimethod and envisions a research space where the generalist researcher, much like the clinical generalist, is trained to focus on a local research problem and view it within its systemic context, not just from a specialized disciplinary perspective.[15,25]

Collection strategies

Qualitative researchers rely on four general types of data collection methods: interviews, observations, recordings, and existing documents. In general, interviews and documents provide an understanding of the perceptions of individuals or groups of individuals; while observations and recordings contribute to insights on behaviours. Depending on the research questions, the investigators may use either individual methods or a combination of methods to get different perspectives.[9,26]

Interviews

Qualitative researchers use a diversity of interviewing techniques, ranging from unstructured key informant interviews to more structured interview questionnaires and pile sorts. The most widely recognized interviewing techniques are formats that use an interview guide, particularly individual depth interviews, focus groups, and life history interviews. These are often used alone as the sole data for a study.[22,23,27]

Focus group interviews have their origins in sociology, although applications in marketing have stimulated widespread dissemination. Focus groups are moderated group interviews that generally follow a semi-structured interview guide and typically last between 1 and 2 h. They are almost always audiotaped and transcribed. A range between 6 and 10 participants appears to provide the best group dynamics, with the number of groups required depending on factors such as the homogeneity of the participants and the goals of the research. Ideally a continual iterative cycle of data collection and analysis is used until new insights are not forthcoming, referred to as *reaching saturation*. Experience has shown that four or five groups are probably a minimum and 6–12 fairly typical. More details on constructing focus groups are widely available.[15,17] Many studies in primary care use focus groups as the primary data collection method. For example, Bertram et al. conducted focus groups of people with physician-diagnosed irritable bowel syndrome (IBS) and found that IBS is perceived as a chronic condition resulting in frustration and social isolation.[27]

There are several types of individual qualitative interviews, including depth interviews, narratives, and life histories. The most widely used are *depth interviews* in which a moderator follows a semi-structured interview guide in order to stimulate a respondent to reflect and expand on fairly focused research questions. Like focus groups, these are almost always audiotaped and transcribed. The depth interview is ideally suited when the research focus is narrow, the respondents are relatively homogeneous, and the respondents' context is already known. Typically, a study will require 6–12 interviews before reaching saturation, with an iterative cycle of data collection and analysis being a critical feature of the method. For example, in the phenomenological study cited earlier,[22] the investigators sampled 11 women within 6 months of initial diagnosis or recurrence of breast cancer.

Narratives are stories of an individual's lived experiences that are often collected through depth interviews, but also come from first person written accounts. For example, to better understand the experience of elderly patients who had experienced a recent hip fracture, Borkan et al. collected injury stories of 80 elderly subjects soon after initial hospitalization.[26] The study identified new narrative prognostic factors for hip fracture rehabilitation. *Life histories* and *diaries* also provide insights into the individual's lived experience. For example, Stensland and Malterud used illness diaries of patients to transform the dialogue in clinical encounters to reflect the patient's own coping resources.[23]

Unstructured *key informant interviews* are seldom used alone, but are incorporated with observational data to provide insights that are not readily observed. Key informants are interviewed at different points in time, with the focus of the interview changing as the researcher's understanding changes. These interviews are seldom taped, but are recorded as notes. Over time, rapport is developed, so more intimate details are disclosed. Key informant interviews were a major source of data for Miller's study of ways family physicians successfully integrate the biopsychosocial model into everyday clinical encounters.[4]

Observation

Participant observation originated in the work of early anthropologists as a way of understanding everyday life from the perspective of those being studied. The observer's task is to collect observational 'fieldnotes' that provide the elements of a good story: *who* is present, *what* is happening, *when* do different activities occur, *where* do activities occur, *why* does it happen, and *how* the activities are organized. To record these details while observing is not possible, so the observer writes short notes or 'jottings' that can serve as reminders for later expansion into more detailed fieldnotes. Some investigators prefer to review their jottings and dictate the fieldnotes for transcription, while others type them directly into the computer.

Recordings

Not surprisingly, the use of *audiotapes* and *videotapes* of outpatient visits are an attractive data source for primary care researchers. Sometimes the original tapes are reviewed, but often a transcript is used for analysis. Content analysis of these data provide insights into the interaction between physicians and patients. The primary advantage of using videotapes is the availability of non-verbal behaviour, but videotapes can be more difficult to obtain in community-based practices. Chen and Britten used audiotaped patient consultations with primary care pharmacists to better understand the role pharmacists might play in providing independent medication advice.[28] To describe the barriers physicians face in evaluating patients for HIV risk behaviours, Epstein et al. videotaped and reviewed outpatient visits of patients who had expressed a concern about HIV infection.[29]

Documents/archives

While archival text documents are not often the primary data in qualitative health research, they are frequently used as supporting evidence. Medical charts, mission statements, procedure manuals, minutes, and flow sheets all provide information on how a practice functions or what the participants value. For example, these were used in a multimethod comparative case study of family practices to document hiring practices.[9]

Sampling strategies

Sampling in qualitative research is designed to maximize the investigator's ability to understand the phenomena they are studying. It is almost always iterative and purposeful—a probability sample is seldom appropriate. That is, the investigators start with an initial understanding of the phenomena based on prior experience and the literature, but gain a better understanding over time that shapes future sampling. In most studies it is not possible to know all the details about who will be studied or the final sample size. Instead the investigators should consider appropriateness and adequacy—is the sample appropriate for the research purpose and is the sample adequate in terms of being responsive to developing interpretations, reaching saturation, and searching for alternative explanations?

Widely used sampling strategies include maximum variation, critical case, theoretical, confirming/disconfirming, and extreme or deviant case.[30] At times, researchers use convenience samples, but this is generally not desirable. For example, in a multimethod comparative case study of family practices, Crabtree et al. selected practices to maximize geographic location (rural, suburban, and urban), size (small and large), and intensity of preventive service delivery (available through a previous study).[9] Once the project was underway, they realized that they also needed to sample on ownership (hospital owned versus private ownership) and they added this to the sampling strategy.

Management strategies

Until the introduction of specialized computer software, data management was a laborious task that required multiple copies of typed fieldnotes, interviews, and index cards. Fortunately, these days are over and there are numerous software programs designed for managing, coding, and retrieving text data. The most widely used are NUDIST, NVivo, Ethnograph, and ATLAS(TM). For some applications, programs not originally designed for qualitative data management can be helpful. For example, Crabtree et al. had collected massive volumes of data in their comparative case study and decided that the best software was FolioViews, a program developed for corporations to manage sales accounts.[9] For smaller studies, the use of a wordprocessing program can be adequate. Regardless, the computer is simply a tool—investigators must read the text and make interpretive decisions.

Interpretive strategies

The interpretive process is a dynamic and iterative process, a dance between the interpreter and the text.[15] The dance changes depending on the type of data, theoretical orientation of the investigators, and stage in the analytic process. The goal of the interpretive process is to make connections in the text that are articulated as themes and patterns. The different research disciplines and traditions have established a multitude of analytic strategies that are often confusing to health care researchers. Fortunately, the interpretive process in most of these strategies follows the same three phases: organizing, connecting, and corroborating/legitimating.[15] Complementary approaches to qualitative interpretation can also be found in the work of Miles and Huberman[31] and Silverman.[32] This latter includes a discussion of conversation analysis.

Organizing refers to the process of identifying relevant text, creating categories, indexing, and sorting. Sometimes this is done with an a priori codebook, but often the analyst reads the text in order to identify possible categories or codes. Connecting is the process whereby the investigators connect various categories in order to discover themes or patterns. There are many strategies for facilitating this process, including the creation of codebooks, the use of data matrices, or the writing of vignettes or short stories from the data. The final phase, corroborating/legitimating, is the process of confirming the themes and patterns. This involves re-entering the data to search for alternative explanations, disconfirming evidence or negative cases. Sometimes this also requires going back to the field to collect additional data.

Verification strategies

There are a number of strategies for enhancing the quality of qualitative research.[33,34] These include prolonged engagement, triangulation (using multiple sources of data, methods, investigators, and theories), negative case analysis, member checks (taking the results back to those being studied for confirmation), and using external auditors. Primary care clinicians and researchers reading a qualitative article should look at the relevance and validity of the research.[34] That is, the study should focus on an outcome that patients and/or clinicians care about, and that is common in clinical practice. The study should also address the following five questions: (i) Was the appropriate method used to answer the question? (ii) Was appropriate and adequate sampling used to get the best information? (iii) Was an iterative process of collecting and analysing data used and saturation achieved? (iv) Was a thorough analysis presented? (v) Are the background, training, and preconceptions of the investigators described?

Conclusions

Qualitative research provides exciting opportunities for primary care. Studies can help understand clinicians and their decision-making process (Quadrant I),[4,11,20,29] as well as providing insights into patients' perceptions and behaviors (Quadrant II).[6,7,10,22,23,26,27] Case studies and ethnographies are especially insightful for understanding practices and the health care system (Quadrant III) in ways not otherwise accessible with more structured approaches.[9,20,24] In addition, qualitative research can enhance clinical trials (Quadrant IV).[6,7] Finally, applications of qualitative research can also provide insights into evidence-based medicine[35] and evaluation.[36]

References

1. **Stange, K.C., Miller, W.L., and McWhinney, I.R.** (2001). Developing the knowledge base of family practice. *Family Medicine* **33**, 286–97.
2. **Epstein, R.M.** (1999). Mindful practice. *Journal of the American Medical Association* **282**, 833–9.
3. **Malterud, K.** (1994). Key questions—a strategy for modifying clinical communication: transforming tacit skills into a clinical method. *Scandinavian Journal of Primary Health Care* **12**, 121–7.
4. **Miller, W.L.** (1992). Routine, ceremony, or drama: an exploratory field study of the primary care clinical encounter. *Journal of Family Practice* **34**, 289–96.
5. **Shaughnessy, A.F., Slawson, D.C., and Bennett, J.H.** (1994). Becoming an information master: a guidebook to the medical information jungle. *Journal of Family Practice* **39**, 489–99.
6. **Nilsson, B. and Westman, G.** (1999). The impact of patients' influence on recovery in a group of patients with dyspepsia. *Family Practice* **16**, 515–21.
7. **Reilly, J. and Kremer, J.** (1999). A qualitative investigation of women's perceptions of premenstrual syndrome: implications for general practitioners. *British Journal of General Practice* **49**, 783–6.
8. **Gallagher, M.** et al. (2001). Managing patient demand: a qualitative study of appointment making in general practice. *British Journal of General Practice* **51**, 280–5.
9. **Crabtree, B.F., Miller, W.L., and Stange, K.C.** (2001). Understanding practice from the ground up. *Journal of Family Practice* **50**, 881–7.
10. **Joosten, A., Mazeland, H., and Meyboom-de Jong, B.** (1999). Psychosocial explanations of complaints in Dutch general practice. *Family Practice* **16**, 245–9.
11. **Dixon-Woods, M. and Critchley, S.** (2000). Medical and lay views of irritable bowel syndrome. *Family Practice* **17**, 108–13.
12. **Thesen, J. and Kuzel, A.J.** (1999). Participatory inquiry. In *Doing Qualitative Research* 2nd edn. (ed. B.F. Crabtree and W.L. Miller), pp. 269–90. Thousand Oaks CA: Sage Publications.
13. **Denzin, N.K. and Lincoln, Y.S.**, ed. *Handbook of Qualitative Research* 2nd edn. Thousand Oaks CA: Sage Publications, 2000.
14. **Murphy, E.** et al. (1999). Qualitative research methods in health technology assessment: a review of the literature. *Health Technology Assessment* **2** (16), 1–276.
15. **Crabtree, B.F. and Miller, W.L.**, ed. *Doing Qualitative Research* 2nd edn. Thousand Oaks CA: Sage Publications, 1999.
16. **Pope, C. and Mays, N.** (1995). Qualitative research: reaching the parts other methods cannot reach: an introduction to qualitative methods in health and health services research. *British Medical Journal* **311**, 42–5.
17. **Mays, N. and Pope, C.** *Qualitative Research in Health Care* 2nd edn. London: BMJ Books, 1999.
18. **Creswell, J.W.** *Qualitative Inquiry and Research Design: Choosing among Five Traditions.* Thousand Oaks CA: Sage Publications, 1998.
19. **Miller, W.L. and Crabtree, B.F.** (2000). Clinical research. In *Handbook of Qualitative Research* 2nd edn. (ed. N.K. Denzin and Y.S. Lincoln), pp. 607–31. Thousand Oaks CA: Sage Publications.
20. **Muller, J.H.** (1992). Shades of blue: the negotiation of limited codes by medical residents. *Social Science and Medicine* **34**, 885–98.
21. **Hannon, P.R., Willis, S.K., and Scrimshaw, S.C.** (2001). Persistence of maternal concerns surrounding neonatal jaundice: an exploratory study. *Archives of Pediatric and Adolescent Medicine* **155**, 1357–63.
22. **McWilliam, C.L., Brown, J.B., and Stewart, M.** (2000). Breast cancer patients' experiences of patient–doctor communication: a working relationship. *Patient Education and Counseling* **39**, 191–204.
23. **Stensland, P. and Malterud, K.** (2001). Unravelling empowering internal voices—a case study on the interactive use of illness diaries. *Family Practice* **18**, 425–9.
24. **Borkan, J.** (1999). Examining American family medicine in the new world order: a study of 5 practices. *Journal of Family Practice* **48**, 620–7.
25. **Crabtree, B.F.** et al., ed. *Exploring Collaborative Research in Primary Care.* Thousand Oaks CA: Sage Publications, 1994.
26. **Borkan, J., Quirk, M., and Sullivan, M.** (1991). Finding meaning after the fall: injury narratives from elderly hip fracture patients. *Social Science and Medicine* **33**, 947–57.
27. **Bertram, S.** et al. (2001). The patients' perspective of irritable bowel syndrome. *Journal of Family Practice* **50**, 521–5.
28. **Chen, J. and Britten, N.** (2000). 'Strong medicine': an analysis of pharmacists consultations in primary care. *Family Practice* **17**, 480–3.
29. **Epstein, R.M.** et al. (1998). Awkward moments in patient–physician communication about HIV risk. *Annals of Internal Medicine* **128**, 435–42.
30. **Patton, M.Q.** *Qualitative Research & Evaluation Methods* 3rd edn. Thousand Oaks CA: Sage Publications, 2001.
31. **Miles, M.B. and Huberman, A.M.** *Qualitative Data Analysis* 2nd edn. Thousand Oaks CA: Sage Publications, 1994.
32. **Silverman, D.** *Interpreting Qualitative Data: Methods for Analysing Talk, Text and Interaction.* London: Sage Publications, 1993.
33. **Mays, N. and Pope, C.** (1995). Qualitative research: rigour and qualitative research. *British Medical Journal* **311**, 109–12.
34. **Malterud, K.** (2001). Qualitative research: standards, challenges, and guidelines. *Lancet* **358**, 483–8.
35. **Green, J. and Britten, N.** (1998). Qualitative research and evidence based medicine. *British Medical Journal* **316**, 1230–2.
36. **Malterud, K.** (1995). Action research—a strategy for evaluation of medical interventions. *Family Practice* **12**, 476–81.

14.3 Methods: quantitative

David P. Weller, Robbie Foy, and Jane Gunn

Overview

In primary care, we have access to many sources of information to help make decisions. Some decisions are, by their nature, quantitative (e.g. how many patients would I need to treat with drug x to bring about an improvement in one?). This chapter provides some examples of the applications of quantitative methods in primary care research, and highlights how these methods can complement other approaches.

General practitioners have been conducting and using quantitative research for a long time. There is a rich history, for example, of GP-epidemiologists such as Clifford Jungfer from South Australia;[1] James Mackenzie from Scotland;[2] and William Pickles from Yorkshire.[3] These early primary care researchers took careful observations, and used their day-to-day work activities to generate research and information that profoundly affected clinical practice. Nowadays, primary care has at its disposal a great deal more information than these early pioneers. Increasingly, computerized data are available on well-defined primary care populations, and this facilitates audit and research. The value of seeking answers to important questions through observation, data gathering, and recording remains unchallenged in quantitative research.

Sources of information for primary care research

Over the previous two decades the importance of high-quality databases for collecting information on activities such as prescribing and morbidity has become increasingly evident in primary and secondary care. Examples include the General Practice Research Database,[4] the THALES study in France,[5] the IPCI database in the Netherlands,[6] and the BEACH study in Australia.[7] Such databases have been greatly assisted by the development of disease-classification systems that are specific to primary care.[8]

Local, well-established health surveys can also provide extensive information dating back many years. Examples include the Trent Health Lifestyle Survey[9] or the South Australian Health Omnibus Survey.[10]

Primary care databases also provide the potential for record linkage.[11] This involves linking, or matching a list of patients (e.g. patients who have participated in a primary care prevention programme) with a broader, population-based dataset (such as a cancer, diabetes, or coronary heart disease (CHD) registry). Record linkage can provide important information on association and causality, and can help verify outcome data.

A thorough search of existing sources of information should be undertaken before embarking on new data-collection strategies. Furthermore, widespread use of existing sources of information by primary care researchers will enhance the quality of the information and its relevance to primary care. Databases should, nevertheless, be used with some caution, paying particular attention to definitions used, and applicability to primary care populations.

General principles of quantitative research

Generating questions and selecting a study design

Research questions should be clinically relevant and/or have the capacity to inform policy. Development of research ideas takes time and should involve careful planning, review of literature, and discussion with colleagues. Clinical practice generates many questions. For example, a patient presenting with a sore throat may prompt questions about prevalence, diagnosis, prognosis, or treatment. How common are the various causes of sore throat in different groups, such as adults and children? How accurate is a clinical assessment alone compared with a clinical assessment and taking a throat swab in identifying bacterial causes of sore throat? In seeking answers to these questions from either available research evidence or doing research, it is helpful to ask a clear focused question. The question should adequately describe characteristics of study subjects, interventions, exposures, and outcomes.

Then, an appropriate research design needs to be chosen. Cross-sectional surveys can provide information on prevalence. Case-control or cohort studies can assess the relationship between risk factors and outcomes. Cohort studies entering similar and representative groups of patients assess prognosis. Diagnostic evaluations need to independently compare one or more tests with an adequate gold standard to assess their accuracy and reliability. Randomized controlled trials are the most appropriate design to address questions regarding the effectiveness of treatments.

Selecting a sample

All primary care quantitative research aims at collecting information from a representative group of individuals drawn from a much larger population of interest. Researchers need to collect information from enough people to be able to generalize the results to the whole population. Obtaining a representative sample is a key component to the conduct of quantitative primary care research. In order to obtain a representative sample, a complete and accurate list of all the members of the population of interest is required (the sampling frame). The representative sample can be drawn from this sampling frame by selecting a:

- random sample of names using a list of random numbers;
- *stratified random sample* of names (to ensure that certain groups within the population are selected in a fixed proportion).

There are many other sampling techniques. For example, it is relatively common in primary care research to use *convenience samples*. Often, researchers gather data from a number of consecutive patients presenting to a general practitioner or community nurse—this involves a trade-off between the convenience and feasibility of the sampling technique, and the generalizability of the sample.

Calculation of sample size

Whatever the research design and sampling technique chosen, a decision will need to be made about the numbers of individuals to include in the study. In descriptive studies, a sample needs to be drawn of sufficient size to be representative of the wider sampling frame. In studies that examine associations between exposures and outcomes, the aim of having adequate sample size (and, hence, statistical power) is to reduce the likelihood of failing to demonstrate a relationship or effect where one truly exists (a 'Type 2' error). Care also needs to be taken to avoid incorrectly detecting a statistically significant difference in the absence of any true effect (a 'Type 1' error, often caused by selecting too many outcomes and comparisons). Power is the probability of detecting a difference between two or more groups when one exists.

Sample size depends upon the desired level of power (80 per cent sometimes 'acceptable'; 90 per cent usually ideal), the likely or clinically important differences expected, and the pre-set significance level (usually 5 per cent but sometimes 1 per cent if it is particularly critical to avoid Type 1 error). Generally, studies aiming to detect small differences need to recruit more participants than those aiming to detect larger differences. Many randomized trials tend to be under-powered, either in the original design or because of insufficient recruitment.

Association and cause–effect

Quantitative research often results in apparent associations between variables (e.g. older general practioners and more satisfied patients, larger practice size, and briefer consultations). Once associations are demonstrated, it is necessary to seek answers to the following questions:

Could it be due to chance alone?

To answer this, we have tests of statistical significance (usually the p-value). Importantly, while a 'significant' p-value (usually set at <0.05) suggests that chance is an unlikely explanation for an association, it cannot take into account study design or the role of bias or confounding.

Is it due to bias?

That is, could the observed association result from an aspect of the design of the study that has introduced a systematic error (bias) into the results. Common forms of bias include *selection bias*, in which differences in characteristics of groups being compared can lead to apparent associations, and *observation bias*, in which study investigators elicit or interpret information differentially (interviewer bias) or study subjects report events in a non-comparable manner (recall bias)—for example, parents of autistic children may be more likely to recall a history of immunization than parents of normal infants.

Is it due to confounding?

We need to consider whether an observed association is due to a mixing of effects between exposure, the outcome, and some third factor that is associated with the exposure but also has an independent effect on the outcome. For example, might an association between older GPs and patient satisfaction be explained by older general practioners spending longer with their patients?

If the association is real, is it most reasonably explained on the basis of a cause–effect relationship?

Primary care research readily provides examples of association from quantitative research, but establishing a cause–effect relationship is often far more difficult. It is reasonable to ask: 'could the outcome or association I have observed reasonably be explained by an activity based in primary care?'. This issue of 'attribution' has been an important question in the development of quality indicators in general practice: 'can lower CHD rates be explained by better primary and secondary prevention in primary care?', or 'does an apparent association between GP-based audit and education activities in region x explain their lower admission rates for asthma?'. The well-established Bradford Hill criteria can provide some useful guidance. These include assessment of factors including the strength of the association, its biological credibility (e.g. could an action undertaken in general practice realistically influence CHD rates at a population level?), consistency with other studies, and dose-response relationship.

Presentation of results

The interpretation of any difference found in a quantitative research study depends upon its size and the precision with which it is estimated. The way in which results are presented can influence clinicians' perceptions of the size of the difference. The presentation of relative rather than absolute benefits tends to be more persuasive.[12] Results can also be presented as the 'number needed to treat' (NNT); for example, for every 33 patients receiving nicotine replacement therapy, one additional patient will quit smoking at 1 year (an NNT of 33). The NNT arguably provides more meaningful information for clinical decision-making.[13]

Confidence intervals provide an estimate of how precise the estimate of the difference is. In the aforementioned trial, the 95 per cent confidence interval for the odds ratio was 1.03–2.11. Hence, the treatment estimate ranges from having almost no effect to more than doubling the chances of quitting.

Descriptive and observational studies

Descriptive studies

Descriptive studies, as the term implies, describe the general characteristics of a sample. These characteristics might include person, place, time, socio-demographic factors, lifestyle variables, etc. They are based on either populations or individuals; population-based descriptive studies typically examine correlations (in classic epidemiological studies they examine correlations between risk factors such as diet and various diseases). While correlational studies can be used in primary care populations, they are typically based on very large samples (often the entire population of a country). They are useful for the formulation of hypotheses but, because they relate to whole populations rather than individuals, it is not possible to link an exposure to occurrence of disease in the same person. Testing of hypotheses requires the design and conduct of analytic studies amongst individuals.

Descriptive studies on individuals comprise *cross-sectional surveys* (which are described later in this chapter), *case reports* (in which individual cases which generate important research or clinical questions might be highlighted), and *case series*. A case series describes the experience of a group of patients with a similar diagnosis, usually highlighting an unusual aspect of a disease or history.[14] Case series may be useful in generating new hypotheses and drawing attention to the start of epidemics, but cannot test the validity of an association; they may suggest that the presence of a risk factor is related to a disease but any link cannot be confirmed in the absence of an appropriate comparison group. Furthermore, case series are usually based upon descriptions of selected patients as seen from the perspective of one individual or group of clinicians. Such selected patients may not be typical of those with the same condition encountered elsewhere.

> *Clinical example:* In 1998, a case series described 12 children diagnosed with ileal-lymphoid-nodular hyperplasia and autism.[15] A temporal link between autism and administration of the measles, mumps, and rubella (MMR) was suggested. However, no causal link between MMR and autism was found in further, more rigorous epidemiological studies.[16,17]
>
> The case series generated fears over possible adverse effects among parents and primary care professionals and had a sustained damaging effect on MMR vaccination programmes.[18]

Hence, case series represent a useful way of highlighting potentially important issues. However, they always require cautious interpretation and should not, in isolation, inform clinical practice and policy.

Observational studies

Observational studies, together with intervention studies (discussed later), form the basis of analytic study designs—that is, designs in which the investigator assembles groups of individuals for the specific purpose of drawing comparisons between groups and testing associations. The two main types of observational study are case–control studies and cohort studies.

Cohort studies (other names: longitudinal, prospective, or incidence studies)

Cohort studies are generally large, population-based studies of individuals exposed to certain risk factors. Comparisons are made between exposed and non-exposed populations.

In cohort studies, a group of people (or cohort) is assembled, none of who has experienced the outcome of interest. At entry, people are classified according to those characteristics that might be related to outcome. Then, the cohort is observed over time to see which of them experience the outcome of interest. An alternative to this prospective design is the retrospective cohort study in which a cohort that existed at some time in the past is assembled, and their outcomes ascertained through existing records.

Advantages

- Best available substitute for a true experiment, when experimentation/manipulation is not possible.
- Only way of establishing incidence.
- Minimize bias in ascertainment of exposure.
- Can examine multiple effects of a single exposure.

Disadvantages

- If prospective, potentially very costly and time consuming.
- If retrospective, requires availability of adequate records.
- Inefficient for evaluation of rare events/outcomes.

With the advent of improved systems of data collection in primary care, there has been a growth in cohort studies based on samples generated within general practice. For example, the RCGP Oral Contraceptive Study provides data on the long-term health effects of oral contraceptive use in UK women.[19]

Case-control studies

These are studies that compare frequency of a purported risk factor in a group of cases and controls. Patients who have the disease and a group of otherwise similar people who do not have the disease are selected and compared.

Advantages

- One of the most important methods used to study rare diseases.
- Investigators can identify cases unconstrained by the natural frequency of disease.
- Relatively inexpensive.
- No need to wait a long time for an answer.

Disadvantages

- Prone to bias.
- Selection of cases and controls.
- Measuring exposure, recall bias.

An example from general practice is a study based on the United Kingdom General Practice Research Database examining children with a possible diagnosis of autism.[20] The vaccination history of cases is compared with controls (also selected from the database) to examine any association between autism and the MMR vaccine. This study is using 'matched' controls, in which, for every case, a number of control subjects are selected who are matched on certain key characteristics.

Intervention studies

Intervention studies involve the assessment of active interventions in study subjects. This section focuses on intervention studies that randomly allocate participants to either treatment or control groups (randomized controlled trials). There is now a widely acknowledged need for relevant, well-designed randomized controlled trials in primary care. Yet randomized trials comprise only a small proportion of published research from primary care.[21] Randomized trials provide the most rigorous evidence of effectiveness of health care interventions compared with other study designs.

In a randomized controlled trial, one group receives the intervention being tested whilst a comparison group receives an alternative intervention. The key is that the likelihood of each participant receiving the trial intervention is determined by chance (random allocation). The nature of the intervention can vary widely and includes specific therapies (e.g. drug treatment, counselling) or any other type of care pathway (e.g. involving the use of diagnostic tests). The alternative intervention may sometimes include the standard treatment or no treatment. The results of the trial are assessed by comparing the outcomes in the different groups.

Many practices in primary care are unsupported by research evidence. New practices are often adopted into routine practice based on evidence from other study designs, or even 'common sense'. When put to randomized evaluations, they may turn out to be ineffective. For example, clinical guidelines, largely derived from hospital-based studies, have in the past recommended adoption of *Helicobacter pylori* testing by general practitioners in young patients to make more efficient use of limited diagnostic services.[22] When tested in a randomized trial in primary care, the strategy proved to be less cost-effective than usual management.[23]

Genuine uncertainty that an intervention works is essential for a randomized trial to be ethically justifiable and feasible to conduct. New treatments rarely have such striking benefits (such as those observed with the introduction of penicillin or insulin), that a randomized trial would not be justifiable.[24] Most treatment effects tend to be relatively modest, although still clinically important. Rigorous research methods are required to reliably detect such effects.

Why is randomization important?

Consider a trial testing whether the prescription of nicotine replacement therapy (NRT) helps smokers quit. In comparing outcomes in the NRT group against those of a placebo group, we would wish to ensure that both groups are as similar as possible. This would enable any differences in outcome to be attributed to NRT rather than other (confounding) factors that might also influence quit rates and complicate interpretation. If the NRT group happened to comprise less-motivated individuals or more smokers who had failed in previous attempts to quit, then any real difference in outcome might be obscured by the imbalance of these factors.

Random allocation distributes potential confounding factors more evenly across the two groups. Any differences in outcome are more likely to be attributable to the treatment alone. Some imbalance in confounding factors between the treatment and control groups can still occur by chance, although this becomes less likely with larger sample sizes. Random allocation safeguards impartiality, so that chance rather than practitioner or patient preference determines who receives the treatment. Non-randomized studies tend to show larger, or even false positive, treatment effects compared with randomized trials.[25]

Important components of randomized control trial design

A patient consults a general practitioner with a request for NRT to help quit smoking. This is a question about therapy and hence most appropriately answered by randomized controlled trials.

Adequate definition of research question

Clearly stating the trial question helps readers decide whether a published study is worth looking at in more detail. A sufficiently focused question considers the characteristics of the study population, the treatment, the control, and the outcomes. Hence, a trial might recruit heavy smokers from general practice lists (the study population) to compare the effectiveness of transdermal patch NRT (the intervention) against a placebo patch (the control) in achieving biochemically verified smoking cessation at 1 year (the outcome).

Randomization

Randomization does not guarantee bias-free results. Attention should be paid to the adequacy of the randomization process and how participants are managed and followed up. Poorer-quality randomized trials produce biased results compared with well-conducted trials.[25] As random allocation aims to prevent selection bias, it is important that the process is free of interference. For example, the use of sealed envelopes containing randomly generated treatment allocations is prone to tampering. A well-meaning practitioner may continue opening envelopes until the preferred treatment for a particular patient is found.

If possible, randomization should occur outside of primary care work places. Remote allocation, whereby the practitioner contacts a centre 'hotline' by telephone or via an Internet website to ascertain the patient's allocation status following consent, can assure the independence of randomization. Hotlines require efficient and flexible running to help minimize disruption during consultations or deal with study entries outside of normal working hours.

Concealment of allocation

Expectations about the effect of a treatment may influence outcomes. Patients who realize they have been allocated to NRT might be more encouraged to quit than controls. General practitioners, aware of the patient's treatment status, may provide more—or even less—support to quit smoking. Researchers may measure effects differently if they know which group a patient is in. In the last case, resultant observation bias is more important when assessing subjective outcomes, such as pain relief, than more objective outcomes, such as death. Poor allocation concealment is associated with bias, usually favouring new treatments being tested.[26]

Concealing which group the patient is allocated to, or 'blinding', can reduce such bias. Blinding can apply to one or more of patients, clinicians, or researchers. Blinding is not always possible, especially for treatments with known side-effects (such as skin irritation associated with use of the NRT patch) or if the intervention is obvious (e.g. counselling). In trials where blinding is desirable, the degree of 'unmasking' can be estimated by asking patients which group they think they were allocated to.

Follow-up and intention-to-treat

Ideally, all patients entering the trial should be accounted for at the end of the study. Attrition bias occurs if patients dropping out of one study arm systematically differ from those in the other arm. Adverse effects or the ineffectiveness of treatment may cause patients to drop out of a treatment arm. Their exclusion from the final analysis will lead to the overestimation of any true treatment effect. Study participants should be analysed in the group to which they were allocated, even if they do not receive the treatment.

Of course, it is not always possible to undertake randomized trials under 'ideal' conditions, particularly in primary care settings, and rigid aherence to randomized control trial criteria may be at the expense of valid results. For example, blinding is important in *explanatory* trials, which measure efficacy—the benefit a treatment produces under ideal conditions.[27] But it may not be desirable in *pragmatic trials*, which measure effectiveness—the benefit the treatment produces in routine clinical practice. Overall assessment of the latter accepts clinician and patient biases as part of their responses to treatment. Pragmatic trials also tend to have broader eligibility criteria. They can enhance transferability by recruiting the relatively heterogeneous mix of patients to whom the treatment will be applied in routine practice. This provides greater reassurance that a treatment will work outside of the trial setting.

Variations on design

There are many variations on the overall design of randomized trials. Three variations will briefly be highlighted here.

In *crossover trials*, patients are randomly allocated to study arms where each arm consists of a sequence of two or more treatments given consecutively. Crossover trials are used most frequently in testing treatments in chronic illness. There is a risk that the effects of one treatment may 'carry over' and alter subsequent responses to the next treatment. For example, some drugs may modify the underlying disease process. Hence, most trials incorporate a 'wash-out' period.

Factorial designs test the effects of combining treatments. In investigating whether patient education adds any benefit to patch NRT, the patients would first be randomized to NRT or control and then randomized again to education or control. Therefore, the effects of NRT and education could be assessed, as well as those of NRT alone, education alone, and no treatment at all. It is possible to analyse the results as if two separate trials were being conducted. However, factorial trials are more difficult to organize and analyse, provide only limited power for head-to-head comparisons (e.g. NRT versus education), and lose power if there is any interaction between the two treatments.

In *cluster randomized trials*, groups of participants are allocated to different treatments. Randomization by individual is inappropriate for interventions taking place at an organizational or geographical level. In testing a computer-driven protocol for primary care professionals to help patients quit smoking, individual randomization at patient level would lead to a substantial risk of contamination. It is likely that physicians' management of control patients would be influenced by what they had learned from following the protocol for treatment patients. Cluster randomization has major implications for design and analysis.[28] Patients within any one cluster are more likely to have similar outcomes; hence, standard statistical analyses assuming that the outcome for one patient would be independent of another no longer hold. Subsequently, larger sample sizes are required, and analysis needs to be based on the cluster as the unit of randomization.

Randomized control trials in primary care: some practical issues

Timeliness

Choosing the optimal time to test an intervention is like a balancing act. On the one hand, the widespread but early adoption of a clinical practice can hinder subsequent attempts to undertake randomized evaluations. A trial of counselling in general practice failed to recruit a sufficient number of patients because practitioners and patients strongly preferred counselling to the option of being randomized to the counselling or control arms.[29] Conversely, failure to work up an intervention sufficiently may lead to a trial demonstrating a lack of effect when further development of the intervention might have improved its effectiveness. An educational intervention for general practitioners would require piloting to test its acceptability and feasibility before undertaking a larger-scale evaluation of a refined approach.[30]

Communication and collaboration

These are essential in designing and running primary care trials. There is a wide range of health professionals, patients, and health care funding agencies; early consultation can enhance the relevance of the research question. Interdisciplinary collaboration helps to ensure rigour in the development of the research question and study protocol. In addition to statistical support and clinical advice, other skills can enhance the value and rigour of a trial.

Recruitment

Most primary care trials require recruitment of patients from more than one practice, sometimes spread over wide geographical areas. They, therefore, need adequate resources and a sound infrastructure to support recruitment and ensure quality control. Poor recruitment rates represent a common problem, leading to a loss of statistical power or premature closure of the trial. The failure to recruit an appropriate spectrum of patients can also limit the transferability of findings. Pilot studies and run-in phases can test anticipated recruitment rates and identify potential improvements. Eligible patients tend to disappear once trials start and investigators may need to consider widening eligibility criteria, with the advantage for pragmatic trials that transferability of findings will also be increased.

Survey design, conduct, and analysis

Surveys are a common primary care research method and can be administered face to face, by mail, by telephone using a paper-based or computer-assisted system, or via the world wide web. Surveys can be used to gain information from both providers and consumers of primary health care and the principles of survey design and implementation are similar in both settings.

Important questions before starting on survey research:

- What is the purpose of the survey, will it influence practice or policy?
- Is there a clear, clinically relevant question?
- Is there a more appropriate way to gather the information that I require?
- Do I have the resources required (time, money, and effort) to obtain responses from a representative sample?

If a study question genuinely warrants a survey in order to gather the required information, we recommend a careful journey of survey design, implementation, analysis, and dissemination of findings.

Choosing the mode of administration

Surveys are usually undertaken to collect information from a representative sample of individuals from the population of interest. This is often a large number of people. This requires a practical method in terms of cost and time.

Postal surveys are easily repeatable, avoid interviewer bias, can be distributed over wide geographical areas with little increase in cost,[31] and result in less 'socially desirable' answers than face-to-face or telephone interviews.[32] The self-administered postal survey is cheaper than telephone or face-to-face interviews,[32] yet it requires high response rates to be achieved if non-response bias is to be minimized.[33] The postal survey is particularly useful when reasonably simple data are required, addresses are known, and the budget is limited.[32]

Face-to-face interviews are expensive and difficult to conduct when the sample size is large, but provide an opportunity to explore issues in greater depth than postal questionnaires. Telephone interviews (which may be computer assisted—CATI) are an alternative to face-to-face interviews, yet need to be used with caution as they tend to under-represent low-income and low-education respondents.[34] The use of CATI and web-based surveys is likely to increase. The way people communicate is undergoing rapid change; the use of mobile phones and the uptake of web-based products bring opportunities and challenges (e.g. privacy issues) to survey research. Internet surveys have the advantages of being 'virtually free', having a quick turn around time, easy follow-up, being simple to complete, and allowing world wide sampling, not constrained by geographical barriers. The main disadvantage of Internet surveys is the selection bias leading to respondents being a more highly educated and better paid group than the general population. It may also be difficult to obtain e-mail addresses and it has been suggested that Internet surveys make impersonation a potential problem.[35]

Maximizing response rates

It would be ideal if 100 per cent of surveys were completed and returned to the researcher, yet this is rare. The higher the response rate, the more likely you are to achieve a representative sample of respondents. There is no 'magic figure' for the best response rate and published research shows that a well-conducted survey can achieve response rates of 65 per cent and higher. Low response rates may lead to biased findings. A UK study, with a response rate of 44 per cent, found that non-responders to a postal survey, about alcohol-misusing patients, differed significantly from responders.[36] Response rates to postal surveys are influenced by the number of follow-up contacts,[37] saliency of the topic, administering institution, length of survey, and target audience,[38] as well as time-period taken for the study[39] and the use of inducements.[38,40,41] Evidence from randomized controlled trials suggests that informing individuals of the forthcoming survey by mail[42,43] or by phone[44] can improve response rates. However, the use of phone prompts are more expensive and do not yield higher response rates than postal prompts.[45] Using financial inducements may accelerate the response rate and reduce follow-up costs[45] and the timing of the inducement may have an impact on the effect on the overall response rate.[40] Difference in response rates according to sex of respondent[40,43,45] have also been noted although the direction of the effect varies between studies and may be related to the study topic. Multivariate analysis of responses to five postal questionnaire surveys indicated that 'serial non-responders' tended to be older, less likely to possess a postgraduate medical qualification, or belong to a training practice.

Implementation research

While not confined to quantitative research methods, studies that examine strategies for improving the quality of primary care by promoting evidence-based practice have attracted growing interest over the last decade. The transfer of research findings into routine practice is unpredictable and tends to be a slow and haphazard process; some interventions are transferred to routine practice despite lack of evidence, while others take years to be transferred to routine practice despite much evidence. Even when primary care researchers find robust evidence that a strategy for changing professional practice and/or promoting quality improvement works, they may encounter many barriers in putting this into practice.

Implementation research involves finding cost-effective approaches to transfer research findings into routine clinical practice. The design and conduct of implementation research add new layers of complexity to more traditional quantitative research methods.

Lessons from systematic reviews

As with clinical care, systematic reviews of rigorous studies can greatly contribute to our knowledge about what works in changing professional and organizational behaviour. Commonly used interventions include the following:[46]

Educational outreach visits (for prescribing in North American settings)—use of a trained person who meets with providers in their practice settings to provide information with the intent of changing the provider's performance. The information given may include feedback on the provider's performance.

Reminders (manual or computerized)—any intervention that prompts the health care provider to perform a patient-specific clinical action.

Multifaceted interventions—a combination that includes two or more of the following: audit and feedback, reminders, local consensus process, marketing.

Interactive educational meetings—participation of health care providers in workshops that include discussion or practice.

Audit and feedback—any summary of clinical performance.

Local opinion leaders—use of providers nominated by their colleagues as 'educationally influential'.

Local consensus process—inclusion of participating providers in discussion to ensure that they agreed that the chosen clinical problem was important and the approach to managing the problem was appropriate.

Patient-mediated interventions—any intervention aimed at changing the performance of health care providers where specific information was sought from or given to patients.

Educational materials—distribution of published or printed recommendations for clinical care, including clinical practice guidelines, audio-visual materials, and electronic publications.

Didactic educational meetings—lectures.

The use of active interventions to promote the use of clinical guidelines, such as reminders or educational outreach, appears to be consistently effective.[47] The evidence is less clear-cut for other interventions. Intuitively, multifaceted interventions should work better than single interventions. But there is no direct evidence of additional effectiveness nor of whether their greater costs are offset by the benefits. In general, effect sizes tend to be relatively modest and are sometimes of uncertain clinical impact. Furthermore, interpretation and subsequent transferability are hindered by the poor methodological quality of primary studies.[48]

There is uncertainty over what factors are important in the relative success or failure of reported strategies because of the lack of an established theoretical framework and inadequate development research. This can lead to premature testing of strategies using a comparative design and in turn 'false-negative' results. Systematic reviews indicate variable effectiveness within the same interventions, such as the use of local opinion leaders (people identified as being educationally influential by their peers). These variations might be attributable to the modifying effects of context: it might be more feasible to identify local opinion leaders in secondary care settings than primary care. Inconsistent findings might also be explained by variations in the intensity or quality of the interventions tested. Although reminders appear to be consistently effective, their frequency and proximity to the point of clinical decision-making may influence the size of their impact.

Study design

Implementation research requires a sound theoretical framework that draws on evidence (often from outstide medicine) about what is likely to change behaviour, a period of careful development work to refine strategies (often incorporating qualitative methods such as focus groups, interview, observation, document, and policy review) and a robust study design—ideally based on random allocation to study groups (to minimize bias).

Cluster trials often represent the most valid design for evaluating interventions that target individual behaviours (e.g. continuing medical education), organizational systems (e.g. information technology), or policies (e.g. financial incentives), and make individual randomization inappropriate (discussed earlier). Weaker designs and poorly controlled evaluations overestimate the effects of interventions.[49] For example, in uncontrolled before-and-after studies, observations are made in one group before and after an intervention (e.g. distribution of a clinical guideline) and observed differences assumed to be due to the intervention. Several potential sources of bias and confounding greatly limit the interpretation of these studies, such as changes in practice occurring over time and independently of any intervention.

Some well-designed, non-randomized studies can provide robust evidence where practical and ethical barriers to conducting randomized studies exist.[50] Time series analyses entail the use of multiple observations before and after an intervention, attempting to detect whether an intervention has had an effect greater than any underlying trends in practice.[51] Conducting an *interrupted* time series analysis requires knowledge of the specific point when an intervention occurred (i.e. looking for the 'interruption' expected in a pattern if an effect is present). Time series analyses may be used in estimating the effects of mass-media campaigns, legislation, or dissemination of national guidelines and, therefore, tend to be opportunistic.[52]

Testing the impact of interventions to change professional practice generally requires greater sample sizes and additional research resources to detect clinically significant changes in the outcome of care. Measuring the process of care is justifiable when evaluating evidence-based recommendations (e.g. from valid guidelines) where link between process and outcome is well understood.

Interventions to change professional or organizational behaviour may have gradual (learning) rather than instant effects. Such effects may decline over time (decay effect), for example, after a period of raised awareness of a recommendation following an educational programme. It is important to measure change over time to identify such effects and quantify their influence.

Priorities in implementation research

Implementation research needs to address a number of issues to improve the transferability and validity of findings: the need for a common descriptive framework; the use of theory in the design and evaluation of strategies; and improving the rigour of evaluations.

Studies require a conceptual framework within which to describe common elements of settings, individuals, targeted behaviours, and interventions. This information would facilitate the comparison of different studies, enhancing the identification of features that influence the likely effectiveness of interventions. Strategies that aim to change professional and organizational behaviour represent complex interventions. Complex interventions require sound theoretical bases and careful exploratory studies to choose and refine interventions before widescale implementation.[53]

Interventions to overcome specific barriers should ideally be tailored to the nature of anticipated local problems.[54] There is a growing body of evidence to support the prior assessment of barriers and needs.[47] Theoretical models of change can be used both to understand the behaviour of health professionals and organizations and to guide the development of interventions to promote change.[55] These theories are derived from a range of disciplines (e.g. applied psychology, management studies) and generally apply to different levels of change, that is, those of individual professionals, teams, and organizations.[56] Qualitative research methods can also provide insights into the processes that contribute to the success or failure of interventions and are increasingly used in parallel to quantitative evaluations.

Newer evaluation methods combine qualitative and quantitative approaches; for example, 'realistic evaluation' begins with theories to describe how mechanisms operate in particular contexts to produce outcomes. Theory is then used to hypothesize about 'what might work for whom in what circumstances' and multimethod data collection and analyses focuses on mechanisms, contexts, and outcomes.[57]

Much scope exists to improve the rigour of evaluations, including greater use of cluster randomized trials.[58] Where effectiveness is consistently demonstrated, those responsible for local implementation need to know as much about the cost-effectiveness of behavioural interventions as they do about that of clinical interventions. Ideally, evaluations should incorporate an economic assessment of either or both of the resource implications of behavioural change strategies per se and of their wider impact on health services.[59]

Summary

In this chapter, we have presented an overview of key methodological concepts in quantitative research. Skills in interpreting the outputs of quantitative research, in areas such as estimating risk and interpreting treatment effects, have progressed in recent years. This quantitative element to decision-making is better understood and better utilized, as is its place amongst other components of decision-making. This chapter brings together some key principles in primary care quantitative research. In many areas, readers will need to seek specific methodological guidance from more detailed texts. Quantitative research designs, in combination with other study designs, will continue to make an important contribution as primary care research progresses over the next decade.

References

1. **Anonymous** (1979). Clifford Jungfer. *Australian Family Physician* **8**, 818–20.
2. **Moorhead, R.** (1999). Sir James Mackenzie (1853–1925): views on general practice education and research. *Journal of Royal Society of Medicine* **92**, 38–43.
3. **Anonymous** (1969). W.N. Pickles. *British Medical Journal* **1**, 719–20.
4. **Walley, T. and Mantgani, A.** (1997). The UK General Practice Research Database. *Lancet* **350**, 1097–9.
5. **Vallancien, G.** (2000). How are lower urinary tract symptoms managed in real life practice? The French experience. *European Urology* **38** (Suppl. S1), 54–9.
6. **van der Linden, P.D.** et al. (1998). Skin reactions to antibacterial agents in general practice. *Journal of Clinical Epidemiology* **51**, 703–8.
7. **Britt, H.C. and Miller, G.C.** (2000). The BEACH study of general practice. *Medical Journal of Australia* **173**, 63–4.
8. **Bentzen, N. and Bridges-Webb, C.** (1995). An international glossary for general/family practice. *Family Practice* **12**, 267.
9. **Roberts, H.** et al. (1997). Unemployment and health: the quality of social support among residents in the Trent region of England. *Journal of Epidemiology and Community Health* **51**, 41–5.
10. **Pilotto, L.S.** et al. (1999). Industry, air quality, cigarette smoke and rates of respiratory illness in Port Adelaide. *Australian & New Zealand Journal of Public Health* **23**, 657–60.
11. **Goldacre, M.** et al. (2000). Use of large medical databases to study associations between diseases. *Quarterly Journal of Medicine* **93**, 669–75.
12. **Naylor, C.D., Chen, E., and Strauss, B.** (1992). Measured enthusiasm: does the method of reporting trial results alter the perception of therapeutic effectiveness? *Annals of Internal Medicine* **117**, 916–21.
13. **Cook, R.J. and Sackett, D.L.** (1995). The number needed to treat: a clinically useful measure of treatment effect. *British Medical Journal* **310**, 452–4.
14. **Hennekens, C.H., Buring, J.E., and Mayrent, S.L.**, ed. Epidemiology in Medicine, 1st edn. Boston: Little, Brown and Company, 1987.
15. **Wakefield, A.J.** et al. (1998). Ileal-lymphoid-nodular hyperplasia, non-specific colitis, and pervasive developmental disorder in children. *Lancet* **351**, 637–41.
16. **Taylor, B.** et al. (1999). Autism and measles, mumps and rubella vaccine: no epidemiological evidence for a causal association. *Lancet* **353**, 2026–9.
17. **Patja, A.** et al. (2000). Serious adverse effects after measles–mumps–rubella vaccination during a fourteen-year prospective follow-up. *Pediatric Infectious Disease Journal* **19**, 1127–34.
18. **Petrovic, M., Roberts, R., and Ramsay, M.** (2001). Second dose of measles, mumps and rubella vaccine: questionnaire survey of health professionals. *British Medical Journal* **322**, 82–5.
19. **Hannaford, P.C. and Kay, C.R.** (1998). The risk of serious illness among oral contraceptive users: evidence from the RCGP's oral contraceptive study. *British Journal of General Practice* **48**, 1657–62.
20. **Smeeth, L.** et al. (2001). A case–control study of autism and mumps–measles–rubella vaccination using the general practice research database: design and methodology. *BMC Public Health* **1**, 2.
21. **Thomas, T., Fahey, T., and Somerset, M.** (1998). The content and methodology of research papers published in three United Kingdom primary care journals. *British Journal of General Practice* **481**, 229–32.

22. **Foy, R., Parry, J.M., Murray, L., and Woodman, C.B.J.** (1998). Testing for *Helicobacter pylori* in primary care: trouble in store? *Journal of Epidemiology and Community Health* **52**, 305–9.
23. **Delaney, B.C., Wilson, S., Roalfe, A., Roberts, L., Redman, V., Wearn, A., and Hobbs, F.D.R.** (2001). Randomised controlled trial of *Helicobacter pylori* testing and endoscopy for dyspepsia in primary care. *British Medical Journal* **322**, 898–901.
24. **Cochrane, A.L.** *Effectiveness and Efficiency: Random Reflections on Health Services.* Nuffield Provincial Hospitals Trust, 1972.
25. **Kunz, R. and Oxman, A.D.** (1998). The unpredictability paradox: review of empirical comparisons of randomised and non-randomised clinical trials. *British Medical Journal* **317**, 1185–90.
26. **Schultz, K.F., Chalmers, I., Hayes, R., and Altman, D.G.** (1995). Empirical evidence of bias. Dimensions of methodological quality associated with estimates of treatment effects in controlled trials. *Journal of the American Medical Association* **273**, 408–12.
27. **Roland, M. and Torgerson, D.J.** (1998). What are pragmatic trials? *British Medical Journal* **316**, 285.
28. **Campbell, M.K.** et al. (2000). Analysis of cluster randomized trials in primary care: a practical approach. *Family Practice* **17**, 192–6.
29. **Fairhurst, K. and Dowrick, C.** (1996). Problems with recruitment in a randomized controlled trial of counselling in general practice: causes and implications. *Journal of Health Services Research and Policy* **1**, 77–80.
30. **Rogers, S.** et al. (2000). Designing trials of interventions to change professional practice in primary care: lessons from an explanatory study of two change strategies. *British Medical Journal* **320**, 1580–3.
31. **Cartwright, A.** (1988). Interviews or postal questionnaires? Comparisons of data about women's experiences with maternity services. *The Milbank Quarterly* **66**, 172–89.
32. **Armstrong, B.K., White, E., and Saracci, R.** *Principles of Exposure Measurement in Epidemiology.* Oxford: Oxford University Press, 1994.
33. **Sibbald, B., Addington-Hall, J., Brenneman, D., and Freeling, P.** (1994). Telephone versus postal surveys of general practitioners: methodological considerations. *British Journal of General Practice* **44**, 297–300.
34. **Marcus, A. and Crane, L.** (1986). Telephone surveys in public health research. *Medical Care* **24**, 97–112.
35. **Mandel, A., Eaden, J., Mayberry, M., and Mayberry, J.** (2000). Questionnaire surveys in medical research. *Journal of Evaluation in Clinical Practice* **6**, 395–403.
36. **Templeton, L.** et al. (1997). Surveying general practitioners: does a low response rate matter? *British Journal of General Practice* **47**, 91–4.
37. **Dillman, D.A.** *Mail and Telephone Surveys: the Total Design Method.* New York: Wiley, 1978.
38. **Heberlein, T. and Baumgartener, R.** (1978). Factors affecting response rates to mailed questionnaires: a quantitative analysis of the published literature. *American Sociological Review* **43**, 447–62.
39. **Parsons, J., Warnecke., R.R.C., Barnsley, J., and Kaluzny, A.** (1994). Factors associated with response rates in a national survey of primary care physicians. *Evaluation Review* **18**, 756–65.
40. **Deehan, A.** et al. (1997). The effect of cash and other financial inducements on the response rate of general practitioners in a national postal study. *British Journal of General Practice* **47**, 87–90.
41. **Goyder, J.** (1982). Further evidence on factors affecting response rates to mailed questionnaires. *American Sociological Review* **47**, 550–3.
42. **Smith, W.** et al. (1995). Increasing response rates in telephone surveys: a randomised trial. *Journal of Public Health Medicine* **17**, 17–22.
43. **Pirotta, M., Gunn, J., Farish, S., and Karabatsos, G.** (1999). Primer postcard improves postal survey response rates. *Australian and New Zealand Journal of Public Health* **23**, 196–7.
44. **Ward, J. and Wain, G.** (1994). Increasing response rates of gynaecologists to a survey: a randomised controlled trial. *Australian Journal of Public Health* **18**, 332–4.
45. **McLaren, B. and Shelley, J.** (2000). Response rates of Victorian general practitioners to a mailed survey on miscarriage: randomised trial of a prize and two forms of introduction to the research. *Australian and New Zealand Journal of Public Health* **24**, 360–4.
46. **Bero, L.A., Grilli, R., Grimshaw, J., Harvey, E., Oxman, A.D., and Thomson, M.A.** (1998). Closing the gap between research and practice: an overview of systematic reviews of interventions to promote the implementation of research findings. *British Medical Journal* **317**, 465–8.
47. **NHS Centre for Reviews and Dissemination.** *Getting Evidence into Practice. Effective Health Care.* University of York, 1999.
48. **Foy, R., Eccles, M., and Grimshaw, J.** (2001). Why does primary care need more implementation research? *Family Practice* **18**, 353–5.
49. **Soumerai, S.B., McLaughlin, T.J., and Avorn, J.** (1989). Improving drug prescribing in primary care: a critical analysis of the experimental literature. *The Milbank Quarterly* **67**, 268–317.
50. **Cook, T.D. and Campbell, D.T.** *Quasi-Experimentation. Design and Analysis Issues for Field Settings.* Boston: Houghton Mifflin Company, 1979.
51. **Campbell, M.K.** et al., ed. (1999). *Changing Professional Practice. Theory and Practice of Clinical Guidelines Implementation.* Design and Statistical Issues in Implementation Research. Copenhagen: Danish Institute for Health Services Research and Development, 1999, pp. 57–76.
52. **Mason, J., Freemantle, N., and Young, P.** (1998). The effect of the distribution of Effective Health Care Bulletins on prescribing selective serotonin reuptake inhibitors in primary care. *Health Trends* **30**, 120–2.
53. **Medical Research Council.** *A Framework for Development and Evaluation of RCTs for Complex Interventions to Improve Health.* London, 2000.
54. **Grol, R.** (1997). Beliefs and evidence in changing clinical practice. *British Medical Journal* **315**, 418–21.
55. **Walker, A.E., Grimshaw, J.M., and Armstrong, E.M.** (2001). Salient beliefs and intentions to prescribe antibiotics for patients with a sore throat. *British Journal of Health Psychology* **6**, 347–60.
56. **Ferlie, E.B. and Shortell, S.M.** (2001). Improving the quality of health care in the United Kingdom and the United States: a framework for change. *The Milbank Quarterly* **79**, 281–315.
57. **Pawson, R. and Tilley, N.** *Realistic Evaluation.* London: Sage Publications, 1997.
58. **Grimshaw, J.M., Campbell, M.K., Eccles, M.P., and Steen, I.N.** (2000). Experimental and quasi-experimental designs for evaluating guideline implementation strategies. *Family Practice* **17** (Suppl.), S11–18.
59. **Sculpher, M.** (2000). Evaluating the cost-effectiveness of interventions designed to increase the utilization of evidence-based guidelines. *Family Practice* **17** (Suppl. 1), S26–31.

14.4 Primary care research networks

Eloy H. van de Lisdonk and David P. Weller

Introduction

Primary care research networks (PCRNs) have an important role to play in building research capacity and output in primary care. Networks have been established in North America for over 20 years, and have recently gained prominence in Europe and Australia. There is a widely perceived need to develop a stronger infrastructure for research in primary care, and PCRNs have played an important developmental role. Further, primary care has at times struggled to establish a strong culture of research and evidence-based practice, and proposals calling for the establishment of networks have highlighted their potential benefits in these areas.[1] Networks have the potential to promote interdisciplinary group participation, and facilitate transfer of knowledge and expertise between research groups and primary care providers.

Despite their recent growth, networks have a long history. Early examples of primary care practices participating in network activities involved in data collection were the 'peilstations', started in the Netherlands in 1967.[2] Morbidity data collection efforts such as these prompted further growth of research activities in primary care, and practice-based research networks developed around the world—particularly in North America, Europe, Australia, and New Zealand.[3–11]

Structure and organization of PCRNs

Networks vary considerably in their organizational structure, and the types of practitioners who participate. Membership may be fixed or flexible; that is participating practitioners may become involved on a long-term basis (e.g. in systematic and continuous data collection and monitoring), or their involvement may be restricted to specific research projects. Networks differ in number of participating practices, clinicians and patients—there is considerable variation between and within countries, depending on the core aims of the network.[12–14]

PCRNs have a broad range of funding arrangements and organizational contexts. For example, most PCRNs in the United States exist within professional independent organizations.[15] In the Netherlands, the converse is true; most PCRNs exist within academic departments (most within departments of family medicine), with relatively few in professional organizations.[13] In the United Kingdom, PCRNs mostly reflect regional activities of the NHS, in some places with connections to university departments.

The establishment of a PCRN is a complex process, and depends on the aims and proposed functions of the network. Table 1 summarizes a number of key organizational issues which networks must address.

Key functions of PCRNs

Establishing and maintaining databases of primary care information

Many PCRNs are principally involved in the collection of data, and the construction of databases available for disease surveillance and research. Primary care is a powerful source of data for such exercises, as it typically provides information which reflects underlying patterns in the general population. For example, the Sentinel Practice Research Network in Australia plays an important role in the ongoing surveillance of infectious and other diseases, and provides data on morbidity and health service utilization which is more representative of the general population than secondary care sources such as hospital statistics.[16] Information typically collected in primary care databases is summarized in Table 2.

While static variables (such as demographic information) need only be recorded once, recording of dynamic variables, necessary for monitoring factors such as morbidity and health service utilization over time, require continuous data-collection systems to be in place, and there is a growing number of such systems.[17] Continuous morbidity recording enables analysis of temporal trends in the population, response to health interventions, and cross-linkage with other databases.

For primary care databases to reach their full potential, standardized recording systems are required. A number of morbidity classification systems now exist—the ICPC (which includes an electronic version) is in widespread usage.[18]

Data held in primary care databases can be analysed at several levels:

- separate contacts between patient and care provider;
- the level of the patient and his/her family;
- the structural level of the practitioner and his/her practice;
- the level of a group of practices, a region, or district.

There are a number of important quality control issues relating to primary care databases, and these are summarized in Table 3.

Amongst the many important functions of primary care databases is feedback and audit for participating primary care providers. The feedback can comprise data on the health of their patients, some of which may reflect individual performance of practitioners. Written newsletters, meetings, and an annual report are traditional ways of providing such feedback. An indication that audit enhanced feedback stimulates motivation comes from France where unpaid clinicians participate in a sentinel network for the surveillance of communicable diseases; their motivations to continue were to share experiences and to self-evaluate by comparison with colleagues.[25] Further, audit can be an incentive to cooperate in a research network as is shown for example by various networks for diabetes care.[26–28]

Networking function

PCRNs have a key role in establishing relationships and building teams. Their success is dependent upon their ability to establish cooperation between groups and individuals from a very wide range of disciplines and backgrounds. Partnerships between service providers and those with academic and research skills are often seen as a positive way forward in primary care research, but require a great deal of investment in building

Table 1 Key organizational issues in establishing a PCRN

Setting goals	PCRNs have a range of potential functions—what will the key goals of the network be?
Responsibility and ownership of data and research outputs	Typically data and research outputs collected within a PCRN are the result of team efforts, involving individuals from a range of organizations and disciplines. It is important to establish 'ownership' of this resource, and responsibility for its use
Management and organizational structure	PCRNs are often complex organizations; there need to be clearly defined systems of management and governance
Infrastructure	The activities of PCRNs need to be supported by appropriate levels of administrative support and IT
Financial arrangements	In order for PCRNs to fulfil their potential they need to have a secure funding base. It is also critical that high-quality mechanisms for financial accountability are in place

Table 2 Information collected in primary care databases

Practice and practitioners	Location and type of practices; age, sex, and experience of the physicians; number of physicians, and number of patients or contacts per physician; type and number of other health care workers in the practice; services and facilities
Patient, his/her family	Demographic variables: date of birth, gender, country of origin, civil status, education, profession, socioeconomic status, ethnic background, address, insurance, family (of origin and actual family)
Health status	Present and previous health problems, disease risk factors, health care variables, family history, allergic status, vaccination status
Health service utilization	Date of entrance in practice, date of departure, number of visits to primary and secondary care services, nature of services, home visits, telephone contacts

Table 3 Important quality control issues in primary care databases

Completeness of the data	This can vary;[19] strategies for checking on completeness include comparison with national statistics and examination of temporal trends
Frequency and duration of data collection	Most networks request reporting on a daily basis. Some PCRNs just require a registration of a few contacts per day, others require a registration of all contacts, some during a certain number of days per year, others throughout the year
Representativeness	In general, larger networks have a greater prospect of providing data which are representative of the wider population of patients and providers. Networks vary in their representativeness; e.g., in the Nijmegen Family Practice Academic Network the network population reflects the composition of the Dutch population in age and social class, but, with eight out of 25 clinicians holding PhDs the clinicians are potentially unrepresentative, with a possible bias towards research[20]
Validity	Strict definitions of the variables used and the use of accepted classification systems enhance validity. Validity can be studied by comparing information in the database with external 'gold standards' if they exist (such as national cancer registries). Validity appears to vary widely; for chronic diseases acceptable validity has been demonstrated in a number of studies[21–23]
Reliability and uniformity	Standardized protocols with clear definitions help enhance reliability. It is suggested that smaller networks can perform better than greater networks as training to adhere to protocol is more feasible.[24] Interdoctor variation is a measure for reliability, however in daily practice a certain degree of interdoctor variation may be normal, probably even desired
Privacy and confidentiality	Patients in PCRNs must be able to give truly informed consent. As PCRNs often function as indices from which cohorts of patients with certain characteristics can be found, privacy enhancing technologies and procedures are needed. There must be a protocol about who has access to the data, how and under what conditions

relationships, establishing new forms of association, and developing new and innovative organization of practices.

Networks require a great deal of trust; the benefits and outputs of research networks must often be shared between many organizations and individuals, and this requires a great deal of clarity over issues such as ownership, territory, and intellectual property. Developing this trust and collaboration must be a central role of a PCRN. Without a sense of goodwill, collegiality, and common purpose a network will not reach its potential and may, indeed, have a negative impact on research capacity and output.

PCRNs have a range of strategies available to them to fulfil this networking function. It requires constant effort from management staff, and needs to make use of all available information-sharing strategies, including regular meetings, newsletters, and IT-based strategies.

Research

There is no 'typical' form of study conducted by a PCRN. Some networks focus, for example, on patient-oriented research (observational, epidemiological, intervention studies), others on health services research (disease management and shared care projects, quality of care, workload, and provision of care).

Observational studies conducted within PCRNs can provide important insights into the nature and practice of primary care. Information can be generated on:

- incidence and prevalence figures of conditions seen in primary care, their natural course and prognosis;
- diagnostic and therapeutic activities;
- satisfaction of professionals and patients;
- health status of patients, and whether these elements are related to each other.

Examples include observational studies on headache, spontaneous abortion, chest pain, otitis media, human immuno-deficiency virus, cough, and carpal tunnel syndrome from ambulatory sentinel practice network (ASPN);[29] studies on childhood morbidity, hypertension, diabetes mellitus, asthma, and depression from the Nijmegen Family Practice Academic Network;[29] the incidence of diabetes in the Netherlands;[30] studies on the quality of care, for example regarding terminally ill persons, diabetes mellitus, and patients in elderly and nursing homes.[5,28,31]

The feasibility, efficiency and effectiveness of preventive, diagnostic, and therapeutic interventions can be examined in PCRN-based research; for example, studies on screening for breast cancer and cholesterol from the Wisconsin Research Network,[32,33] and screening for microalbuminuria in diabetic patients from the Nijmegen Family Practice Academic Network.[34,35] PCRNs can provide important contributions to randomized (controlled) intervention studies as demonstrated in a recent study on aspirin and cardiovascular risk.[36]

Because of the size and nature of PCRNs they have opened up possibilities for enhancing experience in a range of scientific theories, methodologies and analytical techniques. Some examples include:

- Incorporating existing theories from other disciplines such as social theory, network theory, and participatory action research.[37]
- Multilevel analysis techniques, needed for example to estimate the effects of intervention on the level of the practice or the family physician while outcome is measured at the level of the patients. Also, when unit of intervention, measurement, and analysis are not the same and not independent from each other.
- Using information and communication technologies, within the practice or between practices by linking databases.[38,39]

Advantages and disadvantages of PCRNs

With the recent growth of PCRNs, particularly in Europe and Australia, there is now interest in establishing whether networks have made a difference in promoting primary care research. The concept of research networks is appealing; they should be able to achieve economies of scale and enhance output by bringing many dispersed primary care researchers and providers together. They should allow novice researchers to gain access to expertise, and more experienced researchers to access primary care populations. Information collected through PCRNs is potentially of a higher standard than single-institution research; PCRNs are able to define their population at risk, with clearly defined denominators,[40] and many different aspects of co-morbidity can be studied through a broad-based case-mix including many co-morbid diseases.[41,42] Further, they should facilitate the development of research capacity in primary care, and promote research practices, higher degrees, and academic training schemes.

Nevertheless, PCRNs are a long-term, substantial investment which must be weighed up against other strategies for promoting primary care R&D (such as new academic posts and dedicated research funding programmes).[43] They involve considerable cost, time and effort, depending on size and complexity of the network. Strategies for promoting the socialization, openness, teamwork, and development of trust are sometimes difficult to identify; yet they are critical for the successful development of a PCRN.[44] Bringing together multidisciplinary groups, which might include academics, independent practitioners, and social scientists is a complex task, and there are no clear guidelines for PCRN managers. Promoting a sense of ownership amongst people collecting data, and engagement in the aims of the network amongst members are significant challenges.

There are other practical difficulties. PCRNs often involve the recruitment of many small practices, and this can be a significant organizational hurdle. The issues of data protection, ethics, and research governance in PCRN-based organizations are no less relevant than in more 'traditional' modes of research. Yet these concepts must be implemented in a very wide range of organizational settings.

In meeting these challenges, many networks are recognizing the importance of national organizations (e.g. the UK Federation of Primary Care Research Networks). Such organizations can improve discussion and collaboration between PCRNs, and provide opportunities to share strategies for successful networking, training, research, and development.

Evaluation of PCRNs needs to take into account the complex range of tasks of these organizations.[45] While readily measurable outputs such as grants obtained, papers produced, and educational events organized are important, future evaluation efforts will need to take into account these more complex functions if a clear idea of the success of PCRNs is to emerge. Measures which can take into account the degree of shared identification, trust with information and ideas, levels of cooperation, examples of reciprocity, extent to which the PCRN is developing and learning (as opposed to individual members making use of it then moving on) have been suggested.[46] Further, evaluation should be tailored to the objectives of individual PCRNs.

Summary

PCRNs show considerable promise in developing the infrastructure of primary care research and enhancing research capacity. They have undergone considerable growth in recent years, and a number of roles, functions, and organizational structures have emerged.

While PCRNs have many potential advantages, they involve a considerable investment of health resources, and their progress needs to be monitored closely. It is still not known whether PCRNs enhance research activity or promote evidence-based health care, although in theory they have great potential to do so. Evaluation of PCRNs should take into account the range and complexity of tasks faced by these organizations.

References

1. **Mant, D.** *Research and Development in Primary Care: National Working Group Report.* Bristol: NHS Executive South and West, 1997.
2. **Bruins, C.P. and Oeberius Kapteijn, J.C.** (1974). Vier jaar continue morbiditeitsregistratie in de huisartspraktijk door middel van peilstations (Four years continuous morbidity registration in general practice by means of sentinel practices). *Huisarts en Wetenschap* **17**, 407–13.
3. **Green, L.A.** et al. (1984). The ambulatory sentinel practice network: purpose, methods, and policies. *Journal of Family Practice* **18**, 275–80.
4. **Palombi, L.** et al. (1992). A new community-oriented network in Italy for the collection and processing of clinical and epidemiological information. *Journal of Clinical Computation* **20**, 166–75.
5. **Busse, R.** et al. (1998). Sentinel practices in evaluating longer periods of care: quality of life and drug therapy of terminally ill persons in Lower Saxony. *Journal of Epidemiology and Community Health* **52** (Suppl. 1), 56S–60S.
6. **Vega Alonso, A.T., Gill Costa, M., and Ruiz Cosin, C.** (1996). Demand and HIV testing prescriptions in primary care. Registry of the network of sentinel physicians from Castilla y Leon in 1991, 1992, and 1993. *Gac Sanit* **10**, 25–33 (in Spanish).
7. **Maurice, S., Salamon, R., and Dabis, F.** (1989). Telematics and sentinel health information system with general practitioners in Aquitaine, southwest France. *Medical Informatics* **14**, 281–6.
8. **Barrier, J.H., Billaud, E., and Magadur, G.** (1992). Retrospective prevalences and frequencies of Horton's disease and rhizomelic psuedopolyarthritis. Epidemiological study in the Loire-Atlantic department using a general practice research network. *La Revue de Medecine Interne* **13**, 393–6.
9. **Falcão, I.M.** et al. (1998). Programme for the surveillance of influenza in Portugal: results of the period 1990–1996. *Journal of Epidemiology and Community Health* **52** (Suppl. 1), 39S–42S.
10. **Anonymous** (2000). Netting an important database. *Lancet* **357**, 649.
11. **Laurence, C.O.** et al. (2001). Establishing a practice based primary care research network. The University Family Practice Network in South Australia. *Australian Family Physician* **30**, 508–12.
12. **Niebauer, L. and Nutting, P.A.** (1994). Primary care practice-based research networks active in North America. *Journal of Family Practice* **38**, 425–6.
13. **Hart, H.E.** et al. *Huisartsgeneeskundige Registraties in Nederland.* Rotterdam: Instituut Huisartsgeneeskunde, 1996 (in Dutch).
14. www.gprd.com.
15. **Nutting, P.A.** (1996). Practice-based research networks: building the infrastructure of primary care research. *Journal of Family Practice* **42**, 199–203.
16. **Roche, P.** et al. (2001). Annual report of the National Influenza Surveillance Scheme, 2000. *Communicable Diseases Intelligence* **25**, 107–12.
17. **O'Mahony, B.** et al. (2001). Morbidity data collection in general practice: experience in the South Eastern Health Board 1998–1999. *Irish Medical Journal* **94**, 299–302.
18. **Okkes, I.** et al. (2000). ICPC-2-E: the electronic version of ICPC-2. Differences from the printed version and the consequences. *Family Practice* **17**, 101–7.
19. **Pearson, N.** et al. (1996). Collecting morbidity data in general practice: the Somerset morbidity project. *British Medical Journal* **312**, 1517–20.
20. **Van Weel, C., Smith, H., and Beasly, J.W.** (2000) Family practice research networks. Experience from three countries. *Journal of Family Practice* **49**, 938–43.
21. **Schellevis, F.G.** et al. (1993). Validity of diagnoses of chronic diseases in general practice. *Journal of Clinical Epidemiology* **46**, 461–8.
22. **Patchett, P. and Roberts, D.** (1994). Diabetic patients who do not have diabetes: investigation of register of diabetic patients in general practice. *British Medical Journal* **308**, 1225–6.
23. **Van Weel, C.** (1995). Validating long term morbidity recording. *Journal of Epidemiology and Community Health* **49**, 29–32.
24. **Slawson, D.C., Herman, J.M., and Bennett, J.H.** (1993). Single community research networks. The HARNET experience. Harrisburg Area Research Network. *Archives of Family Medicine* **2**, 725–8.
25. **Chauvin, P. and Valleron, A.J.** (1998). Participation of French general practitioners in public health surveillance: a multidisciplinary approach. *Journal of Epidemiology and Community Health* **52** (Suppl. 1), 2S–8S.
26. **Turnbridge, F.K.E.** et al. (1993). Diabetes care in general practice: an approach to audit of process and outcome. *British Journal of General Practice* **43**, 291–5.
27. **Dunn, N.R. and Bough, P.** (1996). Standards of care of diabetic patients in a typical English community. *British Journal of General Practice* **46**, 401–5.
28. **Khunti, K.** et al. (1999). Quality of care of patients with diabetes: collation of data from multi-practice audits of diabetes in primary care. *Family Practice* **16**, 54–9.
29. **Green, L.A., Hames, C.G., and Nutting, P.A.** (1994). Potential of practice-based research networks: experiences from ASPN. *Journal of Family Practice* **38**, 400–6.
30. **Ruwaard, D.** et al. (1996). Is the incidence of diabetes increasing in all age-groups in The Netherlands? Results of the second study in the Dutch Sentinel Practice Network. *Diabetes Care* **19**, 214–18.
31. **Devroey, D., Van Casteren, V., and De Lepeleire, J.** (2001). Revealing regional differences in the institutionalisation of adult patients in homes for the elderly and nursing homes: results of the Belgian network of sentinel GPs. *Family Practice* **18**, 39–41
32. **Love, R.R.** et al. (1993). Frequency and determinants of screening for breast cancer in primary care group practice. *Archives of Internal Medicine* **153**, 2112–17.
33. **McBride, P.** et al. (1998). Primary care practice adherence to national cholesterol program (NCEP) guidelines for patients with coronary heart disease: the HEART project. *Archives of Internal Medicine* **158**, 1238–44.

34. **De Grauw, W.J.C.** et al. (1995). Screening for microalbuminuria in type 2 diabetic patients: the evaluation of a dipstick test in general practice. *Diabetic Medicine* **12**, 657–63.

35. **De Grauw, W.J.C.** et al. (2001). Microalbuminuria in patients with type 2 diabetes mellitus from general practice: course and predictive value. *Diabetic Medicine* **18**, 1–5.

36. **Collaborative Group on the Primary Prevention Project** (2001). Low-dose aspirin and vitamin E in people at cardiovascular risk: a randomised trial in general practice. *Lancet* **357**, 89–95.

37. **Thomas, P.** et al. (2000). Primary care groups and research networks: opportunities for R&D in context. *British Journal of General Practice* **50**, 91–2.

38. **Mettee, T.M., Martin, K.B., and Williams, R.L.** (1998). Tools for community-oriented primary care: a process for linking practice and community data. *Journal of the American Board of Family Practice* **11**, 28–33.

39. **Glasgow, R.E.** et al. (1999). Interactive computer technology, behavioral science, and family practice. *Journal of Family Practice* **48**, 464–70.

40. **Schlaud, M.** et al. (1998). Approaches to the denominator in practice-based epidemiology: a critical overview. *Journal of Epidemiology and Community Health* **52** (Suppl. 1), 13S–19S.

41. **Schellevis, F.G.** et al. (1993). Comorbidity of chronic diseases in general practice. *Journal of Clinical Epidemiology* **46** (5), 469–73.

42. **Van den Akker, M.** et al. (1998). Multimorbidity in general practice: prevalence, incidence, and determinants of co-occuring chronic and recurrent diseases. *Journal of Clinical Epidemiology* **51**, 367–75.

43. **Carter, Y.H., Shaw, S., and Sibbald, B.** (2000). Primary care research networks: an evolving model meriting national evaluation. *British Journal of General Practice* **50**, 859–60.

44. **Fenton, E.** et al. (2001). Reflections from organisation science on the development of primary health care research networks. *Family Practice* **18**, 540–4.

45. **Clement, S.** et al. (2000). Towards a conceptual framework for evaluating primary care research networks. *British Journal of General Practice* **50**, 651–2.

46. **Griffiths, F.** et al. (2000). The productivity of primary care research networks. *British Journal of General Practice* **50**, 913–15.

14.5 Secondary research

Tim Lancaster

Evidence-based practice

The practice of medicine is increasingly driven by research findings, but the quantity of primary research makes it difficult for individual clinicians to keep up, even in specialized fields. The problems in maintaining an evidence-based approach are that much greater in primary care. There is therefore a need for reliable summaries of the evidence to guide clinical practice. The past 15 years have seen an increasingly explicit recognition of the scientific inadequacy of many of the available sources, including textbooks and review articles.(1) A number of studies showed that such summaries were prone to bias and inaccuracy. For example, Lau et al.(2) and Antman et al.(3) used systematic methods to identify and summarize evidence about the value of treatments for myocardial infarction. Using the technique of cumulative meta-analysis, in which each new study alters the summary estimate of effectiveness, they showed that textbooks and review articles had been failing to recommend treatments of proven value for myocardial infarction (most notably thrombolysis) many years after research had shown their benefit. On the other hand, treatments of no value (e.g. prophylactic treatment of arrhythmias) continued to be recommended when there was strong evidence that they were ineffective. They concluded that a more systematic approach to the summarization of clinical research could have saved thousands of lives.

Among a number of initiatives to apply scientific principles to research synthesis, perhaps the most important was the formation of the Cochrane Collaboration in 1992. The aim of this international collaborative effort is to facilitate the preparation, maintenance and dissemination of systematic reviews in all fields of health care.(4,5) In the first decade of its existence, The Cochrane Library has developed into an important source of information on the effects of health care interventions in almost all fields of medicine. Systematic reviews, including Cochrane reviews, increasingly form the evidence base for other tools for evidence-based practice, such as practice guidelines.(6,7)

Although areas of uncertainty and controversy still exist, a number of principles for the better conduct of reviews are now accepted.(8,9) A central aim of the methodology is to minimize the risk of bias in identification and interpretation of data. Reviews conducted according to such methodology are known as systematic reviews, or overviews. Meta-analysis, which may or may not be part of a systematic review, refers to the quantitative synthesis of different studies using statistical techniques. A particular advantage of meta-analysis is that, by increasing the sample size, it can increase the power of existing research to determine the presence or absence of moderate, but clinically significant effects. The techniques of meta-analysis are most well accepted as a method of combining data from randomized trials of medical treatment. They are, however, increasingly applied to observational data, for example, in studies of aetiology, prognosis, and diagnosis.(10)

What are the characteristics of a good systematic review?

Like any scientific inquiry, reviews should set out to answer a question. A review that sets out to give a narrative account of a disease, or even a whole speciality ('dermatology update') is less likely to provide clinically useful information than one whose aim is to address a clearly focused objective, or hypothesis. Most questions in medical research can be articulated in four parts.(11)

1. a patient or problem;
2. an intervention or exposure;
3. the clinical outcomes of interest;
4. a comparison intervention or exposure, when relevant.

For example, a general practitioner might wonder whether she should prescribe bupropion, a drug marketed for smoking cessation, to her patients. In order to judge for whom and when she might use it, she will need to think about the clinical situation in which she is working. For example, the practice may already offer counselling and an offer of nicotine replacement therapy to patients wishing to give up smoking. If so, she might not be particularly interested in the question of whether bupropion is more effective than a placebo tablet. Instead, the question might look more like: in patients who smoke cigarettes (problem), does bupropion (intervention) lead to greater abstinence from cigarettes (outcome) than nicotine replacement and counselling (comparison)? Those conducting systematic reviews should aim to frame the same focused questions that clinicians need to ask themselves.

As with primary research, reviews should include a clear statement of the methods of the study. In order to judge whether the results are valid, we want to know the risk that they may have been affected by bias. To judge whether the results are applicable to our own setting, we want to know about the nature of the intervention, the kinds of people who participated and the way in which outcome was assessed. Review articles should describe both the types of study design to be considered in the review (methodological criteria) and content criteria—a description of the types of participants, interventions, and outcomes to be considered. The practical value of the review will depend on using good judgement at this stage.

The problem of bias

In primary studies, bias can be introduced by failure to consider all the available data. For example, excluding patients lost to follow-up could introduce bias, particularly if the reason for loss to follow-up is related to the treatment. The same bias can occur in reviews when there is a failure to identify all the available studies. Historically, very few review articles included a statement of how studies were identified and included.[1] Such an approach may lead to biased conclusions: authors may selectively cite studies that support their own views, or have been previously prominently cited. For example, Ravnskov showed that studies of the effect of cholesterol lowering on heart disease were far more likely to be cited in reviews if they had positive results than if the results were negative.[12] Other biases in selecting research may result from exclusion of studies in journals that are not easily accessible, especially when they are not published in English. Selective publication represents another threat to the validity of research synthesis.[11] Dickersin et al. showed that clinical trials yielding positive results were more likely to be published than those with negative results—apparently because negative studies were less likely to be written up and submitted for publication.[13] The suppression of negative studies, poses a significant threat to the validity of the conclusions of research synthesis.

How can such bias be reduced? All reviews should include a clear description of the strategy used to identify studies. Although there may be practical difficulties in tracking down every relevant study, this strategy should be as comprehensive as possible. At a minimum, it should include a search of relevant electronic databases stating the search terms used. However, it is important to be aware of the limitations of electronic databases. For example, the most widely used medical database, Medline, indexes only a proportion of the available biomedical literature, and important journals may be missed altogether if this is the sole source. Even when journals are available on Medline, it is easy to miss relevant studies, usually because of the way they were indexed as they entered the database.[14]

Other methods for identifying studies can supplement an electronic search strategy. These include searching reference lists of papers identified by electronic searching, hand-searching specialist journals, and consulting experts in the field. Valuable information may also be found in 'grey literature', for example, as abstracts in conference proceedings, or unpublished theses. The issue of whether to include unpublished data is controversial. Concern over publication bias has to be weighed against the difficulties in ensuring the quality of unpublished data. Prospective registration of trials in progress may ultimately provide a solution to this difficult problem.[15]

Resources may not be available to use all of the available methods. The most important principle is that there is a description of what was done, so that the reader can judge how reliable the search is likely to have been. Figure 1 shows an example of the search strategy used for a Cochrane review of nicotine replacement therapy for smoking cessation.[16]

Having identified the population of studies that will form the data of the review, the next step is to reduce bias in data extraction. Standardized data extraction forms, and systems for entering data and checking for errors are as important in preparing systematic reviews as they are in primary research. Individuals reading papers may make transcriptional or interpretative errors in reading papers. Chalmers et al. suggested that data extraction should be blinded, and occur in duplicate.[17] They suggested a system of differential photocopying. In this method, the methods and results sections of the papers under review are separately copied, and examined by different reviewers. Those assessing the methods are blind to the results, and vice versa. Both are blind to the names and affiliations of the authors.

- A computerized literature search on 7 electronic databases (Medline, Cancerlit, Psych Abstracts, Dissertation Abstracts, Health Planning & Administration, Social Scisearch, and Smoking & Health), using the terms (1) Smoking and (2) Smoking cessation in combination with Randomized Controlled trial or Prospective or Random allocation or Double-blind method
- Scrutiny of published reviews, reference lists from clinical trials, conference abstracts (from primary-care meetings and the World Conferences on Tobacco and Health), smoking and health bulletins, and the bibliography on smoking and health
- Hand-searching of two specialist journals
- Correspondence with pharmaceutical companies to identify unpublished studies

Fig. 1 Methods for searching for randomized trials in smoking cessation.

Although this level of rigour is not always feasible, systematic reviews should at a minimum include some form of double data extraction. Ideally, the results of the review should include a description (and statistical test) of the degree of agreement between the different reviewers.

In the majority of published meta-analyses, tabulated data is extracted from published reports for pooling. A few, however, have attempted to collect individual patient data through cooperation with the investigators on the original studies.[18] Stewart and Parmar studied trials of chemotherapy for ovarian cancer.[19] They showed that meta-analyses based on published data over-estimated the effects of treatment in comparison to an analysis based on individual patient data from the same studies. Publication bias, patient exclusion, length of follow-up, and method of analysis all contributed to this observed difference. They recommended meta-analysis of updated individual patient data as the least biased method of addressing questions not resolved by individual clinical trials. This is a resource-intensive approach, which may nevertheless be justified if it leads to more appropriate treatment for common or serious health care problems.[20]

Data quality

The quality of the underlying data is a central concern in interpreting the results of systematic reviews. An assessment of the validity of the studies included in a review has been recommended as an essential step in the review process.[1] It has, however, proved more difficult to determine which aspects of quality are most important. A number of quality scores for clinical trials have been proposed.[21,22] However, empirical evidence suggests that aggregated scores are less helpful than examining specific elements of methodological quality. For example, Schulz et al. showed that trials that did not contain an adequate description of allocation concealment systematically overestimated the effects of treatment in comparison to those that did report an adequate method.[23] Blinding of outcome assessment and methods for dealing with loss of patients to follow-up are other components of quality that appear to be particularly important.[24]

It is therefore unclear how differences in quality should affect the conclusions of a review. The options are to exclude studies that do not meet quality criteria, to weight the statistical analyses by a quality score,[25] or to perform a 'sensitivity analysis'. Sensitivity analysis assesses whether the results of meta-analysis change significantly when studies of different quality are excluded.

Synthesis of results

Having identified data from the individual studies that are the subject of a review, it is important to have some method for synthesizing the results and arriving at an overall conclusion. In traditional review articles, this process is rarely quantitative, and often apparently intuitive. There are a number of problems with such an approach. First, because it is not explicit, its reproducibility is difficult to determine. It is reasonable for individual reviewers to come to different conclusions about the same set of evidence, but quite unreasonable for the consumer of the review to have no idea how those judgements were reached. A common error is to use a semi-quantitative 'vote counting' approach in which the reviewer compares the number of 'positive' studies with the number of 'negative' studies.[26] With such an approach, a study may be counted as 'positive' in one review and 'negative' in another, depending on how the results are interpreted by the reviewers. There is also a tendency to overlook small but clinically important effects when counting votes, particularly when counting studies with statistically 'non-significant' results as 'negative', and to give equal weight to studies of different size and quality.

Increasingly, therefore, systematic reviews include statistical methods to analyse and summarize data (meta-analysis). By increasing the sample size, meta-analysis can be particularly useful in detecting moderate, but clinically important, differences between groups not detected by individual studies because of inadequate sample size. For example, investigators who had run clinical trials of warfarin to prevent stroke in non-rheumatic atrial fibrillation, performed a collaborative meta-analysis of their data.[27] Although each of the trials was consistent in showing a reduction in risk of stroke with warfarin, individual trials were too small to determine whether treatment efficacy varied by clinical or demographic characteristics. By combining their data, they were able to answer a number of important questions. For example, they showed that the benefits of treatment were seen equally in women and men and in patients with and without diabetes and hypertension. They were also able to identify a set of clinical characteristics that identified a very low risk of stroke.

A frequent complaint about meta-analyses is that they combine 'apples and oranges'. Most studies differ from each other in one or more ways, whether in the nature of the intervention, the population studied, or the outcomes measured. Deciding whether it makes sense to combine them requires judgement. For example, in reviewing the effectiveness of different forms of nicotine replacement, we had to decide whether it made sense to produce a single summary estimates for the different forms available (gum, transdermal patch, inhaler, nasal spray, lozenge). Our solution was to produce both overall estimates, and separate estimates by form: the direction of effect was in fact consistent across the different products.

There are a number of available statistical methods for obtaining a combined estimate of effect for both dichotomous and continuous variables. Usually, the summary estimate is weighted by the inverse of the variance. In other words, larger studies usually contribute more to the summary estimate than smaller studies. The most commonly used are the so-called 'fixed effect' and 'random effects' models. The fixed effect model assumed that the true effect of treatment is the same in each study and differences between study results arise by chance alone. The random effects model includes in the calculation an estimate of between study variation.

Meta-analytic methods typically produce a measure of effect with associated confidence intervals, although there is debate about which summary measure is most informative. For dichotomous outcomes, there are mathematical arguments for using the odds ratio, though some statisticians argue that the risk ratio is a more appropriate measure of the relative effect of treatment.[28] In reporting research there is a strong argument for the clinical applicability of measures based on differences in absolute risk (risk difference and numbers needed to treat), but there are particular difficulties in calculating these in meta-analyses. This is due largely to the widely varying levels of risk in the populations contributing to the meta-analysis. In trials of smoking cessation, for example, the likelihood of quitting without treatment varies from less than 1 per cent to up to 50 per cent, tending to be much lower in primary care populations than in smoking cessation clinics where patients are selected by motivation to quit. Though the relative effects of treatment appear to be constant across these different populations, the absolute effects vary greatly depending on the baseline risk. A relative doubling in quit rates would thus give a risk difference of 1 per cent (NNT 100) with a baseline quit rate of 1 per cent, and a risk difference of 40 per cent (NNT 2.5) with a 40 per cent baseline. Applying the relative effects reported in systematic reviews to the absolute risk level of an individual patient is a better approach to clinical application.

Heterogeneity

A related analytic issue is heterogeneity. Heterogeneity refers to differences in results that are greater than can be explained by the play of chance. If differences are not due to chance, then there must be some true difference between the studies. This may reflect differences in quality—that is, studies are measuring the same underlying effect, but some are more reliable than others. It may also reflect true differences between the studies, either in the nature of the intervention, the participants, or the way the outcomes were measured. Although there are formal statistical tests for heterogeneity, significant heterogeneity is often obvious from examining visual plots of the results of the different studies. If results are going in opposite directions, with little or no overlap of the confidence intervals around the point estimate, heterogeneity is probably present.

There is uncertainty about how best to deal with heterogeneity when it is detected. One suggested approach is to discard the fixed effects model, which assumes no heterogeneity, and calculate the summary statistic using the random effects model.[29] This usually leads to wider confidence intervals around the summary estimate. A more conservative approach is simply to abandon any attempt at calculating a summary estimate in the presence of significant heterogeneity, and rely on a narrative synthesis.

Others argue that heterogeneity should be explored, since it may indicate important clinical differences between studies that can yield useful insights.[30] The objection to this approach is that interpretation is 'post hoc' (inspired by looking at the data). Such interpretation is therefore prone to the problems inherent in retrospective sub-group analysis.[31] If this approach is adopted, it should therefore probably be considered 'hypothesis generating' rather than 'hypothesis testing'.[26]

Since publication bias is such an important threat to the validity of meta-analysis, it may be appropriate to explore possible bias in the analysis. One method is to do a calculation of the number of unpublished studies that would need to exist in the 'file drawer' to overturn the conclusions of the review. If this number is large, it increases our confidence in those conclusions. Another method is to plot the observed effect sizes of the individual sizes against their sample size. This should produce a plot resembling an inverted funnel, with individual studies scattering in a roughly symmetrical fashion around the true underlying value. Gaps in the funnel plot may indicate missing unpublished studies.[32]

Conclusions

The face validity of a systematic approach to research synthesis is now widely accepted. It remains important that the extra investment involved in this approach pays dividends in terms of better quality information about the effects of health care. In the absence of a gold standard, it is difficult to be certain that the conclusions of systematic reviews and meta-analysis are closer to the 'truth'. Perhaps the closest we have to a gold standard is the 'mega-trial', in which the findings of meta-analysis can be compared to the results of studies enrolling many patients according to a single protocol. There is increasing evidence that meta-analysis can yield similar results to 'mega-trials'. The most prominent example of this was the use of thrombolytic therapy for myocardial infarction where a large trial found similar reductions in mortality to those suggested by meta-analysis.[33] However, there have also been a number of examples where meta-analysis and mega-trials have given conflicting results.[9] The use of systematic methods can help to resolve uncertainties in health care, but, like all science, the findings of systematic reviews and meta-analysis are provisional and contingent on new evidence.

References

1. **Mulrow, C.D.** (1987). The medical review article: state of the science. *Annals of Internal Medicine* **106**, 485–8.
2. **Lau, J.** et al. (1992). Cumulative meta-analysis of therapeutic trials for myocardial infarction. *New England Journal of Medicine* **327**, 248–54.
3. **Antman, E.M.** et al. (1992). A comparison of results of meta-analyses of randomized control trials and recommendations of clinical experts. Treatments for myocardial infarction. *Journal of the American Medical Association* **268**, 240–8.
4. **Chalmers, I. and Haynes, B.** (1994). Reporting, updating, and correcting systematic reviews of the effects of health care. *British Medical Journal* **309**, 862–5.

5. **Chalmers, I., Dickersin, K., and Chalmers, T.C.** (1992). Getting to grips with Archie Cochrane's agenda. *British Medical Journal* **305**, 786–8 (editorial).
6. **Silagy, C.A., Lancaster, T., and Stead, L.** (2001). Use of systematic reviews for guideline development: a case study in smoking cessation. *British Medical Journal* **323**, 833–6.
7. **Eccles, M., Freemantle, N., and Mason, J.** (2001). Using systematic reviews in clinical guideline development. In *Systematic Reviews in Health Care Meta-Analysis in Context* (ed. M. Egger, G.D. Smith, and D.G. Altman), pp. 400–9. London: BMJ Publishing Group.
8. **Egger, M., Smith, G.D., and O'Rourke, K.** (2001). Rationale, potentials, and promise of systematic reviews. In *Systematic Reviews in Health Care Meta-Analysis in Context* (ed. M. Egger, G.D. Smith, and D.G. Altman), pp. 3–19. London: BMJ Publishing Group.
9. **Egger, M., Dickersin, K., and Smith, G.D.** (2001). Problems and limitations in conducting systematic reviews. In *Systematic Reviews in Health Care Meta-Analysis in Context* (ed. M. Egger, G.D. Smith, and D.G. Altman), pp. 43–68. London: BMJ Publishing Group.
10. **Egger, M., Smith, G.D., and Schneider, M.** (2001). Systematic reviews of observational studies. In *Systematic Reviews in Health Care Meta-Analysis in Context* (ed. M. Egger, G.D. Smith, and D.G. Altman), pp. 211–27. London: BMJ Publishing Group.
11. **Richardson, W.S.** et al. (1995). The well-built clinical question: a key to evidence-based decisions. *ACP Journal Club* **123**, A-12.
12. **Ravnskov, U.** (1992). Cholesterol lowering trials in coronary heart disease: frequency of citation and outcome (published erratum appears in BMJ 1992 August 29; **305** (6852): 505). *British Medical Journal* **305**, 15–19.
13. **Dickersin, K.** et al. (1987). Publication bias and clinical trials. *Controlled Clinical Trials* **8**, 343–53.
14. **Dickersin, K., Scherer, R., and Lefebvre, C.** (1994). Identifying relevant studies for systematic reviews. *British Medical Journal* **309**, 1286–91.
15. **Dickersin, K.** (1992). Why register clinical trials? *Controlled Clinical Trials* **13**, 170–7.
16. **Silagy, C.** et al. (2002). Nicotine replacement therapy for smoking cessation (Cochrane review). *Cochrane Library* Issue 1. Oxford: Update Software.
17. **Chalmers, T.C.** et al. (1987). Meta-analysis of clinical trials as a scientific discipline. I: Control of bias and comparison with large co-operative trials. *Statistics in Medicine* **6**, 315–28.
18. **Antiplatelet Trialists' Collaboration** (1994). Collaborative overview of randomised trials of antiplatelet therapy. I: Prevention of death, myocardial infarction, and stroke by prolonged antiplatelet therapy in various categories of patients. *British Medical Journal* **308**, 81–106.
19. **Stewart, L.A. and Parmar, M.K.** (1993). Meta-analysis of the literature or of individual patient data: is there a difference? *Lancet* **341**, 418–22.
20. **Clarke, M.J., and Stewart, L.A.** (2001) Obtaining individual patient data from randomised controlled trials. In *Systematic Reviews in Health Care Meta-Analysis in Context* (ed. M. Egger, G.D. Smith, and D.G. Altman), pp. 109–21. London: BMJ Publishing Group.
21. **Emerson, J.D.** et al. (1990). An empirical study of the possible relation of treatment differences to quality scores in controlled randomized clinical trials. *Controlled Clinical Trials* **11**, 339–52.
22. **Chalmers, T.C.** et al. (1981). A method for assessing the quality of a randomized control trial. *Controlled Clinical Trials* **2**, 31–49.
23. **Schulz, K.F.** et al. (1995). Empirical evidence of bias. Dimensions of methodological quality associated with estimates of treatment effects in controlled trials. *Journal of the American Medical Association* **273**, 408–12.
24. **Juni, P., Altman, D.G., and Egger, M.** (2001). Assessing the quality of randomised controlled trials. In *Systematic Reviews in Health Care Meta-Analysis in Context* (ed. M. Egger, G.D. Smith, and D.G. Altman), pp. 87–108. London: BMJ Publishing Group.
25. **Detsky, A.S.** et al. (1992). Incorporating variations in the quality of individual randomized trials into meta-analysis. *Journal of Clinical Epidemiology* **45**, 255–65.
26. **Oxman, A.D.** (1993). Meta-statistics: help or hindrance? *ACP Journal Club* **118**, A-13.
27. **Atrial Fibrillation Investigators** (1994). Risk factors for stroke and efficacy of antithrombotic therapy in atrial fibrillation. Analysis of pooled data from five randomized controlled trials (published erratum appears in Arch Intern Med 1994 Oct 10; 154 (19): 2254). *Archives of Internal Medicine* **154**, 1449–57.
28. **Deeks, J. and Altman, D.G.** (2001). Effect measures for meta-analysis of trials with binary outcomes. In *Systematic Reviews in Health Care Meta-Analysis in Context* (ed. M. Egger, G.D. Smith, and D.G. Altman), pp. 313–35. London: BMJ Publishing Group.
29. **DerSimonian, R. and Laird, N.** (1986). Meta-analysis in clinical trials. *Controlled Clinical Trials* **7**, 177–88.
30. **Thompson, S.G.** (1994). Why sources of heterogeneity in meta-analysis should be investigated. *British Medical Journal* **309**, 1351–5.
31. **Oxman, A.D. and Guyatt, G.H.** (1992). A consumer's guide to subgroup analyses. *Annals of Internal Medicine* **116**, 78–84.
32. **Egger, M. and Smith, G.D.** (1995). Misleading meta-analysis. *British Medical Journal* **310**, 752–4 (editorial).
33. **ISIS-2 (Second International Study of Infarct Survival) Collaborative Group** (1988). Randomised trial of intravenous streptokinase, oral aspirin, both, or neither among 17 187 cases of suspected acute myocardial infarction: ISIS-2. *Lancet* **2**, 349–60.

14.6 Outcomes

Mark Harris

Introduction

There has been considerable attention, in primary care research, to the process and delivery of care. Issues such as access to care, continuity, quality, and coordination of care between providers have been the subject of much research and debate. However, these are not ends in themselves. They are ways of achieving individual and population health goals and at some point need to be evaluated in terms of the health outcomes they produce. Where possible decisions about which interventions or strategies should be supported in primary care should be based on the evidence of outcomes, rather than plausibility or anticipated effects.[1]

We need to be very careful about accepting interventions based on their impact on process of care measures. While measures of quality of primary care may be considered to be important, they do not necessarily result in improved health outcomes. For example, in one study specialist liaison nurses sought to improve communication between hospital and general practice and to ensure structured follow up of patients after admission for myocardial infarction or angina. While the intervention improved follow up in general practice, it failed to improve smoking cessation, lipids, blood pressure, or fitness.[2] The implication is that accepted quality of care measures may not achieve improvements in health status.

What are health outcomes?

The term 'health outcome' was coined in the early 1990s as 'a change in the health of an individual, a group or population, which is attributable to an intervention or series of interventions'.[3] The purpose of measuring these is to re-orientate planning, implementation and evaluation of health and related services towards optimal health outcomes within available resources.[4]

Health has been defined by WHO as 'a state of complete physical, mental, and social well-being and not merely the absence of disease or infirmity'.[5] Health outcomes thus are improvements in this broadly defined health status ranging from mortality to patient reported well-being and quality of life. While all of these outcomes are important, some have more importance in some situations than others. For example, mortality is obviously not a very relevant outcome measure for patients in a terminal illness or for interventions to provide palliation. Measures of quality of life are far more appropriate in this context.

Health outcomes can be considered for individuals, groups, and populations. Population outcomes cannot always be attributed to a particular health service intervention, typically arising from a number of interventions. Some population health outcomes may not have direct counterparts at the individual level. For example, eliminating an infectious disease such as polio is an outcome of considerable import at the population level. At the individual level, however, the risk of this disease may be negligible.

Health outcomes may be difficult to measure because of the length of time or chain of events required to bring them about. For example, declines in mortality due to preventive measures may take decades to achieve. Intermediate measures are measurable indicators of health outcomes over the short term. Physiological or behavioural risk factors such as blood pressure or smoking and some processes of care such as immunization rates are intermediate indicators. Outcomes should be, at least potentially, attributable to the range and scope of health care interventions. They should also be sensitive to change[6] and be based on reliable and valid information.[7]

Not all outcomes of health interventions are health outcomes. Health service outcomes (such as test ordering, prescribing, or admissions) are associated with economic outcomes—the cost of care compared with the benefits of interventions or the cost of other interventions with comparable health outcomes. These may be valid in evaluating the efficiency of care.

Table 1 Criteria for selecting health outcome measures in primary care

Relevance	Does it measure outcomes in patients with multiple diseases? Has the measure been used in long-term community based care (as opposed to episodic care)?
Suitability for primary care	Has it been used in particular primary care settings in multiple countries? Has it been standardized for use with different population groups—for example, language, ethnicity, socio-economic status?
Sensitivity	Has the measure been shown to be sensitive to change over time? Has the measure been demonstrated to be sensitive to change in response to primary care interventions?
Validity	Is there face validity? Is there evidence that this is associated with health status? Is there construct validity? Is the measure able to produce an expected distribution of scores—for example, by age or diagnostic category? Is there criterion validity? How well does the measure perform against a 'gold standard'?
Reliability	Is it internally consistent (the components are related to each other)? Does it give the same result when repeated (test–retest)? Does it give the same result when used by different assessors (inter-rater)?

Health outcome measures in primary care

Primary care is provided to individuals and communities over long periods of time across multiple episodes of illness. Patients are dealt with holistically—considering all the health problems which the patient may have or be at risk of. Contextual factors such as the family and social supports, socio-economic status, and culture, are particularly important. By reaching the majority of the population, primary care can influence population health and help prevent disease or disability.

There are numerous examples where interventions that have been shown to be effective in one population group do not work in another—especially in disadvantaged groups or groups from other cultures. For example, cognitive behavioural interventions have been shown to be relatively ineffective where patients are less compliant or where they have limited comprehension.[8]

While subjective judgement of the outcomes of clinical interventions may be appropriate in clinical settings, in research there is a need to have standardized measures which are reproducible regardless of who is doing the assessment. Standardizing the outcome measure ensures validity and comparability across services and settings and over time. Where possible it is desirable to use established outcomes and indicators and instruments for collecting data.[9] Measures should be acceptable to consumers and providers. They should also be reliable, valid as a measure of the desired outcome, and sensitive to change over time. They also need to be relevant for patients with multiple diseases and apply in different social conditions and at the level of individuals and populations (see Table 1). Common health outcome measures are described in Table 2.

Mortality

In primary care, mortality is relatively rare except where it is expected (as in terminal care). Thus, it is not very useful as a measure of primary care interventions at the local or service level. However at the level of large populations, mortality may still be valuable in the evaluation of primary care systems as has been demonstrated by Shi et al.[33]

Illness or morbidity (incidence, prevalence, duration)

The occurrence of disease is an important health outcome. For example, in the evaluation of an intervention such as influenza vaccination an appropriate health outcome may be the incidence or the number of patients who subsequently developed influenza during that year. The clinical or laboratory definition of influenza needs to be standardized to allow comparison over time or between intervention and control groups.

The outcome being considered may be the prevalence or incidence of the disease. Prevalence (the total number of cases/population) at any point in time is a result of the both the incidence and duration. Interventions to provide early effective management, for example, might be expected to reduce prevalence by decreasing duration. Prevalence is most widely used in chronic disease. Incidence (new cases/population) is a better indicator of the success of preventive interventions and is most frequently used in acute diseases.

Adverse events

Health interventions can produce adverse effects that may manifest as symptoms or more serious complications. These can be important outcomes in themselves. For example, the occurrence of adverse events following procedures or hospitalizations may themselves be reduced by other interventions such as improved communication between hospital and primary care.

Physical, physiological, and behavioural risk factors

Physiological variables may be used as intermediate measures of outcome. These are usually based on direct measurement (e.g. weight or HbA1c). Behavioural risk factors such as smoking or physical inactivity are also intermediate measures. These are usually based on self-report at interview. However, some can be validated by objective measures (e.g. cotinine levels for tobacco smoking). Both types of risk factor may be considered as single risk factors for disease or death or they may be combined using epidemiological data to produce an estimate of the risk of disease or death over

Table 2 Health outcome measures

Type of measures	Available measures
Mortality and fatality	Mortality rate is the number of deaths due to a single or multiple causes in a given population over a period of time. It should be age adjusted Fatality rate is the number of deaths in a group of patients from the time of onset of disease or complication, or the time of a service use or intervention Inverse measures of fatality such as survival times especially for diseases with high mortality (e.g. cancer or HIV-AIDS)
Illness and morbidity	Standardized diagnostic definitions are described in the International Classification of Diseases 10th Edition (ICD 10)[10] or the International Classification of Primary Care (ICPC)[11] (another classification DSMIV is commonly used for psychiatric conditions[12]) Measures of prevalence or incidence should be age standardized Measures of duration are generally from initial diagnosis Measures of severity have been defined for some conditions based on symptoms, signs, exercise tolerance, physiological parameters (e.g. asthma, COPD, cardiac failure, renal failure)
Adverse events	Rates of adverse events or complications from time of intervention or health service provision
Physical, physiological, and behavioural risk factors	These intermediate outcome measures include: Blood pressure Weight, body mass index, skin fold thickness, and abdominal girth Glycaemia (fasting, 2 h post-prandial)—venous, serum, or capillary Serum lipids (total cholesterol, HDL, VLDL, triglycerides) Lung function (PEFR, FEV1, VC, etc.) Smoking (e.g. quantity per day) Alcohol consumption (e.g. standard drinks per week, binge drinking) Physical activity (e.g. time in moderate physical activity per week) Nutrition (e.g. frequency of specific foods) Illicit drug use Other risk-taking behaviour (type, amount, frequency)
Health literacy	The Short Test of Functional Health Literacy in Adults (S-TOFHLA) assesses literacy and numeracy skills involved in self-management. There are two components—a 36-item reading comprehensive test and a 17-item numeracy component[13,14]
Quality of life and functional status measures	Generic examples: Medical Outcomes Study SF-36—The SF-36 is a 36-item self-administered questionnaire which assesses generic symptoms, functioning and quality of life.[45] It has eight multi-item scales—physical functioning, physical role limitation, emotional role limitation, bodily pain, mental health, social functioning, vitality, and general health perceptions. The scale is available in a number of languages and takes about 5–10 min to complete. It can be used as a self-administered questionnaire or administered at interview. Normative data is available for comparison,[16,17] has been validated as a population health measure in a variety of socioeconomic groups[18] and has been used widely in primary care[19] COOP/WONCA charts—The Dartmouth COOP/WONCA charts are six charts with visual representation of the aspects of health status—physical fitness, daily activities, feelings, social activities, change in health, and overall health.[20–22] Patients rate each item on a 1–5 scale. The charts have been specifically developed for easy use in primary care and validated in a number of languages and cultures.[23] The Duke Health Profile is a brief self-administered 17-item measure which is comprised of six health measures—physical, mental, social, general, perceived health, and self-esteem and four dysfunction measures (anxiety, depression, pain, and disability).[24] This has been demonstrated to be responsive to change in a number of studies[25] SIP—The Sickness Impact Profile (SIP) consists of 136 questions on daily functioning in relation to health and illness.[26] These questions are grouped into 12 different categories—sleep and rest, eating, work, home management, recreation and pasttimes, ambulation, mobility, body care and movement, social interaction, alertness, emotional behaviour, and communication. The ambulation, mobility and body care and movement sections can be combined to form a global physical section. It takes about 15 min to administer EQ-5D—The EQ-5D is a generic single index measure developed by the EuroQol Group. It is designed for self completion by patients. It has 15 items across five dimensions—mobility, self-care, usual activities, pain/discomfort, and anxiety/depression each rated on a 1–100 scale. It has been translated into numerous languages and is being used in a wide variety of medical conditions[27] SEIQOL—The schedule for the evaluation of individualized quality of life (SEIQOL) involves interviews where patients specify the five areas of their life that are most important and then rate their current status using a visual analogue scale from 0 to 100[28] WHOQOL-100—The World Health Organization's quality of life profile (WHOQOL-100) is a multilingual multidimensional profile of quality of life for cross-cultural use. It can be self-administered and covers 25 facets of quality of life within six broad domains describing positive and negative aspects of quality of life and the impact of illness[29] Specific measures also exist for respiratory, cardiovascular, musculo-skeletal and neurological conditions. A number of measures have been developed specifically for mental health—such as the GHQ (which is available in a short 12-item form).[30] The Mental Health Inventory (MHI) is the five mental health questions from the SF36 and has been used as a measure on its own. Quality of life measures have also been developed for children[31,32]

a period of time. For example, absolute risk tables or calculators can be used to estimate the risk of cardiovascular disease or death over a 10-year period. The level of this absolute risk can be used an intermediate outcome measure in evaluating the effectiveness of interventions.

Health literacy and self-management

Health literacy has been defined as 'the ability to gain access to, understand, and use information in ways which promote and maintain good health'.[34] It is most frequently considered as a confounding or modifying factor that affects access to health interventions. However, it can also be considered as an intermediate health outcome itself as health literacy has been shown to be related to how people experience illness and to itself be associated with health status.[35,36] Functional health literacy has been shown to be critical to patients acquiring adequate knowledge to self manage chronic diseases such as diabetes and cardiovascular disease.[37]

Functional health status and health-related quality of life (HRQOL)

Functional status and health-related quality of life measures go beyond a purely 'medical' approach to assess physical and psychological well-being or impairment as well as the ability of patients to engage in normal activities—such as walking, climbing stairs, household work, employment, and social interaction. There is overlap between the definitions of functional status and quality of life and instruments commonly used to combine aspects of both.

There are also a large number of measures that are designed to be used in evaluating functional status or quality of life in patients with specific diseases. These are more useful for research in acute care involving single clinical conditions where co-morbidity is of less importance or in more severe or disabling conditions where the more general measures do not provide sufficient sensitivity or responsiveness to change.

Because quality of life and functional status measures rely on self-report, there is some contention that these principally measure subjective well-being rather than objective functioning.[38] However, such self-reports may be to make these more relevant to the needs of patients or local communities. Outcomes of relevance to the patient may not match the outcomes of most concern to health professionals or researchers. They may also reflect a desire to be a more active partner in therapeutic interventions.[39] Concern has been expressed that commonly used quality of life measures describe health status in terms of what health professionals view as important rather than according to the patient's priorities.[40] However, developing a reliable and valid patient centred health outcome measure which can be used in a variety of settings has proven challenging.

Health interventions may also reduce the negative impact of illness or disability on employment social relationships and other forms of participation in family and community life. For example, primary care methadone maintenance has been demonstrated to reduce the impact of depression and drug dependence, respectively, on employment status.[41]

What are the limitations of outcome measures?

Outcome measures, especially health outcome measures, may be confounded by a number of other factors that may also effect the outcome. For example, many outcomes change over time even if there is no intervention. The incidence of infectious diseases such as measles changes in a cyclical manner—dependent on the proportion of individuals who have not recently had the infection and are therefore susceptible.

In primary care, there is often co-morbidity among patients, which may confound disease specific outcome measures.[42] For example, a patient with diabetes may also have musculo-skeletal or psychological conditions which may affect their ability to comply with physical activity programmes and increase their likelihood of weight gain.

Many patient outcomes, such as functional status or even physiological measures, are often the result of a complex chain of events involving the patient, their family, and interventions by other providers. These may need to be controlled for in the analysis. Similarly the context of the patient or population group and the context in which the intervention occurs is also important. Few well-designed studies have demonstrated the effectiveness of interventions in disadvantaged groups.[43]

Some outcomes may be easier to measure than others. For example, physiological measures may be easier than social functioning to measure. This may focus attention on outcomes of importance to health professionals rather than consumers and on the influence of proximal rather than distal determinants of health such as social inequalities.[44]

As has been noted earlier, longer- rather than shorter-term outcomes are likely to be more important in primary care because of its emphasis on chronic and continuing care across multiple episodes. Even intermediate measures may need to be considered over long time frames. For example, the change in blood pressure or physical activity over 6 months or a year may be of more relevance in primary care than shorter term changes.

Can outcomes be determined from routinely collected health data?

There are obvious attractions to using routinely collected health data in outcomes research. Routine data are becoming more available with the increasing development of computer record systems in primary care. Such data collections also avoid the 'Hawthorne effect' where the research process influences how care is provided and is more likely to be 'representative' of primary care. However, there are major problems with such data—the most important being their completeness and quality of recording. Furthermore there may be concerns about their validity and reliability (e.g. whether diagnoses being made according to standard criteria).[45] There may also be privacy and ethical issues to be addressed in accessing even anonymized data.

Potential solutions to these difficulties include:

- Using structured computer health records based on agreed minimum data sets and standardised measures which allow extraction of data. One such agreed minimum data set for primary care of diabetes is the NDOQRIN mimimum data set (described in Table 3).[46]

Table 3 Health outcome measures based on the general practice subset of the NDOQRIN minimum data set for quality improvement for diabetes in primary care[47]

Data item	Values
Behavioural risk factors	
Current smoker	Yes, no
Physiological measures	
Weight	kg
Height	cm
Blood pressure	Systolic and diastolic mmHg
On antihypertensive drug therapy	Yes, no
Visual acuity (right and left)	Acuity at 6 m (e.g. 6/6)
Fasting lipids	mmol/l
Cholesterol	mmol/l
HDL	mmol/l
Triglycerides	mmol/l
On antilipid drug therapy	Yes, no
Glycated Hb (HbA1c)	%
Microalbumen/proteinuria	Time collection or microalbumen/ creatinine ratio
Complications	
Peripheral neuropathy	Yes, no (date)
Peripheral vascular disease	Yes, no (date)
Past history of ulceration	Yes, no (date)
Current foot ulcer	Yes, no (date)
Cerebral stroke	Yes, no (date)
Myocardial infarct	Yes, no (date)
Lower limb amputation	Yes, no (date)
End stage renal disease	Yes, no (date)
CABG/angioplasty	Yes, no (date)
New blindness	Yes, no (date)
Erectile dysfunction	Yes, no (date)

- Using the data for clinical assessment (e.g. absolute risk assessment) monitoring of individual quality of care (e.g. for reminders or recall) and quality assurance reports for groups of patients. These uses provide incentives for clinicians to improve the quality and completeness of such data.
- Adjust the data for confounding such as age and socio-economic status.

Conclusions

In reporting health outcomes, care should be taken to define each outcome and how it has been measured. There are five key components to the evaluation of the outcome of clinical and preventive services and programmes.(48) These involve answers to the questions which link outcomes measurement to continuous quality improvement:(49)

- What is the right thing to do (effectiveness)?
- Did we do the right thing (appropriateness)?
- Did we do the right thing right (performance)?
- Did it have the right result (outcome)?
- Was the right result observed in the right people (equity)?

While outcome measurement is only one component of this approach, it is a critical one. The right result in primary care usually involves change in individual and population outcomes for patients with more than one health problem over long periods of time.

References

1. **Chalmers, I.** (1995). What do I want from health research and researchers when I am a patient? *British Medical Journal* **310**, 1315–18.
2. **Jolly, K., Bradley, F., Sharp, S., Smith, H., Thompson, S., Kinmonth, L., and Mant, D.** (1999). Randomised controlled trial of follow up care in general practice of patients with myocardial infarction and angina: final results of the Southampton heart integrated care project (SHIP). *British Medical Journal* **318**, 706–11.
3. **Commonwealth Department of Human Services and Health.** Better health outcomes for Australians. National goals, targets and strategies for better health outcomes into the next century. Australian Government, 1994.
4. **NSW Health in 1992** (Frommer, Rubin, and Lyle, 1992).
5. **World Health Organization.** Definition of Health. World Health Organization 2001, http://www.who.int.
6. **Leyland, A.H. and Boddy, F.A.** (1998). League tables and acute myocardial infarction. *Lancet* **351**, 555–8.
7. **Mant, J. and Hicks, N.** (1995). Detecting differences in quality of care: the sensitivity of measures of process and outcome in treating acute myocardial infarction. *British Medical Journal* **311**, 793–6.
8. **Schmidt, N.B. and Woolaway-Bickel, K.** (2000). The effects of treatment compliance on outcome in cognitive-behavioural therapy for panic disorder: quality versus quantity. *Journal of Consulting and Clinical Psychology* **68** (1), 13–18.
9. **Dunbar, N.**, ed. Making sense of outcomes: a SERU companion to the implementation guide for outcomes based funding. Integration, Access, Health Promotion and Education SERUs. University of NSW, 1999.
10. **World Health Organization.** *International Classification of Diseases and Related Disorders (ICD-10)*. Geneva: World Health Organization, 1992.
11. **Lamberts, H. and Wood, M.** *International Classification of Primary Care*. Oxford: Oxford University Press, 1987.
12. **Frances, A.J., Widiger, T.A., and Pincus, H.A.** (1989). The development of DSM-IV. *Archives of General Psychiatry* **46**, 373–5.
13. **Parker, R.M., Baker, D.W., Williams, M.V., and Nurss, J.R.** (1995). The test of functional health literacy in adults: a new instrument for measuring patients' literacy skills. *Journal of General Internal Medicine* **10**, 537–41.
14. **Baker, D.W., Williams, M.V., Parker, R.M., Gasmariarian, J.G., and Nurss, J.R.** (1999). Development of a brief test to measure functional health literacy. *Patient Education and Counseling* **38**, 33–42.
15. **Ware, J.E., Snow, K.K., Kosinski, M., and Gadek, B.** *SF-36 Health Survey: Manual and Interpretation Guide*. Boston MA: The Health Institute, New England Medical Centre, 1993.
16. **McCallum, J.** (1995). The SF-36 in an Australian sample: validating a new, generic health status measure. *Australian Journal of Public Health* **19** (2), 160–6.
17. **The Australian Coordinated Care Trials:** Methodological issues in trial design and evaluation. Canberra: Commonwealth Department of Health and Aged Care, 1999, ISBN 0 642 36786 8.
18. **Hemingway, H., Stafford, M., Stansfield, S., Shipley, M., and Marmot, M.** (1997). Is the SF-36 a valid measure of change in population health? Results from the Whitehall II study. *British Medical Journal* **315**, 1273–9.
19. **Brazier, J.E.** et al. (1992). Validating the SF-36 health survey questionnaire: new outcome measure for primary care. *British Medical Journal* **305**, 160–4.
20. **McHorney, C.A.** et al. (1992). The validity and relative precision of the MOS short and long form health status scales and Dartmouth COOP charts. Results from the Medical Outcomes Study. *Medical Care* **30** (Suppl. 5), 253–65.
21. **Kinnersley, P., Peters, T., and Stott, N.** (1994). Measuring functional health status in primary care using the COOP-WONCA charts: acceptability, range of scores, construct validity, reliability and sensitivity to change. *British Journal of General Practice* **44**, 545–9.
22. **Van Weel, C.** et al. *Measuring Functional Health with the COOP/WONCA Charts: A Manual*. Groningen: Northern Centre for Health Care Research, 1995.
23. **Bentsen, B.G., Natvig, B., and Winnem, M.** (1999). Questions you didn't ask? COOP/WONCA Charts in clinical work and research. *Family Practice* **16**, 190–5.
24. **Parkerson, G.R., Broadhead, W.E., and Tse, C.K.** (1990). The Duke Health Profile. A 17 item measure of health and dysfunction. *Medical Care* **28** (11), 1056–72.
25. **Parkerson, G.R., Wilke, R.J., and Hays, R.D.** (1999). An international comparison of the reliability and responsiveness of the Duke Health Profile for measuring health-related quality of life of patients treated with Alprostadil for erectile dysfunction. *Medical Care* **37** (1), 56–67.
26. **Bergner, M.** et al. (1981). The sickness impact profile: development and final revision of a health status measure. *Medical Care* **19**, 787–805.
27. **Kind, P., Dolan, P., Gudex, C., and Williams, A.** (1998). Variations in population health status results from a United Kingdom national questionnaire survey. *British Medical Journal* **316**, 736–41.
28. **Bernheim, J.L.** (1991). How to get serious answers to the serious question: 'How have you been?' subjective quality of life (QOL) as an individual experiential emergent construct. *Bioethics* **13**, 272–87.
29. **Skevington, S.** (1999). Measuring quality of life in Britain. Introducing the WHOQOL-100. *Journal of Psychosomatic Research* **47**, 449–50.
30. **Goldberg, D.** (1992). A classification of psychological distress for use in primary care settings. *Journal of Social Science and Medicine* **35**, 189–93.
31. **Shaffer, D., Gould, M.S., Brasic, J., Ambrosini, P., Fisher, P., Bird, H., and Aluwahlia, S.** (1983). A children's global assessment scale (CGAS). *Archives of General Psychiatry* **40**, 1228–31.
32. **Dossetor, D.R., Liddle, J.L., and Mellis, C.M.** (1996). Measuring health outcome in paediatrics: development of the RAHC measure of function. *Journal of Paediatrics and Child Health* **32**, 519–24.
33. **Shi, L., Starfield, B., Kennedy, B., and Kawachi, I.** (1999). Income inequality, primary care and health indicators. *Journal of Family Practice* **48** (4), 275–84.
34. **Nutbeam, D., Wise, M., Bauman, A., and Harris, E.** *Goals and Targets for Australia's Health in the Year 2000 and Beyond*. Canberra: Australian Government Publishing Service, 1993.
35. **Wagner, E.H.** (1998). Chronic disease management: what will it take to improve care for chronic illness? *Effective Clinical Practice* **1**, 2–4.
36. **Kalischman, S.C. and Rompa, D.** (2000). Functional health literacy is associated with health status and health related knowledge in people living with HIV-AIDS. *Journal of Acquired Immune Deficiency Syndromes* **25**, 337–44.
37. **Williams, M.V., Baker, D.W., Parker, R.M., and Nurss, J.R.** (1998). Relationship of functional health literacy to patient's knowledge of their chronic disease: a study of patients with hypertension and diabetes. *Archives of Internal Medicine* **158**, 166–72.

38. **Gill, T.M. and Feinstein, A.R.** (1994). A critical appraisal of the quality of quality-of-life measurements. *Journal of the American Medical Association* **272**, 619–26.
39. **Little, P., Everitt, H., Williamson, I., Warner, G., Moore, M., Gould, C., Ferrier, K., and Payne, S.** (2001). Preferences of patients for patient centred approach to consultation in primary care: observational study. *British Medical Journal* **322**, 468.
40. **Carr, A.J. and Higginson, I.J.** (2001). Are quality of life measures patient centred? *British Medical Journal* **322**, 1357–60.
41. **Ward, J., Hall, W., and Mattick, R.P.** (1999). Role of maintenance treatment in opioid dependence. *Lancet* **353** (9148), 221–6.
42. **Van Weel, C.** (1996). Chronic diseases in general practice: the longitudinal dimension. *European Journal of General Practice* **2**, 17–21.
43. **Hawe, P. and Shiell, A.** (1995). Preserving innovation under increasing accountability pressures: the health promotion investment portfolio approach. *Health Promotion Journal of Australia* **5** (2), 4–9.
44. **Mackenbach, J.P.** (1995). Public health epidemiology. *Journal of Epidemiology and Community Health* **49**, 333–4 (editorial).
45. **Canto, J.G., Kiefe, C.I., Williams, O.D., Brron, H.V., and Rogers, W.J.** (1999). Comparison of outcomes research with clinical trials using pre-existing data. *American Journal of Cardiology* **84**, 923–7.
46. **Australian Diabetes Society.** National Diabetes Data Working Group. NDOQRIN minimum data set for quality improvement in diabetes care, 2001.
47. **Bonney, M., Burns, J., Harris, M.F., and Priddin, D.** National Divisions Diabetes Program: Recommended GP Subset of the NDOQRIN Data-set and alternate fields from which NDOQRIN fields can subsequently be derived. Sydney: Integration SERU, Centre for GP Integration Studies, School of Community Medicine, UNSW, 1999.
48. **Irwig, L.** (1993). An approach to evaluation of health outcomes. *New South Wales Public Health Bulletin* **4**, 135–6.
49. **Batalden, P.B., Nelson, E.C., and Roberts, J.S.** (1994). Linking outcomes measurement to continual improvement: the serial 'V' way of thinking about improving clinical care. *The Joint Commission Journal on Quality Improvement* **20**, 167–80.

14.7 Publishing primary care research

David Jewell and Roger Jones

Introduction

Publications about primary care appear in a wide range of media, and their content is no less heterogeneous. In this chapter, we concentrate principally on the publication of original research in primary care, but also consider a number of other pertinent topics, including the data sources required to support effective clinical practice, some of the links between publication and professional behaviour change and possible future developments in primary care publishing. We have written from the perspective of two editors of English-language primary care journals. We have tried to offer practical advice on the preparation and submission of papers for publication, together with a description of the processes involved in primary care publishing and a consideration of some ethical challenges.

Overview

The quantity and range of the biomedical literature is vast, and its growth has been fuelled by the increasing specialism that has dominated medicine in the last 50 years. The primary care literature occupies an important niche in this vast array of information. Its content and the media in which it appears reflect the eclecticism of primary medical care and the wide range of methodologies required to address the research agenda. Primary care research can, broadly, be considered as research 'within' primary care or research 'on' primary care. The researchers and authors come from a wide range of disciplines, non-clinical as well as clinical, and from secondary as well as primary care,[1,2] and in the future will, we hope, increasingly encompass the lay voice. Similarly, the primary care literature is in part concentrated in a small number of primary care journals and, in larger part, is distributed throughout a wide range of other journals, varying from those with a focus on the behavioural and social sciences, through health services and operational research journals to those publishing in general medicine and the clinical specialties and journals devoted to epidemiological, ethical, and educational research. For primary care clinicians, the literature also needs to include large quantities of research from secondary and tertiary care that is directly relevant to primary care, such as papers reporting the results of randomized controlled trials of interventions applicable to primary care, secondary research including systematic reviews and the Cochrane library and the 'non-research' literature, including textbooks, informal reviews, guidelines, and protocols.

The primary care literature referred to in this chapter therefore represents only one source of information to which clinicians are likely to turn for help with their clinical problems. Today's clinicians may, reasonably, be sceptical about the immediate value of research currently appearing in the primary care journals. Indeed, although there is some evidence that a substantial proportion of clinical decision-making—over 80 per cent in one retrospective study from the United Kingdom—is based on clinical evidence,[3] it is likely that much of this evidence is contained in the generalist, rather than the primary care, clinical literature. Nevertheless, most would recognize that current clinical practice has been substantially informed by the body of research published in specialist primary care journals over the last 10–20 years.

In much of primary care publishing, the sciences of discovery meet the sciences of implementation; insights into the way that clinicians assimilate evidence of effectiveness—whether of drug therapy, screening, or other interventions—into their clinical practice and the barriers to practising evidence-based medicine have been explored and delineated in primary care research. Indeed, primary care, particularly through the application of qualitative research methodologies, has often led the field in our understanding of the factors that initiate, sustain, and constrain changes in clinical behaviour.

While all stake-holders share an interest in a flourishing primary care literature, their interests are unlikely to coincide for any given article or at any given point in the life cycle of a research area. The publication of papers reporting new methodological approaches and preliminary results of early clinical trials is likely to have little immediate impact on the users of research—clinicians, health care planners, and patients. However, with the accumulation of evidence over time, the replication of results and their incorporation into guidelines, protocols and clinical frameworks, the overlap between authors and 'users' is likely to increase. Journals and their editors need to understand these relationships between the research community and the larger community of research users. For university academics, rapid publication in journals with a high impact factor, as discussed below, may be a priority, while for clinicians or health policy planners, the identification of a useful systematic review, summarizing many years' research, may be the imperative.[4,5]

Primary care publications

Of the 35 000 or so biomedical journals published worldwide, fewer than 20 are English language peer-reviewed primary care journals; four of these are published in Europe (*British Journal of General Practice, Family Practice, Scandinavian Journal of Primary Care*, and *European Journal of General Practice*), three in North America (*Canadian Journal of Family Practice, Journal of Family Practice*, and *Family Medicine*), two in the antipodes

(*New Zealand Journal of Family Practice* and the *Australian Family Physician*), one in Hong Kong (*The Hong Kong Practitioner*), with a number of others in the Asia Pacific region and South Africa. There are other country-specific peer-reviewed primary care journals in Europe, for instance, *Huisaarts en Wetenschap* in the Netherlands, *Attencion Primaria* in Spain, and the *Israel Journal of Family Practice.* These primary care publications share a number of features. First, many of them are more closely linked to the local medical culture and health care systems than are more specialist journals which often share many characteristics throughout the developed world. In this respect, each one reflects the clinical disciplines they represent. The way in which primary care is organized, practised, used by patients, and the position it occupies within the system of medical care are all products of the culture and history of the society in which it is rooted and this varies considerably between countries. The relationship between doctors and patients may be fundamentally different in a system of care where payment is partly by capitation, and where patients have to be registered with doctors, from that in a system where doctors are paid for each consultation and where people are free to consult different doctors as much as they wish. While it is possible to publish international journals of primary care, there will always be a demand for local primary care journals, more relevant to local communities.

The hegemony of English language biomedical publishing means that the primary care journals published in the English-speaking countries gain an advantage over others. While the language may not present an insuperable barrier for many doctors, it is important to remember the ways in which language circumscribes and conditions the understanding of underlying concepts. Papers translated from the original English into other languages must be carefully selected for relevance to other medical cultures.

Finally, the important issues of citation and impact factors require consideration. The impact factor of a journal is an attempt to measure the degree of influence that it exerts. It is based on the number of times each article is cited elsewhere within 2 years of publication, and is also related to the number of articles published in the given journal during that period. Authors, particularly researchers whose careers depend on their publication record, are encouraged to publish in journals with high impact factors. The figures on which impact factors are based are the number of citations published in the Science Citation Index. Numerous problems are associated with the use of impact factors: they particularly favour small research fields, they are sensitive to self-citation and short publication delays, the SCI database has an English language bias and, within that, a bias towards American publications and it is possible to manipulate the figures by, for instance, publishing more reviews than primary research. Worst of all, the impact factors of journals are not directly linked to the citation of the individual articles on which it depends. Bluntly, individual author will gain more prestige from assessors by publishing a poorly cited paper in a high impact journal, than by publishing a frequently cited paper in a low impact journal.(6) Impact factors are, however, likely to be with us for a long time, even while we remain aware of their shortcomings.

Getting into print

Background reading

We think the best way to start a writing career is to have read extensively and critically. In the first place, it will make you familiar with the shape, conventions, and language of biomedical literature. Reading research reports invariably stimulates further questions, often ones that the authors themselves have not thought of. Asking the questions of critical appraisal when reading the work of others will develop the habit of being critical of your own writing and asking yourself all the searching questions before the editor does.

Remember the rules of the game

In a perfect world, every paper that reached the desired scientific standard would be accepted for publication (and in the future, use of electronic media may make this possible). However, at present, journals are constrained by space limitations, and the need to keep delays down to an acceptable level. Papers are therefore in competition with each other to justify taking up journal space. Writers need to make their work as relevant and interesting as possible to editors and readers.

Fit the journal

Getting into print depends on pointing the paper in the right direction. Partly this is a matter of deciding which audience you wish to address. Find out what kind of articles a particular journal is in the habit of publishing. The *British Journal of General Practice* states in its 'Information to Authors' that it does not welcome certain types of articles. *Family Practice* has created a particular niche for itself in the publication of papers describing research methodology. You should not, however, feel too constrained by this: editors may be unhappy at feeling their journal has acquired a particularly restrictive label. Editors of primary care literature may feel they have a duty to readers, authors, and publishers to justify claims that their journals embrace the broad range of primary care.

Start small

For most writers of any description, and that includes almost all doctors, writing is a craft. For a few it may come naturally, but for most of us it is a skill that we develop over a lifetime. Start with shorter pieces. Most journals have spaces for short contributions, most obviously the letters section, but also reviews and case reports.

Take time with the discussion

Writers often fail to do their research justice when it comes to the discussion section. It is easy to err by being both too limited and too grandiose when discussing what the data mean.(7,8) Good writing will never turn a flawed study into a good paper, but careful thought put into the discussion section can show the research study to its best advantage.

Information for authors

All journals have their own 'Information for Authors' to help them define their identity. It may not be essential for submitted papers to observe all the minutiae, particularly when there is, for instance, only a one in six chance of being accepted. However, ignoring them too blatantly, for instance, by exceeding the number of accepted tables or figures, or citing the references in the wrong format may make it too easy for the editor to reject your paper.

Check the citations

With the long gestation involved from original idea, through grant application and ethics committee submission, to completion of the study and writing up the results, it is tempting to rely on the original search for references. However, unless the research is in a field of unparalleled obscurity, the intervening years will have seen other contributions to the literature. Failing to cite such papers, particularly any that have been published in the journal that you are submitting to, is an easily avoidable mistake.

Invite critical comment

At least when you are starting to write, always get someone more experienced whom you trust and respect to read your papers before sending them off to a journal. We all get much too close to our data and our personal agendas while we are completing the work, and an outsider's view can have a vital and cleansing influence.

How to respond to rejection

All successful journals receive more submitted papers than they will have room to publish, and it is highly unlikely that you will always be able to have your papers accepted by the first journal chosen. Rejection should not be taken as a personal judgement of you as a researcher or writer, but as the judgement of a particular piece of work on a particular day, by a process that is agreed to be imperfect. For this reason, if you think your paper has been rejected on the basis of an opinion that is simply wrong you should think about appealing. However, beware: sometimes the editor's letter may not convey the real reason for rejection, either out of sensitivity to your feelings or because it is easier to hide behind the apparently more objective criticisms set out in the referee's.

Processing submitted manuscripts

Because of the volume of papers submitted, most journals use a filtering system, in which an editor checks that they are appropriate to the journal and likely to be of sufficient quality to justify being sent out to peer review. A substantial proportion, as many as half in some journals, are rejected at this stage, often because of authors' failure to select an appropriate journal for their work or because of evident lack of originality, timeliness, or interest. Papers surmounting this initial hurdle are then sent out to a number of reviewers, including an expert statistical reviewer where appropriate. At this point there are still likely to be more positively reviewed papers than the journal has space for, so further editorial judgement is exercised, often supported by a meeting of several editors or 'hanging committee'. At this point, further considerations such as 'fit' with other papers awaiting publication, timeliness, likely policy relevance, and public impact play a part in the final selection of papers for publication. Few papers are accepted without the need for revision, and some require further peer review after extensive revision. This process can be a lengthy one, and a source of frustration for authors; journal editors do their best to minimize the time between submission, a publishing decision, and eventual publication, and the dates of receipt, re-submission, and acceptance of papers are often provided as footnotes so that potential authors can assess the likely lag-times between submitting their work and seeing it in print.

The peer review process

From being a mysterious procedure conducted behind closed doors, the peer review process has gradually come under closer scrutiny.[9] The arguments in favour of the system are straightforward: the process of publishing papers that have been approved by experts in the field gives a guarantee of quality to editors and readers. Recent research has exposed flaws in the system. First, it is not always easy to identify the experts. However expert they are, peer reviewers are no more capable of delivering completely disinterested, objective opinions than anyone else. The system has been criticized as being designed to weed out new and challenging ideas and favour conventional wisdom of the prevailing culture. The more obviously ethical areas of competing interests are particularly of concern to bodies that award grants. In his pioneering study of the peer review system, the then editor of the *British Medical Journal*, Stephen Lock, characterized the system as more of a traffic policeman than a referee, since most papers rejected by the *British Medical Journal* were eventually published elsewhere.[10] This may not apply to those rejected by journals with lesser perceived impact.

The peer review process is intended not only to select papers for publication, but also to improve the presentation of the published research.[11] A more positive view of the process emerges from a study where papers accepted for publication were revised in the light of reports from peer reviewers and then subjected to another round of peer review, using a 34-item peer review instrument. The initial peer review led to an improvement in 33 out of the 34 items, with the largest improvement relating to the discussion sections of the papers.[12] In an accompanying editorial, Stephen Lock stated baldly that peer review cannot guarantee perfection. All it can do is '... detect major defects of originality and scientific credibility, together with commenting on important omissions, the rigor of the arguments, and defects in the writing style'.[13]

Studies have explored the value of blinding reviewers to the authors' identity, and have found no evidence the practice has any effect on the quality of the subsequent reviews.[14,15] The reason is partly the difficulty of hiding the authorship, through both the habit of self-citation and the reviewer's familiarity with the field. One study of papers submitted to seven US journals found they were successful in masking authors' identity in approximately 60 per cent of papers.[16] One of these studies similarly found no benefit in concealing or revealing the reviewers' identities to authors.[14] A subequent study in a specialist psychiatry journal suggested that when reviewers knew their identity was to be revealed to authors the reviews were of higher quality and more courteous. The reviewers took longer over their reports and were less likely to recommend rejection of the articles.[17] While it is easy to criticize these studies on the grounds of size and the quality of the outcome measures used, they currently represent the best evidence available, and give support to those editors who favour openness. Some experienced reviewers have expressed concern that open review will inhibit robust criticism, especially when the authors are senior and influential figures. At the extreme, some have expressed fears that their ability to continue to attract research grants awarded by committees staffed by such senior figures will be compromised. Our view is that the benefits of openness will always outweigh the disadvantages, encouraging reviewers to declare competing interests, and providing them with the easy option of declining to review any paper where they feel unable to express their view honestly.

No system that is self-evidently better has yet been devised. At their best, reviewers offer a superb service, providing clear and cogent arguments, supported by cited references. They crucially give the expert insider's view on the originality and importance of the question being asked. And most of the time they give their time free.

Ethics

Increasing concern over the morality of certain practices in medical publishing has culminated in the formation of the Committee for Publishing Ethics in 1997. This body works as a forum for editors to discuss ethical problems. The annual report contains a sample of the problems that have come up before the committee.[18] The following are some of the ethical problems that we have encountered.

Authorship

The International Committee of Medical Journal Editors (ICMJE) sets out rules for authorship.[19] There are three requirements, all of which have to be fulfilled: conception and design, or acquisition of data, or analysis and interpretation of data; drafting the article or revising it critically for important intellectual content; and final approval of the version to be published. The evidence is that these rules are too restrictive. In particular, they fail to acknowledge that medical research has become a more complex activity relying on substantial teams of researchers from different disciplines to bring studies to completion. Several studies have indicated that they are widely ignored. For instance, a study of papers published in 1996 in six US journals validated authorship on the basis of 17 different activities and identified honorary authorship in 16 per cent of research articles.[20] A number of journals have replaced the concept of authorship with contributorship, with all contributors credited with their specific contributions. A study of research articles published in *The Lancet* after it had made this transition concluded that specifying contributions was feasible, took up little space in the journal, and seems to convey useful information. To emphasize the attraction, the authors also calculated that 44 per cent of contributors did not fulfil a lenient version of the ICMJE's rules for authorship.[21]

Duplicate publication

We have recently received a small number of papers that were obvious duplicates. Identifying these has in each case depended on the vigilance of reviewers. We remain concerned that while we congratulate ourselves for identifying this small number we are almost certain to be missing at least an equal number. Of equal concern is the correct identification and definition of papers on the borders of duplication. Is study 'x', which uses the population, methodology, and data of study 'y', but applies a different analysis, original or not? What may matter most is the claims for originality made by authors, but concerns remain.

Salami publication

For those unfamiliar with the term, salami publication describes taking a single research project and slicing it to generate many papers. Artificially inflating researchers' CVs may not matter; spreading the results of a single study over a wide range probably will. It is important to present to readers as complete a picture as possible, so that, for instance, the qualitative work undertaken to contextualize and explain the quantitative data of an RCT appears in the same paper, or at least alongside it, and not removed in time and space. The salami approach is insidious and difficult to police. The requirement for academics to measure success in terms of volume rather than quality of publications, compounded by the word limits imposed by the journals, all contribute.

Conflicts of interest

In contrast, competing interests and the influence of pharmaceutical companies should be easy to spot. Declaring them is the critical first step. Here again openness is the key, and it is then up to readers to assess the extent to which vested interests may have influenced the findings. Many journals now require both authors and reviewers to complete statements of competing interests. The next step is likely to be a requirement to report the precise nature of any competing interest.

Future of primary care publishing

If we can assume that all the stake-holders will continue to need some form of primary care publishing, can we predict what form it is likely to take in the next 20 years? Electronic publishing has already changed the culture and is likely to become the dominant medium in the future. We do not think this will lead to the death of paper-based journals. Rather, fulfilling the 'Sailing Ship Rule',[1] the paper journals are likely to benefit from the freedom that electronic journals offer to editors to define exactly what the paper journals are intended to achieve.

Electronic publishing offers much more than better storage and access. First, there is the opportunity to become more sophisticated in distinguishing between the needs of casual readers and other researchers. The paper journal can, for instance, carry less data, but carry more commentary that both contextualizes and challenges the paper, and also explains and educates on behalf of the readership. The electronic form is free not only to carry more data but could include complete datasets that would then be available for further analyses.[(22)]

For the most part, editors can only influence the quality of reporting, not of the research that precedes it. However, publication of research protocols, either when the study begins or contemporaneously with the main report could deter some poor research practice.[(23)] The idea arose in response to disquiet about inadequate statistical power of published articles and other deficiencies that may have occurred through changes in protocols taking place in the course of trials. *The Lancet* now publishes some protocols of controlled trials and systematic reviews, offering provisional commitment to publish the primary clinical paper. Advantages could include: reducing publication bias; promoting the successful conduct of trials by encouraging other centres to assist recruitment; and discouraging data dredging by documenting the planned analyses.

There is scope for rapid exchange of ideas among readers once papers have been published, through the medium of an electronic message board. A lively correspondence column in a journal is more than simply a means of challenging and correcting mistakes. At best it can be the tangible expression of a journal's readership, the community being addressed. As with so many other aspects of paper publishing, it is becoming obvious how restrictive hard copy journals can be, creating delays that hamper a lively exchange of ideas and imposing arbitrary space restraints which limit both the number and the length of letters that can be published. Here again the electronic medium liberates and accelerates, although at the potential cost of permitting excess verbiage to clog up cyberspace.

However, electronic publishing has so far failed to throw the slightly closed world of medical publishing open to all. Most journal websites remain accessible only to subscribers in one form or another. For many years there has been a quiet argument between researchers who want their work to be widely available and the publishers who delay publication and then charge exorbitantly for access. The scientific community has long argued that there should be no restriction on access, especially as the funding bodies have already paid for the results and should not have to pay again. The counter argument is that there is a real cost in bringing the material to publication: gathering and responding to the process of peer review, copy editing, printing etc. The arguments are now being tested by the existence of BioMed Central[(24)] which is hoping to bypass existing publishers by taking papers direct from the authors and publishing on the Web.[(25)] Of course there is a cost here too, but this will be borne directly by the funders. It remains to be seen how far this system will undermine traditional publishers.

[1] The Sailing Ship Rule describes the observation that the most successful sailing ships were designed and built in response to the challenge from steam. The first passenger steamers were in service in America in 1807 (the *Clermont*, running between New York and Albany) and in Europe in 1812 (the *Comet*). In contrast, the best known of the tea clippers, the *Cutty Sark*, was launched at Dumbarton in 1869. Clippers continued to ply the route between Europe and Australasia into the twentieth century. Eric Newby described one of the last such commercial voyages in a Finnish four-masted barque in 1938 in his book *The Last Grain Race.*

References

1. **Jones, R.** (1998). Published research in primary care: original papers in the US and UK, 1996. *Family Practice* **15**, 291–5.
2. **Thomas, T., Fahey, T., and Somerset, M.** (1998). The content and methodology of research papers published in three United Kingdom primary care journals. *British Journal of General Practice* **48**, 1229–32.
3. **Gill, P., Dowell, A.C., and Neal, R.D.** (1998). Evidence based general practice: a retrospective study of interventions in one training practice. *British Medical Journal* **312**, 819–21.
4. **McColl, A., Smith, H., White, P., and Field, J.** (1998). General practitioners' perceptions of the route to evidence based medicine: a questionnaire survey. *British Medical Journal* **316**, 361–5.
5. **Salisbury, C., Bosanquet, N., Wilkinson, E., Bosanquet, A., and Hasler, J.** (1998). The implementation of evidence-based medicine in general practice prescribing. *British Journal of General Practice* **48**, 1849–52.
6. **Seglen, P.O.** (1997). Why the impact factor of journals should not be used for evaluating research. *British Medical Journal* **314**, 498–502.
7. **Horton, R.** (1995). The rhetoric of research. *British Medical Journal* **310**, 985–7.
8. **Docherty, M. and Smith, R.** (1999). The case for structuring the discussion of scientific papers. *British Medical Journal* **318**, 1224–5.
9. **Smith, R.** (1997). Peer review: reform or revolution? Time to open up the black box of peer review. *British Medical Journal* **315**, 759–60.
10. **Lock, S.** *A Difficult Balance.* London: The Nuffield Provincial Hospitals Trust, 1985.
11. **Purcell, G.P., Donovan, S.L., and Davidoff, F.** (1998). Changes to manuscripts during the editorial process. *Journal of the American Medical Association* **280**, 227–8.
12. **Goodman, S.N., Berlin, J., Fletcher, S.W., and Fletcher, R.H.** (1994). Manuscript quality before and after peer review and editing at Annals of Internal Medicine. *Annals of Internal Medicine* **121**, 11–21.
13. **Lock, S.** (1994). Does editorial peer review work? *Annals of Internal Medicine* **121**, 60–1.

14. **Van Rooyen, S., Godlee, F., Evans, S., Smith, R., and Black, N.** (1998). Effect of blinding and unmasking on the quality of peer review. *Journal of the American Medical Association* **280**, 234–7.

15. **Justice, A.C., Cho, M.K., Winker, M.A., Berlin, J.A., Rennie, D., and the PEER investigators** (1998). Does masking author identity improve peer review quality? A randomized controlled trial. *Journal of the American Medical Association* **280**, 240–2.

16. **Cho, M.K.** et al. (1998). Masking author identity in peer review. *Journal of the American Medical Association* **280**, 243–5.

17. **Walsh, E., Rooney, M., Appleby, L., and Wilkinson, G.** (2000). Open peer review: a randomised controlled trial. *British Journal of Psychiatry* **176**, 47–51.

18. **Committee on Publication Ethics.** http://www.publicationethics.org.uk.

19. **International Committee of Medical Journal Editors** (1997). Uniform requirements for manuscripts submitted to biomedical journals. *Annals of Internal Medicine* **126**, 36–47.

20. **Flanagin, A.** et al. (1998). Prevalence of articles with honorary authors and ghost authors in peer-reviewed medical journals. *Journal of the American Medical Association* **280**, 222–4.

21. **Yank, V. and Rennie, D.** (1999). Disclosure of researcher contributions: a study of original research articles in the Lancet. *Annals of Internal Medicine* **130**, 661–70.

22. **Davey, S.** (1994). Increasing the accessibility of data. *British Medical Journal* **308**, 1519–20.

23. **Chalmers, I. and Altman, D.G.** (1999). How can medical journals help prevent poor research? Some opportunities presented by electronic publishing. *Lancet* **353**, 490–3.

24. **BioMed Central.** http://www.biomedcentral.com.

25. **Delamothe, T. and Smith, R.** (2001). PubMed Central: creating an Aladdin's cave of ideas. *British Medical Journal* **322**, 1–2.

15

Education and professional development

15 Education and professional development

15.1 Medical education: the contribution of primary care

Robert F. Woollard

The contribution of primary care practitioners to the undergraduate education of physicians is inextricably linked with the perspective of the generalist approach to health and disease. As such the presence and contributions of family physicians/general practitioners in undergraduate curricula has waxed and waned as the twentieth century carried on its prolonged flirtation with the specialist/reductionist approach in the assumption that it was by far the most appropriate to address society's problems.

While this approach has produced undeniable benefits in both the health sector and broader society, the early twenty-first century is coming to realize that this monogamous enterprise has not only produced some noxious and expensive offspring but has failed to effectively address some of the most complex and important factors in the health of both individuals and populations. At all levels of society, from the shop floor to the health care system to the broad issues of social and environmental policy, the instruments of society (legislatures, granting agencies, academies, etc.) are realizing the limits of discipline-specific, single-factor approaches to a wide array of complex problems—some aggravated by the very technological solutions attempting to mitigate them. As a consequence, we see a rising thrust of interdisciplinary research increasingly focused on community/academic partnerships dedicated to joint problem solving. This kind of intermingling of science and community, of physician and patient, has been a hallmark of the generalist perspective since Sir William Osler's nineteenth century admonition to listen to the patient—he is telling you the diagnosis. The educational expression of this perspective can be seen in the evolution of undergraduate medical education towards an increasing emphasis on problem-based learning,(1,2) early clinical exposure and an increasing emphasis on community-based training. That this is a desirable direction has been affirmed by the Education Committee of the General Medical Council in Great Britain.(3) As we shall see, there are a number of reasons why these trends bode well for the increasing integration of the generalist and family practice perspectives in the undergraduate education of twenty-first century physicians. Whether these opportunities come with commensurate resources and respect is another question.(4)

The particular expression of these broad social trends in the realm of medical education has a number of origins, opportunities and intellectual traditions. These must be explored and grasped or the bright possibilities may not be realized. There is real likelihood that community-based generalist teaching will be treated as a convenient return to an apprenticeship mode. This would be tragic because it would represent the loss of a major opportunity for addressing what Ilene Harris calls 'new expectations for professional competence'.(5) In summarizing some of the extensive literature on professionalism and practice as it applies to a variety of professions, Harris notes '… This work suggests that some of the most important problems in practice are characterized by complexity, uniqueness, uncertainty and conflicting values. The goal of practice is wise action. Wise action may involve the use of specialized knowledge, but central to it is judgement in specific situations, with conflicting values about which problems need to be solved and how to solve them'. This might be seen as a pithy description of the lived experience of primary care physicians. Among others, Oswald(6) has moved beyond the description of possible/desirable curricular opportunities to the active exploration of student expectations and responses to formal arrangements for structured clinical encounters and effective debriefing. As we shall see in this chapter, if younger physicians are to develop an effective approach to these 'most important problems', they can hardly be expected to do so by simple observation of the practice of an expert clinician.

The pace of change in the acquisition of new scientific knowledge together with rapid evolution in both the education and expectations of patients dictate real limits to the effectiveness of an unreflective 'see and do' or even a 'see one, do one, teach one' model for the intergenerational transfer of knowledge.

The tendency to an 'overloading of the curriculum … followed by results injurious to the health of students' was noted with concern by the Medical Council as early as 1863(7) and eloquently expressed more than a century ago by Thomas Huxley who derided as a 'disgrace' a 'system of medical education that is actually calculated to obstruct the acquisition of sound knowledge and to heavily favour the crammer and the grinder … ' Increasingly, adult education (of which medical education should be a very high order example) is focused on 'learning how to learn' rather than on a never-ending acquisition of knowledge, of learning how to reflect on rather than simply apply acquired skills. In all of these areas, the generalist/primary care physician has the raw material and experience to make major contributions in an organized, patient-centred curriculum.

Another general opportunity afforded by the place and nature of family practice relates to learning the broad context of health and disease. While technical knowledge and expertise provide an indispensable foundation for any competent practitioner, a profession that aspires to be a 'healing' profession, must intricate that expertise into a broad understanding of the human condition and the values important to the patients they serve. As Oswald observes 'This sort of understanding is something that is helpful for all doctors … '(8) While there is an increasing emphasis on broad education in the pre-medical years(9) it is not clear there is a commensurate commitment to apply this knowledge during the years of medical training. The long tradition of close association between medical schools and universities has served society well. This has been most obviously true in the realm of basic sciences and highly specialized clinical practice when we look at the advent of technological intervention. What is not so obvious is the imperative that we move beyond mere technological interventions to a broader understanding of healing and the meaning of those interventions in the lived lives of patients. As the university/medical school expands its training into this important area, the primary care practice becomes a valuable opportunity. As Armour and Fuhrmann assert 'the intent to develop liberally educated graduates, rather than competent technicians, is what makes a university a university'.[10] As we shall see in this chapter, properly prepared primary care practices can provide remarkable opportunities for the general education of all twenty-first century physicians.

The perspective we bring

Schön[11,12] outlines the foundation for the generalist perspective in medicine under the title of *The Reflective Practitioner*. This requires the physician to simultaneously act and reflect on his/her actions. It is this skill which forms the basis of what Mathers and Rowland[13] call a *post-modern* approach to medicine and education. Weston[14] explicates this distinction in the following way:

> The *modern* view of the world holds that we can 'view the world out there' using the scientific method and assumes this view is uncontaminated by the mind of the knower. A *modern* approach to curriculum design focuses on aims and objectives, content, teaching process and assessment and evaluation. It is linear, mechanistic process akin to the biomedical model. A *post-modern* approach is more fluid and complex. In this approach teachers and students create a dialogue focussed on critical incidents in the curriculum as experienced. In the process of trying to understand and trying to change the problematic aspects of the curriculum they find the right questions to ask and reach a deeper understanding of the learning process and how it needs to change.[15]

While this situates the generalist approach in a broad philosophical tradition, what does it mean we can bring in particular?

One particular set of skills that arises is the application of clinical reasoning in the context of patient-centred care. McWhinney[16] has thought deeply and published extensively on the topic of generalist clinical judgement and the application of evidence in the patient encounter. Figure 1 taken from *Generalist Foundations*[17] summarizes the nature of the hypothetico-deductive process.

This stands on its head the reductionist approach of the dispassionate gathering of evidence until an hypothesis is proven or disproven. It involves a recursive reflection on the current status of a particular clinical approach so that it can be revised by the intrication, not only of evidence from history, physical examination, and investigation but by unexpected cues from the patient and/or his family. The constant revision of an interpolated diagnostic and therapeutic approach, when combined with the longitudinal relationship that is a foundation for family medicine, allows both the best service to the patient and a sustained opportunity for the student to explore the application of their newly acquired biomedical knowledge. The model also leaves room for the evolution of clinical skills with the development of knowledge base and experience as the learner moves through the stages of clinical reasoning defined by Bordage and Zacks[18] and outlined in Fig. 2.

It must be kept in mind that this is one of a rich range of theoretical bases for both clinical reasoning and the ability to acquire and evaluate those skills. Bennett,[19] Fox and Craig,[20] as well as Wales et al.[21] all give useful overviews of the perspectives and challenges in this area. It is not necessary that the role model or practitioner are intimately acquainted with the nuances of theory but rather that they have a shared language and a commitment to using the opportunities in the primary care encounter to think about thinking and to learn about learning.

Other clinical reasoning models can be applied[22] but the point is that having a framework for clinical reasoning allows us to explore *systematic* sources of error with the student. In no other aspect of learning is the concept of 'reflection in action' and 'reflection about action' more important than in the explication of sources of error in diagnostics and management.

By developing these reflective skills the student is able to move beyond the observed (or committed!) error as a basis for learning. This is particularly important given the consequences of medical error. The learning culture in undergraduate medical education has not always been a healthy one. Because of the highly competitive nature of medical school entrance, students may tend to resist admissions of ignorance as this may have proven

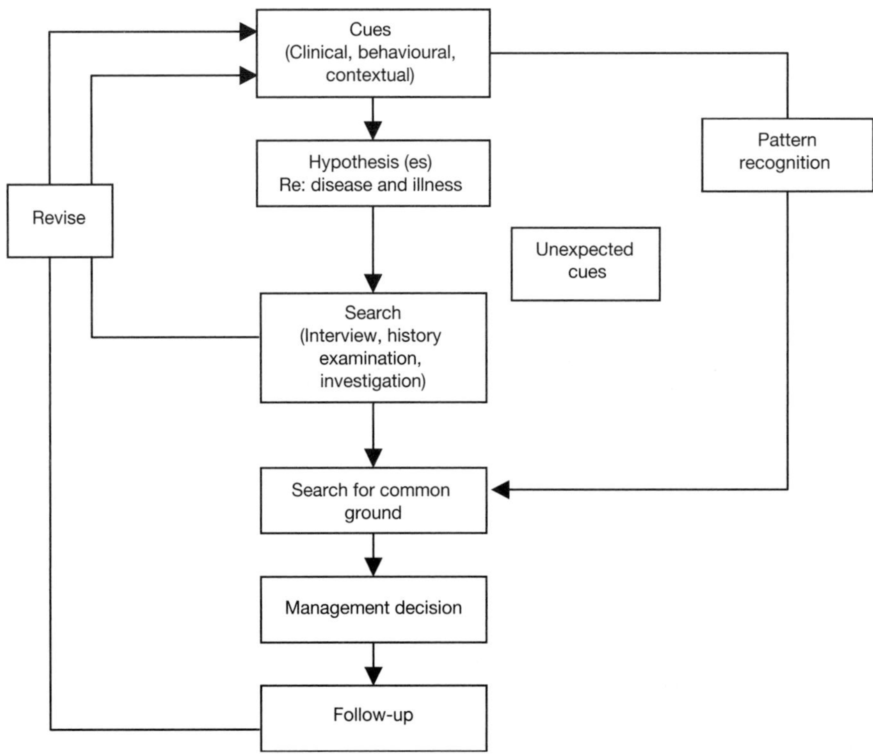

Fig. 1 Model of the Diagnostic Process based on McWhinney.

dangerous in the past. As we shall discuss below, the student must be guided in a transition from this state to one in which errors are seen as raw materials for learning rather than something to be hidden. As they are increasingly involved in clinical decision-making through a graded transfer of responsibility, the hazard moves from them to the patient. During this transition, role models are important but insufficient in themselves if the student is not given a framework by which they can *dissect* the clinical judgement they observe in others and *reflect* on their own capacity.

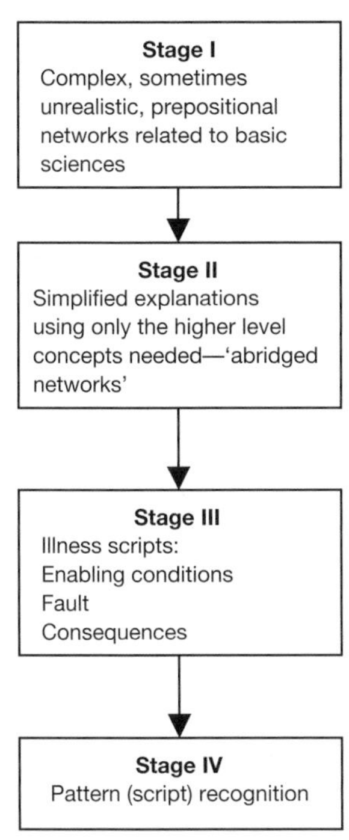

Fig. 2 Stage theory of clinical reasoning. (Bordage and Zacks)

Part of the students armamentarium in this approach is a taxonomy of common errors and Weston's formulation of this can be found in Fig. 3.[23]

The reflective practitioner is also in a position to assist the students in understanding their own progression of learning through medical school. As outlined in Fig. 4, Weston delineates a progression that generalist physicians can encourage in a variety of curricular and extra-curricular ways.

The descriptive power of this model is re-enforced in the qualitative studies of student's perception carried out by Oswald.[25]

Where do/can primary care physicians contribute?

While the general trends outlined in the beginning of this chapter hold true across a variety of medical schools and nations,[26] the precise courses and opportunities for generalist contributions will vary considerably. Notwithstanding, there are a number of particular *topics* and *issues* that are especially amenable to the generalist perspective and/or the opportunities presented in the clinical practice of family medicine. These include but are not confined to:

- communication skills;
- the social and community context of illness;
- evidence-based medicine;
- clinical skills and reasoning;
- health promotion and enhancement;
- exposure to common clinical conditions, etc.

The precise venue in which this subject matter is taught adds a further dimension to student education and underscores another major contribution the generalist/primary care perspective can make to that education. White et al.'s classic study of the ecology of illness[27] has been revisited by Green et al.[28] and has generally confirmed the robustness of the description over 40 years. The description outlines in a succinct fashion (Fig. 5) the places where illness presents and is treated.

This clearly delineates that a medical education based exclusively on patients referred to a university medical centre will be deficient indeed! On the other hand, the primary care practitioner brings not only the broader

Cue blindness:
- Fatigue, personal problems
- Mental set—excessive focus on one type of problem, for example, biological or psychological
- Unfamiliarity with the problem
- System problems, for example, not enough time or resources

Errors in generating hypothesis:
- Focusing on zebras rather than horses (the probability issue)
- Ignoring rare but treatable and serious disorders (the 'payoff' issue)
- Focusing on the wrong kind of problem, for example, ignoring non-disease hypothesis
- Concentrating on one diagnosis too soon—cue blindness or failure to search

Errors in the search:
- Lack of skill in collecting accurate data (interviewing and physical exam skills)
- Over-investigation—seeking unnecessary precision, for example, continuing to test when the pre-test probability is $<10\%$ or $>90\%$
- Inadequate testing
- Focus on 'ruling-in' rather than 'ruling-out'
- Over-reliance on a test of low sensitivity
- Reliance on a test that is often negative early in the illness
- Pressure from a third-party, for example, family, insurance company, institutional policy

Management errors:
- Thinking only of the disease and ignoring the patient's experience of illness and their unique predicament
- Ignoring important variables, for example, ethical issues, risks of treatment, effects on other family members
- Ignoring patient wishes or expectations

Fig. 3 Common errors in clinical reasoning. (Weston)

	From →	To
Focus of learning	Facts Knowledge Practical value	Principles Wisdom Creativity and deeper values
Approach to learning	Passive recipient Errors are to be avoided, denied, punished Dependence Need for certainty Imitation Narrow interests Superficial concerns Amalgamate	Active agent Errors are raw material for learning Independence, interdependence Tolerance of ambiguity Originality Broad interests Deep concerns Integrate
Cognitive style	Dualistic search for the 'right' answer Receiver of meaning	Evolving commitments to better answers Maker of meaning
Personal development	Identity formation Selfishness Boundary maintenance—rigid or vague compartments	Intimacy, early generativity Altruism Boundary maintenance—comfortable and flexible
Professionalization	Sense of self as student Need to prove self Few responsibilities Rescue fantasy Rugged individual	Comfortable in role of doctor Comfortable with strengths and limits Many responsibilities Good enough Team member
Concept of medicine	A 'trade' A dogmatic science A hierarchy MD as expert A job	A 'craft' An art that uses science A contract and a covenant MD also servant A 'calling'

Fig. 4 Progression of learning through medical school. (Weston)

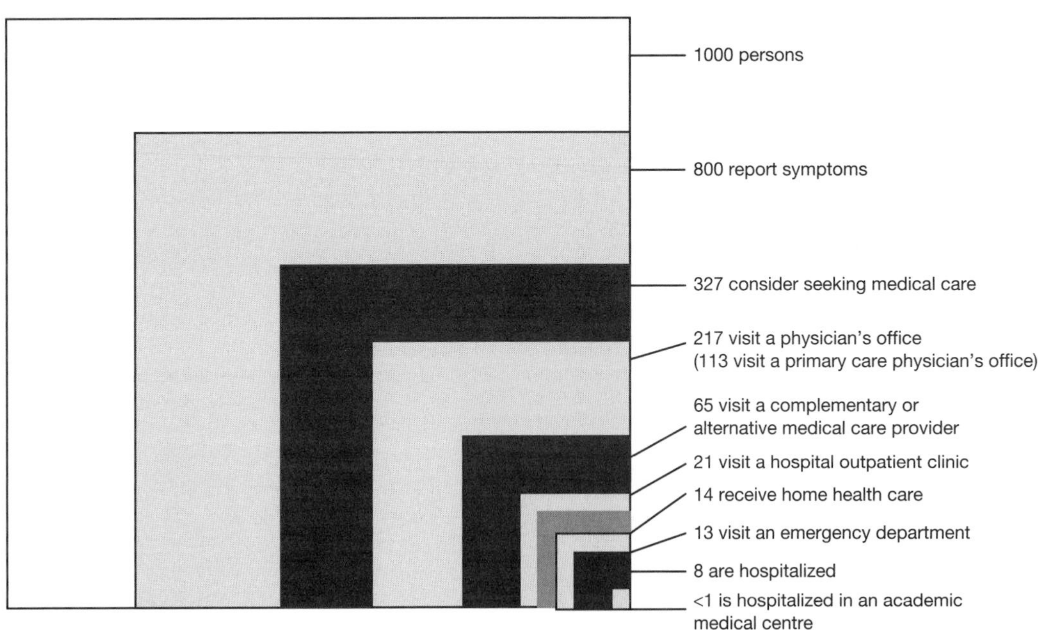
1000 persons
800 report symptoms
327 consider seeking medical care
217 visit a physician's office
(113 visit a primary care physician's office)
65 visit a complementary or alternative medical care provider
21 visit a hospital outpatient clinic
14 receive home health care
13 visit an emergency department
8 are hospitalized
<1 is hospitalized in an academic medical centre

Fig. 5 Results of a re-analysis of the monthly prevalence of illness in the community and the roles of various sources of health care. (*From:* Green, L.A., Fryer, G.E., Yawn, B.P., Lamier, D., and Dovey, S.M. (2001). The ecology of medical care revisited. *New England Journal of Medicine* **344** (26), 2022.)

Home visits
Palliative care
Emergency department
After-hours care
Primary care obstetrics
Long-term, chronic, or senior care
Inpatient care

Fig. 6 Non-office-based components of family medicine clerkships in Canada (1999).[30]

- Physician as medical expert/clinical decision maker
- Physician as communicator/educator/humanist/healer
- Physician as collaborator
- Physician as gate keeper/resource manager
- Physician as health advocate
- Physician as learner
- Physician as scientist/scholar
- Physician as person

Fig. 7 Role of the future physician.

1. The doctor/patient relationship is central to the role of family physician
2. The family physician must be a skilled clinician
3. Family medicine is a community-based discipline
4. The family physician is a resource to a defined practice population

Fig. 8 Four principles of family medicine.

	Doctor/patient relationship	Skilled clinician	Community based	Resource population
Expert/clinician		Y		
Communicator	Y		Y	
Collaborator				
Gate keeper	Y			Y
Health advocate			Y	Y
Learner/scholar		Y		
Scientist		Y		Y
Person			Y	etc.

Fig. 9 The contribution of family medicine to undergraduate education.

Clinical evaluation
Objective structured clinical evaluation (OSCE)
Short answer management (SAM)
Multiple choice questions (MCQs)
Academic project/research project
Key features
Simulated office oral
Oral examination

Fig. 10 Methods of evaluation in family medicine clerkships in Canada (1999).

scope of patients seen in their office but a broader range of patient encounters. In the British context, Oswald[29] as early as 1989, raised the question of the educational opportunities inherent in the physicians office. In the Canadian context, the intervening years have seen the evolution of a variety of venues as outlined in Fig. 6.

It is likely that other venues involving team care and interdisciplinary learning can be afforded in a variety of health care systems.[31]

Physician roles and family medicine

It is important to note that not only are these opportunities available but there is a large and growing body of theory and evidence that there are powerful pedagogic and practical reasons to develop 'community-based education'.[3,28,32] An international partnership of academics devoted to the exploration of the interface between the needs of a society and the education of its physicians has been active for a quarter of a century. More recently, they have assumed the name of *The Network* and have produced a *Handbook of Community-Based Education: Theory and Practices.*[33]

It is worthwhile here to reflect on the various roles that all physicians play in a variety of health care systems. One formulation of these roles established through an intensive public and professional process can be found in Fig. 7.[34,35]

Clearly, this multiplicity of roles applies in varying ways to the full range of physicians in the full range of health care systems. This fact notwithstanding, it is apparent that the generalist/primary care practitioner provides a particularly broad expression of this multiplicity of roles. While the specialist can be appropriately content with a more limited focus on knowledge and expertise, the generalist must practice constantly across the full spectrum and thus in theory can provide opportunities to learn about these roles by all the students—no matter what their speciality destination.

In the Canadian context, family physicians have long promulgated four principles as the basis for their practice and education (Fig. 8).[36]

This formulation has proven to be robust and useful in shaping the curriculum and contribution of family practitioners in both undergraduate and post-graduate teaching. A 'lens' that might situate opportunities for generalist contributions to student education can be constructed by a matrix linking these two important concepts (Fig. 9).[37]

This thinking tool is useful in identifying potential gaps in the curriculum and experience of students as medical schools reflect upon the particular contributions that primary practitioners can make.

Evaluation/assessment

Evaluation rests as a major challenge in teaching situations characterized by distributed venues, multiple roles, varying clinical content and highly complex concepts of health, disease, and healing. It is understandable that educators might look wistfully at situations characterized by simple and measurable knowledge transfer around defined organ systems or diseases in a predictable and time limited institutional contact with a pre-diagnosed patient. In some measure this describes the content of the smallest box in Fig. 5. Since these are not the features of the continuing relationship of a primary care physician with their patients over time, in a variety of settings and across the spectrum of disease, we have had to invoke an armamentarium of evaluative tools extending well beyond a multiple-choice questionnaire. Those outlined in Fig. 10[30] must be tailored to the particular circumstances of particular curricula but provide examples of validated and effective means of determining the quality of the performance of the student, the preceptor and the programme.

An added advantage of the discipline of family medicine in the evaluation of students can be achieved if the teaching relationship continues over an extended period of time.[38] Evolving methods of in-training evaluation nested in this longer-term relationship between learner, teacher, and patient can produce a much more complete evaluation of the skills, and particularly the attitudes, of evolving professionals and highlight interpersonal issues that can readily escape the most scrupulous knowledge testing processes.

As the discipline develops its capacity in a variety of countries[39] and enhances the links between postgraduate and undergraduate curricula and assessment, this important function will be increasingly sought out.

Conclusions

The intellectual basis[16,40] for an expanding role for primary care practitioners in the general medical education of all students must be effectively developed, articulated and used as medicine enters the new millenium. Properly organized and resourced, the contributions of generalists, long-neglected in twentieth century education, can be seen as increasingly important as medicine reinvents itself in a world made increasingly complex by advancing medical knowledge, increasing patient knowledge and evolving patient expectations for both expert and humane care.

The student will be best served if all of these contributions are made in a context in which the patient and their family rather than simply the disease is the unambiguous focus of the both the care and the education. Such an approach in no way diminishes the importance and role for both the specialist's perspective and the understanding of basic sciences central to the practice of scientific, evidence-based medicine. Indeed, there appears to be increasing evidence and opinion that basic science is best learned in a clinically relevant, problem-based milieu. This chapter was written in the hope that specialized clinical medicine might similarly be seen to be best learned with a robust and respectful interplay between the specialist and generalist perspectives as we prepare all medical students to care for patients in the twenty-first century.

References

1. **Albanese, M.A. and Mitchell, S.** (1993). Problem-based learning: a review of literature on its outcomes and implementation issues. *Academic Medicine* **68** (1), 52–81.
2. **Vernon, D.T.A. and Blake, R.L.** Does problem-based learning work? A meta-analysis of evaluative research. *Academic Medicine* **68** (7), 550–63.
3. **General Medical Council.** *Tomorrow's Doctors: Recommendations on Undergraduate Medical Education.* London: General Medical Council, 1993, pp. 33, 42–5.
4. **Woollard, R.F.,** ed. *The Present and Promise of Family Medicine in Undergraduate Education: Generalist Foundations.* Mississauga ON: College of Family Physicians of Canada, 2000.
5. **Curry, L.** et al. *Educating Professionals: Responding to New Expectations for Competence and Accountability* Chapter 2. San Francisco CA: Jossey-Bass, 1993.
6. **Oswald, N.** *Summary Report of Cambridge Community Based Clinical Course (CCBCC)* Chapter 12, pp. 72–6, 1998.
7. **General Medical Council.** *Tomorrow's Doctors: Recommendations on Undergraduate Medical Education.* London: General Medical Council, 1993, p. 3.
8. **Oswald, N.** *Summary Report of Cambridge Community Based Clinical Course (CCBCC)*, Chapter 12, p. 76.
9. **Association of American Medical Colleges.** *Physicians for the Twenty-First Century: The GPEP Report.* Report of the Panel on the General Professional Education of the Physician and College Preparation for Medicine. Washington DC: AAMC, 1984.
10. **Curry, L., Wergin, J.F., and Associates.** *Educating Professionals*, p. 126. San Francisco CA: Jossey-Bass Inc. Publishers, 1993.
11. **Schön, D.A.** *The Reflective Practitioner: How Practitioners Think in Action.* San Francisco CA: Jossey-Bass, 1983.
12. **Schön, D.A.** *Educating the Reflective Practitioner.* San Francisco CA: Jossey-Bass, 1987.
13. **Mathers, N. and Rowland, S.** (1997). General practice—a postmodern speciality? *British Journal of General Practice* **47**, 177–9.
14. **Weston, W.** (2000). In *The Present and Promise of Family Medicine in Undergraduate Education: Generalist Foundations* (ed. R.F. Woollard), p. 52. Mississauga ON: College of Family Physicians of Canada.
15. **Weston, W.** (2000). In *The Present and Promise of Family Medicine in Undergraduate Education: Generalist Foundations* (ed. R.F. Woollard), p. 53. Mississauga ON: College of Family Physicians of Canada.
16. **McWhinney, I.R.** *A Textbook of Family Medicine* 2nd edn. Oxford: Oxford University Press, 1997.
17. **Weston, W.** (2000). In *The Present and Promise of Family Medicine in Undergraduate Education: Generalist Foundations* (ed. R.F. Woollard), p. 45. Mississauga ON: College of Family Physicians of Canada.
18. **Bordage, G. and Zacks, R.** (1984). The structure of medical knowledge in the memories of medical students and general practitioners: categories and prototypes. *Medical Education* **18**, 406–16.
19. **Bennett, N.** (1994). Developmental perspectives in learning. In *The Physician as Learner: Linking Research to Practice* Chapter 5 (ed. D. Davis and R. Fox), Chicago IL: American Medical Association.
20. **Fox, R. and Craig, J.** (1994). Future directions in research on physicians as learners. In *The Physician as Learner: Linking Research to Practice* Chapter 6 (ed. D. David and R. Fox), Chicago IL: American Medical Association.
21. **Curry, L., Wergin, J.F., and Associates.** *Educating Professionals* Chapter 8. San Francisco CA: Jossey-Bass Inc., 1993.
22. **Schmidt, H.G.** et al. (1996). The development of diagnostic competence: comparison of a problem-based, an integrated, and a conventional medical curriculum. *Academic Medicine* **71** (6), 658–64.
23. **Weston, W.** (2000). In *The Present and Promise of Family Medicine in Undergraduate Education: Generalist Foundations* (ed. R.F. Woollard), p. 47. Mississauga ON: College of Family Physicians of Canada.
24. **Weston, W.** (2000). In *The Present and Promise of Family Medicine in Undergraduate Education: Generalist Foundations* (ed. R.F. Woollard), p. 30. Mississauga ON: College of Family Physicians of Canada.
25. **Oswald, N.** *Summary Report of Cambridge Community Based Clinical Course* (CCBCC), p. 73–5, 1998.
26. **General Medical Council.** *Tomorrow's Doctors: Recommendations on Undergraduate Medical Education.* London: General Medical Council, 1993.
27. **White, K.L., Williams, T.F., and Greenberg, B.G.** (1961). The ecology of medical care. *New England Journal of Medicine* **265**, 885–92.
28. **Green, L.A., Fryer, G.E., Yawn, B.P., Lamier, D., and Dovey, S.M.** (2001). The ecology of medical care revisited. *New England Journal of Medicine* **344** (26), 2021–4.
29. **Oswald, N.** (1989). 'Why not base clinical education in general practice?' *Lancet* **43**, 148–9.
30. **Freeman, R.** (2000). In *The Present and Promise of Family Medicine in Undergraduate: Generalist Foundation Education* (ed. R.F. Woolard), p. 16. Mississauga ON: College of Family Physicians of Canada.
31. **Mennin, S.P.** et al. (1996). A Survey of Graduates in Practice from the University of New Mexico's conventional and community-oriented, problem-based tracks. *Academic Medicine* **71** (10), 1079–89.
32. **Jewell, D. and Logan, A.** (2001). *British Journal of General Practice* (editorial) **51**, 89–90.
33. **Schmidt, H., Magzoub, M., Feletti, G., Nooman, Z., and Vluggen, P.,** ed. *Handbook of Community-Based Education: Theory and Practices.* Maastricht: Network Publications, 2000.
34. **Neufeld, V., Maudsley, R., Turnbull, J., Weston, W., Pickering, R., and Brown, M.** (1998). Educating future physicians for Ontario. *Academic Medicine* **73** (11), 1133–48.
35. **Maudsley, R.F., Wilson, D.R., Neufeld, V.R., Hennen, B.K., DeVillaer, M.R., Wakefield, J., MacFadyen, J., Turnbull, J.M., Weston, W.W., Brown, M.G., Frank, J.R., and Richardson, D.** (2000). Educating future physicians for Ontario: phase II. *Academic Medicine* **75** (2), 113–26.
36. **Woollard, R.F.,** ed. *The Present and Promise of Family Medicine in Undergraduate Education: Generalist Foundations.* College of Family Physicians of Canada, 2000, p. 7.
37. **Woollard, R.F.,** ed. *The Present and Promise of Family Medicine in Undergraduate Education: Generalist Foundations.* The College of Family Physicians of Canada, 2000, p. 8.
38. **Oswald, N.** *Summary Report of Cambridge Community Based Clinical Course (CCBCC)*, pp. 73–5.
39. **Alexander, H.G., Jass, J.R., and Campbell, C.B.** (1999). Planning integrated assessment across 12 university departments in a problem-based learning medical course. *Focus on Health Professional Education: A Multi-Disciplinary Journal* **1** (1), 28–33.
40. **Woollard, R.F.** (2000). In *The Present and Promise of Family Medicine in Undergraduate Education: Generalist Foundations*, pp. 5–10. Mississauga ON: College of Family Physicians of Canada.

15.2 Vocational and postgraduate training

Richard Hays

Background

For the purpose of this chapter, the term *primary medical care* is used to include those forms of medical practice that require a capacity to deal, at least initially, with undifferentiated health care problems at the first point of contact patients have with the health care system. Because precise roles depend substantially on the structure and funding of the health care system in which an individual medical practitioner works, this understanding of the term is not necessarily the same in all health care systems. Indeed, systems vary from those that require all patients at entry to be seen by a generalist primary care practitioner to those that allow patients to choose the kind of doctor, generalist, or sub-specialist, that they should consult first. Even where primary care medical practitioners are usually consulted first, the definition of primary care varies. For example, in the United States, paediatricians, general physicians, general surgeons, and obstetricians are included within primary care, whereas in many nations, primary medical care usually includes only general practitioners. Further, national systems vary in the degree to which mandatory postgraduate training and certification assessment is required for that role, from nil to highly structured programmes. The last 30–40 years has seen mandatory training requirements spread to most developed and many developing nations, beginning with the United Kingdom in the 1950s. Hence this chapter will also focus on training arrangements in nations that have strong primary care systems and at least some degree of organized, often mandatory, postgraduate training and assessment of competence to work as a primary medical practitioner.

Why train for primary medical care?

In an era which has seen medical education expand substantially and training programmes become longer and more comprehensive, this is a highly relevant question. In years gone by, graduates felt competent to enter general practice straight from medical school, and then later directly after a 1-year junior hospital experience that offered minimal supervision or training. More recently, few graduates would seriously consider entering unsupervised practice immediately after the junior hospital training, even where this is allowed. This begs an obvious question: has undergraduate medical education failed to help acquire the necessary skills, or has primary medical care become more complex. Although this sounds simplistic, there is truth in both of these questions. The rapid expansion of medical knowledge and technical skills leaves insufficient time to ensure that medical graduates master any more than a limited or 'core' set of skills and knowledge. As hospitals became centres of expensive, complex, high-technology, and short-stay medical care, primary medical care was squeezed out of curricula and assessment nodes.[1] There is now an international swing to correct these deficiencies, as medical schools seek to utilize more community health resources and expose students to more primary care practice issues.[2,3] Such initiatives have arguably been more easily achieved where undergraduate and postgraduate programmes are strongly vertically integrated.[4]

It is also true that primary medical care is now a more complex task. Not long ago, general practitioners could practice simple, reactive, 'presenting complaint' medicine in response to patient requests. It was left to patients to decide how often they presented (if at all) and if they wanted to be immunized and modify lifestyle factors such as obesity, diet, smoking, and alcohol intake. Further, general practice was often a small 'cottage industry', in which individual doctors provided many years of service to a loyal practice population that accepted professional advice with few questions. Primary care doctors now work in an environment of competition for credibility with other medical and even alternative health practitioners, decreasing acceptance of errors of judgement and increasing price sensitivity (in governments, funders, and patients) in a very high-cost industry that consumes 8–14 per cent of gross domestic product (GDP) in developed nations. Increasingly, primary care medical practitioners are expected to play a role in resource management, where duty of care ethics are tested by personal relationships and availability of funds.[5]

These quite complex health care issues cannot be covered sufficiently in any undergraduate course, and so it is now almost universally accepted that a period of postgraduate training specifically in the context of contemporary primary medical care is essential for competent practice with job satisfaction.

What training is needed?

Postgraduate training for general practice picks up where undergraduate education stops, which is usually at a point that enables medical graduates to enter any medical career. In the medical schools of most developed nations, this usually means that graduates entering postgraduate training for general practice have attended lectures or tutorials on the differences between primary care and hospital care. They should also have spent some time in general practices observing and, ideally, participating in the provision of primary care. However, in most cases, the majority of their knowledge and understanding will be based on hospital experiences and culture, as the duration spent in those contexts is much greater.

Hence the challenge of postgraduate training in primary care is to ensure that learners: gain knowledge about the different and additional problems encountered; gain reasonable exposure to primary care patients and problems; improve and broaden consulting skills; can function within the health care system of the relevant nation; and reach the standards required of the relevant certifying authority in the nation or jurisdiction concerned. The term consulting skills is used here to include a wide range of diagnostic, management, and communication skills that define general/ family practice), such as the ability to deal with a wide range of presenting complaints, many of which are rarely seen in hospitals. Further, primary medical practitioners need to know how best to care for many hitherto hospital problems in the community, working as part of a primary health care team.

Principles of postgraduate training for primary medical care

Assuming that entrants to postgraduate training have achieved the core learning objectives for basic registration within their own health care system and nation, postgraduate training programmes should adopt a series of important educational principles. These include: measurable learning objectives; a common curriculum and assessment blueprint; adult learning methods; collaborative supervision; assessment that where possible is performance-based; and evaluation of the training programme from multiple perspectives. Each of these is discussed further below. Please note that I will use consistently the term *learner*, as different terms are used in different systems. For example, *registrar* is the term used for learners in Australia and the United Kingdom, *resident* is used in North America, and the more generic *trainee* is still used in many places.

Measurable learning objectives

While most would assume that training programmes have clear learning objectives, that is not always the case. One of the challenges in primary medical care is that the role description can be very broad, indeed so broad that it may not be possible to ensure that all graduates achieve a set of common educational goals. Hence, many programmes have *core* and *optional* learning objectives that cover a widely agreed set of common tasks that all graduates should master, plus sets of additional tasks that certain primary care practitioners may choose to master.[6] Agreeing on what is core and what is optional is usually an interesting process, as it is difficult to gain agreement at the boundaries of what is core and optional, and there are almost as many opinions as participants. Nevertheless, the discussions, ideally involving other health professionals and patient groups as well as medical practitioners, are essential.

Further, the agreed learning objectives should be measurable as this facilitates sound assessment practices, as described below. This means that the wording of learning objectives is important—the objectives should be in the form of *doing* or some action that can be measured.[7] Furthermore, they should be precise enough to describe discrete and achievable learning objectives, rather than vague expressions suggesting understanding of what might be complex issues. For example, rather than stating 'demonstrates understanding of ethical principles', it is better to state 'can apply ethical principles in the management of clinical conditions that pose a range of common ethical questions' and then try to teach and assess how learners can apply the principles in a range of clinical situations. Finding the right level of precision of learning objectives can be difficult and is best done by groups of individuals with appropriate expertise and, perhaps, differing viewpoints.

A common curriculum and assessment blueprint

Following on from the learning objectives, training programmes should have a clear description of what is to be learned and mastered during training. This is often in the form of a *blueprint*, or a schematic representation of tasks or skills that should be learned, perhaps classified by educational *domains*, patient presentations, age, and gender of patients, context (e.g. rural or urban) or other aspects of health care. Domains are essentially just ways of thinking about curriculum organization and, while they are certainly in vogue at the moment, they are often misused by either being present in name only, rather than in application, or applied too rigidly. In reality, domains are not mutually exclusive and so too rigid application in either teaching or assessment does not make much sense. An important advantage of having a clear curriculum blueprint is that this further facilitates appropriate assessment practices.

Adult learning methods

All postgraduate learners are at least in their early to mid-20s and have experienced many years of formal education. After completion of postgraduate training they will be in a rather open system with less stringent requirements for maintenance of competence than faced during this final period of professional training. Hence, it is essential that training programmes follow not just the rhetoric of adult learning, but ensure its implementation. After this stage, professional development is much more an individual responsibility, although clinical governance strategies will increase the level of accountability that doctors have throughout their whole careers.[8]

In practice as well as theory, adult learning should allow learners a wider choice of, and control over, how and what they will learn. All learners come to postgraduate training with substantial prior educational experience, although perhaps insufficient professional experience to know how to apply that prior knowledge in the real world. Adult learning programmes acknowledge this prior educational achievement and trusts learners to: value their professional development; take responsibility for their learning; learn from experience; reflect on their performance; and learn from errors of judgement.[9]

Hence, the role of teachers of adult learners is to take an active role in assessing the current level of performance of their learners, supporting them through supervised experiences, providing feedback; and providing a safety net so that any errors of judgement do not result in adverse patient outcomes. This is not an easy role description and teachers should possess interest and aptitude for the job, a set of special skills that require training, and a serious time commitment. The roles cannot be done well by busy practitioners who cannot transfer clinical load and who do not receive financial compensation for what is a truly professional role.[10]

Collaborative supervision

Teachers of postgraduate learners should not be seen as teachers in a traditional didactic sense, but rather as experienced senior colleagues of the learners, capable of guiding their learners through the required learning experiences to become at least their equals, if not in time superior practitioners. In a way a 'master–apprentice' relationship exists, except that (as most experienced supervisors know) the apprentice often knows more than the master, although may be less skilled in applying it. Through a process of collaborative supervision the teacher and learner learn from each other, regularly assessing what each knows and how that can be improved, particularly around particular clinical cases.[11] The best teachers are the patients encountered by the learners, so a key element of postgraduate training is ensuring that the clinical caseload provides sufficient breadth and depth of experience to cover curriculum requirements. The next most important teachers are more experienced primary care medical practitioners, as role modelling is a powerful influence on behaviour,[12] but in a system as complex as primary care all health professionals play an important role. Ideally, all learners should learn in a multiprofessional environment that functions well, as that is how primary health care is provided.

Assessment issues

Sound assessment practices are congruent with the curriculum against which learners will be assessed. Hence, as stated previously, sound assessment practices are facilitated by the presence of measurable learning objectives and a common curriculum/assessment framework. Ideally, learners are assessed against the learning objectives through the curriculum/assessment framework, thus ensuring that domains, presentations, age and gender issues and contextual issues etc. are reflected in both teaching and assessment.

Any assessment process should consider the following attributes of assessment: validity (measuring what is intended to be measured); reliability (repeated assessment should achieve the same result); educational impact (assessment that guides learning); feasibility (cost-effectiveness); acceptability (will the profession, community and learners regard it as reasonable); and efficiency (psychometric properties relevant to test length, etc.).[13] In reality, all assessments achieve compromises in the balance between these attributes, but designers should aim high. Of particular interest is the educational impact of assessment. Many educationalists argue that so long as the assessment program is right, any unevenness in curriculum design and implementation will be sorted out as learners prepare for examinations. To paraphrase the oft-despised adage, 'good assessment drives good learning!'. The right balance of assessment should be delivered through a combination of formative and summative assessment, ideally including some in-training assessment that is performance-based.[14]

Evaluation

Responsible training programmes are constantly monitored to ensure that they achieve their stated aims—usually the production of graduates competent for independent primary medical practice. This important attribute is often ignored. Details of evaluation methods are available elsewhere (e.g. see ref. 15).

A brief overview of selected vocational training programmes

This section provides a brief description of established vocational training programmes from selected nations. Their key data are summarized in Table 1.

Table 1 Brief comparison of selected vocational training programmes for primary medical care

Nation	Total duration (years)	Primary medical	Mandatory	Competitive entry	Formal assessment	Public funding[a]	University linked
Australia	3–4	18 months	Yes	Yes	Yes	Yes	No[b]
Canada	2–3	8 months	Yes	Yes	Yes	Yes	Yes
New Zealand	5	1 year	Yes	Yes	Yes	Yes	No
Netherlands	3	2 years	Yes	Yes	Yes	Yes	Yes
Singapore	3	3 years	No	No	Yes	No	Yes
UK	3	1 year	Yes	Yes	Yes	Yes	Varies
USA	3	1 year	Yes	Yes	Yes	Yes	Yes

[a] Funding sources are often mixed.

[b] This may change under the new training arrangements from 2000.

Table 2 Website addresses of colleges of general or family practitioners

College	Website address
Australia	www.racgp.org.au or www.acrrm.org.au
Canada	www.cfpc.ca
Hong Kong	www.hkcfp.org.hk
New Zealand	www.rnzcgp.org.nz
Netherlands	www.nhg.artsennet.nl
Singapore	www.cfps.org.sg
United Kingdom	www.rcgp.org.uk
United States	www.abfp.org
WONCA	www.wonca.org

Programmes are undergoing review or transition in many nations, much of it related to the need to address workforce shortages in regional and rural areas. Readers are advised to seek current information from the relevant college in each nation through the website addresses listed in Table 2. The website addresses of other nations not listed may be obtained through the WONCA website, which is also listed in Table 2.

Australia

Australian vocational training began in the early 1970s as a voluntary 4-year programme (2 years hospital-based, 2 years in general practice). There was no formal end-point examination, although an examination for Fellowship of the Royal Australian College of General Practitioners (RACGP) was available. During the early 1990s, the programme was re-structured to become the RACGP Training Programme, with 3 years (18 months general practice) of more intensive training with mandatory end-point assessment—the re-developed RACGP examination.[16] A fourth year of training is available for those seeking additional skills for rural practice. Because of a marked medical workforce maldistribution,[17] the emphasis in training has moved towards increasing exposure to rural and remote medical practice careers. As of 2002, responsibility for training has moved to an independent Board of General Practice Education and Training (GPET), which contracts out training to regional educational consortia. Consortia are encouraged to include university departments of general practice and must provide local training that meets the standards of both the RACGP and the new Australian College of Rural and Remote Medicine (ACRRM). Graduates must pass a national certification assessment that reflects the requirements of both colleges. Interest in rural careers will be fostered by an expansion of the number of training places in rural areas and the provision of financial incentives to those in rural training.

Canada

Canada has a strong family practice discipline that has provided high quality postgraduate training in a competitive national system. All training programmes must be accredited by the Canadian College of Family Physicians (CCFP) and are provided within university departments of family practice. The standard programme is 2 years in duration, including hospital-based training and a minimum of 8 months of family practice training in a university-affiliated practice, although programmes vary outside of the minimum requirements. An additional 'advanced training' year is available in selected topics (emergency medicine, aged care, palliative care, women's health) for those seeking greater expertise in those topics. Certification as a Family Physician requires satisfactory performance in a national CCFP examination. In recent years, the competition for training places through the national Canadian Residency Matching Service (CARMS) has softened, partly because of an apparent weakening of demand for primary care training overall and an increase in the number of training places available in rural areas. These are regarded by graduates as less desirable, although medical school initiatives are trying to change that culture and rural training programmes, such as the South Western Ontario Rural Medicine (SWORM) programme have succeeded in attracting applicants.[18]

New Zealand

The New Zealand training programme was very like Australia's until the mid-1990s, when government funding restrictions reduced the size of the programme, called the General Practice Education Programme (GPEP), to only 50 entrants per year. This is a well-funded and high-quality programme that places learners in teaching practices for 12 months and funds a seminar programme that prepares them for the PRIMEX examination (essentially a 'part 1' examination). Because competition for places has been so tight, others may find their own general practice place and participate in the seminar series—the 'Seminar Attendee' path—but this has become less popular due to its cost to the individual learner. Following successful performance in PRIMEX, all learners find their own supervised general practice post and participate in the Advanced Vocational Education (AVE) programme, which includes assessment of a series of case studies and audits. Satisfactory completion confers eligibility for Fellowship of the Royal New Zealand College of General Practitioners (RNZCGP), which from July 2001 is a pre-requisite for unsupervised general practice.

Singapore

Training requirements in Singapore provide a reasonably representative sample of systems in South East Asia. In most nations, postgraduate training is voluntary, self-funded, and based in university departments of general practice. Qualifications such as a Diploma in Family Medicine can be achieved after satisfactory participation in professional development programmes. In Singapore, medical graduates must have one prior year of hospital-based training and then participate in flexible delivery modules about common primary care issues. After 1 year, learners qualify for a Diploma in Family Medicine, after a further year for a Masters in Family Medicine, and after a third year for a Fellowship in Family Medicine.

United Kingdom and Western Europe

The United Kingdom was the first nation to introduce mandatory vocational training and (later) assessment for general practice. The programme is managed by an independent Joint Council and is sub-contracted to regional schemes that compete for entrants, who apply directly to the regional scheme of their choice. As elsewhere, the demand for places in regional and rural areas is weaker than in the larger cities. The duration of the programme is 3 years (2 year hospital-based, 1 year in general practice). The level of involvement with undergraduate departments of general practice is variable, but often low. Learners must satisfactorily complete the Summative Assessment Package prior to entering unsupervised practice,[19] after which they may participate in additional professional development and assessment to achieve Membership of the Royal College of General Practitioners (MRCGP) and, with recommendation as a result of substantial seniority or further assessment, Fellowship of the RCGP.

The UK system is now more open to medical graduates from Western Europe, where primary care training is often voluntary, not highly organized, and not linked to end-point assessment. Colleges of general/family practice in each nation generally have a programme of about 3 years, including hospital-based training and general practice experiences. Learners participate in local education programmes that are often peer discussions.[20] Most colleges wish to have training and certification mandated and progress towards this continues. For example, the Netherlands now has a mandatory 3-year programme that includes 2 years in general practice. The programme is managed separately from university departments of general practice, although usually situated adjacent to them. There is no national certification examination, but learners face an assessment of their learning portfolios after the first general practice year before they can proceed to the final year of training.

USA

In the United States, the term 'primary care' includes a range of medical disciplines other than family practice—general internal medicine, obstetrics, paediatrics, psychiatry, and general surgery. However, this discussion is confined to family practice, the nearest match to primary medical care in most other nations. Board certification as a Family Practitioner is not mandatory in some states (passing the three-step US Medical Licensing Examination is), but very few do not seek this. Intending family practitioners apply for specific residency programmes through a national residency matching service. Most, but not all, programmes are based in a university department of family practice. Demand for careers in family medicine has weakened overall, particularly in under-served (inner city and rural) areas, but most applicants will obtain a place, even if not necessarily of first choice. Training programmes are 3 years in duration, with 1 hospital-based year and 2 years of family practice-based training. Board certification hinges on satisfactory performance in national assessment.

Continuing medical education

All colleges and academies of general/family practitioners have continuing medical education (CME) programmes that are intended to maintain competence and, where relevant, certification as a primary care doctor. This is perhaps the most controversial level of medical education, as there is little evidence that traditional CME achieves its lofty aims.[21,22] Most CME programmes have requirements for participation in a variety of practice-based and individual reflection on practice and attendance at education seminars, but there is argument about whether the programmes measure participation or outcomes.

References

1. **Hillman, K.** (1999). The changing role of acute care hospitals. *Medical Journal of Australia* **170**, 325–8.
2. **Jones, R., Higgs, R., de Angelis, C., and Prideaux, D.** (2001). Changing face of medical curricula. *Lancet* **357**, 699–703.
3. **Habbick, B.F. and Leeder, S.R.** (1996). Orienting medical education to community need: a review. *Medical Education* **30**, 163–71.
4. **Snadden, D., Hays, R.B., and Bain, J.** (1999). A tale of two cities: integrating postgraduate and undergraduate general practice education. *Education for General Practice* **9**, 113–18.
5. **General Medical Council.** *The New Doctor.* London: GMC, 1997.
6. **Harden, R.M. and Davis, M.** (1995). The core curriculum with options or special study modules. *Medical Teacher* **17**, 125–48.
7. **Grant, J.** (1999). Measurement of learning outcomes in continuing professional development. *Journal of Continuing Education in the Health Professions* **19**, 214–21.
8. **Campbell, A.** (1999). Clinical governance: the ethical challenge to medical education. *Medical Education* **33**, 870–1.
9. **Knowles, M.** *The Adult Learner: A Neglected Species* 4th edn. Texas: Gulf Publishing Company, 1990.
10. **Hays, R.B.** (1998). Resource implications of shifting medical school education to the community. *Medical Journal of Australia* **169**, 63–4.
11. **Matthews, C.** (2000). Role modelling: how does it influence teaching in Family Medicine. *Medical Education* **34**, 443–8.
12. **Hays, R.B.** *Practice-Based Teaching: A Guide for General Practitioners.* Melbourne: Eruditions Publishing, 1999.
13. **Van der Vleuten, C.P.M.** (1996). The assessment of professional competence: developments, research and practical implications. *Advances in Health Sciences Education* **1**, 41–67.
14. **Hays, R.B. and Wellard, R.** (1998). In-training assessment in postgraduate training for general practice. *Medical Education* **32**, 507–13.
15. **Pitts, J., Percy, D., and Coles, C.** (1995). Evaluating teaching. *Education for General Practice* **6**, 13–18.
16. **Hays, R.B., Van der Vleuten, C., Fabb, W.E., and Spike, N.** (1995). Longitudinal reliability of the FRACGP examination. *Medical Education* **29**, 317–21.
17. **Australian Institute of Health and Welfare.** *A Report of the Australian Medical Workforce Advisory Committee.* Australian Medical Workforce Benchmarks. AMWAC Report 1996. 1. Canberra: Australian Government Publishing Service, 1996.
18. **Rourke, J.** (1999). Postgraduate education for rural family practice. *Canadian Family Physiscian* **45**, 2698–704.
19. **Rhodes, M. and Wolf, A.** (1997). The summative assessment package: a closer look. *Education for General Practice* **8**, 1–7.
20. **Westin, S.** et al. (1988). A group-based training program for general practitioners: a Norwegian experience. *Family Practice* **5**, 244–52.
21. **Oxman, A.D., Thomson, A., Davis, D., and Haynes, R.** (1995). No magic bullets: a systematic review of 102 trials of interventions to improve professional practice. *Canadian Medical Association Journal* **153**, 1423–31.
22. **Cantillon, P. and Jones, R.** (1999). Does continuing medical education in general practice make a difference? *British Medical Journal* **318**, 1276–9.

Further reading

Boaden, N. and Bligh, J. *Community-Based Medical Education.* London: Arnold, 1999.

Hall, M., Dwyer, D., and Lewis, T., ed. *The GP Training Handbook* 3rd edn. Oxford: Blackwell Science, 1999.

Hays, R.B. *Practice-Based Teaching: A Guide for General Practitioners.* Melbourne: Eruditions Publishing, 1999.

15.3 The professional development of the family physician: managing knowledge

David Davis and Michael Francis Evans

> If the physician were to fail to learn after graduation, how sad for [his] patients, how sad for himself
>
> Paraphrased from Sr. Wm. Osler, London, England, 1901

If the quote we have used to begin this chapter were true over a century ago, how much more true we wonder, would it be today?

In this chapter, we discuss the subject of physician learning and change from a variety of perspectives. First, we define pertinent concepts. Second, we examine the self-evident but often underestimated need for continuing education among primary care practitioners. Third, we outline methods to determine physicians' learning needs and the tools to meet them. In particular, we sketch, compare, and contrast many of the current methods of learning. We end by examining the issue of evaluation—how can the primary care practitioner determine if this educational process is effective?

Definitions: the scope of physician learning and change

Several concepts require defining at the outset of this chapter to clarify and contextualize the ideas to be discussed. These terms represent a progression in the evolution of thinking about the learning strategies required by today's primary care practitioners.

Continuing medical education

Continuing medical education (CME) was defined by the American Medical Association in the 1970s, as 'any and all ways by which physicians learn and change'. The term emphasizes the clinical nature of the content of learning and is frequently associated with a lecture or conference format.

Continuing professional development

Continuing professional development (CPD) offers a richer array of educational content and learning activities. In addition to specific clinical subject matter, CPD also encompasses 'non-traditional' topics such as management skills, ethnicity and its role in practice, and ethical decision-making. The growing body of knowledge indicating that further learning in these diverse areas improves patient outcomes in the primary care setting reinforces the need for this expanded approach. The word 'development' implies a broader range of learning activities; not excluding the lecture as an educational medium, CPD may also utilize strategies such as self-reflection, interaction with patients and colleagues, and community-based activities, in which personal learning and growth may occur.

Knowledge translation/management

It has been customary (though incorrect) to view knowledge transfer to practitioners as a linear and simple progression as outlined in Fig. 1.

The first step, research data, resides with basic and applied health science researchers. The second step, the review, distillation, and synthesis of findings, is driven by the work of clinical epidemiologists and other critical appraisal experts, national specialty societies, groups such as the Cochrane Collaborative[1] and the evidence-based care movement itself (see Chapter 14). The third phase, dissemination of information to practitioners, has largely

Research data → Review, distillation, and synthesis of findings → Dissemination
→ Implementation → Improved practitioner performance and health care outcomes

Fig. 1 The knowledge creation to health care outcomes process.

been undertaken by national specialty societies and advocacy groups, through the distribution of paper-based guidelines. This output has been enormous as evidenced by a recent search on congestive heart failure guidelines that produced over 1100 examples,[2] with variable quality.[3] To a lesser extent, continuing professional education (CE or CPE) providers have dissemina-ted findings through venues such as conferences, conventions, and rounds.

It is the fourth step, implementation, that has been widely neglected by both clinicians and continuing education providers.[4] With the exception of the quality improvement collaborative[5] and the outcomes-oriented educational interventions initiative,[6] few concerted efforts to translate knowledge into practice have been undertaken. This phenomenon is reflected in a study of US family doctors, in which participants did not pursue answers to the majority of their clinical questions, and spent on average less than 2 min seeking an answer to those they did.[7] Studies have found that clinical practice guidelines disseminated by traditional means such as mailed materials or didactic lectures have had minimal impact on performance or improved health care outcomes.[8] While the guideline movement has promoted the importance of assessing evidence as a first step and putting it in a well formatted document, guidelines often do little for making the targets set out in the document easier to achieve. The significance of this issue may depend on the topic, as an anti-infective guideline may initiate improved prescribing whereas a diabetes guideline that tells the reader to do systematic foot care does little to enable this activity. In the latter example, a flow chart may be a better intervention (see Chapters 13.4 and 13.5).

Innovative thinking and strategies are needed to address this gap from knowledge to practice. The following terms and definitions delineate this progressive approach to physician learning and change:

- *Knowledge translation* refers to the transfer of evidence-based information into optimal performance and health care outcomes in the primary care setting.
- *Knowledge management* refers to the awareness of gaps between usual and best practice, and the judicious search for, and application of, appropriately packaged evidence-based knowledge products to provide solutions for these gaps.

It is our belief that the clinician who can utilize multiple high quality knowledge products, rather than the 'clinical epidemiologist', will be the foremost evidence-based practitioner in the emerging knowledge management paradigm.[9]

The need for learning: the gap between knowledge and practice

Studies in health services research and continuing professional development demonstrate that a sizable gap exists between the findings of basic and clinical research and actual clinical practice. In cardiology alone, gaps exist in the primary care treatment of congestive heart failure,[10] management of post myocardial infarction,[11] lowering of lipids[12] and in addressing risk factors for cardiac disease.[13] Similar gaps occur in other areas of health care delivery, described by Chassin and Galvin[14] as significant and sizable instances of misuse, underuse, and overuse, yet the cardiology example amplifies the chasm between good and best practice given the many high-quality trials in this field. If we look at other common problems (dizziness, anxiety, medically unexplained symptoms, incontinence, among many) where fewer randomized controlled trials exist, the disparity grows even further. This also reflects the current weighting of resources towards conditions or strategies in which a high agreement and certainty exist;[15]

this may represent the minority, rather than the majority, of primary care practice.[16]

In response to the issues outlined above, it is essential to study new strategies to facilitate knowledge management. For example, an initiative directed at family doctors elucidating the lack of efficacy of antibiotics for common upper respiratory conditions (e.g. bronchitis, pharyngitis), which previously focused on knowledge issues, might also review the evidence regarding the actual problem in the clinic (e.g. perceived patient desire for a prescription, differentiating a high likelihood of a bacterial infection, etc.). Such an approach could include a review of trials on effectiveness of delayed prescriptions[17] or the diagnostic accuracy of a 'strep throat score'.[18] This might be further enhanced by providing enabling tools such as a plastic score card or wallchart, a patient handout, or office systems advice.

Despite the promise of informatics and other innovations, the field characterized by the phrase 'knowledge translation' suffers from numerous difficulties. First, it lacks transdisciplinarity: few fora exist to formulate shared research findings across disciplines such as psychology, computer sciences, electrical/computer engineering, sociology, education, information and communication technologies, health sciences, bioethics, clinical epidemiology. Second, no rigorously tested, common, transtheoretical research framework exists—making comparisons across studies difficult, and progressive, iterative research virtually impossible.

Assessing needs

The journey towards knowledge management, enhanced competence and optimal patient outcomes begins with the first step of determining learning needs. These needs are commonly referred to as gaps in knowledge, skills, or attitudes.[19] They may be small gaps that occur on a regular basis and are easily corrected (e.g. by checking on a drug dosage in a local formulary), or larger gaps that are more difficult to modify. These gaps may be divided into those that are perceived, and those that are unperceived, by the physician. Gaps are not necessarily more evident to content experts or specialists ('if the family doctor only knew what I know they would improve their practice') as the barrier may be of a very different nature. For example, practitioners may be reluctant to jeopardize their relationship with a patient to invoke an evidence-based recommendation.[20] In fact, a recent qualitative study conducted with a random sampling of 50 GPs and 50 consultants by Allery et al.[21] revealed that education was involved in only about a third of changes in clinical practice.

A variety of tools exist to assist primary care physicians identify their needs. Based on a model developed elsewhere,[22] we outline such tools by the degree to which they reflect subjective and objective needs, recognizing that there is a large degree of overlap between these two categories (Fig. 2).

Subjective needs assessment tools

- Practice reflection (e.g. MainPRO-C)
- Continuous quality improvement utilizing informal and more objective methods (below)
- Learning/question logs (MOCOMP examples)[23]
- Use of standard CME materials (conferences, courses, journals) to scan for new information gaps
- Discussion with colleagues, consultants, peers, patients

Objective needs assessment tools

- Chart audit—informal, with/without colleagues[24,25]
- Formal survey methods
- Qualitative methods
- Utilization review (drug prescribing, insurance data, performance review data)
- Patient outcomes—clinical and opinion surveys
- Standardized patient (both blinded and unblinded)

Fig. 2 Tools to help the primary care practitioner to determine learning needs.

Learning strategies

Numerous innovative knowledge management strategies have been studied in an effort to address the gap between knowledge and performance; some, particularly in combination, have shown promise. The problem facing the primary care doctor in selecting a learning method or resource is similar to his or her dilemma in choosing from the amount of information available. The problem is not a lack of methods, rather a plethora. For example, learning resources include printed materials, formal educational conferences and rounds, audiovisual methods, performance feedback, academic detailing, community-based opinion leaders or educational influentials, reminders, and patient-mediated strategies. In addition, initial research on health informatics technologies that bring information to the point of curiosity has demonstrated their potential in closing the evidence-to-practice gaps,[26,27] although questions remain concerning optimal formatting of the evidence to capitalize on the benefits of technology.

The purpose of this section is to help the primary care practitioner choose between the wide variety of learning methods available and to apply the knowledge, skills or attitudes acquired in the process. To provide a framework to this process we explore two models, the PRECEDE model proposed by Green,[28] and the Awareness-to-Adherence model proposed by Pathman.[29]

PRECEDE model

Green et al's model, used in health promotion, describes three stages necessary to produce patient behaviour change. First, the intervention must *predispose* to the change, that is, provide knowledge, skills, or attitudes that provide a scaffold on which the change may be built. Second, the intervention must *enable* the change, that is, facilitate changes in the patient's environment that will support the change. Finally, it must *reinforce* or support the change made. Family physicians are familiar with this model in smoking cessation: an effective patient intervention would educate the patient about the risks of smoking, enlist family and friends in the smoking cessation process, and provide nicotine replacement strategies, and encourage feedback from family and care providers.

This model may be usefully applied to educational methods aimed at the family physician. Thus, to be effective, the strategies must also: predispose to change (by lectures, mailed materials, consultations, etc.), enable or facilitate the change (by providing patient educational materials, flow charts, and other measures), and reinforce the change (e.g. by audit and feedback or reminders). Looking for these components in any educational intervention makes good sense.

The Awareness-to-Adherence model

The Pathman model provides another way to think of educational strategies. This construct suggests that practitioners must: (i) be aware of clinical knowledge; (ii) agree that it is valid and useful; (iii) adopt the information, applying it to practice on a trial or irregular basis; and (iv) adhere to the new practice in usual care on a regular basis. This division of the learning process into four steps is useful in determining the target area for knowledge translation.

Figure 3 outlines the stages developed by Pathman et al. and educational activities that have begun to show promise at each step. Some methods which have demonstrated effectiveness (or not) at each level, and some of our 'best guesses' about which might be of most value are outlined below. While it may seem that the steps in learning and educational methods are clear-cut and non-overlapping, our intuition and common sense tell us that this is not the case.

Awareness

Traditional formal education: conferences, courses, and lectures

While many alternative learning strategies exist, the annual conference, refresher course, hospital round, and other formal CME methods form the cornerstone of most family physicians' educational activities. Several

Awareness ▶	Agreement ▶	Adoption ▶	Adherence
◆ Traditional formal courses ◆ Mailed/distributed materials ◆ Academic detailing ◆ Informatics-based educational approaches	◆ Small groups ◆ Opinion leaders ◆ Other community-based activity	◆ Skills-based workshops ◆ Feedback ◆ Practice enablers	◆ Reminder systems

Fig. 3 Translation of knowledge to practice: the four-stage Pathman model, indicating at what stage educational interventions may work best.

methods further explored elsewhere,[22] but which include examination of the learning objectives, use of handout or reinforcing materials, credibility of the sponsor and other features, can be used to help choose among these ubiquitous activities. Here we will focus on two, more evidence-based methods, interactivity and longitudinality.[30]

There is good evidence that courses that allow at least a modicum of *interactivity* are more successful at changing physician behaviour than those that do not. Such interactivity may take the form of case discussion, extensive question-and-answer or 'meet the professor' sessions, workshops, and hands-on or skill-based sessions. Similarly, course *longitudinality and sequencing*, whereby a course is offered over a period of time—for example, several evening sessions, or two half-day workshops held 1 month apart, appears to effect more change in physicians than one-time-only offerings. The success of these activities may lie in the fact that physicians have an opportunity to 'try on' new skills or knowledge, and can report their success or failure at the next course session.

Mailed materials

Like courses and conferences, mailed materials are commonplace and often ineffective strategies.[31] The trick to making their use more effective appears to reside in two domains—that of the developer and that of the learner/clinician.

In the first instance, successful print media educational resources have brief patient-management summaries that permit quick absorption by the clinician. Further, these summaries may occur in patient-friendly formats, enabling the physician to provide appropriately worded information to his or her patient. From the learner's perspective, the trick is cataloguing and referencing this material in a way that it can be retrieved at the point of need. This process may occur in a variety of ways—by photocopying a relevant summary for a patient chart, keeping file cards referencing materials by disease state or presentation symptom, or by using computer-managed lists, outlined below.

Disseminated computer-based information

Although there are relatively few rigorous studies of computer generated, non-interactive materials, it appears that they exhibit the same problems as printed materials do—dense text, content not always linked to patient problems, information not readily retrievable at the point of care, and other issues explored elsewhere in this chapter. It appears that the successful use of these materials lies in the clinician's familiarity with search strategies coupled with a healthy dose of skeptical, critical appraisal. Many search strategies and methods exist, explored elsewhere.[32]

Other methods

Other ways to disseminate knowledge, which will not be explored in detail but are noted to alert the family physician to their use and occasional effectiveness, include detail visits, audio or videotapes, and teleconferencing. These methods may suffer from deficiencies explored elsewhere in this chapter. For example, a teleconference may be entirely didactic and not based on needs, or a pharmaceutical detail visit may be more promotional than evidence-based or clinically helpful. The wise clinician will know his or her learning style and preferences and will make judicious use of these methods when and where they seem appropriate.

Agreement

Many methods can lead to dialogue and consensus among physicians, including practice reflection and collegial discussion. We explore two relatively common methods here: the use of small group learning activities and opinion leaders or community-based educational influentials.

Small group learning programmes

Small group learning, in which 6–10 family physicians discuss a medical case and apply evidence-based materials, is a well-established learning method in Canada[33] and Ireland,[34] among other countries. In at least one randomized controlled trial these programmes have displayed a positive impact on physician competence[33] and performance.[35] Their success appears to be a function of group interaction and support, availability of resource materials, meshing of research information with the realities of the local setting, with validation in practice. The ability of these groups to generate consensus about the implementation of best practices enhances their adoption.

Opinion leaders, other community-based activities

Less visible in the universe of CME resources are interventions that target communities to promote agreement with, and adoption of, guidelines. Such interventions utilize the natural connectedness and activities of community-based opinion leaders who are respected clinicians with teaching, interpersonal and clinical skill sets.[36] Broader community-based strategies such as public and patient education methods coupled with health professional educational interventions[37] are also used. Recent academic outreach initiatives have linked a local specialist with a family physician to optimize the likelihood of generating practical best practice recommendations.

Adoption

While there are many methods that help or enable family physicians to incorporate new clinical findings into their practices, we have selected two for discussion—practice-based workshops and practice enablers such as flow charts and patient educational materials.

Practice-based workshops

Workshops that provide 'hands-on' experiences to family practitioners have been effective in promoting the adoption of skills learned. Such skills may be technical such as learning to do sigmoidoscopic examinations,[38] or may be interpersonal such as improving communication strategies in health promotion.[39] We believe that the success of such workshops could be attributed to the opportunity for clinicians to 'rehearse' the activity in the safety of the training session, often through role-playing, which in turn increases their comfort and willingness to adopt the technique in the practice setting.

Practice enablers/tools

Practice enablers or tools such as flowcharts and decision aids have shown relative success in promoting behaviour change.[6] These are an often overlooked, but key part, of knowledge interventions. For example, to optimize chronic care of type 2 diabetes it may be more helpful to provide a high-quality and evidence-based flowchart than a guideline (and even more helpful to supply both).[40] The usefulness of each tool is highly topic dependent, and requires the investigator to assess not only the knowledge needs but also the barriers and solutions found in front line care. We suggest the following continuum (Fig. 4).

This figure indicates what we have learned about pathways towards community-oriented primary care, such as the need to get the facts straight, have creative marketing, enlist your end-users right from the beginning, and set realistic goals. Table 1 offers some examples of how educational interventions can be supplemented or modified to improve health care outcomes.

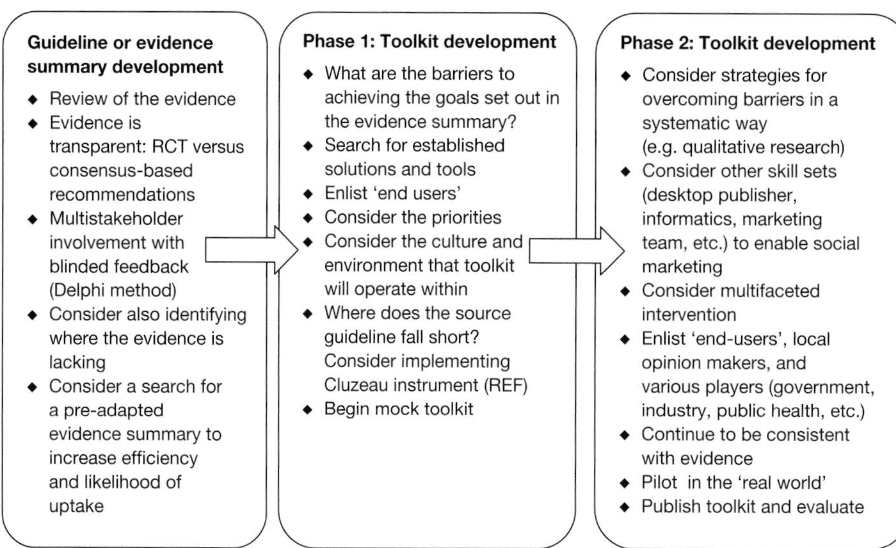

Fig. 4 An evidence-based flowchart.

Table 1 Examples of old and suggested new strategies for making evidence fit the problem

Common problem	Old knowledge intervention	Actual problem in the clinic	Examples of new knowledge intervention(s)
Antibiotics not necessary for the common cold	CME to ↑ physician awareness regarding ↓ effectiveness	Physician perceives ↑ pt. desire for antibiotics Concern that pt. may perceive poor empathy Desire to do something (physician and patient)	Public outreach with town hall meetings Unified approach with other health care givers such as local pharmacists ID new delayed R prescribing strategies (e.g. defer 'cashing in' of R prescription) New 'prescription' that acknowledges problem and gives alternate strategies
Organizing care of Type 2 Diabetes	Guidelines, CME, drug management algorithm, outline of all the systems that need to be screened	Too many things to remember to do and organize Poor patient compliance Minimal support of self management	High quality flowchart by desktop publisher Targets redefined from patient perspective and enabling self-management skills Interactive and graphical representation of guideline targets
Psychological management of depression and anxiety	Training in an inpatient psychiatric unit in residency	Too little time, too much need Opening 'Pandora's box' ↓ Formal training in cognitive–behavioural therapy RCTs do not reflect reality of clinic	Brief CBT training for FP/GPs with interest For the rest: patient-targeted CBT homework series for common problems/symptoms with a physician 'check in' sheet Improved residency training to create skill set that matches typical primary care mental health problems
Should we do a PSA test on all males >50?	Specialists or survivor groups recommending universal screening	Lack of RCT evidence of benefit and none forthcoming for 4+ years. Test has ↑ false +ve rate. However, given above, the test is acceptable to many Personal physician and patient experience with prostate cancer also important factor	Recognizing lack of evidence and developing techniques to deal with uncertainty Experimenting with an information/decision aid for consumer decision-making Encouraging public debate in the media

Adherence

While some may not consider the following methods educational, they form a necessary component of translating knowledge into practice. These interventions recognize that family physicians' practices are busy, multi-dimensional, and complex environments.

Reminders

Reminders are automatic or automated prompts which suggest actions on the part of the clinician. They may be paper-based, placed on the front of patient charts, to promote health promotion activities such as flu shots or mammography or to encourage clinical actions such as checking potassium levels when patients are taking both digitalis and diuretics. Increasingly they may also be computer-based, derived from computerized medical records data. Evidence from randomized controlled trials [41] indicates that these methods are highly effective in changing physician performance and are thus worth the effort required to establish and maintain them in the family practice setting.

Audit/feedback

Similar to reminders in their non-educational and automatic nature, feedback on performance also appears to be an effective method, though perhaps to a lesser degree.[41] Feedback may compare individual performance with that of a group or other individuals, or to established norms. By definition, specified performance indicators (e.g. prescribing rates, utilization of resources such as X-rays, patient data such as length of stay, routine preventive measures) of a peer group are recorded over a particular time period, and then compared.

Although systematic reviews of randomized controlled trials have found that the audit and feedback process is less effective than reminders,[41] they appear to be worth the effort and resources for certain situations such as disease prevention or health promotion.

'The so what?' question—assessing the impact of learning

The process of evaluating whether one's knowledge management strategies have been effective involves the same tools as used in the process of needs assessment. The question here may well be, where to start? There is a hierarchy of evaluative interventions that run the gamut from simple satisfaction surveys to sequential audits or blinded standardized patients. Choice of evaluation strategy is dependent on resources, sophistication of intervention, and outcomes that need to be improved.[42] Our bias is towards measuring outcomes that are most important to primary care clinicians and their patients.[43] We suggest a continuum of evaluation that ranges from pre-intervention qualitative research and practice patterns analysis, documentation of reflective processes in developing the educational intervention and longer-term sequential outcome assessments. These can range from self-report to more generalizable objective measures.

First, *patient outcome evaluation* may be assessed by a variety of means, such as chart audit, case-by-case review, review of errors or untoward outcomes, critical incidents, and institutional measures such as length of stay or infection rates. Second, *clinical process review* refers to physician performance, an assessment of effectiveness of process of care, which can be evaluated, for example, by measuring the percentage of a target population receiving Pap smears, mammograms, flu shots, and other preventive measures. Third, *competency assessment measures* evaluate the physician's knowledge, skills, or attitudes in a test situation. While useful tools, they are measures of what the physician *can* do rather than what he or she *does.* Fourth, a highly useful skill is *practice reflection*, a process of self analysis, which may be applied to specific learning situations, problematic outcomes, daily records, review of consultation letters from specialists, small group peer discussion, and other processes of care.

Each of these interventions should consider not only the evidence, but also the barriers in the average busy clinic. Personalized strategies to overcome these barriers need to be developed and optimized. Although assessing the evidence and barriers and creating local solutions are all keys to success, we would also add that a search for 'toolkits' to enable better practice (e.g. flow chart, decision aid, patient handout, useful website) could be most helpful to translate evidence to practice. This is an area that requires more evaluation and collation, as these types of resources are more difficult to locate using typical searching strategies such as Medline.

Conclusions

Osler's quote, over a century ago, contextualizes the role of continuing education, professional development and knowledge management in the life and career of the primary care physician. Given the rapidly expanding nature of information, the increasing knowledge base of consumers, and the mounting need to apply evidence judiciously and regularly, the family physician is in a unique position to understand and create meaningful knowledge interventions. This chapter has presented various tools to optimize educational interventions, as well as strategies for the primary care professional to maintain his or her competence and to efficiently and effectively manage knowledge, all of which enable positive health care outcomes. The unique location of family physicians at the interface of common problems and the health care consumer combined with the emerging paradigm of interventions that go beyond simply new information, provides extraordinary opportunities to delineate future pathways to improving health education models.

References

1. **Bero, L. and Rennie, D.** (1995). The Cochrane Collaboration. Preparing, maintaining, and disseminating systematic reviews of the effects of health care. *Journal of the American Medical Association* **274** (24), 1935–8.
2. **Woolf, S.H., Grol, R., Hutchinson, A., Eccles, M., and Grimshaw, J.** (1999). Clinical guidelines: potential benefits, limitations, and harms of clinical guidelines. *British Medical Journal* **318** (7182), 527–30.
3. **Shaneyfelt, T.M., Mayo-Smith, M.F., and Rothwangl, J.** (1999). Are guidelines following guidelines? The methodological quality of clinical practice guidelines in the peer-reviewed medical literature. *Journal of the American Medical Association* **281** (20), 1900–5.
4. **Grimshaw, J.M. and Russell, I.T.** (1993). Effect of clinical guidelines on medical practice: a systematic review of rigorous evaluations. *Lancet* **342** (8883), 1317–22.
5. **Batalden, P.B., Mohr, J., Strosberg, M., and Baker, G.R.** (1995). A conceptual framework for learning continual improvement in health administration education programs. *Journal of Health Administration Education* **13** (1), 67–90.
6. **Davis, D.A., Thomson, M.A., Oxman, A.D., and Haynes, R.B.** (1995). Changing physician performance. A systematic review of the effect of continuing medical education strategies. *Journal of the American Medical Association* **274** (9), 700–5.
7. **Ely, J.W., Osheroff, J.A., Ebell, M.H., Bergus, G.R., Levy, B.T., Chambliss, M.L., and Evans, E.R.** (1999). Analysis of questions asked by family doctors regarding patient care. *British Medical Journal* **319** (7206), 358–61.
8. **De Santis, G., Harvey, K.J., Howard, D., Mashford, M.L., and Moulds, R.F.** (1994). Improving the quality of antibiotic prescription patterns in general practice. The role of educational intervention. *Medical Journal of Australia* **160** (8), 502–5.
9. **Evans, M.** (2001). Creating knowledge management skills in primary care residents: a description of a new pathway to evidence-based practice. *ACP Journal Club* **135** (2), A11–12.
10. **Weil, E. and Tu, J.V.** (2001). Quality of congestive heart failure treatment at a Canadian teaching hospital. *Canadian Medical Association Journal* **165** (3), 284–7.
11. **Baillargeon, J.P., Lepage, S., Larrivee, L., Roy, M.A., Landry, S., and Maheux, P.** (2001). Intensive surveillance and treatment of dyslipidemia in the postinfarct patient: evaluation of a nurse-oriented management approach. *Canadian Journal of Cardiology* **17** (7), 767–8.
12. **Bungard, T.J., Ackman, M.L., Ho, G., and Tsuyuki, R.T.** (2000). Adequacy of anticoagulation in patients with atrial fibrillation coming to a hospital. *Pharmacotherapy* **20** (9), 1060–5.
13. **He, J., Ogden, L.G., Bazzano, L.A., Vupputuri, S., Loria, C., and Whelton, P.K.** (2001). Risk factors for congestive heart failure in US men and women: NHANES I epidemiologic follow-up study. *Archives of Internal Medicine* **161** (7), 996–1002.
14. **Chassin, M.R. and Galvin, R.W.** (1998). The urgent need to improve health care quality. Institute of Medicine National Roundtable on Health Care Quality. *Journal of the American Medical Association* **280** (11), 1000–5.
15. **Plsek, P.E. and Greenhalgh, T.** (2001). Complexity science: the challenge of complexity in health care. *British Medical Journal* **323** (7313), 625–8.

16. **McColl, A. and Roland, M.** (2000). Clinical governance in primary care: knowledge and information for clinical governance. *British Medical Journal* **321** (7265), 871–4.
17. **Dowell, J., Pitkethly, M., Bain, J., and Martin, S.** (2001). A randomised controlled trial of delayed antibiotic prescribing as a strategy for managing uncomplicated respiratory tract infection in primary care. *British Journal of General Practice* **51** (464), 200–5.
18. **McIsaac, W.J., Goel, V., To, T., and Low, D.E.** (2000). The validity of a sore throat score in family practice. *Canadian Medical Association Journal* **163** (7), 811–15.
19. **Moore, D.E. Jr.** (1998). Needs assessment in the new health care environment: combining discrepancy analysis and outcomes to create more effective CME. *The Journal of Continuing Education in Health Professions* **18** (3), 133–41.
20. **Freeman, A.C. and Sweeney, K.** (2001). Why general practitioners do not implement evidence: qualitative study. *British Medical Journal* **323** (7321), 1100–2.
21. **Allery, L.A., Owen, P.A., and Robling, M.R.** (1997). Why general practitioners and consultants change their clinical practice: a critical incident study. *British Medical Journal* **314** (7084), 870–4.
22. **Davis, D.A. and Thomson O'Brien, M.A.** (1998). Continuing medical education as a means of lifelong learning. In *Evidence Based Practice in Primary Care* (ed. C. Silagy and A. Haines), London: BMJ Publishing Group.
23. **Campbell, C., Parboosingh, J., Gondocz, T., Babitskaya, G., and Pham, B.** (1999). A study of the factors that influence physicians' commitments to change their practices using learning diaries. *Academic Medicine* **74** (Suppl. 10), S34–6.
24. **Hanna, E., Premi, J., and Turnbull, J.** (2000). Results of remedial continuing medical education in dyscompetent physicians. *Academic Medicine* **75** (2), 174–6.
25. **Bordley, W.C., Chelminski, A., Margolis, P.A., Kraus, R., Szilagyi, P.G., and Vann, J.J.** (2000). The effect of audit and feedback on immunization delivery: a systematic review. *American Journal of Preventive Medicine* **18** (4), 343–50.
26. **Jadad, A.R. and Haynes, R.B.** (1998). The Cochrane Collaboration—advances and challenges in improving evidence-based decision making. *Medical Decision Making* **18** (1), 2–9; discussion 16–18.
27. **Jadad, A.R., Haynes, R.B., Hunt, D., and Browman, G.P.** (2000). The Internet and evidence-based decision-making: a needed synergy for efficient knowledge management in health care. *Canadian Medical Association Journal* **162** (3), 362–5.
28. **Green, L.W., Kreuter, M., Deeds, S., and Partridge, K.** *Health Education Planning: A Diagnostic Approach.* Palo Alto CA: Mayfield Press, 1980.
29. **Pathman, D.E., Konrad, T.R., Freed, G.L., Freeman, V.A., and Koch, G.G.** (1996). The awareness-to-adherence model of the steps to clinical guideline compliance. The case of pediatric vaccine recommendations. *Medical Care* **34** (9), 873–89.
30. **Davis, D., O'Brien, M.A., Freemantle, N., Wolf, F.M., Mazmanian, P., and Taylor-Vaisey, A.** (1999). Impact of formal continuing medical education: do conferences, workshops, rounds, and other traditional continuing education activities change physician behavior or health care outcomes? *Journal of the American Medical Association* **282** (9), 867–74.
31. **Evans, C.E., Haynes, R.B., Birkett, N.J., Gilbert, J.R., Taylor, D.W., Sackett, D.L., Johnston, M.E., and Hewson, S.A.** (1986). Does a mailed continuing education program improve physician performance? Results of a randomized trial in antihypertensive care. *Journal of the American Medical Association* **255** (4), 501–4.
32. **Haynes, R.B., Wilczynski, N., McKibbon, K.A., Walker, C.J., and Sinclair, J.C.** (1994). Developing optimal search strategies for detecting clinically sound studies in MEDLINE. *Journal of the American Medical Informatics Association* **1**, 447–58.
33. **Premi, J., Shannon, S., Hartwick, K., Lamb, S., Wakefield, J., and Williams, J.** (1994). Practice-based small-group CME. *Academic Medicine* **69** (10), 800–2.
34. **Murphy, A.W., Bury, G., and Dowling, E.J.** (1995). Teaching immediate cardiac care to general practitioners: a faculty-based approach. *Medical Education* **29**, 154–8.
35. **Jennett, P.A., Wilson, T.W., Hayton, R.C., Mainprize, G.W., and Laxdal, O.E.** (1989). Desirable behaviors in the office management of hypertension addressed through continuing medical education. *Canadian Journal of Public Health* **80** (5), 359–62.
36. **Stross, J.K.** (1996). The educationally influential physician. *The Journal of Continuing Education in Health Professions* **16** (3), 167–72.
37. **Stewart, J., Dunn, L., and Pilla, J.** (2000). The PACCT project. Pilot study for appropriate anti-infective community therapy. Effect of a guideline-based strategy to optimize use of antibiotics. *Canadian Family Physician* **46** (4), 851.
38. **Perera, D.R., LoGerfo, J.P., Shulenberger, E., Ylvisaker, J.T., and Kirz, H.L.** (1983). Teaching sigmoidoscopy to primary care physicians: a controlled study of continuing medical education. *Journal of Family Practice* **16** (4), 785–8.
39. **Lindsay, E.A., Wilson, D.M., Best, J.A., Willms, D.G., Singer, J., Gilbert, J.R., and Taylor, D.W.** (1989). A randomized trial of physician training for smoking cessation. *American Journal of Health Promotion* **3** (3), 11–18.
40. **Davis, D.A. and Taylor-Vaisey, A.** (1997). Translating guidelines into practice. A systematic review of theoretic concepts, practical experience and research evidence in the adoption of clinical practice guidelines. *Canadian Medical Association Journal* **157** (4), 408–16.
41. **Oxman, A.D., Thomson, M.A., Davis, D.A., and Haynes, R.B.** (1995). No magic bullets: a systematic review of 102 trials of interventions to improve professional practice. *Canadian Medical Association Journal* **153** (10), 1423–31.
42. **Grol, R., Dalhuijsen, J., Thomas, S., Veld, C., Rutten, G., and Mokkink, H.** (1998). Attributes of clinical guidelines that influence use of guidelines in general practice: observational study. *British Medical Journal* **317** (7162), 858–61.
43. **Slawson, D.C. and Shaughnessy, A.F.** (1997). Obtaining useful information from expert based sources. *British Medical Journal* **314** (7085), 947–9.

15.4 Personal growth and professional development

Colin Coles

Introduction

In this chapter, the twin concepts of personal growth and professional development will be examined. In many ways this is timely since governments worldwide are devising largely regulatory ways of 'driving up' and sustaining the quality of health care that health professionals provide.[1] However, a theme running throughout the discussion here will be that political pressure for what has been termed 'accountability' of the professions has led to a distortion of the means whereby this can be realized, and in the process has created a distancing of the professions not just from politicians but through them from society itself, the members of which are the primary focus for any caring professional.

In contrast to this 'top-down' view of professional accountability, arguments will be presented for an alternative approach—one which provides health professionals with the means whereby they are able to give more clearly an account of what it is that makes them truly professional and through that develop their own professional practice.[2]

The chapter draws on a wide range of literature that is both international and burgeoning. It seems that professional people feel they have something to say—and that they must say it now. Throughout the discussion, the term 'professional' will be used to refer to all those who work in this way within a primary care setting.

The nature of professional practice: what do health care professionals actually do?

The starting point for this discussion is an examination of what health care professionals actually do, that is to address the question: what does it mean to practise professionally?

Society asks certain of its members to provide a particular kind of service for them in a professional manner. To be professional is to act in ways that others cannot, or choose not to act. And professionals are able to do this because they have become, through an extended period of development, members of a community. They have taken on the traditions of a profession. As Carr[3] puts it:

> To 'practise'... is always to act within a tradition, and it is only by submitting to its authority that practitioners can begin to acquire the practical knowledge and standards of excellence by means of which their own practical competence can be judged (pp. 68–9).

Another writer has noted.[4]

> Professionalism ... is not just any kind of work ... [It] is esoteric, complex and discretionary in character: it requires theoretical knowledge, skill, and judgement that ordinary people do not possess, may not wholly comprehend and cannot readily evaluate ... The work they do is believed to be especially important for the well-being of individuals or society at large, having a value so special that money cannot serve as its sole measure ... It is the capacity to perform that special kind of work which distinguishes those who are professional from most other workers (p. 200).

Over the past decade or so, many writers have emphasized that professional practice involves dealing with complex, unpredictable situations.[5–7] The kinds of problems that professionals are faced with are often 'indeterminate'—they have no clear or precise solution. It was Schön[5] who coined the term 'the swampy lowlands' to characterize what health professionals only too clearly perceive as their work!

These writers agree that professional practice is located in what some refer to as the 'zone of complexity', where uncertainty is high and agreement low, leading one writer[8] to define professional practice as:

> The exercise of discretion, on behalf of another, in situations of uncertainty.

Now, immediately, this challenges current ideology. Much of today's emphasis on 'quality' in health care assumes that there are clear answers to the problems that patients present. A natural extension of this view is that these 'answers' can be identified, written down, passed on, and 'applied' by health professionals—professionalism by protocol. And if there are no answers at present, then sustained scientific research will eventually find them.

However, the very essence of professional practice is that it involves making judgements. This is not to say that every situation is uncertain—some will be routine. Rather, a professional is required when the situation is not routine, and discretion is required. When one is 'being professional' there are no 'right' answers, only best ones.[7]

Perhaps it is truer to say that professionalism actually begins at the very moment when protocols no longer apply. While some aspects of a professional's practice inevitably entail following protocols, professionalism comes into play precisely at those moments when following the protocol is judged to be inappropriate. These are the moments in which medicine actually happens.[9] Perhaps the high point of professionalism occurs when one decides to take no action or to say nothing in a particular situation. Being professional can often mean choosing to do nothing.

Interestingly (and significantly for this discussion), a recent judicial review[10] in the United Kingdom of a homicide committed by a psychiatric patient (who at the time was being supervised in the community by a psychiatrist) supported this view:

> Each decision made in the care and treatment of a mentally disordered patient involves risk ... There are no simple answers. The complexity and the difficulty of the balancing exercise which clinicians have to make daily as the guardians of the patient's health and the public safety, should not be underestimated ... Clinicians are often placed in an invidious position forced to choose between options which are not ideal ... Even the most eminent can be tested to the utmost of their skill and occasionally fail (p. 2).

With this in mind, it is perhaps encouraging for health professionals in the United Kingdom that the draft proposals by the General Medical Council for revalidation[11] speak of the need for 'a new approach to professionalism ... which ... recognises the inevitability of error in a judgement-based discipline like medicine' (p. 5).

Schön suggested[5] that there are two contrasting views of professional practice in contemporary thinking. On the one hand, there are those who see professionalism as a technical matter (which he calls a 'technical/rational' view of professionalism) whilst on the other hand, there are those who see professionalism as more like artistry. The 'technical/rational' view holds that medicine is an instrumental act, where there are 'right' answers, and clear solutions to clinical problems:

> It views professional practice as a basic matter of delivering a service to clients through a pre-determined set of clear-cut routines and behaviours ... As being able to cut down considerably the risks incurred when professionals make more of their own decisions (ref. 2, pp. 31–2).

The artistry perspective, however, sees this as a deficit view of professional practice:

> Professional practice involves a more complex and less certain 'real world' in which, daily, the professional is involved in making many complex decisions, relying on a mixture of professional judgement, intuition and common sense, and that these activities are not able to be set down in absolute routines, or be made visible in simple terms, and certainly not able to be measured, and which because of this are extremely difficult to teach and to research (ref. 2, p. 32).

The nature of professional knowledge: what enables health professionals to do what they do?

It is now well established[6] that there are different kinds of knowledge. A knowledge of facts—when we 'know' *that* something is the case—is sometimes called 'propositional' knowledge. Skills, on the other hand, require a different kind of knowing, sometimes called 'procedural' knowledge—we know *how* to do something. However, professional judgement— the exercise of discretion in situations of uncertainty—requires yet another kind of knowledge. Epstein describes this in the following way:[12]

> Clinical judgement is based on both explicit and tacit knowledge. Medical decision making ... is often presented only as the conscious application to the patient's problem of explicitly defined rules and objectively verifiable data ... Seasoned practitioners also apply to their practice a large body of knowledge, skills, values and experiences that are not explicitly stated by or known to them ... While explicit elements of practice are taught formally, tacit elements are usually learned during observation and practice. Often, excellent clinicians are less able to articulate what they do than others who observe them (p. 834).

The work of Freidson, cited earlier,[4] also makes clear that a professional's knowledge base may not always be wholly comprehended or readily evaluated. As others too have remarked,[13] much professional knowledge is 'intuitive', and that in a very real sense health professionals may not always know what they are doing!

Referring back to Aristotle's thinking suggests that the kind of knowledge that enables 'making action' (*poesis*) is what he called *techne* (which we would understand today as 'technical knowledge') but that the kind of knowledge that underpins *praxis* (or professional action) is what he called *phronesis* (which today we might term 'practical wisdom').[3] Here, too, the distinction Schön makes between a 'technical/rational' and an 'artistry' view of professionalism is helpful: *Techne* underpins the 'technical/rational' view whilst *phronesis* and 'artistry' are synonymous.

Modern writers[3,7] have revived the concept of 'practical wisdom' to defend (and to some extent to rescue in a world where professionalism appears to be under threat) the notion of being professional. Carr, for example, writes that practical wisdom is ....

> ... a form of reasoning in which choice, deliberation and practical judgement play a crucial role ... [It is] a way of resolving those moral dilemmas which occur when different ethically desirable ends entail different, and perhaps incompatible, courses of action' (ref. 3, pp. 70–1).

Following Aristotle, Carr asserts that practical wisdom is 'the supreme intellectual virtue and an indispensable feature of practice' (ref. 3, p. 71), adding that someone who lacks *phronesis* 'may be technically accountable, but can never be morally answerable'. Carr further suggests that, because of this, professional action is not action that can be proved to be correct in some absolute sense but rather is '*reasoned* action that can be defended discursively in argument and justified as morally appropriate to the particular circumstances in which it was taken' (ref. 3, p. 71).

Put this way, 'practice' (i.e. what a health professional does in the course of his or her practice) and 'theory' (i.e. the knowledge that enables a health professional to practise) are not distinct. They are not 'separate' from one another. Theory does not 'inform' practice. Nor is it 'derived from' practice. And theory cannot be 'applied to' practice. Rather, theory and practice are, as Carr puts it, 'mutually constitutive and dialectically related' (ref. 3, p. 50)—you can only understand your practice by appreciating the theory that, *for you*, underpins it, and you can only understand the theory basis of your practice by appreciating its concrete expressions *in your own practice*. This revelation has profound implications not just for how health professionals practice but more particularly for the discussion here concerning how health professionals *learn* to practise.

The nature of professional development: how do health professionals actually learn to do what they do?

Research over the past decade in North America by Davis and his colleagues has clearly shown that health professionals change their practice[14] and improve health care[15] more as a result of informal educational processes than formal ones. More particularly, health professionals learn through holding professional conversations (where they talk professionally about their practice) with respected peers. These are the moments when professional development actually happens.

Other writers confirm this. Lave and Wenger suggest[16] there is a dynamic process here, which involves what they call absorbing and being absorbed into the practice community. Professionals not only learn *from* hearing others talk but crucially they also learn *to* talk. They acquire an understanding of what is appropriate professional thought (and hence action) in particular situations. Put another way, conversation is crucial to professional development.

A study[17] in the United Kingdom of clinical units that were highly acclaimed by hospital-based medical trainees as places to receive good training (and which the trainees saw as providing high quality health care) showed these units to be characterized by:

- a sense of community—feeling that you belonged there;
- a sense of collegiality—feeling that you were a colleague;
- a sense of criticality—feeling that anything that happened there could be openly and honestly discussed.

All of this suggests that professionals learn in and through their everyday clinical work, and as a result of the many, often informal, contacts with their professional colleagues. Professional development is a natural, and naturally occurring, phenomenon. It is the result of becoming a member of a professional community, of acquiring and accepting the traditions of that profession.

There is, of course, a problem here. If health professionals learn largely through informal means, how can society be reassured that what is being learnt is 'correct'? Carr suggests that

> ... the authoritative nature of a tradition does not make it immune to criticism. The practical knowledge made available through tradition is not mechanically or passively reproduced: it is constantly being reinterpreted and revised through dialogue and discussion about how to pursue the practical goods which constitute the tradition. It is precisely because it embodies this process of critical reconstruction that a tradition evolves and changes rather than remains static or fixed. When the ethical aims of a practice are officially deemed to be either uncontentious or impervious to rational discussion, the notions of practical knowledge and tradition will tend to be used in a wholly negative way (ref. 3, p. 69).

What Carr is arguing for here is of course professional self-regulation, and he is also challenging the competence of people outside the traditions of a profession to determine a profession's practices. There is, however, a wider implication of what he says. His claim for the right of professionals to regulate their own practice rests on an ideal (and perhaps idealized) view of professionalism—one where there is constant reinterpretation and revision of practice through continued dialogue and discussion. In short, he sees professionals developing their professionalism through what he calls 'the critical reconstruction of practice'.

There is strong support in the wider literature for this. What is termed a 'constructivist' (as compared with an 'instructivist') theory of learning[18] holds that all knowledge is 'socially constructed'. Learning occurs through interactions between people when they attempt to make sense of their experiences, clarify their confusions, and correct their misunderstandings. Indeed, learning is a two-way process: as many teachers know, they often learn through the process of teaching.

In particular, constructivist learning theories are thought to be most significant in developing the kind of knowledge that enables people to deal with complexity and uncertainty. Not just this, but these theories suggest that knowledge is temporary and dynamic, and that some things will remain unknowable.[19]

Support for Carr's view that practice develops through its critical reconstruction also comes from a very practical source. The judicial review cited earlier noted:

> ... the importance of clinicians not being so overburdened that they do not have time for mature reflection or to foster appropriately strong links with their teams (ref. 10, p. 3).

However, many health professionals will recognize that this does not always take place. A literature review[20] in the United Kingdom has identified some common features of the failure of many continuing medical education programmes and initiatives to fulfil their potential. These include:

- geographical isolation of health professionals;
- heavy service loads;
- competition with colleagues for inadequate resources;
- lack of time for study;
- CME systems that encourage compliance through external rewards (such as points or payment).

Again, the distinction between a 'technical/rational' and an artistry view of professionalism is helpful. The technical/rational view sees continuing development as 'training'—there are right answers to clinical problems, and health professionals must be told about them. It emphasizes that error is the result of individual failure to follow agreed (and often evidence-based) protocols, and that quality health care can only be achieved through tighter regulations. By contrast, the artistry view is that 'quality' is to be found within professionals, and can only develop when they unearth and explore its basis.

But there is a further and perhaps deeper problem with continuing education, which has already been alluded to here: the kind of knowledge that health professionals need in order to exercise professional judgements is, in part, 'hidden' from them. So how can this be uncovered and developed?

Personal growth and professional development

So far this chapter has shown:

- professional practice involves making judgements in situations of uncertainty;
- this requires practical wisdom;
- which is acquired largely through professional conversations with respected peers.

It has also been noted:

- much contemporary thinking (which is based on a 'technical/rational' view of professionalism) dismisses (or fails to appreciate) any of this;
- and sees the improvement of quality as a need to redress deficits in clinicians' knowledge and skill through remedial training and tighter regulatory frameworks;
- health professionals, however, are often unaware of the nature and magnitude of their acquired practical wisdom;
- and may have difficulty explaining (articulating) this to others.

These matters can be resolved by adopting a developmental rather than a regulatory approach that consciously adopts an 'artistry' view of professionalism and assumes that:

> Quality in patient ... care is not achieved by decree nor by striving to reach standards set by others ... Rather it is achieved by the endless pursuit, by each practitioner, of greater understanding and better practice (ref. 21, p. 181).

On this basis, personal growth and professional development go hand in hand, and these require the appreciation by professionals of the judgements they make in the course of their practice. The thread running through this argument is that professional practice changes when practitioners engage in 'the continuous dialectical reconstruction of knowledge and action' (ref. 3, p. 69)—a process that some writers note involves 'deliberation'.

Deliberation is more than 'reflection' on practice.[2] It is concerned with the critical *construction* of one's practice rather than merely its critical *consideration*. It focuses on 'the contestable *issues* endemic to practising as a professional' (ref. 2, p. 68). As Schwab[22] puts it:

> Deliberation is complex and arduous. It treats both ends and means and must treat them as mutually determining one another. It must try to identify, with respect to both, what facts may be relevant ... Deliberation requires consideration of the widest possible alternatives if it is to be most effective (pp. 318–19).

Deliberation is an important concept in any discussion on personal growth and professional development for three reasons. First, it is concerned with practice 'as a whole', rather than just one's own practice—that is with the critical reconsideration of the *traditions* of one's practice. Second, reconstruction fundamentally involves 'building again', and not merely the mechanical or passive reproduction of practice. Third, critical reconstruction involves a perspective beyond current practice (and even its traditions), and takes the professional into the wider consideration of his or her actions. Here not just other people's views on one's practice but also the accumulated views of the profession itself (made available largely through its literature) are taken into account in reconstructing what one does and says.

Conclusions

This chapter has drawn on current literature to develop the themes of personal growth and professional development, which are necessarily interrelated, through an examination of:

- the nature of professional practice;
- the nature of professional knowledge;
- the nature of professional development.

It has shown that professional practice in health care is often 'messy'[5] and deals with complex situations where uncertainty, fallibility and mystery[9] are the norm. This requires practitioners of all professional groups to exercise their judgement,[2] particularly when the working protocol fails to deal with the particularities of the situation that is being presented. Often in practice there are no right answers in some absolute sense,[3] only best ways of acting.[7] The special kind of knowledge that enables professionals to make these judgements has been termed 'practical wisdom',[3] and this is acquired largely through informal conversations with respected peers rather than through formal educational programmes.[14,15] These informal processes occur 'naturally', and professionals engage in them automatically and largely unknowingly.[12,13] There are, however, countervailing forces that prevent them occurring, and 'top-down' interventions (such as many of those being introduced by governments, often linked with tighter regulatory frameworks) appear to be counter-productive.[20]

Out of this discussion has emerged the need for health professionals to engage in the appreciation of their practice,[2] so as to understand more clearly the judgements they make and the wisdom that underpins them. This process has been described as 'deliberation',[2,3] which involves the critical reconstruction of practice.[3]

The concept of 'critical reconstruction' is well supported in the contemporary learning theory literature reflecting a 'social construction' view, which appears particularly appropriate in dealing with the complexity and uncertainty of clinical practice.[18]

Society needs professional people who can make judgements. Anything less is a disservice. It has been argued here that health care professionals' needs are more likely to be met through education than by regulation, and this requires personal growth linked with their professional understanding.

However, governments and some sections of the media have yet to show in their public utterances and policy frameworks that they appreciate the nature of professional practice. Therefore, it is incumbent upon professionals to give a clearer account of their practice and what fundamentally underpins it. Practical ways of achieving this are described elsewhere.[2]

References

1. For a very full contemporary review see: **Bashook, P.G., Miller, S.H., Parboosingh, J., and Horowitz, S.G.**, ed. *Credentialing Physician Specialists: A World Perspective.* Proceedings of the Conference held in Chicago, 8–10 June 2000. The Royal College of Physicians and Surgeons of Canada, and The American Board of Medical Specialties, 2000.
2. **Fish, D. and Coles, C.** *Developing Professional Judgment in Health Care: Learning through the Critical Appreciation of Practice.* Oxford: Butterworth Heinemann, 1998.
3. **Carr, W.** *For Education: Towards Critical Educational Inquiry.* Buckingham: The Open University, 1995.
4. **Freidson, E.** *Professionalism Reborn: Theory, Prophecy and Policy.* London: Policy Press, 1994.
5. **Schön, D.** *Educating the Reflective Practitioner.* London: Basic Books, 1987.
6. **Eraut, M.** *Developing Professional Knowledge and Competence.* Brighton: The Falmer Press, 1994.
7. **Tyreman, S.** (2000). Promoting critical thinking in health care: phronesis and criticality. *Medicine, Health Care and Philosophy* **3**, 117–24.
8. **Mintzberg, H.** *Structures in Fives.* New York: Prentice Hall, 1983.
9. **Gawande, A.** *Complications: A Surgeon's Notes on an Imperfect Science.* London: Profile Books, 2002.
10. **Bart, A., Kelly, H., and Devaux, M.** *The Report of the Luke Warm Luke Mental Health Inquiry.* Lambeth: Southwark & Lewisham Health Authority, 1998.

11. **General Medical Council.** *The Re-validation of Health Professionals in the United Kingdom (draft).* London: GMC, 2000.
12. **Epstein, R.M.** (1999). Mindful practice. *Journal of the American Medical Association* **282**, 833–9.
13. **Atkinson, T. and Claxton, G.** *The Intuitive Practitioner: On the Value of Not Always Knowing What One is Doing.* Buckingham: The Open University, 2000.
14. **Davis, D.A., Thomson, M.A., Oxman, A.D., and Haynes, R.B.** (1995). Changing physician performance: a systematic review of the effects of continuing medical education strategies. *Journal of the American Medical Association* **282**, 700–5.
15. **Davis. D., O'Brien, M.A.T., Freemantle, N., Wolf, F.M, Mazmaniam, P., and Taylor-Vaisey, A.** (1999). Impact of formal continuing medical education: do conferences, workshops, rounds, and other tratitional continuing education activities change physician behavior or health care outcomes? *Journal of the American Medical Association* **282**, 867–74.
16. **Lave, J. and Wenger, E.** *Situated Learning: Legitimate Peripheral Participation.* Cambridge: Cambridge University Press, 1991.
17. **Coles, C. and Mountford, D.** *Supporting Education in a Service Environment.* Winchester: Wessex Deanery for Postgraduate and Medical Education, 1999.
18. **Fraser, S.W. and Greenhalgh, T.** (2001). Coping with complexity: educating for capability. *British Medical Journal* **323**, 799–803.
19. **Plsek, P. and Greenhalgh, T.** (2001). The challenge of complexity in health care. *British Medical Journal* **323**, 625–8.
20. **Standing Committee for Postgraduate Medical and Dental Education (UK).** *Strategy for Continuing Education and Professional Development for Hospital Health Professionals and Dentists.* London: SCOPME, 1999.
21. **Fish, D. and Twinn, S.** *Quality Clinical Supervision in the Health Care Professions: Principled Approaches to Practice.* Oxford: Butterworth Heinemann, 1997.
22. **Schwab, J.J.** (1970). The practical: a language for curriculum. In *Science, Curriculum, and Liberal Education: Selected Essays* (ed. I. Westbury and N.J. Wilkof), pp. 287–321. Chicago IL: University of Chicago Press.

15.5 Reaccreditation and recertification

Adam Windak

Background

Since the late 1970s, in developed Western countries, there has been a growing concern about the quality of care provided to patients. One of the main issues is the level of competence of clinical staff, particularly of doctors. For this reason, extensive basic medical education, followed by vocational training is aimed at 'production' of competent and safe physicians. Successful completion of the training is an important event for every physician, usually meaning the beginning of a professional career at a higher level. Rapid development of medical science and technology demands from physicians further efforts to keep their knowledge, skills and attitudes up to date. To do this they follow special courses, attend conferences, read medical literature and participate in numerous other activities, termed as Continuing Medical Education (CME). However, the general public expects guarantees that professional standards of all practising physicians are monitored and secured. To answer these needs, the concept of periodic evaluation of physicians' competencies has been developed.

Terms and concepts

Certain confusion exists in the terminology related to the subject. Recertification and reaccreditation are terms used interchangeably in the literature. Revalidation, reregistration and reattestation are other terms also met in the literature, describing the issue in selected countries. Although it seems that 'reaccreditation' would be more properly used in the context of practices rather than physicians, for the purpose of this chapter all above terms will be used in relation to the process of formal recognition of previously fully licensed and vocationally trained general/family practitioners.

Society at large seeks for proof of the competence of individual physicians and of the effectiveness of services provided by them. The public does not have the ability to assess properly the quality of medical care. In general, they have to rely on the judgements of self-regulated organizations of medical professions.[1] Colleges and other professional organizations of physicians are keen to take responsibility for the process. They also want to show their commitment to assuring that the desired quality of care is provided by every physician. However, the interests of both parties can differ.[2] Patients are first of all interested in minimum standards and identification and elimination of doctors who provide services which are risky or not up to date. The profession gives priority to the achievement of optimal standards and continuing improvement of physicians' competence and performance. Although it is claimed that those two purposes need different methods, modern recertification programmes should apply techniques, allowing both—summative and formative assessment.

Recertification is a sensitive issue not only for patients and physicians. Health care administrators, insurance companies, and other payers are also strongly interested in the subject. Although it is generally accepted that professionals should play a key role in the process, other parties should stay involved to maintain transparency and, patients' public accountability. Relevant government agencies, payers' and patients representatives should contribute to the standards setting and agree on the applied methodology.

A separate issue is the credibility of the methodology used for the purpose of recertification. In general, the technique can be regarded credible when it has high validity, reliability, acceptability, feasibility, and an educational impact.[3] Validity answers the question, how far the technique allows the measurement of what it is intended to measure. Reliability means that on two separate measurements done by two independent assessors using the same methodology, identical results can be obtained. Acceptability reflects the level of acceptance of all parties involved in the process of assessment. Feasibility depends on capability to introduce the method on time and with acceptable costs. Educational impact answers the question, how far the method allows the establishment of the educational needs of the person being assessed.

Initial methods only partially fulfilled the above requirements. Written examination, based on multiple choice questions, directly checking knowledge of the physician, is one of the recertification methods widely used in the United States. In other countries, recertification relies mostly on declared or proven minimum involvement in the work in certain professional circumstances and collected credits for participation in accredited or otherwise allowed CME activities. These methods are criticized for their limited or unknown educational value.[4,5] In order to improve, many accrediting bodies give priority to CME activities requiring active participation. More credits are awarded to workshops or other forms of interactive teaching than to traditional lectures. Nevertheless, the impact of CME on daily performance or outcomes remains dubious.[6]

Individual learning portfolios and prior assessment of educational needs are used to better relate CME activities to an individual doctor's needs. However, there are studies arguing that general practitioners are unable to assess properly their knowledge, skills, and competence.[7,8] For that reason, external educational needs assessment as a part of the recertification process has been proposed.[9] Validity of recertification based on CME activities remains very low. Recently a new term—Continuing Professional Development (CPD) has been proposed, fostering the concept of educational activities more related to daily practice needs and aimed rather at enhancement of performance than improvement of competence.

Current approaches to recertification focus entirely on clinical performance, medical outcomes, and communication skills.[10] Review of clinical records, assessment of peers' opinion or patients' satisfaction surveys are techniques better reflecting the physician's performance. Review of the records can give good insight into various aspects of patient management. These include history taking, physical examination, use of diagnostic procedures, laboratory tests, prescription of drugs, or referral behaviour. Review of patients' and peers' opinion are important to assess interpersonal relationships and attitudes. Physicians often are allowed to select the colleagues to be asked for an opinion on their own competence. There is evidence that such a procedure does not affect the validity of the assessment.[11] However, some of the above techniques have been criticized for their limited validity.[12] Direct observation of a single or, even better, several consultations is a method with much higher validity in the assessment of clinicians' performance. Its value in regards to the other required features of good assessment for the purpose of recertification remains questionable. Reliability can be affected by different case-mix in every physician's practice. Acceptability may be low due to the reluctant attitude of evaluated physicians.

In many countries, participation in recertification programmes is voluntary. There are numerous incentives for physicians to take part in it. Higher status within the profession and better payment for provided services are the most direct ones. In some countries reaccreditation is obligatory and is a precondition to keeping rights to practice within specific branches of medicine or to remain on the register of the discipline. However, to reach the aims described above, coverage of all practising physicians in the country is needed. Mandatory recertification of all doctors, especially with the focus on performance, would be expensive and complicated. It seems, however, that a practical solution to this problem has been developed in Canada, where a new, stepwise procedure is proposed.[13] It is expected that the first phase, covering all doctors, would define a group of about 10–20 per cent who are at 'some to moderate risk'. This group would undergo more thorough assessment in the second phase, in order to find about 2 per cent of those at high risk. Having in mind that recertification is done periodically, usually in terms of several years, this approach seems to be feasible.

Examples of existing experience

In 1995, the European Academy of Teachers in General Practice (EURACT) conducted a survey to review the existing recertification procedures in Europe (Table 1).[14] It showed that formal programmes exist in seven out of 20 countries represented in the survey. In Norway, recertification has a relatively long tradition. It was established in 1985 as a voluntary programme. Five years later, recertification was established in the Netherlands. In some countries (Belgium, Norway) financial incentives exist to motivate physicians to take part in it. In others (Estonia, the Netherlands), failure to meet the recertification criteria results in loss of rights to work as a GP. In most countries, the process is based on credits for attendance at courses, teaching, research, quality assurance activities, and/or journal subscriptions. In some countries other formal requirements also exist. In general, recertification is present only in a few European countries and it is designed more to motivate doctors to participate regularly in CME activities than to assess their competence or performance.

In the United States, the Board Certificates, confirming high professional standards of a vocationally trained physician, are time limited, irrespective of the discipline.[15] They are valid for a period of 7–10 years, after which formal recertification is required to maintain the status. In 1969, the American Board of Family Practice was the first board in the United States to issue certificates with an expiry date. In theory, participation in the recertification programmes is voluntary, but failure can result in loss of top reimbursement fees and other privileges. There is also the great pressure of a

Table 1 Examples of recertification in Europe

Country	Responsible institution	Methods used
Belgium	GP organization	Educational credits
Estonia	Government	Recorded work as GP Educational credits Examination
Hungary	University	Educational credits Examination
Israel	GP organization	Educational credits
Norway	GP organization	Recorded work as GP Educational credits
Slovenia	GP organization	Educational credits
The Netherlands	GP organization	Recorded work as GP Educational credits

competitive market, using certification as a one of the key indicators of quality of care. Recertification is usually based on the assessment of knowledge, skills, and performance. Multiple choice question examinations, participation in accredited CME activities, and various forms of performance review are typically used. The latter includes review of medical records, assessment by peers or other health professional and recommendations from different health organizations. There is now a major movement towards the introduction of large scale, computer-based assessment techniques, already widely tested.

The Medical Council of New Zealand requires from all practising physicians proof of participation in continuing medical education.[16] In order to meet this expectation, the Royal New Zealand College of General Practitioners has established the Maintenance of Professional Standards (MOPS) programme. The 3-year programme is available to all vocationally registered general practitioners, irrespective of College membership. Participants are required to collect at least 150 credit points over 3 years. For those joining the programme in the second or third year, requirements are 100 or 50 credits, respectively. Points can be obtained from three categories of activities, namely practice review, CME, or additional professional development. Participation in MOPS is voluntary and submission of the statement, confirming successful completion of the programme, fulfils the Medical Council requirements for recertification.

Reaccreditation of primary health care physicians in Canada is conducted according to the standards set by the College of Family Physicians in Canada. Rules for specialists are established by the Royal College of Physicians and Surgeons of Canada, while standards for basic medical education are the responsibility of the Medical Council of Canada. The maintenance of proficiency programme (MAINPRO) has been established by the College of Family Physicians of Canada and is based on collection of credit points for different type of CME activities. Participation in the programme is obligatory and failure to meet its requirements can result in loss of certification.[13]

Expected development

Periodic evaluation of all vocationally trained and previously fully certified physicians is going to become a reality in many countries in the near future. In the United Kingdom, the decision has been already made. The General Medical Council has decided that after the year 2002, every doctor on the medical register will be evaluated every 5 years in order to assure the public of his/her professional standards.[17] Responsibility for revalidation of general practitioners is in hands of the Royal College of General Practitioners. Not everything has been decided and the discussion is still ongoing. The process is likely to reflect a wide range of aspects of good medical practice. These include professional values, professional relationships with patients, keeping up to date, maintenance of performance, complaints procedures, record keeping, accessibility and availability, teamwork, and effective use of resources. Revalidation is going to be carried out locally, but according to national guidelines. Groups of trained assessors—senior professionals and lay people—will review declarations submitted by physicians, presenting evidence on their good professional and clinical standards. Those who do not meet initial requirements will undergo further evaluation. Cases of severely underperforming doctors will be reported to the General Medical Council, which has the power to remove their names from the register.

Within the ongoing debate on revalidation of physicians in the United Kingdom, McKinley et al.[18] propose a model of reaccreditation combining the assessment of consultation competence and performance review. They strongly focus on the assessment of the consultation as the most important part of every doctor's activity. They recommend a methodology, based on direct observation of the consultation by two trained assessors. Every assessment would conclude with feedback to the physician and the identification of individual educational needs, followed by a plan for improvement and subsequent reassessment. For those who are unable to demonstrate the acquisition of desired competence and satisfactory performance, far-reaching consequences are predicted, including the removal from the register of practising physicians. High validity, reliability, and undoubted educational impact make the proposal interesting. However, questionable or at least unknown feasibility and acceptability make the credibility of the proposal vulnerable. Nevertheless, the scientifically founded proposal of recertification based on actual assessment of physicians in their day to day practice, deserves attention and further discussion in other countries as well.

Another development is taking place in the United States, where periodic examination is a routine part of the recertification process. Several boards, including the American Board of Family Practice, developed computer-based recertification programmes.[19] Computer-based techniques are not merely electronic versions of paper tests. They allow wide use of videotaped materials and virtual reality environments. This latter technology was originally developed to train doctors to perform minor surgery and other invasive procedures. Nowadays the same technique can be used to assess the skills of physicians.[15] Another advantage of computer-based assessment is the immediate response given to the physician being assessed.

Costs of the process

Recertification usually is very expensive. It can result in high costs to governments, purchasers of care, physicians or their associations. It is not clear how these costs should be divided between different stakeholders. Even relatively simple procedures, based on CME, require extra resources for maintenance of the accrediting bodies and databases of participating physicians. Recertification based on any direct assessment of physicians' knowledge, competence or performance is even more expensive. For example, in the United States, participation in the written examination alone, depending on the speciality, costs roughly 600–1200 dollars, paid by the physician applying for recertification.[15] Training of assessors, their remuneration, development of assessment tools, and application of the assessment techniques need serious resources, especially if the recertification is to cover all practising physicians. The expected high expenditures related to the coming revalidation in the United Kingdom, has given grounds for criticism.[20] It is foreseen that more regional advisers will be needed. Locum cover paid to general practitioners acting as assessors and costs of the time devoted by all doctors should be also taken into account.[7] In general, however, costs of recertification can be seen as a justified investment to enhance medical services and as proof of the commitment of all the parties involved to assure the public about the efforts to provide high quality of care.

The way forward

Although different concepts and solutions are discussed and often criticized, the need for recertification seems to be well understood by doctors in many countries.[21,22] Gradually patients and governments will increase the pressure to introduce it in many countries now considering the concept.

Box 1 Desired features of modern recertification programmes

- Mandatory for all practising physicians
- Based on explicit, reliable, and valid standards
- Focused on physicians' performance and medical outcomes
- Accepted by physicians, patients, and decisions makers
- Conducted in a formative manner with an exceptional use of penalties

Some desired features of recertification programmes are given in Box 1. Aims and rules should be agreed between physicians, patients, and decision makers. The profession should take a responsibility and lead the process. Input from lay people is essential to assure its credibility. Recertification should be mandatory for all practising physicians. Methods can vary from typical continuing medical education to direct assessment. In any form of assessment the focus should be on performance and medical outcomes, wherever possible. Explicit standards, criteria, and indicators must be developed, announced, and approved by all the stakeholders. Recertification must be conducted in a non-threatening, formative manner, creating the opportunity for all doctors to better recognize and answer their educational needs. Those who need it should have a chance to improve their knowledge, competence, or performance. Those severely and continuously underperforming may be penalized, in extreme cases even rejected to practice further independently.

Implementation of recertification procedures in different countries may depend on cultural, political, organizational, or financial conditions. Their exact impact on different aspects of quality of care require further research. However, it is obvious that well-designed, sensible recertification programmes can have a meaningful impact on physicians' behaviour, protecting patients from poor performance.

References

1. **Buckley, G.** (1999). Revalidation is the answer. *British Medical Journal* **319**, 1145–6.
2. **Newble, D.** (2001). GMC's proposals for revalidation. *British Medical Journal* **322**, 358.
3. **Van der Vleuten, C.P.M.** (1996). The assessment of professional competence: developments, research and practical implications. *Advances in Health Sciences Education* **1**, 41–67.
4. **Hayes, T.M.** (1995). Continuing medical education: a personal view. *British Medical Journal* **310**, 994–6.
5. **Cantillon, P. and Jones, R.** (1999). Does continuing medical education in general practice make a difference? *British Medical Journal* **318**, 1276–9.
6. **Richards, T.** (1995). Recertifying general practitioners. *British Medical Journal* **310**, 1348–9.
7. **Jansen, J.J.M., Tan, L.H.C., van der Vleuten, C.P.M., van Luijk, S.J., Rethans, J.J., and Grol, R.P.T.M.** (1995). Assessment of competence in technical clinical skills of general practitioners. *Medical Education* **29**, 247–53.
8. **Tracey, J., Arroll, B., Barham, P., and Richmond, D.** (1997). The validity of general practitioners' self assessment of knowledge: cross sectional study. *British Medical Journal* **315**, 1426–8.
9. **Norcini, J.J.** (1994). Recertification in the medical specialities. *Academic Medicine* **69**, S90–3.
10. **Wasserman, S.I., Kimball, H.R., and Duffy, F.D.** (2000). Recertification in internal medicine: a program of continuous professional development. Task Force on Recertification. *Annals of Internal Medicine* **133**, 202–8.
11. **Ramsey, P.G., Wenrich, M.D., Carline, J.D., Inui, T.S., Larson, E.B., and LoGerfo, J.P.** (1993). Use of peer ratings to evaluate physician performance. *Journal of the American Medical Association* **269**, 1655–60.

12. **Baker, R.** (1997). Pragmatic model of patient satisfaction in general practice: progress towards a theory. *Quality Health Care* **6**, 201–4.
13. **Dauphinee, W.D.** (1999). Revalidation of doctors in Canada. *British Medical Journal* **319**, 1188–90.
14. **Windak, A.** Survey of current reaccreditation and recertification procedures in Europe. Cambridge: EURACT Council, 1995.
15. **Bashook, P.G. and Parboosingh, J.** (1998). Continuing medical education: recertification and the maintenance of competence. *British Medical Journal* **316**, 545–8.
16. **Newble, D., Paget, N., and McLaren, B.** (1999). Revalidation in Australia and New Zealand: approach of Royal Australian College of Physicians. *British Medical Journal* **319**, 1185–8.
17. **Southgate, L. and Pringle, M.** (1999). Revalidation in the United Kingdom: general principles based on experience in general practice. *British Medical Journal* **319**, 1180–3.
18. **McKinley, R., Fraser, R.C., and Baker, R.** (2001). Model for directly assessing and improving clinical competence and performance in revalidation of clinicians. *British Medical Journal* **322**, 712–15.
19. **Summer, W., Truszczynski, M., and Marek, V.W.** (1996). A formal model of family medicine. *Journal of the American Board of Family Practice* **9**, 41–52.
20. **Wakeford, R.** (2000). GMC's proposals for revalidation would not be accurate, economical, or fair. *British Medical Journal* **321**, 1220.
21. **Sylvester, S.H.H.** (1993). General practitioners' attitudes to professional reaccreditation. *British Medical Journal* **306**, 912–14.
22. **Tracey, J.M., Arroll, B., and Richmond, D.E.** (1999). Attitudes to recertification measured over time using a validated semantic differential scale. *Medical Education* **33**, 327–33.

15.6 Multi-professional education

Yvonne Steinert

> It is hardly surprising that professionals who have been almost exclusively trained in isolation find it difficult to come to terms with sharing care when they finally emerge in practice.[1]

Changing patterns in clinical practice and health care delivery have led to an increasing need for integration of health and social services, and a renewed emphasis on collaboration and teamwork among health care professionals.[2] Technological and educational advances have led to significant changes in professional roles,[3] and overlapping skills and competencies have become increasingly common. Within this changing context, there is a need to produce practitioners who are able to collaborate and work together as a team, to best serve the complex needs of patients, their families, and their communities.

The goal of this chapter is to provide an overview of multi-professional education. If education is the key to expanding and changing clinical practice methods within the health care community,[4] approaches to preparing students for collaborative practice at each level of the educational spectrum must be explored.

The spectrum of multi-professional education

Multiple terms have been used to describe the concept of multi-professional education (MPE). These terms have included: multi-disciplinary education, multi-professional education, interdisciplinary education, interprofessional education, shared learning, and transprofessional education, to name a few. Although it is not the intent of this chapter to dwell on this 'terminological quagmire',[5] it is important to recognize that the different nomenclatures result, in part, from the fact that the educational philosophies underpinning the different terms comprise a range of different concepts and approaches whereby different professionals can, in some way, learn together.[6]

For the purpose of this discussion, we have chosen to use the term MPE, recognizing that the above-mentioned terms can be used interchangeably, and that the following principles are key:

1. MPE is not an end in itself, but rather a means of ensuring that health professionals can work together to meet the needs of patients and their families.[7]
2. MPE is not one entity, but should be viewed as a continuum, with a number of clearly identifiable steps.[6]
3. MPE is predicated on the belief that teamwork and collaborative practice is needed to best serve the needs and interests of the patient and the community.[8]

The World Health Organization (WHO) has defined MPE as 'the process by which a group of students (or workers) from the health-related occupations with different educational backgrounds learn together during certain periods of their education, with interaction as an important goal, to collaborate in providing promotive, preventive, curative, rehabilitative and other health-related services'.[7] Although this definition mostly refers to students working together, the value of students learning from teachers of different professional backgrounds cannot be underestimated.[6] MPE can also refer to physicians of different specialties learning together,[9] and can occur at each level of the educational spectrum: undergraduate, postgraduate, and continuing professional education.

Harden[10] has described different approaches to integrated teaching and learning with 11 steps on a continuum, from discipline or subject-based teaching at one end of the spectrum to integrated or multi-disciplinary teaching at the other. The stages in this continuum can be related to the specific learning situation and to whether students from different professions are taught together or separately. When applied to MPE, one moves along the continuum from 'a different content for each discipline, through an emphasis on similar content, to an appreciation of comparative content and the differences and similarities between the professions'.[6] In addition, one also moves from passive learning to interaction between the different professions, from theoretical learning to experience-based clinical practice, and from an awareness of the role of other professions to an appreciation of the other professions.[6] Harden's model is useful for conceptualizing the spectrum of MPE and as a tool in curriculum planning and evaluation.

In this chapter, MPE will refer to students learning together and separately, with teachers of a similar or different background, in a variety of settings and contexts, at different levels of training, with one goal in mind—to learn together in order to work together in the best interests of patients, their families, and their communities.

The goals of MPE

The need for MPE has been highlighted by many different stakeholders, which include diverse professional bodies such as the WHO and the World Federation for Medical Education (WFME). One of the key recommendations of the WFME stated that: 'MPE establishes and enhances the ethos of teamwork, and the essential collaboration of medicine with allied health personnel ... MPE will produce more effective doctors who can work as members of health care teams, with enhanced respect for colleagues, and for the benefit of patients and communities'.[11] It follows, therefore, that the primary goals of MPE are to develop:

1. Collaborative skills and the ability to work together as a team.
2. Positive attitudes and perceptions among different health care professionals.

3. A better understanding of the roles and responsibilities of other health care professionals, and an appreciation of health care delivery from diverse perspectives.
4. A common language, that will facilitate collaboration among the different members of the healthcare team and help to begin to break down certain professional boundaries.
5. Core competencies common to the different professions (e.g. skills relating to teamwork, collaboration, and communication).

In general, MPE tries to foster positive attitudes and skills related to collaboration with other health professionals[12] and the promotion of teamwork, a reality in the health care setting. It is clear that MPE is intended complement—and not replace—existing curricula, and that ideally, it will enhance and foster multi-professional *care*.

MPE at the undergraduate and postgraduate level

The literature on MPE describes diverse programmes and courses, primarily at the undergraduate and postgraduate level for students of all the health professions. Important considerations in the development of such programmes have included the setting for MPE; common content areas; learning strategies and formats; and the 'appropriate' stage of learning. Each of these issues will be addressed in some detail as they impact on programme design and delivery.

The setting for MPE

MPE programmes and activities occur in both the university and the clinical setting, using a variety of educational formats and methodologies to achieve stated goals and objectives. University based initiatives provide an opportunity for reflection and theoretical analysis,[3] and range from 1-h lectures on multi-professionalism to an entire curricula based on shared learning. Clinical (work-based) initiatives tend more towards specific tasks, and they often occur on an ad hoc basis.[3] These educational endeavours are often conducted in general and specialist practices, in the hospital and outpatient setting, and in community sites, with significant attention paid to the primary care team.[6]

Common content areas

Common content areas include knowledge (e.g. of what the other professions do), attitudes (e.g. respect, trust), and skills (e.g. communication). Not surprisingly, there has been an emphasis to date on topics where teamwork plays an important part in clinical practice and on areas or themes that cut across the boundaries of different professions.[6] Examples of such themes include medical ethics, health promotion, and palliative care. An emphasis on teamwork,[13] that includes the importance of respect, the building of trust, and the development of interpersonal skills needed to work together as a team, has also been highlighted by many authors. Other content areas of interest include population-based health, evidence-based medicine, quality assurance, medical informatics, and life-long learning skills.[9]

Learning strategies/formats

As in other areas of health professional education, the key learning strategies include: large class lectures and written materials; small group discussions; observations of clinical practice, and visits to community sites; simulation-based learning; and practice-based-initiatives.[14] Clinical skills laboratories[15] distance learning and computer-based modules[16] have also been used, but in a more limited fashion. Small group discussions are usually theme-based (e.g. focusing on the roles of health professionals or the management of pain) or case-based, promoting problem-solving and reflective skills. Practice-based learning initiatives occur more frequently at the postgraduate level and often require students to undertake assignments in their place of work.[2] Multi-disciplinary rounds and team meetings are viewed as a fundamental learning strategy for practice-based learning, as are month-long rotations or electives.

At the undergraduate level, problem-based learning initiatives have offered particular attractions as a context for MPE as they promote co-operation rather than competition among the students.[17] At the later stages of training, practice-based initiatives, with appropriate role models, have clearly been the 'method of choice'.[18] As Barr[14] has said, university-based MPE can predispose students towards collaborative practice by modifying attitudes and perceptions, whereas work-based MPE can result directly in collaborative practice, in a specific context. Practice-based initiatives also rely on what has often been called 'opportunistic teaching',[3] in that teachers must take advantage of the clinical situation and ensure that educational objectives are met in the context of patient care.

Throughout the literature, it is clear that the choice of learning strategy and format will vary with the intended goals and outcomes,[6] and the level of the student. In fact, choosing the best time for MPE continues to be a hotly debated topic.

The appropriate 'stage of learning'

As the WHO Study Group[7] has highlighted, MPE can be introduced and used with advantage at all phases of education, ranging from undergraduate to postgraduate to continuing professional education. Some educators believe that it is best to promote MPE at the beginning of undergraduate training. These health care professionals feel that it is important to start early in order to cultivate positive attitudes, limit the development of negative stereotypes,[19,20] and prevent students from becoming entrenched in a conventional professional role. As Areskog[21] has said, 'there is a belief that starting shared learning as early as possible in undergraduate courses will change negative attitudes or prevent stereotyped views from forming and that students will be better prepared for team work and collaboration after qualification'. However, others believe that students in different health professions need time to learn the basic elements of their own fields and to acquire their separate professional identities before engaging in multi-professional learning.[22] These educators suggest that MPE take place later in postgraduate training.

At present, there is little evidence to determine the most appropriate stage at which to introduce MPE.[3] Although shared learning is recognized as having short-term value through course evaluation and learner satisfaction, there is little evidence to suggest that shared learning skills can be transferred to professional practice. However, based on the limited evidence to date, it appears that formal MPE should be introduced early in undergraduate education, and that it needs to be continued—and reinforced—in postgraduate and continuing professional education, where there is a greater emphasis on 'on-the-job learning and healthcare delivery'.[6] Moreover, the integration of MPE throughout a curriculum can help to ensure continuity and a gradual progression from the simple to the more complex.[23]

The need for continuing professional development

Although the literature is replete with examples of MPE at the undergraduate and postgraduate levels of training, few professional development programmes are described; and yet, without appropriate and effective role models, teaching in this area is bound to fail.

In 1988, the WHO Study Group reported that structured teacher training programmes concerned with educational principles and application of MPE are relatively rare.[7] The situation has not changed significantly more than a decade later, and the need remains to provide teachers, in both the clinical and the classroom setting, with the knowledge, skills, and attitudes to foster MPE. In particular, training faculty for MPE needs to focus on a change in attitudes,[7] increased understanding of the roles and responsibilities of other health care professionals, and skill acquisition in the areas being taught to students. As Byrne[24] has pointed out, most teachers are products of an educational system whose perspective is limited to that of their own discipline. The majority have not trained in a multi-professional approach and many do not practice within one either. As a result, teachers may be either uncomfortable with this approach to teaching and learning or not sufficiently knowledgeable to teach within it. Faculty development programmes, in which teachers of different health professions, learn together—about teaching methods and the content of MPE—is a critical ingredient to success in this area. As the WHO Study Group has said, MPE cannot meet its desired goal or objective without first focusing on faculty development. If teachers are not given an opportunity to learn the necessary educational skills, they will revert to more conventional methods already familiar to them.[7]

Continuing professional education is closely linked to faculty development. In CME in particular, the call has gone out to general practitioners to promote team learning to meet the demands of general practice.[25] Courses have ranged from 1 h to 1 year, with the major focus being on clinical competencies.[26] Other initiatives have included modules on research methods and project work in a multi-professional context. One interesting example involves a multi-professional problem-based learning programme that was delivered to physicians, nurses, dieticians, pharmacists, and social workers, in heart health promotion.[27] This programme was developed in primary health care and its evaluation showed the benefits for collaborative teamwork and for acquiring greater understanding of the content area among all of the participants.

In reviewing the current literature, it is clear that there is a need to develop ongoing programmes in continuing professional development and to 'develop a working context in which learning together becomes a vital part of working together'.[26]

The 'evidence' for MPE

Research regarding outcomes of successful initiatives in MPE has been limited to date, and the gap between ideology and evidence has not yet been closed.[6] Currently, there is little evidence to show that when different health care professionals learn together they will be able to work together more effectively in clinical practice.[28,29] In addition, there is a lack of evidence to indicate the value of MPE to health and social care organizations and to those using them.[29]

However, currently available data do suggest that well-designed courses are able to bring about changes in knowledge, attitudes and skills at the undergraduate (pre-qualifying) level. In particular, MPE can change attitudes in a direction favourable to collaboration and teamwork,[20] can break down negative stereotypes,[21,22] and can increase understanding about the roles and responsibilities of other professionals.[30–32] Freeth and Nicol[15] have also shown that effective and well-evaluated learning of clinical skills can occur in mixed groups of medical students and nurses. However, although a change in attitudes can be achieved, it is unknown whether these changes, in fact, translate into clinical practice. This observation has been further underscored by Parsell et al.,[31] who stated that unless there is support and reinforcement of new knowledge by regular, practical experience or further shared learning, the initial gain in knowledge and skill will disappear.

Hammick[28] noted that MPE at the in-service level (where the students are qualified practitioners) is more likely to change clinical practice or benefit patients. Her review of the literature highlighted the importance of work-based initiatives, as did that of Pirrie and her colleagues.[2,22] This qualitative study found that both course organizers and students felt that MPE had its greatest 'impact' at post-registration (postgraduate and continuing professional education), when health care professionals could reflect on their practice in a clinical context.

Despite an increasing number of interesting initiatives, the literature is hampered by a lack of systematic evaluations of MPE. Many of the studies are short and often 'one off'[3] in nature, and their impact on longer-term behaviour change is impossible to verify. In fact, the majority of MPE programmes are often ad hoc and not evidence based. Clearly, there is a need for more systematic and rigorous evaluations. In addition, educators should move beyond the question of whether a particular programme is effective, and systematically assess the components of the educational process in order to determine which variables may affect outcome (e.g. location, stage of learning, student readiness).[14] As Hammick[28] has pointed out, studies must examine 'who is learning what, in what context, and with whom'. Collaboration in evaluating outcomes is also needed, and programmes must be assessed across paradigms and disciplines.[28]

In summary, there is a lack of evidence to support the assumptions that multi-professional learning in undergraduate courses will improve collaborative teamwork in practice, or that it will improve quality of care. Moreover, it appears easier to adduce evidence for the impact of MPE on attitudes (towards patient care and collaborative practice) than on outcomes (such as improved patient care).[22] However, as Hammick[28] has said, the lack of evidence of effectiveness does not imply ineffectiveness, and instead of abandoning programmes in this area, MPE initiatives must be more systematically planned and evaluated.

Examples of MPE 'in action'

As stated earlier, there are different models of MPE in undergraduate curricula, which span the continuum between total separation of disciplines through to 'true transprofessionality' where disciplines are not distinguished.[33] Important lessons can be learned from these initiatives, and several of these programmes will be described in order to demonstrate the diversity of programmes currently in place.

Pomeroy and Philp[8] developed a 1-day workshop for first-year students from nursing, medicine, occupational therapy, physiotherapy, and podiatry that focused on teamwork as an important aspect of health care delivery. During the workshop, students considered their different professional roles, how these integrated in the delivery of service, and how the team worked together to form clinical management plans. Preliminary assessment of this workshop, which was given eight times to 170 students, showed that the stated goals were achieved and that the students were very positive about this experience. In fact, they requested more joint learning activities.

Parsell and et al.[31] developed a 2-day pilot course for 28 undergraduate students from seven health care professionals in the Faculty of Medicine in Liverpool. Using small multi-professional groups, final-year students explored professional roles and clinical problem solving using a theme-based approach, with the goal of increasing the students' knowledge and understanding of the roles and attitudes of other professions. The evaluation of this course showed benefits of increased knowledge and understanding of other professionals and the development of more positive attitudes. Students also reported that they believed that early opportunities for shared learning should be an essential component of undergraduate courses. In a follow-up study, Leaviss[19] found that students' knowledge of the other professions was maintained, but that the negative attitudes towards other professionals formed in the early years of their education were not changed by this course. Changes only started to occur once the students started their clinical practices.

Freeth and Nicol[15] developed an innovative four-session course of shared learning in acute care for final-year medical students and newly qualified nurses. Student learning took place in a clinical skills laboratory and was based on a patient scenario, pertinent to the students' clinical experiences. The course was taught by teachers in medicine and in nursing, and focused on issues related to communication skills and the management of clinical problems (e.g. diabetes, pain management, cardiac arrest). Evaluations of this programme indicated short-term achievement of the educators' goals and high student and teacher satisfaction. The intensive nature of the training and time constraints were also highlighted.

A new Faculty of Health Sciences was established in 1986 in Linköping University in Sweden.[23,33] An integrated approach using problem-based learning as its main teaching method was used to deliver a multi-professional course to students from six health care disciplines. For the first 10 weeks of their courses, and prior to discipline-based studies, students from medicine, nursing, physiotherapy, occupational therapy, laboratory medicine, and social work learned together about *Man in Society*. The course was oriented towards the social and behavioural sciences in the context of health promotion, disease prevention, and a holistic view of health care. Additional shared learning occurred in the following three semesters when separate days of shared learning were arranged around common themes. Practical training also provided opportunities for students to learn together. Throughout this course, students learned through problem-based learning, using real-life clinical scenarios as the trigger for learning. Following this initiative, the course planners decided to extend this shared learning programme to the final year.

In another initiative in Linköping, Wahlström and Sanden[34] developed a programme that consisted of training in a clinical ward with orthopaedic patients where students representing all of the programmes at the Faculty of Health Sciences jointly took a major share of the primary responsibility for the examination, diagnosis, treatment, and rehabilitation of patients. This model demonstrated that education delivered in a multi-professional training ward enabled the participants to gain team-working skills.

Based on these examples, it can be seen that successful programmes build on the current practice environment, with an eye to what the future might be like, and gather support from all levels, from the leaders among the faculty to the trainees and support staff. In addition, ongoing improvements are an integral part of implementation at each institution, as barriers are recognized and addressed, as problems are acknowledged and solutions are proposed, and as the practice environment changes in response to market pressure.[9]

General educational principles

The opportunities for designing and delivering MPE programmes have clearly been highlighted in the literature. The challenges for implementing such programmes have also been described. As in all other educational endeavors, it is important to develop clear learning outcomes, to design appropriate teaching and learning strategies, and to create appropriate methods of evaluation—of both the students and the curriculum. It is equally important to integrate theory with practice, and to ensure that the learning is perceived as relevant to the work setting and to the profession. Learning should be interactive, participatory, and experientially based, using the students' previous learning and experience as a starting point. Detailed planning and organization, involving all stakeholders become even more important in this context,[31] as does institutional support for the curricular programme and learning objectives. A positive learning environment (communicating respect and understanding of similarities and differences), and 'equal' participation of all the participants, is also essential,[35] as is student 'readiness'[36] and teacher 'buy in' and commitment.

When designing MPE programmes, it is critical that teaching not occur in a vacuum and that the students (at whatever level) see the learning and teaching as 'real'. Students need to witness teams in action, to participate in clinical and community experiences, and to observe appropriate role models. As Carpenter and Hewstone[35] have so eloquently said, 'students must observe other professionals working as equals, and they must view the members of the team as typical, not just exceptions to the stereotype'. At a more global level, it is important that the health care delivery system reinforce the educational mission, and that the educational programme supports the health care system.

Finally, it is important to overcome commonly encountered difficulties. Common obstacles have been identified as organizational, structural, and attitudinal,[36] with attitudes being the most difficult to change. However, for a course or curriculum to succeed, organizers must pay scrupulous attention to logistical details[3] that are often used as a reason not to engage in MPE.

The ingredients for success include institutional support, 'equal status' of the participants, positive expectations, a cooperative atmosphere, and concern for differences and similarities.[3] However, putting ideology and theory into practice remains a challenge.

Conclusions

MPE is based on the assumption that bringing students together will enhance their future collaborative practices.[22] It is widely assumed that learning together is a necessary and sufficient precondition for working together. However, although the rationale for MPE appears self-evident, the evidence for its effectiveness in clinical practice is lacking. There is clearly a need for increased evaluations of programme initiatives, as changes in the delivery of health care require greater collaboration across different health professions.

Although the most appropriate 'timing' for MPE has not yet been determined, it appears that training in teamwork, collaboration, and communication is key. Training modalities should include more didactic formats, to provide a basic foundation, and experiential learning, to allow the individual to integrate the knowledge, attitudes, and skills required to practice in a collaborative fashion.[9] The educational system needs to prepare students at every level of the continuum to meet the challenges of the future. MPE is one way by which to achieve this goal, as it encourages health care professionals to learn together and to work together in order to meet the needs and interests of patients, their families, and their communities.

References

1. **Gray, P.** (1986). (Preface) *Working Together—Learning Together* (ed. R. Jones), Exeter: Royal College of General Practitioners, Occasional Paper No. 33.
2. **Pirrie, A.** et al. *Evaluating Multidisciplinary Education in Health Care*. Edinburgh: Scottish Council for Research in Education, 1998.
3. **Cable, S.** (2001). Multi-professional education. In *A Practical Guide for Medical Teachers* (ed. J.A. Dent and R.M. Harden), pp. 180–91. Edinburgh: Churchill Livingstone.
4. **Majumdar, B., Dye, P., and Ellis, S.** (1998). The use of problem-based learning within a multi-professional curriculum. *Newsletter of the Network of Community Orientated Educational Institutions for Health Sciences* **28**, 20–1.
5. **Leathard, A.** (1991). Going interdisciplinary. *Nursing* **4**, 9–11.
6. **Harden, R.M.** (1998). AMEE guide no. 12: Multi-professional education: Part 1—effective multi-professional education: a three-dimensional perspective. *Medical Teacher* **20**, 402–8.
7. **World Health Organization.** *Learning Together to Work Together for Health*. Report of a WHO Study Group on multi-professional education of health personnel: the team approach. WHO Technical Report Series 769, Geneva: WHO, 1988.
8. **Pomeroy, V.M. and Philp, I.** (1994). Healthcare teams: an interdisciplinary workshop for undergraduates. *Medical Teacher* **16**, 341–6.
9. **Ramsbottom-Lucier, M., Pregler, J., and Gomez, A.G.** (1999). Challenges in medical education: training physicians to work collaboratively. *Journal of General Internal Medicine* **14** (Suppl. 1), S21–5.
10. **Harden, R.M.** (2000). The integration ladder: a tool for curriculum planning and evaluation. *Medical Education* **34**, 551–7.
11. **The World Summit on Medical Education** (1993). Recommendations. *Medical Education* **28** (Suppl. 1), 142–9.
12. **Wahlström, O., Sanden, I., and Hammar, M.** (1997). Multi-professional education in the medical curriculum. *Medical Education* **31**, 425–9.

13. **Parsell, G. and Bligh, J.** (1998). Interprofessional learning. *Postgraduate Medical Journal* **74**, 89–95.
14. **Barr, H.** (1996). Ends and means in interprofessional education: towards a typology. *Education for Health* **9**, 341–52.
15. **Freeth, D. and Nicol, M.** (1998). Learning clinical skills: an interprofessional approach. *Nurse Education Today* **18**, 455–61.
16. **Stumpf, S.H. and Clark, J.Z.** (1999). The promise and pragmatism of interdisciplinary education. *Journal of Allied Health* **28**, 30–2.
17. **Brandon, J.E. and Majumdar, B.** (1997). An introduction and evaluation of problem-based learning in health professions education. *Family Community Health* **20**, 1–15.
18. **Barr, H. and Waterton, S.** *Interprofessional Education in Health and Social Care in the United Kingdom.* London: The UK Center for the Advancement of Interprofessional Education, 1996.
19. **Leaviss, J.** (2000). Exploring the perceived effect of an undergraduate multi-professional educational intervention. *Medical Education* **34**, 483–6.
20. **Horder, J.** (1996). The Centre for the Advancement of Interprofessional Education. *Education for Health* **9**, 397–400.
21. **Areskog, N.H.** (1988). The need for multi-professional health education in undergraduate studies. *Medical Education* **22**, 251–2.
22. **Pirrie, A.** et al. (1998). AMEE guide no. 12: Multi-professional education: Part 2—promoting cohesive practice in health care. *Medical Teacher* **20**, 409–16.
23. **Areskog, N.H.** (1994). Multi-professional education at the undergraduate level: the Linköping experience. *Journal of Interprofessional Care* **8**, 279–82.
24. **Byrne, C.** (1991). Interdisciplinary education in undergraduate health sciences, *Pedagogue* **3**, 1–3.
25. **Irvine, D.** (1993). Educating general practitioners. *British Medical Journal* **307**, 696–7.
26. **Parsell, G. and Bligh, J.** (1998). Educational principles underpinning successful shared learning. *Medical Teacher* **20**, 522–9.
27. **Mann, K.** et al. (1996). Multidisciplinary learning in continuous professional education: the Heart Health Nova Scotia experience. *Journal of Continuing Education in the Health Professions* **16**, 50–60.
28. **Hammick, M.** (2000). Interprofessional education: evidence form the past to guide the future. *Medical Teacher* **22**, 461–7.
29. **Zwarenstein, M.** et al. (1999). A systematic review of interprofessional education. *Journal of Interprofessional Care* **13**, 417–24.
30. **Carpenter, J.** (1995). Interprofessional education for medicine and nursing students: evaluation of a programme. *Medical Education* **29**, 265–72.
31. **Parsell, G., Spalding, R., and Bligh, J.** (1998). Shared goals, shared learning: evaluation of a multi-professional course for undergraduate students. *Medical Education* **32**, 304–11.
32. **Roberts, C., Howe, A., Winterburn, S., and Fox, N.** (2000). Not so easy as it sounds: a qualitative study of a shared learning project between medical and nursing undergraduate students. *Medical Teacher* **22**, 386–91.
33. **Davidson, L. and Lucas, J.** (1995). Multi-professional education in the undergraduate health professions curriculum: observations from Adelaide, Linköping and Salford. *Journal of Interprofessional Care* **9**, 163–76.
34. **Wahlström, O. and Sanden, I.** (1998). Multi-professional training ward at Linköping University: early experience. *Education for Health* **11**, 225–31.
35. **Carpenter, J. and Hewstone, M.** (1996). Shared learning for doctors and social workers: evaluation of a programme. *British Journal of Social Work* **26**, 239–57.
36. **Parsell, G. and Bligh, J.** (1999). The development of a questionnaire to assess the readiness of health care students for interprofessional learning (RIPLS). *Medical Education* **33**, 95–100.

15.7 Addictions and mental illness in physicians

Peter E. Mezciems

Introduction

Physicians worldwide are under increased professional stress. The field of medical knowledge is expanding as never before, as is accessibility to sources of this knowledge. Patients are armed with information and misinformation, often from potentially unreliable sources such as the Internet. In British Columbia, Canada, a job satisfaction survey of rural physicians revealed a self reported burn-out rate of 55 per cent.[(1)] A Norwegian survey found a lifetime prevalence of 'feeling that life was not worth living' of 51.1 per cent in active physicians and a 1.6 per cent rate of attempted suicide.[(2)] German physicians were found to have an increased rate over the general population of suicide, divorce, and addiction.[(3)] Similar figures have been reported in primary and secondary care in the United Kingdom. The effects of this increasing stress ripple outwards from the physician to involve family, friends, colleagues, and the ability to work.

Categories of problem physicians

Talbott, in a report to the Georgia Composite State Board of Medical Examiners,[(4)] reflects the North American experience and has put forward 12 categories of problem physicians:

1. Substance abuse;
2. Substance abuse relapse;
3. Psychiatric disorders;
4. Disruptive behaviour;
5. Sexual misconduct;
6. Dyscompetence (fading competence);
7. Inappropriate prescribing;
8. Ethical violations;
9. Physical/medical disability;
10. Age-related issues;
11. Pain and disability;
12. Infectious disease (blood borne infections—AIDS, hepatitis).

I will discuss the first three categories with brief reference to the fifth. I include all 12 categories primarily to indicate the scope of possible problems, for as Loevenich states, 'The phenomenon of mentally ill physicians is hardly noticed in Germany today—a fact that possibly indicates a taboo'.[(3)] The literature and personal communication (from physicians in Canada, the United Kingdom, Italy, and Australia), support this idea. Much of the population would prefer to deny the reality that trusted physician caretakers may suffer from emotional illness, and physicians themselves are often reluctant to become patients.[(5)]

The lifetime risk of addiction to alcohol in physicians is at least equal to that of the general population, about 6–8 per cent.[(6)] Talbott reports that the rate is higher, perhaps above 14 per cent when drug addiction is included.[(4)] The rate of mental illness in physicians seems to parallel that of the general population. Unfortunately, we are rarely taught that physicians become emotionally ill, let alone given tools to deal with stress and emotional illness in our colleagues or ourselves.

Physician-patients: rules to follow

Physicians can both cause and suffer stress when they present as patients. As the treating physician, I may feel pressured when dealing with a colleague.

I may feel inhibited by my physician-patient's medical knowledge, we may socialize together, we may share consults and patients. Rather than giving the benefit of a proper office visit, I may indulge in a hallway or backroom 'exam'. I may not appreciate that my physician-patient is likely feeling particularly 'exposed, vulnerable, and dependent'.[7]

Schneiderman[7] has recommended four rules when dealing with physicians as patients:

1. Talk to the patient, not the doctor. (We must not assume that the physician-patient is knowledgeable about illnesses.)
2. If possible, take a history from the patient's spouse as well as the patient. (Physicians tend to self-diagnose and self-treat before seeking help, and often deny or minimize their symptoms.)
3. Be clear and supportive about hospitalization. ('Suddenly being the one lying down rather than the one standing up can come as a shock to even the most experienced doctor.'[7])
4. Be frank about consultation. (Physicians will often request a degree of secrecy, particularly in cases of mental illness. This generally comes from a deep feeling of shame and fear at being perceived as inadequate or defective as a result of alcoholism, drug addiction, or other mental illness.)

Risk factors in physicians

These risk factors for susceptibility to mental illness or alcohol/drug abuse result from the demands of the medical profession as illustrated in Table 1.

The stresses from these traits and behaviour patterns increase the risk of mental illness, and abuse of, or addiction to, drugs and alcohol.

Table 1 Risk factors in physicians

A. Denial of basic needs	Sleep deprivation, excessive fatigue Meal skipping Social isolation Insufficient exercise Insufficient leisure pursuits Lack of spiritual development Valuing intellectual achievement over balanced emotional growth
B. Medical personality traits	Perfectionistic Obsessive compulsive Narcissistic Altruistic Medical idealism Intellectualization Denial
C. Professional demands	Patient care responsibility Ongoing need to accumulate knowledge Increasing knowledge base in patient population Peer competition rather than support Increasing demands, decreasing remuneration Malpractice concerns Professional role in conflict with personal life roles
D. Exposure to mood altering chemicals	Office and hospital samples of, or access to, mood altering drugs Patient returns of 'leftover' medications House calls—patients medications left out, medications in doctor's bag Direct administration of medications—emergency room, anaesthesia
E. Environment of denial	Personal – 'It can't happen to me', 'I am what I do' Family, institutional—people don't want to see Colleagues and coworkers—'the conspiracy of silence' Legal status minimizes consequences License, livelihood, sense of self perceived to be at risk
F. Poor self-care	Pattern of self-diagnosis and treatment No personal family doctor 'Corridor consultation' with colleagues Self-prescribing Resist patient role Pressures to treat family/friends

Prevention

> Mental illness is universally thought to be caused by one of three things: biological events, experiential events, or metaphysical events. The first two are the foundation for Western therapy, the third for therapy elsewhere in the world. The difference is one of degree, however. All are found in some form in almost every culture in the world. Biological causes widely believed in by people in Western cultures include genetic damage, inborn constitutional factors, biochemical and metabolic disturbances, infections, drug toxicity, and damage to the brain... Experiential causes, especially experiences in childhood, are the hallmark of psychotherapy and treatment consists of an exploration of these events... Metaphysical causes are the most important ones in most of the world: the loss of the soul; the intrusion of a spirit into the body; sorcery; angering God.[8]

In the biological realm,[8] there are things that we need to do. Regular habits—exercise, nutrition, sleep—must be a primary goal. In the real world, lives do go out of balance: babies do not wait to be delivered; emergencies do happen; on call schedules need to be covered. However, if one is living a life in balance, then there is an emotional reserve to deal with these issues, and, when appropriate, the ability to bring life back into a healthier place.

Experiential issues affect the emotional stability that we try so hard to establish. Vaillant et al. found that physicians who developed addiction to drugs or alcohol perceived their upbringing as emotionally cold and distant.[9] A universal thread in addiction and mental illness is emotional isolation from colleagues and friends.[4,9,10] In many years with my colleagues I found that the talk in the doctor's lounge centred around 'safe' topics: clinical cases, material achievement, sports, and entertainment—rarely did we discuss personal struggles. We are dedicated to taking care of others, but need to ask ourselves a simple question: 'Who takes care of me?'

The suffering physician should ask: 'When I am tired, emotionally and spiritually drained, to whom can I turn for intimate support and help? If I do not have these resources in place, why not? Do I need to pay someone as a therapist to be my intimate confidant until I develop the emotional ability to invite others into my life?' Emotional isolation begets loneliness, which intensifies psychic pain.

Socrates is thought to have been the first to say: 'the unexamined life is not worth living'. McWhinney adds insight, stating that spiritual growth 'requires self-knowledge, the most difficult and painful knowledge of all'.[11]

Healing the experiential issues is also linked with the metaphysical—healing our spirit. In Western society, the metaphysical aspect is perhaps most poorly dealt with. In your medical school, as a student or faculty, or in the school you attended years ago, how was your spirit nurtured? In the above-referenced convocation address, McWhinney quotes from a book published in 1852 by John Henry Newman, in which Newman prophesied (in reference to universities) that separation of the life of the mind from the life of the spirit would have adverse effects on both. We must periodically take time to replenish our souls—with *our* time, undisturbed, for meditation, recreation, retreats. We need to take the risk of finding out for ourselves what enables us to recharge.

Our task, if we wish to live in balance within our selves, with our fellows, and with our professional and natural worlds, is to nurture and heal our biological, experiential, and metaphysical selves. This is an inextricably linked triad—neglect of one part affects the others; improved health on one part helps heal the others. The trap is that we can neglect parts of this triad for a long time and it appears that nothing happens. Preventative work helps us to avoid this trap.

Recognition and intervention

Addiction medicine consultants talk about a 'conspiracy of silence' when it comes to our physician colleagues, meaning that when a colleague shows signs of alcoholism, drug addiction, or mental illness, we often tend to avoid, minimize, and deny these signs.

We need first to know the signs and symptoms to look for. Problems tend first to develop in intimate relationships such as the family, next evolve to affect social activities, and last show up in the workplace. The converse is that if one sees problems at work, then there has been pain and dysfunction in the family for some time.

Signs and symptoms of dysfunction

The signs and symptoms of dysfunction in physicians are illustrated in Table 2. These then are issues to be sensitive to in our colleagues and in ourselves. None of them are diagnostic of illness, but we need to be alert to the process that may be underlying the behaviour that we see. MacMillan says: 'the more unlovable and the more crazy and the more off-putting are the actions of the active addict—the more he or she *yearns* to be heard, to be understood, to be loved—and it is at this level, no other, that a therapeutic exchange may occur . . .'.

In addiction and emotional illness, as in other areas of life, change does not happen until the consequences of behaviour mount up. However, because of the issue of public safety in a physician who may have the effects of his/her illness manifest on patient care, sometimes consequences have to be put into place by colleagues, friends and family, or licensing bodies.

Talbott, in his programme in Atlanta, Georgia, was one of the earliest to codify the principles of intervention.[12,13] The entire process of intervention is described more fully in the book: *Healing the Healer*.[14] Salient points are that:

- Intervention is caring and should not be considered punitive.
- The process should wherever possible be carried out by two leaders, with objective information from, and perhaps participation by, family, friends, and colleagues.
- The goals must be clear to everyone, with a well thought out assessment and treatment plan.
- Objective relating of incidents and consequences of the individual's behaviour will have far more impact than emotional opinions.
- Denial, anger, and minimization by the individual should be anticipated.
- The intervention must be carried out in a neutral setting without external time constraints.

If this process is carried out in a caring and non-judgemental fashion, then instead of the impaired physician being shamed, he or she will emerge with some level of hope for the future. It is important that there are family or friends to support the person afterward, as this process can also be traumatic, and there is often an increase in depression with some risk of suicide until treatment can be put in place.

The family

We can view the family as the prime unit of personal interaction, usually seen either as biologic (family of origin), or consensual (nuclear family). It is important to include single parent families, same sex parents, step families, etc. In families, behaviour tends to be circular and self-reinforcing, in that one family member's behaviour impacts all of the other members in some way.

Cermak has eloquently delineated the core traits of a healthy, well-functioning family.[15] These are safety, open communication, self-care, individualized roles, continuity, respect for privacy, and focused attention.

When emotional trauma such as mental illness or addiction invades this unit, then bit by bit, the safety and support unravel.

Table 2 Signs and symptoms of dysfunction in physicians

A. In the hospital	Late rounds Poor presentations, charts, etc. Physician offers to administer medications to patients Over-prescription of medications Staff report concerns about the physician's behaviour Reports that the physician is unavailable when on call, hard to locate, or responds slowly to telephone calls or pages Reluctant to discuss self, issues, 'closed' or evasive Heavy drinking at staff functions
B. In the office	Appointments and schedule become disorganized; there is chronic lateness Hostile, withdrawn, unreasonable with staff/patients Much time 'behind locked doors' Writes prescriptions for self/office, excessive 'office supplies' of drugs Patient complaints increase Frequent absences; unexplained or frequent illness
C. In physical condition	Looks tired Eyes do not look right, bloodshot Personal care, hygiene deteriorates Smells of alcohol Tremulous or sweaty Agitated or irritated Frequent bathroom breaks Weight loss
D. In the community	Withdrawal from church, friends, leisure, hobbies, peers Embarrassing behaviour at parties, meetings Impaired driving, role discordant behaviour Unreliable, unpredictable behaviour at community and social activities Unpredictable personal behaviour—excessive spending, risk taking
E. In the family	Withdrawal from family activities Spouse becomes a caretaker Increased, dysfunctional anger Spouse becomes angry, tries to control use of alcohol/drugs There may be child abuse Children start to assume inappropriate adult roles Children develop antisocial behaviours Sexual problems emerge, affairs occur Spouse disengages, abuses drugs or alcohol, or enters recovery Separation, divorce

- *Safety:* I no longer know what to expect—one day mom's happy and nothing fazes her, and the next day she yells at me for nothing.[16] My parents are emotionally unavailable, sometimes lose control, and fail to protect me from hazards.
- *Open communication:* If I fear rejection, if I experience sudden, unexplained shifts of mood and response, I learn not to talk and not to trust. I hide my feelings and have secrets to keep the peace.
- *Self-care:* I can no longer care for myself and my needs if I am being a parent to my parent when he or she is drunk, or if I spend my time covering up my parent's behaviour to my friends. The sick family member's needs come first.
- *Individualized roles:* All the roles blur and become distorted if I have to shift from being a child to parenting my siblings to being 'the adult of the house' to being mom or dad's confidant. The family's needs dictate the roles, and they become rigid at times of stress.
- *Continuity:* I can no longer trust that things will feel the same from one day to the next. 'I worry if dad's going to get drunk and fall into the Christmas tree; I worry that mom's going to be spaced out on her pills and not care when I get home.'[14] There is chaos and may eventually be dissolution of the family.
- *Respect for privacy:* 'Is dad going to get mad and charge into my room again?'[16] Secrets become confused with privacy; there may not be respect for individual differences.
- *Focused attention:* 'Nobody cares about me anymore, we spend all our time trying to keep from getting dad mad.'[16]

As the situation worsens, the physician's spouse, who often early in the marriage fits the role of being a caretaker,[14] goes through various phases. First there is denial; then, an increase in the intensity of the caretaking role. There may be some early benefit, but as the illness worsens, there are ever increasing angry attempts at control, particularly with alcoholic or drug-addicted physicians. The spouse goes through intense feelings: anger (just get over it, why can't you stop?), shame (what if someone finds out?), guilt (if only I were better as a wife/husband . . .). Eventually, the spouse may join the physician in alcohol/drug abuse, may separate, or may enter a recovery process of his/her own.

Wegscheider-Cruse[17] has described roles that the children in a dysfunctional family fall into:

- *Family hero:* This is usually the eldest child, who is regarded as capable and required to behave as an adult, often repressing feelings.
- *Scapegoat:* The traditional butt of the frustrations and conflicts in the family; often showing feelings through disruptive behaviour.
- *Lost child:* Neither the eldest nor youngest, suffers most from role conflicts, because his or her identity is completely ambiguous.
- *Mascot:* Generally the youngest, often overprotected, safe by being 'cute' or funny, often lacks independence.

A tragic part of this family's slow disintegration is that through much of this process the outward appearance to society will be that of the perfect physician-led family unit.[14,16,17]

Special issues for female physicians

It is important to note that impaired female physicians have issues of their own. There are extra layers of shame and guilt, ongoing demands of childcare or the 'homemaker's' role, and there is profound loneliness and isolation.[14] There is an increased suicide rate, one study showing a fourfold elevation over non-physicians.[18] Alcoholic and addicted women physicians tend to be stigmatized more than men, and male colleagues tend to diagnose them as neurotic or depressed rather than alcoholic.[14,19] Female physicians tend to deal with these demands by becoming 'supermom'.[14]

These issues deserve a more in depth discussion, and I would refer the interested reader to *Healing the Healer*, by Talbott et al.[14]

Process addictions

Issues of behaviour that from a psychiatric viewpoint have been classed as compulsive[20] are increasingly being viewed as an addictive process.[21] Regardless of the pathologic process, these must be mentioned, if briefly.

Many physicians who come to treatment for mental illness or addiction have problems with compulsive (addictive) gambling[14] or sexual behaviour.[10,14] These behaviours are potentially devastating professionally and to the family. If undiagnosed and untreated, they are frequently a cause of relapse to alcohol or drugs.[10,14] These behaviours frequently respond to an addiction treatment model as will be discussed below. There may also be a need for psychiatric treatment including medication. In some physicians, the sexual behaviour has spilled over into the medical practice and has become exploitative of patients.[10] There may be regulatory and licensing consequences. Irons and Schneider deal in depth with the difficult issue of inappropriate sexual behavior in their book *The Wounded Healer—Addiction Sensitive Approach to the Sexually Exploitative Professional.*[10]

Treatment

Psychiatric treatment for mental illness has steadily expanded the range of treatment options, from psychoactive medications to varied psychotherapies. In regards to alcoholism/addiction, Pelton et al. studied physicians in a monitored recovery programme and found that over 5 years, the recovering physicians had fewer practice problems than a control group.[22]

The focus in this section is on treatment for addiction, but it is important to keep in mind the issue of concurrent diagnosis—29 per cent of patients with a mental disorder have an addiction diagnosis, 22 per cent of alcoholics and 53 per cent of drug dependent patients have a psychiatric diagnosis.[23] In this situation, both diagnoses must be treated.

Talbott and Angres,[14] Graham,[24] Cunningham,[25] and others have found that inpatient treatment for the majority of addicted physicians is a critical component of long-term recovery. Within these programmes there is education, time for reflection, and support—all to deal with the demoralization and isolation that is core to the process of addiction. Fair but firm confrontation of the manipulative processes of denial and minimization is essential. Emotional pain is involved in such self-awareness, but without this component, there is no true recovery or emotional growth.[26] If the family is willing, a family treatment track is available.

Physicians graduated from such treatment programmes in North America are placed on recovery agreements that span 5 years. The core components follow, although individual programmes will have far more detailed agreements.

Weekly after-care programmes (generally for 1 year) give time for change in behaviour to be reinforced; they give support to deal with the life stresses that triggered abuse/addiction and may still be risks for relapse. Some treatment centres have 'refresher' weekends several times a year for more intense recovery and family work.

Ongoing 12-step recovery work in Alcoholics Anonymous or Narcotics Anonymous continues to be a recommendation of most treatment centres. There unfortunately is great misunderstanding as to the nature of these movements. Perhaps the best way to illustrate the need for this fellowship is through the words of Dr M.M., an intelligent top of the class medical student who became addicted:

> Although I had perfected my outer persona, I still experienced excruciating inner pain, but I never revealed it to anyone. Rarely a day went by when I didn't experience terror, loneliness, paranoia, and confusion, and I remained preoccupied with death. I just got loaded continuously to cover it all up.[27]

Addicted physicians repeatedly describe an emptiness of spirit at the core of their being. The 12 steps of these movements help to heal the wounded, empty spirit—without this work there may be abstinence from mood altering chemicals, but rarely is there peace.

A vital recovery support that started in North America with Talbott and Martin[28] and has since been adopted by many other programmes,[24,25] is that of a weekly facilitated health professionals recovery group, commonly known as a Caduceus Group. Issues of shame and guilt associated with addiction, return to work, licensing, and dealing with access to addictive drugs in one's work can be addressed.

Another necessary support is having a family physician of one's own. An informal survey in our Caduceus Group revealed that upwards of 60 per cent of our physician-patients did not have a personal family physician on entry to treatment. Instead physicians relied on self-treatment, or hallway consultation with colleagues. We also insist on the recovering physician meeting with an addiction-knowledgeable physician on a regular basis, at least every 3 months for the duration of the recovery agreement. Urine testing for drugs of abuse, including alcohol, is instituted on a random basis, for the duration of the recovery agreement.

Many jurisdictions now have formal programmes to assist impaired physicians in recovery. Kaufmann in Ontario, Canada, has published details of the Physician Health Programme.[29] These programmes typically offer preliminary assessment, intervention coordination, referral for counselling and clinical services, recovery monitoring, case management, family support, and advocacy.

Regulatory issues

Regulatory and licensing bodies vary widely. Generally, the prime mandate is protection of the public from unhealthy or malevolent physicians. Some forward-thinking regulatory bodies are also finding that the public protection is enhanced in the long run if they include support and monitoring of recovering physicians, rather than punitive measures, as part of their mandate. Recovering physicians are generally enrolled in a formal recovery agreement for at least 5 years. In Ontario, we strongly feel that a physician who is conscientiously following a programme of recovery with ongoing monitoring *deserves* to practice his/her profession. In the year 2000, of 56 patients enrolled, two left prematurely and *none* have had to go to a fitness to practice hearing at the College of Physicians of Ontario.[29]

Conclusions

Denial is not solely the province of the sick physician. Family, society, medical associations, regulatory bodies, and, most painful of all, our colleagues, have their own issues of denial and minimization. Physicians do become ill; they become ill from causes many of us do not like to think about, such as mental illness and addiction. However, *they can and do recover*. It behoves us to examine ourselves and our own attitudes; we must no longer leave our colleagues to suffer alone.

References

1. **Thommasen, H.V.** et al. (2001). Mental health, job satisfaction, and intention to relocate—opinions of physicians in rural British Columbia. *Canadian Family Physician* **47**, 737–44.
2. **Hem, E.** et al. (2000). The prevalence of suicidal ideation and suicidal attempts among Norwegian Physicians. Results from a cross-sectional survey of a nationwide sample. *European Psychiatry* **3**, 183–9.
3. **Loevenich, A., Schmidt, R., and Schifferdecker, M.** (1996). Physicians as patients—on the problem of the mentally ill physician. *Fortschritte der Neurologie-Psychiatrie* **64** (9), 344–52.
4. **Talbott, D.**, ed. *Problem Physicians: A National Perspective.* A report to the Georgia Composite State Board of Medical Examiners, 2001. http://www.talbottcampus.com/Perspective.PDF.
5. **Thompson, W.T.** et al. (2001). Challenge of culture, conscience, and contract to general practitioners' care of their own health: qualitative study. *British Medical Journal* **323**, 728–31.
6. **Kaufmann, M.** (2001). Physician burnout: part 1. *Ontario Medical Review* **11**, 48–9.
7. **Schneiderman, G.** (2001). The physician as psychiatric patient. *Ontario Medical Review* **11**, 31–3.
8. **Torrey, E.F.** *Witchdoctors and Psychiatrists.* New York: Harper and Row, 1986.
9. **Vaillant, G., Sobowale, N., and McArthur, C.** (1972). Some psychological vulnerabilities of physicians. *New England Journal of Medicine* **287**, 372–5.
10. **Irons, R. and Schneider, J.** *The Wounded Healer.* London: Jason Aronson Inc., 1999.
11. **McWhinney, I.R.** Convocation address. The University of Western Ontario, June 7, 2000.
12. **Talbott, D.** (1982). The impaired physician and intervention; a key to recovery. *Journal of the Florida Medical Association* **69**, 793–7.
13. **Talbott, D. and Gallegos, K.V.** (1990). Intervention with health professionals. *Addiction and Recovery* **10** (3), 13–16.
14. **Talbott, D., Angres, D., and Bettinardi-Angres, K.** *Healing the Healer—The Addicted Physician.* Madison: Psychosocial Press, 1998.
15. **Cermak, T.** *A Time to Heal.* Los Angeles: Tarcher, 1988.
16. **Peltoniemi, T.** Children in violent and alcohol abusing families. *Ninth Annual Congress on Child Abuse and Neglect.* Chicago IL, 1992.
17. **Wegscheider-Cruse. S.** *Another Chance: Hope and Health for the Alcoholic Family.* Palo Alto: Science and Behaviour Books, 1981.
18. **Blachly, P., Disher, W., and Roduner, G.** (1968). Suicide by physicians. *Bulletin of Suicidology,* 1–18.
19. **Bissell, L. and Skorina, J.** (1987). One hundred alcoholic women in medicine. *Journal of the American Medical Association* **257**, 2939–44.
20. **Diagnostic and Statistical Manual of Mental Disorders** 4th edn. Washington DC: American Psychiatric Association, 1994.
21. **The National Council on Sexual Addiction and Compulsivity.** (2002). http://www.ncsac.org/index.htm.
22. **Pelton, C.** et al. (1993). Physician diversion program: experiences with successful graduates. *Journal of Psychoactive Drugs* **25** (2), 159–65.
23. **Epidemiologic Catchment Area Study.** US Department of Health and Human Services, National Institute of Human Health, 1981–5.
24. **Graham, D.** Physician support program of British Columbia, annual outcome data. Presented at the *Canadian Society of Addiction Medicine Annual Scientific Meeting.* Vancouver, 1992.
25. **Cunningham, G.** (1994). A treatment program for physicians impaired by alcohol and other drugs. *Annals RCPSC* **27** (4), 219–21.
26. **Longhurst, M.** (1988). Physician self-awareness: the neglected insight. *Canadian Medical Association Journal* **139**, 121–4.
27. **Morrison, M.** *White Rabbit.* New York: Berkley, 1989.
28. **Talbott, D. and Martin, C.** (1986). Treating impaired physicians: fourteen keys to success. *Virginia Medical Journal* **113**, 94–9.
29. **Kaufmann, M.** *Physician Health Program Annual Report.* Toronto: Ontario Medical Association, 2000.

16

Ethics and law

16 Ethics and law

16.1 Ethics in primary care

Len Doyal

Practicing primary care as a family doctor can be one of the most rewarding careers within medicine.[1] Like other clinicians, general practitioners (GPs) should pride themselves on the help that they are able to provide to others. And GPs have the added advantage of being able to witness the real benefits of their help on the lives of their patients. Because of their role as the doctors of families, GPs may also play a part in the fascinating interpersonal dynamics between family members and may be personally and professionally valued as a result. Finally, because much of their work with patients takes place without professional collaboration, GPs are often able to take personal pride in their clinical successes.

Yet, there is a downside. Long-term relationships with patients and families, accompanied by the potential isolation of primary clinical responsibility, can create heavy burdens. This chapter will explore these potential problems, showing how they set the stage generally for some of the important ethico-legal issues in primary care. It will do so through:

- outlining the accepted duties of care associated with good clinical practice;
- illustrating how the institutional environment of acute hospital care leads to an oversimplified interpretation of these duties;
- exploring the reasons why the demands of primary care do not lend themselves to such simplicity;
- assessing how this can lead to stress and uncertainty in ethico-legal and other clinical decision-making.

The chapter argues that because of these uncertainties, GPs can face ethico-legal challenges that are more dramatic than those of clinicians working in acute hospital care.[2] It will conclude with some suggestions for managing such uncertainty.

The primary duties of care: the problem of interpretation

There is widespread agreement that good medical practice would be impossible without the trust of patients. Such trust is proportional to the degree to which patients believe that clinicians will treat them in conformity with established duties of care.[3] Here, we will focus on the duties to:

- protect the life and health of patients to an acceptable professional standard that is underwritten by expert opinion;
- respect the autonomy of patients to the same standard, especially as regards the disclosure of appropriate information for informed choices about treatment options and the control of access of others to confidential medical information.

Aside from professional guidelines, each of these clinical duties is reflected in the law of many countries.[4]

These duties may be clear in principle but in practice they require interpretation when applied to individual cases. Yet, interpretations may conflict, despite agreement about the general meaning of the duties of care. This may be because of differences in moral belief. For example, clinicians may all accept that they should respect autonomy. However, those who take individual rights seriously (e.g. the right to information about prognosis) will interpret this duty with less paternalism than clinicians who place moral priority on minimizing distress.[5,6] Equally, the institutional environment within which the duties of care are applied can also lead to different interpretations. For example, hospital clinicians who work in intensive care are sometimes more aggressive in their interpretation of the duty to protect life and health than those who work in general medicine or surgery.[7]

The role of the institutional environment in shaping interpretations of the duties of care will be the primary focus of this chapter. Whatever differences may exist between clinical specializations in acute care within hospitals, there is usually agreement about the ways in which the duties of care are interpreted within them. These similarities go to the heart of explaining why it can be argued that GPs can have a harder ethico-legal time of it than many hospital clinicians.

Ethics in a slice of time: hospital medicine

In the acute sector of hospital medicine, many clinical consultations occur in what might be called slices of time.[2] Temporally, the professional relationship between clinicians and patients is highly structured and constrained. Both parties understand that their time together is limited, that efforts must be concentrated on the diagnosis and delivery of treatment, and that, aside from perhaps a few follow-up appointments, they may never see each other again. The same applies to whatever professional relationship exists between clinicians and the relatives of patients. Further, the focus of the duty of care is entirely on the patient. Depending on the legal jurisdiction, relatives may have some or no rights as regards influencing the course of treatment.

These environmental factors influence the way in which ethico-legal problems may be posed and resolved within hospitals. Beginning with the duty of care to respect autonomy, the right of patients to consent to and refuse treatment calls for a highly focused interpretation when located within severe temporal constraints. For example, the appropriate response to a competent refusal of treatment by an adult is to accept it, no matter how much it may compromise what are believed to be the patient's best interests.[8] When time is sliced within acute care, whatever negotiation and debate occurs between clinicians and patients is short-lived and is essentially between strangers. Since clinicians know that they will usually have limited future contact with patients or their families, this will inevitably influence their communication and management of conflict. They will focus on the facilitation of immediate therapeutic goals rather than their impact on future professional relationships.

It is commonly accepted that clinical medicine contains a great deal of scientific uncertainty in the face of difficult cases. This same uncertainty applies to respect for autonomy. While generally acknowledging their acceptance of the substantive principle of such respect, clinicians can still dramatically disagree about its practical interpretation—about, say, the amount of information that should be disclosed for obtaining informed consent and how much consultation should occur with relatives about the future course of a patient's care. The fact that such professional conflict must be resolved in short slices of time simply adds to the uncertainty. Yet, this is counterbalanced by the collectivity of much clinical and ethico-legal decision-making within a hospital environment. This ensures that uncertainty and conflict of interpretation can be resolved as rationally as possible through the collaboration of experts as in management meetings, ward rounds, case conferences.[9]

Ethics in the long run: general practice

While the difficulty and complexity of ethico-legal issues in acute care should not be underestimated, there are three reasons why GPs can face even more serious challenges.[2] First, they do not treat patients in a slice of time but over much longer periods. This means that they can develop a more detailed and evolving understanding of their patients and their physical and emotional needs than is possible in a hospital setting. With this understanding comes special responsibilities that lead to more morally textured and complex interpretations of the duty of care to respect autonomy. GPs know that their contact with patients will usually be long-term, where judgements, beliefs, and decisions can be negotiated in depth and, if necessary, reconsidered.

For example, while respect for autonomy in acute care usually means straightforward acceptance of patients' choices, within primary care, this may take the form of more extended discussion and debate. Thus, if a patient refuses advice, say, about smoking or diet, it will be natural for good GPs to revisit this issue on a regular basis and not simply accept the choice tout court. Indeed, GPs may rightly feel it appropriate to apply gentle educational and emotional pressure on patients who are placing themselves at risk—more as one might do with a friend rather than a 'patient' construed in the institutional context of a hospital.[10] This observation is not intended to suggest that respect for autonomy is ultimately any different for GPs than for hospital clinicians. It does mean, however, that the experience of taking on these extra responsibilities—of quasi-friend, counsellor, educator, and even surrogate parent—can look, feel, and be understood to be quite different.

Further, primary care is quintessentially family medicine. Each family member is owed the same duty of care. Combined with long-term relationships, this can lead to severe moral tensions relatively unknown where the focus of clinical duty is on just one patient in a slice of time. Nothing illustrates this tension better than dilemmas surrounding the duty to respect confidentiality in primary care.[11] On the one hand, GPs are obliged to show such respect. Yet, on the other hand, they also have an obligation to act in the best interests of patients. When both duties are combined in the context of conflicts of interest within families (e.g. one relative taking medication or receiving other forms of treatment that relatives wish to know about) the GP can often become the focal point of such conflict. The maintenance of a successful clinical relationship with all parties requires negotiation that balances tact, interpersonal skill, and moral flexibility with a sustained commitment to respect for the right of each family member to confidentiality. The challenge and risks of failure associated with the achievement of such balance should not be underestimated: sometimes GPs do collude with relatives in ways that constitute a technical breach of confidentiality.[12,13]

Therefore, like hospital clinicians, GPs face ethico-legal uncertainties in their professional lives. However, unlike in their case, these can be increased by the intellectual and emotional complexities of long-term relationships with patients and families.[14] In these circumstances, it may be unclear how best to proceed at any particular point in time since patients can demonstrate different levels of autonomy over time, inviting different types of ethico-legal responses (e.g. more encouragement to alter damaging behaviour in some instances and to respect immediate choice in others).[2] Yet, GPs do not usually have access to the same patterns of collective decision-making as hospital doctors and appeals to substantive ethico-legal principles may in themselves be of little help in resolving related uncertainty. Again, interpretations of such principles may conflict—especially with difficult cases—and it is this conflict that creates the uncertainty. Therefore, one must look to procedural rather than substantive means for its resolution.[15]

It has been argued that hospital clinicians are fortunate in having access to environmental infrastructures of collective debate and decision-making that are designed to optimize the rationality of otherwise uncertain clinical judgements. GPs are often deprived of such resources, either because they are single practitioners or, more likely, because their group practices have not incorporated regular opportunities for such collective deliberation into their organizational structures. The result is that GPs must cope with ethico-legal uncertainty either on their own, with all of the obvious scientific and emotional difficulties that this can pose for them and their patients, or through ad hoc communication with others. The latter is better than nothing but it does not constitute an environment of collaborative communication designed to minimize uncertainty through maximizing rationality.

Conclusion: what is to be done?

This chapter has set the stage for more detailed discussions of ethico-legal questions in primary care. It has done so through focusing on three reasons why such questions can be particularly complex and uncertain for GPs: long-term relationships with patients, potential family conflicts, and lack of access to established frameworks of collective decision-making. For reasons of space, this analysis is in no sense exhaustive. No reference has been made, for example, to the further duty of care to protect life and health and to respect autonomy fairly in accordance with good principles of distributive justice.[3] Adherence to this duty raises just as much ethico-legal uncertainty as the others. Equally, the importance of collaborative decision-making is just as applicable to the resolution of uncertainty in clinical diagnosis and treatment as it is in dealing with moral and legal uncertainty (e.g. in the management of chronic illness or the non-provision or withdrawal of life-sustaining treatment).

To counter these problems, GPs should try to remain as reflective as possible about all aspects of their clinical practice.[16] In particular, they should:

- Ensure through regular professional audit and further training that their clinical skills do not become out-dated or diminished.
- Make themselves knowledgeable about the standard literature on professional ethics within medicine in general and primary care in particular. They should also be aware of the basic legal constraints within their respective national jurisdictions. Accessible professional literature exists to satisfy these needs.
- Review the organization of their practice to improve the opportunities for collective debate and decision-making. One indicator of success or failure will be the relative amount of time in planning and management meetings spent on business issues and a discussion of difficult clinical cases.

It is equally clear, however, that GPs should be realistic about the ethico-legal burdens that they face. For example, busy and often under-resourced GPs can only do so much to correct the educational, emotional, and environmental problems that place limitations on the autonomy of their patients. The stress of dealing professionally with resulting uncertainties in primary care and of sustaining a viable professional relationship with patients and families can be difficult enough without setting moral goals that are unattainable in practice.[17] As long as GPs do their best to attain a reasonable standard of care while embracing acceptable systems of quality control, this is all that patients can morally expect of them and all that they should morally expect of themselves.

References

1. **Heath, I.** *The Mystery of General Practice.* London: Nuffield Provincial Hospitals Trust, 1995.
2. **Doyal, L.** (1999). Ethico-legal dilemmas within general practice: moral indeterminacy and abstract morality. In *General Practice and Ethics* (ed. C. Dowrick and L. Frith), pp. 45–61. London: Routledge.
3. **Chantler, C. and Doyal, L.** (2000). Medical ethics: the duties of care in principle and practice. In *Clinical Negligence* (ed. M. Powers and N. Harris), pp. 549–72. London: Butterworths.
4. **de Cruz, P.** *Comparative Health Care Law.* London: Cavendish, 2001.
5. **Higgs, R.** *Truth Telling, Lying and the Doctor–Patient Relationship.* London: Wiley, 1994, pp. 499–509.
6. **Leydon, G.M.** et al. (2000). Cancer patients' information needs and information seeking behaviour: in depth interview study. *British Medical Journal* **319**, 909.
7. **Hanson, L.D., Danis, M., Garrett, J.M., and Multran, E.** (1996). Who decides? Physicians' willingness to use life-sustaining treatment. *Archives of Internal Medicine* **156**, 785–9.
8. **Kennedy, I. and Grubb, A.** *Medical Law.* London: Butterworths, 2000, pp. 910–62.
9. **Doyal, L.** (1990). Medical ethics and moral indeterminacy. *Journal of Law and Society* **17** (1), 1–16.
10. **Toon, P.** (1987). Promoting prevention and patient autonomy. *Journal of the Royal Society of Medicine* **80** (26), 502–4.
11. **Orme-Smith, A. and Spicer, J.** *Ethics in General Practice.* Oxford: Radcliffe Medical Press, 2001, pp. 35–62.
12. **Lako, C.J., Huygen, F.J., Lindenthal, J.J, and Persoon, J.M.** (1990). Handling of confidentiality in general practice: a survey among general practitioners in the Netherlands. *Family Practitioner* **7**, 34–8.
13. **Lako, C.J. and Lindenthal, J.J.** (1991). The management of confidentiality in general practice: a comparative study in the USA and the Netherlands. *Social Science and Medicine* **32**, 153–7.
14. **Nelson, H.L. and Nelson, J.L.** *The Patient and the Family.* New York: Routledge, 1995.
15. **Doyal, L. and Gough, I.** *A Theory of Human Need.* London: Macmillan, 1991, pp. 116–26.
16. **Toon, P.** *What is Good General Practice.* London: Royal College of Practitioners, 1994.
17. **Caplan, R.P.** (1994). Stress, anxiety and depression in hospital consultants, general practitioners and senior health service managers. *British Medical Journal* **309**, 1261–3.

16.2 The doctor–patient relationship—ethical perspectives

W. Wayne Weston

The relationship between patient and physician is central to good medical care—it is the medium for exploring the patient's problems, establishing a diagnosis, and providing treatment. But more than this, the relationship itself has intrinsic value as the expression of our determination to care even when we have nothing else to offer. Simply 'being there' and offering comfort and support may be the source of the placebo effect and healing. Even when our science and our caring have no observable impact on outcomes we have a moral obligation to our sick and injured brethren to be with them in a deep and personal way.

In the past 25 years we have witnessed, in the West, a major shift in our perceptions of the patient–physician relationship. In the past, physicians were encouraged to distance themselves from their patients—to preserve a detached objectivity thought to be important for avoiding subjective bias. We now recognize that subjectivity is inevitable and that detachment results in poor communication, poor understanding of the patient, and inferior outcomes. In addition, physicians were taught to be paternalistic—to take charge of clinical decisions always with the patient's best interests in mind. Later, the focus shifted from beneficence to autonomy—physicians were admonished to respect patient's self-determination on the basis that decisions about medical care involve so many considerations and trade-offs that no one except the patient is in a position to decide what is best. Recently, we have experienced a shift away from principle-based ethics, especially its preoccupation with autonomy, to a variety of perspectives that provide a broader context for exploring the ethical dimensions of the patient–physician relationship.

In this chapter, I will focus on several of these perspectives. First, I will outline the special features of family practice that have a bearing on the ethical dimensions of the relationship. Next, I will review the issues of autonomy, beneficence, and paternalism. Then, I will raise issues related to unconscious features of the relationship. Subsequently, I will comment on narrative approaches, and, finally, provide practical examples about how to incorporate these understandings into our conversations with patients.

Special features of family practice

The relationship between patients and their personal physicians is different from their relationships with consultant physicians whom they see only once or twice.[1–3] Some have argued that principle-based ethics, and its fixation on autonomy, grew out of patients' 'suspicion that physicians were perhaps neither so omniscient nor infallible in their fiduciary actions as the public might hope' (ref. 4, p. 22). It is much harder for patients to be confident of the good intentions of strangers[5] and understandable that they would wish to have more involvement in decisions about their medical care when their association has no track record. The relationship with a family physician is different in several important aspects. First, 'family physicians are committed to the person rather than to a particular body of knowledge, group of diseases, or special technique' (ref. 2, p. 13).

Consequently, the patient can feel confident that the physician's focus will be on their concerns, no matter what they are; and, because of continuity of care with their personal physician, patient and physician will already have a relationship, which, if based on trust and mutual respect, will make it easier for the patient to reveal concerns, fears, and personal preferences. Also, the physician will have built up considerable knowledge of the patient over time that will assist him or her to understand the patient's particular concerns and wishes. Because of comprehensiveness of care and care for the whole family, patient and physician may have been through a variety of illnesses together, and shared in significant family milestones such as births, family crises, and deaths. These shared experiences create a special bond between patients and physicians that facilitates the discussion of intensely personal matters such as family secrets and spiritual struggles. The topics for these conversations are not bounded by a limited notion of 'medical issues'. Anything can be addressed in such a relationship. Of course, physicians need to remember that their expertise is in medicine and not in all of the issues that patients bring them. However, this need not limit their discussions with patients. The physician's role in such conversations is to act as a sounding board, to ask questions that will encourage the patient to explore his or her values more deeply, to provide encouragement and moral support, but most of all to listen intently as if nothing else mattered in that moment except the patient. But a nagging question remains—how can patients and physicians share decisions about care and remain focused on the patients' best interests? Let us start by exploring the contribution of principle-based ethics to this question.

Autonomy, beneficence, and paternalism

The literature on the ethics of the doctor–patient relationship often seems obsessed with autonomy and paternalism.[1,6] This may be a reaction to the tendency of physicians to keep patients in the dark and to make all the decisions on their behalf. This tradition was well established even in the time of Hippocrates who admonished physicians to:

> [p]erform [these duties] calmly and adroitly, concealing most things from the patient while you are attending to him. Give necessary orders with cheerfulness and serenity, turning his attention away from what is being done to him; sometimes reprove sharply and emphatically, and sometimes comfort with solicitude and attention, revealing nothing of the patient's future or present condition.[7]

In the modern era, patients are expected to be better informed and to be more actively involved in decisions about their own care. This is a response to increasing emphasis on individualism and to the increased amount of chronic sickness where the focus is on learning to cope with sickness rather than on being rescued from acute illness. It may also be a reaction to the increased number of people involved in providing health care. No longer is care received from a single practitioner who is well known and trusted; instead, a whole team of experts is involved and it is harder to develop the same degree of confidence. Patients often prefer to be called clients, consumers, customers, or users of health care—terms that reflect a desire for greater control and respect. Medical ethics responded by focusing on patient autonomy and the need to limit physician power—'to render the relationship doctor-proof'.[6] In its simplest terms, autonomy is the right of self-determination and paternalism is any action that reduces autonomy in the name of protecting the best interests of the patient. Expressed in such stark, black and white terms, it is hard to find any good reason to defend paternalism. However, it is not so simple. First, autonomy is defined in a number of different, and sometimes conflicting, ways. Seedhouse[8] argues that it is erroneous to think of autonomy as a right that 'trumps' all other values such as patient welfare. 'Indeed, if doctors think respecting autonomy merely means saying "over to you" whenever there are hard clinical decisions to be taken, they have things badly wrong' (p. 183). Instead, Seedhouse urges us to consider autonomy to be a quality: 'the ability to adapt to life's changing circumstances' (p. 180). In this sense, concern for patient autonomy can be consistent with a concern for patient welfare. Consider the case of a patient who refuses life-saving surgery. In the name of respecting autonomy as a right, patients should not be prevented from making a decision that would likely lead to their death. However, if autonomy is only one among many important values, then the physician has an obligation to intervene to protect patients from making a serious error, not only by providing information, but also by challenging the patient's assumptions and even trying to change the patient's mind.

Quill and Brody[9] argue that the pendulum has swung too far from 'the coerciveness of paternalism' to the 'remoteness of... independent choice'. They present an enhanced autonomy model that 'assumes that an open dialogue, in which the physician frankly admits his or her biases, is ultimately a better protector of the patient's right to autonomous choice than artificial neutrality would be' (p. 765). An open debate between patient and physician would lead both parties to a better understanding of the issues and values. 'Final choices belong to patients, but these choices gain meaning, richness, and accuracy if they are the result of a process of mutual influence and understanding between physician and patient'.

Traditionally, physicians have felt an obligation to make decisions on behalf of their patients. It was generally believed that such decisions were far too complex for patients to make especially when their ability to think clearly was impaired by their diseases. Individuals stricken by illness were considered to be more like children than adults and such paternal, or parental, behaviour was justified by the principle of beneficence—concern for patient welfare. Preliminary research by Cassell et al.[10] showed that, in sicker hospitalized patients, performance on seven Piagetian tasks of judgement was similar to that among children younger than 10 years of age. For example, patients were presented with two identical containers with an equal amount of water in each. Then, in full view of the patient, one of the containers was emptied into a tall thin container. Only 33.3 per cent of sicker patients were able to correctly state that both containers held an equal amount of water compared to 76.9 per cent of less sick patients and 85.7 per cent of controls. This could be used as an argument in favour of paternalism. But perhaps this study should challenge us instead to find more effective ways to converse with patients in a manner that recognizes the potential impact of illness on their cognitive abilities. Family physicians are in the best position to recognize how their patients have been changed by their illnesses and to provide support and guidance that reduces the risk that patients will make unwise decisions. Even if patients remains technically competent, it may be advisable to involve other family members to help with important medical decisions.

Katz points out a similar dilemma raised by recognition of unconscious and irrational elements in everyday thinking, not only of patients but of physicians too. Katz summarizes physicians' obligations succinctly:

> If I am correct, then individual freedom should be equated neither with simply permitting patients to do what they initially desire nor with requiring them simply to make complete sense to their physicians. Instead, and above all, respect for freedom would demand respectful conversation. True freedom entails constant struggle and anguish with oneself and with others. This is the lesson of psychoanalysis and its theories about human conduct and interactions.[11]

Such a conversation would be difficult with a stranger and would be unlikely to be repeated with a series of physicians—another argument for a personal doctor.

Unconscious factors

It is important for physicians to recognize how unconscious factors such as transference can affect patient's choices and physician's responses. Autonomy has little meaning if unconscious forces hijack the patient's ability to react to the current situation free of undue influences from the past. Transference is a universal phenomenon in human relationships—the unconscious process of projecting expectations, hopes, fears, love, and hatred that belong in one relationship (often the early relationship with a parent) onto another relationship (often a relationship with an authority figure such as a physician). Unresolved issues in earlier relationships are often the source of transference in the patient–physician relationship and the process becomes more intense when persons are ill. Because the projection is unconscious and irrational, the patient may react towards the physician as if he or she were, in reality, the patient's parent—patients may expect too much in a magical wish for the parent surrogate to 'make it all better' and be bitterly disappointed when the physician inevitably fails to measure up. The process unleashes strong feelings that may interfere with a rational analysis of the true situation.

Caught up in a strong transference, the patient is at the mercy of these primitive, irrational forces and may make serious errors of judgement. It behoves the physician to help the patient to recognize the source of the feeling or, at least, to recognize that he or she is overreacting to the physician. Anna Freud offers this wise advice:

> ... [t]he patient... will do his best to push you into the place of parental authority, and he will make use of you as a parental authority to the utmost. You must understand that. On the other hand, you must not be tempted to treat him as a child. You must be tolerant towards him as you would be towards a child and as respectful as you would be towards a fellow adult because he has only gone back to childhood as far as he's ill. He also has another part of his personality which has remained intact, and that part of him will resent it deeply, if you make too much use of your authority.[12]

Freud's comments alert us to the importance of counter-transference—the unconscious reaction of the physician to the patient's transference arising out of significant relationships in the physician's past. Self-awareness is a crucial skill to minimize the risk that counter-transference will lead to poor care. There are several clues of counter-transference. Physicians may find themselves not listening attentively, interpreting too soon, becoming too active in offering advice, engaging in power struggles, consistently going overtime, over-identifying with the patient's problem, or thinking too much about a patient.(13) For example, when physicians find themselves frustrated and angry with uncooperative patients, this may reflect the reality that such situations are inherently difficult. But, if this happens repeatedly, or the reaction is extreme, it could reflect unresolved issues in the physicians' own families—either related to their own early struggles with their parents or their unresolved struggles with their own teenagers.

When a physician reacts strongly towards a patient, it may be a clue about other important relationships in the patient's life—others may be reacting to this patient in the same way. This may help physicians to understand some of their patients' current struggles. Human behaviour is never random; what patients say and how they say it (and what they leave out) all have meaning. 'Thus, by continually asking ourselves such questions as "Why is he telling me this?" or "Why did she use that particular phrase?" we can identify clues pertaining to the deeper levels of the patient's story.'(14) These deeper connections are unlikely unless the relationship is continuous.

Narrative approaches

In a text of readings on the social dimensions of bioethics, Hoffmaster points out the deficiencies of traditional ethics preoccupied with 'providing "good reasons" for judgements':

> Bioethics, in this view, is situated in rationality and generality. It prescinds the messy details and attachments that give our lives meaning and vigour, the nagging contradictions that make us squirm and struggle, and the social, political, and economic arrangements that simultaneously create and constrain us. Because they are yoked to the abstractions of reason and theory, judgments about matters of bioethics frequently outstrip the contexts that generate and shape those matters and ignore the agonizing experiences of the people who grapple with them.(15)

Patients' stories of their encounters with physicians reveal much about the nature and importance of their relationships with physicians. These first-person narratives admit us to the worlds of real persons struggling with their experiences of serious illness and help us to understand their flesh and blood daily struggles to cope. Common to many of these stories is a concern about the shortcomings of modern medicine. Anatole Broyard, an editor and literary critic dying of prostate cancer, reflected on the qualities he looked for in a physician:

> I wouldn't demand a lot of my doctor's time. I just wish he would brood on my situation for perhaps five minutes, that he would give me his whole mind just once, be bonded with me for a brief space, survey my soul as well as my flesh to get at my illness, for each man is ill in his own way... Just as he orders blood tests and bone scans of my body, I'd like my doctor to scan me, to grope for my spirit as well as my prostate. Without some such recognition, I am nothing but my illness.(16)

Regarding his first physician, he commented:

> He was such an innocuous looking man that he didn't seem intense enough or wilful enough to prevail over something powerful and demonic like illness. He was bland, hearty and vague, polite where politeness was irrelevant. I felt that he would be polite even to my illness, whatever it might be... There was no sign of a tragic sense of life in him that I could see, no furious desire to oppose himself to fate. I realized of course, that what I was looking for was unreasonable, that I was demanding nothing less than an ideal doctor. I sat there in this poor man's office and compared him to a heroic model I had summarily imagined (ref. 17, p. 36).[1]

Another author-patient, Arthur Frank, a medical sociologist, described his experiences of cancer:

> Critical illness leaves no aspect of life untouched. The hospitals and other special places we have constructed for critically ill persons have created the illusion that by sealing off the ill person from those who are healthy, we can also seal off the illness in that ill person's life. This illusion is dangerous. Your relationships, your work, your sense of who you are and who you might become, your sense of what life is and ought to be—these all change, and the change is terrifying... My questions end up being phrased in disease terms, but what I really want to know is how to live with illness... After five years of dealing with medical professionals in the context of critical illness, as opposed to the routine problems I had had before, I have accepted their limits, even if I have never become comfortable with them. Perhaps medicine should reform itself and learn to share illness talk with patients instead of imposing disease talk on them. Or perhaps physicians and nurses should simply do what they already do well—treat the breakdowns—and not claim to do more... To talk about illness you must go elsewhere (ref. 18).[2]

Both patient-authors found doctors competent in the technical realm but empty-handed when the patient wished to discuss the meaning of their illness experiences. Both suggest that perhaps they expected too much. But they continued to long for a connection with someone who would understand their unique plight and take the time to listen. Such narratives are powerful reminders of the human dimensions of health care and our obligation to enter into our patients' worlds in such a way that our patients realize that the physician has at least tried to comprehend their suffering. Would these stories be different if they each had a personal physician? Are family doctors too busy to provide this kind of care? Is medicine too preoccupied with attending to the grave biological needs of patients to be able to sit and listen to the existential concerns of patients? Shortage of family physicians in many countries and organizational arrangements such as managed care in the United States threaten long-term personal relationships that are essential to meet the needs of such patients.

Practical applications

Health care is inherently a moral enterprise because of its impact on persons—health care can enhance or diminish the quality and quantity of life. According to Seedhouse:

> Health work, in its most complete sense, is work aimed at preventing or eliminating obstacles that might or do stand in the way of individuals' biological and chosen potentials (so long as achievement of these potentials causes no intentional harm to other human beings) (ref. 8, p. 47).

Even such an apparently simple decision to prescribe or not prescribe penicillin for pharyngitis is a moral, as well as a medical, decision. Patients may request, or even demand, penicillin based on their belief that it will provide a quick cure of their sore throat. When physicians suggest that penicillin is not needed, patients may believe that, although penicillin would help, the physician does not think their condition 'worthy enough' to treat with antibiotics; penicillin should be reserved for sicker patients. They may even recognize the role of over-prescribing of antibiotics on the development of resistant organisms. They may be willing to take the small risk of an allergic reaction to get rid of the pain and inconvenience. Faced with such a patient, physicians have a number of choices, all of which have ethical implications.

First, they can 'give in' to the patient's wishes, reasoning that even if penicillin has no pharmacological effect, it may have a placebo effect, is unlikely to cause harm, and is quicker and easier than a fruitless discussion or argument with the patient that could damage their relationship. Since the physician has not explored the patient's reasoning—because of being rushed or assuming the patient must be wrong—he or she will not understand the patient's rationale. Alternatively, physicians can refuse to prescribe unless a throat swab grows streptococci and insist that the patient put up with it or use analgesics until then. This also assumes that the only possible justification for antibiotics is a clear-cut diagnosis of streptococcal pharyngitis.

A third approach(19) is to provide information to the patient about the causes and treatment of sore throat and the clinical cues that suggest a streptococcal versus a viral aetiology. In addition, physicians could use

[1] Excerpts from Broyard, A. *Intoxicated by my Illness and Other Writings on Life and Death.* New York: Clarkson Potter, 1992.

[2] Excerpts from Frank, A. *At the Will of the Body: Reflections on Illness.* Boston: Houghton Mifflin, 1991.

Table 1 Decision-making options and effect on doctor–patient relationship

Option	Moral issues	Effect on the relationship	Comments
I 'Give in'— patient decides	Supports patient's autonomy. But lacks respect for the patient's reasoning. Unnecessary risk of harm from allergic reactions	Ironically, this approach may create dependency and childlike demanding behaviour	This is a simplistic notion of autonomy—'getting one's way'—which encourages future expectation of penicillin
II Refuse—physician decides	Paternalistic—focuses on patient welfare and protecting the community from penicillin resistance	Creates mutual antagonism and disrespect. Alternatively, patients may become dependent on the physician's judgement without any understanding of the rationale for treatment	Without an explanation, patients may be angry, more demanding, and may 'doctor shop' until they get what they feel they need. Or they may give up and bow to the physician's authority
III Shared decision-making—find common ground	Focuses on patient welfare but also enhances autonomy in a deeper sense	Collaboration among adults who treat each other with respect. Decision not just on biomedical grounds. Builds trust which enhances future work together	The patient will be able to take a more active role with future sore throats

a decision aid that can provide an actual calculation of the patient's chances of having a streptococcal pharyngitis. The physician will be prepared to prescribe antibiotics, even if the likelihood of streptococcal infection is low, after considering the risks and benefits from the patient's perspective. Physicians should not set aside standards of care lightly, but the patient's unique situation and personal imperatives may be more relevant to the treatment decision than a standard guideline. This approach may take much longer than the other options but, in the long run, by providing patients with a tool to decide when they need to see a physician, it could cut down on future visits.

In Table 1, the shared decision model is preferred. But there are situations where other models may be favoured. In acute emergencies where patients are so sick that they cannot think clearly and there is no time for deliberation, the physician will decide after providing enough information to satisfy the requirements for informed consent. With regard to issues related to lifestyle, for example, whether of not to exercise or start a diet, or for conditions where there is no clearly recommended treatment, the patient will decide after being informed about the pros and cons of various options. The shared decision-making approach involves active participation and true dialogue between patient and physician. Each is willing to learn from the other in a mutual process of finding the best approach for *this* patient at *this* time.

The Patient-Centred Clinical Method,[20] developed at the University of Western Ontario since 1972, is a model of care rooted in the belief that patients should have an opportunity for active involvement in any medical decisions about their care. Although there is growing evidence[21,22] that a patient-centred approach improves outcomes of care for both patients and physicians, the Western Ontario group argues that, even without such evidence, physicians have a moral obligation to enter into their patients' worlds to connect with them in a manner in which they feel understood, cared for, and respected. This approach transforms the clinical method because it involves the patient in the whole process of exploring and understanding their problems and not just at the end when decisions must be made about investigation and treatment. The traditional history of the disease and the functional inquiry is expanded to include the patient's experience of their illness—their feelings about being ill, their ideas about what is wrong, how it affects their day-to-day function, and their expectations of the physician.

For example, in the patient with sore throat mentioned above, the physician will ask about onset, associated symptoms, and current family illness. In addition, the doctor will inquire about the patient's experience of this illness. He may have had numerous sore throats before and often received penicillin for them; it would be natural that he would expect penicillin again. A friend may have developed infectious mononucleosis and been too sick to attend school for 6 months; it is understandable that he would want some form of treatment to prevent this from happening to him. He may have an important school exam coming up in 3 days and feel desperate to be treated so that he can perform at his best. A simple explanation about how viruses and bacteria are treated, although helpful, is insufficient. Patients need to know that the physician understands their plight and their needs before they are willing to listen to the physician's explanation. These issues become even more imperative when patients fear that they have a more serious illness. Simply providing excellent biomedical care is inadequate in such situations. Often, there is no treatment that will alter the natural history of the patient's condition but physicians must still offer understanding, compassion, and hope. Withholding such basic human responses to suffering, based on insufficient evidence of effectiveness, would be unconscionable.

A central feature of the patient-centred clinical method is the task of finding common ground between patient and physician, especially regarding the nature of the patient's problems, the goals of treatment, and the respective roles of patient and physician in management. In a recent study, this was the key to the effectiveness of the method for improved patient satisfaction with care, reduced concerns, fewer tests and referrals, and improved physiological outcome.[23] One of the communication strategies for finding common ground is motivational interviewing, a method based on a model of stages of change.[24] The model is based on the theory that persons change their behaviours in predictable stages and they are more likely to succeed if they are helped by a counsellor who tailors his or her interventions to the person's particular stage of change. Motivational interviewing strategies are often recommended for addictive behaviours such as smoking. A person may desire to be a non-smoker but be unwilling or unable to tolerate the struggle to quit. The traditional intervention of a physician is to point out the dangers of smoking, make a recommendation to quit and provide pharmacological aids such as nicotine patches, sticks, or bupropion. Special interviewing techniques to change behaviour might be viewed with suspicion as some form of mind control or coercion. But leaving patients to their own devices to fight off the disabling effects of addiction is not supporting their free choice of treatment. Supporting autonomy is not simply leaving all decisions up to the patient but rather providing whatever assistance is needed to learn how to cope and to strengthen motivation.

Another clinical example of the complexity of ethical decision-making and informed consent in practice is the treatment of prostate cancer. At the time of writing, there is insufficient evidence to support a preference for surgery, radiation, or watchful waiting for clinically localized prostate cancer.[25] How is a patient with prostate cancer to decide? How much information is needed for informed consent? One approach is to provide information, let the patient think it over on his own, and return when he has reached a decision. This could be supplemented with an opportunity to ask questions or to meet with a self-help group. But with such a complex issue, where physicians often disagree, this may leave the patient even more confused. The patient may benefit from someone helping him to consider his own values and how these might influence his decision. For example, if his sex life is still very important to him, it may be more in keeping with his values to opt for watchful waiting or radiation, which have lower risks of impotence than surgery. On the other hand, if he wants to do everything possible to prolong his life, even if it means greater risk, then surgery may be his preferred choice. The patient's comfort with uncertainty and preference for *doing* rather than *waiting* also need to be considered. The physician might ask: 'Are you the kind of person who would find it very hard to just wait and see what happens and would want us to do everything we can to get rid of this cancer even if we can't prove that the treatment is effective? Or are you the kind of person who feels it is better to leave well enough alone unless we have good evidence that treatment will do more good than harm?' Such questions open up discussion of the possible benefits and harms of treatment as well as the patient's preferred approach to management in the face of uncertainty.

Buckman urges physicians to ask similar questions before breaking bad news: 'If this condition turns out to be something serious, are you the sort of person who likes to know exactly what's going on? Would you like me to tell you the full details of the diagnosis? ... Or would you prefer to hear just about the treatment plans? Do you like to know exactly what's going on or would you prefer me to give you the outline only? ... Would you like me to tell you the full details of your condition—or is there somebody else you'd like me to talk to?'.[26] These questions reflect sensitivity to individual preferences of patients and highlight the complexity of sharing information with them. If a particular patient prefers to be told only about treatment options and the physician goes into great detail about the patient's disease and poor prognosis, the patient may suffer from additional anxiety and will lose confidence in the physician's willingness to respect the patient's wishes.

Because patients trust and respect their family physicians, there is a danger of physicians having undue influence. It is very easy to take advantage of this power in a busy practice where it is quicker and easier to give advice than to help patients explore their alternatives, especially when patients are so appreciative of the advice. However, patients are expressing a desire for more information about their conditions and a wish to be more involved in decisions about their care although there remain a significant number of patients who favour a more passive role in treatment decisions. The preferred role depends on age, presenting problem, social class, and educational level of the patient.[27] The Informed Shared Decision Making Model[28] provides an approach to involving patients in their own care to the extent that they wish to be involved. In this model, physicians determine their patients' preferences for learning more about their condition (e.g. pamphlets, Internet, videotapes, or support groups) and their preferences for role in decision-making (e.g. talking to other family members, relying on the doctor's advice, being self-reliant, comfort with risk taking). Discussing how patients prefer to handle decisional conflict—what they do when they are confronted with opposing ideas and uncertainty—may help them to resolve such dilemmas. It is important to understand that, in this model, the physician is not simply a servant doing whatever the patient requests but rather a partner who brings medical expertise and evidence to the discussion about management. In addition, family physicians will bring a wealth of knowledge about the patient and their previous choices and outcomes in similar situations. Towle and Godolphin argue that being explicit about these issues enhances patients' opportunities for an effective partnership with physicians as they explore choices together and come to a mutual decision that best matches patients' preferences and is congruent with the best available evidence and clinical wisdom. They urge the profession to enhance the communication skills of clinicians and also to provide opportunities for patients to develop skills to interact more effectively with physicians. Doyal points out that this is particularly important for the poor who will remain disadvantaged by these changes in the roles of patients and physicians unless they can be empowered by 'much more profound social and political change'.[29]

The commonest argument against a shared model of decision-making is the lack of time. Such an approach, it is argued, requires more time than is available for good care. It is true that involving patients in a meaningful discussion of choices can be time consuming. But such an approach has a number of benefits that may reduce physicians' time in the long run. Patients are more satisfied with care, are less likely to sue their physicians, have reduced concerns, better physiological outcomes, and fewer referrals and laboratory investigations.[22] Family physicians have an advantage—because of their long-term relationships, they already know the preferences of many of their patients. Time spent educating patients about their chronic conditions will pay dividends over the years as patients take on more responsibility for their care. Because adherence to care is enhanced when communication is effective, patients are more likely to follow the treatment plan and to avoid complications thus further reducing demands on physicians' time. Lijas and Lahdensuo[30] demonstrated the cost-effectiveness of guided self-management of asthma using written treatment plans and an approach that emphasized the importance of forming a partnership for care with the patient. Every $1 (£1.60) spent on this programme saved $11.22 (£7) mostly from reduced unscheduled visits to their physicians and emergency departments and hospitalizations.

Conclusions

I have explored a number of related concepts to examine the ethical dimensions of the patient–physician relationship in family medicine. Principle-based ethics, focusing on patient autonomy, proved inadequate to guide our care of patients who often are too sick to take charge of decision-making in the short time available to be well informed. Their autonomy is already weakened by the impact of cognitive impairment that accompanies their illnesses and also by unconscious factors that may emerge. Additionally, this approach is often based on a stunted notion of autonomy—as simply getting one's way regardless of the results. Narrative approaches take us into the personal experiences of our patients and help us to understand their plight, especially their need to be acknowledged as fellow human beings who are seeking to find meaning in their suffering and to retain some semblance of normal life. Family physicians have an advantage over their hospital colleagues because of the opportunity to see their patients when they are relatively healthy as well as when ill—this affords an opportunity to discuss personal preferences for care and to help them develop skills in self-care. The patient-centred clinical method provides a framework for effective shared decision-making between patients and physicians—an approach that attempts to avoid the dangers of paternalism on the one hand and abandonment of the patient to their own devices on the other hand. The special features of family medicine—the intimate knowledge that builds up after many years of continuous care, especially in the context of personal crises—make it easier to share decisions and imposes an obligation on family physicians to challenge the forces that threaten the survival of personal doctoring. In many countries, family physicians are finding it harder to fill their traditional roles because of increased paperwork and regulations imposed by third-party payers. The poor are particularly disadvantaged by their increased risk of disease, reduced access to care, and diminished sense of their own ability to influence medical decisions. The splintering of care among several specialists, emergency physicians, and walk-in clinics makes it harder to build a relationship and to coordinate care. Never has it been more important to have a personal doctor to help patients navigate an increasingly complex medical system.

References

1. **Christie, R. and Hoffmaster, B.** *Ethical Issues in Family Medicine.* Oxford: Oxford University Press, 1986.
2. **McWhinney, I.R.** *A Textbook of Family Medicine* 2nd edn. Oxford: Oxford University Press, 1997.

3. **Doyal, L.** (1999). Ethical–legal dilemmas within general practice. Moral indeterminacy and abstract morality. In *General Practice and Ethics: Uncertainty and Responsibility* (ed. C. Dowrick and L. Firth), p. 49. London: Routledge.
4. **Tauber, A.I.** *Confessions of a Medicine Man—An Essay in Popular Philosophy.* Cambridge MA: The MIT Press, 1990.
5. **Rothman, D.J.** *Strangers at the Bedside.* New York: Basic Books, 1992.
6. **Brody, H.** *The Healer's Power.* New Haven: Yale University Press, 1992.
7. **Hippocrates, Decorum, trans. W. Jones** (Cambridge: Harvard University Press, 1967, p. 297), quoted in Katz, J. *The Silent World of Doctor and Patient.* New York: The Free Press, 1984.
8. **Seedhouse, D.** *Ethics: The Heart of Health Care* 2nd edn. Toronto: John Wiley and Sons, 1998.
9. **Quill, T.E. and Brody, H.** (1996). Physician recommendations and patient autonomy: finding a balance between physician power and patient choice. *Annals of Internal Medicine* **125**, 763–9.
10. **Cassell, E.J., Leon, A.C., and Kaufman, S.G.** (2001). Preliminary evidence of impaired thinking in sick patients. *Annals of Internal Medicine* **134**, 1120–3.
11. **Katz, J.** *The Silent World of Doctor and Patient.* New York: The Free Press, 1984.
12. **Freud, A.** Unpublished manuscript based on a lecture to students at Case Western Reserve Medical School (29 October 1964). Reprinted in Katz, J. The Silent World of Doctor and Patient. Baltimore: The Johns Hopkins University Press, reprint edn., 2002.
13. **Dubovsky, S.L.** *Psychotherapeutics in Primary Care.* New York: Grune and Stratten, 1981.
14. **Matthews, D.A., Suchman, A.L., and Branch, W.T.** (1993). Making 'connexions': enhancing the therapeutic potential of patient–clinician relationships. *Annals of Internal Medicine* **118**, 973–7.
15. **Hoffmaster, B.,** ed. *Bioethics in Social Context.* Philadelphia: Temple University Press, 2001.
16. **Broyard, A.** *New York Times Magazine,* 26 August 1990.
17. **Broyard, A.** *Intoxicated by my Illness and Other Writings on Life and Death.* New York: Clarkson Potter, 1992.
18. **Frank, A.** *At the Will of the Body: Reflections on Illness.* Boston: Houghton Mifflin, 1991.
19. **Charles, C., Whelan, T., and Gafni, A.** (1999). What do we mean by partnership in making decisions about treatment? *British Medical Journal* **319**, 780–2.
20. **Stewart, M., Brown, J.B., Weston, W.W., McWhinney, I.R., McWilliam, C.L., and Freeman, T.R.** *Patient-Centered Medicine: Transforming the Clinical Method* 2nd edn. Abingdon: Radcliffe Medical Press, 2003.
21. **Stewart, M.A.** (1995). Effective physician–patient communication and health outcomes: a review. *Canadian Medical Association Journal* **152**, 1423–33.
22. **Stewart, M., Brown, J.B., Boon, H., Galajda, J., Meredith, L., and Sangster, M.** (1999). Evidence on patient–doctor communication. *Cancer Prevention and Control* **3**, 25–30.
23. **Stewart, M., Brown, J.B., Donner, A., McWhinney, I.R., Oates, J., Weston, W.W., and Jordan, J.** (2000). The impact of patient-centred care on outcomes. *Journal of Family Practice* **49**, 796–804.
24. **Rollnick, S., Mason, P., and Butler, C.** *Health Behavior Change: a Guide for Practitioners.* Edinburgh: Churchill Livingstone, 1999.
25. **Jones, G.,** ed. *Clinical Evidence* Issue 8. London: BMJ Publishing Group, 2002.
26. **Buckman, R. and Kason, Y.** *How to Break Bad News; A Guide for Health Care Professionals.* Toronto: University of Toronto Press, 1992.
27. **McKinstry, B.** (2000). Do patients wish to be involved in decision making in the consultation? A cross sectional survey with video vignettes. *British Medical Journal* **321**, 867–71.
28. **Towle, A. and Godolphin, W.** (1999). Framework for teaching and learning informed shared decision making. *British Medical Journal* **319**, 766–9.
29. **Doyal, L.** (2001). Informed consent: moral necessity or illusion? *Quality in Health Care* **10** (Suppl. 1), i29–33.
30. **Lijas, B. and Lahdensuo, A.** (1997). Is asthma self-management cost-effective? *Patient Education and Counseling* **32**, 97–104.

16.3 Truth-telling in family medicine

Eugene Bereza

Introduction

The truth, the whole truth, and nothing but the truth . . . so help you . . .

This well-known adage would seem to set the ideal and self-evident standard for truth-telling in family medicine. Yet, Katz, Bok, and others believe that physicians' attitudes to straying from this ideal are often cavalier and all too pervasive. Brody has observed the irony in our choice of labelling this controversial topic in medical ethics as 'truth-telling' rather than 'lying', as if it is the former that requires ethical justification.[1] Clinicians and philosophers have long appreciated, however, that the concept of truth-telling, as well as its application in family medicine, is far more complex.

The current consensus acknowledges both realities. As a guiding principle of medical ethics, physicians should be truthful with their patients. However, the complexities of modern-day family practice have contributed numerous qualifications of this general rule.

The first challenge for family physicians is to learn to identify and analyse ethical issues in truth-telling, in order to differentiate appropriate exceptions to full disclosure from unacceptable abuses. Secondly, physicians must transfer these skills to the realities of family practice by communicating effectively when contributing their perspectives to that of patients and families.

'How should family physicians arrive at morally acceptable and clinically pragmatic judgments?' In an attempt to answer this question, traditional arguments and innovative approaches to the ethics of truth-telling will be reviewed. Perhaps more importantly, the physician will be urged to go beyond knowledge-based learning of ethical theory and 'extract critical methodological skills of ethical analysis' appropriate to the clinical context.

Truth, truthfulness, and truth-telling

The primordial question that underlies truth-telling concerns the nature of 'truth' itself. Most clinicians and many philosophers have argued that 'truth', as an idealized concept, cannot be achieved in reality. Furthermore, they agree that there are ethically justifiable exceptions to full disclosure. The philosopher Henry Sidgwick commented:

> . . . it does not seem clearly agreed whether Veracity is an absolute and independent duty, or a special application of some higher principle. . . . reflection seems to show that the rule of Veracity . . . cannot be elevated into a definite moral axiom: . . . it is contrary to Common Sense to exact absolute candour under all circumstances . . .[2]

The physician Richard Cabot wrote:

> What is sometimes called the simple truth, the 'bald truth' or the 'naked truth' is often practically false—as unrecognizable as Lear naked upon the moor. It needs to be explained, supplemented, modified.[3]

L.J. Henderson echoed these sentiments over 30 years later when he added:

> The idea that the truth, the whole truth, and nothing but the truth can be conveyed to the patient is an example of false abstraction. . . . since telling the truth is impossible, there can be no sharp distinction between what is true and what is false.[4]

However, the issues of truth-telling cannot be so simply dismissed or reduced to a choice between truth and falsehood. Bok responds to this kind of critique by suggesting that a relevant distinction between 'truth' and 'falsehood' involves the concept of 'truthfulness'. She asserts that 'truthfulness can be required even where full "truth" is out of reach' (ref. 2, p. 13).

Family physicians have come to appreciate that while 'truthfulness' is a prerequisite for a therapeutic patient–physician relationship, it is only meaningful when considered in the context of an individual patient's unique life narrative. This narrative typically includes critical relationships with family and intimate friends. A physician's goal is to ceaselessly strive to help patients achieve an appreciation of such a truth. This task can be as daunting as that of the mythological Sisyphus.

Traditional issues

In her classic book *Lying: Moral Choice in Public and Private Life*,(2) Bok examines the anatomy of lies and deceptions. Her list includes clearly intended lies ('the most sharply etched forms of duplicity'), 'white lies', breaching pledges of confidentiality, diagnostic use of placebos, excuses, and the 'noble' lie. There are also more marginal strategies used in undermining truth-telling, such as evasion, euphemism, exaggeration, and sudden changes of subject. The specific problems encountered in medicine, as well as the corresponding ethics analysis, have been well documented by Hebert and coworkers.(5,6)

Much of the original literature focused on providing 'bad' information to patients in medical crises, or divulging diagnoses and prognoses of terminal illness. The predominant communication strategy in such cases is silence. In his book, *The Silent World of Doctor and Patient*, Katz asserts that such silence is the hallmark of current medical practice. He goes on to generalize that there is 'contemporary and historical evidence that patients' participation in decision making is an idea alien to the ethos of medicine'.(7)

Is there evidence to support such assertions? Anecdotal clinical experience supports the impression that truth-telling must occasionally be compromised in pursuing patients' best interests. This impression is hardly 'evidence based'. In the United States, the President's Commission concluded that there was little documentation to support claims of the alleged harms of truth-telling, particularly when such communication was done skillfully.(8)

The evidence suggests that physicians in North America disclose 'truth' more than they did a few decades ago.(9,10) This may be the result of the formal introduction of ethics into medical school curricula, or the changing legal standard for disclosure from a 'professional disclosure standard' to the 'reasonable patient standard'. However, it is difficult to be confident about reports of changing trends. A Canadian survey in 1991 indicated that most patients were satisfied with the way physicians communicated with them, whereas a study at the University of Chicago a decade later concluded that doctors 'gave terminal patients frank estimates of how long they could expect to live in just 37% of the cases... investigated'.(11)

The evidence also supports the conclusion that the practice of disclosure by physicians in different parts of the world can vary significantly, with physicians generally disclosing less to patients in Italy and Japan, compared with the United States.

Conventional arguments

To the extent that 'truth' can be known, truth-telling in family medicine is all too often compromised. There are two main reasons for this. Physicians can undermine truth-telling for interests other than those of patients—their own, family members', or for the public good. Hopefully, the more prevalent reason is that physicians often view complete disclosure as potentially harmful to patients and, therefore, not in their best interests.

A physician's duty to be judicious with respect to truth-telling can be traced as far back as Hippocrates. This ancient code is still echoed in the most recent medical texts. In the last edition of Harrison's *Principles of Internal Medicine*, Lo writes:

> Physicians may consider withholding a serious diagnosis, misrepresenting it, or limiting discussions of prognosis or risks out of fear that a patient will develop severe anxiety or depression or refuse needed care.(12)

In addition to these conceptual considerations, physicians face many practical constraints that undermine truth-telling. These include uncertainty of medical information and lack of time to optimize communication. In addition, patients' ability to assimilate and understand complex medical information when ill may vary considerably. Even cognitively competent patients are often vulnerable and compromised by virtue of suffering physical, emotional, or psychological trauma. These factors support Pellegrino's conclusion that the 'amount, manner, and timing of truth telling or truth withholding are crucial factors for which there is no ready formula'.(13)

Nevertheless, physicians should appreciate that there are many serious risks associated with invoking 'therapeutic privilege'. These include basing judgements on intuitive moral reflexes that may be arbitrary, idiosyncratic, systemically conditioned, and not subject to rigorous ethical reflection.

The potential harms to patients are significant. In the absence of complete information, patients cannot appreciate how their health care problems may affect the rest of their lives and those of their family. As a result, they cannot make fully informed decisions about their health care and initiate appropriate lifestyle changes.

Another kind of harm affects the very nature of the therapeutic relationship between patient and physician. When truth-telling is compromised, there is significant risk that the trust upon which this fiduciary relationship is based will be broken and irrevocably lost. The potential harms here are to the patient, the physician, and the medical profession.

Appreciating these risks, Bok suggests that we:

> set a severely restricted and narrowed paternalistic view—that some patients cannot understand, some do not want, and some may be harmed by, knowledge of their condition, and that they ought not to have to be treated like everyone else if this is not in their best interest. Such a view is persuasive... Concealment, evasion, withholding of information may at times be necessary. But if someone contemplates lying to a patient or concealing the truth, the burden of proof must shift. It must rest... on those who advocate it... (ref. 2, p. 238).

Evolving approaches to ethics analysis

Ethics theory has provided the foundation for medical ethics by elucidating fundamental arguments and, perhaps more importantly, providing the tools for reasoned argumentation. The publication of *Principles of Biomedical Ethics* ushered in the modern era of medical ethics discourse. The authors articulated four founding principles—autonomy, non-maleficence, beneficence, and justice.(14) The hallmark of such analysis is the translation of practical medical problems into moral dilemmas that are characterized as competing values or principles.

Thus, many of the conventional arguments in bioethics concerning truth-telling revolve around two allegedly competing values—patient autonomy and benevolent medical paternalism. The former requires an appreciation and respect for each individual's right to full self-determination. The latter assumes that there are justifiable situations where one individual assumes a paternalistic attitude toward another, ostensibly as a means of protecting the vulnerable one from harm.

Effective as this methodology is, many find its application to clinical medicine inadequate. The limiting preoccupation in bioethics with the juxtaposition of patient autonomy and physicians' paternalism may be due, in part, to the fact that the

> ethical questions that have attracted the most attention are the controversial 'headline' issues such as euthanasia, abortion, human experimentation, and genetic engineering. The more mundane, but more pervasive, problems that arise in the daily practices of family physicians have been left aside... (ref. 3, p. xi).

The practical resolution of such 'mundane' issues as truth-telling in family medicine defies such polarizing dichotomies. More innovative contributions to bioethics have incorporated a richer tapestry of visions that focus on moral qualifiers related to relationships, culture, and community.

A significant contribution to modern bioethics was the publication in 1988 of *The Abuse of Casuistry*. Jonsen and Toulmin argued that there was an indiscriminate emphasis in bioethics debate on 'matters of principle'. 'Too often the resulting argumentation has boiled down to pure head-butting' with the result 'that on the practical level the only possible outcome is deadlock'.(15)

The authors characterized this phenomenon as 'the tyranny of principles' and suggested that

> . . . ethics deals with a multitude of particular concrete situations, which are themselves so variable that they resist all attempts to generalize about them in universal terms. In short . . . ethics . . . is a field of experience that calls for a recognition of significant particulars and for informed prudence: for what [Aristotle] called *phronesis*, or 'practical wisdom' (ref. 15, p. 19).

This philosophical tradition, with its roots in antiquity and its heyday in the sixteenth century, fell into disrepute when its methodology was abused by some to provide argumentation and justifications for untenable moral conclusions. Nevertheless, physicians welcomed the newly rediscovered casuistry as analogous to their own familiar method of 'case-based' analysis, which considers the particular and unique elements of each situation in the ethical analysis.

Thus, casuists would be less interested in proclaiming a universal rule which determined that patient autonomy ranked as a higher principle than medical beneficence, or vice versa. Instead, they would be more interested in the ethical analysis of a specific case, recognizing that, as in medicine, no two cases are identical.

As the world evolves into the 'global village', family physicians are increasingly faced with the challenge of providing care to patients from a range of cultural backgrounds. They are often confronted by apparently conflicting social norms and values. Bioethicists have recently redirected their attention to this issue. Turner critiques the limitations of conventional principlism and casuistry by pointing out how both traditions rely upon the assumption of a common morality.

> Both casuists and principlists . . . rely upon 'commonsense' understandings of morality that presume an expansive beachhead of shared moral experience . . . [they] fail sufficiently to address the significance of distinctive patterns of enculturaltion for the variable evaluation of what is regarded as 'reasonable' . . . A better awareness of the diversity of moral traditions can help . . . recognize the limitations of . . . common methodological tools of reasoning and justification.[16]

He goes on to say:

> . . . Instead of exploring the basic norm of truth-telling, current debates tend to address the more nuanced question of the extent to which prognostic information ought to be made available to patients. In contrast, within nations such as Japan and Italy, it is still common for physicians and family members to conceal diagnoses of cancer . . . from patients. These practices of deception and non-disclosure receive justification from several sources. First, patient autonomy is not accepted as an obvious, 'commonsensical' norm. To the contrary, physicians and family members are expected to fulfil their familial, communal, and professional obligations by assuming responsibility for making decisions (ref. 16, p. 129).

As a variety of other ethics theories, including feminist theory, the 'ethic of caring', and communitarianism contributed new perspectives to bioethics, Beauchamp and Childress addressed what they referred to as 'convergence across theories' and the need for interdisciplinarity.

> Any solidly grounded discipline of ethics involves obtaining relevant factual information, assessing its reliability, and mapping out alternative solutions to problems that have been identified. This mapping sometimes entails presenting and defending reasons in support of factual, conceptual, and moral claims, while at the same time analyzing and assessing basic assumptions and commitments. Ethical theory, then, is but one vital contributor among the disciplines, including medicine, nursing, public health, law, and the social sciences (ref. 14, p. 40).

This rich diversity of ethical theories could easily overwhelm the busy family physician trying to appreciate the ethical dimensions of truth-telling. Which theory is best? How should a family physician apply ethics theories in daily practice? As Beauchamp and Childress point out, '. . . we stand to learn from all of these theories. Where one theory is weak in accounting some part of the moral life, another is often strong' (ref. 14, p. 111). While mastery of philosophy is not a realistic goal for most, physicians who strive to practice ethically will benefit from a basic understanding of the strengths and limitations of these ethical traditions, and integrate the lessons with effective communication skills in clinical practice.

The therapeutic relationship as a foundation for truth-telling

One of the distinguishing features of family medicine is how much it emphasizes the intrinsic value of the long-term, therapeutic, patient–physician relationship. It is often referred to as a 'fiduciary' relationship based on mutual trust and respect. Brennan, in characterizing Paul Ramsay's covenant-fidelity model of medical ethics, writes that

> the moral worth of the doctor–patient relationship is contained within the relationship itself, not in the possible end of the relationship . . . The goodness must reside in the immediate interaction of doctor and patient.[17]

Christie and Hoffmaster have argued that

> knowing that the relationship itself can be a therapeutic tool makes it morally incumbent on family physicians to try to cultivate close, caring, trusting relationships with their patients (ref. 3, p. 29).

Good communication and appropriate attitudes of honesty and respect are required for nurturing such a relationship. Successful communication is dependent on many other variables, including an accurate knowledge of the patient's medical condition. Perhaps more importantly, it requires a comprehensive and sophisticated appreciation of the patient as a unique individual enmeshed in the dynamics of family relationships.

To care for the patient in the context of the family is one thing: to turn the family in to the object of care is another.[18] Pellegrino sees the union of these two concepts as another distinguishing feature of family medicine. In this context, the ethics of family medicine goes beyond the traditional principles of modern bioethics to include the key values of duty and caring. Ironically, this vision of family medicine is both the source of additional dilemmas as well as the foundation for their resolution.

Conventional bioethics discourse focuses on the typical paradigm of a competent, informed, autonomous adult. Within the constellation of a single family, however, a physician may be caring for patients of different ages and capacities, and in varying stages of the life-cycle.

The implicit grey zones of autonomous capacity and familial interdependency profoundly complicate the controversy surrounding disclosure of private medical information. Patients rightly assume that there is an implicit pledge of confidentiality about the personal information they share with their physicians. When physicians breach this pledge, they are effectively lying and violating a patient's privacy. In many family situations, however, physicians might presume patients' consent to relevant disclosure, and such sharing of information would be considered appropriate and even required in many cultures.

The neonate or infant child, as well as the parent with end-stage dementia, may be perceived as completely vulnerable, dependent on family, and lacking autonomy. Here, the issue of truth-telling cannot be polarized into competing values of patient autonomy and physician paternalism. Moral judgements about truth-telling will necessarily be shared not only between physician and patient, but also with responsible family members. The issues become even more complex when addressing the needs of patients in the transitional phases of autonomous living namely the maturing adolescent and the deteriorating elder.

Another kind of truth-telling issue arises when there are inherently conflicting interests and demands among family members, and the physician's role as patient advocate is challenged by potentially conflicting allegiances. The classic scenario of a physician responding to a patient's demands that his sexual infidelity not be divulged to his spouse has been extensively discussed in the literature.[19]

One strategy for defusing some of these tensions is for the family physician to establish a 'contractual' relationship with family members at the outset. By suggesting parameters for information sharing, physician and family members can explicitly agree to reasonable and ethically acceptable boundaries of confidentiality.

The complexities of family dynamics may complicate truth-telling. Nevertheless, it is also the extensive experiential knowledge that comes from the long-term, extensive relationships with patients in a family context, which allows the family physician to lay solid foundations for ethical truth-telling.

Clinical applications

The truth may be brutal, but 'the telling of it should not be'.[20]

When family physicians run into conflicts with patients and family members over issues of truth-telling, the complaints they usually face involve critiques of attitude or action. Physicians may be seen as 'unethical' because they are perceived as uncaring, insensitive, egotistical, or unavailable. They may be accused of telling too much truth, not enough truth, the wrong kind of truth, or revealing truth at the wrong time, in the wrong place, to the wrong people, and in the wrong way. Rarely do patients accuse their physicians of being unethical on the basis of perceived inadequacies in formal skills of ethics analysis. Is the answer to the problem of truth-telling simply one of good communication and not of ethical discernment?

In the clinical setting, the importance of attitude and communication skills cannot be overstated. Yet, analytical skills in ethics and communication skills at the bedside are not unrelated. As Brody points out in his description of the deductive model of ethical justification, our actions are derived from specific decisions, which are in turn derived from moral rules and fundamental values (ref. 1, p. 341). How we act towards others is very much a reflection of our ethical foundations. The key to ethical practice is the successful integration of carefully examined ethical reflection with effective communication strategies.

Resources for training communication skills in medicine are rapidly expanding. As Kurtz et al. states, 'For most people working in this area, the question is no longer whether to teach and assess communication skills and attitudes but, rather, how to do so most efficiently and effectively'.[21] The authors then proceed to identify specific strategies for teaching communication skills and describe a wide variety of available resources on the subject.

One of the most effective strategies in determining the scope and timing of truth-telling was recognized early in the palliative care movement, and later described by Freedman.[22] Skillful communication often begins with sensitive listening. The physician then proceeds to 'offer truth' in logical, sequential phases. By carefully asking sensitive questions, the skilled communicator can effectively determine what the patient's needs and wishes are with respect to truth-telling at any given time.

Such an approach, properly implemented, can untangle the orthodox dilemma between patient autonomy and medical paternalism. The physician can navigate the delicate route between providing as much 'truth' as possible, while respecting the patient's own assessment of his capacity to deal with it safely. Objections from family members and friends can be similarly defused when they see that truth-telling is a shared experience between patient and physician, with the physician providing guidance and cues, and the patient providing direction.

The skills required to navigate such complex ethical waters on a case-by-case basis may appear daunting. Consider the following clinical scenarios.

> Two patients are diagnosed with inoperable cancer. They are both surrounded by loving and caring family members who insist that the truth about their illness and prognosis be withheld on the grounds that it would do them irreparable harm. Both patients are weak and frail. Both are competent, but exhibit initial signs of cognitive impairment, including memory loss, poor concentration, and questionable judgement. Their families firmly believe that the patients' best interests can only be met if the quality and length of their lives is maximized, and both of these would be compromised if the truth were known. In both cases, a single family member approaches you and suggests that it would be inappropriate to withhold the truth, as the patient has a right to be aware of and understand his situation, and be able to plan the rest of his life accordingly.

One of the advantages of family medicine is that the physician is likely to have a long-term relationship with these patients, and is able to appreciate their life narratives as richly textured and unique experiences. Using this privileged information, the family physician can be particularly sensitive to any stated or implied questions that would indicate an interest in knowing the truth. In the absence of such clues, the physician may gently raise a succession of questions, ranging from the very general to the more specific, to gauge patients' willingness and ability to explore the truth.

Patient 'A' never raises the issue of diagnosis and prognosis, despite the fact that his symptoms are increasing in frequency and intensity, and more visits to the physician are required. He consistently deflects any general questions from the physician regarding his condition, maintains a determined and stoic disposition, and begins to request that his son accompany him on all future visits. Eventually, it becomes obvious to all parties that the patient's condition has deteriorated significantly within a relatively short period of time.

> 'Is there anything else you want to ask me about that we haven't already discussed?' his physician asks once again.
>
> 'Doctor, where I come from, family takes care of each other, through thick and thin, no matter what. We've been through some pretty bad times, but we've always been there for each other. Thanks for all your help, but I'll be O.K. My son is here. He'll be there for me when I need him. I'll see you next week.'

Patient 'B', on the other hand, is accompanied on all visits by his ever-present and protective spouse, who answers almost all questions the physician poses to the patient. The patient himself looks forlorn and withdrawn. The physician respectfully asks the spouse to leave as he starts examining the patient. During the examination, the physician remarks on how uncharacteristically quiet the patient has been. The patient says nothing, but looks at the physician with pleading eyes.

> 'You know we haven't had much time to talk about things like we did before,' the physician offers.
>
> 'What is there to talk about?' the patient counters.
>
> 'Well, there could be lots of things. I'm sure you must have a lot of questions.'
>
> 'No one wants to tell me anything.'
>
> 'Illness can be a very scary thing. Perhaps your family is having a great deal of difficulty talking about it. But I can promise that I'll answer any questions you may have as honestly as I can. I can also help your wife with what must be a difficult situation.'
>
> Patient B silently squeezes his doctor's hand and nods his head.
>
> 'Is there anything you would like to ask me now?...'

Patient 'A' died several months later without ever hearing the word 'cancer' spoken to him. Patient 'B' died having had explicit discussions with his physician and family about his diagnosis and prognosis. The family physician monitored both patients very closely to make clinical judgements on the scope and timing of truth-telling. The physician's role was to follow each patient's directives about truth-telling, by interpreting those directives in the context of the knowledge garnered from the long-term patient–doctor relationship. Ultimately, both patients learned and knew the truth in a way that was most meaningful for them.

One can imagine other clinical scenarios where the ethical choices are even more challenging. Consider patient 'C', who is in a similar predicament to the previous two patients. However, he has had a long history of severe, refractory depression, punctuated by numerous episodes of attempted suicide. His current illness has further undermined his psychological coping abilities. He is also a highly individualistic, somewhat eccentric artist, who confronts the physician and insists that he be told 'the truth, the whole truth, and nothing but the truth'. Without an appreciation of this patient's life narrative, it would be almost impossible to judge which action would produce the greatest good and the least harm—to tell or not to tell.

It would be difficult to justify denying this patient his request. Traumatic as the truth might be for the patient and his family, many would argue that the patient has an overarching and fundamental right to know the truth about his life. The physician's role would be to tell the truth while mitigating the potential harms.

In even more extreme situations, however, physicians have invoked the concept of 'therapeutic privilege', where they judge the potential harms of disclosure to be so high and so grossly disproportionate to any anticipated benefit, that the truth is withheld from the patient even in the face of an explicit demand for it. Increasingly, this notion of 'therapeutic privilege' is being narrowly defined to limit the dangers associated with paternalism.

These clinical vignettes illustrate an important point. While physicians must appreciate the value of guiding ethical principles, there is no ready-made algorithm or hierarchy of values that can be universally applied to all clinical situations. The complexity of the human condition and the uniqueness of each clinical situation seem to defy such simplicity. Instead, the ethical physician is required to make moral *judgements* by interpreting the guiding principles in the context of the patient's life narrative. The long-standing nature of the patient–physician relationship in family medicine is critical to the appreciation of that life narrative.

Conclusions

The practicing family physician may be overwhelmed and intimidated by the exaggerated complexity of a seemingly simple topic. The following summary is intended to help extract key lessons.

The two major conclusions of this chapter are:

1. Family physicians must learn to identify and analyse ethical issues in truth-telling in order to differentiate appropriate exceptions to full disclosure from unacceptable abuses.
2. Family physicians must integrate ethics analysis with effective communication skills in order to achieve a meaningful clinical application.

In order to achieve these objectives, the following points may prove useful:

1. Truth-telling is not an idealized, comprehensive, and immutable list of information. It is meaningful when interpreted in the context of a patient's life narrative. This includes references to family and intimate friends.
2. Compromises to truth-telling should be considered as exceptions to the general rule of full and meaningful disclosure.
3. The burden of proof in justifying exceptions falls to the physician.
4. Ethical justification derives from a careful, interdisciplinary analysis involving philosophy, theology, medicine, nursing, law, etc.
5. Philosophy has contributed numerous theories of ethics analysis. Each has strengths and limitations, and the prudent physician will apply the best of each theory with the specificity required by a given case.
6. Autonomy, non-maleficence, beneficence, and justice are the cornerstone principles of modern bioethics. This framework helps us convert the clinical problem of 'tell or do not tell' into an appreciation of the competing principles of patient autonomy and medical beneficence.
7. Casuistry offers a case-based approach that emphasizes the qualifiers that are unique to each situation and facilitates a practical resolution.
8. Sensitivity to cultural differences may facilitate a better awareness of the diversity of moral traditions and diminish the risk of 'cultural imperialism'.
9. Many resources now exist for teaching physicians communications skills. Effective communication requires a respectful attitude and active listening. The dilemma of competing values of patient autonomy and medical beneficence may be substantially defused by invoking techniques such as 'offering the truth' in a logical, sequential manner where the physician guides and the patient directs.
10. Despite the daunting challenges, family physicians may capitalize on their long-standing therapeutic relationships with their patients and access rich life narratives that reveal meaningful contexts for truth-telling.

References

1. **Brody, H.** *Ethical Decisions in Medicine* 2nd edn. Boston: Little, Brown and Company, 1981, p. 48.
2. **Bok, S.** *Lying: Moral Choice in Public and Private Life.* New York: Vintage Books, 1989, pp. 272–5.
3. **Christie, R.J. and Hoffmaster, C.B.** *Ethical Issues in Family Medicine.* Oxford: Oxford University Press, 1986, p. 98.
4. **Sheldon, M.** (1982). Truth telling in medicine. *Journal of the American Medical Association* **247** (5), 652.
5. **Hebert, P.** (1994). Truth-telling in clinical practice. *Canadian Family Physician* **40**, 2105–13.
6. **Hebert, P., Hoffmaster, B., Glass, K., and Singer, P.** (1997). Bioethics for clinicians: truth telling. *Canadian Medical Association Journal* **156** (2), 225–8.
7. **Katz, J.** *The Silent World of Doctor and Patient.* New York: The Free Press, 1986, p. xvi.
8. **Beauchamp, T. and McCullough, L.** *Medical Ethics: the Moral Responsibilities of Physicians.* New Jersey: Prentice-Hall, 1984, p. 59.
9. **Miyaji, N.** (1993). The power of compassion: truth-telling among American doctors in the care of dying patients. *Social Science and Medicine* **36** (3), 249–64.
10. **Novack, D.** et al. (1989). Physicians' attitudes toward using deception to resolve difficult ethical problems. *Journal of the American Medical Association* **261** (20), 2980–5.
11. **Newsbriefs** (1991). *Canadian Medical Association Journal* **145** (5), 490.
12. **Lo, B.** (1998). Ethical Issues in Clinical Medicine. *Harrison's Principles of Internal Medicine* 14th edn. New York: McGraw-Hill, p. 3.
13. **Pellegrino, E.** (1992). Is truth telling to the patient a cultural artifact? *Journal of the American Medical Association* **268** (13), 1735.
14. **Beauchamp, T. and Childress, J.** *Principles of Biomedical Ethics* 4th edn. Oxford: Oxford University Press, 1994.
15. **Jonsen, A. and Toulmin, S.** *The Abuse of Casuistry.* Berkeley: University of California Press, 1988, p. 4.
16. **Turner, L.** (1998). An anthropological exploration of contemporary bioethics: the varieties of common sense. *Journal of Medical Ethics* **24**, 127.
17. **Brennan, T.** *Just Doctoring: Medical Ethics in the Liberal State.* Berkeley: University of California Press, 1991, p. 34.
18. **Carmichael, L.P.** (1976). The family in medicine, process or entity? *Journal of Family Practice* **3**, 562.
19. **Doyal, K. and Hurwitz, B.** (1987). Respecting confidentiality and telling the truth in general practice. *The Practitioner* **231**, 1067–71.
20. **Jonsen, A., Siegler, M., and Winslade, W.** *Clinical Ethics.* New York: Macmillan Publishing Co., 1992, p. 53.
21. **Kurtz, S.** et al. (1999). Medical education initiatives in communication skills. *Cancer Prevention & Control* **3** (1), 37.
22. **Freedman, B.** (1993). Offering truth: one ethical approach to the uninformed cancer patient. *Archives of Internal Medicine* **153** (5), 572–6.

16.4 Confidentiality

Roger Higgs

Of course, everybody knows that what they say to their doctor is confidential. A medical secret is safe with the clinician: it is part of the professional ethos, protected and policed by professional bodies world-wide. The tradition is ancient, the assumptions deep. The problem is, does it work that way? If it does not, should it? If it does, is it always for the best? Might there be real hazards or are there limits to its application? Is confidentiality especially difficult in community practice, primary care or family medicine? If things are going to change, how should they be thought through and how negotiated? It will not be possible to give complete answers to any of these questions which will satisfy everybody. Ethical thinking is always work in progress, and to be anywhere near half satisfactory must be contextual and iterative as well as coherent and rational. But, as Kirkegaard said, in moral thinking, like sewing, it is necessary to knot the end of the thread.[1] We must start with the central concept.

The medical secret

Clinicians invade the privacy of a person who comes to them as a patient out of the demands of their task. For some patients, medical care necessitates revealing a part of the body never since childhood seen by anyone else, perhaps not even by a sexual partner. For others, it may involve discussing or demonstrating symptoms which risk being seen as shameful, ludicrous, or disgusting. Part of the very process of understanding such symptoms may be a discussion of issues the patient has never shared with anyone else before: a sexual infidelity, or an antisocial desire. The patient is deeply vulnerable: dignity, sense of self, special relationships may be at risk. The atmosphere of trust, within which such things must be handled, is precious: it may have taken a lot on both sides to establish, both within the history of that relationship and in the development of the surrounding society. The promise of that trust (implicit or explicit), once broken, may be impossible to rebuild. Patients may never return. Thus, everyone has an interest in preserving the possibility of confidential discussion in health care. This interest is strong enough to be maintained by law, so strong that in some countries (like France and Belgium) it is enshrined in the criminal law.[2] As a commitment, it could be seen as a 'guarantee of fairness in medical actions',[3] and in some areas of work, such as with sexually transmitted diseases, this is so important as to be an absolute commitment, or 'as so near absolute as makes no difference'.[4]

But this secret hides a deeper secret

We do not need philosophers of language, however, to tell us that anything which is near but not absolute could be trumped, and that this *will* make a difference, somewhere, sometime for someone. Were we to be able to say that confidentiality (or any other major concept in ethics and law for that matter) was absolute, then this would be the end of the discussion. But this is neither logically nor practically a possibility. Logically, to admit to any other issues being able to challenge or negate a concept renders it something less than absolute. Practically, it may be difficult to maintain when there are coherent societal interests in disclosure (as vital in some circumstances it seems, as those commanding confidentiality); and then impossible in many cases because modern medical work simply cannot and should not be undertaken by one person alone. The details of the latter were so overwhelming to lawyer Paul Sieghart that, when he saw how many people working in hospital had legitimate access to patients' files, he called confidentiality a 'decrepit concept'.[5] The theoretical principal enacted in practice had simply fallen to pieces in his hands. The differences in primary care are of degree only. General practitioners, nurses, receptionists, and secretaries all have legitimate access, at some level or other, to the medical records of patients as part of their job. This is not widely understood by the public. In a qualitative study Carman and Britten[6] showed that British patients even had concerns about other doctors' access to their records, let alone non-medical staff. There were concerns too about computer-held records. 'There seemed to be a hope that confidentiality would be maintained by indifference', the authors conclude. Shortly after this was published, the current writer talked to a medical student just returned from staying in a country practice. She described the handling within that community of the information that one of their early teenage patients had tested positive for gonorrhoea. 'As an outsider it was alarming to see who got to know about it. The information proved much more infectious and transmissible than the disease.' The gay community at the beginning of the AIDS epidemic in the United Kingdom had some hard lessons to learn about the 'leakiness' of general practice and many lost faith in the system.[7] In spite of all the fine words, confidential issues are still poorly handled in many circumstances both within hospitals and in primary care. The profession has moved from the Hippocratic to the hypocritical. It is an accident waiting to happen.

The practicalities

What can be done? One logical response would be to abandon the pretence altogether, and acknowledge that the decrepit concept should be allowed to die—last rites for lost rights. Everyone would then be clear in whose hands the responsibility lay. Without a commitment by professionals to confidentiality, proposed Warwick, the patient would be left as 'absolute guardian of his/her own personal privacy and autonomy'.[8] It would be up to each ill person to decide, between privacy and health, which was the more important to them. Such a clear-cut approach might appeal to purists but would be a hard experiment for the medical world to conduct in isolation from society in general. Whilst shame, blame, and loss of face exist in human relationships worldwide, it would be paradoxical for a kind or fair doctor to offer this type of decision, which Gillon likens to a surgeon offering an operation but refusing to provide an anaesthetic. Even if respect for autonomy has wide appeal as an underpinning principle, most patients would still probably choose 'optimal treatment including disclosure of necessary private information but in the context of confidentiality'.[9] Like partners stuck in an old and battered marriage, it appears we must make do.

Part of that 'making do' is to make the system do what it should in the way it should. Slipshod practice has no defence. Currently professional medical organizations in primary care work on the basis that there is a *cordon of confidentiality* around those who need to work within medical teams. Those who are about to move into this cordon should receive proper training. Sanctions are real: transgression is a serious offence, and could lead to an employee being dismissed. But not all who need to join a team are in a contractual relationship with that team. Some may be in training, such as medical or nursing students, while some may be part of other teams, such as social work or voluntary sector workers: these must sign up to the same standards. In the context of any individual's health care, a distinction has to be made between groups that form round an organization and those that form round an individual. The latter may include neighbours or members of the family: in primary care, the key carer may be a close relative. Lines have to be drawn, but where and how? Strict or stringent criteria in these circumstances may be hard to negotiate or maintain. Where the main patient belongs to a small linguistic minority group, for instance, a translator may be part of the caring team but may also be a close relative with different or unknown allegiances. A process to determine how we should proceed is now desperately needed. What is the legal and moral thinking which underpins the arguments? How can these ideas be negotiated in practice?

The concept and its backing

What does the law say? The legal nature of the obligation may vary from country to country: but a limited conditional right to confidentiality is a basic human right recognized by most legal systems. In the English system, its basis has been described by two experts as 'a bizarre cocktail of tort, equity, contract, property and downright judicial imagination... arguing about the obligation is a waste of time: the obligation exists and has well known characteristics'.[10] Thus, the law imposes the duty of confidentiality on clinicians (and others); but the public interest in disclosure may override it. The boot may then be on the other foot: a clinician who does not disclose may be at fault. As Justice Tobriner famously declared in 1976, finding against the University of California when a threat from a patient to kill a young woman was not properly declared by the psychotherapy services, 'The protective privilege ends where the public peril begins'.[11] While 'public peril' may be the key concept, the shift in word from 'duty' to 'privilege' of confidentiality shows something of the delicate but in individual cases decisive nature of this balance. The clinician or manager is not let off the hook. However much professional agencies, such as the British General Medical

Council[12], may publish guidelines, the individual clinician with a confidence must still make a proper assessment of the arguments, and make her justifications clear, explicitly and in writing in difficult cases. What can guide that clinician?

Roles and rules

With danger and the threat of harm may come a consideration of the role that the clinician is in. While all of us as citizens may have a duty to prevent harm coming to others, a clinician may have a very clear protective role, say to save a child from abuse or the public from a dangerous driver. In the role of a teacher, researcher, employer, or friend these duties may be less immediately clear or differently balanced: but issues of clinical governance will undoubtedly be there at second hand. While some people are used to juggling different roles informally as a parent or spouse, some roles, such as that of occupational health physician, formally carry explicit dual responsibilities. In these circumstances, specific arrangements have to be made to control the boundaries of information in both directions: to ensure, say, that the patient is fully warned about the purpose of procedures and the limits of confidentiality, and to ensure that the employer respects the doctor–patient relationship and trusts the doctor to act in good faith. A physician asked to work in such an environment without the rules being clear would be as unwise to sign up for the job as the patient would be to disclose to the physician.

Disclosure—agreed, minimal, justified and with consent

Where there is a balance to be struck between the harm of danger and the harm of disclosure, the key issue allowing disclosure remains permission from an informed autonomous subject (with respect given to individual autonomy even if that autonomy may be compromised or in question). This should permeate and direct both policies and promises, but should always include the clear understanding that in extreme circumstances disclosure without permission may be forced upon the professional. The first part is core, but the second part is the small print which needs often to be enlarged. The first dictates that the preferred route is always through discussion, exploration, negotiation, education, and persuasion: where possible permission should always be explicit. This may need time, both in the sense of requiring professional attention and in the passing of time for ideas and information to 'sink in' and be processed by the patient. Medical emergencies may preclude this, but a judgement that the harm is so serious or that personal autonomy is at risk is an emergency in its own right and should be given proper attention. Second or third opinions may be necessary, with their own 'rules of engagement'. Throughout these processes, practical considerations must be given proper place. Nothing more should be told than needs to be told. All data should be anonymized wherever possible. This should allow an individual professional to discuss whether or not to disclose with suitable other nominated individuals within the cordon of confidentiality or to go outside it without breaking trust while the issue is under consideration.

Working practices

In practice, this means that every professional should have someone to whom she could turn, and that teams must have discussion time built into busy working lives to enable education and debate to take place as well as sharing information. No one should be surprised or put out if the 'need to know' includes a 'need not to know' or be excluded. It may be vital for a receptionist, observing a child and a parent in a waiting room for longer than a clinician might have available, to know that there was a suspicion of abuse, but it would almost certainly not be necessary for either the receptionist or clinician to know of the fantasies the mother might have told the practice counsellor in a bereavement session. Different professionals within that team may have differing views of potential harms and so different professional boundaries. But these differences should be recognized and the

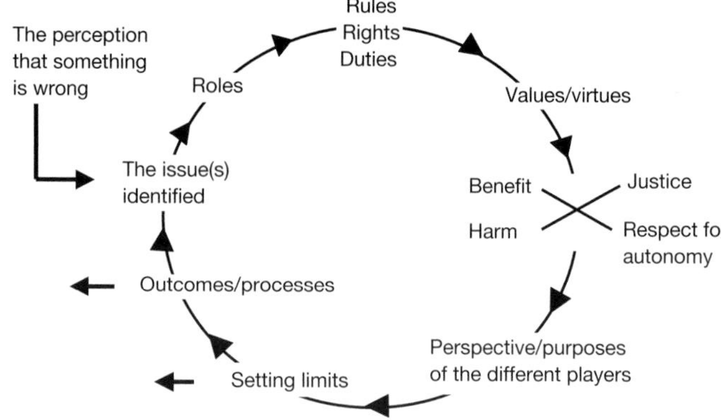

Fig. 1 The formal process of reasoning.

rules clear. Working with the mind or sexual relationships may rightly raise the threshold for sharing information, whereas working with children or families may require the reverse. Clinicians often assume that they are the pinnacle of such a process within a primary care team, but the present author, in training workshops with teams, has come across situations where a receptionist, say, felt it unfair to share a particular observation or perception with a clinician, on the grounds that it might undermine the doctor–patient relationship. The clinicians were surprised, some appalled, to be excluded: but most equally agreed that the decision was reasonable. The dilemmas are not just in the practice of health care. Are the arguments we use sound ones?

Thinking it through

Most of us learn whether to tell or not to tell through living in families and surviving in the playground. Studies of people making difficult decisions suggest that some go through a formal process of reasoning, while others consider the effects on all the people relevant to the decision.[13] The formal process may be seen as a circle, entering different argument 'modes' and using different approaches (Fig. 1). But while a judgement may be inadequate when only one point of view is considered, it may be impossible to do justice to all. A decision has to be made: in health care, there is seldom the luxury of staying permanently on the fence. Sometimes a final decision will be made against a background of intuition, instinct, 'common sense' or emotion we may not (yet) be aware of—though becoming aware may be one of the important outcomes of reflection. Equally, we may be guided by outside forces, in terms of tradition, authority, or consensus. Finally we may wish to bring together the tools we know (or think we know) we use—rational theory, logic, experience and professional judgement or even guesswork.[14]

All this may be happening when we bring to bear professional and interpersonal processes in a nuanced way on moral reasoning in practice, and questions of confidentiality should be no different. The routines we have will have to be of the best, but it's unlikely that 'one size will fit all'. Contextual thinking using key concepts appropriately and consistently is hard but a skill which can be developed.

Some traps

Gossip

While proper communication within teams is essential, the most common interchange in practice is usually of a different sort: gossip, letting off steam, casual talk between individuals which means no harm and usually causes none until it leaks out. In an institution like a hospital chat between professionals has its own rhythm, language, and containment, but in community practice it may be more problematic for many reasons. One is geographical.

European Data Protection Act 1998 involves three main parties:
- Data subject
- Data controller (the professional)
- Data Protection Commissioner (who has a register)

Principles include: personal data
- may only be processed fairly and lawfully
- shall be adequate, relevant, not excessive
- shall be accurate and up-to-date
- shall not be kept for any longer than necessary for the purpose
- shall be protected by adequate technical and organizational measures to prevent unauthorized processing, loss, damage, destruction

Fig. 2 The European Data Protection Act 1998 and its principles.

People can overhear what is said behind the reception desk. Staff live locally, next to, or related to patients. Carers or translators may be relatives. Much maybe learnt by someone sitting in a waiting room by the demeanour of those who come and go, and by how long is a consultation, what specimens are handed across the desk, which pills are collected. One side of a telephone conversation may reveal both.

But gossip is a word which has come down in the world. A gossip originally was 'God's sib or sibling'. It is due perhaps for some rehabilitation. In all walks of life the grapevine, informal exchange of information, is valued: it may increase social effectiveness, and it may create cohesion in a group: to be out of its hearing is to be out of circulation, 'out of the loop'.[15] Like trade, there has to be a two-way flow of information or there is no exchange. Confidentiality poses an insurmountable barrier here, but there is no doubt that primary care workers do risk losing important information about clients, about the effectiveness (or rather, the ineffectiveness) of their treatments, about people's real motivations, joys, or suffering by not joining in informal discussions. But the temptation to gossip may come from a deeper compulsion. Morally difficult situations, revealed to clinicians, cannot but raise anxiety. Most people deal with this by sharing what they have heard with someone else, both for guidance and to compare and diffuse. Total elimination of such contact between clinicians would therefore come at a price unless there are other ways in which such debriefing can happen. Doctors appear to be one of the last remaining groups delivering personal care in Western society who are expected to cope on their own, and to have no supervision or guidance from any other defined individual. With major responsibilities in a complex society this may simply be beyond the capacity of other than exceptional individuals. The results, in terms of breakdown or bad behaviour are there for all to see. Doctors are human and need professional support like others.[16] Better professional supervision would be more likely to improve than dilute patient confidentiality.

Data protection

The media show no sign of reducing their interest in the medical details of whoever is deemed newsworthy at the time: columnists more and more depend on high technology. While new technology may assist data protection in some ways, it raises specific problems for a professional. The principles of data protection are not in question, but the implications may be changing almost as quickly as the data systems themselves. The European Data Protection Act of 1998 (Fig. 2) is likely to become influential: wide definitions may even lead to the inclusion of oral data under legal scrutiny.[10]

Dilemmas of the new medical ethics

If ordinary clinical work in primary care were not difficult enough within the rubric of confidentiality, some other areas stand out where practice is changing rapidly.

Designer genes

Confidentiality about an individual is one thing, but where the implications involve a family or a group, lines become very blurred. A clinician discovers the couple is infertile because the wife is a feminized male. Genetic testing of a child suggests that the father could not be biologically related. An aunt hides her breast cancer from a niece: the niece asks for guidance about her own genetic risk. These are the sort of issues that are as common crises in primary care as heart failure or intestinal obstruction, yet receive surprisingly little attention. What is germane here is that the usual arguments for disclosure, such as public danger, the patient's best interests, administration or emergency do not apply, and yet there are parties with strong interests who might come to harm. None of this undermines the usual practice of confidentiality, but family doctors may have to learn watertight procedures that respect individuals but allow a measure of disclosure to groups.[17] In that way, community practice acknowledges that there are other strands of thought or ways of constructing morality, which are common currency in some cultures but submerged in the west, such as communitarian thinking which values interdependence as highly as independence. Some, reporting on other cultures, are clear that the West will have to change.[18]

Crossing to safety

The balance between protecting confidences and protecting the vulnerable may be more difficult to strike at times of transition. Children becoming adults or adults becoming dependent elderly may pose moral problems for the safe and sensitive clinician. An unwanted pregnancy in an early teenager will only be revealed out of necessity or in conditions of trust, and it is vital to respect the confidences of children just as much as of adults. Yet the father may turn out to be an abusive adult and so a great deal of sensitive work may be needed to enable the child to open up about this and seek proper protection.[19] A dementing old lady may be falling in her daughter's home but might be being pushed by someone at the end of her tether. Care is at risk either way, and the confidences of each party may reside in different quarters. Discussion held within the cordon of confidentiality where care not condemnation is the guiding principle may be the only way forward.

Standards and whistle-blowing

Anonymized data or largely depersonalized information for administration purposes, research, or publication have long been a justified form of disclosure, but the concern that confidentiality could hide bad practice has until recently been largely a theoretical concern. Taking quality monitoring seriously however means that professional or managing agencies have to be able to know something about treatment details. Where this raises concerns about the health of a member of staff, the balance of information flow becomes particularly delicate and should be handled by someone with skills and standing in occupational health. By their very nature groups in primary care may not have access to such agencies, or may be providing their own healthcare to staff internally, creating a structured problem where none should exist.

Mental health and public safety

As secondary and tertiary care increasingly takes on the care of psychotic illness, primary care finds itself in many countries taking up a key role in providing psychotherapy, counselling and guidance in areas of behaviour and lifestyle. Where individuals express interests or have fantasies about behaviour which may create a public threat, the responses of law-makers and keepers increasingly place an onus on therapy to prevent as well as cure. The difficulty of doing either in areas such as child abuse or family violence has not diminished the enthusiasm of the public to pursue potential perpetrators or, if that is impossible, those in whom those potential perpetrators place their trust. It may be very hard for a clinician or therapist to know when a fantasy becomes a plan, and a plan a reality. Discussion with a supervisor in total confidentiality has been a method of working, yet courts in some countries show signs of wishing to subpoena notes and get evidence from supervisors as well as therapists. Our commitment to holistic and narrative practice and the imperative to be in contact with new forms of distress may be deflected. A solution, such as the creation of an inviolable 'third space', or extending the protection rights of confidentiality of legal counsel to specific supervisors provide some possible ways forward.[20]

The way ahead

The modern concept of confidentiality in practice may now be seen to be emerging. We have moved from an abused absolute principle to a realistic clinical process held in dynamic balance within a group mutually and strictly committed to the ideals of privacy and safety. This suggests that a new dialogue between clinicians and society is required.[21] As well as informing the public of the realities of information-passing in modern medical care, explicit agreements based on mutual education seem to be needed. Anonymized data, consent to disclose, the cordon of confidentiality, and proper training in the justifications for disclosure are a good start but may not be enough. Information is a gift, and should be received and handled with due respect. This respect will always have to include evaluation and re-evaluation of how to preserve and strengthen both public safety and private sanctuaries. This balance can never be done by rote. As Nussbaum has reminded us, what we value most may also be most vulnerable.[22] Value and risk inhabit the same space.

References

1. **Kirkegaard, S.** Quoted in Murdoch, I. *Metaphysics as a Guide to Morals.* London: Penguin, 1993.
2. **Mason, J. and McColl Smith, R.** *Law and Medical Ethics.* London: Butterworth, 1987.
3. **Kottow, M.** (1986). Medical confidentiality: an intransigent and absolute obligation. *Journal of Medical Ethics* **12**, 117–22.
4. **Pinching, A.J.** (1994). AIDS: Health care ethics and society. In *Principles of Health Care Ethics* (ed. R. Gillon), pp. 903–15. Chichester UK: Wiley.
5. **Siegler, M.** (1982). Confidentiality in medicine: a decrepit concept. *New England Journal of Medicine* **307**, 1518–21.
6. **Carman, D. and Britten, N.** (1995). Confidentiality of medical records: the patient's perspective. *British Journal of General Practice* **45**, 485–8.
7. **Pinching, A.J., Higgs, R., and Boyd, K.M.** (2000). The impact of AIDS on medical ethics. *Journal of Medical Ethics* **26**, 3–8.
8. **Warwick, S.J.** (1989). A vote for no confidence. *Journal of Medical Ethics* **15**, 183–5.
9. **Gillon, R.** (1998). Confidentiality. In *A Companion to Bioethics* (ed. H. Kuhse and P. Singer), pp. 425–31. Oxford: Blackwell.
10. **Foster, C. and Peacock, N.** *Clinical Confidentiality.* Sudbury UK: Monitor Press, 2000.
11. **California Supreme Court** (1994). Tarasoff versus Regents of the University of California. In *Contemporary Issues in Bioethics* (ed. T.L. Beauchamp and L. Watters), pp. 174–8. Belmont CA: Wadsworth.
12. **General Medical Council.** *Confidentiality: Protecting and Providing Information.* London: GMC, 2000.
13. **Gilligan, C.** *In a Different Voice: Psychological Theory and Women's Development.* Cambridge MA: Harvard University Press, 1993.
14. **Lloyd, D., Maycock, A., and Nixon, J.** Personal communication, 2001.
15. **Ben-Ze'ev, A.** (1994). The vindication of gossip. In *Good Gossip* (ed. R.F. Goodman and A. Ben-Ze'ev). Kansas: University Press.
16. **Higgs, R.** (1994). Doctors in crisis: creating a strategy for mental health in health care work. *Journal of the Royal College of Physicians London* **28**, 538–40.
17. **Skene, L.** (2001). Genetic secrets and the family: a response to Bell and Bennett. *Medical Law Review* **9**, 162–9.
18. **Schweder, R.A.** et al. (1997). The 'big three' of morality (autonomy, community, diversity) and the 'big three' explanations of suffering. In *Morality and Health* (ed. A.M. Brandt and P. Rozin). New York: Routledge.
19. *Confidentiality and Young People: Improving Teenagers' Uptake of Sexual and other Health Advice.* London: Royal College of General Practitioners and Brook, 2000.
20. **Cordess, C.** (2001). Confidentiality and contemporary practice. In *Confidentiality and Mental Health* (ed. C. Cordess). London: Jessica Kingsley Publishers.
21. **Boyd, K., Callaghan, B., Gillon, R., Higgs, R., and Hoffenberg, R.** (2002). Wanted: a social contract for the practice of medicine (editorial). *British Medical Journal* **323**, 64.
22. **Nussbaum, M.C.** *The Fragility of Goodness: Luck and Ethics in Greek Tragedy and Philosophy.* Cambridge UK: Cambridge University Press, 2001.

16.5 Ethics of research

Anne Slowther and Tony Hope

The fundamental ethical principles underpinning the conduct of medical research are the same in primary, secondary, or tertiary care. Where the research takes place does not affect the standards laid down in national and international guidelines for good practice in medical research. However, the application of these guidelines, and their underlying principles, may have specific implications for particular types of research carried out in primary care, and for a primary care physician's role in the research (Table 1).

The amount of research carried out in primary care is increasing. Many conditions are dealt with wholly in primary care and others have a spectrum of severity, only part of which is seen in secondary care where most clinical research is done. There is increasing emphasis on providing care for chronic disease such as diabetes and asthma in primary care. This means that the research focus for these conditions will also shift from secondary to primary care, if only because too few patients are seen in secondary care. New models of health care delivery based in primary care need research evidence of their effectiveness. Similarly, the impact of the proliferation of 'evidence-based guidelines' for managing disease in primary care needs evaluating (see Section 14).

The expansion of research in or on primary care requires more than transposing traditional clinical trials or epidemiological methodology into a different setting. New methods are required for looking at the complex clinical and social situations seen in primary care. There has been some discussion in the literature around the theoretical and practical problems of research in primary care and approaches to developing high-quality, relevant research. There has been less discussion of the ethical issues raised by this research. Research in primary care may place a different perspective on

Table 1 Five different roles for primary care physicians in research

Principal researcher responsible for designing and conducting research
Secondary researcher carrying out research on behalf of a larger research organization
Provider of patients by recruiting participants for research carried out by others
Providers of information for epidemiological studies
Research participant in studies where the intervention is at an individual or practice-based level, e.g. implementation of guidelines or introduction of a new service

common ethical issues in medical research, including the nature of consent, what is considered a harm, and how important is confidentiality.

In this chapter, we shall first consider the ethical framework within which all medical research should be undertaken and then focus on some specific issues relevant to primary care.

Historical perspective of ethics in medical research

There are historical reasons why the regulation of medical research involving patients differs from the regulation of normal clinical practice.

The appalling experiments conducted by some doctors under the Nazi regime led to the first internationally agreed guidelines on research involving people, the Nuremberg Code (1949).[(1)] This consisted of 10 principles that were incorporated by the World Medical Association into the Declaration of Helsinki, first published in 1964 and last updated in 2000.[(2)] The Declaration provides an internationally agreed ethical framework for the conduct of medical research involving humans. It is the basis for the various more detailed national guidelines that have been developed by many countries. Thus, whereas the regulation of good medical practice has developed, to a large extent, separately in each country and has generally emerged upwards from medical practice, the regulation of medical research has developed 'top-down', from an internationally agreed approach. Medical practice broadly assumes that the doctor and the patient both want what is best for the patient. Despite the emphasis on patient autonomy in recent decades, modern models of the doctor–patient relationship emphasize a collaborative approach to decision-making.[(3–5)] The regulation of research ethics, because of its origins in the Nuremberg code, focuses on protecting research participants. The central concern is to ensure that the interests of society, or the enthusiasm of the researcher, do not override the interests of the individual. These differences in the origins and perspectives of the regulation of clinical and research practice account for much of the tension that can arise between a medical researcher and a research ethics committee.

Ethical framework

The guidelines, and ethical debate, around research involving people highlight four main issues: respect for the autonomy of the potential participants; the risk of harm; the value and quality of the research; and aspects of justice. The first two issues are of particular importance and are the issues most likely to cause a research protocol to be rejected by an ethics committee (Table 2).

Table 2 Checklist of specific ethical issues in medical research

Respect for autonomy	Consent
	Competent
	Informed
	Voluntary
	Confidentiality
	Patient contact details
	Information from medical records
	Research data and results
Risk of harm to participants	Physical
	Psychological
	Therapeutic/non-therapeutic research
Value and quality of the research	Are the aims worthwhile?
	Is the methodology appropriate to the aims?
	Are the outcomes clinically significant?
	Are the outcomes patient centred?
Justice	Are the inclusion and exclusion criteria appropriate (see text)

Respect for the autonomy of potential research participants

Respecting the autonomy of potential research participants has implications for both the consent procedure and confidentiality. From this perspective, for consent to be valid the potential participant should be properly informed about those issues relevant to making a decision; and completely free from any coercion or pressure to take part. In addition, the potential participant should have the capacity to understand the relevant information and make a decision. Respecting autonomy also emphasizes the importance of confidentiality. On this view, personal information should not normally be shared without the explicit consent of the person to whom it relates.

One approach to the ethics of research would be to give almost exclusive weight to respecting patient autonomy. This is the libertarian position. It has some interesting implications.

1. If a potential research subject is fully informed, competent, and not coerced, then that person has a right to take part in even very dangerous research. In defence of this position, libertarians might point out that we allow people to take considerable risks, for example, in the pursuit of dangerous sports.

   This position is not that endorsed in the guidelines for research ethics, which emphasize that research subjects should not normally be put at more than minimal risk.
2. Should payments be given to participants as inducement to improve recruitment? Such inducements are often analysed in terms of their acting as a form of coercion for subjects to take part in the research and are, therefore, seen as unethical. This would not be the libertarian position that would see it as a matter entirely for the potential subject to decide for himself/herself. Again, this position is not that given in the relevant guidelines.[(6,7)]
3. The libertarian would give a great deal of weight to a potential participant's right of confidentiality and right to withhold consent to take part even when the benefit of the research is great and there is no harm to the participant. Thus, epidemiological research involving anonymized data obtained from individual patient records without consent would be problematic. The issue for the libertarian is not that no harm results but that patients have the right to control access to information about themselves.
4. Research on those who do not have the capacity to give consent (e.g. young children or those suffering from cognitive impairment) is problematic for the libertarian, as such people are not able to express an autonomous view.
5. The opportunity to participate in research, on the libertarian view, should not be restricted by a third party. A primary care physician, for example, should not be able to prevent a researcher from asking one of her patients to participate in a research study on the grounds that the research, or the request, would harm the patient.

The risk of harm

A different ethical perspective emphasizes the importance of the risk of harm to the potential research subject. Almost exclusive concern for such risk gives rise to what might be called the paternalistic position. Thus, the paternalist holds the following views:

1. If the research involves more than minimal harm then it should not normally be carried out even if the potential subject gives fully informed consent, and wishes to take part in such research.
2. If the research does not involve harm or risk of harm then the subject could be enrolled into the research without consent. A breach of confidentiality that does not result in actual harm is of little importance and is readily justified if it would be difficult to obtain specific consent.
3. The paternalist position would probably be against financial inducements in order to protect participants from harm.

Table 3 Summary of international and national guidelines on research ethics

Research participants should not be put at more than minimal risk of harm as a result of taking part in research. Guidelines suggest that some balancing between risk of harm and other considerations is appropriate. However, even if the research is likely to lead to enormous benefit to others, the risk to participants should be small. The only possible exception is in some therapeutic research (see text)
Potential research participants should be fully informed about both the purpose of the study and what will be involved in taking part, including an honest account of risks and benefits
It is difficult or even impossible to carry out some research with individual consent from participants, e.g. some research using data from case notes or clinical databases. Ethics committees will need to be satisfied that such research is of sufficient value to justify the breach of autonomy (confidentiality) and that the research cannot be satisfactorily carried out in any other way
No coercion must be brought to bear on people to take part in research. Care must be taken to ensure that the potential participant does not feel an obligation to take part in the research. It must be made clear to patients that their clinical care (outside the research study) will not be affected by refusing to take part in research
Payments may be made to patients only to offset reasonable costs and must not be such as to act as inducement for the person to take part in the research
Patients who are not competent to give consent for research may be eligible to take part in research. Ethics committees will need to be satisfied that: The risk of harm is very low, probably lower than the risk that is acceptable in the case of competent participants That the research aims cannot be achieved by other means That the research is of considerable value That a relevant person (usually a close relative) gives valid consent

Value and quality of the research

The main purpose of medical research is to gain knowledge that will benefit people in the future. Three issues arise relevant to the ethics of research:

1. Is the research itself of good quality? If the aims of the research are of no value, or the methodology is poor, then the research is unlikely to benefit people in the future and may even be harmful. The Declaration of Helsinki states:

   > Medical research involving human subjects must conform to generally accepted scientific principles and should be based on adequately performed laboratory and animal experimentation and on a thorough knowledge of the scientific literature (s. B11).[2]

2. If the research poses some risk of harm to participants but potential benefit to people in the future, how should these be balanced? Some ethical perspectives would give equal weight to the interests of all those potentially affected, that is, to research participants and to those who might benefit from the research results in the future. The Declaration of Helsinki and national guidelines reject this position. The interests of research participants are given much greater weight than the interests of people in the future who might gain from the research.
3. The general presumption of research ethics guidelines is that participating in research is potentially harmful, or at least burdensome. However, at least for some therapeutic research, participants may benefit simply from participating in the research, because the standard of clinical care may be better within a funded research project. Different views about the value of the research to participants can be a source of friction between researcher and research ethics committee.

Justice

Questions of justice are increasingly the focus for ethical discussion in research ethics. Commonly, women of child-bearing age or older people have been excluded from medical research because of the danger of harming a foetus or because elderly people may be at more risk from the research. Similarly, people with a poor command of English, or who are less likely to comply with a research protocol, such as the homeless, may be excluded because their inclusion would have practical difficulties for carrying out the research. However, as a result of this there are fewer data on which to base management decisions for people in these, often excluded, categories.

A more recent concern has arisen around research funded from rich countries but carried out in poor countries. In randomized controlled trials, for example, should the control 'arm' include best standard care as provided in rich countries or best standard care as provided in the country in which the research is being carried out? There has been much debate in the medical literature on this subject, as well as discussion by national and international regulatory bodies.[2,8–11]

Most guidelines emphasize the rights of people not to take part in research. However, it could be argued that if we wish to benefit from medical research, now or in the future, then we have a moral obligation to take part, or at least allow data from our medical records to be used (Table 3).

Research ethics committees

The Declaration of Helsinki stipulates that research involving human subjects should be reviewed by a properly constituted ethics committee or institutional review board. As a result, many countries now have regulations governing the formation and procedure of research ethics committees. Some, such as the Netherlands, Belgium, and the United States, have specific legislation in this area.[12–14] Others, such as the United Kingdom, have a regulatory system controlled by government but not legislation. In the United Kingdom, research ethics committees are situated in health authorities and run by either the health authority (local research ethics committees, LRECs) or the Department of Health (multicentre research ethics committees, MRECs). A research study involving participants in localities covered by two or more LRECs requires approval from an MREC. Approval by an MREC covers the whole of the United Kingdom. The relevant LRECs then consider specific local issues, such as local environment, local population, and the suitability of local researchers (see ref. 7 for latest guidelines).

The independence of the REC from the researchers and the sponsors of research is seen as a fundamental requirement of research governance.[15] It is helpful for researchers to understand that members of research ethics committees must operate within the relevant guidelines.

Ethical considerations for research in primary care arising from the framework

Consent to participate in a research study

The Declaration of Helsinki states:

> . . . the physician should obtain the subject's freely given informed consent, preferably in writing (B22).[2]

For consent to be valid, the person must be competent to give the consent, be properly informed, and be free from coercion.

Competence

Research guidelines give little guidance on how to assess competence. The legal approach in the United Kingdom to assessing capacity to consent to medical treatment emphasizes three issues:

- does the patient understand the relevant information;
- is he able to believe it; and
- is he able to weigh up the information and come to a decision?

The assessment of competence is specific to each decision. It should not be assumed that someone with cognitive impairment is necessarily incompetent to consent to take part in research.

The position regarding patients who are not competent to consent to research is problematic. In English law, no one can give consent for medical treatment on behalf of an incompetent adult. Doctors should treat such patients in their best interests. It will be in the best interests of some patients to take part in research, particularly in therapeutic research. This is not necessarily true in non-therapeutic research.

The European Commission's guidelines on Good Clinical Practice for Trials of Medicinal Products in the European Community state:

> Consent must always be given by the signature of the subject in a non-therapeutic study i.e. when there is no direct clinical benefit to the subject.[16]

However, the UK Department of Health's guidelines to local research ethics committees state:

> Proposals for research where capacity to consent is impaired will need particularly careful consideration by the LREC (local research ethics committee), with regard to its acceptability in terms of the balance of benefits, discomfort and risk to the patient and the need to advance knowledge so that people with mental disorder may benefit.[17]

This suggests that non-therapeutic research on incompetent adults *may* be acceptable. In the United Kingdom, a research ethics committee may allow non-therapeutic research on incompetent adults but only if there is a strong argument that the research could not be done in any other group of people. Furthermore, the consent of a relevant person (usually a close relative) would normally be necessary. Countries, particularly those that give powers of consent to a proxy, may differ in their approach.

Whether children are competent to consent to participate in medical research, and when they become competent, is not clear cut, as children's competence will vary depending on their age, intellectual ability, and the nature of the research. Also, different countries have different legal requirements governing consent in children. In England, a child over the age of 16 years would be able to give consent to medical treatment, and possibly therapeutic research, in the same way as an adult.[18] Under the age of 16 years a child may be competent to give consent to treatment or research but it would depend on their level of understanding of the particular procedure. Guidance for researchers in the United Kingdom issued by multicentre research ethics committees, while acknowledging that children under 16 *may* give consent to research, advises that it would be unwise to allow participation of such a child in research where parental consent was not forthcoming.[7]

For research on children who are not competent to give consent, the parent or guardian must give consent, and in consenting must act in the child's best interests. This essentially means that they can consent to some therapeutic research. Non-therapeutic research cannot usually be said to be in the child's best interests. The British Paediatric Association's guidelines advise that non-therapeutic research can only be validly consented to if:

> the risks are sufficiently small to mean that the research can be reasonably said not to go against the child's interests.[19]

Information

The information required to be given to someone recruited into a research study is greater than that which is required for someone consenting to medical treatment. Several researchers have argued that these 'double standards' are applied to therapeutic research without good reason.[20] The main argument in defence of a 'double standard' is that, in a research situation, the doctor has an interest in ensuring that the study achieves its objective. This interest may interfere with the professional requirement to act in the patient's best interests.

The International Conference on Harmonisation of Technical Requirements for Registration of Pharmaceuticals for Human Use (ICH) guidelines on good clinical practice includes detailed specification of what information should be given to participants in clinical trials. These guidelines have been adopted by both the European Union and the Food and Drug Administration in the United States. The guidance for researchers published by the UK Central Office for Research Ethics Committees complies with the ICH guidelines.[6] This guidance does not only apply to clinical trials and is relevant for all research considered by research ethics committees.

Freedom from coercion

In therapeutic research, the potential participants are also patients. The doctor who is treating the patient may be enthusiastic to enrol him/her for the research. The patient may be keen to please his/her doctor, and may also assume that the doctor will only be acting in his/her best interests. Researchers, and research ethics committees, need to ensure that the recruitment method protects patients from pressures to take part in the research. In particular, it must be made clear that any medical treatment will not be affected by whether the patient takes part in the research, except to the extent that the research may involve treatment not available outside the research setting. In addition, ethics committees will be concerned that undue pressure may be brought to bear on patients to take part in the research if doctors receive payment for the research according to the number recruited. The ICH guidelines specify that any payment to researchers should be stated in the patient information sheet.[6] The issue of paying people to take part in research has been discussed above and is summarized in Table 3.

Particular concerns around consent in research in primary care

The relationship between GPs and their patients is often more long term and far reaching than that between hospital doctors and their patients. Thus, patients may feel less able to decline to take part in a research study when it is suggested by their GP than by a specialist registrar or consultant whom they have only seen once or twice. Particular care must be taken to ensure that there is no element of coercion in the consent process.

Some research in primary care may be non-therapeutic and the participant has simply been identified randomly from those patients registered for treatment. However, because the invitation to participate comes from the GP, the person may feel an obligation to 'help out' by participating.

Payment of primary care physicians by pharmaceutical companies and other sponsors of research can introduce a conflict of interest between their duty to act in the best interests of their patient and their own financial interests. There could be a temptation to 'talk up' the benefits of participating in the research in order to boost recruitment and increase payment. Potential participants need to be made aware of any payment to their doctor for the research as part of an informed consent process.

Cluster randomized trials pose particular problems for researchers required to obtain informed consent from research participants. They are increasingly common in primary care, especially when a complex intervention is being studied. Such trials involve randomization, not at the level of an individual patient but at the level of a 'cluster', for example, a general practice or health authority. Individual patients may not be asked to give consent to take part in the research although their care may be affected by the research. There has been some debate about the ethics of cluster randomized trials.[21,22] To justify conducting a trial without the informed consent of some of those participating it would be necessary to show that the research could not be carried out in another way, and that the benefits of the research were sufficiently great to outweigh the breach of autonomy.

Harm to the research participant

The Declaration of Helsinki states:

> In medical research on human subjects, considerations related to the well-being of the human subject should take precedence over the interests of science and society (A7).[2]

A central ethical position taken by international and national guidelines is that research participants must be protected from being at much risk of harm, even if the benefit of the research to people in the future is considerable. The term minimal risk is often used. The Royal College of Physicians (UK) describes minimal risk as either 'a small chance of a reaction which itself is trivial, for example, a mild headache or feeling of lethargy', or 'a very remote chance of serious injury or death'. The latter risk to the healthy volunteer would be comparable to that of flying as a passenger in a scheduled aircraft.[23]

There are some situations where more than minimal risk to a research participant would be ethically acceptable, for example, therapeutic research in patients with serious disease where the risk of the disease itself is great.[23]

Harm to the participants in medical research is not only obvious physical harm. The UK Royal College of Physicians guidelines state:

> ...it is important that when risk is assessed, harms other than serious injury or danger to life should be included. Thus the risk of any discomfort or other physical effects, such as the possibility of psychological disturbance, breach of confidentiality and even simple inconvenience must all be considered (5.18).[24]

Another consideration that is becoming more common is the risk of disclosure of genetic information as a result of the research.

Particular considerations around the issue of harm in research in primary care

It is important for primary care researchers to recognize that the concept of harm is much broader than obvious physical harm. Psychological distress may be particularly important in questionnaire surveys on patients accessed via their GP but not currently under medical care.

Liability for compensation in the event of harm occurring to the research participants is important for all researchers but is something that the primary care clinician particularly needs to be aware of as they are unlikely to belong to a medical or research institution that has insurance against such liability. International and national guidelines specify that researchers should make appropriate arrangements to compensate research participants if they suffer harm as a consequence of taking part in the research. Medical defence organizations do not normally indemnify for non-negligent harm, so additional insurance may be needed.

Confidentiality

Most medical research involves collecting patient data that should be kept confidential. A researcher could be found negligent if reasonable precautions were not taken to ensure that information gained is stored in a secure manner. Furthermore, information should normally be passed on to another person only with the explicit consent of the research subject. This requirement is underpinned by the ethical principle of respect for autonomy.

Particular considerations around confidentiality for research in primary care

Much research in primary care involves access to patient records and this has specific implications for patient confidentiality. Two particular scenarios are common.

Access to patient details for recruitment for studies

An increasing number of epidemiological and community based research in the United Kingdom use general practitioner practice registers as a sampling frame. Approaching patients to invite them to take part in the research, and selecting an appropriate sample, may require researchers to have access to either the names and addresses of all patients in a particular group, or to have further patient details so that a more specific sampling can occur. If this information is given to researchers by the general practitioner (or primary care physician) patient confidentiality will be breached.

Access to patient records for epidemiological research

Some research studies do not involve direct contact with patients but are based on collection and analysis of existing information in medical records. The General Medical Council (UK) guidelines state:

> Where research projects depend on using identifiable information or samples, and it is not practicable to contact patients to seek their consent, this fact should be drawn to the attention of a research ethics committee, so that it can consider whether the likely benefits of the research outweigh the loss of confidentiality.[25]

The UK Medical Research Council (MRC) has published guidance for researchers conducting studies funded by the MRC that involve access to confidential information.[26]

Conclusion

Research in and on primary medical care is an increasingly important area of medical research. It is essential that such research is of a high scientific and ethical standard. As the scientific methodology needs to be appropriate to primary care, the ethical principles need to be considered in the context of primary care. Some ethical issues common to research in secondary care may be less relevant, but other issues may raise specific problems for primary care research. Knowledge of the ethical framework that should underpin all medical research and of the specific context of primary care is essential for all researchers wishing to undertake good medical research in primary care.

References

1. **Nuremberg Code,** 1949 (www.fuente.de/bioethik/nuremb.htm), accessed August 2001.
2. **World Medical Association.** *Declaration of Helsinki: Ethical Principles for Medical Research Involving Human Subjects.* Edinburgh, Scotland: World Medical Association, 2000 (www.wma.net/e/policy/17-c_e.html), accessed July 2001.
3. **Braddock, C.H., Edwards, K.A., Hasenberg, N.M., Laidley, T.L., and Levinson, W.** (1999). Informed decision making in outpatient practice. *Journal of the American Medical Association* **282**, 2313–20.
4. **Elwyn, G., Edwards, A., and Kinnersley, P.** (1999). Shared decision making in primary care: the neglected second half of the consultation. *British Journal of General Practice* **49**, 477–82.
5. **Towle, A. and Godolphin, W.** (1999). Framework for teaching and learning informed shared decision making. *British Medical Journal* **319** (7212), 766–71.
6. **International Conference on Harmonisation of Technical Requirements for Registration of Pharmaceuticals for Human Use.** *Good Clinical Practice Consolidated Guideline E6.* Geneva, 1996 (www.ifpma.org/ich.html), accessed July 2001.
7. **UK Central Office for Research Ethics Committees.** Multi-Centre Research Ethics Committees, Guidance for Researchers, 2000 (www.corec.org.uk).
8. **Angell, M.** (2000). Investigators' responsibilities for human subjects in developing countries. *New England Journal of Medicine* **342**, 967–9.
9. **Lurie, P. and Wolfe, S.M.** (1997). Unethical trials of interventions to reduce perinatal transmission of the human immunodeficiency virus in developing countries. *New England Journal of Medicine* **337**, 853–6.
10. **National Bioethics Advisory Commission.** *Ethical and Policy Issues in International Research: Clinical Trials in Developing Countries.* Bethesda MD: National Bioethics Advisory Commission, 2001.
11. **Shapiro, H.T. and Meslin, E.M.** (2001). Ethical issues in the design and conduct of clinical trials in developing countries. *New England Journal of Medicine* **345**, 139–42.

12. **Medical Research Involving Human Subjects Act.** *Regulations on Medical Research Involving Human Subjects*, Netherlands, 1998 (www.ccmo.nl), accessed August 2001.
13. Arreté royal du 12 aout 1994 modifant l'Arreté royal du 23 Octobre 1964, fixant les normes auxelles les hospitaux et leurs services doivent répondre. Ministere de la Santé Publique et de l'Environment, Moniteur belge, 27 Septembre 1994.
14. **Code of Federal Regulations Part 46.** *Protection of Human Subjects* (www.ohrp.osophs.dhhs.gov/humansubjects/guidance/statute.htm), accessed July 2001.
15. **Department of Health.** *Research Governance Framework for Health and Social Care*, 3.12.4. London: Department of Health, 2001 (http://www.doh.gov.uk/research/rd3/nhsrandd/researchgovernance.htm), accessed August 2001.
16. **Working Party on Efficacy of Medicinal Products of the Committee for Proprietary Medicinal Products of the European Community** (1991). Good clinical practice for trials on medicinal products in the European Community. In *Manual for Research Ethics Committees* 4th edn. (ed. C. Foster), pp. V.1.1–1.4. London: Centre for Medical Law and Ethics, King's College.
17. **Department of Health.** Local research ethics committees (HSG) (91)5. London: DOH, 1991, s4.11
18. **Family Law Reform Act 1969 s8.**
19. **British Paediatric Association.** *Guidelines for the Ethical Conduct of Medical Research Involving Children*, V.27.1. London: British Paediatric Association, 1994, p. 12.
20. **Chalmers, I. and Lindley, R.I.** (2001). Double standards on informed consent to treatment. In *Informed Consent in Medical Research* (ed. L. Doyal and J.S. Tobias), pp. 266–76. London: BMJ Books.
21. **Edwards, S.J., Braunholtz, D.A., Lilford, R.J., and Stevens, A.J.** (1999). Ethical issues in the design and conduct of cluster randomised controlled trials. *British Medical Journal* **318**, 1407–9.
22. **Hutton, J.L.** (2001). Are distinctive ethical principles required for cluster randomised controlled trials? *Statistics in Medicine* **20** (3), 473–8.
23. **Royal College of Physicians.** *Guidelines on the Practice of Ethics Committees in Medical Research Involving Human Subjects* 2nd edn. London: Royal College of Physicians, 1990.
24. **Royal College of Physicians.** *Research Involving Patients* (5.26). London: Royal College of Physicians, 1990.
25. **General Medical Council.** *Confidentiality: Protecting and Providing Information* (s31). London: General Medical Council, 2000.
26. **Medical Research Council.** *Personal Information in Medical Research*, MRC Ethics Series. London: Medical Research Council, 2001 (www.mrc.ac.uk), accessed July 2001.

16.6 Ethics of resource allocation

Colin Bradley

Introduction

Historically, doctors did not concern themselves much with how resources were allocated in the health system beyond, perhaps, seeking to maximize those allocated to their own area of activity. The process of allocating the nation's resources was seen as either the task of government or as the outcome of market forces. The distribution of health care resources, for instance, between geographical regions and health care sectors—a process referred to as 'macro-allocation'[1]—was seen as a responsibility of those in charge of health care funding. However, everyone providing health care uses resources; hence, all clinicians have a responsibility for the allocation of whatever resources are placed at their disposal by the macro-allocation process. Clinicians, as well as managers, have an ethical responsibility to ensure that resources are allocated fairly and used wisely.

The day-to-day choices made in the use of health care resources constitute a micro-allocation process that mirrors the macro-allocation process and which ought to be governed by broadly similar ethical considerations. While this has always been true, there are now a number of developments in health care systems in developed countries which seek to make more explicit to physicians the inter-relationship between micro-allocation decisions and their macro-allocation consequences. Examples include the indicative drug budgeting system in the United Kingdom[2] and managed care in the United States.[3] Other initiatives, such as the Primary Care Trusts in the United Kingdom,[4] go further and seek to involve primary care physicians more directly in macro-allocation processes themselves. These trends, combined with an ever-increasing scrutiny of professionals' decision-making that is part of a general trend towards demanding greater accountability, require that doctors should be clear about the basis of their resource allocation decisions and are able to defend them if challenged. To these ends, it is important that one can explicate the ethical underpinnings of resource allocation decisions made.

Resources, in this context, are sometimes seen exclusively in terms of money. However, the resources distributed by primary care physicians include their own time and energies, those of other primary health care professionals, the technologies used in the investigation of patients' problems, and the drugs used in their treatment. In many health care systems primary care physicians also exert a degree of control of access to secondary care resources.[5] Doctors often see decisions about the use of all these resources as purely clinical, albeit increasingly informed by health economic considerations. However, such day-to-day decisions about the use of resources do have important ethical dimensions. Furthermore, these ethical aspects go beyond the more familiar territory of maximizing good and minimizing harm that dominate much of doctors' routine ethical thinking. As well as striking a balance between risks and benefits doctors are also required to balance the needs and wishes of individual patients against the needs of society as a whole. One of the requirements of society is that everyone be treated fairly, which is an expression of the justice principle. The justice principle is one of the most difficult and elusive in ethics. In health care ethics, the type of justice at play is virtually always 'distributive' justice.

Distributive justice in health care

Distributive justice is concerned with the fair distribution of benefits and burdens within society.[1] The finite nature of resources often compels us to make trade-offs between the competing interests of individuals and groups in society. These trade-offs need to be governed by principles of equity or fairness. They also need to be based on principles of material justice such that the grounds on which benefits and burdens are distributed are material, that is, morally relevant and reasonable. There are several candidates for material principles that could or should be used in determining equity between groups or individuals. The many candidate material principles can be gathered into one of four main groups. These are needs-based principles; maximizing principles; egalitarian principles; and libertarian principles.

Needs-based principles

That health care should be provided on the basis of need is the traditional foundation of several health care systems in Europe, including the UK NHS. However, there are difficulties in applying the broad principle that health care resources should be distributed according to 'need'. Difficulties arise in agreeing what constitutes need and how conflicting or competing needs are to be resolved or met. The first step is often to try and distinguish between needs and wants. Needs are defined by clinicians and usually relate to their perception of the patient's problem. Clinicians tend to consider patients' needs as relating to problems that are reasonably serious, involve pain and/or suffering and possibly a threat to life and for which the clinician feels there is a remedy available. Wants, while often overlapping with needs, are defined by patients and may include desires for treatments to make them feel better even when they are not suffering as such or where the treatment is one deemed less than suitable by their doctor. Distinguishing these is not always as easy as it might sound. Doctors may differ in what they recognize as suffering and in what treatments they see as appropriate. Patients may vary in how they present their complaint such that it may sound like a need when it is really only a want (or vice versa).

Even if it is agreed to allocate resources only on the basis of need and to deny those that appear only as wants, there are still issues regarding how need should be measured in order to adjudicate between competing needs. Health need may relate to the immediacy of any threat to life, in which case patients at risk of dying without treatment would receive priority. This way of assessing health need can be broadened to include immediate threats to health and well-being rather than threats to life alone but defining and quantifying such needs becomes more difficult. If one further broadens the definition of need to include future or lifetime risks to life or health, deciding on the allocation of resources in the face of competing needs becomes even more of a problem.

An alternative approach is to define need in terms of capacity to benefit from treatment rather than in terms of the initial degree of ill health.(6) Capacity to benefit depends on many factors of which the availability of health care resources is but one. Benefit achieved can be measured as health gain which is, at a minimum, measured in terms of morbidity and mortality. However, benefit may also be measured in terms of social gain, enhancement of quality of life, enablement, or on a number of other parameters. The measurement of all of these is fraught with methodological difficulty.(7) Distinguishing need, defined as capacity to benefit, from wants is also exceedingly difficult as it relates, in part, to the many different conceptions of what constitutes health. Certain treatments, such as cosmetic surgery and infertility treatments, are particularly controversial with regard to whether they meet legitimate needs or simply fulfil desires. Treatments provided for conditions characterized by a substantial psycho-social component or that are associated with what are considered social rather than health gains are particularly likely to be seen as controversial.

Furthermore, needs, and, hence, potential health gains, are not just present or absent but are graded. Thus the process of resource allocation may not be about giving to some categories of patient and not to others (as it is sometimes construed) but rather it is likely to be about allocating to the most needy (i.e. likely to gain the most) within different categories and across categories. This often entails comparing quite dissimilar health problems and disparate potential gains. There have been attempts, using various quality of life measures, to provide a common denominator for such comparisons but such comparisons remain difficult and require considerable skill and judgement. This graded approach of allocating resources to the most needy in each possible category is designed to maximize the benefits from health care expenditure and so is also governed by maximizing principles (see below).

Maximizing principles

Maximizing principles are closely related to utilitarianism,(8) the difference being that utilitarianism is concerned with maximizing human happiness whereas the application of maximizing principles of distributive justice in the allocation of health care resources is concerned with maximizing the health gain of the population. The consequences of this approach will greatly depend on how health gain is measured, what indirect impacts of health interventions are considered and the time-frame over which gain is considered. Measuring health gain is very difficult especially when trying to compare quite different interventions in different health areas. How does one compare the health gains associated with smoking cessation interventions, say, with health gains associated with cardiac surgery? Quality of life measures such as the Quality Adjusted Life Year (QALY) are one attempt but, as noted above, these are methodologically challenging and are really designed for comparisons across populations rather than making decisions about resource allocation between individuals. Clinicians usually end up having to make educated guesses regarding comparative health gains. In doing so it is important to consider lifetime health gain rather than, perhaps, short term gains (in which case smoking cessation therapies would win out) and also indirect gains in terms of reduced burdens to the health services and/or relatives as well as direct health gains.

Another type of maximizing principle that is sometimes argued for is that of societal worth. This is certainly accepted as a basis for the just distribution of other of society's goods. Thus, people of high societal worth, such as doctors, may be rewarded with higher pay without this being seen as unjust. The approach is sometimes seen in health care, too, with high-profile individuals such as political leaders accorded enormous health care resources that might not be so readily available for ordinary citizens. However, this approach applied on a routine basis would be questionable, as it would involve doctors assigning to people a relative worth. Some resource allocation decisions, for instance decisions to prioritize young patients over older patients, may appear to be according greater worth to the young. This would not generally be acceptable. However, the same outcome may be more defensible if based on maximization principles.

Egalitarian principles

Egalitarian principles start from the premise that every one should be treated equally. With many goods the most egalitarian distribution is to give every one the same amount—the same shares approach, but in health care this does not make much sense. As one commentator has put it, one does not find ordinary people queuing for heart by-pass operations of which they have no need.(9) Thus, rather than seeking to treat everyone the same, in health care egalitarianism leads to a quest to allocate resources so as to reduce inequalities in health. One form of this approach is the 'fair innings' approach which would distribute resources with the aim of ensuring everyone has an equally long and healthy life. Another way of looking at egalitarianism would give greater priority to someone who had made fewer demands on the health service in the past than to someone who has already made substantial use of them. Yet another approach would be to prioritize people who have tried to maintain their own health and have avoided behaviours that might threaten their health over those who have led unhealthy lifestyles. This is a principle based on relative effort and has been advocated as grounds to deny priority in health care resource allocation to people who smoke or drink or adopt other unhealthy lifestyles. However, such an approach is questionable in deeming someone lower priority on the basis of whether or not they have 'earned' it by behaving themselves. It also implies a degree of victim blaming. The argument hinges on the extent to which one believes people with unhealthy lifestyles exercise choice in their lifestyle. Given the strong association of such unhealthy lifestyles with social deprivation it is difficult to maintain the stance that such lifestyles are freely chosen by completely autonomous individuals. Hence, such disparities of apparent effort should not be used as a basis for resource allocation.

The fair opportunity rule

One proponent of egalitarian principles, Daniels, has argued for the application of a fair opportunity rule.(10) The fair opportunity rule states that no person should be granted social benefits on the basis of undeserved advantageous properties and that no person should be denied social benefits on the basis of undeserved disadvantageous properties. This rule seeks to exclude the use of such properties as IQ, race, gender, etc. to exclude people from equality of access to health care and other resources. Many studies have provided evidence that women, the socially deprived, and ethnic minorities do receive less than their fair share of health care resources and the fair opportunity rule challenges health care professionals and the health system to address these inequities. Older patients are also vulnerable to being denied equitable access to health care resources but, as noted above, this might be justifiable on maximization principles and possibly even on egalitarian principles as long as access is not denied simply because they are old.

Libertarian principles

Libertarian principles are based on an understanding of justice that gives prominence to free choice and focuses on the application of fair procedures rather than on concern about the outcomes produced. Libertarians are typically strong proponents of the free market. They would contend that the best health care system, in terms of quality and value for money, will emerge from allowing market forces, particularly competition, to determine who provides health care and at what price. Libertarians recognize that not everybody will be capable of providing for their own health care needs and that provision may have to be made by society to cover their health care costs. How this provision is made, though, they argue should be a matter of free choice and so they oppose tax-based systems or compulsory insurance.[11] However, all those who can, free marketers believe, should become consumers and be enabled to use their consumer power to shape the health care market place.

From an ethical viewpoint, if capitalism and the free market are not of themselves immoral, then it might constitute reasonable mechanism for allocating health care resources. However, unchecked, free market forces seem unlikely to distribute health care resources according to any of the other principles above. A free market in health care will not allocate resources according to need or in a way that reduced inequalities or, possibly, not even in a way that maximizes benefit. The only determinant in a free market is ability to pay. It could be argued, though, that as long as there are mechanisms to deal with the requirements to meet needs and address inequalities a free market system could be ethically acceptable. It would be unlikely to maximize benefits but this would not matter so much as the excess resources spent would be coming from people's disposable incomes rather than the public purse and is thus, arguably, of less ethical concern. The reality is, though, that mechanisms to meet needs and address inequalities are rarely, if ever, adequate.

Combination of principles

As each of these material principles seems ethically reasonable, the most equitable distribution would seem to need to take each of them, or as many as seem to apply in any particular situation, into account.[6] The challenge is not so much in deciding on which of these grounds health care resources should be distributed, but rather how much weighting should be given to any one of them. In other words, each case needs to be judged on its own particular merits. It helps, though, to have a moral framework within which each judgement is made and with which decisions can subsequently be justified.

The rule of rescue

One of the challenges to any system devised for the fair distribution of resources will be what to do in situations where there is a very visible high risk to an identifiable individual. This is particularly a problem where a potential intervention is available which has chance of saving or rescuing the individual but only at the cost of consuming resources that would otherwise have been available to effect an even greater health gain in a less visible way in other as yet unidentified individuals. The norm in such situations, and they are not that uncommon, is for resources to be poured in to saving the identified individual and this is referred to as the 'rule of rescue'. However, whether this is the most ethical thing to do in the circumstances is, at least, questionable. Wishing to attempt to rescue identifiable individuals is a basic human instinct and in the age of modern media, the demands of the individual in the situation can be graphically highlighted in a way that gets us all to identify with the individual. However, these are emotional responses and if we are to be reasonable and ethical it is important that we make the value judgements we are required to on thought-out ethical grounds. Many of the grounds on which the rule of rescue is advocated do not stand up to close scrutiny.[12] Primary care physicians are particularly prone to the effects of the rule of rescue as our philosophical predisposition is towards the care of the individual. As more preventive interventions become available and make more demands on ever more clearly limited resources we are likely to become more and more frequently challenged to resist the claims of individual patients for rescue in order to conserve resources for the less visible but more valid claims of our populations.

Thus, for example, GPs may be pressurized to give expensive treatment, such as growth hormone, to individuals for whom it is not clinically indicated even though it can sometimes be of limited value. The need to resist this demand is made particularly pressing if one has a fixed prescribing budget and the prescribing of this treatment would reduce the resources available for the prescribing of lipid lowering drugs to patients whose cardiovascular risk profile suggests they might benefit.

The roles of the primary care physician

Therapist versus Steward

Primary care physicians have a number of roles of which the allocation of health care resources is only one. Some of the ethical problems that arise in resource allocation do so because of difficulties in reconciling conflicts in these roles. Thus, the primary role of the physician is as a therapist in which capacity he/she is expected to provide the patient with whatever treatment he/she deems appropriate to his/her condition. However, he/she also has a role in ensuring that the maximum benefit is achieved from whatever health care resources are available if for no other reason than ensuring that these resources are available when another needy patient comes seeking help. This tension between a role as a therapist for individual patients and a responsibility to ensure the fair allocation of resources can be seen as a conflict between responsibility for stewardship of resources on behalf of the whole community and loyalty or fidelity to patients.

The general view would be that physicians owe their primary loyalty to individual patients but the requirement of justice are that the claims of others are at least taken into consideration in making resource allocation decisions. The point has already been made that all clinical decisions are, in effect, resource allocation decisions. Thus, for example, in the treatment of migraine there are now treatments available that are highly effective but rather costly, compared to older treatments. One could easily justify prescribing these treatments to all patients with migraine (who do not have clinical contraindications) but this would have implications for one's prescribing budget with possible consequences for prescribing to other patient groups. However, many patients still respond quite well to more traditional and cheaper treatment and so there is a good ethical case for prescribing the newer treatments only to patients for whom the older treatments are unsuitable or ineffective. Indeed, there is a general case for saying that doctors should adopt all newer treatments in a highly selective way applying them only to patients for whom they provide a worthwhile benefit over existing treatments. Very new drugs also have unproven safety records and there may be further ethical grounds for limiting their use, especially in the primary care situation, where the marginal benefit is less likely to be manifest and where the marginal risk may be a more important consideration.

An even more common, but more subtle, example of primary care physicians' allocation of resources relates to how they allocate their time between different patients. Time given to one patient can be time denied to another. If when seeing patients booked at 10-minute intervals, as would be common in the British Isles, one spends longer than this with patients at the beginning of a consultation session, those at the end may suffer from a rushed consultation and sub-optimal care. Howie et al. have demonstated how consultation length may be positively associated with quality of care.[13] They have also demonstrated how doctors who do not manage their time in consultations with patients well become stressed themselves, which may lead to a further deterioration in the quality of care they are able to provide. That said, some patients, may, because of the nature of their complaint or the urgency of their clinical need, require more time be given to their care even if this is at the expense of less immediately needy patients. However, this needs to be carefully judged and certainly there is an ethical imperative on doctors to ensure that they use their time carefully, applying as best they can, the principles of providing care according to need, maximizing benefit, ensuring equity of treatment of different patients and using fair procedures for allocation of their time.

Gate keeper

In many health care systems primary care physicians occupy a position of 'gate keeper' in that access to the secondary health care system is only available through a referral from them.[5] There are many advantages for the health care system, for primary and secondary care doctors and for patients from such a system. However, it does place special ethical responsibilities on such primary care physicians to ensure that their referral decisions lead to an equitable distribution of the resources involved. The rule of fair opportunity implies that all patients be treated equally and referred appropriately regardless of race, gender, IQ, or other characteristics.[14] While doctors would rarely deny patients access on these grounds deliberately, there is evidence that these groups do not always get equal treatment. For example, there is evidence that women with ischaemic heart disease are referred less frequently than men for work-up and evaluation for possible coronary artery by-pass grafting.[15] This may be based on a mistaken belief that women are less likely to benefit from such procedures but it may also be informed, sub-consciously possibly, by a tendency to see women as less deserving of consumption of health care resources.

The gate keeper role, as well as requiring doctors to ensure all patients gain fair access to necessary treatment, also requires that doctors deny access to others whose case is deemed not to justify use of secondary care. This may be because their medical need falls below a threshold allowed for within existing resource or because their gaining access would deny access to others who are even more needy. For example, doctors may have to deny some patients with headache, who are pressing to have an MRI scan, access to this expensive investigation with limited availability, in order that other patients whose condition more adequately justifies this test can have more ready access to it.

This is a very uncomfortable role for doctors and some commentators would argue that it is not an appropriate role for physicians as it places them in unnecessary conflict between their duties to individual patients and the needs of society to achieve cost containment in the health care system.[16] While it might seem an attractive idea for the doctor not to concern her or himself with the costs of health care, and, therefore, to always be able to recommend what he or she believes to be the best treatment for the patient regardless of cost, this is unrealistic. Such judgements have to be made in all health care systems and it is, arguably, better that such decisions are made by doctors than by others without reference to doctors. Increasingly, there are attempts, at least at the macro-allocation level, to have these difficult decisions made by a group or panel of people rather than by a single physician. Given the need to balance conflicting demands, it probably is helpful to include a range of perspectives in decision making. However, it is vitally important that the decision making process is grounded in identifiable justice principles and is transparent. In the end, though, primary care physicians still have to make referral decisions on a daily basis and, as all such decisions have resource implications, doctors also have to have workable and transparent procedures for ensuring that their decisions are ethical.

Patient advocate

Another important role for primary care physicians is that of patient advocate. Patients depend on us to look after their interests and sometimes this will require us to challenge the health care system and resource allocation decisions made therein. In managed care systems, physicians may be pressurized to deny certain costly treatments to particular patients or groups of patients. This may be reasonable if there are equally effective but cheaper alternatives. Indeed, as is argued above, it behoves doctors to use the least costly treatment that is effective for any given patient. However, if a treatment is effective and the alternatives are not satisfactory for a particular patient, the doctor's role may change to become one of advocating for his or her patient and insisting that the treatment be made available. This does not, as it might appear, contradict the arguments for doctors to accept the gate-keeping or stewardship roles described above. Accepting the gate-keeping role is done for the sake of patients or potential patients and not for the sake of the system.

It is important that doctors remain clear about the reasons for their resource allocation decisions and are prepared to defend them under scrutiny from either health care funders or patients. Patients need to be able to trust that their physicians are safe-guarding their fundamental interests. Most patients are accepting of the need to use health care resources wisely and appreciate that such prudence may be to their benefit on another occasion. Such trust is, admittedly, more difficult to maintain in a cost contained and managed health care system but the effort must be made. If doctors should ever prioritize the needs of the system over the needs of patients or are seen to do so, trust, which is so vital to effective doctor–patient relationships, comes under serious threat.

Thus, if in a physician's judgement an individual patient's needs are sufficiently great as to justify a diversion of a proportion of total resources towards that patient, this should be allowable. A system which does not allow this under any circumstances must be challenged. Indeed, it is also part of the role of primary care physicians to advocate for a sufficiency of resources being made available in the first place to meet the largest possible proportion of reasonable medical need. However, doctors must also be alert to the rule of rescue (see above) and ensure that their advocacy is deployed in favour of the most appropriate patients. These will often be the least vocal and most deprived members of society rather than the ones who agitate the most for a greater share of health care resources.

Conclusions

All clinical decisions, including the day-to-day decisions of primary care physicians, have implications for the allocation of health care resources. It is important, therefore, that all clinicians, and not just those directly and overtly involved in resource allocation decisions, understand and apply the appropriate ethical principles to these decisions. The ethical principles are those of distributive justice. A multitude of potential principles of material justice are promoted and making decisions may require the application of several of these, but the principles of medical need and of reducing health inequalities deserve special attention. Primary care physicians have several important, sometimes apparently conflicting, roles among which are those of therapist, gate keeper, and patient advocate. While duties to individual patients will tend to predominate, duties to the community of potential patients should not be denied or ignored. Finding the correct balance between these different roles should be aided by a good understanding of the underlying ethical issues.

References

1. **Beauchamp, T.L.** (1999). Justice in the distribution of health care. In *Contemporary Issues in Bioethics* 5th edn. (ed. T.L. Beauchamp and L. Walters), pp. 355–61. Belmont CA: Wadsworth.
2. **Department of Health.** *Improving Prescribing.* London: HMSO, 1990.
3. **Emanuel, E.J. and Dubler, N.N.** (1999). Preserving the physician–patient relationship in the era of managed care. In *Contemporary Issues in Bioethics* 5th edn. (ed. T.L. Beauchamp and L. Walters), pp. 387–93. Belmont CA: Wadsworth.
4. **Secretary of State for Health.** *The New NHS.* London: Stationery Office, 1997.

5. **Starfield, B.** *Primary Care: Balancing Health Needs, Services and Technology.* Oxford: Oxford University Press, 1998.
6. **Cookson, R. and Dolan, P.** (2000). Principles of justice in health care ratioining. *Journal of Medical Ethics* **26**, 322–9.
7. **Bowling, A.** *Measuring Disease: A Review of Disease-specific Quality of Life Measurement Scales.* Buckingham: Open University Press, 1995.
8. **Beauchamp, T.L. and Childress, J.F.** (1993). Utilarianism: consequences-based theory. In *Principles of Biomedical Ethics*, pp. 47–55. Oxford: Oxford University Press.
9. **Draper, H. and Tunna, K.** *Ethics and Values for Commissioners.* Leeds: Nuffield Institute for Health, 1996.
10. **Daniels, N. and Sabin, J.** (1997). Limits to health care: fair procedures, democratic deliberation and the legitimacy problem for insurers. *Philosophy and Public Affairs* **26**, 305–50.
11. **Engelhardt, T.** (1999). Rights to health care, social justice and fairness in health care allocations: frustrations in the face of finitude. In *Contemporary Issues in Bioethics* 5th edn. (ed. T.L. Beauchamp and L. Walters), pp. 380–7. Belmont CA: Wadsworth.
12. **Hope, T.** (2001). Rationing and life-saving treatments: should identifiable patients have higher priority? *Journal of Medical Ethics* **27**, 179–85.
13. **Howie, J.G.R., Heaney, D.J., and Maxwell, M.** *Measuring Quality in General Practice.* Occasional Paper 75. London: Royal College of General Practitioners, 1997.
14. **Beauchamp, T.L. and Childress, J.F.** (1993). Fair opportunity. In *Principles of Biomedical Ethics*, pp. 341–8. Oxford: Oxford University Press.
15. **Giles, W.H., Anda, R.F., Casper, M.L., Escobedo, L.G., and Taylor, H.A.** (1995). Race and sex differences in rates of invasive cardiac procedures in US hospitals. Data from the National Hospital Discharge Survey. *Archives of Internal Medicine* **155**, 318–24.
16. **Levinsky, N.G.** (1984). The doctor's master. *New England Journal of Medicine* **311**, 1573–5.

16.7 End-of-life decisions

Howard Brody, Karen S. Ogle, and Gregg K. VandeKieft

Introduction

The revolution in bioethics which has occurred since the 1960s has focused particularly on ethical decisions at the end of life—to the extent that some used to feel that the 'institutional ethics committees' that have developed in US hospitals and other inpatient facilities ought to be renamed 'end of life care committees'. Prior to the development of the medical technology of the post-World-War-II period, physicians all too often simply lacked the capacity to extend life beyond the relatively early stages of many terminal and degenerative illnesses. The question therefore seldom arose of whether one ought to forgo the use of some life-prolonging intervention, because continued life under treatment might actually be worse for the individual than a quicker and more peaceful death. Today, many people who are informed about modern medical technology fear dying while 'tied to machines' and seek assurances that their physicians will not subject them to such an end, while others continue to demand life-prolonging treatment even after physicians have given up hope that the treatment can change the outcome. Thus, explicit ethical decision-making at the end of life has become relatively commonplace within a few decades.

We will offer an overview of this issue for the primary care physician by focusing first on developments in US medical practice. The bioethics revolution started in the United States, and many other cultures, even if they generally do not share the basic worldview of the American culture, have been increasingly influenced by the US ethical approach. We will then refine this American-dominated view of end of life decisions by sketching briefly the alternative cultural views which remain prevalent in other nations (and in subcultures within the United States itself). We will indicate a few lessons that US bioethics might learn from these other cultural traditions.

Two limits to our overview require mention. The laws of most countries are relatively permissive regarding how physicians manage care at the end of life. Occasionally one encounters significant interjurisdictional differences, such as the legal acceptance of active euthanasia in the Netherlands but nowhere else, and the legalization of physician-assisted suicide in Oregon alone among the US states. The popular idea, however, that the law imposes considerable restrictions on US medical practice in the forgoing of life-prolonging therapy has been clearly revealed to be a myth.(1) We will, therefore, have few things to say about legal issues at the end of life, and defer to the legal discussion in Chapter 16.8. Also in US practice, many issues in end-of-life care have been heavily influenced by concerns about rising health care costs and the fair allocation of resources. Since that issue is addressed in Chapter 16.6, we will again avoid focusing upon it in our discussion.

Central bioethical concepts at the end of life

We describe a consensus view of ethical decisions at the end of life which, while hardly accepted unanimously by American physicians and ethicists, has nevertheless proven extremely influential in both law and medical practice. Still, it is important to recall that some concepts widely agreed upon among bioethicists may not be accepted by physicians and nurses in practice.(2)

Sanctity of life versus individual autonomy

The view that life itself has predominant moral value in medical practice, while still supported by some religious traditions, has been largely replaced by the notion that the ultimate goal of medicine is service to the patient according to the patient's own values and preferences. While many older physicians were trained in an era when the decision to employ or to forgo a treatment that might extend life was presumed to be a medical decision within the physician's exclusive purview, younger physicians have been educated to view such behaviour as unwarranted medical paternalism, in which the physician inappropriately takes upon himself the role of deciding what is in the patient's best interests. It follows that the ideal end-of-life-care decision is one made by the patient himself, based on his/her own values. This model also presumes a fully informed patient who knows his/her own diagnosis and prognosis, and also the medical options available to manage his/her case. Respect for patient autonomy is fully consistent with the physician offering guidance, counsel, and emotional support.(3,4)

Hospice and palliative care

Experience with the autonomy model has shown that many patients near death will choose a medical course which maximizes comfort and ability to enjoy the company of friends and family, rather than a course which maximizes the length of biological life. Thus, the autonomy model has developed hand in hand with the hospice and palliative care movements, designed to offer comfort-oriented alternatives to the dying patient.(5)

Improved understanding of palliative care has de-emphasized one ethical concern of long standing—the so-called issue of double effect. So long as it was believed that adequate relief of terminal pain by opiate medication carried with it a significant risk of shortening life via respiratory depression, ethical analysis was required to explain how a physician could, in good conscience, administer such agents and thereby risk being the cause of the patient's premature death. 'Double effect' (the argument that some consequences that were foreseen but unintended, and that were the only available means to other good consequences, might be ethically acceptable under circumscribed conditions) was usually invoked to permit the compassionate relief of pain in these circumstances. New research has revealed that the actual risk of respiratory depression when opiates are properly used for pain relief has been greatly exaggerated, making it unnecessary to appeal to 'double effect' to justify good pharmacologic pain management.[6] (Double effect remains pertinent, however, to more extreme palliative measures such as terminal sedation.[7,8])

Advance care planning

The model of individual autonomy has proven so attractive that it has even guided ethical thinking about the dying patient who currently lacks the capacity to make decisions about medical treatment. Rather than saying that autonomy no longer applies, the dominant bioethics consensus is that one can make good decisions by appealing to the patient's prior autonomy. This can be done most explicitly when the patient has anticipated the later terminal course of illness and has left instructions, either in writing or verbally, about medical treatment he/she would or would not wish to receive. These instructions have been termed *advance directives*. Earlier ways of thinking about advance directives led to the unfortunate result that physicians and other workers focused too much on the *product* (such as a written document or 'living will') rather than the quality of the *process* of communication among patient, physician, and other family members by which the decision was made. The term *advance care planning* was therefore introduced by some who hoped to refocus attention on the ideal communication process, and to signal that the autonomous person ought to think ahead to the entire range of medical care choices that his/her family might later face on his/her behalf—decisions about location of care, for example (home, nursing facility, or acute care hospital) as well as whether the patient would wish life prolonged by medical technology in various disease states.[9]

Bioethicists have disagreed about how advance care planning should be structured. Some urge patients to think in terms of specific disease-treatment pairs and to accept or refuse treatment in each instance (e.g. whether one would wish a blood transfusion to prolong life if one was suffering from advanced dementia). Others argue that this approach focuses too much on medical technology and not enough on what matters to patients. The alternative proposal calls for the patient to indicate a threshold quality of life or functional level—for example, to say that he/she would wish life-prolonging treatment if the end result would be that he/she would be alert and able to converse with his/her family, even if bedbound; but he/she would not want such therapy if he/she would end up cognitively impaired to the point of being unable to recognize and communicate with family members. It is important to focus on the *process* of advance care planning since it is normal for patients' wishes on such matters to undergo change during the course of a chronic, terminal illness.

Relatively small percentages of US patients have gone through the process of advance care planning and have left specific instructions. One response to this fact is to admit that many of us do not know in advance, with any confidence or precision, what we would want done in the event of later severe illness. It makes more sense therefore to focus on the legal notion of *durable power of attorney for health care*, asking all patients to designate the person or persons they most trust to make such decisions on their behalf. Arguably, such a designation is more likely to remain stable over time than specific wishes about specific disease–treatment pairs. For the appointed agent or proxy to do the ideal job of deciding on behalf of the patient according to the patient's own values (the goal enshrined in American law as well as ethics as 'substituted judgement'), some conversation is usually required about the patient's basic treatment preferences and related values. Many families still shy away from explicit discussions of these matters until a health crisis actually occurs and forces the issue. However, demonstration projects have shown that most people in a community will engage in advance care planning if health care facilities join forces with other community institutions and train a cadre of lay helpers to assist people in the planning process.[10]

Futility

Futility remains a relatively contested area within bioethics. Some question the wisdom of labelling a category of treatments as 'futile' with the implication that physicians may ethically withhold such treatments even if patients or families request or demand them. For some, such unilateral physician decision-making seems too threatening to the concept of patient autonomy.[11] However, medical decision-making on the basis of futility is widespread, even if it is disguised as 'clinical judgment' or mere common sense rather than as an explicit ethical decision. In most medical systems around the world, and even in the United States, a mode of medical therapy widely believed by physicians not to be efficacious for the patient's disease is simply never brought up as an option. When patients in a given culture are less well informed about treatment alternatives, and more used to deferring to the physician's recommendations, explicit disputes over medical futility are unlikely to arise. When such disputes do arise, the most practical solution appears to be careful attention to the process of communication between the physician and the family or patient.[12]

Controversial end-of-life practices

Also highly contested are practices designed to hasten death rather than simply to allow the patient to die of the underlying disease. The major controversy has settled upon active euthanasia in Europe and physician-assisted suicide in the United States. Even in the majority of jurisdictions, where these acts remain illegal, surveys suggest that a minority of physicians occasionally help patients to die by these means.[13,14] Other practices debated in the bioethics literature include terminal sedation in the hospice setting, which is argued by some to be merely a means to relieve terminal suffering and by others to be a form of 'slow euthanasia';[15] and voluntary cessation of eating and drinking, which could be construed alternatively as a refusal of treatment by an autonomous patient or as a slower form of physician-assisted suicide.[8]

British guidelines

Support for the claim that the dominant US view has become a sort of international standard comes from a review of recent guidelines published by the British Medical Association (BMA).[16] The BMA endorses the competent patient's right to refuse life-prolonging therapy, and to make such decisions by means of 'advance statements'. The BMA recognizes a category of futile interventions, and includes artificial nutrition and hydration among modalities that may be withdrawn. The guidelines endorse a concern for the quality of life of terminal patients and call for improved palliative care practices.[17] At this point we discern little substantive disagreement between the British guidelines and the dominant American view of bioethics at the end of life. One difference in the legal climate, however, is that British and Scottish courts have been less accepting of the doctrine of substituted judgement than their American counterparts, creating a greater level of uncertainty in the face of a relative's request that life-prolonging therapy be withdrawn.

Competency for the primary care physician

The bioethics agenda as outlined above suggests in turn a set of skills which primary physicians ought to master, in order to assist their patients in optimal management of end-of-life issues:

- Bringing up advance care planning during routine or preventive visits before a serious illness occurs, in a non-threatening manner, and aiding patients to clarify their own wishes and communicate them to family members.

- When a health crisis occurs, informing the patient of the true diagnosis and prognosis in a compassionate, supportive way which facilitates the patient's involvement in key treatment decisions.
- Advising terminally ill patients of all reasonable care choices, including hospice care; being able to implement the basic measures needed for comfort care, and consulting or referring when more complex palliative care needs are encountered.
- Convening a family conference to discuss treatment decisions for the patient incapable of choosing, offering emotional support to family members facing such a decision, and helping them to determine what the patient would most likely want in the current circumstances.
- Consulting with a formal institutional ethics committee, or informally consulting with appropriate colleagues across health care disciplines, when facing a difficult or unprecedented ethical decision in one's practice.
- Dealing compassionately and sensitively with a patient's request for euthanasia or assisted suicide, determining if this request is a clue to unmet palliative care needs, and counselling patients about the options available depending on the laws and professional practice standards in one's community.(18)

Primary care physicians are uniquely situated within the health system by virtue of their long-standing relationships with their patients, the frequency with which they also know other family members, and their understanding of the practices and conditions within the community. Knowing the patient and the family well over time, however, will not by themselves substitute for the relevant skills in communication and in medical management. Fortunately, medical education in primary care increasingly focuses upon such skills today, and relatively brief training programmes can bring older practitioners up to speed.(19,20)

Studies of international and cross-cultural comparisons

In past years, bioethicists have been too often seduced by the vision that their conclusions are the result of pure reason and logic and betray no evidence of any cultural bias. More recently, a greater humility has become evident and bioethicists accept that it will be impossible for Americans (for instance) to judge end-of-life issues without inserting some peculiarly American values. Some empirical data help to illustrate these international and cross-cultural tensions in bioethics. Anthropological perspectives reveal marked differences across cultures in some of the 'common sense' concepts that underlie issues such as disclosure of a grim prognosis, informed consent, euthanasia, and brain death followed by organ transplantation.(21) Significant differences exist in the law and medical guidelines regarding the care of seriously ill neonates among eight European countries.(22) Geriatricians in the United States, Germany, and Japan differ in a number of ways in how they would care for a typical elderly person with early or advanced Alzheimer dementia.(23)

The following criticisms have been directed against the dominant consensus in bioethics described in the previous section:

- The stress on individual free choice and on rationally planning the course of one's life in advance is much greater in American culture than in the belief systems of many other nations.
- The stress on direct verbal communication about a dire prognosis is a similarly American aberration. In many cultures, politeness and respect for others demand indirect communication and often the concealment of such information. In extreme cases, asking a patient about future treatment wishes in the event of a terminal illness is viewed by the culture as tantamount to the physician's magically casting an evil spell.(24)
- The bioethical consensus severely limits the role of family members, to the extent that they serve as little more than conduits to report the patients' previously formed personal values.(25) Many other cultures place considerably more value on family decision-making and see the individual's own interests as to some extent subservient to (if not in fact defined by) the interests of the family as a unit.
- The bioethical consensus tends to assume ready access to a wide range of life-extending technologies. In some other cultures, limited resources will severely restrict the availability of these technologies. Those cultures may find it more in keeping with social cohesion and stability to allow non-treatment decisions to be made implicitly by a system short of resources, rather than explicitly by frank physician and family dialogue.

Two provisos should be appended to these observations. First, while traditional views in many cultures run counter to the American-dominated bioethical consensus, those cultures are not static, and many are evolving in directions that will bring them in the future more in line with Western and American values.(26,27) It is common, for instance, for first-generation immigrants to cling tightly to the practices of their country of birth, while second-generation immigrants seek to become more assimilated into the culture of their adopted country. Second, disparity between the bioethical consensus and a traditional cultural belief does not automatically mean that the bioethical consensus should be rejected in that setting. For example, a cultural practice in which the dominant male clan member makes a decision on medical treatment for a female relative without informing her of the options may reflect a history of unjust gender exploitation which should at least be called into question.

Lessons for bioethics from cross-cultural research

In time, more detailed studies of cross-cultural variation in ethical views may lead to the modification of portions of the dominant bioethical stance in the United States. We may, for example, see less focus on individual autonomy and more emphasis on respect for family relationships. Bioethics may come to have more respect for the views of some previously marginalized groups, such as persons with disabilities.(28)

The more pressing concern for today's practitioner is a strategy for negotiating differences that arise when caring for patients and families who represent a cultural group different from that of the physician and medical staff. It is difficult to give firm guidance because some cases seem to require a deeper respect for the practices of the 'foreign' culture, while others seem to demand imposing the values and attitudes of our own culture. One proposal for a negotiation strategy calls for a three-step process of identifying the patient's and family's goals, trying to find mutually agreeable strategies that address those goals while still meeting minimal criteria for acceptable medical care, and finally acknowledging and accepting overriding ethical constraints that limit the extent to which the physician can agree with the patient's or family's request. If this strategy produces an impasse, the physician should be willing to re-examine personal ethical values, for it may be that only when we see how our values play themselves out in the lives of others do we realize that we had perhaps been inflexible or shortsighted in drawing our lines where we did. Finally, if all else fails, it may be necessary to agree on a fair adjudication procedure.(29) One of the most valuable resources for the primary care physician in such cases is the 'cultural broker'. Such an individual has credibility with both sides of the dispute. The person knows enough about the dominant system of medical care to be able to correct any misinformation the patient or family may be labouring under. The person also knows the patient's culture well enough to advocate for the patient's point of view in language that the medical staff can readily understand. Another resource that is absolutely indispensable in resolving cross-cultural disputes is the medically trained and non-related translator. Too often, busy physicians rely on family members to translate, which severely limits the ability to transmit complicated medical information back and forth, and places the relative in an inherently conflicted role. Making medically trained translators available when needed should be a high priority for any medical clinic or hospital seeking to improve its capacity for culturally sensitive care.

Conclusions

We have reviewed a number of specific skills necessary to deliver high-quality care for patients at the end of life. But a good deal of end-of-life care depends on basic attitudes—commitment to effective communication; interest in the patient as a whole person and in the patient's familial and community environment; and concern for quality of life and relief of symptoms even when the underlying disease cannot be cured. Traditionally, primary care physicians have exhibited these attitudes more than physicians in most other specialties—and physicians who especially value these aspects of practice have tended to be drawn to primary care as a specialty choice. Primary care physicians ought therefore to excel in the care of the dying patient.[30]

One of the things the dying patient fears most is abandonment. It is the very nature of other specialties to abandon their patients. Oncologists stop seeing patients who can no longer benefit from chemotherapy, surgeons no longer care for patients who do not need surgery, and so on. Primary care physicians, by contrast, define their role in terms of continuous and comprehensive care, and pride themselves on both the duration and intensity of their relationships with their patients. Primary physicians are specialists in non-abandonment. The willingness to be there for the patient represents one of the unique contributions that primary care can make to the effective management of the end of life.

References

1. **Meisel, A.** (1991). Legal myths about terminating life support. *Archives of Internal Medicine* **151**, 1497–1502.
2. **Dickenson, D.L.** (2000). Are medical ethicists out of touch? Practitioner attitudes in the US and UK towards decisions at the end of life. *Journal of Medical Ethics* **26**, 254–60.
3. **Emanuel, E.J. and Emanuel, L.L.** (1992). Four models of the physician–patient relationship. *Journal of the American Medical Association* **267**, 2221–6.
4. **Quill, T.E. and Brody, H.** (1996). Physician recommendations and patient autonomy: finding a balance between physician power and patient choice. *Annals of Internal Medicine* **125**, 763–9.
5. **Doyle, D., Hanks, G.W.C., and MacDonald, N.**, ed. *Oxford Textbook of Palliative Medicine*. London: Oxford University Press, 1998.
6. **Fohr, S.A.** (1998). The double effect of pain medication: separating myth from reality. *Journal of Palliative Medicine* **1**, 315–28.
7. **Quill, T.E., Dresser, R., and Brock, D.W.** (1997). The rule of double effect—a critique of its role in end-of-life decision making. *New England Journal of Medicine* **337**, 1768–71.
8. **Quill, T.E., Lo, B., and Brock, D.W.** (1997). Palliative options of last resort: a comparison of voluntarily stopping eating and drinking, terminal sedation, physician-assisted suicide, and voluntary active euthanasia. *Journal of the American Medical Association* **278**, 2099–104.
9. **Teno, J.M., Nelson, H.L., and Lynn, J.** (1994). Advance care planning: priorities for ethical and empirical research. *Hastings Center Report* **24** (6), S32–6.
10. **Hammes, B.J. and Rooney, B.L.** (1998). Death and end-of-life planning in one midwestern community. *Archives of Internal Medicine* **158**, 383–90.
11. **Gillon, R.** (1997). 'Futility': too ambiguous and pejorative a term? *Journal of Medical Ethics* **23**, 339–40.
12. **Council on Ethical and Judicial Affairs, American Medical Association** (1999). Medical futility in end-of-life care. *Journal of the American Medical Association* **281**, 937–41.
13. **Kuhse, H.** et al. (1997). End-of-life decisions in Australian medical practice. *Medical Journal of Australia* **166**, 191–6.
14. **Back, A.L., Wallace, J.I., Starks, H.E., and Pearlman, R.A.** (1996). Physician-assisted suicide and euthanasia in Washington State. Patient requests and physician responses. *Journal of the American Medical Association* **275**, 919–25.
15. **Billings, J.A. and Block, S.D.** (1996). Slow euthanasia. *Journal of Palliative Care* **12** (4), 21–30.
16. **British Medical Association.** *Withholding and Withdrawing Life Prolonging Medical Treatment: Guidance for Decision Making*. London: BMJ, 1999. http://www.bmjpg.com/withwith/ww.htm.
17. **British Medical Association.** *End of Life Decisions—Views of the BMA* (online ethics), 2001. http://www.bma.org.uk/homepage.nsf/htmlpagevw/ethics.
18. **Emanuel, L.L.** (1998). Facing requests for physician-assisted suicide: toward a practical and principled clinical skill set. *Journal of the American Medical Association* **280**, 643–7.
19. **The EPEC Project: Education for Physicians on End-of-Life Care.** http://www.epec.net.
20. **The Michigan Physician Guide to End-of-Life Care.** Michigan State Medical Society/Michigan Department of Community Health, 2001. http://www.msms.org/peml/elc/elc.html
21. **Turner, L.** (1998). An anthropological exploration of contemporary bioethics: the varieties of common sense. *Journal of Medical Ethics* **24**, 127–33.
22. **McHaffie, H.E.** et al. (1999). Withholding/withdrawing treatment from neonates: legislation and official guidelines across Europe. *Journal of Medical Ethics* **25**, 440–6.
23. **Lynn, J.** et al. (1999). Dementia and advance-care planning: perspectives from three countries on ethics and epidemiology. *Journal of Clinical Ethics* **10**, 271–85.
24. **Carrese, J.A. and Rhodes, L.A.** (1995). Western bioethics on the Navajo reservation: benefit or harm? *Journal of the American Medical Association* **274**, 826–9.
25. **Nelson, H.L. and Nelson, J.L.** *The Patient in the Family*. New York: Routledge, 1995.
26. **Surbone, A.** (1992). Truth telling to the patient. *Journal of the American Medical Association* **268**, 1661–2.
27. **Emura, S.** et al. (2001). A surveillance of patients' preferences in truth-telling at the Department of General Medicine, Saga Medical School. *Japanese Journal of Primary Care* **24**, 138–43.
28. **Parens, E. and Asch, A.** (1999). The disability rights critique of prenatal genetic testing: reflections and recommendations. *Hastings Center Report* **29** (5), S1–22.
29. **Jecker, N.S., Carrese, J.A., and Pearlman, R.A.** (1995). Caring for patients in cross-cultural settings. *Hastings Center Report* **25** (1), 6–14.
30. **Ogle, K.S. and Plumb, J.D.** (1996). The role of the primary care physician in the care of the terminally ill. *Clinics in Geriatric Medicine* **12**, 267–78.

16.8 Medico-legal issues

Brian Hurwitz

> We live in and by the law. It makes us what we are: citizens and employees and doctors and spouses. It is sword, shield and menace: we insist on our wage, or refuse to pay our rent, all in the name of what the law has decreed. And we argue about what it has decreed. We are subjects of law's empire, liegemen to its methods and ideals.
>
> Ronald Dworkin[1]

Introduction

Law impinges on medicine most visibly when things go wrong. Patients turn increasingly to legal remedies if harmed physically, psychologically, or in perception only, in search of compensation, reparation, emotional vindication, justice, and deterrence. By this process the law gives legal form to many facets of doctor–patient relationships, including the diversity of duties primary care teams owe to patients; confidentiality of health information and rules governing access to it by patients, parents, clinicians, and researchers; and provision of particular health services such as abortion and contraception.

The law comes into play not only when things go wrong; it also *creates and maintains* the framework of medical practice in which things go right. Such legal frameworks differ widely between countries, yet case law, case series, and empirical research into claims and patient safety world-wide yield congruent findings: primary care errors are frequently multifactorial in origin and associated with poor communication, prescription errors, failure to diagnose, investigate, monitor, or to refer patients in a timely fashion.

Complaints and claims against GPs are rising

Complaints lodged in the year 2000 with the UK regulatory body, the General Medical Council, alleged misconduct or poor performance on the part of 4470 doctors (half of them GPs), a 49 per cent increase on the preceding 12 months.[2] In the same year, there were 23 000 outstanding clinical negligence claims associated with an estimated liability in the United Kingdom of over £4 billion.[3] Despite studies showing claims are growing at a pace faster than the increase in health care activity,[4] many patients fail to make a claim; they remain unaware of having sustained harm and/or of the grounds for taking action,[3] a situation matched by findings in the United States.[5]

Data on claims relating to primary care are based on less robust studies than for hospital claims but paint a similar picture: between 1989 and 1998, the Medical Protection Society observed a 10-fold increase in the number of claims it dealt with on behalf of its GP membership, estimating that 3.6 per cent of its GP members would face legal action as a result of work undertaken in the previous 12 months.[6] The annual incidence of written complaints submitted to the NHS concerning GPs' behaviour or the organization of primary health care is also rising. In 2001, there were over 44 000 complaints related to GPs and community dentists, an increase of 12 per cent on the previous year and an overall increase of 20 per cent since the current complaints procedure was implemented in 1996.[7]

Yet, claims for negligence against UK primary care physicians have a relatively low profile—to date systematic studies of their frequency are few and when complainants (formerly plaintiffs in the United Kingdom) sue GPs successfully they are generally awarded lower damages than successful actions against secondary care physicians. World-wide, however, 45 per cent of all new claims cases opened by the Medical Protection Society in 1997 involved GPs, with obstetricians and gynaecologists accounting for the next highest number (11 per cent of the total). The highest pay-out recorded by 1997 was 4.8 million Australian Dollars (in an obstetric case) compared to the highest award against a GP of 1.65 million Irish pounds (failure to diagnose meningitis),[8] figures which translate into lower premiums for malpractice insurance for GPs than for hospital doctors.

Nevertheless, GPs admit to adopting defensive medical practices—ordering or avoiding treatments, tests, or procedures primarily for the purpose of protecting themselves from criticism rather than for purposes of diagnosis or treatment. Some of these defensive practices could be either beneficial or harmful to patient care, and include more diagnostic testing, increased referrals, more intensive follow-up, more detailed patient explanations and note-taking, avoiding treating certain conditions in general practice, and not prescribing unnecessary drugs.[9]

The reasons usually adduced for a relatively low rate of claims against GPs include the belief that arrangements for primary care and its quality are still accorded a measure of esteem by the public. It is said that patients enjoy a more personal relationship with their GP—lasting on average for some 10 years—than they do with hospital doctors. As a consequence, mistakes may be more likely to be overlooked or accepted as part and parcel of such a relationship; patients may not wish to put a doctor they know well—and who perhaps has dealt satisfactorily with many previous medical episodes (together with those experienced by close relatives)—'into the dock'.[10] Serious criminal cases in which physicians have been accused (and in some cases convicted) of assault and murder show how difficult it can be for patients to become aware not only of substandard primary care but of serious criminal wrongdoing by GPs.[11–13]

UK data reveal the vast majority claims—up to 78 per cent—are abandoned prior to issuance of formal proceedings; 9–16 per cent are settled out of court, a further 1–20 per cent are settled after a writ has been served, with 1–3 per cent reaching trial stage.[14] Findings such as these mean that many of the principles of medical law holding sway over health care emanate, for the most part, from the tiny percentage of claims that reach the court rooms, claims, moreover, which have proved difficult to resolve without formal adjudication. What can be learned from case law and case series is different from what can be learned from empirical research and risk management studies. From case law we can learn principles of law related to medical practice and the general approach of courts to deciding whether care provided has been substandard. From empirical research arise understandings of how commonly people suffer avoidable health care harms, what sort of doctors are more likely to face legal claims, why patients sue, and which areas of practice are especially risky for patients.

Negligence

The *Oxford English Dictionary* defines negligence as 'a want of attention to what ought to be done or looked after'. It is a concept potentially applicable to almost any human action that may be dubbed 'negligent' if performed inadequately compared to a desirable, achievable standard of performance.

The majority of claims against doctors are actions alleging negligence and although their positive effects elude quantification, such actions are believed to play a role in the maintenance of health care standards. In common law jurisdictions these actions conform to a similar pattern illustrated here with reference to the United Kingdom.

To prove negligence in a court of law, a plaintiff (complainant in the United Kingdom)—the person bringing the action—must show that:

- the defendant doctor owed the plaintiff a *duty of care*;
- the doctor *breached* this duty of care by failing to provide the *required standard of medical care*; and
- on the balance of probabilities this failure actually *caused* the plaintiff harm.

Duty of care and its breach

Once a doctor–patient relationship clearly exists, common law holds doctors to have a *duty of care* towards their patients. The broad nature and scope of this duty arises from patients' reliance upon doctors and was spelt out in 1925 in a case in which a doctor was accused of criminal negligence in performing a traumatic forceps delivery:

> If a person holds himself out as possessing special skill and knowledge, and he is consulted as possessing such skill and knowledge, by or on behalf of a patient, he owes a duty to the patient to use due caution in undertaking the treatment. If he accepts the responsibility and undertakes the treatment and the patient submits to his discretion and treatment accordingly, he owes a duty to the patient to use diligence, care, knowledge, skill and caution in administering treatment. No contractual relation is necessary, nor is it necessary that the service be rendered for reward.
>
> (*R v Bateman 1925*)

The duty of care is imposed by law and its standard is determined by the courts after hearing expert evidence. Since a doctor's duty of care consists of an obligation to provide treatment of a fair and reasonable standard, breach of this standard consists in providing treatment that falls below such a standard.

What is a reasonable standard of care? The standard of treatment a doctor generally owes to a patient derives from the case of *Bolam v Friern Hospital Management Committee (1957)*. In the words of Mr Justice McNair:

> the test is the standard of the ordinary skilled man exercising and professing to have that special skill.
>
> (*Bolam v Friern Hospital Management Committee 1957*)

Doctors are required to act in a manner judged reasonable and proper by a body of other responsible doctors. The degree of care and skill that can reasonably be expected of a prudent practitioner is judged by a 'peer-review process' formulated as follows by Judge McNair:

> A doctor will not be guilty of negligence if he has acted in accordance with a practice accepted as proper by a responsible body of medical men skilled in that particular art.

In UK law, historically influential upon US and Commonwealth common law too, this test has become known as the 'Bolam test'. Expert testimony helps courts to ascertain what is accepted and proper practice in specific cases, which generally ensures professionally generated standards are applied, rather than standards originating from elsewhere.

Legal standards of care

The Bolam test appears to be a 'state-of-the-art' descriptive test about what *is* done in practice, rather than a normative one about what *ought* to be done. As a legal standard it is derived—on a case-by-case basis—from professionally defined standards. Lord Woolf, now Lord Chief Justice of England, speaking extra-judicially to the Royal College of Physicians of London about legal standards of care explained that:

> The general approach of the courts is to apply the standards that the medical profession adopts. Thus we judge whether there has been negligence in the treatment of a patient by asking whether or not the medical treatment, which is the subject of complaint, accords with standards which *any* recognised section of the medical profession regards as acceptable . . . By adopting this standard the courts have managed to hold the balance fairly between the interests of the patient and the interest of the profession. By striking the right balance, the courts reduce the risk of proper medical practice being undermined by fear of litigation and recognise the need for compensation to be paid where treatment is of an unacceptable standard. In addition, the courts do not impose their ethical standards upon the medical professions. Wisely, they leave the medical profession to determine what is, and what is not, ethical behaviour' (emphasis added).[15]

In an evidence-linked era this test may be thought to demand too little to encourage higher standards of care as it appears to licence any treatment a body of responsible practitioners testifies should be adopted in the circumstances. On one reading the test turns on whether doctors can be found who are prepared to testify that they themselves would provide similar care in the circumstances before a court. Condemned as 'a blot on English medical law', a mere sociological criterion at the heart of legal decision-making, it has been disparaged as reflecting undue judicial deference to medical opinion. However, the Bolam test is no longer as influential as it once was on medico-legal cases in north American and Australian jurisdictions, which are more sensitive to patients' rights and the paramountcy of health care consumers than is UK law.

Some judges maintain that application of the Bolam test—particularly in cases concerning how much information about risks and benefits of proposed treatment patients are entitled to receive to give valid consent—does not involve handing over to the medical profession the crucial matter of deciding which standard of care a conduct in question is to be judged by (*Sidaway v Board of Governors of the Bethlem and the Maudsley Hospital 1985*) and assert courts are free to examine the substance and rationale of treatments provided, not merely the fact that others can be found to support them (*Chapman v Rix 1959* reported in 1994).[16] Such a view has been strengthened by the *Bolitho v City and Hackney Health Authority case (1997)*, in which the House of Lords adopted a modified Bolam test, allowing expert opinions that cannot be logically supported to be disregarded by judges.

In respect of standards of disclosure—the information patients are entitled to in order to give valid consent to a procedure—UK courts have generally adopted a Bolam approach, basing their decisions on what a responsible body of doctors would have disclosed in the circumstances. In the 1970s, US case law formulated a more patient-oriented test, allowing courts to ignore what reasonable doctors would have told patients in such circumstances and to ask, instead, what a reasonable patient would want to know in the circumstances (*Canterbury v Spence 1972*). Australian courts have gone further, ruling that doctors should disclose all material risks that the reasonable patient is likely to regard as being significant (*Rogers v Whittaker 1992*). There are indications that UK courts are moving towards adopting a reasonable patient test rather than deferring to what a body of doctors says it would divulge in the circumstances (*Pearce v United Bristol Healthcare Trust 1999*).[17]

Framework of practice

Legal cases concerning GPs are influenced not only by the law of negligence but by the framework of medical practice as well, and the increasingly complex regulations by governments of the practice of family medicine merit, in the view of one expert, legal textbooks of their own.[10] Since frameworks of practice differ widely between countries, the UK situation will be described illustratively.

In the United Kingdom, the majority of GP principals are doctors who work as self-employed, independent contractors providing general medical services to registered patients in accordance with the National Health Service Act 1977. Principals gain inclusion to the Medical List of a Primary Care Trust by undertaking approved, certified training and clinical experience, and by signing a contract binding them to nationally agreed Terms of Service which are governed by statute. Since the Primary Care Act 1997, a growing number of GPs have been employed as employees of Trusts, Health authorities, or general practices, many to provide very similar services to those offered by the majority of GPs but under differing regulations. GP Terms of Service state that: 'a doctor shall not . . . be expected to exercise a higher degree of skill, knowledge and care than . . . that which general practitioners as a class may reasonably be expected to exercise'.[18] Judgement in the Bolam case referred to doctors 'skilled in that particular art' and in subsequent legal cases this has been taken to indicate that the standard of care required from one sort of practitioner could be different from that required from another sort (see *Hucks v Cole 1968*). Lord Bridge reiterated the point in 1985 in his House of Lords judgement in the case of *Sidaway v Governors of Bethlem Royal Hospital*:

> The language of the *Bolam* test clearly requires a different degree of skill from a specialist in his own field than from a general practitioner.

Some successful actions in negligence against GPs

In this chapter, it is possible to refer only to a tiny fraction of case law pertaining to primary care.[19–21] Courts have long recognized that GPs have responsibilities to monitor the effectiveness of treatments (*Farquar v Murray 1901*), to investigate, and refer patients to specialists where there is doubt about diagnosis and treatment, or where patients are likely to benefit from particular specialist expertise (see Box 1).

Common law cases point to particular areas of risk in creating liability in primary care: maintenance of adequate records and ensuring effective communication with hospitals and community pharmacies (*Coles v Reading and District HMC 1963*); failure to record and hand on information about patients (*Farquar v Murray 1901, Chin Keow v Government of Malaysia 1967, Hucks v Cole 1968*); prescription errors (*Dwyer v Rodrick 1983, Prendergast v Sam and Dee Ltd 1990*), failure to diagnose, investigate, or

Box 1 Case law defined GP responsibilities

In *Connolly v Rubra (1937)* a patient's GP treated him for bronchitis while he complained of night sweats and a productive bloody cough, but Dr Rubra did not request a chest X-ray or sputum analysis. The patient's condition worsened and when finally seen by a specialist he was diagnosed as suffering from tuberculosis, from which he died. Dr Rubra was found negligent in not making further examination of the patient, and not referring him earlier to a specialist.

Dwyer v Rodrick (1983) concerned a GP who had diagnosed migraine and had prescribed too large a dose of Migril tablets (6–8 per day) containing the vasoconstrictor, ergotamine. Without noticing the error a qualified pharmacist dispensed the tablets to the unsuspecting patient. Three days later another GP from the same practice visited the patient because she was vomiting but the doctor did not have her clinical notes with him and did not realize she was taking Migril. After a further 3 days he visited again by which time she had suffered gangrene of her toes and peripheral nerve damage. The trial judge held all three defendants liable for damages (£100 000) and apportioned liability at 45% to Dr Rodrick, 15% to his partner GP, and 40% to the dispensing chemist. On appeal, the second GP was exculpated and liability adjusted to 45% to Dr Rodrick and 55% to the chemist.

Prendergast v Sam and Dee Ltd (1990) concerned an asthmatic patient, Mr Prendergast, who visited his GP fearing he was developing a chest infection. He was prescribed Amoxil (branded form of antibiotic amoxycillin) 250 mg to be taken three times a day. The GP's handwriting was so poor that the dispensing chemist thought the GP had prescribed Daonil (branded oral antidiabetic medication, glibenclamide 2.5 mg) for reducing blood sugar and dispensed this drug with instructions to take it three times a day, the patient suffering brain damage as a result. The Court of Appeal (*Prendergast v Sam and Dee Ltd 1990*) upheld the finding of the judge at first instance that both doctor (25%) and pharmacist (75%) were liable, as the GP should have foreseen that poor handwriting of a prescription could mislead a pharmacist into dispensing a dangerous drug; the pharmacist was liable because the dosage and other medications on the prescription should have alerted him to the fact that the GP did not intend to prescribe Daonil.

In *Langley v Campbell (1985)* a patient visited his GP after returning from East Africa with a 9-day history of fever. The GP diagnosed influenza and 6 days later the patient died of malaria. The GP was found liable for failing to consider, and to test for, malaria after having been told by the patient of his recent return from a part of the world where the disease was prevalent (see Chapter 13.4).

refer patients for diagnosis (*Connolly v Rubra 1937*, *Langley v Campbell 1985*), vicarious GP liability for failures of communication on the part of reception staff about, for example, the urgency of a patient's medical condition (*Lobely v Going 1985*).

Case series of serious drug-related errors in primary care

Medical defence organizations providing malpractice insurance to family physicians hold data on the content of all claims against their membership. Because the vast majority of these claims are abandoned or settled out of court, these data offer potentially valuable insights into aspects of practice where patients perceive family physicians are failing in ways they believe cause harm. Analysis of 1000 consecutive claims lodged against GP members of the Medical Protection Society after July 1996 reveals that by far the most frequently perceived cause (63.1 per cent) involves failure/delay in diagnosis, one-fourth of which concern malignant disease. Of the 1000 claims, 19.3 per cent relate to alleged prescribing mistakes, the commonest of which involve failure to recognize or to monitor adverse medication effects.[22,23] Eighteen per cent involve prescription of incorrect or inappropriate medication, 12.5 per cent contraindicated drugs, and 12 per cent wrong doses of medication. In terms of drug groupings, steroids account for a fifth, other named groups (antibiotics, phenothiazines, hormone replacement, oral contraception, antiepilepsy, opiates and lithium, non-steroidal anti-inflammatories, and warfarin) each amount to a few per cent of the total of prescribing-related claims. In addition, 45 per cent of the 1000 claims related to failure to:

- refer for hospital admission, 11.8 per cent;
- refer to another speciality, 11.6 per cent;
- examine adequately, 6.9 per cent;
- maintain adequate medical records, 6.6 per cent;
- investigate adequately, 5.2 per cent;
- monitor adequately, 4.5 per cent;
- arrange an X-ray/scan, 3.7 per cent;
- act on an abnormal finding, 21 per cent;
- visit a patient at home, 1.7 per cent.

The importance of prescribing safely is reinforced by findings from a systematic review and meta-analysis of 15 descriptive studies which concluded that 7 per cent of all hospital admissions are drug-related, approximately half of which could be considered preventable.[24]

Physician-related factors to claims

Several US studies have sought to delineate risk factors for claims; their results, though suggestive, are not definitive. Amongst primary care physicians in Colorado and Oregon, the relationship between communication skills and malpractice claims for doctors without versus with (two or more) claims against them was studied; physicians without claims had significantly longer consultations (18.3 versus 15 min), employed more orientating statements (explaining what's likely to happen next), more facilitating statements (asking patient opinions and checking understanding), laughed more, and used more humour in consultations than did the no-claims physicians.[25] Consultation length and physician affect (particularly laughter and behaviour demonstrative of concern, approval, and empathy) were found to predict physician claims status.

A study using a large malpractice database in Florida, containing information over a 13-year period, found doctors with a favourable claims profile to be older but no more likely to have more prestigious professional credentials, to have qualified in the United States or Canada, be in solo or group practice, or to be involved in research or teaching, than doctors with an unfavourable claims profile.[26] Using the same database, a subsequent study involving family physicians found a host of measures traditionally associated with doctor quality (graduation from US or Canadian medical school, specialty board certification, holding American Medical Association Physician's Recognition Award, and Alpha Omega Honor Society membership) were significant risk factors for being sued. The authors were surprised by these findings, and comment that their findings have been confounded by major unstudied differences between claim and no-claim physicians in patient complexity (case mix) and physician's interpersonal skills.[27]

Incident monitoring

An observational study conducted over 21 months in a non-random selection of Australian general practices (involving 324 GPs) collected data on adverse incidents of potential or actual harm to patients and evaluated possible causes.[28] Incidents were broadly defined as events, no matter how

Table 1 Contributory and mitigating factors in genesis of adverse incidents in Australian General Practice

	Rate per 100 incidents (*n* = 805)
Contributory factors	
Poor communication between patient and health professionals	23
Action of others (not GP or patient)	23
Error in judgement	22
Poor communication between health professionals	19
Patient consulted other medical officer	15
Failure to recognize signs and symptoms	15
Patient's history not adequately reviewed	13
Omission of checking procedure	10
GP tired/rushed/running late	10
Patient misunderstood problem/treatment	10
Inadequate patient assessment	10
Administrative inadequacies	9
Mitigating factors	
Plain good fortune	23
Patient's good physical condition	19
Patient's good psychological condition	11
Early intervention by	
Reporting GP	22
Patient	9
Relative/carer	6
Another non-GP health professional	5
Another GP	4
Pharmacist	2

Adapted from: Bhasale, A., Miller, G., Reid, S., and Britt, H. (1998). *Medical Journal of Australia* **169**, 73–6.

seemingly trivial or commonplace, which could have harmed (near misses) or actually did harm patients. GPs reported free text descriptions of incidents and structured their reports to include estimates of preventability, potential for harm, immediate consequences, predictable long-term outcomes, type of incident, and factors contributing and mitigating the causes of incidents.

Eight hundred and five incidents were reported, 76 per cent of which were judged preventable, 27 per cent potentially harmful. For 66 per cent of incidents no long-term harm was predicted. Fifty-one per cent incidents related to pharmacological management, 41 per cent to non-pharmacological management, 34 per cent to diagnosis, and 5 per cent to equipment. The two commonest contributory factors to their inception were poor communication between patients and health professionals (23/100) and errors of judgement (22/100). Additional contributing factors are listed in Table 1, including mitigating factors. Particularly noteworthy is that adverse incidents were more frequently mitigated by chance than by systematic fail-safe or preventive procedures.

Although the study is likely to have under-sampled adverse events in primary care, it successfully characterized their diversity. Together with the experiences of the aviation and oil industries in scrutiny of organizational and human factors associated with errors, studies such as these have contributed to determination on the part of the US and British governments to support programmes of research and development designed to log, study, and learn from medical errors and near misses.(29–32)

Medical error and culpability

The most influential researcher into human error, James Reason, has put forward a widely accepted definition of error that places the accent on planning that has gone awry: 'all errors', he states, 'involve some kind of deviation understood as occasions in which a planned sequence of mental or physical activities fails to achieve its intended outcome'.(33) He divides errors into those caused by problems with *physical execution*—such as slips,

Box 2 *Hucks v Cole and another (1968)*

Mrs Hucks developed a septic finger just prior to confinement in 1963. Her GP, Dr Cole, neither treated the finger nor informed the maternity unit about its condition. When admitted to hospital, Mrs Hucks was found to be septicaemic and was therefore treated with a 5-day course of tetracycline. After discharge her septic lesions recurred, but Dr Cole failed to institute a further course of antibiotics and Mrs Hucks suffered permanent impairment as a result. At trial, Dr Cole argued—and produced expert witness to support his claim—that his practice had been in line with that of a responsible body of medical opinion; he contended that Mrs Hucks had been treated properly but had been unlucky in suffering an adverse outcome. Nevertheless, he was found negligent in allowing his patient to enter hospital with an untreated septic finger, for failing to notify the hospital about her condition, and for failing to treat her with a second course of antibiotics after her discharge.

lapses, trips, and fumbles, usually associated with attention or memory failures—and mistakes related to *planning* or *problem-solving*, in which actions are performed correctly but fail to achieve their purpose because of inadequate plans, faulty formulation, poor judgement, or problem-solving. Clearly, many errors have the potential to lead to harmful consequences but not all do so—quite serendipitously, harm may be averted (near misses).

Two ethnographic studies conducted amongst US,(34) UK, and Swedish doctors(35) found many clinicians believe medical errors to be insufficiently acknowledged in health care systems and that even when recognized errors are frequently believed to be dealt with too informally. Recurrent themes identified by these studies include: a belief that mistakes are only to be expected since medicine is inherently uncertain and its practitioners are clearly fallible; that clinicians feel vulnerable to error, identify strongly with those who make mistakes, and look to colleagues for understanding and forgiveness in the event of making mistakes themselves; and that despite overlap in the types of errors made practitioners recognize different sorts of mistake, such as errors of judgement, technique, or moral conduct.

Rosenthal singled out a tendency for doctors to see themselves in the tragedy of each other's mistakes, and quoted the views of an experienced UK GP:

> We're all entitled to make mistakes aren't we? We're all vulnerable. 'There but for the grace of God go I'...I remember making that mistake myself. We are all human. There are problems in our lives that are not our fault. As long as you can say: 'That could happen to me', you are going to be sympathetic. You have to look at actual cases; we all have the right to err. But the excessively repeated error is something else. A minority of doctors are repeating major errors and the formal system catches only some of them. A lot are never caught because it is hard to identify errors and patients may not complain.

In the United States, family doctors in Iowa associated the cause of errors in 91 per cent of cases with physician stress (being hurried or distracted), process of care factors in 91 per cent, lack of physician knowledge in 62 per cent, and patient-related factors (e.g. misleading but in the event normal findings) in 72 per cent of errors.(36) Given the multifactorial nature of harm causation and the role of factors such as chance in determining whether harm from certain errors transpires, questions are posed as to whether some errors ought to attract the censure that a finding of negligence implies. Instead, certain medical errors might no longer usefully be viewed as the result of morally relevant wrong-doing. Such a change will require reform of medical negligence systems to ensure not only apportionment of 'fair blame' where negligence is proved, but also—as in New Zealand and (for some cases only) in Florida and Virginia—compensation for the much larger number of patients who are non-negligently harmed by health care.(37,38)

Even though chance can play a decisive role in whether harm eventuates from error, the law of negligence tends to ignore intercalation of chance factors and the effects of random intra- and interdoctor variability. In a case involving a GP with a diploma in obstetrics (see Box 2), a senior UK judge, Lord Denning, sought to draw a legal distinction between errors of judgement and negligence.

Denning stated:

> A doctor is not to be held negligent simply because something has gone wrong. He is not liable for mischance or misadventure; or for an error of judgment. He is only liable when he falls below the standard of a reasonably competent practitioner in the field.
>
> (*Hucks v Cole and another 1968*)

Twelve years later he reiterated the point:

> We must say firmly, that, in a professional man, an error of judgment is not negligent. To test it, I would suggest that you ask the average competent and careful practitioner: 'Is this the sort of mistake that you yourself might have made?' If he says 'Yes, even doing the best I could, it might have happened to me', then it is not negligent.
>
> (*Whitehouse v Jordan 1980*)

This formulation was subsequently rejected by the Law Lords, who insisted that errors of judgement must be seen as potentially negligent:

> Merely to describe something as an error of judgment tells us nothing about whether it is negligent or not; it depends on the nature of the error. If it is one that would not have been made by a reasonably competent professional man professing to have the standard and skill that the defendant held himself out as having, and acting with ordinary care, then it is negligent. If, on the other hand, it is an error that a man, acting with ordinary care, might have made, then it is not negligence
>
> (Per Lord Fraser in *Whitehouse v Jordan 1981*)

In common law, negligence remains a binary concept; when found it implies fault based on transgression of a reasonable standard of care which has caused the patient harm. It aportions blame and a transfer of resources from negligent agents (or their insurers) to the injured party. Empirical research indicates that many claimants wish for a wider range of remedies than litigation can provide. Patients desire a complex amalgam consisting of admission of fault, apology, full explanation of how the injury came about, serious investigation of the cause of the injury and evidence of steps taken to prevent recurrence.[(39)] Desires motivating many claims—for explanation, retribution, evidence of prevention of recurrence—are frequently disappointed, even when complainants are successful in the courts, as the adversarial aspect of litigation often hinders satisfaction of such motives. In some countries, alternative resolution approaches are under consideration and aim to settle claims within the framework of a clinical dispute rather than a demand solely for money. Such approaches would allow a package of responses to be developed and offered to claimants, including, for example, apology, explanation, access to remedial treatment, counselling, meeting with medical staff to learn about what went wrong, explanation of action taken to prevent recurrence, provision of on going support.

Growth in numbers of legal claims against doctors and complaints about them—whether procedural or clinical—took place world-wide in the second half of the twentieth century and shows little sign of abating in the twenty-first century. This growth has variously been attributed to patients as a body becoming more rights oriented, possibly more litigious, more demanding, and consumerist in health care attitudes and therefore more dissatisfied than hitherto with health care received.

Case law, case series, and empirical research into primary care claims and patient safety show considerable congruence of findings. Primary medical care errors are frequently multifactorial in origin, and poor communication, prescription errors, failure to diagnose, investigate, monitor, or to refer patients are perennially implicated in claims. Yet, despite the growth in such claims, a substantial number of patients suffering preventable harm at the hands of doctors remain unaware of it, or of the grounds upon which they could make a claim. In these circumstances, numbers of claims alleging medical negligence against primary care physicians and teams are likely to continue to grow.

References

1. **Condensed from: Dworkin, R.** *Law's Empire*. London: Fontana Press, 1986, p. 7.
2. **GMC Council Minutes.** May 2000. Section 9. http://www.gmc-uk.org.
3. **Report by the Comptroller and Auditor General.** *Handling Clinical Negligence Claims in England*. HC 403 Session 2000–2001. London: The Stationery Office, 2001.
4. **Fenn, P., Diacon, S., Gray, A., Hodges, R., and Rickman, N.** (2000). Current cost of medical negligence in NHS hospitals: analysis of claims. *British Medical Journal* **320**, 1567–71.
5. **Meyers, A.R.** (1987). 'Lumping it': the hidden denominator of the medical malpractice crisis. *American Journal of Public Health* **77**, 1544–8.
6. **Dyer, C.** (1999). GPs face escalating litigation. *British Medical Journal* **318**, 830.
7. http://www.doh.gov.uk/complaints.
8. **Medical Protection Society Review.** London: Medical Protection Society, 1997, p. 7.
9. **Summerton, N.** (1995). Positive and negative factors in defensive medicine: a questionnaire study of general practitioners. *British Medical Journal* **310**, 27–9.
10. **Brazier, M.** *Medicine, Patients and the Law*. London: Pelican Books, 1992, p. 354.
11. **Dyer, C.** (2001). Shipman inquiry to investigate 466 deaths. *British Medical Journal* **322**, 1018.
12. **Devlin, P.** *Easing the Passing*. London: Faber and Faber, 1985.
13. **O'Neill, B.** (2000). Doctor as murderer. *British Medical Journal* **320**, 329–30.
14. **Mulcahy, L.** (2000). Threatening behaviour: the challenge of medical negligence claims. In *Law and Medicine* (ed. M. Freeman and A. Lewis), pp. 81–105. Oxford: Oxford University Press.
15. **The Right Honorable Lord Woolf** (1997). Medics, lawyers and the courts. *Journal of the Royal College of Physicians, London* **31**, 686–93.
16. **Newdick, C.** *Who Should We Treat?* Oxford: Clarendon Press, p. 86, 1995.
17. **Skene, L. and Smallwood, R.** (2002). Informed consent: lessons from Australia. *British Medical Journal* **324**, 39–41.
18. **Statutory Instruments 1992 No. 635, The National Health Service (General Medical Services) Regulations.** London: HMSO, 1992.
19. **Nelson-Jones, R. and Burton, F.** *Medical Negligence Case Law*. London: Butterworths, 1995.
20. **Scott, W.** *The General Practitioner and the Law*. London: Cavendish Publishing Ltd., 1995.
21. **Drury, M., ed.** *Clinical Negligence in General Practice*. Abingdon: Radcliffe Medical Press, 2000.
22. **Silk, N.** (2000). What went wrong in 1000 negligence claims. In *Health Care Risk Report*, pp. 14–16. London: Medical Protection Society.
23. **Silk, N.** (2001). Findings from 1000 negligence claims—part two. In *Health Care Risk Report*, pp. 13–15. London: Medical Protection Society.
24. **Winterstein, A.G., Sauer, B.C., Hepler, C.D., and Poole, C.** (2000). The incidence of preventable drug-related hospital admissions. *Pharmacoepidemiology and Drug Safety* **9**, S147–8.
25. **Levinson, W.** et al. (1997). Physician–patient communication. The relationship with malpractice claims among primary care physicians and patients. *Journal of the American Medical Association* **277**, 553–9.
26. **Sloan, F.A.** et al. (1989). Medical malpractice experience of physicians. *Journal of the American Medical Association* **262**, 3291–7.
27. **ly, J., Dawson, J., Young, P., Doebbeling, B., Goerdt, C., Elder, N., and Olick, J.** (1999). Malpractice claims against family physicians. Are the best doctors sued more? *Journal of Family Practice* **48**, 23–9.
28. **Bhasale, A., Miller, G., Reid, S., and Britt, H.** (1998). Analysing potential harm in Australian general practice: an incident monitoring study. *Medical Journal of Australia* **169**, 73–6.
29. **The Federal Aviation Administration Aviation System.** http://nasdac.faa.gov/aviation_studies/safety_data
30. **Kohn, L.T., Corigan, J.M., and Donaldson, M.S.** (1999). Error reporting systems. In *To Err is Human: Building a Safer Health System* (ed. L.T. Kohn,

J.M. Corigan, and M.S. Donaldson), pp. 86–108. Washington DC: National Academy Press.

31. **Department of Health.** *An Organisation with a Memory.* London: Stationery Office, 2000.
32. **Department of Health.** *Building a Safer NHS.* London: Stationery Office, 2001.
33. **Reason, J.** (2001). Understanding adverse events: the human factor. In *Clinical Risk Management* (ed. C. Vincent), pp. 9–30. London: BMJ Books.
34. **Bosk, C.L.** *Forgive and Remember.* Chicago IL: Chicago University Press, 1981.
35. **Rosenthal, M.M.** *The Incompetent Doctor.* Buckingham: Open University Press, 1995.
36. **Ely, J.W.** et al. (1995). Perceived causes of family physicians' errors. *Journal of Family Practice* **40**, 337–44.
37. **Britsol Royal Infirmary Inquiry**. *Learning from Bristol.* Bristol: Bristol Royal Infirmary Inquiry, 2001.
38. **Merry, A. and McCall Smith, A.** *Errors, Medicine and the Law.* Cambridge: Cambridge University Press, 2001.
39. **Vincent, C., Young, M., and Phillips, A.** (1994). Why do people sue their doctors? A study of patients and relatives taking legal action. *Lancet* **343**, 1609–13.

Index

Main index entries are given in **bold**.
Page numbers in *italics* refer to tables.